Pathophysiology of Disease:
An Introduction to Clinical Medicine

Sixth Edition

Edited by

Stephen J. McPhee, MD
Professor of Medicine
Division of General Internal Medicine
Department of Medicine
University of California, San Francisco
San Francisco, California

Gary D. Hammer, MD, PhD
Millie Schembechler Professor of Adrenal Cancer
Director, Endocrine Oncology Program
Comprehensive Cancer Center
University of Michigan
Ann Arbor, Michigan

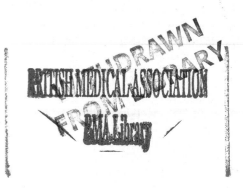

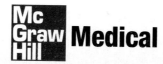
McGraw Hill Medical

New York Chicago San Francisco Lisbon London Madrid Mexico City
Milan New Delhi San Juan Seoul Singapore Sydney Toronto

Pathophysiology of Disease: An Introduction to Clinical Medicine, Sixth Edition

1 2 3 4 5 6 7 8 9 0 CTP/CTP 14 13 12 11 10 9

ISBN 978-0-07-162167-0
MHID 0-07-162167-9
ISSN 1079-6185

Notice

Medicine is an ever-changing science. As new research and clinical experience broaden our knowledge, changes in treatment and drug therapy are required. The authors and the publisher of this work have checked with sources believed to be reliable in their efforts to provide information that is complete and generally in accord with the standards accepted at the time of publication. However, in view of the possibility of human error or changes in medical sciences, neither the authors nor the publisher nor any other party who has been involved in the preparation or publication of this work warrants that the information contained herein is in every respect accurate or complete, and they disclaim all responsibility for any errors or omissions or for the results obtained from use of the information contained in this work. Readers are encouraged to confirm the information contained herein with other sources. For example and in particular, readers are advised to check the product information sheet included in the package of each drug they plan to administer to be certain that the information contained in this work is accurate and that changes have not been made in the recommended dose or in the contraindications for administration. This recommendation is of particular importance in connection with new or infrequently used drugs.

This book was set in Minion Pro by Silverchair Science + Communications, Inc.
The editors were James F. Shanahan and Robert Pancotti.
The production supervisor was Catherine Saggese.
The illustration manager was Armen Ovsepyan.
Project management was provided by Jeff Houck, Progressive Publishing Alternatives.
The text designer was Elise Lansdon; the cover designer was Margaret Webster-Shapiro.
Cover photo: Whole body MRI. Colored magnetic resonance imaging (MRI) scan of the whole body of a woman, in coronal (frontal) section. The head is seen in side (sagittal) section. Various parts of the anatomy of the human body are visible. The skeleton is seen as long bones of the limbs and vertebra of the spine. At top, the brain is pink in the skull. In the chest, the lungs are dark. In the abdomen, lobes of the liver are blue/green, while the rounded bladder is in the pelvis. This whole body image is the product of a number of MRI scans made along the length of the body and combined. MRI scanning uses radio waves and magnetic fields to produce "slice" images through the body. (Credit: Simon Fraser/Photo Researchers, Inc. Image and text copyright © 2009 Photo Researchers, Inc. All rights reserved.)
Smaller images: Credit: Images copyright © 2009 Photo Researchers, Inc. All rights reserved.
China Translation & Printing Services, Ltd. was printer and binder.

This book is printed on acid-free paper.

McGraw-Hill books are available at special quantity discounts to use as premiums and sales promotions, or for use in corporate training programs. To contact a representative, please e-mail us at bulksales@mcgraw-hill.com.

International Edition ISBN 978-0-07-163850-0; MHID 0-07-163850-4
Copyright © 2010. Exclusive rights by The McGraw-Hill Companies, Inc., for manufacture and export. This book cannot be reexported from the country to which it is consigned by McGraw-Hill. The International Edition is not available in North America.

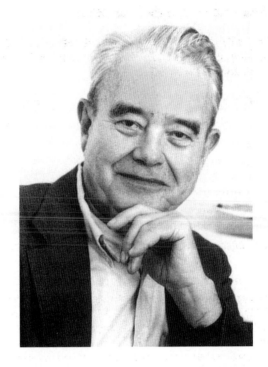

The editors and contributors wish to dedicate this sixth edition of *Pathophysiology of Disease: An Introduction to Clinical Medicine* to William Francis ("Fran") Ganong, MD, former Jack and DeLoris Lange Professor of Physiology, University of California San Francisco, who died at age 83 during the early planning for the sixth edition. Dr. Ganong joined Stephen J. McPhee, MD, and Viswanath R. Lingappa, MD, PhD, as an editor for the first five editions of *Pathophysiology of Disease*, and contributed a new chapter on vascular disease beginning with the second edition. Fran, widely renowned as the author of the popular Lange series book, *Review of Medical Physiology*, willingly read, amended, and corrected every chapter for the first five editions of *Pathophysiology*. Although he had re-tired as Chairman of the Department of Physiology at UCSF in 1987, Fran continued to read widely in the field of physiology and related disciplines and thus made a superb editor in querying and clarifying the science in this book. When Dr. Lingappa left UCSF in 2002, Fran and Steve edited the fifth edition together. Finally, Fran was enthusiastic about the idea of bringing on as coeditor, Gary D. Hammer, MD, PhD, Millie Schembechler Professor of Adrenal Cancer and Director of the Endocrine Oncology Program in the Comprehensive Cancer Center at the University of Michigan. Thus, this sixth edition of *Pathophysiology* is the result, in many ways, of Fran's work. We miss him.

Key Features of the Sixth Edition of
Pathophysiology of Disease

- **Case-based reviews of the essentials of pathophysiology** – covering the signs and symptoms of 100 diseases commonly encountered in medical practice

- **Logically organized** by body system and organ

- **NEW full-color illustrations** enrich the text

- **NEW sections** in the chapters on liver disease and inflammatory rheumatic diseases and a completely rewritten chapter on male reproductive tract disorders

- **111 case studies (22 new ones)** provide an opportunity to test your understanding of the pathophysiology of each disease discussed

- **A complete chapter** devoted to detailed analyses of cases

- **"Checkpoint" review questions** appear in every chapter

- **Numerous tables and diagrams** encapsulate important information

- **References** are included for each chapter topic

NEW full-color illustrations enhance the content

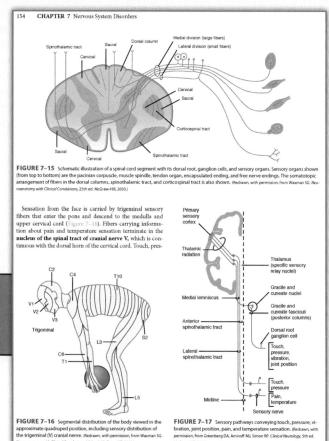

154　**CHAPTER 7** Nervous System Disorders

FIGURE 7–15 Schematic illustration of a spinal cord segment with its dorsal root, ganglion cells, and sensory organs. Sensory organs shown (from top to bottom) are the pacinian corpuscle, muscle spindle, tendon organ, encapsulated ending, and free nerve endings. The somatotopic arrangement of fibers in the dorsal columns, spinothalamic tract, and corticospinal tract is also shown. (Redrawn, with permission, from Waxman SG. *Neuroanatomy with Clinical Correlations,* 25th ed. McGraw-Hill, 2003.)

Sensation from the face is carried by trigeminal sensory fibers that enter the pons and descend to the medulla and upper cervical cord (Figure 7–18). Fibers carrying information about pain and temperature sensation terminate in the **nucleus of the spinal tract of cranial nerve V,** which is continuous with the dorsal horn of the cervical cord. Touch, pres-

FIGURE 7–16 Segmental distribution of the body viewed in the approximate quadruped position, including sensory distribution of the trigeminal (V) cranial nerve. (Redrawn, with permission, from Waxman SG. *Neuroanatomy with Clinical Correlations,* 25th ed. McGraw-Hill, 2003.)

FIGURE 7–17 Sensory pathways conveying touch, pressure, vibration, joint position, pain, and temperature sensation. (Redrawn, with permission, from Greenberg DA, Aminoff MJ, Simon RP. *Clinical Neurology,* 5th ed. McGraw-Hill, 2002.)

Valuable case studies in every chapter

"Checkpoint" review questions appear in every chapter

Tables encapsulate important information

---

animals, induction of intestinal inflammation induces visceral hyperalgesia and altered intestinal motility and secretion that persists many months after the inflammation is resolved. A similar mechanism may occur in a subset of patients who develop irritable bowel syndrome after an infection causes intestinal inflammation.

CHECKPOINT

69. List three characteristics of irritable bowel syndrome.
70. What are possible factors in the pathogenesis of the irritable bowel syndrome?

CASE STUDIES

Eva M. Aagaard, MD, & Yeong Kwok, MD

(See Chapter 25, p. XXX for Answers)

CASE 57

A 60-year-old man presents to the clinic with a 3-month history of gradually worsening dysphagia (difficulty swallowing). At first, he noticed the problem when eating solid food such as steak, but now it happens even with drinking water. He has a sensation that whatever he swallows becomes stuck in his chest and does not go into the stomach. He has also developed worsening heartburn, especially upon lying down, and has had to prop himself up at night to lessen the heartburn. He has lost 10 kg as a result of his swallowing difficulties. His physical examination is unremarkable. A barium swallow x-ray reveals a decrease in peristalsis of the body of the esophagus along with dilatation of the lower esophagus and tight closure of the lower esophageal sphincter. There is a beaked appearance of the distal esophagus involving the lower esophageal sphincter. There is very little passage of barium into the stomach.

Questions

A. What is the likely diagnosis in this patient, and what is the underlying pathophysiology of this condition?
B. Botulinum toxin can be used to treat this disorder. How does it help ameliorate the symptoms?
C. What are the possible complications of this disorder, and how do they arise?

CASE 58

A 32-year-old woman presents to her primary care provider complaining of a persistent burning sensation in her chest and upper abdomen. The symptoms are worse at night when she is lying down and after meals. She has tried drinking hot cocoa to help her sleep. She is a smoker and frequently relies on benzodiazepines for insomnia. She notes a sour taste in her mouth every morning. Physical examination is normal.

Questions

A. What is the pathogenetic mechanism of her GI disorder?
B. How may her lifestyle impact her symptoms?
C. What are some complications of chronic esophageal reflux disease?

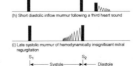

FIGURE 7–21 Syringomyelia (the presence of a cavity in the spinal cord resulting from breakdown of gliomatous new formations, presenting clinically with pain and paresthesias followed by muscular atrophy of the hands) involving the cervicothoracic portion of the cord. (Redrawn, with permission, from Waxman SG. *Neuroanatomy with Clinical Correlations*, 25th ed. McGraw-Hill, 2003.)

impair all primary sensation contralateral to the lesion. Because sensory fibers converge at the thalamus, lesions there tend to cause fairly equal loss of pain, temperature, and proprioceptive sensation on the contralateral half of the face and body. Lesions of the sensory cortex in the parietal lobe impair discriminative sensation on the opposite side of the body, whereas detection of the primary modalities of sensation may remain relatively intact.

CHECKPOINT

19. What fibers carry pain, and how are they segregated from fibers that carry proprioception information in the spinal cord?
20. What are the differences in characteristics of sensory loss at different levels of the nervous system?
21. What is the function of the sensory cortex in the parietal lobe, and what are the clinical features of damage to this region?

VISION & CONTROL OF EYE MOVEMENTS

The visual system provides our most important source of sensory information about the environment. The visual system and pathways for the control of eye movements are among the best characterized pathways in the nervous system. Familiarity with these neuroanatomic features is often extremely valuable in localization of neurologic disease.

Anatomy

The cornea and lens of the eye refract and focus images on the photosensitive posterior portion of the retina. The posterior retina contains two classes of specialized photoreceptor cells, **rods** and **cones**, which transduce photons into electrical signals. At the retina, the image is reversed in the horizontal and vertical planes so that the inferior visual field falls on the superior portions of the retina and the lateral field is detected by the nasal half of the retina.

Fibers from the nasal half of the retina traverse the medial portion of the optic nerve and cross to the other side at the **optic chiasm** (Figure 7–22). Each **optic tract** contains fibers from the same half of the visual field of both eyes. The optic tracts terminate in the **lateral geniculate nuclei** of the thalamus. Lateral geniculate neurons send fibers to the primary visual cortex in the occipital lobe (area 17, **calcarine cortex;** see Figure 7–9). These fibers form the **optic radiations,** which extend through the white matter of the temporal lobes and the inferior portion of the parietal lobes.

Eye movements are produced by the extraocular muscles, which function in pairs to move the eyes along three axes (Figure 7–23). These muscles are innervated by the **oculomotor** (III), **trochlear** (IV), and **abducens** (VI) nerves. The oculomotor nerve innervates the ipsilateral **medial, superior,** and **inferior rectus muscles** and the **inferior oblique muscles.** It also supplies the ipsilateral levator palpebrae, which elevates the eyelid. The oculomotor nerve also carries parasympathetic fibers that mediate pupillary constriction (see later discussion). Trochlear nerve fibers decussate before leaving the brainstem, and each trochlear nerve supplies the contralateral **superior oblique muscle.** The abducens nerve innervates the **lateral rectus muscle** of the same side.

Cortical and brainstem gaze centers innervate the extraocular motor nuclei and provide for supranuclear control of gaze. A **vertical gaze center** is located in the midbrain tegmentum, and **lateral gaze centers** are present in the pontine paramedian reticular formation. Each lateral gaze center sends fibers to the neighboring ipsilateral abducens nucleus and, via the **medial longitudinal fasciculus,** to the contralateral oculomotor nucleus. Therefore, activation of the right lateral gaze center stimulates conjugate deviation of the eyes to the right. Rapid **saccadic eye movements** are initiated by the **frontal eye fields** in the premotor cortex that stimulate conjugate movement of the eyes to the opposite side. Slower eye movements involved in pursuit of moving objects are controlled by parieto-occipital gaze centers, which stimulate conjugate gaze

---

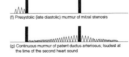

(a) Aortic systolic ejection murmur following an ejection click and ending before the second heart sound

(b) Long pulmonary systolic ejection murmur in severe pulmonary stenosis lasting through left ventricular systole and ending before a delayed and diminished pulmonary have closure

(c) Pansystolic murmur of mitral or tricuspid regurgitation or of ventricular septal defect

(d) Immediate diastolic murmur of aortic or pulmonary regurgitation

(e) Delayed diastolic murmur of mitral stenosis following the opening snap

(f) Presystolic (late diastolic) murmur of mitral stenosis

(g) Continuous murmur of patent ductus arteriosus, loudest at the time of the second heart sound

(h) Short diastolic inflow murmur following a third heart sound

(i) Late systolic murmur of hemodynamically insignificant mitral regurgitation

S_1 S_2
Systole   Diastole

FIGURE 10–21. The timing of the principal cardiac murmurs. (Redrawn, with permission, from Wood P. *Diseases of the Heart and Circulation*, 3rd ed. Lippincott, 1968.)

Once symptoms occur, the prognosis is poor if the obstruction is untreated, with average life expectancies of 2, 3, and 5 years for angina pectoris, syncope, and heart failure, respectively.

On physical examination, palpation of the carotid upstroke reveals a pulsation (pulsus) that is both decreased (parvus) and late (tardus) relative to the apical impulse. Palpation of

the chest reveals an apical impulse that is laterally displaced and sustained. On auscultation, a midsystolic murmur is heard, loudest at the base of the heart, and often with radiation to the sternal notch and the neck. Depending on the cause of the aortic stenosis, a crisp, relatively high-pitched aortic ejection sound can be heard just after the first heart sound. Finally, a fourth heart sound (S_4) is often present.

Etiology

Various causes of aortic stenosis are listed and described in Table 10–4.

Pathophysiology

The normal aortic valve area is approximately 3.5–4.0 cm². Critical aortic stenosis is usually present when the area is less than 0.8 cm². At this point, the systolic gradient between the left ventricle and the aorta can exceed 150 mm Hg, and most patients are symptomatic (Figure 10–22a). The fixed outflow obstruction places a large afterload on the ventricle. The compensatory mechanisms of the heart can be understood by examining Laplace's law for a sphere, where wall stress (T) is proportionate to the product of the transmural pressure (P) and cavitary radius (r) and inversely proportionate to wall thickness (W):

$$T \propto P \times \frac{r}{W}$$

In response to the pressure overload (increased P), left ventricular wall thickness markedly increases—while the cavitary radius remains relatively unchanged—by parallel replication of sarcomeres. These compensatory changes, termed "concentric hypertrophy," reduce the increase in wall tension observed in aortic stenosis (see Aortic Regurgitation). Analysis of pressure-volume loops reveals that, to

TABLE 10–4. Causes of aortic stenosis.

Type	Pathology	Clinical Presentation
Congenital	The valve can be unicuspid, bicuspid, or tricuspid with partially fused leaflets. Abnormal flow can lead to fibrosis and calcification of the leaflets.	Patient usually develops symptoms before age 30 years.
Rheumatic	Tissue inflammation results in adhesion and fusing of the commissures. Fibrosis and calcification of the leaflet tips can occur because of continued turbulent flow.	Patient usually develops symptoms between ages 30 and 70 years. Often the valve will also be regurgitant. Accompanying mitral valve disease is frequently present.
Degenerative	Leaflets become inflexible because of calcium deposition at the bases. The leaflet tips remain relatively normal.	The most likely cause of aortic stenosis in patients older than 70 years. Particularly prevalent in patients with diabetes or hypercholesterolemia.

Contents

Authors

Eva M. Aagaard, MD
Associate Professor of Medicine, University of Colorado Denver School of Medicine, Aurora, Colorado
Case Studies and Answers

Gregory Barsh, MD, PhD
Professor of Pediatrics and Genetics, Stanford University School of Medicine
gbarsh@stanford.edu
Genetic Disease

Douglas C. Bauer, MD
Professor of Medicine, Epidemiology and Biostatistics, Division of General Internal Medicine, University of California, San Francisco
Dbauer@psg.ucsf.edu
Thyroid Disease

Karen C. Bloch, MD, MPH
Assistant Professor, Infectious Diseases and Preventive Medicine, Vanderbilt University Medical Center
karen.bloch@vanderbilt.edu
Infectious Diseases

Nigel Bunnett, PhD
Professor, University of California, San Francisco
nigel.bunnett@ucsf.edu
Gastrointestinal Disease

J. Ben Davoren, MD, PhD
Clinical Professor of Medicine, University of California San Francisco; Director, Clinical Informatics, San Francisco VA Medical Center
Ben.davoren@va.gov
Blood Disorders

Tobias Else, MD
Metabolism, Endocrinology & Diabetes, Department of Internal Medicine, University of Michigan, Ann Arbor
telse@umich.edu
Disorders of the Adrenal Medulla; Disorders of the Hypothalamus & Pituitary Gland; Disorders of the Adrenal Cortex

Mikkel Fode
PhD trainee, Department of Urology, Herlev Hospital, Herlev, Denmark
mikkelfode@hotmail.com
Disorders of the Male Reproductive Tract

Jonathan D. Fuchs, MD, MPH
Assistant Clinical Professor of Medicine, Department of Medicine, University of California, San Francisco; Director, Vaccine Studies, HIV Research Section, San Francisco Department of Health, San Francisco, California
Case Studies and Answers

Janet L. Funk, MD
Associate Professor of Medicine, University of Arizona, Tucson, Arizona
Jfunk@u.arizona.edu
Disorders of the Endocrine Pancreas

Allan C. Gelber, MD, MPH, PhD
Associate Professor of Medicine; Director, Rheumatology Fellowship Program, Johns Hopkins University School of Medicine
agelber@jhmi.edu
Inflammatory Rheumatic Diseases

Gary D. Hammer, MD, PhD
Millie Schembechler Professor of Adrenal Cancer; Director, Endocrine Oncology Program; Comprehensive Cancer Center, University of Michigan, Ann Arbor, Michigan
ghammer@umich.edu
Disorders of the Adrenal Medulla; Disorders of the Hypothalamus & Pituitary Gland; Disorders of the Adrenal Cortex

Joachim H. Ix, MD
Assistant Professor, Division of Nephrology, Department of Medicine, University of California San Diego, The Veteran Affairs San Diego Healthcare Systems, San Diego, California
joeix@ucsd.edu
Renal Disease

Mandana Khalili, MD
Associate Professor of Medicine, University of California San Francisco, San Francisco, California; Department of Medicine, Director of Clinical Hepatology, San Francisco General Hospital, San Francisco, California
mandana.khalili@ucsf.edu
Liver Disease

Jeffrey L. Kishiyama, MD
Associate Clinical Professor of Medicine, University of California, San Francisco
jeff.kishiyama@ucsf.edu
Disorders of the Immune System

Fred M. Kusumoto, MD
Associate Professor of Medicine, Director of Electrophysiology and Pacing, Division of Cardiovascular Diseases, Department of Medicine, Mayo Clinic, Jacksonville, Florida
Kusumoto.Fred@mayo.edu
Cardiovascular Disorders: Heart Disease

Yeong Kwok, MD
Assistant Professor of Medicine, Division of General Medicine, Department of Medicine, University of Michigan
ykwok@med.umich.edu
Case Studies and Answers

Stuart M. Levine, MD
Assistant Professor of Medicine, Division of Rheumatology; Co-Director, The Johns Hopkins Vasculitis Center, Johns Hopkins University School of Medicine, Baltimore, Maryland
slevine@jhmi.edu
Inflammatory Rheumatic Diseases

Charles E. Liao, MD
University of California at San Francisco, School of Medicine; San Francisco General Hospital
c_liao@hotmail.com
Liver Disease

Catherine Lomen-Hoerth, MD, PhD
Associate Professor of Neurology, Director, ALS Center, Department of Neurology, University of California, San Francisco
catherine.lomen-hoerth@ucsf.edu
Nervous System Disorders

Timothy H. McCalmont, MD
Professor of Clinical Pathology & Dermatology, University of California, San Francisco, San Francisco, California
tim.mccalmont@ucsf.edu
Diseases of the Skin

Stephen J. McPhee, MD
Professor of Medicine, Division of General Internal Medicine, Department of Medicine, University of California, San Francisco
smcphee@medicine.ucsf.edu
Disorders of the Adrenal Medulla; Disorders of the Exocrine Pancreas; Thyroid Disease; Disorders of the Adrenal Cortex; Disorders of the Male Reproductive Tract

Robert O. Messing, MD
Professor of Neurology, University of California San Francisco; Senior Associate Director, Ernest Gallo Clinic and Research Center, Emeryville, California
Robert.Messing@ucsf.edu
Nervous System Disorders

Jason C. Mills, MD, PhD
Assistant Professor, Department of Pathology & Immunology, Washington University School of Medicine, St. Louis, Missouri
jmills@pathology.wustl.edu
Gastrointestinal Disease

Igor Mitrovic, MD
Associate Professor, Director of Professional School Education, Department of Physiology, University of California, San Francisco
imitrov@phy.ucsf.edu
Cardiovascular Disorders: Vascular Disease

Mark M. Moasser, MD
Associate Professor of Medicine, Helen Diller Family Comprehensive Cancer Center, University of California, San Francisco
mmoasser@medicine.ucsf.edu
Neoplasia

Tung T. Nguyen, MD
Clinical Professor of Medicine, Division of General Internal Medicine, University of California, San Francisco
Liver Disease

Dana A. Ohl, MD
Professor of Urology, University of Michigan, Ann Arbor, Michigan
daohl@med.umich.edu
Disorders of the Male Reproductive Tract

Benjamin D. Parker, MD
Division of Nephrology, Department of Medicine, University of California, San Diego, The Veteran Affairs San Diego Healthcare Systems, San Diego, California
bdparker@ucsd.edu
Renal Disease

Thomas J. Prendergast, MD
Associate Professor of Medicine, Pulmonary & Critical Care Medicine, Oregon Health & Science University, Portland; Staff Physician, Portland Veterans' Affairs Medical Center
thomas.prendergast@va.gov
Pulmonary Disease

Karen J. Purcell, MD, PhD
Fertility Physicians of Northern California, San Jose, California
cjpurcell@pol.net
Disorders of the Female Reproductive Tract

Antony Rosen, MB, ChB, BSc (Hons)
Mary Betty Stevens Professor of Medicine, Professor of Pathology; Director, Division of Rheumatology, Johns Hopkins University School of Medicine, Baltimore, Maryland
arosen@jhmi.edu
Inflammatory Rheumatic Diseases

Stephen J. Ruoss, MD
Associate Professor of Medicine, Pulmonary and Critical Care Medicine, Stanford University School of Medicine
ruoss@stanford.edu
Pulmonary Disease

Eric J. Seeley, MD
Fellow in Pulmonary and Critical Care, Department of Medicine, University of California, San Francisco
eric.seeley@ucsf.edu
Pulmonary Disease

Deborah E. Sellmeyer, MD
Department of Medicine/Endocrinology, Johns Hopkins University School of Medicine, Baltimore, Maryland; Department of Medicine/Endocrinology, Johns Hopkins Bayview Medical Center, Baltimore, Maryland
dsellme1@jhmi.edu
Disorders of the Parathyroids & Calcium & Phosphorus Metabolism

Dolores M. Shoback, MD
Professor of Medicine, University of California, San Francisco; Staff Physician, San Francisco Department of Veterans Affairs Medical Center
dolores.shoback@ucsf.edu
Disorders of the Parathyroids & Calcium & Phosphorus Metabolism

Diane M. Simeone, MD
Lazar J. Greenfield Professor of Surgery and Professor of Molecular and Integrative Physiology; Chief, Gastrointestinal Surgery, University of Michigan
simeone@umich.edu
Disorders of the Exocrine Pancreas

Jens Sønksen, MD, PhD
Professor of Urology; Head, Section of Male Infertility and Microsurgery, Department of Urology, Herlev Hospital, Herlev, Denmark; University of Copenhagen, Copenhagen, Denmark
jens@sonksen.dk
Disorders of the Male Reproductive Tract

Christopher J. Sonnenday, MD, MHS
Assistant Professor of Surgery, University of Michigan School of Medicine, Ann Arbor, Michigan; Assistant Professor of Health Management & Policy, University of Michigan School of Public Health, Ann Arbor, Michigan
csonnend@umich.edu
Disorders of the Exocrine Pancreas

Thaddeus S. Stappenbeck, MD, PhD
Assistant Professor, Department of Pathology & Immunology, Washington University School of Medicine, St. Louis, Missouri
stappenb@pathology.wustl.edu
Gastrointestinal Disease

Robert N. Taylor, MD, PhD
Vice Chair for Research, Department of Gynecology and Obstetrics, Emory University School of Medicine
robert.n.taylor@emory.edu
Disorders of the Female Reproductive Tract

Sunny Wang, MD
Hematology/Oncology Fellow, University of California, San Francisco
sunny.wang@ucsf.edu
Blood Disorders

Preface

One of Dr. Jack Lange's goals late in life was to add a pathophysiology text to the Lange series of unique basic and clinical books that have had such a great impact on health science education all over the world. *Pathophysiology of Disease: An Introduction to Clinical Medicine* is the result, and until he died in 1999, Dr. Lange was one of its editors. The goal of this book is outlined in the introductory chapter (Chapter 1)—to introduce students to clinical medicine by reviewing the pathophysiologic basis of the symptoms and signs of various common diseases.

The book has proved useful as a text for both pathophysiology and introduction to clinical medicine courses in medical schools, and it has been popular in similar courses in nursing schools and allied health programs. It is valuable to students early in their medical school years by highlighting the clinical relevance of their basic science courses and in preparation for their USMLE Step 1 examinations. The book is also helpful to students engaged in their internal medicine and surgery clerkships and to house officers as an up-to-date summary of relevant physiology and a source of key references. Practitioners (both internists and specialists who provide generalist care) will find it beneficial as a refresher text, designed to update their knowledge of the mechanisms underlying diseases. Nurses and other allied health practitioners have found that its concise format and broad scope facilitate their understanding of basic disease entities.

Pathophysiology of Disease has been translated into Spanish, Italian, Chinese, Japanese, Greek, Turkish, Albanian, Macedonian, Portuguese, and Indonesian. It is also available along with other Lange books on the Internet, at www.accessmedicine.com, an online version of McGraw-Hill's many medical textbooks.

In preparation for this sixth edition, the editors and authors reviewed the entire book. There have been many revisions aimed at updating information, improving clarity, and eliminating minor errors. References have also been updated, with emphasis on valuable reviews. "Checkpoints," collections of review questions, continue to appear throughout the chapters.

New to This Edition

Sadly, between publication of the fifth edition and start of work on this sixth edition, Dr. William "Fran" Ganong, one of the book's editors for the previous 5 editions, died after a long illness. This sixth edition is dedicated to him (see Dedication). Thus, a major change with this new edition is the introduction of a new title page editor, Gary D. Hammer, MD, PhD. While attending on the wards at the University of California, San Francisco, Dr. Stephen McPhee first met Dr. Hammer when he was a resident in internal medicine there. Dr. Hammer is now Millie Schembechler Professor of Adrenal Cancer and Director of the Endocrine Oncology Program at the Comprehensive Cancer Center, and Associate Professor in the Department of Internal Medicine in the Metabolism, Endocrinology, and Diabetes Section and Associate Professor, Department of Molecular and Integrative Physiology, at the University of Michigan. The combination of his expertise in molecular and integrative physiology and his clinical proficiency in endocrinology and metabolism make him an ideal editor for this text, which is intended as a bridge between basic science and clinical understanding. Dr. Hammer's energy and enthusiasm are apparent in the look and feel of this new edition.

With this sixth edition, the authorship of several chapters has evolved and transitioned—the editors wish to welcome aboard the following new contributors and thank the following past contributors who are now departing the book:

- Sunny Wang, MD, has joined J. Ben Davoren, MD, PhD, as the coauthor of Chapter 6: Blood Disorders;
- Catherine Lomen-Hoerth, MD, PhD, joins Robert O. Messing, MD, for the current revision of Chapter 7: Nervous System Disorders, and will take over the chapter in future editions;
- Eric J. Seeley, MD, has joined Thomas J. Prendergast, MD, and Stephen J. Ruoss, MD, as a coauthor for Chapter 9: Pulmonary Disease;
- Igor Mitrovic, MD, has taken over revision of Dr. Fran Ganong's Chapter 11: Cardiovascular Disorders: Vascular Disease;
- Tobias Else, MD, and Dr. Hammer, join Dr. McPhee for the current revisions of Chapter 12: Disorders of the Adrenal Medulla, and Chapter 21: Disorders of the Adrenal Cortex, and will henceforth take over the updating of these chapters;
- Jason C. Mills, MD, PhD, and Thaddeus S. Stappenbeck, MD, PhD, have taken on and revised Chapter 13: Gastrointestinal Disease as Nigel Bunnett, PhD, and Vishwanath Lingappa, MD, PhD, have retired from the book;

- Mandana Khalili, MD, working with Charles E. Liao, MD, produced the current revision of Chapter 14: Liver Disease by Tung T. Nguyen, MD, who will retire from the book;
- Christopher J. Sonnenday, MD, and Diane M. Simeone, MD, join Dr. McPhee for the current revision of Chapter 15: Disorders of the Exocrine Pancreas, and will henceforth take over the chapter from him;
- Benjamin D. Parker, MD, has joined Joachim H. Ix, MD, as coauthor of Chapter 16: Renal Disease;
- Mikkel Fode, Jens Sønksen, MD, PhD, and Dana A. Ohl, MD, join Dr. McPhee for the current revision of Chapter 23: Disorders of the Male Reproductive Tract, and will henceforth take over the chapter; and
- Stuart M. Levine, MD, joins Allan C. Gelber, MD, MPH, PhD, and Antony Rosen, MB, ChB, BSc, as a coauthor of Chapter 24: Inflammatory Rheumatic Diseases.

With these transitions, the content of almost half of the book has benefited from the new contributors' viewpoint and input.

In addition, as with previous editions, each chapter ends with a collection of Case Studies. These clinical problems give students an opportunity to test their understanding of the pathophysiology of each clinical entity discussed and to apply their knowledge to exemplar clinical situations. With this edition, an additional 22 Case Studies have been added by Yeong Kwok, MD, bringing the total number to 111; in this effort, Dr. Kwok joined his work to that of Eva M. Aagaard, MD, and Jonathan D. Fuchs, MD, MPH, who prepared the cases for the previous editions. Drs. Aagaard and Fuchs have now handed on to Dr. Kwok the task of adding to and maintaining this valuable learning tool. The editors and chapter authors are indebted to Drs. Aagaard and Fuchs for their work on the previous five editions. As before, detailed analyses of the cases appear in Chapter 25: Case Study Answers; Dr. Kwok has added answers to the new Case Studies and updated the existing answers to reflect the changes made by chapter authors in their revisions.

Finally, the sixth edition of *Pathophysiology of Disease: An Introduction to Clinical Medicine* also introduces an attractive new design with four-color illustrations and layout.

With publication of this sixth edition, the editors want to extend special thanks, not only to the contributors old and new, but also to the students and colleagues who have offered helpful comments and criticisms for each of the previous editions. The authors and editors continue to welcome comments and recommendations for future editions, in writing or via electronic mail. The editors' and authors' institutional and e-mail addresses are given in the Authors section.

Stephen J. McPhee, MD
San Francisco, California

Gary D. Hammer, MD, PhD
Ann Arbor, Michigan
October 2009

Introduction

Stephen J. McPhee, MD, &
Gary D. Hammer, MD, PhD

"A man cannot become a competent surgeon without the full knowledge of human anatomy and physiology, and the physician without physiology and chemistry flounders along in an aimless fashion, never able to gain any accurate conception of disease, practicing a sort of popgun pharmacy, hitting now the malady and again the patient, he himself not knowing which."

Sir William Osler (1849–1919)

Osler expresses particularly well the relation between the basic sciences and clinical medicine in the aphorism cited above. Indeed, ever since the Middle Ages, wise physicians and others concerned with the sick and their care have realized that most human disease may be understood in a real sense as disordered physiology (pathophysiology). Something (eg, a mutation in a gene or invasion by a bacterial organism) triggers an illness, and the body reacts with molecular, cellular, and systemic responses that are the symptoms and signs of the disease. Therefore, with proper knowledge of normal structure and function, and the ways in which these can become disordered, comes the ability to understand disease and to design rational and effective treatment. In addition, of course, the relation between pathophysiology and disease is a two-way street. Diseases may be viewed as "experiments of nature" that may uncover previously unknown or unappreciated physiologic mechanisms, and the investigation of these physiologic mechanisms in normal individuals advances our fundamental biomedical knowledge. Therefore, it is important that students understand normal structure and function, and how they can become disordered, and apply this knowledge to disease.

The aim of this book is to provide students with an introduction to clinical medicine through the study of diseases as manifestations of pathophysiology. The authors (all experts in their respective fields) have provided a brief review of the relevant normal structure and function of each system in the body, followed by a description of the underlying pathophysiologic mechanisms that underlie several common diseases related to that system. With this approach comes an explication of the symptoms and signs of each disease state and an essential framework for the student's later mastery of treatment strategies. Several subject areas that are not restricted to a single body system are also covered (eg, neoplasia and infectious disease), but the same approach is used in these instances as well. In general, diagnosis and treatment are not covered here but are left for later, more detailed study and textbooks such as *Current Medical Diagnosis & Treatment*. No attempt is made here to be comprehensive or complete. The aim is to introduce students to diseases as manifestations of disordered function and to start them thinking about symptoms and signs in terms of their pathophysiologic basis.

Genetic Disease

Gregory Barsh, MD, PhD

Mechanisms of cellular and tissue dysfunction in genetic diseases are as varied as the organs they affect. To some extent, these mechanisms are similar to those that occur in nonheritable disorders. For example, a fracture resulting from decreased bone density in osteoporosis heals in much the same way as one caused by a defective collagen gene in osteogenesis imperfecta, and the response to coronary atherosclerosis in most individuals does not depend on whether they have inherited a defective low-density lipoprotein (LDL) receptor. Thus, the pathophysiologic principles that distinguish genetic disease focus not so much on the affected organ system as on the mechanisms of mutation, inheritance, and molecular pathways from genotype to phenotype.

This chapter begins with a discussion of the terminology used to describe inherited conditions, the prevalence of genetic disease, and some major principles and considerations in medical genetics. Important terms and keywords used throughout the chapter are defined in Table 2–1.

Next, a group of disorders caused by mutations in collagen genes is discussed (ie, **osteogenesis imperfecta**). Although osteogenesis imperfecta is often considered a single entity, different mutations and different genes subject to mutation lead to a wide spectrum of clinical phenotypes. The different types of osteogenesis imperfecta exhibit typical patterns of autosomal dominant or autosomal recessive inheritance and are, therefore, examples of so-called **mendelian conditions.** To show how environmental factors can influence the relationship between genotype and phenotype, I discuss another mendelian condition, **phenylketonuria.** This serves as a paradigm for newborn screening programs and treatment of

genetic disease. Several genetic conditions have been found to depend not only on the gene being inherited but also on the phenotype or the sex of the parent. As an example of a condition that exhibits nontraditional inheritance, **fragile X-associated mental retardation syndrome** is discussed. This syndrome not only is the most common inherited cause of mental retardation but also illustrates how different types of mutations can explain the perplexing phenomenon of **genetic anticipation,** where the severity of a mendelian syndrome appears to progress with every generation of inheritance. Another group of disorders that depend on the phenotype and sex of the parent consists of those that affect the mitochondrial genome. As examples, **Leber's hereditary optic neuropathy** (LHON) and **myoclonic epilepsy with ragged red fibers** (MERRF) are considered. These illustrate the principles of mitochondrial inheritance and its pathophysiology. **Aneuploidy** is discussed as one of the most common types of human genetic disease that does not affect DNA structure but instead alters the normal chromosome content per cell. The example that is considered, **Down syndrome,** has had a major impact on reproductive medicine and reproductive decision making and serves to illustrate general principles that apply to many aneuploid conditions. Finally, I consider how the Human Genome Project is improving our understanding of pathophysiology for many diseases. With the completion of the human genome sequence and the rapid accumulation of sequence variation from different human populations, prospects are at hand to identify genetic components of any human phenotype.

UNIQUE PATHOPHYSIOLOGIC ASPECTS OF GENETIC DISEASES

Although the phenotypes of genetic diseases are diverse, their causes are not. The primary cause of any genetic disease is a change in the sequence or cellular content of DNA that ulti-

mately deranges gene expression. Most genetic diseases are caused by an alteration in DNA sequence that alters the synthesis of a single gene product. However, some genetic diseas-

TABLE 2–1   Glossary of terms and keywords.

Term	Definition
Acrocentric	Refers to the terminal location of the centromere on chromosomes 13, 14, 15, 21, and 22.
Allelic heterogeneity	The situation in which multiple alleles at a single locus can produce one or more disease phenotypes.
Amorphic	Refers to mutations that cause a complete loss of function for the respective gene and, therefore, yield the same phenotype as a complete gene deletion.
Aneuploidy	A general term used to denote any unbalanced chromosome complement.
Antimorphic	Refers to mutations that, when present in heterozygous form opposite a nonmutant allele, will result in a phenotype similar to homozygosity for loss-of-function alleles.
Ascertainment bias	The situation in which individuals or families in a genetic study are not representative of the general population because of the way in which they are identified.
Autosomal	Located on chromosomes 1–22 rather than X or Y.
CpG island	A segment of DNA that contains a relatively high density of 5′-CG-3′ dinucleotides. Such segments are frequently unmethylated and located close to ubiquitously expressed genes.
Dictyotene	The end of prophase during female meiosis I in which fetal oocytes are arrested prior to ovulation.
Dominant	A pattern of inheritance or mechanism of gene action in which the effects of a variant allele can be observed in the presence of a nonmutant allele.
Dominant negative	A type of pathophysiologic mechanism that occurs when a mutant allele interferes with the normal function of the nonmutant gene product.
Dosage compensation	Mechanism by which a difference in gene dosage between two cells is equalized. For XX cells in mammals, decreased expression from one of the two X chromosomes results in a concentration of gene product similar to an XY cell.
End-product deficiency	A pathologic mechanism in which absence or reduction in the product of a particular enzymatic reaction leads to disease.
Epigenetic	Refers to a phenotypic effect that is heritable, through somatic cell division and/or across organismal generations, but that does not depend on variation in DNA sequence. Instead, epigenetic inheritance is associated with alterations in chromatin structure such as DNA methylation or histone modification that can be transmitted during cell division.
Expressivity	The extent to which a mutant genotype affects phenotype, including the tissues that are affected, and the severity of those effects.
Fitness	The effect of a mutant allele on an individual's ability to produce offspring.
Founder effect	One of several possible explanations for an unexpectedly high frequency of a deleterious gene in a population. If the population was founded by a small ancestral group, it may have, by chance, contained a large number of carriers for the deleterious gene.
Gamete	The egg or sperm cell that represents a potential reproductive contribution to the next generation. Gametes have undergone meiosis and so contain half the normal number of chromosomes found in zygotic cells.
Gene dosage	The principle that the amount of product expressed for a particular gene is proportionate to the number of gene copies present per cell.
Genetic anticipation	A clinical phenomenon in which the phenotype observed in individuals carrying a deleterious gene appears more severe in successive generations. Possible explanations include ascertainment bias or a multistep mutational mechanism such as expansion of triplet repeats.
Haplotype	A set of closely linked DNA sequence variants on a single chromosome.
Hemizygous	A term referring to the presence of only one allele at a locus, either because the other allele is deleted or because it is normally not present, eg, X-linked genes in males.
Heterochromatin	One of two alternative forms of chromosomal material (the other is euchromatin) in which chromosomal DNA is highly condensed and usually devoid of genes that are actively transcribed.
Heteroplasmy	The mixture of mutant and nonmutant mitochondrial DNA molecules in a single cell.
Heterozygote advantage	One way to explain an unexpectedly high frequency of a recessively inherited mutation in a particular population. During recent evolution, carriers (ie, heterozygotes) are postulated to have had a higher fitness than homozygous nonmutant individuals.

(continued)

TABLE 2–1 Glossary of terms and keywords. (Continued)

Term	Definition
Heterozygous	Having two alleles at the same locus that are different.
Homozygous	Having two alleles at the same locus that are the same.
Hypermorphic	Refers to a mutation that has an effect similar to increasing the number of normal gene copies per cell.
Hypomorphic	Refers to a mutation that reduces but does not eliminate the activity of a particular gene product.
Imprinting	Most commonly, the process whereby expression of a gene depends on whether it was inherited from the mother or the father.
Linkage disequilibrium	A condition in which certain combinations of closely linked alleles, or haplotypes, are present in a population at frequencies not predicted by their individual allele frequencies.
Locus heterogeneity	A situation in which mutations of different genes produce similar or identical phenotypes. Also referred to as genetic heterogeneity.
Mendelian	A form of inheritance that obeys Mendel's laws, ie, autosomal dominant, autosomal recessive, X-linked dominant, or X-linked recessive.
Mosaicism	A situation in which a genetic alteration is present in some but not all the cells of a single individual. In germline or gonadal mosaicism, the alteration is present in germ cells but not somatic cells. In somatic mosaicism, the genetic alteration is present in some but not all of the somatic cells (and is generally not present in the germ cells).
Monosomy	A reduction in zygotic cells from two to one in the number of copies for a particular chromosomal segment or chromosome.
Neomorphic	Refers to a mutation that imparts a novel function to its gene product and consequently results in a phenotype distinct from an alteration in gene dosage.
Nondisjunction	Failure of two homologous chromosomes to separate, or disjoin, at metaphase of meiosis I, or the failure of two sister chromatids to disjoin at metaphase of meiosis II or mitosis.
Penetrance	In a single individual of a variant genotype, penetrance refers to whether or not the variant genotype can be inferred on the basis of defined phenotypic criteria. In a population, reduced penetrance refers to the rate at which individuals of a variant genotype cannot be recognized according to specific phenotypic criteria.
Phenotypic heterogeneity	The situation that pertains when mutations of a single gene produce multiple different phenotypes.
Postzygotic	A mutational event that occurs after fertilization and that commonly gives rise to mosaicism.
Premutation	A genetic change that does not result in a phenotype itself but has a high probability of developing a second alteration—a full mutation—which does cause a phenotype.
Primordial germ cell	The group of cells set aside early in development that go on to give rise to gametes.
Recessive	A pattern of inheritance or mechanism of gene action in which a particular mutant allele causes a phenotype only in the absence of a nonmutant allele. Thus, for autosomal conditions, the variant or disease phenotype is manifest when two copies of the mutant allele are present. For X-linked conditions, the variant or disease phenotype is manifest in cells, tissues, or individuals in which the nonmutant allele is either inactivated (a heterozygous female) or not present (a hemizygous male).
RFLP	Restriction fragment length polymorphism—a type of DNA-based allelic variation in which different alleles at a single locus are recognized and followed through pedigrees based on the size of a restriction fragment. The locus is defined by the segment of DNA that gives rise to the restriction fragment; the different alleles are generally (not always) caused by a single change in DNA sequence that creates or abolishes a site of restriction enzyme cleavage.
Robertsonian translocation	A type of translocation in which two acrocentric chromosomes are fused together with a single functional centromere. A carrier of a robertsonian translocation with 45 chromosomes has a normal amount of chromosomal material and is said to be euploid.
SNP	Single nucleotide polymorphism—the most common type of genetic variation. There are approximately 1 million SNPs in the human genome. Most do not affect protein structure but may serve as valuable markers for determining the effect of genetic variation on complex and common diseases and disorders such as diabetes, heart disease, hypertension, and obesity.
Substrate accumulation	A pathogenetic mechanism in which deficiency of a particular enzyme causes disease because the substrate of that enzyme accumulates in tissue or blood.
Triplet repeat	A three-nucleotide sequence that is tandemly repeated many times—ie, $(XYZ)_n$. Alterations in length of such simple types of repeats (dinucleotide and tetranucleotide as well) occur much more frequently than most other kinds of mutations; in addition, alteration in the length of trinucleotide repeats is the molecular basis for several heritable disorders.
Trisomy	An abnormal situation in which there are three instead of two copies of a chromosomal segment or chromosome per cell.

es are caused by (1) chromosomal rearrangements that result in deletion or duplication of a group of closely linked genes or (2) abnormalities during mitosis or meiosis that result in an abnormal number of chromosomes per cell. In most genetic diseases, every cell in an affected individual carries the mutated gene or genes as a consequence of its inheritance via a mutant egg or sperm cell (**gamete**). However, mutation of the gametic cell may have arisen during its development, in which case somatic cells of the parent do not carry the mutation and the affected individual is said to have a "new mutation." In addition, some mutations may arise during early embryogenesis, in which case tissues of the affected individual contain a mixture, or **mosaic,** of mutant and nonmutant cells. Depending on the time of embryogenesis and cell type in which a new mutation arises, an individual may carry the mutation in some but not all of their germ cells (**germline mosaicism**), some but not all of their somatic cells (**somatic mosaicism**), or both.

It is helpful to begin with a brief review of terms that are commonly used in discussing genetic disease with patients and their families. Although genes were recognized and studied long before the structure of DNA was known, it has become common usage to regard a **gene** as a short stretch of DNA, usually but not always <100,000 base pairs (bp) in length, that encodes a product (usually protein) responsible for a measurable trait. DNA length is typically measured in base pairs, kilobase pairs (kb), or megabase pairs (Mb); chromosomes vary in length from about 46–245 Mb. The **locus** is the place where a particular gene lies on its chromosome. A gene's DNA sequence nearly always shows slight differences when many unrelated individuals are compared, and the variant sequences are described as **alleles**. A **mutation** is a biochemical event such as a nucleotide change, deletion, or insertion that has produced a new allele. Many changes in the DNA sequence of a gene, such as those within introns or at the third "wobble" position of codons for particular amino acids,

do not affect the structure or expression of the gene product; therefore, although all mutations result in a biochemical or molecular biologic phenotype (ie, a change in DNA), only some of them result in a clinically abnormal phenotype. The word **polymorphism** denotes an allele that is present in 1% or more of the population. At the biochemical level, polymorphic alleles can be recognized by their effect on the size of a restriction fragment (**restriction fragment length polymorphism [RFLP]**), the length of a short but highly repetitive region of DNA (a **simple sequence length polymorphism [SSLP]**), or a **single nucleotide polymorphism** (**SNP**). On the other hand, at the clinical level, polymorphic alleles are recognized by their effect on a phenotype such as HLA type or hair color. For an autosomal gene (those that lie on chromosomes 1–22, carried in two copies per cell), individuals carrying identical copies are **homozygous,** whereas individuals whose two copies differ from each other are **heterozygous.** These terms—homozygous and heterozygous—can apply to the DNA sequence, the protein product, or the clinical phenotype. In other words, an individual may be heterozygous for a SNP that does not alter the protein product, heterozygous for a deletion that causes a genetic disease, or heterozygous for a DNA sequence alteration that causes a change in protein structure but does not cause disease.

This discussion helps to illustrate the use of the word **phenotype,** which refers simply to any characteristic that can be measured, with the type of measurement depending on the characteristic. Hair color and height are phenotypes readily apparent to a casual observer that are not obviously associated with disease. Diabetes mellitus and coronary artery disease are disease phenotypes that typically require clinical investigation to be recognized, whereas RFLPs, SSLPs, and SNPs are molecular biologic phenotypes that can only be detected with a laboratory test.

PENETRANCE & EXPRESSIVITY

One of the most important principles of human genetics is that two individuals with the same mutated gene may have different phenotypes. For example, in the autosomal dominant condition called type I osteogenesis imperfecta, pedigrees may occur in which there is both an affected grandparent and an affected grandchild even though the obligate carrier parent is asymptomatic (Figure 2–1). Given a set of defined criteria, recognition of the condition in individuals known to carry the mutated gene is described as **penetrance.** In other words, if 7 of 10 individuals older than 40 years with the type I osteogenesis imperfecta mutation have an abnormal bone density scan, the condition is said to be 70% penetrant by that criterion. Penetrance may vary both with age and according to the set of criteria being used; for example, type I osteogenesis imperfecta may be 90% penetrant at age 40 years when the conclusion

is based on a bone density scan in conjunction with laboratory tests for abnormal collagen synthesis. **Reduced penetrance** or **age-dependent penetrance** is a common feature of dominantly inherited conditions that have a relatively high **fitness** (the extent to which individuals carrying a mutant allele produce offspring relative to individuals who do not carry a mutant allele); Huntington's disease and polycystic kidney disease are examples.

Although the presence of a mutated gene can be observed in many individuals, their phenotypes may still be different. For example, blue scleras and short stature may be the only manifestations of type I osteogenesis imperfecta in a particular individual, whereas a sibling who carries the identical mutation may be confined to a wheelchair as a result of multiple fractures and deformities. The mutation is penetrant in

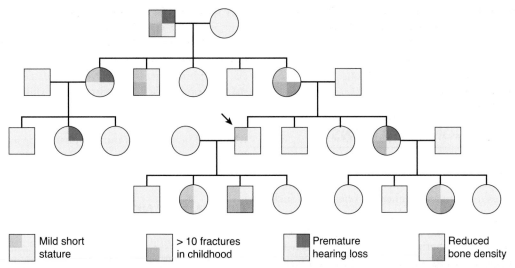

| | Mild short stature | | > 10 fractures in childhood | | Premature hearing loss | | Reduced bone density |

FIGURE 2–1 Penetrance and expressivity in type I osteogenesis imperfecta. In this schematic pedigree of the autosomal dominant condition type I osteogenesis imperfecta, nearly all of the affected individuals exhibit different phenotypic features that vary in severity (variable expressivity). As is shown, type I osteogenesis imperfecta is fully penetrant, because every individual who transmits the mutation is phenotypically affected to some degree. However, if mild short stature in the individual indicated with the arrow had been considered to be a normal variant, then the condition would have been nonpenetrant in this individual. Thus, in this example, judgments about penetrance or nonpenetrance depend on the criteria for normal and abnormal stature.

both individuals, but its effects vary, a phenomenon referred to as **variable expressivity.** Both reduced penetrance and variable expressivity may occur in individuals who carry the same mutated allele; therefore, phenotypic differences between these individuals must be due to the effects of other "modifier" genes, to environmental interactions, or to chance.

MECHANISMS OF MUTATION & INHERITANCE PATTERNS

Mutations can be characterized both by their molecular nature—nucleotide deletion, insertion, substitution—or by their effects on the gene product (ie, no effect [neutral], complete loss of function [amorphic mutation], partial loss of function [hypomorphic mutation], gain of function [hypermorphic mutation], or acquisition of a new property [neomorphic mutation]). Geneticists who study experimental organisms frequently use specific deletions to ensure that a mutated allele causes a loss of function, but human geneticists rely on biochemical or cell culture studies. Amorphic and hypomorphic mutations are probably the most frequent type of mutation in human genetic disease because there are many ways to interfere with a protein's function.

For autosomal genes, the fundamental difference between dominant and recessive inheritance is that, with dominant inheritance, the disease state or trait being measured is apparent when one copy of the mutated allele and one copy of the normal allele are present. With recessive inheritance, two copies of the mutated allele must be present for the disease state or trait to be apparent. However, for genes that lie on the X chromosome, the situation is slightly different because females have two X chromosomes and males have only one. X-linked dominant inheritance occurs when one copy of a mutant gene causes the disease phenotype (in males and females); X-linked recessive inheritance occurs when two copies of a mutant gene cause the disease phenotype (in females). Because most mutations are amorphic or hypomorphic, however, one copy of an X-linked mutant allele in males is not "balanced" with a nonmutant allele, as it would be in females; therefore, in X-linked recessive inheritance, one copy of a mutant allele is sufficient to produce a disease phenotype in males, a situation referred to as **hemizygosity.**

RECESSIVE INHERITANCE & LOSS-OF-FUNCTION MUTATIONS

As mentioned, most recessive mutations are due to loss of function of the gene product, which can occur from a variety of different causes, including failure of the gene to be transcribed or translated and failure of the translated gene product to function correctly. There are two general principles to keep in mind when considering loss-of-function mutations. First, because expression from the nonmutant allele usually does not change (ie, there is no **dosage compensation**), gene expression in a heterozygous carrier of a loss-of-function allele is reduced to 50% of normal. Second, for most biochemical pathways, a 50% reduction in enzyme concentration is not sufficient to produce a disease state. Thus, most diseases resulting from enzyme deficiencies such as phenylketonuria (Table 2–2) are inherited in a recessive fashion.

DOMINANT INHERITANCE & LOSS-OF-FUNCTION MUTATIONS

If 50% of a particular product is not enough for the cell or tissue to function normally, then a loss-of-function mutation in this gene produces a dominantly inherited phenotype. Such mutations often occur in structural proteins; an example is type I osteogenesis imperfecta, which is considered in detail later. Most dominantly inherited phenotypes are actually **semidominant,** which means that an individual who carries two copies of the mutant allele is affected more severely than someone who carries one mutant and one normal copy. However, for most dominantly inherited conditions, homozygous mutant individuals are rarely observed. For example, inheritance of achondroplasia, the most common genetic cause of very short stature, is usually described as autosomal dominant. However, rare matings between two affected individuals have a 25% probability of producing offspring with two copies of the mutant gene. This results in homozygous achondroplasia, a condition that is very severe and usually fatal in the perinatal period; thus, achondroplasia exhibits semidominant inheritance. Huntington's disease, a dominantly inherited neurologic disease, is the only known human condition in which the homozygous mutant phenotype is identical to the heterozygous mutant phenotype (sometimes referred to as a "true dominant").

DOMINANT NEGATIVE GENE ACTION

A special kind of pathophysiologic mechanism, referred to as dominant negative, occurs frequently in human genetic diseases that involve proteins that form oligomeric or polymeric complexes. In these disorders, the mutant allele gives rise to a structurally abnormal protein that interferes with the function of the normal allele. Note that any molecular lesion (ie, dele-

TABLE 2–2 Phenotype, inheritance, and prevalence of selected genetic disorders.

Disorder	Phenotype	Genetic Mechanism	Incidence
Down syndrome	Mental and growth retardation, dysmorphic features, internal organ anomalies	Chromosomal imbalance; caused by trisomy 21	≈ 1:800; increased risk with advanced maternal age
Fragile X-associated mental retardation	Mental retardation, characteristic facial features, large testes	X-linked; progressive expansion of unstable DNA causes failure to express gene encoding RNA-binding protein	≈ 1:1500 males; can be manifested in females; multistep mechanism
Sickle cell anemia	Recurrent painful crises, increased susceptibility to infections	Autosomal recessive; caused by a single missense mutation in beta-globin	≈ 1:400 blacks
Cystic fibrosis	Recurrent pulmonary infections, exocrine pancreatic insufficiency, infertility	Autosomal recessive; caused by multiple loss-of-function mutations in a chloride channel	≈ 1:2000 whites; very rare in Asians
Leber's hereditary optic neuropathy	Acute or subacute blindness, occasional myopathy or neurodegeneration	Mutation of electron transport chain encoded by mtDNA	≈ 1:50,00–1:10,000
Myoclonic epilepsy with ragged red fibers	Uncontrolled periodic jerking, muscle weakness	Mutation of mitochondrial tRNA in mtDNA	≈ 1:100,000–1:50,000
Neurofibromatosis	Multiple café-au-lait spots, neurofibromas, increased tumor susceptibility	Autosomal dominant; caused by multiple loss-of-function mutations in a signaling molecule	≈ 1:3000; ≈ 50% are new mutations
Duchenne's muscular dystrophy	Muscular weakness and degeneration	X-linked recessive; caused by multiple loss-of-function mutations in muscle protein	≈ 1:3000 males; ≈ 33% are new mutations
Osteogenesis imperfecta	Increased susceptibility to fractures, connective tissue fragility, blue scleras	Phenotypically and genetically heterogeneous	≈1:10,000
Phenylketonuria	Mental and growth retardation	Autosomal recessive; caused by multiple loss-of-function mutations in phenylalanine hydroxylase	≈ 1:10,000

tion, nonsense, missense, or splicing) can produce a loss-of-function allele. However, only molecular lesions that yield a protein product (ie, splicing, missense, or nonsense mutations) can result in a dominant negative allele. Type II osteogenesis imperfecta, described later, is an example of a dominant negative mutation.

Although the terms "dominant" and "recessive" are occasionally used to describe specific mutations, a DNA sequence alteration itself cannot, strictly speaking, be dominant or recessive. The terms are instead appropriate to the effect of a mutation on a particular trait. Therefore, in characterizing a particular mutation as "recessive," one is referring to the effect of the mutation on the trait being studied.

MUTATION RATE & THE PREVALENCE OF GENETIC DISEASE

At the level of DNA sequence, nucleotide mutations (substitutions, small insertions, or small deletions) in humans occur at a rate of approximately 2×10^{-8} per nucleotide per human generation, or 150 new mutations per diploid genome. However, only about 5% of the human genome is functional, so most new mutations have no effect. Still, with approximately 23,000 genes in the human genome and an estimated deleterious "per locus" mutation rate of 10^{-5} per generation, the chance of a new deleterious mutation in any one individual is about 20%. Furthermore, assuming 10 billion new births in the last millennium, every gene in the human genome has probably been mutated (in a deleterious manner) about 100,000 different times. However, from a clinical perspective, only about 5000 single-gene disorders have been recognized to cause a human disease. In considering possible explanations for this disparity, it seems likely that deleterious mutations of many single genes are lethal very early in development and thus not clinically apparent, whereas deleterious mutations in other genes do not cause an easily recognizable phenotype. The overall frequency of disease attributable to defects in single genes (ie, mendelian disorders) is approximately 1% of the general population.

Table 2–2 lists the major symptoms, genetic mechanisms, and prevalence of the diseases considered in this chapter as well as of several others. The most common conditions, such as neurofibromatosis, cystic fibrosis, and fragile X-associated mental retardation syndrome, will be encountered at some time by most health care professionals regardless of their field of interest. Other conditions such as Huntington's disease and adenosine deaminase deficiency, although of intellectual and pathophysiologic interest, are not likely to be seen by most practitioners.

Many common conditions such as atherosclerosis and breast cancer that do not show strictly mendelian inheritance patterns have a genetic component evident from familial aggregation or twin studies. These conditions are usually described as **multifactorial,** which means that the effects of one or more mutated genes and environmental differences all contribute to the likelihood that a given individual will manifest the phenotype.

ISSUES IN CLINICAL GENETICS

Most patients with genetic disease present during early childhood with symptoms that ultimately give rise to a diagnosis such as fragile X-associated mental retardation or Down syndrome. The major clinical issues at presentation are arriving at the correct diagnosis and counseling the patient and family regarding the natural history and prognosis of the condition. It is important to assess the likelihood that the same condition will occur again in the family and determine whether it can be diagnosed prenatally. These issues are the subject matter of genetic counseling by medical geneticists and genetic counselors.

Understanding the pathophysiology of genetic diseases that interfere with specific metabolic pathways—so-called inborn errors of metabolism—has led to effective treatments for selected conditions such as phenylketonuria, maple syrup urine disease, and homocystinuria. Many of these diseases are rare, but efforts are underway to develop treatments for common single-gene disorders such as

Duchenne's muscular dystrophy, cystic fibrosis, and hemophilia. Some forms of therapy are directed at replacing the mutant protein, whereas others are directed at ameliorating its effects.

CHECKPOINT

1. Define gene, locus, allele, mutation, heterozygosity, hemizygosity, polymorphism, and phenotype.
2. How is it possible for two individuals with the same mutation to have differences in the severity of an abnormal phenotype?
3. Explain the pathophysiologic difference between mutations that act via loss of function and those that act via dominant negative gene action.

PATHOPHYSIOLOGY OF SELECTED GENETIC DISEASES

OSTEOGENESIS IMPERFECTA

Osteogenesis imperfecta is a condition inherited in mendelian fashion that illustrates many principles of human genetics. It is a heterogeneous and pleiotropic group of disorders characterized by a tendency toward fragility of bone. Advances in the last two decades demonstrate that nearly every case is caused by a mutation of the *COL1A1* or *COL1A2* genes, which encode the subunits of type I collagen, pro1(I) and proα2(I), respectively. More than 100 different mutant alleles have been described for osteogenesis imperfecta; the relationships between different DNA sequence alterations and the type of disease (genotype-phenotype correlations) illustrate several pathophysiologic principles in human genetics.

Clinical Manifestations

The clinical and genetic characteristics of osteogenesis imperfecta are summarized in Table 2–3, in which the timing and severity of fractures, radiologic findings, presence of additional clinical features, and family history are used to discriminate among four different subtypes. All forms of osteogenesis imperfecta are characterized by increased susceptibility to fractures ("brittle bones"), but there is considerable phenotypic heterogeneity, even within individual subtypes. Individuals with type I or type IV osteogenesis imperfecta present in early childhood with one or a few fractures of long bones in response to minimal or no trauma; x-ray films reveal mild osteopenia, little or no bony deformity, and often evidence of earlier subclinical fractures. However, most individuals with type I or type IV osteogenesis imperfecta do not have fractures in utero. Type I

and type IV osteogenesis imperfecta are distinguished by the severity (less in type I than in type IV) and by scleral hue, which indicates the thickness of this tissue and the deposition of type I collagen. Individuals with type I osteogenesis imperfecta have blue scleras, whereas the scleras of those with type IV are normal or slightly gray. In type I, the typical number of fractures during childhood is 10–20; fracture incidence decreases after puberty, and the main features in adult life are mild short stature, a tendency toward conductive hearing loss, and occasionally dentinogenesis imperfecta. Individuals with type IV osteogenesis imperfecta generally experience more fractures than those with type I and have significant short stature caused by a combination of long bone and spinal deformities, but they often are able to walk independently. Approximately one fourth of the cases of type I or type IV osteogenesis imperfecta represent new mutations; in the remainder, the history and examination of other family members reveal findings consistent with autosomal dominant inheritance.

Type II osteogenesis imperfecta presents at or before birth (diagnosed by prenatal ultrasonography) with multiple fractures, bony deformities, increased fragility of nonbony connective tissue, and blue scleras and usually results in death in infancy. Two typical radiologic findings are the presence of isolated "islands" of mineralization in the skull (wormian bones) and a beaded appearance to the ribs. Nearly all cases of type II osteogenesis imperfecta represent a new dominant mutation, and there is no family history. Death usually results from respiratory difficulties.

Type III osteogenesis imperfecta presents at birth or in infancy with progressive bony deformities, multiple fractures, and blue scleras. It is intermediate in severity between types II

TABLE 2–3 Clinical and molecular subtypes of osteogenesis imperfecta.

Type	Phenotype	Genetics	Molecular Pathophysiology
Type I	**Mild:** Short stature, postnatal fractures, little or no deformity, blue scleras, premature hearing loss	Autosomal dominant	Loss-of-function mutation in proα1(I) chain resulting in decreased amount of mRNA; quality of collagen is normal; quantity is reduced twofold
Type II	**Perinatal lethal:** Severe prenatal fractures, abnormal bone formation, severe deformities, blue scleras, connective tissue fragility	Sporadic (autosomal dominant)	Structural mutation in proα1(I) or proα2(I) chain that has mild effect on heterotrimer assembly; quality of collagen is severely abnormal; quantity often reduced also
Type III	**Progressive deforming:** Prenatal fractures, deformities usually present at birth, very short stature, usually nonambulatory, blue scleras, hearing loss	Autosomal dominant[1]	Structural mutation in proα1(I) or proα2(I) chain that has mild effect on heterotrimer assembly; quality of collagen is severely abnormal; quantity can be normal
Type IV	**Deforming with normal scleras:** Postnatal fractures, mild to moderate deformities, premature hearing loss, normal or gray scleras, dental abnormalities	Autosomal dominant	Structural mutation in the proα2(I), or, less frequently, proα1(I) chain that has little or no effect on heterotrimer assembly; quality of collagen is usually abnormal; quantity can be normal

[1]Autosomal recessive in rare cases.

and IV; most affected individuals will require multiple corrective surgeries and lose the ability to ambulate by early adulthood. Unlike other forms of osteogenesis imperfecta, which are nearly always due to mutations that act dominantly, type III can be inherited in either a dominant or (rarely) recessive fashion. From a biochemical and molecular perspective, type III osteogenesis imperfecta is the least well understood form.

Although different subtypes of osteogenesis imperfecta can often be distinguished biochemically, the classification presented in Table 2–3 is clinical rather than molecular, and the disease phenotypes for each subtype show a spectrum of severities that overlap one another. For example, a few individuals diagnosed with type II osteogenesis imperfecta based on the presence of severe bony deformities in utero will survive for many years and thus overlap the type III subtype. Similarly, some individuals with type IV osteogenesis imperfecta have fractures in utero and develop deformities that lead to loss of ambulation. Distinguishing this presentation from type III osteogenesis imperfecta may be possible only if other affected family members exhibit a milder course.

Additional subtypes of osteogenesis imperfecta have been suggested for individuals that do not match types I–IV, and there are additional disorders associated with congenital fractures that are usually not considered to be "classic" osteogenesis imperfecta. In some cases, mutations of type I collagen genes have been excluded as potential causes of these additional disorders. However, the approach to clinical classification depicted in Table 2–3 is helpful for most affected individuals in predicting the course and inheritance pattern of the illness. The classification also serves as an important framework within which to correlate molecular abnormalities with disease phenotypes.

Pathophysiology

Osteogenesis imperfecta is a disease of type I collagen, which constitutes the major extracellular protein in the body. It is the major collagen in the dermis, the connective tissue capsules of most organs, and the vascular and GI adventitia and is the only collagen in bone. A mature type I collagen fibril is a rigid structure that contains multiple type I collagen molecules packed in a staggered array and stabilized by intermolecular covalent cross-links. Each mature type I collagen molecule contains two α1 chains and one α2 chain, encoded by the *COL1A1* and *COL1A2* genes, respectively (Figure 2–2). The *COL1A1* and *COL1A2* genes have 51 and 52 exons, respectively, of which exons 6–49 encode the entire triple-helical domain. The α1 and α2 chains are synthesized as larger precursors with amino and carboxyl terminal "propeptide" extensions, assemble with each other inside the cell, and are ultimately secreted as a heterotrimeric type I procollagen molecule. During intracellular assembly, the three chains wind around each other in a triple helix that is stabilized by interchain interactions between hydroxy proline and adjacent carbonyl residues. There is a dynamic relationship between the posttranslational action of prolyl hydroxylase and assembly of the triple helix, which begins at the carboxyl terminal end of the molecule. Increased levels of hydroxylation result in a more stable helix, but helix formation prevents further prolyl hydroxylation. The nature of the triple helix causes the side chain of every third amino acid to point inward, and steric constraints allow only a proton in this position. Thus, the amino acid sequence of virtually all collagen chains in the triple-helical portion is $(Gly\text{-}X\text{-}Y)_n$, where Y is proline about one third of the time.

The fundamental defect in most individuals with type I osteogenesis imperfecta is reduced synthesis of type I collagen resulting from loss-of-function mutations in *COL1A1*. In most cases, the mutant *COL1A1* allele gives rise to greatly reduced (partial loss-of-function) or no (complete loss-of-function) mRNA. Because the nonmutant *COL1A1* allele continues to produce mRNA at a normal rate (ie, there is no dosage compensation), heterozygosity for a complete loss-of-function mutation results in a 50% reduction in the total rate of proα1(I) mRNA synthesis, whereas heterozygosity for a partial loss-of-function mutation results in a less severe reduction. A reduced concentration of proα1(I) chains limits the production of type I procollagen, leading to (1) a reduced amount of structurally normal type I collagen and (2) an excess of unassembled proα2(I) chains, which are degraded inside the cell (Figure 2–3).

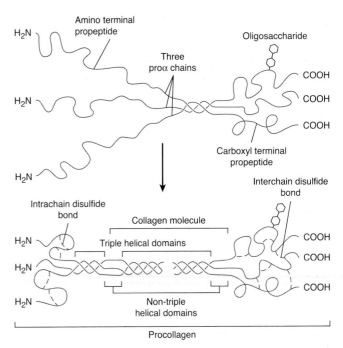

FIGURE 2–2 Molecular assembly of type I procollagen. Type I procollagen is assembled in the endoplasmic reticulum from three proα chains that associate with each other beginning at their carboxyl terminals. An important requirement for proper assembly of the triple helix is the presence of a glycine residue at every third position in each of the proα chains. After secretion, the amino and carboxyl terminal propeptides are proteolytically cleaved, leaving a rigid triple helical collagen molecule with very short non-triple-helical domains at both ends. (Redrawn, with permission, from Alberts BA. *Molecular Biology of the Cell*, 3rd ed. Garland, 1994.)

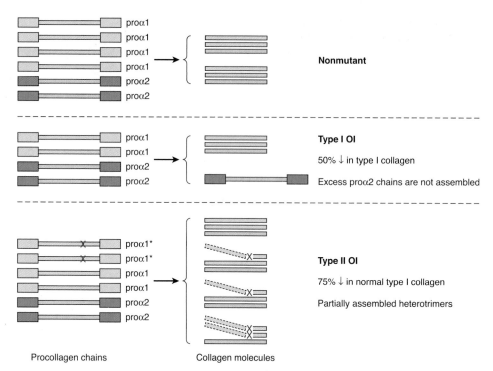

Procollagen chains   Collagen molecules

FIGURE 2–3 Molecular pathogenesis of type I and type II osteogenesis imperfecta (OI). The *COL1A1* gene normally produces twice as many proα chains as the *COL1A2* gene. Therefore, in nonmutant cells, the ratio of proα1 to proα2 chains is 2:1, which corresponds to the ratio of α1 and α2 chains in intact collagen molecules. In type I osteogenesis imperfecta, a mutation (X) in one of the *COL1A1* alleles (*) results in failure to produce proα1 chains, leading to a 50% reduction in the total number of proα1 chains, a 50% reduction in the production of intact type I collagen molecules, and an excess of unassembled proα2 chains, which are degraded inside the cell. In type II osteogenesis imperfecta, a mutation in one of the *COL1A1* alleles results in a structural alteration that blocks triple-helix formation and secretion of partially assembled collagen molecules containing the mutant chain. (Redrawn from Thompson MW et al. *Genetics in Medicine,* 5th ed. Saunders, 1991.)

There are several potential molecular defects responsible for *COL1A1* mutations in type I osteogenesis imperfecta, including alterations in a regulatory region leading to reduced transcription, splicing abnormalities leading to reduced steady state levels of RNA, and deletion of the entire *COL1A1* gene. However, in many cases, the underlying defect is a single base pair change that creates a premature stop codon (also known as a "**nonsense mutation**") in exons 6–49. In a process referred to as "nonsense-mediated decay," partially synthesized mRNA precursors that carry the nonsense codon are recognized and degraded by the cell. With collagen and many other genes, production of a truncated protein (as might be predicted from a nonsense mutation) would be more damaging to the cell than production of no protein at all. Thus, nonsense-mediated decay, which has been observed to occur for mutations in many different multiexon genes, serves as a protective phenomenon and is an important component of genetic pathophysiology.

An example of these principles is apparent from considering type II osteogenesis imperfecta, which is caused by structurally abnormal forms of type I collagen and is more severe than type I osteogenesis imperfecta. Mutations in type II osteogenesis imperfecta can be caused by defects in either *COL1A1* or *COL1A2* and usually are missense alterations of a glycine residue that allow the mutant peptide chain to bind to

normal chains in the initial steps of trimer assembly (Figure 2–3). However, triple-helix formation is ineffective, often because amino acids with large side chains are substituted for glycine. Ineffective triple-helix formation leads to increased posttranslational modification by prolyl hydroxylase and a reduced rate of secretion. These appear to be critical events in the cellular pathogenesis of type II osteogenesis imperfecta, because glycine substitutions toward the carboxyl terminal end of the molecule are generally more severe than those at the amino terminal end.

These considerations help to explain why type II osteogenesis imperfecta is more severe than type I and exemplify the principle of dominant negative gene action. The effects of an amino acid substitution in a proα1(I) peptide chain are amplified at the levels of both triple-helix assembly and fibril formation. Because every type I procollagen molecule has two proα1(I) chains, only 25% of type I procollagen molecules will contain two normal proα1(I) chains even though only one of the two *COL1A1* alleles is mutated. Furthermore, because each molecule in a fibril interacts with several others, incorporation of an abnormal molecule can have disproportionately large effects on fibril structure and integrity.

Collagen mutations that cause type III and type IV osteogenesis imperfecta are diverse and include glycine substitutions in the amino terminal portion of the collagen triple helix, a few internal deletions of *COL1A1* and *COL1A2* that do not significantly disturb triple helix formation, and some unusual alterations in the non–triple-helical extensions at the amino and carboxyl terminals of proα chains.

Genetic Principles

As already described, most cases of type I osteogenesis imperfecta are caused by partial or complete loss-of-function mutations in *COL1A1*. However, in approximately one third of affected individuals, the disease is caused by a new mutation; in addition, there are many ways in which DNA sequence alterations can reduce gene expression. Consequently, there is a wide range of mutant alleles (ie, **allelic heterogeneity**), which represents a challenge for the development of molecular diagnostic tests. In a family in which type I osteogenesis imperfecta is known to occur clinically and a proband seeks a diagnostic test for the purposes of reproductive planning, it is possible in most cases to use linkage analysis at the *COL1A1* locus. In this approach, one distinguishes between chromosomes that carry the mutant and nonmutant *COL1A1* alleles using closely linked DNA-based polymorphisms, even though the causative molecular defect is not known. Once this information is established for a particular family, inheritance of the mutant allele can be predicted in future pregnancies.

For types III and IV osteogenesis imperfecta, mutations can occur in *COL1A1* or *COL1A2* (ie, **locus heterogeneity**), and in this situation linkage analysis is more difficult because one cannot be sure which locus is abnormal.

For both type I and type IV osteogenesis imperfecta, the most important question in the clinical setting often relates to the natural history of the illness. For example, reproductive decision making in families at risk for osteogenesis imperfecta is influenced greatly by the relative likelihood of producing a child who will never walk and will require multiple orthopedic operations versus a child whose major problems will be a few long bone fractures and an increased risk of mixed sensorineural and conductive hearing loss in childhood and adulthood. As evident from the prior discussion, both different mutant genes and different mutant alleles, as well as other genes that modify the osteogenesis imperfecta phenotype, can contribute to this **phenotypic heterogeneity**. When allelic rather than locus heterogeneity is operative, as in type I osteogenesis imperfecta, comparison of interfamilial with intrafamilial variability allows one to assess the relative contribution of different mutant alleles to phenotypic heterogeneity. For most genetic diseases, including type I osteogenesis imperfecta, intrafamilial variability is less than interfamilial variability.

In type II osteogenesis imperfecta, a single copy of the mutant allele causes the abnormal phenotype and, therefore, has a dominant mechanism of action. Although the type II phenotype itself is never inherited, there are rare situations in which a phenotypically normal individual harbors a *COL1A1* mutant allele among his or her germ cells. These individuals with so-called **gonadal mosaicism** can produce multiple offspring with type II osteogenesis imperfecta (Figure 2–4), a

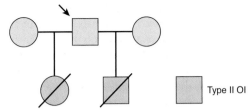

FIGURE 2–4 Gonadal mosaicism for type II osteogenesis imperfecta. In this idealized pedigree, the phenotypically normal father (indicated with the arrow) has had two children by different mates, each of whom is affected with autosomal dominant type II osteogenesis imperfecta (OI). Analysis of the father showed that some of his spermatozoa carried a *COL1A1* mutation, indicating that the explanation for this unusual pedigree is germline mosaicism. (Redrawn from Cohn DH et al. Recurrence of lethal osteogenesis imperfecta due to parental mosaicism for a dominant mutation in a human type I collagen gene [*COL1A1*]. Am J Hum Genet. 1990;46:591.)

pattern of segregation that can be confused with recessive inheritance. In fact, many other mutations, including Duchenne's muscular dystrophy, which is X linked, and type 1 neurofibromatosis, which is autosomal dominant, also occasionally show unusual inheritance patterns explained by gonadal mosaicism.

CHECKPOINT

4. When and how does type II osteogenesis imperfecta present? To what do these individuals succumb?
5. What are two typical radiologic findings in type II osteogenesis imperfecta?
6. Explain how nonsense-mediated decay can help protect individuals affected by a genetic disease.

PHENYLKETONURIA

Phenylketonuria presents one of the most dramatic examples of how the relationship between genotype and phenotype can depend on environmental variables. Phenylketonuria was first recognized as an inherited cause of mental retardation in 1934, and systematic attempts to treat the condition were initiated in the 1950s. The term "phenylketonuria" denotes elevated levels of urinary phenylpyruvate and phenylacetate, which occur when circulating phenylalanine levels, normally between 0.06 and 0.1 mmol/L, rise above 1.2 mmol/L. Thus, the primary defect in phenylketonuria is **hyperphenylalaninemia,** which itself has a number of distinct genetic causes.

The pathophysiology of phenylketonuria illustrates several important principles in human genetics. Hyperphenylalaninemia itself is caused by **substrate accumulation**, which occurs when a normal intermediary metabolite fails to be eliminated properly and its concentrations become elevated to levels that are toxic. As described later, the most common cause of hyperphenylalaninemia is deficiency of the enzyme phenylalanine hydroxylase, which catalyzes the conversion of phenylalanine to tyrosine. Individuals with mutations in phenylalanine hydroxylase usually do not suffer from the absence of tyrosine because this amino acid can be supplied to the body by mechanisms that are independent of phenylalanine hydroxylase. In other forms of phenylketonuria, however, additional disease manifestations occur as a result of **end-product deficiency,** which occurs when the downstream product of a particular enzyme is required for a key physiologic process.

A discussion of phenylketonuria also helps to illustrate the rationale for, and application of, population-based screening programs for genetic disease. More than 10 million newborn infants per year are tested for phenylketonuria, and the focus today in treatment has shifted in several respects. First, "successful" treatment of phenylketonuria by dietary restriction of phenylalanine is, in general, accompanied by subtle neuropsychologic defects that have been recognized only in the last decade. Thus, current investigations focus on alternative treatment strategies such as somatic gene therapy as well as on the social and psychologic factors that affect compliance with dietary management. Second, a generation of females treated for phenylketonuria are now bearing children, and the phenomenon of **maternal phenylketonuria** has been recognized in which in utero exposure to maternal hyperphenylalaninemia results in congenital abnormalities regardless of fetal genotype. The number of pregnancies at risk has risen in proportion to the successful treatment of phenylketonuria and represents a challenge to public health officials, physicians, and geneticists in the future.

Clinical Manifestations

The incidence of hyperphenylalaninemia varies among different populations. In African Americans, it is about 1:50,000; in Yemenite Jews, about 1:5000; and in most Northern European populations, about 1:10,000. Postnatal growth retardation, moderate to severe mental retardation, recurrent seizures, hypopigmentation, and eczematous skin rashes constitute the major phenotypic features of untreated phenylketonuria. However, with the advent of widespread newborn screening programs for hyperphenylalaninemia, the major phenotypic manifestations of phenylketonuria today occur when treatment is partial or when it is terminated prematurely during late childhood or adolescence. In these cases, there is usually a slight but significant decline in IQ, an array of specific performance and perceptual defects, and an increased frequency of learning and behavioral problems.

Newborn screening for phenylketonuria is performed on a small amount of dried blood obtained at 24–72 hours of age. From the initial screen, there is about a 1% incidence of positive or indeterminate test results, and a more quantitative measurement of plasma phenylalanine is then performed before 2 weeks of age. In neonates who undergo a second round of testing, the diagnosis of phenylketonuria is ultimately confirmed in about 1%, providing an estimated phe-nylketonuria prevalence of 1:10,000, although there is great geographic and ethnic variation (see prior discussion). The false-negative rate of phenylketonuria newborn screening programs is approximately 1:70; phenylketonuria in these unfortunate individuals is usually not detected until developmental delay and seizures during infancy or early childhood prompt a systematic evaluation for an inborn error of metabolism.

Infants in whom a diagnosis of phenylketonuria is confirmed are usually placed on a dietary regimen in which a semisynthetic formula low in phenylalanine can be combined with regular breast feeding. This regimen is adjusted empirically to maintain a plasma phenylalanine concentration at or below 1 mmol/L, which is still several times greater than normal but similar to levels observed in so-called **benign hyperphenylalaninemia** (see later discussion), a biochemical diagnosis which is not associated with phenylketonuria and has no clinical consequences. Phenylalanine is an essential amino acid, and even individuals with phenylketonuria must consume small amounts to avoid protein starvation and a catabolic state. Most children require 25–50 mg/kg/d of phenylalanine, and these requirements are met by combining natural foods with commercial products designed for phenylketonuria treatment. When dietary treatment programs were first implemented, it was hoped that the risk of neurologic damage from the hyperphenylalaninemia of phenylketonuria would have a limited window and that treatment could be stopped after childhood. However, it now appears that even mild hyperphenylalaninemia in adults (> 1.2 mmol/L) is associated with neuropsychologic and cognitive deficits; therefore, dietary treatment of phenylketonuria should probably be continued indefinitely.

As an increasing number of treated females with phenylketonuria reach childbearing age, a new problem—fetal hyperphenylalaninemia via intrauterine exposure—has become apparent. Newborn infants in such cases exhibit microcephaly and growth retardation of prenatal onset, congenital heart disease, and severe developmental delay regardless of the fetal genotype. Rigorous control of maternal phenylalanine concentrations from before conception until birth reduces the incidence of fetal abnormalities in maternal phenylketonuria, but the level of plasma phenylalanine that is "safe" for a developing fetus is 0.12–0.36 mmol/L—significantly lower than what is considered acceptable for phenylketonuria-affected children or adults on phenylalanine-restricted diets.

Pathophysiology

The normal metabolic fate of free phenylalanine is incorporation into protein or hydroxylation by phenylalanine hydroxylase to form tyrosine (Figure 2–5). Because tyrosine, but not phenylalanine, can be metabolized to produce fumarate and acetoacetate, hydroxylation of phenylalanine can be viewed both as a means of making tyrosine a nonessential amino acid and as a mechanism for providing energy via gluconeogenesis during states of protein starvation. In individuals with muta-

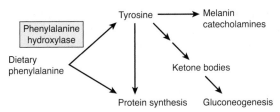

FIGURE 2–5 Metabolic fates of phenylalanine. Because catabolism of phenylalanine must proceed via tyrosine, the absence of phenylalanine hydroxylase leads to accumulation of phenylalanine. Tyrosine is also a biosynthetic precursor for melanin and certain neurotransmitters, and the absence of phenylalanine hydroxylase causes tyrosine to become an essential amino acid.

tions in phenylalanine hydroxylase, tyrosine becomes an essential amino acid. However, the clinical manifestations of the disease are caused not by absence of tyrosine (most people get enough tyrosine in the diet in any case) but by accumulation of phenylalanine. Transamination of phenylalanine to form phenylpyruvate normally does not occur unless circulating concentrations exceed 1.2 mmol/L, but the pathogenesis of CNS abnormalities in phenylketonuria is related more to phenylalanine itself than to its metabolites. In addition to a direct effect of elevated phenylalanine levels on energy production, protein synthesis, and neurotransmitter homeostasis in the developing brain, phenylalanine can also inhibit the transport of neutral amino acids across the blood-brain barrier, leading to a selective amino acid deficiency in the cerebrospinal fluid. Thus, the neurologic manifestations of phenylketonuria are felt to be due to a general effect of substrate

accumulation on cerebral metabolism. The pathophysiology of the eczema seen in untreated or partially treated phenylketonuria is not well understood, but eczema is a common feature of other inborn errors of metabolism in which plasma concentrations of branched-chain amino acids are elevated. Hypopigmentation in phenylketonuria is probably caused by an inhibitory effect of excess phenylalanine on the production of dopaquinone in melanocytes, which is the rate-limiting step in melanin synthesis.

Approximately 90% of infants with persistent hyperphenylalaninemia detected by newborn screening have typical phenylketonuria caused by a defect in phenylalanine hydroxylase (see later discussion). Of the remainder, most have benign hyperphenylalaninemia, in which circulating levels of phenylalanine are between 0.1 mmol/L and 1 mmol/L. However, approximately 1% of infants with persistent hyperphenylalaninemia have defects in the metabolism of tetrahydrobiopterin (BH_4), which is a stoichiometric cofactor for the hydroxylation reaction (Figure 2–6). Unfortunately, BH_4 is required not only for phenylalanine hydroxylase but also for tyrosine hydroxylase and tryptophan hydroxylase. The products of these latter two enzymes are catecholaminergic and serotonergic neurotransmitters; thus, individuals with defects in BH_4 metabolism suffer not only from phenylketonuria (substrate accumulation) but also from absence of important neurotransmitters (end-product deficiency). Affected individuals develop a severe neurologic disorder in early childhood manifested by hypotonia, inactivity, and developmental regression and are treated not only with dietary restriction of phenylalanine but also with dietary supplementation with BH_4, dopa, and 5-hydroxytryptophan.

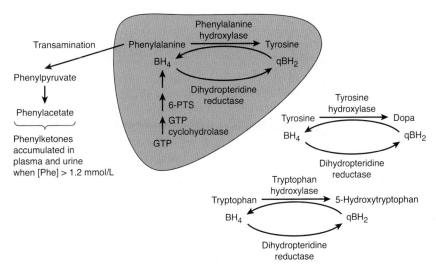

FIGURE 2–6 Normal and abnormal phenylalanine metabolism. Tetrahydrobiopterin (BH_4) is a cofactor for phenylalanine hydroxylase, tyrosine hydroxylase, and tryptophan hydroxylase. Consequently, defects in the biosynthesis of BH_4 or its metabolism result in a failure of all three hydroxylation reactions. The absence of phenylalanine hydroxylation has phenotypic effects because of substrate accumulation, but the absence of tyrosine or tryptophan hydroxylation has phenotypic effects as a result of end-product deficiency. (6-PTS, 6-pyruvoyltetrahydrobiopterin synthetase; qBH_2, quinonoid dihydrobiopterin.)

Genetic Principles

Phenylketonuria is one of several mendelian conditions that have a relatively high incidence, others being cystic fibrosis, Duchenne's muscular dystrophy, neurofibromatosis type 1, and sickle cell anemia (Table 2–2). These conditions share no single feature; some are recessive, some dominant, some autosomal, and some X linked, and some are lethal in early childhood but others have very little effect on reproduction (and transmission of mutant genes to subsequent generations). In fact, the incidence of a mendelian condition is determined by a balance of factors, including the rate at which new mutations occur, and the likelihood that an individual carrying a mutation will transmit it to his or her offspring. The latter characteristic—the probability, compared with the general population, of transmitting one's genes to the next generation—is called **fitness.** Reduced fitness exhibited by many genetic conditions such as Duchenne's muscular dystrophy or type 1 neurofibromatosis is balanced by an appreciable **new mutation rate,** so that the incidence of the condition remains constant in successive generations.

For recessive conditions such as phenylketonuria or sickle cell anemia (or X-linked recessive conditions such as Duchenne's muscular dystrophy), another factor that can influence disease incidence is whether heterozygous carriers experience a selective advantage or disadvantage compared with homozygous nonmutant individuals. For example, the relatively high incidence of sickle cell anemia in individuals of West African ancestry is due in part to **heterozygote advantage,** conferring resistance to malaria. Because the detrimental effects of homozygosity for the hemoglobin B sickle allele (HBB^S) are balanced by the beneficial effects of heterozygosity, the overall frequency of the HBB^S allele has increased over time in populations where malaria is endemic.

A final factor that may contribute to the high incidence of a mendelian disease is **genetic drift,** which refers to the fluctuation of gene frequencies due to random sampling over many generations. The extent of fluctuation is greatest in very small populations. A related phenomenon is the **founder effect,** which occurs when a population founded by a small number of ancestors has, by chance, a high frequency of a deleterious mutation. A founder effect and genetic drift can operate together to produce large changes in the incidence of mendelian diseases, especially in small populations founded by a small number of ancestors.

In the case of phenylketonuria, the fitness of affected individuals has until recently been very low, and new mutations are exceedingly rare; however, population genetic studies provide evidence for both a founder effect and heterozygote advantage.

Phenylketonuria is also representative of a class of mendelian conditions for which efforts are under way to develop gene therapy, such as hemophilia and ornithine transcarbamoylase deficiency. A thorough understanding of the pathophysiology of these conditions is an important prerequisite to developing treatments. Each of these conditions is caused by loss of function for an enzyme expressed specifically in the liver; therefore, attempts to deliver a normal gene to affected individuals have focused on strategies to express the gene in hepatocytes. However, as is the case for benign hyperphenylalaninemia, individuals with very low levels of enzymatic activity are clinically normal, and successful gene therapy might, therefore, be accomplished by expressing the target gene in only a small proportion of hepatic cells.

CHECKPOINT

7. What are the primary defects in phenylketonuria?
8. Why is dietary modification a less than satisfactory treatment of this condition?
9. Explain how strategies of dietary treatment for inborn errors of metabolism depend on whether the pathophysiology is caused by substrate accumulation or end-product deficiency.
10. Explain the phenomenon of maternal phenylketonuria.

FRAGILE X-ASSOCIATED MENTAL RETARDATION SYNDROME

Fragile X-associated mental retardation syndrome produces a combination of phenotypic features that affect the CNS, the testes, and the cranial skeleton. These features were recognized as a distinct clinical entity more than 50 years ago. A laboratory test for the syndrome was developed during the 1970s, when it was recognized that most affected individuals exhibit a cytogenetic abnormality of the X chromosome: failure of the region between bands Xq27 and Xq28 to condense at metaphase. Instead, this region appears in the microscope as a thin constriction that is subject to breakage during preparation, which accounts for the designation "fragile X." Advances in the past decade have helped to explain both the presence of the fragile site and the unique pattern of inheritance exhibited by the syndrome. In some respects, fragile X-associated mental retardation syndrome is similar to other genetic conditions caused by X-linked mutations: Affected males are impaired more severely than affected females, and the condition is never transmitted from father to son. However, the syndrome breaks the rules of mendelian transmission in that at least 20% of carrier males manifest no signs of it. Daughters of these nonpenetrant but "transmitting males" are themselves nonpenetrant but produce affected offspring, male and female, with frequencies close to mendelian expectations (Figure 2–7). About a third of carrier females (those with one normal and one abnormal X chromosome) exhibit a significant degree of mental retardation. These unusual features of the syndrome were explained when the subchromosomal region spanning the fragile site was isolated and shown to contain a segment in which the triplet sequence CGG was repeated many times: $(CGG)_n$. The number of triplet repeats is very polymorphic but normally less

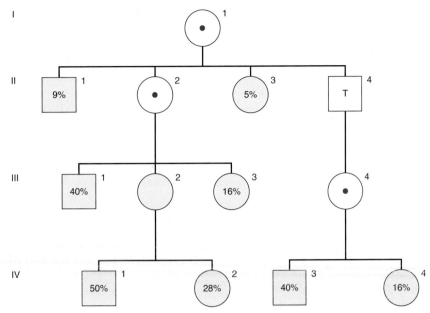

FIGURE 2–7 Likelihood of fragile X-associated mental retardation syndrome in an artificial pedigree. The percentages shown indicate the likelihood of clinical manifestation according to position in the pedigree. Because individuals carrying the abnormal X chromosome have a 50% chance of passing it to their offspring, penetrance is twice that of the values depicted. Penetrance increases with each successive generation owing to the progressive expansion of a triplet repeat element (see text). Expansion is dependent on maternal inheritance of the abnormal allele; thus, daughters of normal transmitting males (indicated with a T in II-4) are nonpenetrant. Obligate carrier females are indicated with a central dot.
(Redrawn, with permission, from Nussbaum RL, Ledbetter DH. Fragile X syndrome: a unique mutation in man. Annu Rev Genet. 1986;20:109.)

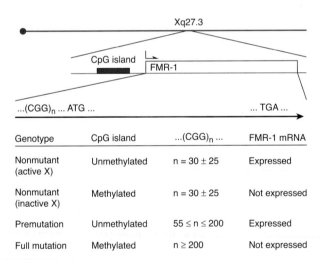

Genotype	CpG island	...(CGG)$_n$ ...	FMR-1 mRNA
Nonmutant (active X)	Unmethylated	n = 30 ± 25	Expressed
Nonmutant (inactive X)	Methylated	n = 30 ± 25	Not expressed
Premutation	Unmethylated	55 ≤ n ≤ 200	Expressed
Full mutation	Methylated	n ≥ 200	Not expressed

FIGURE 2–8 Molecular genetics of fragile X-associated mental retardation syndrome. The cytogenetic fragile site at Xq27.3 is located close to a small region of DNA that contains a CpG island (see text) and the *FMR1* gene. Within the 5′ untranslated region of the *FMR1* gene lies an unstable segment of repetitive DNA 5′–(CGG)$_n$–3′. The table shows the methylation status of the CpG island, the size of the triplet repeat, and whether the FMR1 mRNA is expressed depending on the genotype of the X chromosome. Note that the inactive X chromosome in nonmutant females has a methylated CpG island and does not express the FMR1 mRNA. The methylation and expression status of *FMR1* in premutation and full mutation alleles applies to males and to the active X chromosome of females; premutation and full mutation alleles on the inactive X chromosome of females exhibit methylation of the CpG island and fail to express the FMR1 mRNA.

than 60. A repeat size between 60 and 200 does not cause a clinical phenotype or a cytogenetic fragile site but is unstable and subject to additional amplification, leading to typical features of the syndrome (Figures 2–8 and 2–9).

Clinical Manifestations

Fragile X-associated mental retardation syndrome is usually recognized in affected boys because of developmental delay apparent by 1–2 years of age, small joint hyperextensibility, mild hypotonia, and a family history of mental retardation in maternally related males. Affected females generally have either mild mental retardation or only subtle impairments of visuospatial ability, and the condition may not be evident or diagnosed until it is suspected after identification of an affected male relative. In late childhood or early adolescence, affected males begin to exhibit large testes and characteristic facial features, including mild coarsening, large ears, a prominent forehead and mandible, a long face, and relative macrocephaly (considered in relation to height). The syndrome is extremely common and affects about 1:1500–1:1000 males. Virtually all affected males are born to females who are either affected or carry the premutation, and there are no well-recognized cases of new premutations in males or females.

The inheritance of fragile X-associated mental retardation syndrome exhibits several unusual features and is often described in terms of empiric risk figures (Figure 2–7). In particular, the likelihood that an individual carrying an abnormal chromosome will manifest clinical features depends

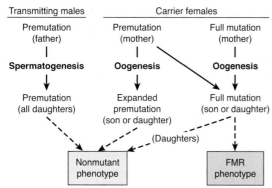

FIGURE 2–9 Transmission and amplification of the fragile X-associated mental retardation triplet repeat. The heavy arrows show expansion of the triplet repeat, which is thought to occur postzygotically after the premutation or full mutation is transmitted through the female germline. The dashed arrows represent potential phenotypic consequences. Daughters with the full mutation may not express the fragile X-associated mental retardation phenotype, depending on the proportion of cells in which the mutant allele happens to lie on the inactive X chromosome. (Redrawn from Tarleton JC, Saul RA. Molecular genetic advances in fragile X syndrome. J Pediatr. 1993;122:169.)

on the number of generations through which the abnormal chromosome has been transmitted and the sex of the transmitting parent. For example, nonpenetrant transmitting males tend to occur in the same sibship with each other and with nonpenetrant carrier females. This is reflected in low risk figures for brothers and sisters of transmitting males: 9% and 5%, respectively, compared with 40% and 16% for their maternal grandsons and granddaughters. This latter observation, in which the penetrance or expressivity (or both) of a genetic disease seems to increase in successive generations, is sometimes referred to more generally as **genetic anticipation.**

Genetic anticipation in fragile X-associated mental retardation syndrome is caused by progressive expansion of the triplet repeat. A similar phenomenon occurs in several neurodegenerative disorders such as Huntington's disease and spinocerebellar ataxia (ie, grandchildren are affected more severely than grandparents). The neurodegenerative disorders are caused by production of abnormal proteins; fragile X-associated mental retardation is caused by failure to produce a normal protein. Although the biochemical mechanisms are different, the underlying molecular causes of genetic anticipation are identical and involve progressive expansion of an unstable triplet repeat.

In addition to triplet repeat expansion, genetic anticipation can be caused by **bias of ascertainment,** which occurs when a mild or variably expressed condition first diagnosed in grandchildren from a three generation pedigree is then easily recognized in siblings of the grandchildren who are available for examination and testing. In contrast to genetic anticipation caused by expansion of a triplet repeat, anticipation caused by bias of ascertainment affects the *apparent* rather than the actual penetrance.

Pathophysiology

Amplification of the $(CGG)_n$ repeat at the fraXq27.3 site affects both methylation and expression of the *FMR1* gene. This gene and the unstable DNA responsible for the expansion were isolated on the basis of their proximity to the cytogenetic fragile site in Xq27.3. *FMR1* encodes an RNA-binding protein that regulates translation of mRNA molecules carrying a characteristic sequence in which four guanine residues can form intramolecular bonds, a so-called G quartet structure.

The $(CGG)_n$ repeat is located in the 5′ untranslated region of the *FMR1* gene (Figure 2–8). This segment is highly variable in length; the number of repeats, n, is equal to about 30 ± 25 in individuals who are neither affected with nor carriers for fragile X-associated mental retardation syndrome. In transmitting males and in unaffected carrier females, the number of repeats is usually between 70 and 100. Remarkably, alleles with fewer than 50 repeats are very stable and almost always transmitted without a change in repeat number. However, alleles with 55 or more repeats are unstable and often exhibit expansion after maternal transmission; these individuals are said to carry a **premutation.** Although premutation carriers do not develop a typical fragile X-associated mental retardation syndrome, studies indicate that female premutation carriers exhibit a 20% incidence of premature ovarian failure, whereas male premutation carriers are at increased risk for a tremor/ataxia syndrome. In both cases, the mechanism is likely to be explained by somatic expansion of the premutation (see later discussion). The degree of expansion is related to the number of repeats; premutation alleles with a repeat number less than 60 rarely are amplified to a full mutation, but premutation alleles with a repeat number greater than 90 are usually amplified to a full mutation. The number of repeats in the full mutation—observed both in affected males and in affected females—is always greater than 200 but is generally heterogeneous, suggesting that once this threshold is reached, additional amplification occurs frequently in somatic cells.

Expansion from a premutation to a full mutation has two important effects: *FMR1* gene transcription is shut off, and DNA surrounding the transcriptional start site of the *FMR1* gene becomes methylated. The clinical phenotype is caused by failure to produce FMR1; in addition, methylation of surrounding DNA has important implications for molecular diagnosis. Methylation occurs in a so-called **CpG island,** a several hundred base pair segment just upstream of the *FMR1* transcriptional start site that contains a high frequency of 5′-CG-3′ dinucleotides compared with the rest of the genome. Methylation of the CpG island and expansion of the triplet repeat can be easily detected with molecular biologic techniques, which are the basis of the common diagnostic tests for individuals at risk.

Genetic Principles

In addition to the tendency of $(CGG)_n$ premutation alleles to undergo further amplifications in length, the molecular genetics of fragile X-associated mental retardation syndrome exhibit several unusual features. As described previously, each phenotypically affected individual carries a full mutation defined by a repeat number greater than 200, but the exact repeat number exhibits considerable heterogeneity in different cells and tissues.

Diagnostic testing for the number of CGG repeats is usually performed on approximately 10^7 lymphocytes taken from a small amount of peripheral blood. In individuals who carry a repeat number less than 50, each of the 10^7 cells has the same number of repeats. However, in phenotypically affected males or females (ie, those with a repeat number greater than 200), many of the 10^7 cells may have a different number of repeats. This situation, often referred to as **somatic mosaicism,** indicates that at least some of the amplification is **postzygotic,** meaning that it occurs in cells of the developing embryo after fertilization. In addition to the DNA methylation associated with an abnormal *FMR1* gene, methylation of many genes is a normal process during development and differentiation that helps to regulate gene expression. Cells in which a particular gene should not be expressed frequently shut off that gene's expression by methylation. For example, globin should be expressed only in reticulocytes; albumin should be expressed only in hepatocytes; and insulin should be expressed only by pancreatic B cells. During gametogenesis and immediately after fertilization, specific patterns of methylation characteristic of differentiated cells are erased, only to be reestablished in fetal development. Thus, methylation provides a reversible change in gene structure that can be inherited during mitosis of differentiated cells yet erased during meiosis and early development. This type of alteration—a heritable phenotypic change that is not determined by DNA sequence—is broadly referred to as **epigenetic.**

Analysis of fragile X-associated mental retardation syndrome pedigrees reveals that one of the most important factors influencing whether a premutation allele is subject to postzygotic expansion is the sex of the parent who transmits the premutation allele (Figures 2–7 and 2–9). As discussed, a premutation allele transmitted by a female expands to a full mutation with a likelihood proportionate to the length of the premutation. Premutation alleles with a repeat number between 52 and 60 rarely expand to a full mutation, and those with a repeat number greater than 90 nearly always expand. In contrast, a premutation allele transmitted by a male rarely if ever expands to a full mutation regardless of the length of the repeat number.

The notion that alleles of the same DNA sequence can behave very differently depending on the sex of the parent who transmitted them is closely related to the concept of **gametic imprinting,** which is used to describe the situation that occurs when expression of a particular gene depends on the sex of the parent who transmitted it. Gametic imprinting affects a handful of genes involved in fetal or placental growth, including insulin-like growth factor 2 (IGF2) and the type 2 IGF receptor (IGF2R); for example, the *IGF2* gene is expressed only on the paternally derived chromosome, whereas in some individuals the *IGF2R* gene is expressed only on the maternally derived chromosome. The mechanisms responsible for gametic imprinting depend on biochemical modifications to the chromosome that occur during gametogenesis; these modifications do not affect the actual DNA sequence but are stably transmitted for a certain number of cell divisions (ie, they are epigenetic and contribute to the pathogenesis of certain types of cancer).

CHECKPOINT

11. Explain why fragile X-associated mental retardation syndrome exhibits an unusual pattern of inheritance.

12. What is genetic anticipation? What are two explanations for it?

13. What is an epigenetic change?

LEBER'S HEREDITARY OPTIC NEUROPATHY, MITOCHONDRIAL ENCEPHALOMYOPATHY WITH RAGGED RED FIBERS, & OTHER MITOCHONDRIAL DISEASES

In nearly every cell in the body, the indispensable job of turning nutrients into energy takes place in mitochondria, ubiquitous subcellular organelles with their own genomes and unique rules of gene expression. Over the last decade, defects in mitochondrial function have become increasingly recognized as important human causes of diseases, from rare conditions whose study has led to a deeper understanding of pathophysiologic mechanisms to common conditions such as diabetes and deafness. On one level, the consequences of defective mitochondrial function are predictable and nonspecific: Inability to generate sufficient adenosine triphosphate (ATP) leads to accumulation of lactic acid, weakness, and, eventually, cell death. However, every mitochondrion contains multiple mitochondrial genomes; every cell contains multiple mitochondria; the requirements for energy production vary from one tissue to another; and, most importantly, mutations in mitochondrial DNA affect only a fraction of mitochondrial genomes within a given individual. Because of these characteristics, defects in mitochondrial function present clinically with symptoms and signs that are both specific and protean. In addition, mitochondrial DNA is transmitted by eggs but not by sperm, leading to a unique and characteristic pattern of inheritance.

Clinical Manifestations

First described by a German physician in 1871, Leber's hereditary optic neuropathy (LHON) presents as painless bilateral loss of vision that occurs in young adults, more commonly in males. Loss of vision can be sudden and complete or subacute and progressive, proceeding from central scotomas to blindness over 1–2 years and usually affecting both eyes within 1–2 months. The condition is occasionally associated with neurologic findings, including ataxia, dysarthria, or symptoms of demyelinating disease, and may be associated also with cardiac conduction abnormalities. Ophthalmologic examination shows peripapillary telangiectasia, microangiopathy, and vascular tortuosity; in patients with neurologic findings (and some without), CNS imaging studies may reveal abnormalities of the basal ganglia and corpus striatum.

By contrast to LHON, mitochondrial encephalomyopathy with ragged red fibers (MERRF) was recognized as a distinct clinical entity relatively recently. The presenting symptoms are usually periodic jerking and progressive skeletal weakness, but the onset and severity of the symptoms are variable. The term "ragged red fibers" refers to the histologic appearance of muscle from affected individuals, in which abnormal mitochondria accumulate and aggregate in individual muscle fibers. Other symptoms may include sensorineural hearing loss, ataxia, cardiomyopathy, and dementia.

Pathophysiology

The central energy-producing machinery of the mitochondria, complexes I–V of the electron transport chain, contains approximately 90 polypeptides. The majority are encoded by the nuclear genome and—like proteins required for replication, transcription, and translation of the mitochondrial genome—they are imported into the mitochondria after translation. The mitochondrial genome itself (mtDNA) is 16,569 bp in length and encodes 13 polypeptides that are transcribed and translated in mitochondria; mtDNA also encodes mitochondrial ribosomal RNA and 22 mitochondrial tRNA species. Complexes I, III, IV, and V of the electron transport chain contain subunits encoded by both mtDNA and the nuclear genome, whereas the proteins that form complex II are encoded entirely in the nuclear genome.

LHON and MERRF are both caused by mutations in mtDNA; LHON is caused by mutations in a component of the electron transport chain, whereas MERRF is caused by mutations of mitochondrial tRNA, usually tRNA^{Lys}. Thus, from a biochemical perspective, LHON is caused by a specific inability to generate ATP, whereas MERRF is caused by a general defect in mitochondrial protein synthesis. However, the pathophysiologic mechanisms that lead from defective mitochondrial function to specific organ abnormalities are not completely understood. In general, organ systems affected by mitochondrial diseases are those in which ATP production plays a critical role, such as skeletal muscle and the central nervous system. In addition, defects in electron transport can cause excessive production of toxic free radicals, leading to oxidative damage and cell death, and may contribute to age-related dementia. Finally, several proteins that normally reside within mitochondria play key roles in the control of apoptosis; thus, primary abnormalities in mitochondrial integrity can contribute to disease both by decreasing energy production and by increasing programmed cell death.

Genetic Principles

For mitochondrial proteins encoded by the nuclear genome and imported into mitochondria after translation, defects that cause disease are inherited in a typical mendelian fashion. mtDNA, however, is transmitted by the egg and not the sperm, in part because the egg contains more than 1000 times more mtDNA molecules than the sperm. Therefore, for diseases like LHON and MERRF caused by defects in mtDNA, the conditions show a characteristic pattern of maternal inheritance (Figure 2–10) in which all offspring of an affected female are at risk but affected males never transmit the condition.

A second unique feature of diseases caused by mutations in mtDNA is the mosaic nature of the mutation within individual cells. Typically, a single cell contains 10–100 separate mtDNA molecules; in the case of an mtDNA mutation, only a fraction of the molecules carry the mutation, a situation referred to as **heteroplasmy.** The levels of heteroplasmy may vary considerably among different individuals and among different tissues; furthermore, a female primordial germ cell with a mixture of normal and mutated mtDNA molecules can transmit different proportions to daughter eggs (Figure 2–11). For both LHON and MERRF, levels of mutant mtDNA may vary from about 50% to about 90%; in general, the severity of the condition correlates with the extent of heteroplasmy.

A final principle that is apparent from the pathophysiology of mitochondrial diseases is genetic interaction between the nuclear and mitochondrial genomes. One of the best examples is the sex difference in LHON, which affects four to five times as many males as females. This observation suggests that there may be a gene on the X chromosome that modifies the severity of a mitochondrial tRNA^{Lys} mutation and underscores the observation that, even though mtDNA itself encodes for a set of key mitochondrial components, most mitochondrial proteins are encoded by the nuclear genome.

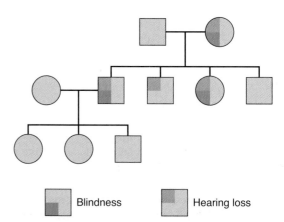

FIGURE 2–10 Maternal inheritance. An idealized pedigree illustrating maternal inheritance, which occurs in disease caused by mutations in mitochondrial DNA. Mothers transmit the mutated mtDNA to all of their offspring, but fathers do not. Variable expressivity and reduced penetrance are a consequence of different levels of heteroplasmy.

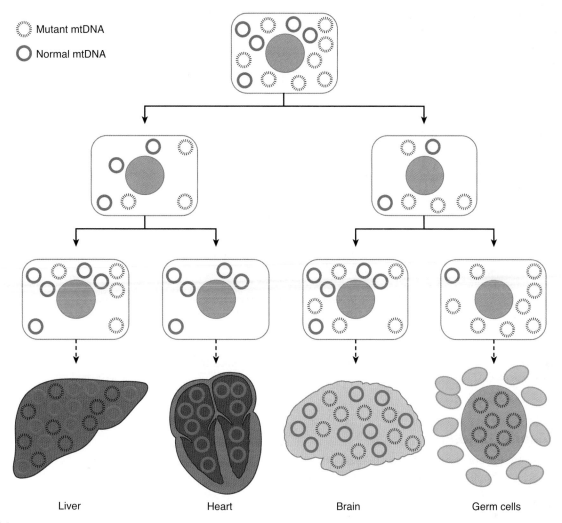

Mutant mtDNA

Normal mtDNA

Liver Heart Brain Germ cells

FIGURE 2–11 Heteroplasmy and variable expressivity. The fraction of mutated mtDNA molecules within a cell is determined by a combination of random chance and selection at the cellular level during embryonic development. Adult tissues are mosaic for cells with different fractions of mutated mtDNA molecules, which helps to explain why mitochondrial dysfunction can produce different phenotypes and different levels of severity.

DOWN SYNDROME

The clinical features of Down syndrome were described over a century ago. Although the underlying cause—an extra copy of chromosome 21—has been known for more than 4 decades, the nearly complete DNA sequence of chromosome 21—some 33,546,361 base pairs—was determined only 4 years ago, and the relationship of genotype to phenotype is just beginning to be understood. Down syndrome is broadly representative of **aneuploid** conditions, or those that are caused by a deviation from the normal chromosome complement (**euploidy**). Chromosome 21, which contains a little less than 2% of the total genome, is one of the **acrocentric** autosomes (the others are 13, 14, 15, and 22), which means one in which nearly all the DNA lies on one side of the centromere. In general, aneuploidy may involve part or all of an autosome or sex chromosome. Most individuals with Down syndrome have 47 chromosomes (ie, one extra

chromosome 21, or **trisomy 21**) and are born to parents with normal karyotypes. This type of aneuploidy is usually caused by **non-disjunction** during meiotic segregation, which means failure of two homologous chromosomes to separate (disjoin) from each other at anaphase. In contrast, aneuploid conditions that affect part of an autosome or sex chromosome must at some point involve DNA breakage and reunion. DNA rearrangements are an infrequent but important cause of Down syndrome and are usually evident as a karyotype with 46 chromosomes in which one chromosome 21 is fused via its centromere to another acrocentric chromosome. This abnormal chromosome is described as a **robertsonian translocation** and can sometimes be inherited from a carrier parent (Figure 2–12). Thus, Down syndrome may be caused by a variety of different karyotypic abnormalities, which have in common a 50% increase in **gene dosage** for nearly all of the genes on chromosome 21.

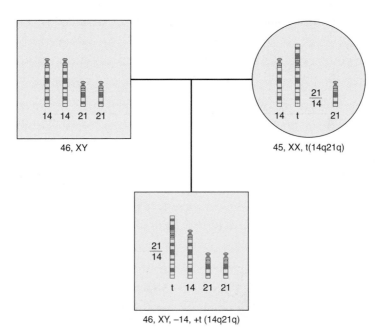

FIGURE 2–12 Mechanisms leading to Down syndrome. A pedigree in which the mother is phenotypically normal yet is a balanced carrier for a 14;21 robertsonian translocation. She transmits both the translocation chromosome and a normal chromosome 21 to her son, who also inherits a normal chromosome 21 from his father. Three copies of chromosome 21 in the son cause Down syndrome. (Redrawn from Thompson MW et al. *Genetics in Medicine,* 7th ed. Saunders, 2007.)

Clinical Manifestations

Down syndrome occurs approximately once in every 700 live births and accounts for approximately one third of all cases of mental retardation. The likelihood of conceiving a child with Down syndrome is related exponentially to increasing maternal age. However, screening programs detect most Down syndrome pregnancies in pregnant women older than 35 years (Figure 2–13). This fact, combined with the inverse relationship of maternal age to overall birth rate, means that most children with Down syndrome are now born to women younger than 35 years. The condition is usually suspected in the perinatal period from the presence of characteristic facial and dysmorphic features such as brachycephaly, epicanthal folds, small ears, transverse palmar creases, and hypotonia (Table 2–4). Approximately 50% of affected children have congenital heart defects that come to medical attention in the immediate perinatal period because of cardiorespiratory problems. Strong suspicion of the condition on clinical grounds is usually confirmed by karyotyping within 2–3 days.

A great many minor and major abnormalities occur with increased frequency in Down syndrome, yet two affected individuals rarely have the same set of abnormalities, and many single abnormalities can be seen in unaffected individuals. For example, the incidence of a transverse palmar crease in Down syndrome is about 50%, ten times that in the general population, yet most individuals in whom transverse palmar creases are the only unusual feature do not have Down syndrome or any other genetic disease.

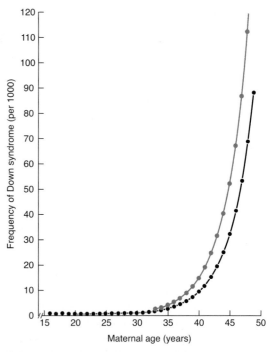

FIGURE 2–13 Relationship of Down syndrome to maternal age. The frequency of Down syndrome rises exponentially with increasing maternal age. The frequency at amniocentesis (blue symbols) is slightly higher than in live-born infants (black symbols) because miscarriages are more likely in fetuses with Down syndrome. (Data from Scriver CR et al [editors]. *The Metabolic and Molecular Bases of Inherited Disease,* 8th ed. McGraw-Hill, 2001.)

TABLE 2–4 Phenotypic features of trisomy 21.

Feature	Frequency
Upslanting palpebral fissures	82%
Excess skin on back of neck	81%
Brachycephaly	75%
Hyperextensible joints	75%
Flat nasal bridge	68%
Wide gap between first and second toes	68%
Short, broad hands	64%
Epicanthal folds	59%
Short fifth finger	58%
Incurved fifth finger	57%
Brushfield spots (iris hypoplasia)	56%
Transverse palmar crease	53%
Folded or dysplastic ear	50%
Protruding tongue	47%

Data from Scriver CR et al (editors). *The Metabolic and Molecular Bases of Inherited Disease*, 7th ed. McGraw-Hill, 1995.

The natural history of Down syndrome in childhood is characterized mainly by developmental delay, growth retardation, and immunodeficiency. Developmental delay is usually apparent by 3–6 months of age as failure to attain age-appropriate developmental milestones and affects all aspects of motor and cognitive function. The mean IQ is between 30 and 70 and declines with increasing age. However, there is a considerable range in the degree of mental retardation in adults with Down syndrome, and many affected individuals can live semi-independently. In general, cognitive skills are more limited than affective performance, and only a minority of affected individuals are severely impaired. Retardation of linear growth is moderate, and most adults with Down syndrome have statures 2–3 standard deviations below that of the general population. In contrast, weight growth in Down syndrome exhibits a mild proportionate increase compared with that of the general population, and most adults with Down syndrome are overweight. Although increased susceptibility to infections is a common clinical feature at all ages, the nature of the underlying abnormality is not well understood, and laboratory abnormalities can be detected in both humoral and cellular immunity.

One of the most prevalent and dramatic clinical features of Down syndrome—premature onset of Alzheimer's disease—is not evident until adulthood. Although frank dementia is not clinically detectable in all adults with Down syndrome, the incidence of typical neuropathologic changes—senile plaques and neurofibrillary tangles—is nearly 100% by age 35 years.

The major causes of morbidity in Down syndrome are congenital heart disease, infections, and leukemia. Life expectancy depends to a large extent on the presence of congenital heart disease; survival to ages 10 and 30 years is approximately 60% and 50%, respectively, for individuals with congenital heart disease and approximately 85% and 80%, respectively, for individuals without congenital heart disease.

Pathophysiology

The advent of molecular markers for different portions of chromosome 21 provided considerable information about when and how the extra chromosomal material arises in Down syndrome; and the Human Genome Project has provided a list of the approximately 230 genes found on chromosome 21. In contrast, much less is known about why increased gene dosage for chromosome 21 should produce the clinical features of Down syndrome.

For trisomy 21 (47,XX+21 or 47,XY+21), cytogenetic or molecular markers that distinguish between the maternal and paternal copies of chromosome 21 can be used to determine whether the egg or the sperm contributed the extra copy of chromosome 21. There are no obvious clinical differences between these two types of trisomy 21 individuals, which suggests that gametic imprinting does not play a significant role in the pathogenesis of Down syndrome. If both copies of chromosome 21 carried by each parent can be distinguished, it is usually possible to determine whether the nondisjunction event leading to an abnormal gamete occurred during anaphase of meiosis I or meiosis II (Figure 2–14). Studies such as these show that approximately 75% of cases of trisomy 21 are caused by an extra maternal chromosome, that approximately 75% of the nondisjunction events (both maternal and paternal) occur in meiosis I, and that both maternal and paternal nondisjunction events increase with advanced maternal age.

Several theories have been proposed to explain why the incidence of Down syndrome increases with advanced maternal age (Figure 2–13). Most germ cell development in females is completed before birth; oocytes arrest at prophase of meiosis I (the **dictyotene** stage) during the second trimester of gestation. One proposal suggests that biochemical abnormalities that affect the ability of paired chromosomes to disjoin normally accumulate in these cells over time and that, without a renewable source of fresh eggs, the proportion of eggs undergoing nondisjunction increases with maternal age. However, this hypothesis does not explain why the relationship between the incidence of trisomy 21 and advanced maternal age holds for paternal as well as maternal nondisjunction events.

Another hypothesis proposes that structural, hormonal, and immunologic changes that occur in the uterus with advanced age produce an environment less able to reject a developmentally abnormal embryo. Thus, an older uterus would be more likely to support a trisomy 21 conceptus to term regardless of which parent contributed the extra chromosome. This hypothesis can explain why paternal nondisjunction errors increase with advanced maternal age.

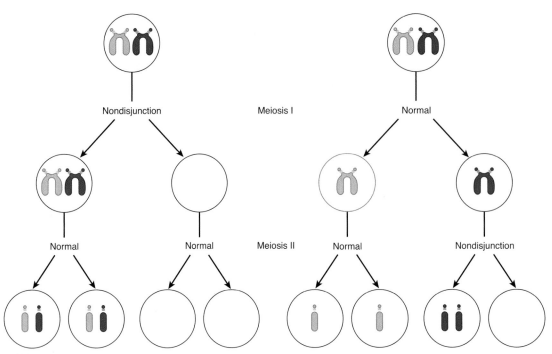

FIGURE 2–14 Nondisjunction has different consequences depending on whether it occurs at meiosis I or meiosis II. The abnormal gamete has two copies of a particular chromosome. When nondisjunction occurs at meiosis I, each of the copies originates from a different chromosome; however, when nondisjunction occurs at meiosis II, each of the copies originates from the same chromosome. Both cytogenetic and molecular polymorphisms can be used to determine the stage and the parent in which nondisjunction occurred. (Redrawn, with permission, from Thompson MW et al. *Genetics in Medicine,* 7th ed. Saunders, 2007.)

However, it does not explain why the incidence of Down syndrome resulting from chromosomal rearrangements (see later discussion) does not increase with maternal age.

These and other hypotheses are not mutually exclusive, and it is possible that a combination of factors is responsible for the relationship between the incidence of trisomy 21 and advanced maternal age. A number of environmental and genetic factors have been considered as possible causes of Down syndrome, including exposure to caffeine, alcohol, tobacco, radiation, and the likelihood of carrying one or more genes that would predispose to nondisjunction. Although it is difficult to exclude all of these possibilities from consideration as minor factors, there is no evidence that any of these factors play a role in Down syndrome.

The recurrence risk for trisomy 21 is not altered significantly by having had previous affected children. However, approximately 5% of Down syndrome karyotypes have 46 rather than 47 chromosomes as a result of robertsonian translocations that usually involve chromosomes 14 or 22. As described, this type of abnormality is not associated with increased maternal age; however, in about 30% of such individuals, cytogenetic evaluation of the parents reveals a so-called balanced rearrangement such as 45,XX,+t(14q;21q). Because the robertsonian translocation chromosome can pair with both of its component single acrocentric chromosomes at meiosis, the likelihood of segregation leading to unbalanced gametes is significant (Figure 2–15), and the recurrence risk to the parent with the abnormal karyotype is

much higher than for trisomy 21 (Table 2–5). Approximately 1% of Down syndrome karyotypes show mosaicism in which some cells are normal and some abnormal. Somatic mosaicism for trisomy 21 or other aneuploid conditions may initially arise either pre- or postzygotically, corresponding to nondisjunction in meiosis or mitosis, respectively. In the former case (one in which a zygote is conceived from an aneuploid gamete), the extra chromosome is then presumably lost mitotically in a clone of cells during early embryogenesis. The range of phenotypes seen in mosaic trisomy 21 is great, ranging from mild mental retardation with subtle dysmorphic features to "typical" Down syndrome, and does not correlate with the proportion of abnormal cells detected in lymphocytes or fibroblasts. Nonetheless, on average, mental retardation in mosaic trisomy 21 is generally milder than in nonmosaic trisomy 21.

Genetic Principles

A fundamental question in understanding the relationship between an extra chromosome 21 and the clinical features of Down syndrome is whether the phenotype is caused by abnormal gene expression or an abnormal chromosomal constitution. An important principle derived from studies directed at this question is that of **gene dosage,** which states that the amount of a gene product produced per cell is proportionate to the number of copies of that gene present. In other words, the amount of protein produced by all or nearly all genes that

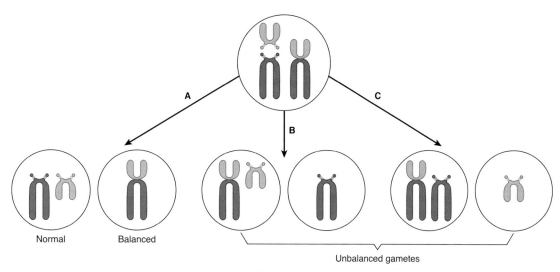

FIGURE 2–15 Types of gametes produced at meiosis by a carrier of a robertsonian translocation. In a balanced carrier for a robertsonian translocation, different types of segregation at meiosis lead to several different types of gametes, including ones that are completely normal (A), ones that would give rise to other balanced translocation carriers (B), and ones that would give rise to aneuploid progeny (C).

lie on chromosome 21 is 150% of normal in trisomy 21 cells and 50% of normal in monosomy 21 cells. Thus, unlike the X chromosome, there is no mechanism for dosage compensation that operates on autosomal genes.

Experimental evidence generally supports the view that the Down syndrome phenotype is caused by increased expression of specific genes and not by a nonspecific detrimental effect of cellular aneuploidy. Rarely, karyotypic analysis of an individual with Down syndrome reveals a chromosomal rearrangement (usually an unbalanced reciprocal translocation) in which only a very small portion of chromosome 21 is present in three copies per cell (Figure 2–16). These observations suggest that there may be a critical region of chromosome 21, which, when present in triplicate, is both sufficient and necessary to produce Down syndrome.

The idea that altered gene dosage of a group of closely linked genes can produce a distinct clinical phenotype is also supported by the observation that several multiple congenital

anomaly syndromes are due to small interstitial deletions of particular autosomes, often mediated by homologous segments of DNA that lie at both ends of the deletion breakpoints. These deletions, which often are detectable only with special cytogenetic or molecular techniques, result in monosomy for the genes located within the deleted segment. Such **contiguous gene syndromes,** described in Table 2–6, are generally rare, but they have played important roles in understanding the pathophysiology of aneuploid conditions.

TABLE 2–5 Risk for Down syndrome depending on parental sex and karyotype.

	Risk of Abnormal Live-Born Progeny	
Karyotype of Parent	Female Carrier	Male Carrier
46,XX or 46,XY	0.5% (at age 20) to 30% (at age 30)	< 0.5%
Rb(Dq;21q) (mostly 14)	10%	< 2%
Rb(21q;22q)	14%	< 2%
Rb(21q;21q)	100%	100%

Data from Scriver CR et al (editors). *The Metabolic and Molecular Bases of Inherited Disease,* 7th ed. McGraw-Hill, 1995.

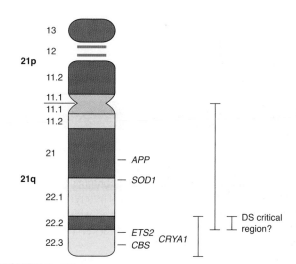

FIGURE 2–16 Down syndrome (DS) critical region. Rarely, individuals with Down syndrome will have chromosomal rearrangements that cause trisomy for just a portion of chromosome 21. The *APP, SOD1, ETS2, CRYA1,* and *CBS* genes encode proteins (amyloid precursor, superoxide dismutase, the Ets2 transcription factor, crystallin, and cystathionine beta-synthase, respectively) that may play a role in the pathogenesis of Down syndrome. Analysis of two sets of individuals (indicated by the two vertical lines) suggests that the genes responsible for Down syndrome lie in the region of overlap. (Redrawn, with permission, from Thompson MW et al. *Genetics in Medicine,* 5th ed. Saunders, 1991.)

TABLE 2–6 Phenotype and karyotype of some contiguous gene syndromes.

Syndrome	Phenotype	Deletion
Langer-Gideon	Mental retardation, microcephaly, bony exostoses, redundant skin	8q24.11–q24.3
WAGR	Wilms' tumor, aniridia, gonado-blastoma, mental retardation	11p13
Prader-Willi	Mental and growth retardation, hypotonia, obesity, hypopig-mentation	15q11–q13
Miller-Dieker	Severe mental retardation, absence of cortical gyri (lissenceph-aly) and corpus callosum	17p13.3

Carriers for robertsonian translocations that involve chromosome 21 can produce several different types of unbalanced gametes (Figure 2–15). However, the empiric risk for such a carrier bearing an infant with Down syndrome is higher than for other aneuploid conditions, in part because embryos with other types of aneuploidies are likely to result in miscarriages early in development. Thus, the consequences of trisomy for embryonic and fetal development are proportionate to the number of genes expressed to 150% of their normal levels. Because monosomy for chromosome 21 (and other autosomes) is virtually never seen in live-born infants, a similar line of reasoning suggests that a 50% reduction in gene expression is more severe than a 50% increase. Finally, female robertsonian translocation carriers exhibit much higher empiric recurrence risks than male carriers, which suggests that (1) selective responses against aneuploidy can operate on gametic as well as somatic cells and (2) spermatogenesis is more sensitive to aneuploidy than oogenesis.

CHECKPOINT

14. What are the common features of the variety of different karyotypic abnormalities resulting in Down syndrome?

15. What are the major categories of abnormalities in Down syndrome, and what is their natural history?

16. Explain why trisomy 21 is associated with such a wide range of phenotypes from mild mental retardation to that of "typical" Down syndrome.

IMPACT OF THE HUMAN GENOME PROJECT & HUMAN GENETIC VARIATION ON PATHOPHYSIOLOGY

The major goal of the Human Genome Project is to determine the identity and gain understanding of all the genes of human beings and to apply this information to the diagnosis and treatment of human disease. An international collaboration, in which U.S. efforts were coordinated by the National Human Genome Research Institute, achieved a primary milestone in 2003 when the approximately 3 billion nucleotide human genome DNA sequence was determined.

Understanding the function of all of the genes of human beings has been facilitated by determining genome sequences for other living organisms. Some are closely related to humans on an evolutionary time scale, such as the chimpanzee, whose genome is approximately 98% the same as humans, and whose last common ancestor with humans lived approximately 6 million years ago. Others are more distantly related such as the laboratory mouse, the fruit fly, or bakers' yeast, but nonetheless serve as valuable model organisms for experimental biologists. Even the laboratory mouse, whose last common ancestor with humans lived approximately 100 million years ago, shares more than 95% of its genes with the human genome. These considerations underscore the important genetic principle that the processes of evolution have left valuable molecular footprints that can be used to learn more about human biology.

One of the most important advances of the Human Genome Project in the last few years has been a catalog of common human genetic variation, usually referred to as the HapMap (for Haplotype Map), in which more than 3 million SNPs have been genotyped among individuals of diverse genetic ancestry, including populations from Asia, Africa, the Americas, and Europe. Because common genetic differences are a major determinant of susceptibility to conditions such as diabetes mellitus, hypertension, obesity, and schizophrenia, a principal goal of the HapMap is to develop a molecular understanding of those determinants.

The idea that measuring human genetic variation on a genome-wide scale could provide insight into common diseases such as hypertension, schizophrenia, and cancer underscores the perspective that there is a spectrum of genetic disease from rare conditions inherited in a mendelian fashion (which have been the major subject of this chapter) to so-called complex genetic or multifactorial conditions, for which the incidence of the disease is influenced by a combination of genes, environment, and chance. Identifying genetic components of multifactorial conditions is an important goal of the field of genetic epidemiology, in which epidemiology-based study designs are applied to populations whose familial structure is uncertain or unknown, and the measurement of SNPs in candidate genes are treated as hypothetical risk factors. For example, the epsilon 4 allele of the apolipoprotein E gene (*APOE 4*), is found in approximately 15% of the population and increases the risk of both atherosclerosis and late-onset Alzheimer disease. However, *APOE4* is just one of many genes that influence susceptibility to these important conditions, and a major goal of the HapMap is to identify and characterize those genes, both to develop new treatments and to provide as much information as possible to physicians and their patients regarding disease susceptibility as a function of genetics.

Indeed, there is much excitement today about the potential of personalized genetic medicine, in part due to recent advances in several different areas. First, technological advances now make it possible to efficiently measure variation at millions of SNPs in individual patient samples as a routine laboratory test. These kinds of tests have been applied to thousands of individuals in so-called case-control studies to identify particular SNPs that occur more or less frequently in cases versus controls. Second, advances in the design and analysis of this type of approach, known as a **genome-wide association study** or GWAS, have recently been very successful in identifying new genetic determinants for obesity, diabetes mellitus, inflammatory bowel disease, coronary artery disease, and other common conditions. Finally, availability of the human genome sequence (without which the millions of SNPs could not have been identified in the first place) together with the HapMap catalog of common human genetic variation makes it possible to predict DNA sequence variation for specific segments of the genome, even when that sequence has not been measured directly. The underlying reason is that in most cases, closely linked SNPs are not independently distributed among humans, but are nonrandomly associated in clusters known as haplotype blocks. For example, if two closely linked SNPs are each found at a frequency of 30%, chromosomes that carry both SNPs may exist at a frequency considerably different from 9%, which would be the prediction if the two SNPs were completely independent. This phenomenon, referred to as allelic association or **linkage disequilibrium,** is due to human evolutionary and population history; the extent to which new SNPs (that arise by mutation) become separated from closely adjacent SNPs (by recombination) depends on the distance between adjacent SNPs and the effects of population history on the chances for recombination.

The future of genetic medicine will be greatly informed by these advances; many scientists envision that powerful but inexpensive laboratory tests that measure genetic variation across the entire genome will soon be used routinely to predict individual susceptibility to common diseases and take appropriate steps to intervene and/or modify the course of those conditions. For example, individuals at high risk for certain types of cancer may benefit from aggressive screening programs.

Common genetic differences may also help identify subgroups of patients whose course is likely to be more or less severe and who may respond to a particular treatment. The latter approach is part of the larger field of pharmacogenomics, in which sequence variation in the hundreds of genes that influence drug absorption, metabolism, and excretion is a major determinant of the balance between pharmacologic efficacy and toxicity. One might imagine, for example, that tests for specific nucleotide differences in a set of genes unique to a particular situation might be used to help predict the pathophysiologic response to alcoholic liver damage, type of regimen used to treat leukemia, and course of infectious diseases such as tuberculosis or HIV infection. The latter example already has some support, because certain alleles of the chemokine receptor genes *CCR5* and *CCR2,* found in 10–25% of the population, may delay the progression of HIV-associated diseases.

CASE STUDIES

Eva M. Aagaard, MD, & Yeong Kwok, MD

(See Chapter 25, p. 671 for Answers)

CASE 1

A 4-year-old boy is brought in with pain and swelling of the right thigh after a fall in the home. An x-ray film reveals an acute fracture of the right femur. Questioning of the mother reveals that the boy has had two other known fractures—left humerus and left tibia—both with minimal trauma. The family history is notable for a bone problem during childhood in the boy's father that got better as he grew into adulthood. A diagnosis of osteogenesis imperfecta is entertained.

Questions

A. What are the four types of osteogenesis imperfecta? How are they genetically transmitted?

B. Which two types are most likely in this patient? How might they be distinguished clinically?

C. Further workup results in a diagnosis of type I osteogenesis imperfecta. What clinical features may the boy expect in adult life?

D. What is the pathogenesis of this patient's disease?

CASE 2

A newborn girl tests positive for phenylketonuria (PKU) on a newborn screening examination. The results of a confirmatory serum test done at 2 weeks of age are also positive, establishing the diagnosis of PKU.

Questions

A. What are the metabolic defects in persons with PKU?
B. How do these defects lead to clinical disease in persons not treated with dietary restrictions appropriate for PKU?
C. What is the genetic pattern of inheritance, and what are some possible explanations on why the gene for the condition has persisted in the gene pool despite the obvious disadvantages for the affected individuals?

CASE 3

A young woman is referred for genetic counseling. She has a 3-year-old boy with developmental delay and small joint hyperextensibility. The pediatrician has diagnosed fragile X-associated mental retardation. She is currently pregnant with her second child at 14 weeks of gestation. The family history is unremarkable.

Questions

A. What is the genetic mutation responsible for fragile X-associated mental retardation? How does it cause the clinical syndrome of developmental delay, joint hyperextensibility, large testes, and facial abnormalities?
B. Which parent is the probable carrier of the genetic mutation? Explain why this parent and the grandparents are phenotypically unaffected.
C. What is the likelihood that the unborn child will be affected?

CASE 4

A 16-year-old boy presents with worsening vision for the past 2 months. He first noticed that he was having trouble with central vision in his right eye, seeing a dark spot in the center of his visual field. The dark spot had gotten larger over time, and he had also developed a central loss of vision in his left eye. Two of his maternal uncles had loss of vision, but his mother and another maternal uncle and two maternal aunts had no visual difficulties. No one on his father's side was affected. Physical examination reveals microangiopathy and vascular tortuosity of the retina. Genetic testing confirms the diagnosis of Leber's hereditary optic neuropathy.

Questions

A. What is the central defect in Leber's hereditary optic neuropathy (LHON)?
B. How is this disorder inherited, and what is the principle of heteroplasmy?
C. What explains the fact that males are much more likely to be affected than females?

CASE 5

A 40-year-old woman, recently married and pregnant for the first time, comes to the clinic with a question about the chances of having "a Down syndrome baby."

Questions

A. What is the rate of occurrence of Down syndrome in the general population? What are some of the common clinical features?
B. What major genetic abnormalities are associated with Down syndrome? How might these abnormalities lead to the clinical features of the syndrome?
C. How might this woman's age contribute to her risk of having a child with Down syndrome?

CASE 6

A newborn girl of Yemenite Jewish descent presents in pediatric clinic. The results of a screening test for phenylketonuria were suspicious for the disease.

Questions

A. What is the incidence of phenylketonuria in the general population? How does the risk differ among ethnic groups?

B. What is the primary defect in phenylketonuria?

C. What are the clinical manifestations of phenylketonuria? What is the pathophysiology underlying them?

D. How can phenylketonuria be treated?

E. When this child is of childbearing age, what should she be told about the risks to her baby should she become pregnant?

REFERENCES

Osteogenesis Imperfecta

Cheung MS et al. Osteogenesis imperfecta: Update on presentation and management. Rev Endocr Metab Disord. 2008 Jun;9(2):153–60. [PMID: 18404382]

Martin E et al. Osteogenesis imperfecta: Epidemiology and pathophysiology. Curr Osteoporos Rep. 2007 Sep;5(3):91–7. [PMID: 17925189]

Rauch F et al. Osteogenesis imperfecta. Lancet. 2004 Apr 24;363(9418):1377–85. [PMID: 15110498]

Phenylketonuria

Blau N et al. New approaches to treat PKU: How far are we? Mol Genet Metab. 2004 Jan;81(1):1–2. [PMID: 14728984]

Hanley WB. Adult phenylketonuria. Am J Med. 2004 Oct 15;117(8):590–5. [PMID: 15465508]

Santos LL et al. The time has come: A new scene for PKU treatment. Genet Mol Res. 2006 Mar 31;5(1):33–44. [PMID: 16755495]

Fragile X-Associated Mental Retardation

Debacker K et al. Fragile sites and human disease. Hum Mol Genet. 2007 Oct 15;16 Spec No. 2:R150–8. [PMID: 17567780]

Garber KB et al. Fragile X syndrome. Eur J Hum Genet. 2008 Jun;16(6):666–72. [PMID: 18398441]

Penagarikano O et al. The pathophysiology of fragile X syndrome. Annu Rev Genomics Hum Genet. 2007;8:109–29. [PMID: 17477822]

Reiss AL et al. Fragile X syndrome: Assessment and treatment implications. Child Adolesc Psychiatr Clin N Am. 2007 Jul;16(3):663–75. [PMID: 17562585]

LHON, MERFF, & Mitochondrial Diseases

Haas RH et al. Mitochondrial disease: A practical approach for primary care physicians. Pediatrics. 2007 Dec;120(6):1326–33. [PMID: 18055683]

McFarland R et al. Mitochondrial disease—Its impact, etiology, and pathology. Curr Top Dev Biol. 2007;77:113–55. [PMID: 17222702]

Pieczenik SR et al. Mitochondrial dysfunction and molecular pathways of disease. Exp Mol Pathol. 2007 Aug;83(1):84–92. [PMID: 17239370]

Down Syndrome

Antonarakis SE et al. Chromosome 21 and Down syndrome: From genomics to pathophysiology. Nat Rev Genet. 2004 Oct;5(10):725–38. [PMID: 15510164]

Irving C et al. Twenty-year trends in prevalence and survival of Down syndrome. Eur J Hum Genet. 2008 Nov;16(11):1336–40. [PMID: 18596694]

Rachidi M et al. Mental retardation in Down syndrome: From gene dosage imbalance to molecular and cellular mechanisms. Neurosci Res. 2007 Dec;59(4):349–69. [PMID: 17897742]

The Human Genome Project and Human Genetic Variation

Guttmacher AE et al. Genomic medicine—A primer. N Engl J Med. 2002 Nov 7;347(19):1512–20. [PMID: 12421895]

Scheuner MT et al. Delivery of genomic medicine for common chronic adult diseases: A systematic review. JAMA. 2008 Mar 19;299(11):1320–34. [PMID: 18349093]

Zondervan KT et al. The complex interplay among factors that influence allelic association. Nat Rev Genet. 2004 Feb;5(2):89–100. [PMID: 14735120]

Disorders of the Immune System

Jeffrey L. Kishiyama, MD

The function of the immune system is to protect the host from invasion of foreign organisms by distinguishing "self" from "nonself." Such a system is necessary for survival. A well-functioning immune system not only protects the host from external factors such as microorganisms or toxins but also prevents and repels attacks by endogenous factors such as tumors or autoimmune phenomena. Dysfunction or deficiency of components of the immune system leads to a variety of clinical diseases of varying expression and severity, ranging from atopic disease to rheumatoid arthritis, severe combined immunodeficiency, and cancer. This chapter introduces the intricate physiology of the immune system and abnormalities that lead to diseases of hypersensitivity and immunodeficiency.

NORMAL STRUCTURE & FUNCTION OF THE IMMUNE SYSTEM

ANATOMY

Cells of the Immune System

The immune system consists of both antigen-specific and nonspecific components that have distinct yet overlapping functions. The antibody-mediated and cell-mediated immune systems provide specificity and memory of previously encountered antigens. The nonspecific natural defenses include epithelial barriers, mucociliary clearance, phagocytic cells, and complement proteins. Despite their lack of specificity, these components are essential because they are largely responsible for natural immunity to a vast array of environmental threats and microorganisms. Knowledge of the components and physiology of normal immunity is essential for understanding the pathophysiology of diseases of the immune system.

The major cellular components of the immune system consist of monocytes and macrophages, lymphocytes, and the family of granulocytic cells, including neutrophils, eosinophils, and basophils.

Mononuclear phagocytes play a central role in the immune response. Tissue macrophages are derived from blood monocytes and play a central role in antigen processing, tissue repair, and secretion of mediators vital to initiation of specific immune responses. In response to antigenic stimulation, macrophages engulf the antigen (phagocytosis) and then process and present that antigen in a form recognizable to T lymphocytes. Activated macrophages secrete proteolytic enzymes, active metabolites of oxygen (including superoxide anion and other oxygen radicals), arachidonic acid metabolites, cyclic adenosine monophosphate (cAMP), and cytokines such as interleukin (IL)-1, IL-6, IL-8, and tumor necrosis factor (TNF), among others. Many epithelial **dendritic cells** (eg, Langerhans' cells, oligodendrocytes, Kupffer cells) may share a common hematopoietic precursor and function to process and transport antigen from skin, respiratory, and GI surfaces to regional lymphoid tissues.

Lymphocytes are responsible for the specific recognition of antigen and for immunologic memory, features of the adaptive immunity. They are functionally and phenotypically divided into bursa-derived B lymphocytes and thymus-derived T lymphocytes. Morphologically, B and T lymphocytes cannot be distinguished visually from each other under the microscope, but flow cytometry and immunophenotyping through recognition of cell surface markers and clusters of differentiation (CD markers) can distinguish between the two. Approximately 75% of circulating blood lymphocytes are T lymphocytes and 10–15% B lymphocytes; the remainder are neither B nor T lymphocytes and are often referred to as "null cells."

Null cells probably include a number of different cell types, including a group called **natural killer (NK) cells**. These cells appear distinct from other lymphocytes in that they are slightly larger, with a kidney-shaped nucleolus, and have a granular appearance (large granular lymphocytes), express

ADA	Adenosine deaminase	**JC**	Jakob–Creutzfeldt
ADCC	Antibody-dependent cell-mediated cytotoxicity	**LAK cell**	Lymphokine-activated killer cell
AIDS	Acquired immunodeficiency syndrome	**LPS**	Lipopolysaccharide
APC	Antigen-presenting cell	**MAC**	*Mycobacterium avium* complex
BCR	B-cell receptor	**MHC**	Major histocompatibility complex
BTK	Bruton's tyrosine kinase	**NADPH**	Nicotinamide adenine dinucleotide phosphate
C1, C2, etc	Complement factor 1, complement factor 2, etc	**NK**	Natural killer cells
cAMP	Cyclic adenosine monophosphate	**PAF**	Platelet-activating factor
CCR5	CC-subfamily chemokine receptor 5	**PGD**	Prostaglandin D
CD	Clusters of differentiation	**PNP**	Purine nucleoside phosphorylase
CD4	Helper T-cell subset	**PTK**	Protein tyrosine kinase
CD8	Cytotoxic T-cell subset	**RAG**	Recombination-activating gene
CTL	Cytotoxic lymphocyte	**RANTES**	Chemokine regulated on activation normal T expressed and secreted
CXCR5	CXC-subfamily chemoreceptor 5		
F(ab)	Antigen-binding fragment	**RAST**	Radioallergosorbent test
Fc	Crystallizable fragment	**SCID**	Severe combined immunodeficiency disease
FcɛRI	High-affinity IgE receptor	**TAME**	*N*-α-*p*-tosyl-L-arginine methylester-esterase
FcγR	Fc gamma receptor	**TCR**	T-cell receptor
GM-CSF	Granulocyte-macrophage colony-stimulating factor	T_H1	Helper T 1 subset
HBV	Hepatitis B virus	T_H2	Helper T 2 subset
HCV	Hepatitis C virus	T_H17	Helper T subset secreting IL-17
HIV	Human immunodeficiency virus	T_{REG}	Helper T subset with regulatory function
HPV	Human papillomavirus	**Tr1**	Regulatory T-cell subset
HSV	Herpes simplex virus	**TLR**	Toll-like receptor
HZV	Herpes zoster virus	**TNF**	Tumor necrosis factor
ICAM-1	Intercellular adhesion molecule-1	**TSH**	Thyroid-stimulating hormone
IFN-γ	Interferon-γ	**V-CAM-1**	Vascular cell adhesion molecule-1
Ig	Immunoglobulin	**VIP**	Vasoactive intestinal peptide
IVIG	Intravenous immunoglobulin	**XLA**	X-linked agammaglobulinemia
IL-1, IL-2, etc	Interleukin-1, interleukin-2, etc.	**XSCID**	X-linked severe combined immunodeficiency disease
JAK	Janus kinase	**ZAP-70**	Protein tyrosine kinase ZAP-70

distinct cell surface markers (CD56, CD161), but lack antigen-specific T-cell receptors (CD3 or TCRs). Recruited to sites of inflammation, NK cells possess membrane receptors for the immunoglobulin G (IgG) molecules (FcγR), facilitating antibody-dependent cell-mediated cytotoxicity (ADCC). Binding of an antibody-coated cell or foreign substance triggers release of perforin, a pore-forming protein that causes cytolysis. Other NK cell functions include antibody-independent cellular killing, induction of apoptosis in Fas-expressing cells, and immunomodulation of responses to viruses, malignancy, and transplanted tissue through a potent release of interferon-γ (IFN-γ), TNF, and other key cytokines.

Polymorphonuclear leukocytes (neutrophils) are granulocytic cells that originate in the bone marrow and circulate in blood and tissue. Their primary function is antigen-nonspecific phagocytosis and destruction of foreign particles and organisms. They contain cytoplasmic granules filled with degradative enzymes and can also produce oxidative metabolites with potent antimicrobial properties like hydrogen peroxide, superoxide, and hypohalous acid. The presence of complement and Fcγ receptors on the surface of neutrophils also facilitates the clearance of opsonized microbes through the reticuloendothelial system.

Eosinophils are often found in inflammatory sites or at sites of immune reactivity and play a crucial role in the host's defense against parasites. Despite many shared functional similarities to neutrophils, eosinophils are considerably less efficient than neutrophils at phagocytosis. However, in the airway inflammatory response in asthma, eosinophil-derived cytotoxic proteins, including major basic protein, lipid mediators (eg, leukotriene C4), oxygen radicals, and cytokines (eg, IL-3) can induce damage to airway epithelium and potentiate the allergic response.

Basophils play an important role in both immediate- and late-phase allergic responses. These cells release many of the potent mediators of allergic inflammatory diseases, including histamine, leukotrienes, prostaglandins, and platelet-activating factor (PAF), all of which have significant effects on the vasculature and on the inflammatory response. Basophils are present in the circulation, possess high-affinity receptors for IgE (FcεRI), and mediate immediate hypersensitivity (allergic) responses.

Organs of the Immune System

Several tissues and organs play roles in host defenses and are functionally classified as the immune system. In mammals, the primary lymphoid organs are the thymus and the bone marrow.

All cells of the immune system are originally derived from **bone marrow**. Pluripotent stem cells differentiate into lymphocyte, granulocyte, monocyte, erythrocyte, and megakaryocyte populations. In humans, B lymphocytes, which are the antibody-producing cells, undergo early antigen-independent maturation into immunocompetent cells in the bone marrow. Deficiency or dysfunction of the pluripotent stem cell or the various cell lines developing from it can result in immune deficiency disorders of varying expression and severity.

The **thymus,** derived from the third and fourth embryonic pharyngeal pouches, functions to produce T lymphocytes and is the site of initial T-lymphocyte differentiation. Its reticular structure allows a significant number of lymphocytes to migrate through it to become fully immunocompetent thymus-derived cells. Developing T cells in the thymic cortex are first positively selected for their ability to recognize self-peptides (ie, major histocompatibility complex [MHC]). In subsequent negative selection, T cells that avidly recognize self-peptides are destroyed, thus removing deleterious self-reactive clones. In some murine models, autoimmune diseases such as systemic lupus erythematosus may develop in mice with defective apoptotic (programmed cell death) pathways in T cells recognizing self-antigen. The thymus also regulates immune function by secretion of multiple hormones that promote T-lymphocyte differentiation and are essential for T-lymphocyte-mediated immunity.

In mammals, the **lymph nodes, spleen,** and **gut-associated lymphoid tissue** are secondary lymphoid organs connected by blood and lymphatic vessels. Lymph nodes are strategically dispersed throughout the vasculature and are the principal organs of the immune system that localize antigen, promote cell-cell interaction and lymphocyte activation, and prevent the spread of infection. Lymph nodes have a framework of reticular cells and fibers that are arranged into a **cortex** and **medulla**. B lymphocytes, the precursors of antibody-producing cells, or **plasma cells**, are found in the cortex (the follicles and germinal centers) as well as in the medulla. T lympho-

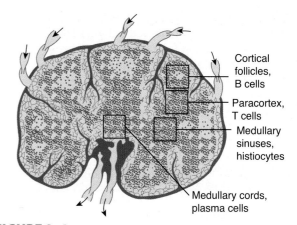

FIGURE 3–1 Anatomy of a normal lymph node. (Redrawn, with permission, from Chandrasoma P, Taylor CR: *Concise Pathology*, 3rd ed. Originally published by Appleton & Lange. Copyright © 1998 by the McGraw-Hill Companies, Inc.)

cytes are found chiefly in the medullary and paracortical areas of the lymph node (Figure 3–1).

The spleen is functionally and structurally divided into B-lymphocyte and T-lymphocyte areas similar to those of the lymph nodes. The spleen filters and processes antigens from the blood.

Gut-associated lymphoid tissue includes the tonsils, Peyer's patches of the small intestine, and the appendix. Like the lymph nodes and spleen, these tissues exhibit separation into B-lymphocyte–dependent and T-lymphocyte–dependent areas. Mucosal immune responses tend to generate antigen-specific IgA, and with some orally administered antigens, T-cell anergy or tolerance may occur rather than immune stimulation.

Inflammatory Mediators

Mediators are released or generated during immune responses to coordinate and regulate immune cell activities to generate physiological or cytotoxic responses. The **complement cascade** consists of plasma proteins that are activated by immune complex (antigen-antibody) formation or triggered by certain microbial surface proteins. By proteolytic activation, the complement cascade generates proteins that enhance opsonization, phagocytosis, and cytolysis of microbes. Interestingly, inherited deficiencies of the early components of the classic complement cascade (C1, C4, C2) are associated with immune-complex–mediated autoimmune disease. Deficiencies of C3 in particular are associated with increased risk of infection, and deficiencies of the late classic components (C5–C9) are associated with recurrent *Neisseria* sp. infections. Hereditary angioedema (HAE) occurs when an inherited deficiency of C1 esterase inhibitor leads to recurrent episodes of subcutaneous or submucosal swelling. HAE highlights the interplay between and overlap of immunomodulatory factors, which regulate the complement, kinin, and fibrinolytic pathways. **Cytokines** are soluble polypeptide signaling mediators, produced after immune stimulation, that direct and regulate immune and inflammatory reactions. They target many diverse cell types, can have antiviral, proinflammatory, or anti-inflammatory activities, act locally or systemically, and can be redundant in their actions (Table 3–1). A group of chemotactic factors (**chemokines**) regulate homing and migration of immune cells to sites of inflammation. HIV may exploit certain chemokine receptors to infect host cells and natural mutations in these same chemokine coreceptors may confer a susceptibility or resistance to infection.

CHECKPOINT

1. What are the specific and nonspecific components of the cellular and noncellular limbs of the immune system?

2. What is the role of macrophages in the immune system, and what are some of the products they secrete?

3. What are the categories of lymphocytes, and how are they distinguished?

4. What is the role of lymphocytes in the immune system, and what are some of the products they secrete?

5. What is the role of eosinophils in the immune system, and what are some of the products they secrete?

6. What is the role of basophils in the immune system, and what are some of the products they secrete?

7. What is the role of epithelial cells in the immune system, and what are some of the products they secrete?

8. What are the primary and secondary lymphoid organs, and what roles do they play in the proper functioning of the immune system?

PHYSIOLOGY

1. Innate & Adaptive Immunity

Living organisms exhibit two levels of response against external invasion: an **innate system** of natural immunity and an **adaptive system** that is acquired. Innate immunity is present from birth, is rapidly mobilized, and is nonspecific in its activity. The skin and epithelial surfaces serve as the first line of defense of the innate immune system, whereas enzymes, the alternative complement system pathway, acute-phase proteins, phagocytic, NK cells, and cytokines provide additional layers of protection. Microbial cell walls or nucleic acids contain nonmammalian patterns or motifs that can bind to **toll-like receptors** (**TLRs**) on innate immune cells including macrophages and dendritic cells. Their structure is highly conserved and each TLR binds to specific microbial products, such as lipopolysaccharide (LPS or bacterial endotoxin), viral RNA, microbial DNA and yeast wall mannon proteins. Binding of TLR and ligand triggers transcription of proinflammatory factors and cytokine synthesis. Higher organisms have evolved an adaptive immune system, which is triggered by encounters with foreign agents that have evaded or penetrated the innate immune defenses. The adaptive immune system is characterized both by **specificity** for individual foreign

TABLE 3–1 **Cytokines and their functions.**

Cytokine	Major Cellular Source	Principal Effect
IFN-α	Macrophages, dendritic cells	Inhibit viral replication
IFN-β	Virally infected cells	
IFN-γ	T cells, NK cells	Upregulation of adhesion and MHC molecules, increased macrophage and antigen-presenting cell (APC) activity
IL-1	Macrophage	Endogenous pyrogen, endothelial cell activation, induces acute-phase reactants
IL-2	T cells	T-cell growth factor and regulatory factor, B-cell and NK cell activation
IL-3	T cells	Hematopoietic growth factor
IL-4	T cells, mast cells	Induces IgE synthesis, T_H2 responses
IL-5	T cells	Eosinophil activation and growth factor, B-cell activation factor
IL-6	Macrophages, T cells, endothelial cells	Induces Ig synthesis and acute-phase reactants
IL-7	Bone marrow	B-cell and T-cell growth and differentiation factor
IL-8	Macrophage, neutrophils, endothelial, and epithelial cells	Leukocyte chemotactic factor
IL-10	T cells, macrophages	Inhibits antigen presentation, cytokine responses
IL-12	Macrophage	Induces T_H1 responses
IL-13	T cells, mast cells	Induces IgE responses
GM-CSF	Macrophages, T cells	Hematopoietic growth factor for neutrophils, eosinophils, and macrophages
TGF-β	Platelets	Immune modulator for leukocytes, tissue growth factor for wound healing
TNF	Macrophage, T cell	Endogenous pyrogen; activates neutrophils, endothelial cells, and acute-phase reactants; promotes angiogenesis and coagulation

agents and by **immunologic memory,** which makes possible an intensified response to subsequent encounters with the same or closely related agents. The presentation of antigen by **antigen-presenting cells** (**APCs**) to T lymphocytes triggers the adaptive immune response with production of antibodies and effector T cells, and ultimately elimination of the inciting agent.

2. Antigens (Immunogens)

Foreign substances that can induce an immune response are called **antigens,** or **immunogens.** Antigenicity (immunogenicity) implies that the substance has the ability to react with products of the adaptive immune system (ie, antibodies or TCRs). Complex foreign agents possess distinct and multiple immunogenic components. It is estimated that the human immune system can respond to 10^7–10^9 different antigens, an amazingly diverse repertoire. Most antigens are proteins, although pure carbohydrates may be antigenic as well.

3. Immune Response

The primary role of the immune system is to discriminate self from nonself and to eliminate the foreign substance. The physiology of the normal immune response to antigen is summa-

rized in Figure 3–2. A complex network of specialized cells, organs, and biologic factors is necessary for the recognition and subsequent elimination of foreign antigens. These complex cellular interactions require specialized microenvironments in which cells can collaborate efficiently. Both T and B cells need to migrate throughout the body to increase the likelihood that they will encounter an antigen to which they have specificity. Soluble antigens are transported to regional lymph tissues through afferent lymphatic vessels, while other antigens are carried by phagocytic dendritic cells. Regional, peripheral lymphoid organs and the spleen are sites for concentrated immune responses to antigen by recirculating lymphocytes and APCs. Antigens encountered via inhaled or ingested routes activate cells in the mucosa-associated lymphoid tissues. The major pathways of antigen elimination include the direct killing of target cells by a subset of T lymphocytes called **cytotoxic T**

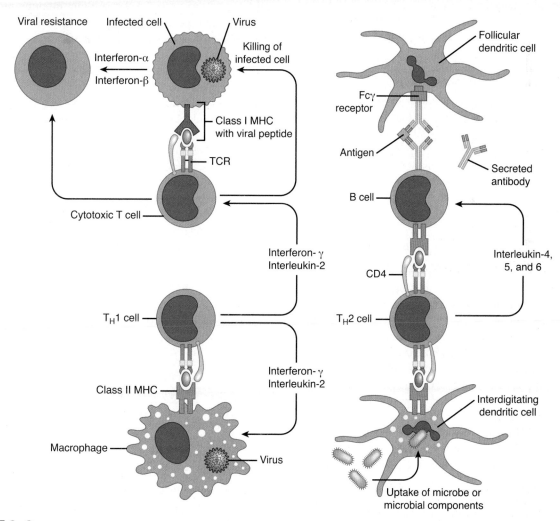

FIGURE 3–2   The normal immune response. Cytotoxic T-cell response is shown on the left side of the figure and the helper T-cell response on the right side. As depicted on the left, most CD8 T cells recognize processed antigen presented by MHC class I molecules and destroy infected cells, thereby preventing viral replication. Activated T cells secrete interferon-γ that, along with interferon-α and interferon-β secreted by infected cells, produces cellular resistance to viral infection. On the right and at the bottom, CD4 helper cells (T$_H$1 and T$_H$2 cells) recognize processed antigen presented by MHC class II molecules. T$_H$1 cells secrete interferon-γ and interleukin-2, which activate macrophages and cytotoxic T cells to kill intracellular organisms; T$_H$2 cells secrete interleukin-4, -5, and -6, which help B cells secrete protective antibodies. B cells recognize antigen directly or in the form of immune complexes on follicular dendritic cells in germinal centers. (Redrawn, with permission, from Delves PJ, Roitt IM: The immune system: Second of two parts. N Engl J Med. 2000;343:113.)

lymphocytes (**cellular response**) and the elimination of antigen through antibody-mediated events arising from T- and B-lymphocyte interactions (**humoral response**). The series of events that initiate the immune response includes antigen processing and presentation, lymphocyte recognition and activation, cellular or humoral immune responses, and antigenic destruction or elimination.

Antigen Processing & Presentation

Most foreign immunogens are not recognized by the immune system in their native form and require capture and processing by professional **APCs,** which constitutively express class II MHC molecules and accessory costimulatory molecules on their surfaces. Such specialized cells include macrophages, dendritic cells in lymphoid tissue, Langerhans' cells in the skin, Kupffer cells in the liver, microglial cells in the nervous system, and B lymphocytes. Dendritic cells in the spleen and lymph nodes may be the primary APCs during a primary immune response. Following an encounter with immunogens, the APCs internalize the foreign substance by phagocytosis or pinocytosis, modify the parent structure, and display antigenic fragments of the native protein on its surfaces in association with MHC class II molecules (see later discussion). T-cell–independent antigens such as polysaccharides can activate B cells without assistance from T cells by binding to B-cell receptors (BCRs, or surface-bound antibody), leading to rapid IgM responses, without generation of memory cells or long-lived plasma cells. Most antigens, however, require internalization and processing by B cells or other APCs with subsequent recognition by CD4 T cells.

T-Lymphocyte Recognition & Activation

The recognition of processed antigen by specialized T lymphocytes known as **helper T (CD4) lymphocytes** and the subsequent activation of these cells constitute the critical events in the immune response. The helper T lymphocytes orchestrate the many cells and biologic signals (cytokines) that are necessary to carry out the immune response. Activated CD4 T lymphocytes are mainly cytokine-secreting helper cells, whereas CD8 T lymphocytes are mainly cytotoxic killer cells. A number of subsets of CD4 helper T lymphocytes have been identified, differing in their phenotypic patterns of cytokine synthesis and release. T_H1 cells develop in the presence of IL-12, secreted from activated macrophages, especially in the presence of infection with intracellular microbes. T_H1 cells elaborate IFN-γ and TNF-β but not IL-4 and IL-5 and have been found to participate in cell-mediated immunity and type IV delayed hypersensitivity reactions. T_H2 cells develop in the presence of IL-4, secrete IL-4, IL-5, and IL-13, but not IFN-γ and TNF-β, which facilitates humoral responses but has also been implicated in response to allergens and helminths. A number of additional T helper subsets have been discovered that contribute to immune regulation. T_H17 cell subsets appear to boost early phagocytic cell responses through their elaboration of IL-17 and may play a role in autoimmune diseases. T_{reg} CD4+ cells express high-affinity receptors for IL-2 (CD25) and FOXP3, a transcription factor that may suppress autoimmune disease. Mutations of FOXP3 have been associated with inflammatory autoimmune disease, immune dysregulation, polyendocrinopathy, X-linked syndrome (IPEX). Other T-regulatory cells (**Tr1, T_H3**) appear to secrete inhibitory cytokines IL-10 and TGF-1, respectively.

Helper T lymphocytes recognize processed antigen displayed by APCs only in association with polymorphic cell surface proteins called the **major histocompatibility complex (MHC)**. During cell-cell contact between T helper cells and APCs, the process of dual recognition is referred to as **MHC restriction.** Exogenous foreign antigens that require an antibody-mediated response are expressed in association with **MHC class II** structures. Only the specialized APCs can express MHC class II. The genes encoding MHC distinguish self from nonself, thereby determining immune responsiveness to foreign agents, enabling graft rejection, and conferring susceptibility to certain autoimmune disorders.

The antigen-MHC class II complex forms the epitope that is recognized by antigen-specific **TCRs** on the surface of the CD4 molecules. The TCR is composed of six gene products, TCR α- and β-subunits, CD3 (γ-, δ-, and two ε-subunits), and ζ_2 chains. Besides binding to modified antigen, activation of T cells depends on the costimulation of **accessory molecules.** Accessory molecules on T cells bind to ligands found on APCs, epithelial cells, vascular endothelium, and extracellular matrix, controlling the subsequent T-cell function or homing (Table 3–2). In the absence of such signals, the T cell may be "tolerized" or may undergo apoptosis instead of being activated. (*Tolerization* refers to induction of tolerance by low-avidity engagement of the TCR in which, eg, oral administration of small quantities of agonist peptides induces immunologic tol-

TABLE 3–2 T-cell and APC surface molecules and their interactions.

T-Cell Surface Receptor	APC Counter-Receptor	Function and Effect
T-cell receptor (CD3)	Processed antigen + MHC complex	Antigen presentation
CD4	MHC class II	Presentation of antigen to helper T cell by APC
CD8	MHC class I	Presentation of antigen to cytotoxic T cell
CD40 ligand (CD154)	CD40	T-cell–induced B-cell activation
CD28	B7	T-cell proliferation and differentiation
CTLA-4	B7	T-cell anergy
LFA-1	ICAM-1	Adhesion

erance.) Biologic products that block some of these costimulatory pathways are currently being investigated as potential therapeutic agents to prevent organ rejection in transplantation and in the management of some autoimmune diseases.

Before an activated T cell can differentiate, proliferate, produce cytokines, or participate in cell killing, the activation signal must be transduced into the cytoplasm or nucleus of the cell. The principal signaling molecules in the TCR complex appear to be the CD3 and the ζ homodimer or heterodimer. The presence of immunoreceptor tyrosine activation motifs associated with each TCR complex facilitates amplification of signaling. The binding of ZAP-70, a Syk-family protein tyrosine kinase (PTK), to CD3ε and ζ subunits after they are phosphorylated is critical for downstream signaling. Another important enzyme in the activation of T cells is CD45, a protein tyrosine phosphatase. The critical nature of these enzymes in lymphocyte development is underscored by the discovery of ZAP-70 and CD45 deficiency syndromes, disorders that result in various forms of severe combined immunodeficiency disease (**SCID**, see Primary Immunodeficiency Diseases).

Activation of T cells does not occur in isolation but is also dependent on the cytokine milieu. In true autocrine fashion, the APCs involved in antigen presentation release **IL-1,** which induces the release of both **IL-2** and **IFN**-γ from CD4 cells. IL-2 feeds back to stimulate the expression of additional **IL-2 receptors** on the surface of the CD4 cells and stimulates the production of various cell growth and differentiation factors (**cytokines**) by the activated CD4 cells. Induction of IL-2 expression is particularly critical for T cells. Cyclosporine and tacrolimus (FK506), two immunosuppressive agents used for prevention of organ transplant rejection, function by downregulating IL-2 production by T cells.

CD8 Effector Cells (Cellular Immune Response)

Cytotoxic T lymphocytes (**CTLs**) eliminate target cells (virally infected cells, tumor, or foreign tissues), thus constituting the cellular immune response. CTLs differ from helper T lymphocytes in their expression of the surface antigen CD8 and by the recognition of antigen complexed to cell surface proteins of **MHC class I.** Pathogenic microorganisms whose proteins gain access to the cell cytoplasm (eg, malarial parasites) or by de novo gene expression in the infected cell cytoplasm (eg, viruses) stimulate CD8 class I MHC-restricted T-cell responses. All somatic cells can express MHC class I molecules. Two major mechanisms for killing target cells have been described. One mechanism involves the secretion of perforin, a molecule related to C9 that inserts in the plasma membrane of target cells along with serine proteases called granzymes, which lead to osmotic lysis. A second mechanism involves the expression of the Fas ligand on the surface of CTLs that bind to Fas on the target cell membrane to induce apoptosis. In addition to killing infected cells directly, CD8 T cells can elaborate a number of cytokines, including TNF and lymphotoxin. Memory CTLs may be long-lived to provide "recall" responses and immunity against latent or persistent viral infections. A subset of CD8+ T-regulatory cells may suppress potentially self-reactive T cells in the periphery.

Activation of B Lymphocytes (Humoral Immune Response)

Like T-cell activation, B-lymphocyte activation is triggered after antigen binds to B-cell receptors (BCRs; ie, surface-bound immunoglobulin) and is regulated through concomitant coreceptor binding. In secondary lymphoid tissues, release of cytokines IL-2, IL-4, IL-5, and IL-6 by activated helper T lymphocytes promotes the proliferation and terminal differentiation of B cells into high-rate antibody-producing cells called plasma cells, which secrete antigen-specific **immunoglobulin.** If complement fragments bind B-cell surface complement receptors at the same time antigen engages BCRs, cellular responses are heightened. T cells also modulate humoral immunity through their activation-dependent membrane expression of **CD40 ligand** protein. Through direct T- and B-cell contact, CD40 ligand binds to the **CD40 receptor** on the surface of B cells, inducing apoptosis (programmed cell death) or activation of immunoglobulin synthesis, depending on the situation. The importance of CD40 ligand-CD40 binding in normal humoral immunity is highlighted by the congenital immunodeficiency, X-linked hyper-IgM syndrome. A defect in the synthesis of CD40 ligand on activated T cells results in impaired "isotype switching" and hyper-IgM, with subsequent deficient production of IgG, IgA, and impaired humoral immunity.

Although their primary function is synthesis of immunoglobulin, B lymphocytes may also bind and internalize foreign antigen directly, process that antigen, and present it to CD4 T lymphocytes. A pool of activated B lymphocytes may differentiate into **memory cells,** which respond more rapidly and efficiently to subsequent encounters with identical or closely related antigenic structures.

Antibody Structure & Function

Antibodies (immunoglobulins) are proteins that possess "specificity," enabling them to combine with one particular antigenic structure. Antigen-binding sites for immunoglobulin will recognize three-dimensional structures, whereas TCR will bind short peptide segments without tertiary structure. Humoral (antibody-mediated) immune responses result in the production of a diverse repertoire (estimated 10^9–10^{11}) of antibody specificities, providing the ability to recognize and bind with a broad range of antigens. This diversity is a function of somatic recombination of gene segments within B lymphocytes early in ontogenetic development. Somatic mutations occurring after antigenic stimulation lead to affinity maturation, ie, average affinity of antibody binding increases throughout the immune response. Somatic recombination in both T and B cells is dependent on recombination-activating genes (RAG1 and RAG2), the deficiency of which leads to a lack of T and B lymphocytes, an autosomal recessive form of SCID.

All immunoglobulin molecules share a four-chain polypeptide structure consisting of two heavy and two light chains (Figure 3–3). Each chain includes an amino terminal portion, containing the **variable (V) region,** and a carboxyl terminal portion, containing four or five **constant (C) regions.** V regions are highly variable structures that form the antigen-binding site, whereas the C domains support effector functions of the molecules. The five classes (**isotypes**) of immunoglobulins are **IgG, IgA, IgM, IgD,** and **IgE** and are defined on the basis of differences in the C region of the heavy chains. The isotype expressed by a particular B lymphocyte is dependent on the state of cellular differentiation and "isotype switching," a process characterized by splicing of heavy chain mRNA prior to translation. Different isotypes contribute to different effector functions on the basis of the ability of the molecule to bind to specific receptors and their efficiency in fixing serum complement.

Humoral Mechanisms of Antigen Elimination

Antibodies may induce the elimination of foreign antigen through a number of different mechanisms. Binding of antibody to bacterial toxins or foreign venoms may cause neutralization or promote elimination of these antigen-antibody immune complexes through the reticuloendothelial system.

Antibodies may coat bacterial surfaces, enhancing phagocytosis by macrophages in a process known as opsonization. Some classes of antibodies may complex with antigen and activate the complement cascade ("complement fixation"), culminating in lysis of the target cell. Finally, the major class of antibody, IgG, can bind to NK cells that subsequently complex with target cells and release cytotoxins (see prior discussion of antibody-dependent cellular cytotoxicity). IgG passes transplacentally, providing passive immunization of neonates.

After the successful elimination of antigen, the immune system uses several mechanisms to return to basal homeostasis. IgG can switch off its own response to antigen through the binding of immune complexes that transmit inhibitory signals into the nuclei of B cells.

Mechanisms of Inflammation

Elimination of foreign antigen by cellular or humoral processes is integrally linked to the inflammatory response, in which cytokines and antibodies trigger the recruitment of additional cells and the release of endogenous vasoactive and proinflammatory enzymatic substances (**inflammatory mediators**).

Inflammation may have both positive and deleterious effects. Tight control of inflammatory mechanisms promotes efficient elimination of foreign substances, killing of microbes, infected cells, and tumors, as well as prevention of

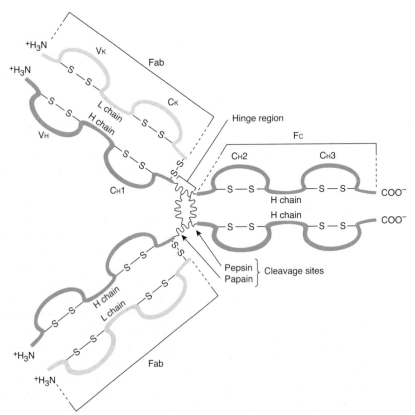

FIGURE 3–3 Structure of a human IgG antibody molecule. Depicted are the four-chain structure and the variable and constant domains. (V, variable region; C, constant region. The sites of pepsin and papain cleavage are shown.) (Redrawn, with permission, from Stites DP, Terr AL, Parslow TG: *Basic & Clinical Immunology,* 9th ed. Originally published by Appleton & Lange. Copyright © 1997 by the McGraw-Hill Companies, Inc.)

autoimmune disease or hypersensitivity reactions. However, uncontrolled lymphocyte activation and unregulated antibody production can lead to tissue damage and organ dysfunction. Pathogenic immune dysfunction is responsible for hypersensitivity reactions, immunodeficiency, and many of the clinical effects of autoimmunity. Imbalances in the inflammatory system may result from genetic defects, infection, neoplasms, and exposure to environmental triggers, although precise mechanisms that promote abnormal regulation and persistence of inflammatory processes are complex and poorly understood.

Hypersensitivity Immune Responses

Gell and Coombs classified the mechanisms of immune responses to antigen into four distinct types of reactions to allow for clearer understanding of the immunopathogenesis of disease.

A. Type I

Clinical allergy represents IgE-mediated hypersensitivity response arising from deleterious inflammation in response to the presence of normally harmless environmental antigens. Anaphylactic or immediate hypersensitivity reactions occur after binding of antigen to IgE antibodies attached to the surface of the mast cell or basophil and result in the release of preformed and newly generated inflammatory mediators that produce the clinical manifestations. Examples of type I–mediated reactions include anaphylactic shock, allergic rhinitis, allergic asthma, and allergic drug reactions.

B. Type II

Cytotoxic reactions involve the binding of either IgG or IgM antibody to antigens covalently bound to cell membrane structures. Antigen-antibody binding activates the complement cascade and results in destruction of the cell to which the antigen is bound. Examples of tissue injury by this mechanism include immune hemolytic anemia and Rh hemolytic disease in the newborn. Another example of the type II–mediated disease process without cell death is autoimmune hyperthyroidism, a disorder in which thyroid-stimulating antibodies stimulate thyroid tissue.

C. Type III

Immune complex–mediated reactions occur when immune complexes are formed by the binding of antigens to antibodies with fixation of complement. Complement-bound immune complexes facilitate opsonization by phagocytes and ADCC. Complexes are usually cleared from the circulation in the reticuloendothelial system. However, deposition of these complexes in tissues or in vascular endothelium can produce immune complex–mediated tissue injury by leading to complement activation, anaphylatoxin generation, chemotaxis of polymorphonuclear leukocytes, mediator release and tissue injury. Cutaneous Arthus reaction, systemic serum sickness,

some aspects of clinical autoimmunity, and certain features of infective endocarditis are clinical examples of type III–mediated diseases.

D. Type IV

Cell-mediated immunity is responsible for host defenses against intracellular pathogenic organisms, although abnormal regulation of this system may result in delayed-type hypersensitivity. Type IV hypersensitivity reactions are mediated not by antibody but by antigen-specific T lymphocytes. Classic examples are tuberculin skin test reactions and contact dermatitis.

Synthesis of IgE in Allergic Reactivity

Allergic hypersensitivity results from the inappropriate and sustained production of IgE in response to allergen. T_H2 cytokines IL-4 and IL-13 are critical to isotype switching through induction of germline transcription of IgE heavy chain genes. IL-13 has about 30% structural homology with IL-4 and shares much of the activities of IL-4 on mononuclear cells and B lymphocytes. There is a strong genetic predisposition toward the development of atopic disease. Evidence has been found for the linkage of 5q31.1 and the IL-4 gene, suggesting that IL-4 or a nearby gene in this chromosome locale regulates overall IgE production.

In contrast, T_H1-generated IFN-γ inhibits IL-4–dependent IgE synthesis in humans. Thus, an imbalance favoring IL-4 over IFN-γ may induce IgE formation. In one study, reduced cord blood IFN-γ at birth was associated with clinical atopy at age 12 months.

In allergic inflammatory processes, T_H2 lymphocytes represent a source of IL-4 as well as secondary signals necessary to drive the production of IgE by B lymphocytes. Another T_H2 cytokine, IL-5, promotes maturation, activation, chemotaxis, and prolongation of survival in eosinophils. In situ hybridization analysis of T-cell mRNA in airway mucosal biopsies from allergic rhinitis and asthma patients show a distinct T_H2 pattern. The demonstration of allergen-specific T-cell lines that proliferate and secrete large amounts of IL-4 on exposure to relevant antigen in vitro further supports the existence of specific T_H2-like clones. The original source of the IL-4 responsible for T_H2 differentiation is unclear, although some observations suggest that there exists a T_H2 bias during fetal development in both atopic and nonatopic individuals. The "hygiene hypothesis" posits that environmental exposures, possibly to bacterial products such as endotoxin or bacterial DNA, encourage a shift toward T_H1 and subsequent reduced risk of clinical atopic disease. Mononuclear phagocytes are the major source of IL-12, suggesting a mechanism whereby antigens more likely to be processed by macrophages, including bacterial antigens and intracellular pathogens, produce T_H1 responses. Epidemiologic studies of children suggest those exposed to daycare at early ages and those with numerous siblings are at reduced risk for atopy and asthma.

Since the discovery of IgE more than 3 decades ago, scientists have considered various therapeutic strategies to selectively inhibit IgE antibody production and action. Research has focused on understanding the mechanisms controlling IgE production, including the molecular events of B-cell switching to IgE synthesis, IL-4 and IL-13 signaling, T- and B-cell surface receptor interactions, and the mechanisms driving T_H2 differentiation. Soluble cytokine receptors and genetically engineered monoclonal antibodies are currently under development for the purpose of cytokine neutralization in allergic diseases. Many of these specifically target IL-4, IL-5, IL-13, or CD23 (a low-affinity IgE receptor). Other experimental strategies include treatment with agents such as DNA oligonucleotides that are biased toward T_H1 immune responses. Conventional and modified immunotherapy may work by eliminating ("anergize") rather than stimulating T_H2 responses to environmental allergen. Besides conventional immunotherapy (allergy shots), the only other U.S. Food and Drug Administration (FDA)–approved immunomodulatory strategy for treatment of allergic disease is omalizumab or "anti-IgE." Omalizumab is a humanized monoclonal antibody directed against the region of IgE heavy chain involved in the interaction with IgE receptors. Clinical trials in asthma patients have shown that this antibody is well tolerated and can reduce symptoms and medication requirements in patients with allergic asthma.

CHECKPOINT

9. What are the components of and distinctions between the innate and adaptive forms of immunity?
10. Indicate the primary role of the immune system and the major classes of events by which this is accomplished.
11. What is the phenomenon of MHC restriction?
12. What signals are necessary for activation of helper T lymphocytes?
13. What two signals are necessary for activation of cytotoxic T lymphocytes?
14. What are the common structural features of antibodies?
15. Name four different mechanisms by which antibodies can induce the elimination of foreign antigens.
16. What are the four types of immune reactions in the Gell and Coombs classification scheme, and what are some examples of disorders in which each is involved?
17. What is the critical factor in switching Ig synthesis to the IgE isotype? What are some secondary factors that contribute to, or inhibit, IgE synthesis?

PATHOPHYSIOLOGY OF SELECTED IMMUNE DISORDERS

ALLERGIC RHINITIS

Clinical Presentation

Allergic airway diseases such as allergic rhinitis and asthma are characterized by local tissue damage and organ dysfunction in the upper and lower respiratory tract arising from an abnormal hypersensitivity immune response to normally harmless and ubiquitous environmental allergens. Allergens that cause airway disease are predominantly seasonal tree, grass, and weed pollens or perennial inhalants (eg, house dust mite antigen, cockroach, mold, animal dander, and some occupational protein antigens). Allergic disease is a common cause of pediatric and adult acute and chronic airway problems. Both allergic rhinitis and asthma account for significant morbidity, and atopic disorders have increased in prevalence over the past few decades. In a Danish survey, the prevalence of skin test–positive allergic rhinitis in persons 15–41 years of age increased from 12.9% in 1990 to 22.5% in 1998. Allergic rhinitis is discussed here as a model for the pathophysiology of IgE-mediated allergic airway disease.

Etiology

Allergic rhinitis implies the existence of type I (IgE-mediated) immediate hypersensitivity to environmental allergens that impact the upper respiratory mucosa directly. Particles larger than 5 μm are filtered almost completely by the nasal mucosa. Because most pollen grains are at least this large, few intact particles would be expected to penetrate the lower airway when the nose is functioning normally. The allergic or atopic state is characterized by an inherited tendency to generate IgE antibodies to specific environmental allergens and the physiologic responses that ensue from inflammatory mediators released after the interaction of allergen with mast cell-bound IgE. The clinical presentation of allergic rhinitis includes nasal, ocular, and palatal pruritus, paroxysmal sneezing, rhinorrhea, and nasal congestion. A personal or family history of other allergic diseases such as asthma or atopic dermatitis supports a diagnosis of allergy. Evidence of nasal eosinophilia or basophilia by nasal smear or scraping may support the diagnosis also. Confirmation of allergic rhinitis requires the demonstration of specific IgE antibodies to common allergens by in vitro tests such as the radioallergosorbent test or in vivo (skin) testing in patients with a history of symptoms with relevant exposures.

Pathology & Pathogenesis

Inflammatory changes in the airways are recognized as critical features of both allergic rhinitis and chronic asthma. Cross-linking of surface-bound IgE by antigen activates tissue mast cells and basophils, inducing the immediate release of preformed mediators and the synthesis of newly generated mediators. Mast cells and basophils also have the ability to synthesize and release proinflammatory cytokines, growth and regulatory factors that interact in complex networks. The interaction of mediators with various target organs and cells of the airway can induce a **biphasic allergic response:** an early phase mediated chiefly by release of histamine and other stored mediators (tryptase, chymase, heparin, chondroitin sulfate, and TNF), whereas late-phase events are induced after generation of arachidonic acid metabolites (leukotrienes and prostaglandins), platelet-activating factor and *de novo* cytokine synthesis.

The **early-phase response** occurs within minutes after exposure to an antigen. After intranasal challenge or ambient exposure to relevant allergen, the allergic patient begins sneezing and develops an increase in nasal secretions. After approximately 5 minutes, the patient develops mucosal swelling leading to reduced airflow. These changes are secondary to the effects of vasoactive and smooth muscle constrictive mediators, including histamine, N-α-p-tosyl-L-arginine methylester-esterase (TAME), leukotrienes, prostaglandin D_2 (PGD_2), and kinins and kininogens from mast cells and basophils. Histologically, the early response is characterized by vascular permeability, vasodilatation, tissue edema, and a mild cellular infiltrate of mostly granulocytes.

The **late-phase allergic response** may follow the early-phase response (dual response) or may occur as an isolated event. Late-phase reactions begin 2–4 hours after initial exposure to antigen, reach maximal activity at 6–12 hours, and usually resolve within 12–24 hours. If the exposure is frequent or ongoing, however, the inflammatory response becomes chronic. The late-phase response is characterized by erythema, induration, heat, burning, and itching and microscopically by a significant cellular influx of mainly eosinophils and mononuclear cells. Changes consistent with airway remodeling and tissue hyperreactivity may also occur.

Mediators of the early-phase response—except for PGD_2—reappear during the late-phase response in the absence of antigen rechallenge. Absence of PGD_2, an exclusive product of mast cell release, in the presence of continued histamine release suggests that basophils and not mast cells are an important source of mediators in the late-phase response. There is an early accumulation of neutrophils and eosinophils, with later accumulation of activated T cells, synthesizing T_H2 cytokines. Inflammatory cells infiltrating tissues in the late response may further elaborate cytokines and histamine-releasing factors that may perpetuate the late-phase response, leading to sustained hyperresponsiveness, mucus hypersecretion, IgE production, eosinophilia, and disruption of the target tissue (eg, bronchi, skin, or nasal mucosa).

There is strong circumstantial evidence that eosinophils are key proinflammatory cells in allergic airway disease. Eosinophils are frequently found in secretions from the nasal mucosa of patients with allergic rhinitis and in the sputum of asthmatics. Products of activated eosinophils such as major basic protein and eosinophilic cationic protein, which are destructive to airway epithelial tissue and predispose to persistent airway reactivity, have also been localized to the airways of patients with allergic disease.

The recruitment of eosinophils and other inflammatory cells to the airway is largely a product of activated **chemokines** and **adhesion molecules.** There are two subfamilies of chemokines, which differ in the cells they primarily attract and in the chromosome location of their genes. The C-C chemokines, including RANTES, MCP-1, MCP-3, and eotaxin, are located on chromosome segment 7q11-q21 and selectively recruit eosinophils. Leukocytes attach to vascular endothelial cells through receptor-ligand interaction of cell surface **adhesion molecules** of the integrin, selectin, and immunoglobulin supergene family. The interaction of these adhesion molecules and their counterreceptors mediates a sequence of events that includes margination of leukocytes along the walls of the microvasculature, adhesion of leukocytes to the epithelium, transmigration of leukocytes through vessel walls, and migration along a chemotactic gradient to reach tissue compartments. Both chemokine production and adhesion molecule expression are upregulated by soluble inflammatory mediators. For instance, endothelial cell adhesion molecule receptors, ICAM-1, VCAM-1, and E-selectin, are upregulated by IL-1, TNF, and LPS.

Clinical Manifestations

The clinical manifestations of allergic airway disease (Table 3–3) arise from the interaction of mast cell and basophil mediators with target organs of the upper and lower airway. The symptoms of allergic rhinitis appear immediately after exposure to a relevant allergen (early-phase response), although many patients experience chronic and recurrent symptoms on the basis of the late-phase inflammatory response. Complications of severe or untreated allergic rhinitis include sinusitis, auditory tube dysfunction, dysosmia, sleep disturbances, asthma exacerbations, and chronic mouth breathing.

TABLE 3–3 Clinical manifestations of allergic rhinitis.

Symptoms and signs
Sneezing paroxysms
Nasal, ocular, palatal itching
Clear rhinorrhea
Nasal congestion
Pale, bluish nasal mucosa
Transverse nasal crease
Infraorbital cyanosis ("allergic shiners")
Serous otitis media
Laboratory findings
Nasal eosinophilia
Evidence of allergen-specific IgE by skin or RAST testing

A. Sneezing, Pruritus, Mucus Hypersecretion

Patients with allergic rhinitis develop chronic or episodic paroxysmal sneezing; nasal, ocular, or palatal pruritus; and watery rhinorrhea triggered by exposure to a specific allergen. Patients may demonstrate signs of chronic pruritus of the upper airway, including a horizontal nasal crease from frequent nose rubbing ("allergic salute") and palatal "clicking" from rubbing the itching palate with the tongue. Many tissue mast cells are located near terminal sensory nerve endings. Pruritus and sneezing are caused by histamine-mediated stimulation of these C fibers. Mucus hypersecretion results primarily from excitation of parasympathetic-cholinergic pathways. Early-phase symptoms are best treated with avoidance of relevant allergens and oral or topical antihistamines, which competitively antagonize H_1 receptor sites in target tissues. Anti-inflammatory treatment can reduce cellular inflammation during the late phase, providing more effective symptom relief than antihistamines alone. Allergen immunotherapy (hyposensitization) has shown effectiveness in reducing symptoms and airway inflammation by inhibiting both early- and late-phase allergic responses. Diverse mechanisms of immunotherapy have been observed, including reduction of seasonal increases in IL-4 and allergen-specific IgE, induction of allergen-specific IgG_1 and IgG_4 (blocking antibodies), modulation of T-cell cytokine synthesis by enhancing T_H1 and inhibiting T_H2 responses, upregulation of $\mathbf{T_{reg}}$ and downregulation of eosinophilic and basophilic inflammatory responses to allergen. One trial found that immunotherapy administered to patients with grass-pollen allergy for 3–4 years induced prolonged clinical remission accompanied by a persistent alteration in immunologic reactivity that included sustained reductions in the late skin response and associated T-cell infiltration and IL-4 mRNA expression.

B. Nasal Stuffiness

Symptoms of nasal obstruction may become chronic as a result of persistent late-phase allergic mechanisms. Nasal mucous membranes may appear pale blue and boggy. Children frequently show signs of obligate mouth breathing, including long facies, narrow maxillae, flattened malar eminences, marked overbite, and high-arched palates (so-called adenoid facies). These symptoms are not mediated by histamine and are, therefore, poorly responsive to antihistamine therapy. Oral sympathomimetics that induce vasoconstriction by stimulation of α-adrenergic receptors are often used in conjunction with antihistamines to treat nasal congestion. Topical decongestants may be used to relieve acute congestion but have limited value in patients with chronic allergic rhinitis because frequent use results in rebound vasodilation (rhinitis medicamentosa).

C. Airway Hyperresponsiveness

The phenomenon of heightened nasal sensitivity to reduced levels of allergen after initial exposures to the allergen is known as priming. Clinically, priming may be observed in patients who develop increased symptoms late in the pollen season compared with early in the season. Late-phase inflammation induces a state of nasal airway hyperresponsiveness to both irritants and allergens in patients with chronic allergic rhinitis and asthma. Airway hyperreactivity can cause heightened sensitivity to both environmental irritants such as tobacco smoke and noxious odors as well as to allergens such as pollens. There are no standardized clinical tools to accurately assess late-phase hyperresponsiveness in allergic rhinitis as there are for asthma (methacholine or histamine bronchoprovocation challenge). Genetic markers for bronchial airway hyperresponsiveness, however, have been identified. It also appears that late-phase cellular infiltration and eosinophil by-products may inflict airway epithelial damage, which in turn can predispose to upper and lower airways hyperreactivity.

Accumulating evidence supports a relationship between allergic rhinitis and asthma. Many patients with rhinitis alone demonstrate nonspecific bronchial hyperresponsiveness, and prospective studies suggest that nasal allergy may be a predisposing risk factor for developing asthma. Treatment of patients with allergic rhinitis may result in improvement of asthma symptoms, airway caliber, and bronchial hyperresponsiveness to methacholine and exercise. Finally, mechanistic studies of airway physiology have demonstrated that nasal disease may influence pulmonary function via both direct and indirect mechanisms. Such mechanisms may include the existence of a nasal-bronchial reflex (with nasal stimulation causing bronchial constriction), postnasal drip of inflammatory cells and mediators from the nose into the lower airways, absorption of inflammatory cells and mediators into the systemic circulation and ultimately to the lung, and nasal blockage and subsequent mouth breathing, which may facilitate the entry of asthmagenic triggers to the lower airway.

D. In Vivo or In Vitro Measurement of Allergen-Specific IgE

This is the primary tool for the confirmation of suspected allergic disease. *In vivo* skin testing with allergens suspected of causing hypersensitivity constitutes an indirect bioassay for the presence of allergen-specific IgE on tissue mast cells or basophils. Percutaneous or intradermal administration of dilute concentrations of specific antigens elicits an immediate wheal-and-flare response in a sensitized individual. This response marks a "local anaphylaxis" resulting from the controlled release of mediators from activated mast cells. Positive skin test results to airborne allergens, combined with a history and examination suggestive of allergy, strongly implicate the allergen as a cause of the patient's symptoms. Negative skin test results with an unconvincing allergy history argue strongly against an allergic origin. Major advantages to skin testing include simplicity, rapidity of performance, and low cost.

In vitro tests provide quantitative assays of allergen-specific IgE in the serum. In these assays, patient serum is reacted initially with antigen bound to a solid-phase material and then labeled with a radioactive or enzyme-linked anti-IgE antibody. These immunoallergosorbent tests show a 70–80% correlation with skin testing to pollens, dust mites, and danders and are useful in patients receiving chronic antihistamine therapy who are unable to undergo skin testing and in patients with extensive dermatitis.

E. Complications of Allergic Rhinitis

Serous otitis media and sinusitis are major comorbidities in patients with allergic rhinitis. Both conditions occur secondarily to the obstructed nasal passages and sinus ostia in patients with chronic allergic or nonallergic rhinitis. Complications of chronic rhinitis should be considered in patients with protracted rhinitis unresponsive to therapy, refractory asthma, or persistent bronchitis. Serous otitis results from auditory tube obstruction by mucosal edema and hypersecretion. Children with serous otitis media can present with conductive hearing loss, delayed speech, and recurrent otitis media associated with chronic nasal obstruction.

Sinusitis may be acute, subacute, or chronic depending on the duration of symptoms. Obstruction of osteomeatal drainage in patients with chronic rhinitis predisposes to bacterial infection in the sinus cavities. Patients manifest symptoms of persistent nasal discharge, cough, sinus discomfort, and nasal obstruction. Examination may reveal chronic otitis media, infraorbital edema, inflamed nasal mucosa, and purulent nasal discharge. Radiographic diagnosis by x-ray film or computed tomographic (CT) scan reveals sinus opacification, membrane thickening, or the presence of an air-fluid level. Effective treatment of infectious complications of chronic rhinitis requires antibiotics, systemic antihistamine and decongestants, and perhaps intranasal or systemic corticosteroids.

CHECKPOINT

18. What are the major clinical manifestations of allergic rhinitis?

19. What are the major etiologic factors in allergic rhinitis?

20. What are the pathogenetic mechanisms in allergic rhinitis?

PRIMARY IMMUNODEFICIENCY DISEASES

There are many potential sites where developmental aberrations in the immune system can lead to abnormalities in immunocompetence (Figure 3–4; Tables 3–4 and 3–5). When these defects are genetic in origin, they are referred to as primary immunodeficiency disorders. This is in contrast to compromised immunity secondary to pharmacologic therapy, HIV, malnutrition, or systemic illnesses such as systemic lupus erythematosus or diabetes mellitus.

Clinical investigations of various congenital defects have helped characterize many aspects of normal immune physiology. The very nature of a defect in host immune responses places the susceptible individual at high risk for a variety of infectious, malignant, and autoimmune diseases and disorders. The nature of the specific functional defect will significantly influence the type of infection that affects the host. Table 3–5 lists some of the typical organisms causing infection in patients with various immunodeficiency disorders. Any immunopathogenic mechanism that impairs T-lymphocyte function, or **cell-mediated immunity,** predisposes the host to the development of serious chronic and potentially life-threatening opportunistic infections with viruses, mycobacteria, fungi, and protozoa involving any or all organ systems. Similarly, immunopathogenic dysfunction of B lymphocytes resulting in **antibody deficiency** will predispose the host to pyogenic sinopulmonary and mucosal infections. As the molecular bases of many primary immunodeficiency disorders are being discovered, it has become apparent that different molecular defects can result in common clinical phenotypes.

The T lymphocyte plays a central role in inducing and coordinating immune responses, and dysfunction can be associated with an increased incidence of autoimmune phenomena. These include diseases clinically similar to rheumatoid arthritis, systemic lupus erythematosus, and immune hematologic cytopenias. Patients with impaired immune responses are also at greater risk for certain malignancies than the general population. The occurrence of cancer may be related to an underlying impairment of tumor surveillance, dysregulation of cellular proliferation and differentiation, chromosomal translocations during defective antigen

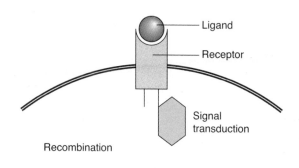

FIGURE 3–4 Simplified schema of defects in cell surface receptor-dependent activation leading to different primary immunodeficiency disorders. In Table 3–4 are listed the syndromes and immunologic deficits seen with a variety of these humoral, cellular, neutrophil, or combined immunodeficiency disorders.

TABLE 3–4 Primary immunodeficiency disorders.

Combined immunodeficiency		
XSCID	Deficiency of common γ chain	Defective cytokine signaling
ZAP-70 deficiency	Defective TCR signaling	CD8 T-cell lymphopenia, CD4 T-cell dysfunction
SCID-ADA deficiency	Enzyme defect	T cell (−), B cell (−), NK cell (−)
P56^{lck} deficiency	Defective T-cell receptor–associated tyrosine kinase	T cell (+), B cell (+), NK cell (+)
JAK-3 deficiency	Defective cytokine signaling	T cell (−), B cell (+), NK cell (+)
RAG1 deficiency	Recombination defect	T cell (−), B cell (−), NK cell (+)
RAG2 deficiency		
PNP deficiency	Enzyme defect	T cell (−)
MHC class I deficiency	Defect in transporter associated with antigen presentation (TAP)	Bare lymphocyte syndrome, no MHC class I expression
MHC class II deficiency	Defective transcription of MHC class II genes	Bare lymphocyte syndrome, no MHC class II expression
Humoral immunodeficiency		
X-linked agammaglobulinemia	Defect in BTK	Arrested maturation of B-cell lineage
Common variable immunodeficiency	Abnormal proliferation and differentiation of B cells or abnormal regulatory cell function[1]	Heterogeneous disorder with agammaglobulinemia
Hyper-IgM syndrome	Defective CD40-ligand binding	Abnormal immunoglobulin isotype switching
Cellular immunodeficiency		
DiGeorge syndrome	Most have chromosome 22q11 deletion	Complete or partial T-cell deficiency
Phagocytic cell disorders		
Chronic granulomatous disease	Defective NADPH oxidase	Abnormal oxidative metabolism
Leukocyte adhesion deficiency	Defect in CD18 subunit of β$_2$-integrin molecule	

[1]Variable defects, although the most common is in terminal differentiation of B lymphocytes.

TABLE 3–5 Relationship of various pathogens to infection in primary immunodeficiency disorders.

	Pyogenic Bacteria	Mycobacteria	Fungi		Viruses	Parasites		
			Pneumocystis jiroveci	Other Fungi		*Giardia lamblia*	*Toxoplasma gondii*	*Cryptosporidium, Isospora*
SCID	+	+	+	+	+	−	−	−
Thymic hypoplasia	−	+	−	+	+	−	−	−
X-linked agamma-globulinemia	+	−	−	−	−	+	−	−
Common variable immunodeficiency	+	−	−	−	−	+	−	−
Complement deficiency	+	−	−	−	−	−	−	−
Phagocytic defects	+	−	−	−	−	−	−	−

Key: + = association; − = no association.

receptor gene rearrangement, or the presence of infectious agents predisposing to or causing cellular transformation. Non-Hodgkin's lymphoma or B-cell lymphoproliferative disease, skin carcinomas, and gastric carcinomas are the most frequently occurring tumors in patients with immunodeficiency.

Traditionally, the primary immunodeficiencies are classified according to which component of the immune response is principally compromised: the humoral response, cell-mediated immunity, complement, or phagocytic cell function (Table 3–4). Distinct developmental stages characterize the maturation and differentiation of the cellular components of the immune system. The underlying pathophysiologic abnormalities leading to primary immunodeficiency are diverse and include the following: (1) early developmental defects in cellular maturation, (2) specific enzyme defects, (3) abnormalities in cellular proliferation and functional differentiation, (4) abnormalities in cellular regulation, and (5) abnormal responses to cytokines.

COMBINED IMMUNODEFICIENCY

Severe Combined Immunodeficiency Disease

Clinical Presentation

Clinically, many primary immunodeficiency disorders present early in the neonatal period. In patients with SCID, there is an absence of normal thymic tissue, and the lymph nodes, spleen, and other peripheral lymphoid tissues are devoid of lymphocytes. In these patients, the complete or near-complete failure of development of both the cellular and the humoral component of the immune system results in severe infections. The spectrum of infections is broad because these patients may also suffer from overwhelming infection by opportunistic pathogens, disseminated viruses, and intracellular organisms. Failure to thrive may be the initial presenting symptom, but mucocutaneous candidiasis, chronic diarrhea, and pneumonitis are common. Vaccination with live viral vaccines or bacillus Calmette-Guerin (BCG) may lead to disseminated disease. Without immune reconstitution by bone marrow transplantation, SCID is inevitably fatal within 1–2 years.

Pathology & Pathogenesis

SCID is a heterogeneous group of disorders characterized by a failure in the cellular maturation of lymphoid stem cells, resulting in reduced numbers and function of both B and T lymphocytes and hypogammaglobulinemia. The molecular basis for many types of SCID have been discovered (Table 3–4). The genetic and cellular defects can occur at many different levels, starting with surface membrane receptors but also including deficiencies in signal transduction or metabolic biochemical pathways. Although the different molecular defects may cause clinically indistinguishable phenotypes, identification of specific mutations allows for improved genetic counseling, prenatal diagnosis, and carrier detection. Moreover, specific gene transfer offers hope as a future therapy.

1. Defective cytokine signaling—X-linked SCID (XSCID) is the most prevalent form, resulting from a genetic mutation in the common γ chain of the trimeric ($\alpha\beta\gamma$) IL-2 receptor. This defective chain is shared by the receptors for IL-4, IL-7, IL-9, and IL-15, leading to dysfunction of all of these cytokine receptors. Defective signaling through the IL-7 receptor appears to block normal maturation of T lymphocytes. Defective IL-2 responses inhibit proliferation of T, B, and NK cells, explaining the combined immune defects seen in XSCID patients. A defect in the α chain of the IL-7 receptor can also lead to an autosomal recessive form of SCID through mechanisms similar to XSCID but with intact NK cells.

2. Defective T-cell receptor signaling—The genetic defects for several other forms of the autosomal recessive SCID have also been identified. **A deficiency of ZAP-70** (zeta-associated protein 70), a protein tyrosine kinase important in signal transduction through the T-cell receptor, leads to a total absence of CD8 T lymphocytes. ZAP-70 plays an essential role in thymic selection during T-cell development. Consequently, these patients possess functionally defective CD4 T lymphocytes and no circulating CD8 T lymphocytes but normal B-lymphocyte and NK cell activity.

Deficiencies of both p56^{lck} and Jak3 (Janus kinase 3) can also lead to SCID through defective signal transduction. P56^{lck} is a T-cell receptor–associated tyrosine kinase that is essential for T-cell differentiation, activation, and proliferation. Jak3 is a cytokine receptor–associated signaling molecule.

3. Defective receptor gene recombination—Patients have been identified with **defective recombination-activating gene (*RAG1* and *RAG2*)** products. RAG1 and RAG2 initiate recombination of antigen-binding proteins, immunoglobulins, and T-cell receptors. The failure to form antigen receptors leads to a quantitative and functional deficiency of T and B lymphocytes. NK cells are not antigen specific and for that reason are unaffected.

4. Defective nucleotide salvage pathway—Approximately 20% of SCID cases are caused by a **deficiency of adenosine deaminase** (ADA), which is an enzyme in the purine salvage pathway, responsible for the metabolism of adenosine. Absence of the ADA enzyme results in an accumulation of toxic adenosine metabolites within the cells. These metabolites inhibit normal lymphocyte proliferation and lead to extreme cytopenia of both B and T lymphocytes. The combined immunologic deficiency and clinical presentation of this disorder, known as **SCID-ADA,** is identical to that of the other forms of SCID. Skeletal abnormalities and neurologic abnormalities may be associated with this disease.

CELL-MEDIATED IMMUNODEFICIENCY

Congenital Thymic Aplasia (DiGeorge Syndrome)

Clinical Presentation & Pathogenesis

The clinical manifestations of **DiGeorge syndrome** reflect the defective embryonic development of organs derived from the third and fourth pharyngeal arches, including the thymus, parathyroids, and cardiac outflow tract. Occasionally, the first and sixth pharyngeal pouches may also be involved. Cytogenetic abnormalities, most commonly chromosome 22q11 deletions, are associated with DiGeorge syndrome, especially in patients manifesting cardiac defects. DiGeorge syndrome is classified as complete or partial depending on the presence or absence of immunologic abnormalities. In this syndrome, the spectrum of immunologic deficiency is wide, ranging from immune competency to conditions in which there are life-threatening infections with organisms typically of low virulence. Patients affected by the complete syndrome have a profound T lymphocytopenia resulting from thymic aplasia with impaired T-lymphocyte maturation, severely depressed cell-mediated immunity, and decreased suppressor T-lymphocyte activity. B lymphocytes and immunoglobulin production are unaffected in most patients, although in rare instances patients may present with mild hypogammaglobulinemia and absent or poor antibody responses to neoantigens. In this subset of patients, inadequate helper T function as a result of dysfunctional T- and B-cell interaction and inadequate cytokine production leads to impaired humoral immunity.

DiGeorge syndrome is truly a developmental anomaly and can be associated with structural abnormalities in the cardiovascular system such as truncus arteriosus or right-sided aortic arch. Parathyroid abnormalities may lead to hypocalcemia, presenting with neonatal tetany or seizures. In addition, it is common for patients to exhibit facial abnormalities such as micrognathia, hypertelorism, low-set ears with notched pinnae, and a short philtrum.

HUMORAL IMMUNODEFICIENCY

X-Linked Agammaglobulinemia

Clinical Presentation

Formerly called Bruton's agammaglobulinemia, **X-linked agammaglobulinemia** (XLA) is thought to be pathophysiologically and clinically more homogeneous than SCID. It is principally a disease of childhood, presenting clinically within the first 2 years of life with multiple and recurrent sinopulmonary infections caused primarily by pyogenic bacteria and, to a much lesser extent, viruses. Because encapsulated bacteria require antibody binding for efficient opsonization, these humorally immune-deficient patients suffer from sinusitis, pneumonia, pharyngitis, bronchitis, and otitis media secondary to infection with *S pneumoniae,* other streptococci, and *H influenzae.* Although infections from fungal and opportunistic pathogens are rare, patients display a unique susceptibility to a rare but deadly enteroviral meningoencephalitis.

Pathology & Pathogenesis

Patients with XLA are pan-hypogammaglobulinemic, with decreased levels of IgG, IgM, and IgA. They exhibit poor to absent responses to antigen challenge even though virtually all demonstrate normal functional T-lymphocyte responses to *in vitro* as well as *in vivo* tests (eg, delayed hypersensitivity skin reactions). The basic defect in this disorder appears to be arrested cellular maturation at the pre-B-lymphocyte stage. Indeed, normal numbers of pre-B lymphocytes can be found in the bone marrow, although in the circulation B lymphocytes are virtually absent. Lymphoid tissues lack fully differentiated B lymphocytes (antibody-secreting plasma cells), and lymph nodes lack developed germinal centers. The gene that is defective in XLA has been isolated. The defective gene product, BTK (Bruton's tyrosine kinase), is a B-cell–specific signaling protein belonging to the cytoplasmic tyrosine kinase family of intracellular proteins. Gene deletions and point mutations in the catalytic domain of the *BTK* gene block normal BTK function, necessary for B-cell maturation.

Common Variable Immunodeficiency

Clinical Presentation

This disorder is often referred to as acquired or adult-onset hypogammaglobulinemia. It is the most common serious primary immune deficiency disorder in adults. In North America, for example, it affects an estimated 1:75,000 to 1:50,000 individuals. The clinical spectrum is broad, and patients usually present within the first 2 decades of life. Affected individuals commonly develop recurrent sinopulmonary infections, including sinusitis, otitis, bronchitis, and pneumonia. Bronchiectasis can be the result of recurrent serious respiratory infections, can lead to infection with more virulent pathogens, and can change the long-term prognosis. A number of important noninfectious disorders are commonly associated with common variable immunodeficiency, including GI malabsorption, autoimmune disorders, and neoplasms. The most frequently occurring malignancies are lymphoreticular, but gastric carcinoma and skin cancer also occur. Autoimmune disorders occur in 20–30% of patients and may precede the recurrent infections. Autoimmune cytopenias occur most frequently, but rheumatic diseases can also be seen. Serologic testing for infectious or autoimmune disease is unreliable in hypogammaglobulinemia. Monthly infusions of intravenous immunoglobulin can reconstitute humoral immunity, decrease infections, and improve quality of life.

Pathology & Pathogenesis

Common variable immunodeficiency is a heterogeneous disorder in which the primary immunologic abnormality is a marked reduction in antibody production. The vast majority of patients demonstrate an *in vitro* defect in terminal differentiation of B lymphocytes. Peripheral blood lymphocyte phenotyping demonstrates normal or reduced numbers of circulating B lymphocytes, but antibody-secreting plasma cells are conspicuously sparse in lymphoid tissues. In sharp contrast to XLA, no single gene defect can be held accountable for the multitude of defects known to cause common variable immunodeficiency. In approximately 80% of patients, the defect is intrinsic to the B-lymphocyte population. In the rest, a variety of T-cell abnormalities lead to immune defects with subsequent impairment of B-cell differentiation. These rare T-lymphocyte abnormalities include increased suppressor T-lymphocyte activity, decreased production of IL-2 and other cytokines, and defective synthesis of B-lymphocyte growth factors such as IL-4 and IL-6. In some patients, there is also evidence of defective cytokine gene expression in T cells, decreased T-cell mitogenesis, and deficient lymphokine-activated killer cell function. More than 50% of patients also have some degree of T-lymphocyte dysfunction as determined by absent or diminished cutaneous responses to recall antigens. Immune dysregulation may contribute to the morbidity and the myriad autoimmune manifestations associated with common variable immunodeficiency.

Hyper-IgM Immunodeficiency

Clinical Presentation

In patients with hyper-IgM immunodeficiency, serum levels of IgG and IgA are very low or absent, but serum IgM (and sometimes IgD) levels are normal or elevated. Inheritance of this disorder may be autosomal, although it is most often X-linked. Clinically, this syndrome is manifested by recurrent pyogenic infections and an array of autoimmune phenomena such as Coombs-positive hemolytic anemia and immune thrombocytopenia.

Pathology & Pathogenesis

The principal abnormality is the defective expression of CD154, a T-lymphocyte activation surface marker (also known as CD40-ligand or gp39). In the course of normal immune responses, CD154 interacts with CD40 on B-cell surfaces during cellular activation, initiating proliferation and immunoglobulin isotype switching. In hyper-IgM syndrome, defective CD40 coreceptor stimulation during T- and B-cell interactions leads to impairment of B-cell isotype switching and subsequent production of IgM but no production of IgG or IgA.

Selective IgA Deficiency

This is the most common primary immunodeficiency in adults, with a prevalence of 1:700 to 1:500 individuals. Most affected individuals have few or no clinical manifestations, but there is an increased incidence of upper respiratory tract infections, allergy, asthma, and autoimmune disorders. Whereas serum levels of the other immunoglobulin isotypes are typically normal, serum IgA levels in these individuals are markedly depressed, often less than 5 mg/dL.

As in common variable immunodeficiency, the primary functional defect is an inability of B cells to terminally differentiate to IgA-secreting plasma cells. An associated deficiency of IgG subclasses (mainly IgG$_2$ and IgG$_4$) and low-molecular-weight monomeric IgM is not uncommon and can be clinically significant. Because of the role of secretory IgA in mucosal immunity, patients with this immunodeficiency frequently develop significant infections involving the mucous membranes of the gut, conjunctiva, and respiratory tract. There is no specific therapy, but prompt antibiotic treatment is necessary in patients with recurrent infections. A subset of patients may recognize IgA as a foreign antigen. These patients are at risk for transfusion reactions to unwashed red blood cells or other blood products containing trace amounts of IgA.

PHAGOCYTIC CELL DISORDERS

Defective phagocytic cell function presents with infections at sites of interface between the body and the outside world. Recurrent skin infections, abscesses, gingivitis, lymphadenitis, and poor wound healing are seen in patients with macrophage or neutrophil disorders. More difficult to assay, clinical immunodeficiency can occur through defects in phagocytic cell migration, adhesion, opsonization, or killing.

Chronic Granulomatous Disease

Clinical Presentation

Chronic granulomatous disease is typically X-linked and characterized by impaired granulocyte function. This disorder of phagocytic cell function presents with recurrent skin infections, abscesses, and granulomas at sites of chronic inflammation. Abscesses can involve skin or viscera and may be accompanied by lymphadenitis. Catalase-positive organisms predominate; *S aureus* is thus the most common pathogen, although infections with gram-negative bacteria and *Aspergillus* species also occur. Sterile noncaseating granulomas resulting from chronic inflammatory stimuli can lead to GI or genitourinary tract obstruction. Chronic granulomatous disease typically presents in childhood, although cases in adulthood are occasionally reported.

Pathology & Pathogenesis

Defects in the gene coding for nicotinamide adenine dinucleotide phosphate (NADPH) oxidase inhibit oxidative metabolism and severely compromise neutrophil killing activity. NADPH oxidase is assembled from two membrane and two cytosolic components after phagocytic cell activation, leading to catalytic conversion of molecular oxygen into superoxide. Oxidative burst and intracellular killing rely on production of superoxide, which is later converted to hydrogen peroxide and sodium hypochlorite (bleach). In patients with chronic granulomatous disease, other neutrophil functions such as chemotaxis, phagocytosis, and degranulation remain intact but microbial killing is deficient. Catalase-negative bacteria are effectively killed because microbes produce small amounts of peroxide, concentrated in phagosomes, leading to microbial death. Catalase-positive organisms scavenge these relatively small amounts of peroxide and are not killed without neutrophil oxidative metabolism. X-linked inheritance is most frequently seen, but autosomal recessive forms and spontaneous mutations can also lead to clinical disease.

Leukocyte Adhesion Deficiency, Type 1

Integrins and selectins are specialized molecules that play a role in leukocyte homing to sites of inflammation. These adhesion molecules facilitate cell-cell and cell–extracellular matrix interactions, allowing circulating leukocytes to stick and roll along endothelial cell surfaces prior to diapedesis into extravascular tissues. In leukocyte adhesion deficiency, type 1, defective expression of β_2-integrin (CD11/CD18) adhesion molecules results in recurrent infections and poor wound healing. Leukocytosis occurs because cells cannot exit the circulation and recurrent infections of skin, airways, bowels, perirectal area, and gingival and periodontal areas are common.

Hyper-IgE Immunodeficiency

Clinical Presentation

This disorder is often referred to as "Job's syndrome" because affected individuals suffer from recurrent boils like the tormented biblical figure. The initial description of this immunodeficiency disorder was in two fair-skinned girls with recurrent staphylococcal "cold" skin abscesses associated with furunculosis, cellulitis, recurrent otitis, sinusitis, pneumatoceles, and a coarse facial appearance. The predominant organism isolated from sites of infection is *S aureus,* although other organisms such as *H influenzae,* pneumococci, gram-negative organisms, *Aspergillus sp* and *C albicans* are often identified also. Characteristically, patients have a chronic pruritic eczematoid dermatitis, growth retardation, coarse facies, osteopenia, and hyperkeratotic fingernails. Extremely high IgE levels (> 3000 IU/mL) have also been observed in patients' serum.

Pathology & Pathogenesis

The high IgE levels are thought to be a consequence of dysregulated immunologic responsiveness to cytokines, yet it is unclear whether they contribute to the observed susceptibility to infection. Other immunopathologic states can be associated with elevated IgE levels, including graft-versus-host disease, AIDS, and Wiscott-Aldrich syndrome. Several immune defects have been described, but the primary defect remains unknown. Humoral immunodeficiency is suggested by poor antibody responses to neoantigens, deficiency of IgA antibody against *S aureus,* and low levels of antibodies to carbohydrate antigens. T-lymphocyte functional abnormalities are suggested by decreased absolute numbers of suppressor T lymphocytes, poor *in vitro* proliferative responses, and defects in cytokine production. Several reports have also documented highly variable abnormalities in neutrophil chemotaxis.

CHECKPOINT

21. What are the major clinical manifestations of each of the five categories of primary immune deficiency?
22. What are the major pathogenetic mechanisms in each category of primary immune deficiency?

AIDS

AIDS is the most common immunodeficiency disorder worldwide, and HIV infection is one of the greatest epidemics in human history. AIDS is the consequence of a chronic retroviral infection that produces severe, life-threatening CD4 helper T-lymphocyte dysfunction, opportunistic infections, and malignancy. Retroviruses contain viral RNA that is transcribed by viral reverse transcriptase into double-stranded DNA, which is integrated into the host genome. Cellular activation leads to transcription of HIV gene products and viral replication. AIDS is defined by serologic evidence of HIV infection with the presence of a variety of indicator diseases associated with clinical immunodeficiency. Table 3–6 lists criteria for defining and diagnosing AIDS. HIV is transmitted by exposure to infected body fluids or sexual or perinatal contact. Transmissibility of the HIV virus is related to subtype virulence, viral load, and immunologic host factors.

Acute HIV infection may present as an acute, self-limited, febrile viral syndrome characterized by fatigue, pharyngitis, myalgias, rash, lymphadenopathy, and significant viremia without detectable anti-HIV antibodies. After an initial viremic phase, patients seroconvert and a period of clinical latency is usually seen. Lymph tissues become centers for massive viral replication during a "silent," or asymptomatic, stage of HIV infection despite an absence of detectable virus in the peripheral blood. Over time, there is a progressive decline in CD4 T lymphocytes, a reversal of the normal CD4:CD8 T-lymphocyte ratio, and numerous other immunologic derangements. The clinical manifestations are directly related to HIV tissue tropism and defective immune function. Development of neurologic complications, opportunistic infections, or malignancy signal marked immune deficiency. The time course for progression varies, but the median time before appearance of clinical disease is about 10 years. Approximately 10% of those infected manifest rapid progression to AIDS within 5 years after infection. A minority of individuals are "long-term nonprogressors." Genetic factors, host cytotoxic immune responses, and viral load and virulence appear to impact susceptibility to infection and the rate of disease progression.

TABLE 3–6 1993 revised classification system for HIV infection and expanded AIDS surveillance case definition for adolescents and adults.

I. Clinical and lymphocyte categories

| | Clinical Categories | | |
CD4 T-Cell Categories	(A) Asymptomatic, Acute (Primary) HIV or PGL[1]	(B) Symptomatic, Not (A) or (C) Conditions	(C) AIDS-Indicator Conditions
(1) ≥ 500/µL	A1	B1	C1
(2) 200–499/mL	A2	B2	C2
(3) < 200/mL	A3	B3	C3

II. Conditions included in the 1993 AIDS surveillance case definition:

- Candidiasis of the esophagus, bronchi, trachea, or lungs

- Cervical cancer, invasive

- Coccidioidomycosis, disseminated or extrapulmonary

- Cryptococcosis, extrapulmonary

- Cryptosporidiosis, chronic intestinal (> 1-month duration)

- Cytomegalovirus disease (other than liver, spleen, or nodes); cytomegalovirus retinitis (with loss of vision)

- Encephalopathy, HIV related

- Herpes simplex: chronic ulcers (> 1-month duration); or bronchitis, pneumonitis, or esophagitis

- Histoplasmosis, disseminated or extrapulmonary

- Isosporiasis, chronic intestinal (> 1-month duration)

- Kaposi's sarcoma

- Lymphoma, Burkitt's (or equivalent term); immunoblastic lymphoma (or equivalent term); primary brain lymphoma

- *Mycobacterium avium* complex or *Mycobacterium kansasii*, disseminated or extrapulmonary

- *Mycobacterium tuberculosis,* any site (pulmonary or extrapulmonary)

- *Mycobacterium*, other species or unidentified species, disseminated or extrapulmonary

- *Pneumocystis jiroveci* pneumonia

- Pneumonia, recurrent

- Progressive multifocal leukoencephalopathy

- *Salmonella* septicemia, recurrent

- Toxoplasmosis of brain

- Wasting syndrome resulting from HIV

III. Clinical categories:

A. Category A consists of one or more of the conditions listed below in an adolescent (> 13 years) or adult with documented HIV infection. Conditions listed in categories B and C must not have occurred.

- Asymptomatic HIV infection

- Persistent generalized lymphadenopathy

- Acute (primary) HIV infection with accompanying illness or history of acute HIV infection

(continued)

TABLE 3–6 **1993 revised classification system for HIV infection and expanded AIDS surveillance case definition for adolescents and adults. (Continued)**

III. Clinical categories
B. Category B consists of symptomatic conditions in an HIV-infected adolescent or adult that are not included among conditions listed in clinical category C and that meet at least one of the following criteria: (a) the conditions are attributed to HIV infection or are indicative of a defect in cell-mediated immunity; or (b) the conditions are considered by physicians to have a clinical course or to require management that is complicated by HIV infection.
Examples of conditions in clinical category B include but are not limited to:
• Bacillary angiomatosis
• Oropharyngeal candidiasis (thrush)
• Vulvovaginal candidiasis, persistent, frequent, or poorly responsive to therapy
• Cervical dysplasia (moderate or severe) or cervical carcinoma in situ
• Constitutional symptoms, such as fever (38.5 °C) or diarrhea lasting > 1 month
• Hairy leukoplakia
• Herpes zoster (shingles), involving at least two distinct dermatomes or more than one episode
• Idiopathic thrombocytopenic purpura
• Listeriosis
• Pelvic inflammatory disease, particularly if complicated by tuboovarian abscess
• Peripheral neuropathy
• For classification purposes, category B conditions take precedence over those in category A. For example, someone previously treated for oral or persistent vaginal candidiasis (and who has not developed a category C disease) but who is now asymptomatic should be classified in clinical category B.
C. Category C includes the clinical conditions listed in the AIDS surveillance case definition (section II above). For classification purposes, once a category C condition has occurred, the person will remain in category C.

Including the expanded AIDS surveillance case definition. Persons with AIDS-indicator conditions (category C) as well as those with AIDS-indicator CD4 T-lymphocyte counts < 200/μL (categories A3 or B3) have been reportable as AIDS cases in the United States and Territories since January 1, 1993. Modified from MMWR Morb Mortal Wkly Rep. 1992;41[RR-17]. Sections II and III of this table are modified and reproduced, with permission, from Lawlor GL Jr, Fischer TJ, Adelman DC (editors). *Manual of Allergy and Immmunology.* Little, Brown, 1994.

[1]PGL, persistent generalized lymphadenopathy. Clinical category A includes acute (primary) HIV infection.

Pathology & Pathogenesis

Chemokines (chemoattractant cytokines) regulate leukocyte trafficking to sites of inflammation and have been discovered to play a significant role in the pathogenesis of HIV disease. During the initial stages of infection and viral proliferation, virion entry and cellular infection requires binding to two coreceptors on target T lymphocytes and monocyte/macrophages. All HIV strains express the envelope protein gp120 that binds to CD4 molecules, but different viral strains display tissue "tropism" or specificity on the basis of the coreceptor they recognize. These coreceptors belong to the chemokine receptor family. Changes in viral phenotype during the course of HIV infection may lead to changes in tropism and cytopathology at different stages of disease. Viral strains isolated in early stages of infection (eg, R5 viruses) demonstrate tropism toward macrophages. X4 strains of HIV are more commonly seen in later stages of disease. X4 viruses bind to chemokine receptor CXCR4, more broadly expressed on T cells, and are associated with syncytium formation. A small percentage of individuals possessing nonfunctional alleles for the polymorphic chemokine receptor CCR5 appear to be highly resistant to HIV infection or display delayed progression of disease.

Mathematical models estimate that during HIV infection billions of virions are produced and cleared each day. The reverse transcription step of HIV replication is error prone; mutations occur frequently, and even within an individual patient, HIV heterogeneity develops rapidly. The development of antigenically and phenotypically distinct strains contributes to progression of disease, clinical drug resistance, and lack of efficacy of early vaccines.

Cellular activation is critical for viral infectivity and reactivation of integrated proviral DNA. Although only 2% of mononuclear cells are found peripherally, lymph nodes from HIV-infected individuals can contain large amounts of virus sequestered among infected follicular dendritic cells in the germinal centers. The marked decline in CD4 T-lymphocyte counts—characterizing HIV infection—is due to several mechanisms, including the following: (1) direct HIV-mediated destruction of CD4 T lymphocytes, (2) autoimmune destruction of virus-infected T cells, (3) depletion by fusion and formation of multinucleated giant cells (syncytium formation), (4) toxicity of viral proteins to CD4 T lymphocytes and hematopoietic precursors, and (5) induction of apoptosis (programmed cell death). CD8 CTL activity is initially brisk and effective at controlling viremia through elimination of virus and virus-infected cells. Ultimately, viral proliferation outpaces host responses, and HIV-induced immunosuppression leads to disease progression. Loss of viral containment occurs with lack of adequate helper T function and decreased IL-2 production leading to diminution of CD8+ T-cell–dependent cytotoxic responses. Subsequently, there is an accumulation of viral escape mutations with general cytokine dysregulation detrimental to maintenance of lymphatic organs, bone marrow integrity, and effective immune responses.

In addition to the cell-mediated immune defects, B-lymphocyte function is altered such that many infected individuals have marked hypergammaglobulinemia but impaired specific antibody responses. Both anamnestic responses and those to neoantigens can be impaired. However, the role of humoral immunity in controlling viremia or slowing disease progression is unclear.

The development of assays to measure viral burden (plasma HIV-RNA quantification) has led to a better understanding of HIV dynamics and has provided a tool for assessing response to therapy. It is now well recognized that viral replication continues throughout the disease, and immune deterioration occurs despite clinical latency. The risk of progression to AIDS appears correlated with an individual's viral load after seroconversion. Data from several large clinical cohorts have shown that there is a direct correlation between the CD4 T-lymphocyte count and the risk of AIDS-defining opportunistic infections. Thus, the viral load and the degree of CD4 T-lymphocyte depletion serve as important clinical indicators of immune status in HIV-infected individuals. Prophylaxis for opportunistic infections such as pneumocystis pneumonia is started when CD4 T-lymphocyte counts reach the 200–250 cells/μL range. Similarly, patients with HIV infection with fewer than 50 CD4 T lymphocytes/μL are at significantly increased risk for cytomegalovirus (CMV) retinitis and *Mycobacterium avium* complex (MAC) infection.

Cells other than CD4 T lymphocytes contribute to the pathogenesis of HIV infection. Monocytes, macrophages, and dendritic cells can be infected with HIV and facilitate transfer of virus to lymphoid tissues and immunoprivileged sites, such as the CNS. HIV-infected monocytes will also release large quantities of the acute-phase reactant cytokines, including IL-1, IL-6, and TNF, contributing to constitutional symptomatology. TNF, in particular, has been implicated in the severe wasting syndrome seen in patients with advanced disease. Concomitant infections may serve as cofactors for HIV infec-

tion, increasing expression of HIV through enhanced cytokine production, coreceptor surface expression, or increased cellular activation mechanisms.

Clinical Manifestations

The clinical manifestations of AIDS are the direct consequence of the progressive and severe immunologic deficiency induced by HIV. Patients are susceptible to a wide range of atypical or opportunistic infections with bacterial, viral, protozoal, and fungal pathogens. Common nonspecific symptoms include fever, night sweats, and weight loss. Weight loss and cachexia can be due to nausea, vomiting, anorexia, or diarrhea. They often portend a poor prognosis.

The incidence of infection increases as the CD4 T lymphocyte number declines. **Lung infection** with *Pneumocystis jiroveci* is the most common opportunistic infection, affecting 75% of patients. Patients present clinically with fevers, cough, shortness of breath, and hypoxemia ranging in severity from mild to life threatening. A diagnosis of pneumocystis pneumonia can be made by substantiation of the clinical and radiographic findings with Wright-Giemsa or silver methenamine staining of induced sputum samples. A negative sputum stain does not rule out disease in patients in whom there is a strong clinical suspicion of disease, and further diagnostic maneuvers such as bronchoalveolar lavage or fiberoptic transbronchial biopsy may be required to establish the diagnosis. Complications of pneumocystis pneumonia include pneumothoraces, progressive parenchymal disease with severe respiratory insufficiency, and, most commonly, adverse reactions to the medications used for treatment and prophylaxis.

As a consequence of chronic immune dysfunction, HIV-infected individuals are also at high risk for other pulmonary infections, including bacterial infections with *S pneumoniae* and *H influenzae*; mycobacterial infections with *M tuberculosis* or *M avium-intracellulare* (MAC); and fungal infections with *C neoformans*, *H capsulatum*, or *C immitis*. Clinical suspicion followed by early diagnosis of these infections should lead to aggressive treatment.

The development of active tuberculosis is significantly accelerated in HIV infection as a result of compromised cellular immunity. The risk of reactivation is estimated to be 5–10% per year in HIV-infected patients compared with a lifetime risk of 10% in those without HIV. Furthermore, diagnosis may be delayed because of anergic skin responses. Extrapulmonary manifestations occur in up to 70% of HIV-infected patients with tuberculosis, and the emergence of multidrug resistance may compound the problem. MAC is a less virulent pathogen than *M tuberculosis*, and disseminated infections usually occur only with severe clinical immunodeficiency. Symptoms are nonspecific and typically consist of fever, weight loss, anemia, and GI distress with diarrhea.

The presence on physical examination of **oral candidiasis (thrush)** and **hairy leukoplakia** is highly correlated with HIV infection and portends rapid progression to AIDS. Abnormal outgrowth of *Candida* from normal mouth flora is the cause of persistent oral candidiasis, whereas Epstein-Barr virus is the cause of hairy leukoplakia. HIV-infected individuals with oral candidiasis are at much greater risk for esophageal candidiasis, which may present as substernal pain and dysphagia. This infection and its characteristic clinical presentation are so common that most practitioners treat with empiric oral antifungal therapy. Should the patient not respond rapidly, other explanations for the esophageal symptoms should be explored, including herpes simplex and CMV infections.

Persistent diarrhea, especially when accompanied by high fevers and abdominal pain, may signal **infectious enterocolitis.** The list of potential pathogens in such cases is long and includes bacteria, MAC, protozoans (cryptosporidium, microsporidia, *Isospora belli, Entamoeba histolytica, Giardia lamblia*), and even HIV itself. HIV-associated gastropathy and malabsorption are commonly noted in these patients. Because of their reduced gastric acid concentrations, patients have an increased susceptibility to infection with *Campylobacter, Salmonella,* and *Shigella.* Co-infection with viral hepatitis (HBV, HCV, CMV) can lead to end-stage liver disease, but fortunately, institution of highly active antiretroviral therapy (HAART) can lead to a reduction in clinical HBV disease.

Skin lesions commonly associated with HIV infection are typically classified as infectious (viral, bacterial, fungal), neoplastic, or nonspecific. Herpes simplex virus (HSV) and herpes zoster virus (HZV) may cause chronic persistent or progressive lesions in patients with compromised cellular immunity. HSV commonly causes oral and perianal lesions but can be an AIDS-defining illness when involving the lung or esophagus. The risk of disseminated HSV or HZV infection and the presence of molluscum contagiosum appear to be correlated with the extent of immunoincompetence. Seborrheic dermatitis caused by *Pityrosporum ovale* and fungal skin infections (*Candida albicans,* dermatophyte species) are also commonly seen in HIV-infected patients. *Staphylococcus* including methacillin-resistant *S aureus* can cause the folliculitis, furunculosis, and bullous impetigo commonly observed in HIV-infected patients, which require aggressive treatment to prevent dissemination and sepsis. **Bacillary angiomatosis** is a potentially fatal dermatologic disorder of tumor-like proliferating vascular endothelial cell lesions, the result of infection by *Bartonella quintana* or *Bartonella henselae.* The lesions may resemble those of Kaposi's sarcoma but respond to treatment with erythromycin or tetracycline.

CNS manifestations in HIV-infected patients include infections and malignancies. **Toxoplasmosis** frequently presents with space-occupying lesions, causing headache, altered mental status, seizures, or focal neurologic deficits. Cryptococcal meningitis commonly manifests as headache and fever. Up to 90% of patients with cryptococcal meningitis exhibit a positive serum test for *Cryptococcus neoformans* antigen.

HIV-associated cognitive-motor complex, or **AIDS dementia complex,** is the most frequently diagnosed cause of altered mental status in HIV-infected patients. Patients typically have difficulty with cognitive tasks, poor short-term memory, slowed motor function, personality changes, and waxing and waning dementia. Up to 50% of patients with AIDS suffer from this disorder, perhaps caused by glial or macrophage infection by HIV resulting in destructive inflammatory changes within the CNS. The differential diagnosis can be broad, including metabolic disturbances and toxic encephalopathy resulting from drugs. Other causes of altered mental status include neurosyphilis, CMV or herpes simplex encephalitis, lymphoma, and **progressive multifocal leukoencephalopathy,** a progressive demyelinating disease caused by a JC papovavirus.

Peripheral nervous system manifestations of HIV infection include sensory, motor, and inflammatory polyneuropathies. Almost 33% of patients with advanced HIV disease develop peripheral tingling, numbness, and pain in their extremities. These symptoms are likely to be due to loss of nerve axons from direct neuronal HIV infection. Alcoholism, thyroid disease, syphilis, vitamin B_{12} deficiency, drug toxicity (ddI, ddC), **CMV**-associated ascending polyradiculopathy, and transverse myelitis also cause **peripheral neuropathies.** Less commonly, HIV-infected patients can develop an inflammatory demyelinating polyneuropathy similar to Guillain-Barré syndrome; however, unlike the sensory neuropathies, this inflammatory demyelinating polyneuropathy typically presents before the onset of clinically apparent immunodeficiency. The origin of this condition is not known, although an autoimmune reaction is suspected. **Retinitis** resulting from CMV infection is the most common cause of rapidly progressive visual loss in HIV infection. The diagnosis can be difficult to make because *Toxoplasma gondii* infection, microinfarction, and retinal necrosis can all cause visual loss.

HIV-related malignancies commonly seen in AIDS include Kaposi's sarcoma, non-Hodgkin's lymphoma, primary CNS lymphoma, invasive cervical carcinoma, and anal squamous cell carcinoma. Impairment of immune surveillance and defense and increased exposure to oncogenic viruses appear to contribute to the development of neoplasms.

Kaposi's sarcoma is the most common HIV-associated cancer. In San Francisco, 15–20% of HIV-infected homosexual men develop this tumor during the progression of their disease. Kaposi's sarcoma is uncommon in women and children for reasons that are not clear. Unlike classic Kaposi's sarcoma, which affects elderly men in the Mediterranean, the disease in HIV-infected patients may present with either localized cutaneous lesions or disseminated visceral involvement. It is often a progressive disease, and pulmonary involvement can be fatal. Histologically, the lesions of Kaposi's sarcoma consist of a mixed cell population that includes vascular endothelial cells and spindle cells within a collagen network. Human herpesvirus 8 is associated with Kaposi's sarcoma in patients with AIDS. HIV itself appears to induce cytokines and growth factors that stimulate tumor cell proliferation rather than causing malignant cellular transformation. Clinically, cutaneous Kaposi's sarcoma typically presents as a purplish nodular skin lesion or painless oral lesion. Sites of visceral involvement include the lung, lymph nodes, liver, and GI tract. In the GI tract, Kaposi's sarcoma can produce chronic blood loss or acute hemorrhage. In the lung, it often presents as coarse nodular infiltrates bilaterally, frequently associated with pleural effusions.

Non-Hodgkin's lymphoma is particularly aggressive in HIV-infected patients and usually indicative of significant immune compromise. The majority of these tumors are high-grade B-cell lymphomas with a predilection for dissemination. The CNS is frequently involved either as a primary site or as an extranodal site of widespread disease.

Anal dysplasia and **squamous cell carcinoma** are also more commonly found in HIV-infected homosexual men. These tumors appear to be associated with concomitant anal or rectal infection with human papillomavirus (HPV). In HIV-infected women, the incidence of HPV-related **cervical dysplasia** is as high as 40%, and dysplasia can progress rapidly to **invasive cervical carcinoma.**

Adherence to multidrug regimens remains a challenge, but clearly antiretroviral therapy improves immune function. For reasons that are not clear, HIV-infected patients have an unusually high rate of adverse reactions to a wide variety of antibiotics and frequently develop severe debilitating cutaneous reactions. Drug hypersensitivity and toxicity can be severe, potentially life-threatening, and limiting with certain agents. **Immune reconstitution syndrome** is a described reaction occurring days to weeks after initiation of HAART. Clinical relapse or worsening of mycobacterial, pneumocystis, hepatitis, or neurological infections occurs as a result of a resurgence of immune activity, causing paradoxical worsening of inflammation, possibly as residual antigens or subclinical pathogens are attacked.

Other complications of HIV-infection include arthritides, myopathy, GI syndromes, dysfunction of the adrenal and thyroid glands, hematologic cytopenias, and nephropathy. Since the disease was first described in 1981, medical knowledge of the underlying pathogenesis of AIDS has increased at a rate unprecedented in medical history. This knowledge has led to the rapid development of therapies directed at controlling HIV infection as well as the multitude of complicating opportunistic infections and cancers.

CHECKPOINT

23. What are the major clinical manifestations of AIDS?
24. What are the major steps in development of AIDS after infection with HIV?

CASE STUDIES

Eva M. Aagaard, MD, & Yeong Kwok, MD

(See Chapter 25, p. 674 for Answers)

CASE 7

A 2-month-old child is admitted to the ICU with fever, hypotension, tachycardia, and lethargy. The medical history is notable for a similar hospitalization at 2 weeks of age. Physical examination is notable for a temperature of 39 °C, oral thrush, and rales in the right lung fields. Chest x-ray film reveals multilobar pneumonia. Given the history of recurrent severe infection, the pediatrician suspects an immunodeficiency disorder.

Questions

A. What is the most likely immunodeficiency in this child? Why?
B. What are the underlying genetic and cellular defects associated with this disease?
C. What is the overall prognosis for patients with this disorder?

CASE 8

An 18-month-old boy is brought to the emergency department by his parents with a high fever, shortness of breath, and cough. The boy was well until he was 6 months old. Since then, he has had four bouts of otitis media, and because of their severity and recurrence, he was placed for several months on prophylactic antibiotics. He was recently taken off the antibiotics to see how he would do. The day before presentation, he developed a cough that has quickly progressed into an illness with high fevers and lethargy. Both of his parents are healthy, and he has a healthy older sister. His father's family history is unremarkable, but his maternal uncle died of pneumonia in infancy. Examination is remarkable for a normally developed toddler who is lethargic and tachypneic. His temperature is 39 °C, and he has decreased breath sounds at both lung bases. Chest x-ray film shows consolidation of the right and left lower lobes, as well as bilateral pleural effusions. He is admitted to the hospital, and the boy's blood cultures grow out *Streptococcus pneumoniae* the next day. Immunologic testing shows very low levels of IgG, IgM, and IgA antibodies in the serum, and flow cytometry shows the absence of circulating B lymphocytes.

Questions

A. What is the likely diagnosis in this patient and why?

B. What is the primary pathophysiologic defect in the condition, and how does it lead to this clinical presentation?

C. Why are the affected children generally fine until they reach 4–6 months of age?

CASE 9

An 18-year-old man presents with complaints of fever, facial pain, and nasal congestion consistent with a diagnosis of acute sinusitis. His medical history is notable for multiple sinus infections, two episodes of pneumonia, and chronic diarrhea, all suggestive of primary immunodeficiency syndrome. Workup establishes a diagnosis of common variable immunodeficiency.

Questions

A. What are the common infectious manifestations of common variable immunodeficiency?

B. What are the underlying immunologic abnormalities responsible for these infectious manifestations?

C. What other diseases is this patient at increased risk for?

D. What treatment is indicated?

CASE 10

A 31-year-old male injection drug user presents to the emergency department with a chief complaint of shortness of breath. He describes a 1-month history of intermittent fevers and night sweats associated with a nonproductive cough. He has become progressively more short of breath, initially only with exertion, but now he feels dyspneic at rest. He appears to be in moderate respiratory distress. His vital signs are abnormal, with fever to 39 °C, heart rate of 112 bpm, respiratory rate of 20/minute, and oxygen saturation of 88% on room air. Physical examination is otherwise unremarkable but notable for the absence of abnormal lung sounds. Chest x-ray film reveals a diffuse interstitial infiltrate characteristic of pneumocystis pneumonia, an opportunistic infection.

Questions

A. What is the underlying disease most likely responsible for this man's susceptibility to pneumocystis pneumonia?

B. What is the pathogenesis of the immunosuppression caused by this underlying disease?

C. What is the natural history of this disease? What are some of the common clinical manifestations seen during its progression?

REFERENCES

General

Abbas AK et al (editors). *Cellular and Molecular Immunology*, 6th edition. Saunders, 2007.

Chaplin DD. Overview of the human immune response. J Allergy Clin Immunol. 2006 Feb;117(2 Suppl Mini-Primer):S430–5. [PMID: 16455341]

DeFranco AL et al. *Immunity, The Immune Response in Infectious and Inflammatory Disease*. New Science Press Ltd, 2007.

Jiang H et al. Regulation of immune responses by T cells. N Engl J Med. 2006 Mar 16;354(11):1166–76. [PMID: 16540617]

Middleton E et al (editors). *Allergy: Principles and Practice*, 7th edition. Mosby, 2008.

Mosmann TR et al. Two types of murine helper T cells clone: I. Definition according to profiles of lymphokine activities and secreted proteins. J Immunol. 1986 Apr 1;136(7):2348–57. [PMID: 2419430]

Orange JS et al. Natural killer cells in human health and disease. Clin Immunol. 2006 Jan;118(1):1–10. [PMID: 16337194]

Prussin C et al. IgE, mast cells, basophils and eosinophils. J Allergy Clin Immunol. 2006 Feb;117(2 Suppl Mini-Primer):S450–6. [PMID: 16455345]

Schwartz RS. Shattuck lecture: Diversity of the immune repertoire and immunoregulation. N Engl J Med. 2003 Mar 13;348(11):1017–26. [PMID: 12637612]

Allergic Rhinitis

Broide DH. The pathophysiology of allergic rhinoconjunctivitis. Allergy Asthma Proc. 2007 Jul-Aug;28(4):398–403. [PMID: 17883906]

Cruz AA et al. Common characteristics of upper and lower airways in rhinitis and asthma: ARIA update, in collaboration with GA(2)LEN. Allergy. 2007;62(Suppl 84):1–41. [PMID: 17924930]

Durham SR et al. Long-term clinical efficacy of grass-pollen immunotherapy. N Engl J Med. 1999 Aug 12;341(7):468–75. [PMID: 10441602]

James LK et al. Update on mechanisms of allergen injection immunotherapy. Clin Exp Allergy. 2008 Jul;38(7):1074–88. [PMID: 18691292]

Miyahara S et al. Contribution of allergen-specific and nonspecific nasal responses to early-phase and late-phase nasal responses. J Allergy Clin Immunol. 2008 Mar;121:718–24. [PMID: 18155286]

Kirtsreesakul V et al. Role of allergy in rhinosinusitis. Curr Opin Allergy Clin Immunol. 2004 Feb;4(1):17–23. [PMID: 15090914]

Primary Immunodeficiency Diseases

Bonilla FA et al. Update on primary immunodeficiency diseases. J Allergy Clin Immunol. 2006 Feb;117(2 Suppl Mini-Primer):S435–41. [PMID: 16455342]

Buckley RH: Primary immunodeficiency diseases due to defects in lymphocytes. N Engl J Med. 2000 Nov 2;343(18):1313–24. [PMID: 11058677]

Lekstrom-Himes JA et al. Immunodeficiency diseases caused by defects in phagocytes. N Engl J Med. 2000 Dec 7;343(23):1703–14. [PMID: 11106721]

Primary immunodeficiency diseases. Report of a WHO scientific group. Clin Exp Immunol. 1997 Aug;109(Suppl 1):1–28. [PMID: 9274617]

Sánchez-Ramón S et al. Memory B cells in common variable immunodeficiency: Clinical associations and sex differences. Clin Immunol. 2008 Sep;128(3):314–21. [PMID: 18620909]

Stiehm ER (editor). *Immunologic Disorders in Infants and Children*, 5th edition. Saunders, 2004.

AIDS

Boassa A et al. Chronic innate immune activation as a cause of HIV-1 immunopathogenesis. Clin Immunol. 2008 Mar;126(3):235–42. [PMID: 17916442]

Grossman Z et al. Pathogenesis of HIV infection: What the virus spares is as important as what it destroys. Nat Med. 2006 Mar;12(3):289–95. [PMID: 16520776]

Levy J. *HIV and the Pathogenesis of AIDS*. ASM Press, 2007.

Mientjes G et al. Tuberculosis-associated immune reconstitution inflammatory syndrome: Case definitions for use in resource-limited settings. Lancet Infect Dis. 2008 Aug;8(8):516–23. [PMID: 18652998]

Moir S et al. Pathogenic mechanisms of B-lymphocyte dysfunction in HIV disease. J Allergy Clin Immunol. 2008 Jul;122(1):12–9. [PMID: 18547629]

Zolopa A et al. HIV infection. In: *Current Medical Diagnosis and Treatment 2008*. McPhee SJ, Papadakis M (editors). McGraw-Hill, 2009.

1993 revised classification system for HIV infection and expanded surveillance case definition for AIDS among adolescents and adults. MMWR Morb Mortal Wkly Rep. 1992;41(RR-17):1.

Infectious Diseases

Karen C. Bloch, MD, MPH

Infectious diseases cause significant morbidity and mortality, especially in individuals who are most vulnerable to illness: the very young, the elderly, the immunocompromised, and the disenfranchised.

The pathogenesis of infectious diseases is dependent on the relationship among the human host, the infectious agent, and the external environment. Figure 4–1 portrays a host-agent-environment paradigm for the study of infectious diseases. The infectious agent can be either **exogenous** (ie, not normally found on or in the body) or **endogenous** (ie, one that may be routinely cultured from a particular anatomic site but that does not normally cause disease in the host). Infection results when an exogenous agent is introduced into a host from the environment or when an endogenous agent overcomes innate host immunity to cause disease. Host susceptibility plays an important role in either of these settings.

The environment includes **vectors** (insects and other carriers that transmit infectious agents) and **zoonotic hosts** or **reservoirs** (animals that harbor infectious agents and often act to amplify the infectious agent). For example, the white-footed mouse (*Peromyscus leucopus*) serves as an animal reservoir for *Borrelia burgdorferi*, the bacterium that causes Lyme disease. The *Ixodes* tick serves as an insect vector. Infection in the mouse is asymptomatic, and the bacteria can multiply to high levels in this animal. When the tick larva feeds on an infected mouse, it becomes secondarily infected with *B burgdorferi*, and this infection persists when the tick molts into a nymph. Subsequently, when an infected nymph feeds on a human, the bacterium is transmitted into the host bloodstream, causing disease.

The study of infectious diseases requires understanding of pathogenesis at the level of the population, the individual, the cell, and the gene. For example, at the population level, the spread of tuberculosis in the community is related to the social interactions of an infectious human host. Outbreaks of tuberculosis have occurred in homeless shelters, prisons, bars, and nursing homes when an index case comes in close contact with susceptible persons. At the individual level, tuberculosis results from inhalation of respiratory droplets containing airborne tubercle bacilli. At the cellular level, these bacilli activate T cells, which play a critical role in containing the infection. Individuals with an impaired T-cell response (eg, those infected with HIV) are at particularly high risk for primary tuberculosis at the time of the initial infection or for reactivation of latent tuberculosis as their immunity wanes. Finally, at the genetic level, individuals with specific polymorphisms in a macrophage protein gene may be at significantly higher risk for pulmonary tuberculosis.

Specific microorganisms have a tendency to cause certain types of infections: *Streptococcus pneumoniae* commonly causes pneumonia, meningitis, and bacteremia but rarely causes endocarditis (infection of the heart valves); *Escherichia coli* is a common cause of GI and urinary tract infections; *Plasmodium* species infect red blood cells and liver cells to cause malaria; *Entamoeba histolytica* causes amebic dysentery, liver abscesses, and so on. Table 4–1 presents a clinical approach to taking a patient history that considers features of the host and the environment in identifying the most likely microorganisms associated with specific clinical syndromes.

HOST DEFENSES AGAINST INFECTION

The human body has the ability to control infection through a number of different mechanisms. Physical barriers impede the entry of bacteria from the external environment and from normally colonized sites in the body into sterile anatomic areas. When these physical defenses are breached, the immune system is activated (Figure 4–2). **Constitutive** or **innate im-**

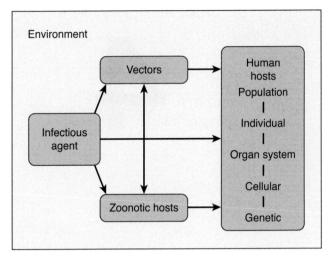

FIGURE 4–1 The fundamental relationships involved in the host-agent-environment interaction model. In the host, pathogenetic mechanisms extend from the level of populations (eg, person-to-person transmission) to the level of cellular and molecular processes (eg, genetic susceptibility).

munity, provided by preformed proteins (eg, complement) and immune cells (eg, phagocytes) that are activated by nonspecific foreign proteins, allows an immediate response to foreign material. **Induced** or **adaptive immunity** includes both early and late adaptive responses activated by specific antigenic proteins (eg, production of antibodies active against the specific strains of *S pneumoniae* contained in the pneumococcal vaccine in a previously vaccinated individual). Induction of these specific immune receptor cells may take several days in the immunologically naive host. **Protective immunity,** which occurs after initial exposure (infection or vaccination) through generation of memory lymphocytes and pathogen-specific antibody, allows a much more rapid response to reinfection. These components of the immune response are discussed in detail later.

NORMAL MICROBIAL FLORA

The human body harbors numerous species of bacteria, viruses, fungi, and protozoa. The great majority of these are **commensals,** or **"normal flora,"** defined as organisms that live

TABLE 4–1 Obtaining a history in the diagnosis of infectious diseases.

Component of History	Host-Specific History	Environmental Features	Agent-Specific History
History of present illness	Age Sex Symptoms: duration, severity, pattern	Site of acquisition: home, nursing home, hospital Season	*Listeria* meningitis in elderly and neonates, but rare in other age groups; influenza epidemics in winter months
Medical history (including medications, allergies, and immunizations)	Immunocompromise (eg, HIV, transplant, steroid use, chemotherapy, asplenia). Comorbid disease (eg, chronic obstructive lung disease, diabetes, alcohol abuse).	Exposure to infectious agents (eg, recent hospitalization, blood transfusion)	*Pneumocystis jirovecii* pneumonia in HIV-infected individuals; *Clostridium difficile* colitis with recent antibiotics
Habits and exposures	Substance use (eg, alcohol, cigarettes, type and route of illicit drug use)	Sexual contacts Outdoor exposure (arthropod-borne infections) Pets	Infections or infectious agents associated with host-specific habits (eg, *S aureus* endocarditis in injection drug users)
Social history	Occupation	Congregated living facility: dormitory, prison, shelter, barracks Homelessness Travel	Hepatitis B virus in a phlebotomist; meningococcal meningitis in a freshman living in a college dormitory
Family history	Tuberculosis, immune deficiency syndromes	Household contacts	Reactivation of latent tuberculosis
Review of systems	Symptoms by organ system: constitutional (fever, chills, night sweats, weight loss); CNS (headache, confusion); cardiovascular system (palpitations); lung (cough, shortness of breath); genitourinary (discharge, dysuria); GI system (abdominal pain, diarrhea); skin (rash)	Break in skin integrity (blood draw, trauma, scratch, acupuncture), prosthetic device (Foley catheter, intrauterine device), dental procedure (cleaning, extraction), endoscopy	Endocarditis after dental manipulation; tetanus infection after piercing with nonsterile needle; acute mononucleosis in patient with fever and sore throat

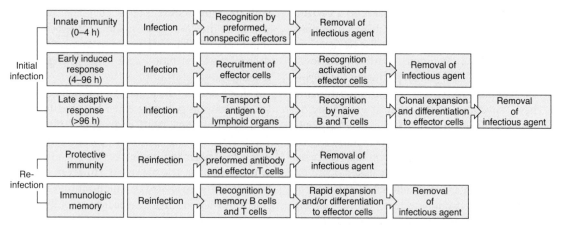

FIGURE 4–2 Phases of the host response to infection. During the earliest stage of initial infection, nonspecific mediators (complement, phagocytes) predominate. Adaptive immunity (production of antibody, stimulation of lymphocytes) requires clonal expansion after recognition of specific antigens. Once immunity toward a specific agent is induced, the immune response remains primed so that the response to reinfection is much more rapid.

symbiotically on or within the human host but rarely cause disease (Figure 4–3). Anatomic sites where bacteria are normally found include the skin (staphylococci and diphtheroids), oropharynx (streptococci, anaerobes), large intestine (enterococci, enteric bacilli), and vagina (lactobacilli).

Determining when an isolate is a component of the normal flora rather than an invasive pathogen may be difficult. For example, culture of staphylococci from a blood sample may represent skin contamination at the time of phlebotomy or may indicate a potentially life-threatening bloodstream infec-

tion. Helpful clues include symptoms and signs of infection (eg, cough, fever) and the presence of inflammatory cells (eg, polymorphonuclear cells in the sputum and an increased proportion of immature neutrophils in the blood). Isolation of an **obligate pathogen** such as *Mycobacterium tuberculosis* from any site is diagnostic of infection. Fortunately, few microorganisms are absolute pathogens. For example, *Neisseria meningitidis*, a major bacterial cause of meningitis, can be cultured from the oropharynx of as many as 10% of asymptomatic individuals, in which case it represents transient normal

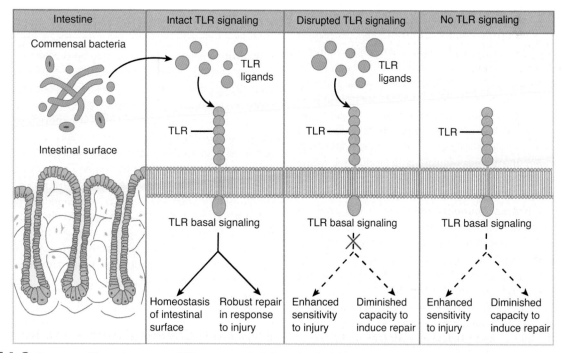

FIGURE 4–3 Commensal bacteria secrete toll-like receptor (TLR) ligands, which bind to TLR on the surface of normal intestinal tissue. This interaction stimulates basal signaling, which protects against cellular injury. Disruption of TLR signaling or antibiotic associated eradication of commensal bacteria result in compromised ability of the intestinal epithelium to withstand injury and repair cell damage. (Redrawn, with permission, from Madara J. Building an intestine—Architectural contributions of commensal bacteria. N Engl J Med. 2004;351:1686.)

flora. Even if asymptomatic, the host can serve as a **carrier,** transferring bacteria to susceptible individuals. Infections resulting from commensals that rarely cause disease (eg, *Candida albicans*) or organisms ubiquitous in the environment that are generally not considered human pathogens (eg, *Mycobacterium avium* complex; MAC) are termed **opportunistic infections.** These infections occur almost exclusively in **immunocompromised hosts** such as HIV-infected patients or transplant recipients. The agents are opportunists in that they take advantage of impaired host immunity to cause infection but rarely cause disease in a healthy host.

The site from which an organism is cultured is important in differentiating colonization from infection. Growth of any microorganism from a normally sterile site such as blood, cerebrospinal fluid, synovial (joint) fluid, or deep tissues of the body is diagnostic of infection. For example, *Bacteroides,* the predominant genus of bacteria in the colon, may cause intra-abdominal abscesses and sepsis when the integrity of the colonic mucosa is breached. *Staphylococcus epidermidis,* a common skin commensal, can cause bacteremia after intravascular catheter placement. Knowledge of the common endogenous flora may be useful in determining the cause of an infection and may aid in the choice of empiric antibiotic therapy.

When the delicate symbiosis between the commensal and the host is disturbed, the normal flora may be overgrown by either endogenous or exogenous organisms. This phenomenon, which may be transient or persistent, is called **colonization.** For example, broad-spectrum antibiotics will destroy normal vaginal flora, such as lactobacilli, and allow overgrowth of *Candida* (yeast) species. When replacement of the normal flora occurs in the hospital environment, the colonizers are said to be **nosocomially acquired.** The distinction between hospital-acquired and community-acquired infections has blurred in recent years, because of an increase in medical care in the home or skilled nursing facility among patients who previously would have required long-term hospitalization. For this reason, the broader term "healthcare-associated infections" is used to encompass both hospitalized patients and patients with frequent medical interactions (eg, residence in nursing home, outpatient hemodialysis, home intravenous antibiotics). Healthcare-associated infections are significant because the organisms are often resistant to multiple antibiotics. Not uncommonly, colonization will progress to symptomatic infection. For example, individuals hospitalized for extended periods often become colonized with gram-negative bacteria such as *Pseudomonas aeruginosa.* These individuals are then at increased risk for life-threatening infections such as pseudomonas pneumonia.

Host defense mechanisms that serve to inhibit colonization by pathogenic bacteria include (1) mechanical clearance, (2) phagocytic killing, and (3) depriving organisms of necessary nutrients. Successful colonizers have adapted to evade or overcome these defenses. For example, gonococci, the bacteria that cause gonorrhea, avoid excretion in the urine by adhering to the mucosal epithelium of the urogenital tract

with pili. Pneumococci resist phagocytosis by encapsulation within a slime layer that impairs uptake by neutrophils. Some staphylococci elaborate enzymes known as hemolysins that destroy host red blood cells, thus giving them access to a needed source of iron.

Colonization of sites that are normally sterile or have very few microbes is generally easier because there is no competition for nutrients from endogenous flora. However, host defenses at these sites are often vigorous. For instance, the stomach is normally sterile because few microbes can survive at the normal gastric pH of 4.0. However, if antacids are used to decrease gastric acidity, colonization of the stomach and trachea with gram-negative bacteria rapidly occurs.

The normal flora prevents colonization through numerous mechanisms. These organisms often have a selective advantage over colonizers in that they are already established in an anatomic niche. This means that they are bound to receptors on the host cell and are able to metabolize local nutrients. Many species of the normal flora are able to produce bacteriocins, proteins that are toxic to other bacterial strains or species. Finally, the normal flora promotes production of antibodies that may cross-react with colonizing organisms. For instance, an antibody produced against *E coli*, a gram-negative bacterium normally found in the large intestine, cross-reacts with the polysaccharide capsule of a meningitis-producing strain of *N meningitidis.* When the normal flora is altered (eg, by the administration of broad-spectrum antibiotics), one bacterial species may predominate or exogenous bacteria may gain a selective advantage, permitting colonization and predisposing the host to infection.

CONSTITUTIVE DEFENSES OF THE BODY

Constitutive defenses of the human body are nonspecific barriers against infectious diseases that do not require prior contact with the microorganism. These defenses consist of simple physical (eg, skin) and chemical (eg, acidic gastric secretions) barriers that prevent easy entry of microorganisms into the body. Some infectious agents use a vector (such as an insect) to bypass structural barriers and gain direct access to the blood or subcutaneous tissues of the body. Once an agent has entered the body, the major constitutive defenses are the acute inflammatory response and the complement system. These defenses can neutralize the agent, recruit phagocytic cells, and induce a more specific response through humoral and cell-mediated immunity. The constitutive defenses of the body are important from an evolutionary perspective in enabling humans to encounter and adapt to a variety of new and changing environments.

Physical & Chemical Barriers to Infection

The squamous epithelium of the skin is the first line of defense against microorganisms encountered in the outside world. As keratinized epithelial surface cells desquamate, the skin maintains its protective barrier by generating new epithelial cells beneath the surface. The skin is also bathed with oils and moisture from the sebaceous and sweat glands. These secretions contain fatty acids that inhibit bacterial growth. Poor vascular supply to the skin may result in skin breakdown and increased susceptibility to infection. For example, chronically debilitated or bedridden patients may suffer from decubitus ulcers as a result of constant pressure on dependent body parts, predisposing to severe infections by otherwise harmless skin flora.

The mucous membranes also provide a physical barrier to microbial invasion. The mucous membranes of the mouth, pharynx, esophagus, and lower urinary tract are composed of several layers of epithelial cells, whereas those of the lower respiratory tract, the GI tract, and the upper urinary tract are delicate single layers of epithelial cells. These membranes are covered by a protective layer of mucus, which traps foreign particles and prevents them from reaching the lining epithelial cells. Because the mucus is hydrophilic, many substances produced by the body easily diffuse to the surface, including enzymes with antimicrobial activity such as lysozyme and peroxidase.

Inflammatory Response

When a microorganism crosses the epidermis or the epithelial surface of the mucous membranes, it encounters other components of the host constitutive defenses. These responses are constitutive because they are nonspecific and do not require prior contact with the organism to be effective. Clinically, signs of inflammation (heat, erythema, pain, and swelling) are the characteristic features of localized infection, secondary tissue injury, and the body's response to this injury. Blood supply to the affected area increases in response to vasodilation, and the capillaries become more permeable, allowing antibodies, complement, and white blood cells to cross the endothelium and reach the site of injury. An important consequence of inflammation is that the pH of the inflamed tissues is lowered, creating an inhospitable environment for the microbe. The increased blood flow to the area allows continued recruitment of inflammatory cells as well as the necessary components for tissue repair and recovery.

When a microorganism enters host tissue, it activates the complement system and components of the coagulation cascade and induces the release of chemical mediators of the inflammatory response. These mediators result in the increased vascular permeability and vasodilation characteristic of inflammation. For example, the anaphylatoxins C3a, C4a, and C5a, produced by the activation of complement, stimulate the release of histamine from mast cells. Histamine dilates the blood vessels and further increases their permeability. Bradykinin is also released, increasing vascular permeability.

Proinflammatory cytokines include interleukin-1 (IL-1), IL-6, tumor necrosis factor, and interferon-γ. These factors, singly or in combination, promote fever, produce local inflammatory signs, and trigger catabolic responses. During severe infection, hepatic synthesis of proteins is altered, lead-

ing to an increase in proteins described as "**acute-phase** reactants." Typically, serum albumin concentration is reduced, whereas rheumatoid factor, C-reactive protein, ferritin, and various proteinase inhibitors increase. Serum levels of zinc and iron decrease at the same time, and the erythrocyte sedimentation rate, a nonspecific marker of inflammation, rises. A catabolic state is further augmented by simultaneous increases in levels of circulating cortisol, glucagon, catecholamines, and other hormones.

Mild to moderate inflammatory responses serve important host defense functions. For example, elevated body temperature may inhibit viral replication. Inflammatory hyperemia and systemic neutrophilia optimize phagocyte delivery to sites of infection. The decreased availability of iron inhibits the growth of microbes such as *Yersinia* that require this element as a nutrient. However, when the inflammatory responses become extreme, extensive tissue damage can result, as in the case of sepsis.

Complement System

The complement system is composed of a series of plasma protein and cell membrane receptors that are important mediators of host defenses and inflammation (Figure 4–4). Most of the biologically significant effects of the complement system are mediated by the third component (C3) and the terminal components (C5–9). To carry out their host defense and inflammatory functions, C3 and C5–9 must first be activated. Two pathways of complement activation have been recognized and have been termed the **classic** and **alternative** pathways. The classic pathway is activated by antigen-antibody complexes or antibody-coated particles, and the alternative pathway is activated by mechanisms independent of antibodies, usually by interaction with bacterial surface components. Both pathways form C3 convertase, which cleaves the C3 component of complement, a key protein common to both pathways. The two pathways then proceed in identical fashion to bind late-acting components to form a membrane attack complex (C5–9), which results in target cell lysis.

Once activated, complement functions to enhance the antimicrobial defenses in several ways. Complement facilitates phagocytosis through proteins called **opsonins,** which coat invading microorganisms, making them susceptible to engulfment and destruction by neutrophils and macrophages. The complement-derived membrane attack complex inserts itself into the membrane of a target organism, leading to increased permeability and subsequent lysis of the cell. Complement also acts indirectly through production of substances that are chemotactic for white blood cells and through promotion of the inflammatory response.

Inherited disorders of complement are associated with an increased risk of bacterial infection. The specific infections seen in complement-deficient patients relate to the biologic functions of the missing component (Figure 4–4). Patients with a deficiency of C3 or of a component in either of the two pathways necessary for the activation of C3 typically

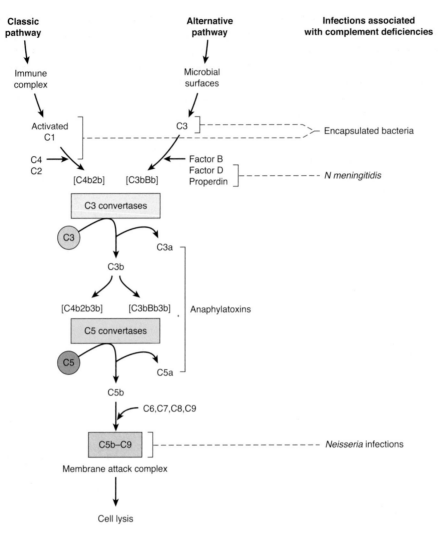

FIGURE 4–4 Complement reaction sequence and infections associated with deficiency states. (Redrawn, with permission, from Nairn R. Immunology. In: *Jawetz, Melnick, and Adelberg's Medical Microbiology,* 23rd ed. Brooks GF, Butel JS, Morse SA [editors]. McGraw-Hill, 2004.)

have increased susceptibility to infections with encapsulated bacteria such as *S pneumoniae* and *Haemophilus influenzae*. In contrast, patients with deficiencies of C5–9 have normal resistance to encapsulated bacteria because C3b-mediated opsonization is intact. These patients, however, are unusually susceptible to life-threatening infections with *N meningitidis* and *N gonorrhoeae* because they are unable to form a membrane attack complex and, therefore, cannot lyse the *Neisseria* cell membrane.

Phagocytosis

After the natural barriers of the skin or mucous membranes have been penetrated, the phagocytic cells—neutrophils, monocytes, and macrophages—constitute the next line of host defense. The process of internalizing organisms by these cells (**phagocytosis**) involves attachment of the organism to the cell surface. This triggers extension of a pseudopod to enclose the bacterium in an endocytic vesicle, or **phagosome.** The circu-

lating polymorphonuclear neutrophil (PMN) is an important component of the host immune response that in the absence of infection circulates in a quiescent state. When chemotactic factors, arachidonic acid metabolites, or complement cleavage fragments interact with specific PMN membrane receptors, the neutrophil rapidly becomes activated and moves toward the chemoattractants. After phagocytosis, the mechanisms by which the phagolysosome destroys the microorganism can be divided into oxygen-independent and oxygen-dependent processes. Functional defects or quantitative deficiencies of neutrophils are important risk factors for infection.

Neutropenia, defined as an absolute neutrophil count of < 1000 cells/μL, is a common predisposing factor for life-threatening bacterial and fungal infections. The risk of infection is inversely proportionate to the number of neutrophils, rising significantly with neutrophil counts < 500 cells/μL. The longer the duration of profound neutropenia, the greater is the risk of infection. At the first sign of infection (eg, fever), these patients should be given broad-spectrum antibacterial agents to cover gram-negative bacterial pathogens. In addition to impaired immunity, neutropenic hosts often have additional risk factors for infection such as the need for long-term indwelling central venous catheters (predisposing to staphylococcal and candidal infection) and the frequent use of hyperalimentation (predisposing to fungal infection due to *Malassezia furfur*).

Several inherited disorders of neutrophil function have been described. **Chédiak-Higashi syndrome** is a rare autosomal recessive hereditary disorder in which the neutrophils have a profound defect in the formation of intracellular granules. Opsonized bacteria such as *S aureus* are ingested normally, but viable bacteria persist intracellularly, presumably because of the inability of the neutrophil's intracellular granules to fuse with phagosomes to form phagolysosomes. Patients with Chédiak-Higashi syndrome experience recurrent bacterial infections, most frequently involving the skin and soft tissues and the upper and lower respiratory tracts.

Myeloperoxidase deficiency is the most common neutrophil disorder, with a prevalence of one case per 2000 individuals. In this disorder, phagocytosis, chemotaxis, and degranulation are normal, but microbicidal activity for bacteria is delayed. In general, these patients do not suffer from recurrent infections. In contrast, **chronic granulomatous disease** is a genetically heterogeneous group of inherited disorders characterized by the failure of phagocytic cells to produce superoxides. The defect involves neutrophils, monocytes, eosinophils, and some macrophages. Oxygen-dependent intracellular killing is impaired, and these patients are susceptible to recurrent, often life-threatening infections. Patients with chronic granulomatous disease also tend to form granulomas in tissues, particularly in the lungs, liver, and spleen, and are particularly susceptible to infection with *S aureus* and *Aspergillus* species.

INDUCED DEFENSES OF THE BODY

Although constitutive host defenses against infectious agents are generally nonspecific and do not require prior exposure to the invading agent, induced defenses are highly specific and are qualitatively and quantitatively altered by prior antigenic exposure. Details of the pathophysiology of the host immune system are covered in Chapter 3. Infections associated with common defects in the induced immune response are shown in Table 4–2.

ESTABLISHMENT OF INFECTIOUS DISEASES

An infectious disease occurs when a pathogenic organism causes inflammation or organ dysfunction. This may be caused directly by the infection itself, as when the etiologic agent

TABLE 4–2 **Infections associated with common defects in humoral and cellular immune response.**

Host Defect in Immune Response	Examples of Immune Defect States	Common Etiologic Agents of Infections
T-lymphocyte deficiency or dysfunction	Thymic aplasia, hypoplasia	*Listeria monocytogenes, Mycobacterium tuberculosis, Candida, Aspergillus, Cryptococcus neoformans,* herpes simplex, herpes zoster
	Solid organ transplant	
	Corticosteroid use	
	Pregnancy	
	AIDS	*Pneumocystis jiroveci,* cytomegalovirus, herpes simplex, *Mycobacterium avium* complex, *C neoformans, Candida*
B-cell deficiency or dysfunction	Bruton's X-linked agammaglobulinemia	*Streptococcus pneumoniae,* other streptococci, *Haemophilus influenzae, Neisseria meningitidis, Staphylococcus aureus, Klebsiella pneumoniae, Escherichia coli, Giardia lamblia, P jiroveci,* enteroviruses
	Agammaglobulinemia	
	Chronic lymphocytic leukemia	
	Multiple myeloma	
	Selective IgA deficiency	*G lamblia,* hepatitis viruses, *S pneumoniae, H influenzae*
Mixed T- and B-cell deficiency or dysfunction	Common variable hypogammaglobulinemia	*P jiroveci,* cytomegalovirus, *S pneumoniae, H influenzae,* various other bacteria
	Ataxia-telangiectasia	*S pneumoniae, H influenzae, S aureus, G lamblia*
	Severe combined immunodeficiency	*S aureus, S pneumoniae, Candida albicans, P jiroveci,* varicella virus, rubella virus, cytomegalovirus

Modified and reproduced, with permission, from Madoff LC, Kasper DL. Introduction to infectious diseases: Host-parasite interaction. In: *Harrison's Principles of Internal Medicine,* 14th ed. Fauci AS et al (editors). McGraw-Hill, 1998.

multiplies in the host, or indirectly as a result of the host's inflammatory response. Many infections are subclinical, not producing any obvious manifestations of disease. To cause overt infection, all microorganisms must go through the following stages (Table 4–3): The microorganism must (1) **encounter** the host, (2) **gain entry** into the host, (3) **multiply and spread** from the site of entry, and (4) **cause host tissue injury,** either directly (eg, cytotoxins) or indirectly (host inflammatory response). The severity of infection ranges from asymptomatic to life threatening, and the course may be characterized as acute, subacute, or chronic. Whether infection is subclinical or overt, the outcome is either (1) resolution (eg, eradication of the infecting pathogen), (2) chronic active infection (eg, HIV or hepatitis), (3) prolonged asymptomatic excretion of the agent (eg, carrier state with *Salmonella typhi*), (4) latency of the agent within host tissues (eg, latent tuberculosis), or (5) host death from infection.

Except for **congenital infections** (acquired in utero) caused by agents such as rubella virus, *T pallidum*, and cytomegalovirus, human beings first encounter microorganisms at birth. During parturition, the newborn comes into contact with microorganisms present in the mother's vaginal canal and on her skin. Most of the bacteria the newborn encounters do not cause harm, and for those that might cause infection, the newborn usually has **passive immunity** through antibodies acquired from the mother in utero. For example, neonates are protected against infection with *H influenzae* by maternal antibodies for the first 6 months of life until passive immunity wanes and the risk of infection with this bacterium increases. On the other hand, newborns whose mothers are vaginally colonized with group B streptococci are at increased risk in the perinatal period for serious infections such as sepsis or meningitis with this organism.

Direct entry into the host (ie, bypassing the usual chemical and physical barriers) occurs via **penetration.** This may occur when (1) an insect vector directly inoculates the infectious agent into the host (mosquitoes transmitting malaria), (2) bacteria gain direct access to host tissues through loss of integrity of the skin or mucous membranes (trauma or surgical wounds), or (3) microbes gain access via instruments or catheters that allow communication between usually sterile sites and the outside world (eg, indwelling venous catheters). **Ingression** occurs when an infectious agent enters the host via an orifice contiguous with the external environment. This primarily involves inhalation of infectious aerosolized droplets (*M tuberculosis*) or ingestion of contaminated foods (salmonella, hepatitis A virus).

Other infectious agents directly infect mucous membranes or cross the epithelial surface to cause infection. This commonly occurs in sexually transmitted diseases. For example, HIV can cross vaginal mucous membranes by penetration of virus-laden macrophages from semen.

After the initial encounter with the host, the infectious agent must successfully multiply at the site of entry. The process whereby the newly introduced microorganism successfully competes with normal flora and is able to multiply is termed **colonization** (eg, pneumococci colonizing the upper respiratory tract). When the microorganism multiplies at a usually sterile site, it is termed **infection** (eg, pneumococci multiplying

TABLE 4–3 The establishment and outcome of infectious diseases.

Stage of Infection	Factors Influencing Stage of Infection
Encounter	Host immune state
	Exogenous (colonization)
	Endogenous (normal flora)
Entry	Ingress
	Inhalation
	Ingestion
	Mucous membrane entry
	Penetration
	Insect bites
	Cuts and wounds
	Iatrogenic (intravenous catheters)
Multiplication and spread	Inoculum size
	Physical factors
	Microbial nutrition
	Anatomic factors
	Microbial sanctuary
	Microbial virulence factors
Injury	Mechanical
	Cell death
	Microbial product induced
	Host induced
	Inflammation
	Immune response
	Humoral immunity
	Cellular immunity
Course of infection	Asymptomatic versus life threatening
	Acute versus subacute versus chronic
Outcome of infection	Resolution (self-limited)
	Chronic
	Carrier state (saprophytic versus parasitic)
	Latent → Reactivation
	Death

Adapted in part, with permission, from Schaechter M, Medoff G, Eisenstein BI (editors). *Mechanisms of Microbial Disease,* 3rd ed. Lippincott Williams & Wilkins, 1999.

in the alveoli, causing pneumonia). Factors that facilitate the multiplication and spread of infection include inoculum size (the quantity of infectious organisms introduced), host anatomic factors (eg, impaired ciliary function in children with cystic fibrosis), availability of nutrients for the microbe, physicochemical factors (eg, gastric pH), microbial virulence factors, and microbial sanctuary (eg, abscesses). An abscess is a special case in which the host has contained the infection but is unable to eradicate it, and these localized infections generally require surgical drainage. Once introduced, infections can spread along the epidermis (impetigo), along the dermis (erysipelas), along subcutaneous tissues (cellulitis), along fascial planes (necrotizing fasciitis), into muscle tissue (myositis), along veins (suppurative thrombophlebitis), into the blood (bacteremia, fungemia, viremia, etc), along lymphatics (lymphangitis), and into organs (eg, pneumonia, brain abscesses, hepatitis).

Infections cause direct injury to the host through a variety of mechanisms. If organisms are present in sufficient numbers and are of sufficient size, **mechanical obstruction** can occur (eg, children with roundworm GI infections may present with bowel obstruction). More commonly, pathogens cause an intense secondary **inflammatory response,** which may result in life-threatening complications (eg, children with *H influenzae* epiglottitis may present with mechanical airway obstruction secondary to intense soft tissue swelling of the epiglottis). Some bacteria produce **neurotoxins** that affect host cell metabolism rather than directly causing cell damage (eg, tetanus toxin antagonizes inhibitory neurons, causing unopposed motor neuron stimulation, manifested clinically as sustained muscle rigidity). Host cell death can occur by a variety of mechanisms. *Shigella* produces a **cytotoxin** that causes death of large intestine enterocytes, resulting in the clinical syndrome of dysentery. Poliovirus-induced cell lysis of the anterior horn cells of the spinal cord causes flaccid paralysis. Gram-negative bacterial **endotoxin** can initiate a cascade of cytokine release, resulting in sepsis syndrome and septic shock.

The time course of an infection can be characterized as **acute, subacute,** or **chronic,** and its severity may vary from asymptomatic to life threatening. Many infections that begin as mild and easily treatable conditions readily progress without prompt treatment. Small, seemingly insignificant skin abrasions superinfected with toxic shock syndrome toxin (TSST-1)-producing *S aureus* can result in fulminant infection and death. Even indolent infections, such as infective

endocarditis resulting from *Streptococcus viridans*, can be fatal unless they are recognized and appropriately treated.

There are three potential outcomes of infection: recovery, chronic infection, and death. Most infections resolve, either spontaneously (eg, rhinovirus, the leading cause of the common cold) or with medical therapy (eg, after treatment of streptococcal pharyngitis with penicillin). Chronic infections may be either **saprophytic,** in which case the organism does not adversely affect the health of the host; or **parasitic,** causing tissue damage to the host. An example of the former is *Salmonella typhi*, which may be harbored asymptomatically in the gallbladder of about 2% of individuals after acute infection. Chronic infection with the hepatitis B virus may be either saprophytic, in which case the human host is infectious for the virus but has no clinical evidence of liver damage, or parasitic, with progressive liver damage and cirrhosis. A final form of chronic infection is tissue **latency.** Varicella-zoster virus, the agent causing chickenpox, survives in the dorsal root ganglia, with reactivation causing a dermatomal eruption with vesicles or shallow ulcerations, commonly known as shingles. When the ability of the immune system to control either the acute or the chronic infection is exceeded, the infection may result in **host death.** Table 4–4 summarizes some microbial strategies to overcome host immune defenses. A unifying theme is that all infectious agents, regardless of specific mechanisms, must successfully reproduce and evade host defense mechanisms. This knowledge helps the physician to prevent infections (eg, vaccinate against influenza virus); when infection occurs, to treat and cure (eg, antibiotics for *E coli* urinary tract infection); and when infection cannot be cured, to prevent further transmission, recurrence, or reactivation (eg, barrier protection to reduce the sexual spread of genital herpes simplex infection).

CHECKPOINT

1. By what three general mechanisms do hosts resist colonization by pathogenic bacteria?

2. What are three ways in which the normal flora contributes to the balance between health and disease?

3. Which specific host defenses against infection do not require prior contact with the infecting organism?

4. What are the categories of outcomes from an infection?

PATHOPHYSIOLOGY OF SELECTED INFECTIOUS DISEASE SYNDROMES

INFECTIVE ENDOCARDITIS

Clinical Presentation

Infective endocarditis refers to a bacterial or, rarely, a fungal infection of the cardiac valves. Infection of extracardiac endothelium is termed "endarteritis" and can cause disease that is

clinically similar to endocarditis. The most common predisposing factor for infective endocarditis is the presence of structurally abnormal cardiac valves. Consequently, patients with a history of rheumatic or congenital heart disease, mitral valve prolapse with an audible murmur, a prosthetic heart valve, or a history of prior endocarditis are at increased risk for infective endocarditis. Infection involves the left side of the

TABLE 4–4 Selection of microbial strategies against host immune defenses.

Host Defense Action	Microbial Counteraction	Example
Complement actions	Masking of complement-activating substances	*Staphylococcus aureus,* surface capsule
		Meningococcus, coating with IgA
	Inhibition of surface complement activation	*Schistosoma mansoni,* decay-accelerating factors
	Inhibition of action of membrane attack complex	*Salmonella,* long surface O antigen
	Inactivation of complement chemotaxin C5a	*Pseudomonas aeruginosa*
Phagocytic actions	Inhibition of phagocyte recruitment	*Bordetella pertussis,* toxin paralysis of chemotaxis
	Microbial killing of phagocytes	*P aeruginosa,* leukocidins
	Escape from phagocytosis	Staphylococci, surface protein A
	Survival after phagocytosis	Trypanosomes, enter cytoplasm
		Rickettsiae, enter cytoplasm
		Mycobacterium tuberculosis, inhibit lysosome fusion
		Chlamydia psittaci, inhibit lysosome fusion
		Legionella, inhibit lysosome fusion
	Inhibition of phagocyte oxidative pathway	Staphylococci, catalase production against H_2O_2
Cell-mediated immunity	CD4 T-cell depletion	HIV
	Decreased B-cell immunoglobulin production	Measles virus
	Inhibition of lymphokine synthesis	Leishmania
Humoral-mediated immunity	Changing of surface antigens	Influenza virus
		Neisseria gonorrhoeae
		Trypanosoma brucei
	Proteolysis of antibodies	*Haemophilus influenzae,* IgA proteases
Humoral and cell-mediated immunity	DNA incorporation into host genome	Herpes simplex
		Herpes zoster

Modified and reproduced, with permission, from Schaechter M, Eisenstein BI, Engleberg NC (editors). The parasite's way of life. In: *Mechanisms of Microbial Disease,* 3rd ed. Lippincott Williams & Wilkins, 1999.

heart (mitral and aortic valves) almost exclusively, except in patients who are injection drug users or, less commonly, in patients with valve injury from a pulmonary artery (Swan-Ganz) catheter, in whom infection of the right side of the heart (tricuspid or pulmonary valve) may occur.

Etiology

The most common infectious agents causing native valve infective endocarditis are gram-positive bacteria, including *Streptococcus viridans, S aureus,* and enterococci. The specific bacterial species causing endocarditis can often be anticipated on the basis of host factors. Injection drug users commonly introduce *S aureus* into the blood when nonsterile needles are used or the skin is not adequately cleaned before needle insertion. Patients with recent dental work are at risk for transient bacteremia with normal oral flora, particularly *S viridans,* with subsequent endocarditis. Genitourinary tract infections with enterococci may lead to bacteremia and subsequent seeding of damaged heart valves. Patients with prosthetic heart valves are also at increased risk for infective endocarditis resulting from skin flora such as *S epidermidis* or *S aureus.* Before the availability of antibiotics, infective endocarditis was a progressively fatal disease. Even with antibiotics, the case fatality rate for endocarditis approaches 25%, and definitive cure often requires both prolonged antibiotic administration and urgent surgery to replace infected cardiac valves.

Pathogenesis

Several hemodynamic factors predispose patients to endocarditis: (1) a high-velocity jet stream causing turbulent blood flow, (2) flow from a high-pressure to a low-pressure chamber, and (3) a comparatively narrow orifice separating the two chambers that creates a pressure gradient. The lesions of infective endocarditis tend to form on the surface of the valve in the cardiac chamber with the lower pressure (eg, on the ventricular surface of an abnormal aortic valve and on the atrial surface of an abnormal mitral valve). Endothelium damaged by turbulent blood flow results in exposure of extracellular matrix proteins, promoting the deposition of fibrin and platelets, which form sterile vegetations (**nonbacterial thrombotic endocarditis or marantic endocarditis**). Infective endocarditis occurs when microorganisms are deposited onto these sterile vegetations during the course of bacteremia (Figure 4–5). Not all bacteria adhere equally well to these sites. For example, *E coli*, a frequent cause of bacteremia, is rarely implicated as a cause of endocarditis. Conversely, virulent organisms such as *S aureus* can invade intact endothelium, causing endocarditis in the absence of preexisting valvular abnormalities.

Once infected, these vegetations continue to enlarge through further deposition of platelets and fibrin, providing the bacteria a sanctuary from host defense mechanisms such as polymorphonuclear leukocytes and complement. Consequently, once infection takes hold, the infected vegetation continues to grow in a largely unimpeded fashion. Prolonged administration (4–6 weeks) of bactericidal antibiotics is required to penetrate the vegetation and cure this disease. Bacteriostatic antimicrobial agents, which inhibit but do not kill the bacteria, are inadequate. Surgical removal of the infected valve is sometimes required for cure, particularly for infections with gram-negative bacilli or fungi, if there is mechanical dysfunction of the valve with resultant congestive heart failure, or in prosthetic valve infections.

A hallmark of infective endocarditis is persistent bacteremia, which stimulates both the humoral and cellular immune systems. A variety of immunoglobulins are expressed, resulting in immune complex formation, increased serum levels of rheumatoid factor, and nonspecific hypergammaglobulinemia. Immune complex deposition along the renal glomerular basement membrane may result in the development of acute glomerulonephritis and renal failure.

Clinical Manifestations

Infective endocarditis is a multisystem disease with protean manifestations. For these reasons, the symptoms can be nonspecific and the diagnosis may not be initially included in the differential diagnosis. Table 4–5 summarizes the important features of the history, physical examination, laboratory results, and complications of infective endocarditis. Cutaneous findings suggestive of endocarditis include Osler's nodes, painful papules on the pads of the fingers and

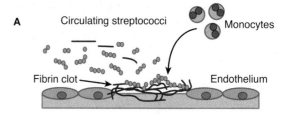
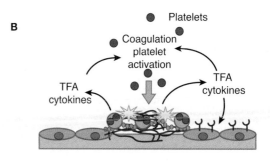
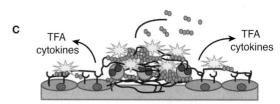

FIGURE 4–5 Pathogenesis of bacterial valve colonization. Viridans group streptococci adhere to fibrin-platelet clots that form at the site of damaged cardiac endothelium (**A**). The fibrin-adherent streptococci activate monocytes to produce tissue factor activity (TFA) and cytokines (**B**). These mediators activate the coagulation pathway, resulting in further recruitment of platelets and growth of the vegetation (**C**). (Redrawn, with permission, from Moreillon P et al. Pathogenesis of streptococcal and staphylococcal endocarditis. Infect Dis Clin North Am. 2002;16:297.)

toes thought to be secondary to deposition of immune complexes; and Janeway lesions, painless hemorrhagic lesions on the palms and soles caused by septic microemboli (Figure 4–6). Symptoms and signs of endocarditis may be acute, subacute, or chronic. The clinical manifestations reflect primarily (1) hemodynamic changes from valvular damage; (2) end-organ symptoms and signs from septic emboli (right-sided emboli to the lungs, left-sided emboli to the brain, spleen, kidney, and extremities); (3) end-organ symptoms and signs from immune complex deposition; and (4) persistent bacteremia with metastatic seeding of infection (abscesses or septic joints). Death is usually caused by hemodynamic collapse or by septic emboli to the CNS, resulting in brain abscesses or mycotic aneurysms and intracerebral hemorrhage. Risk factors for a fatal outcome include left-sided valvular infection, bacterial etiology other than *S viridans*, medical comorbidities, complications from endocarditis (congestive heart failure, valve ring abscess, or embolic disease), and, in one study, medical management without valvular surgery.

TABLE 4–5 Diagnosis of infective endocarditis and its complications.

History	Physical Examination	Laboratory Data	Complications
Fever, chills, fatigue, malaise (nonspecific constitutional symptoms; can be acute, subacute, or chronic)	"Ill appearing"	Positive blood cultures	**Systemic**
	Fever	↑ White blood cell count	Persistent bacteremia
	Tachycardia	↑ Erythrocyte sedimentation rate	Sepsis syndrome
	Hypotension	↑ Rheumatoid factor	
Headaches	Papilledema	Head CT or MRI	**CNS**
Back pain	Focal vertebral spinal tenderness	Spinal MRI	Cerebral emboli
Focal weakness	Focal neurologic exam (weakness, hyperreflexia, positive Babinski's sign, etc)		Mycotic aneurysm (with or without hemorrhage)
			Vertebral osteomyelitis
			Epidural abscess
Dyspnea	↑ Jugular venous pressure	Chest radiograph	**Cardiovascular (with left-sided endocarditis)**
Orthopnea	Cardiac murmurs	Electrocardiogram	Mitral regurgitation
Pedal edema	Quincke's pulses (AR)	Transthoracic echocardiogram	Aortic regurgitation
	Water-hammer pulses (AR)	Transesophageal echocardiogram	Congestive heart failure
	Rales		Valve ring abscess
	Hepatojugular reflux		Pericarditis
Pleuritic chest pain, cough	Crackles	Chest radiograph	**Pulmonary (with right-sided endocarditis)**
	Pleural rub		Septic pulmonary emboli
Flank pain	Flank tenderness	↑ BUN, ↑ creatinine	**Renal**
Discolored (brown) urine		Pyuria	Immune-complex glomerulonephritis
Oliguria		Hematuria	
		Renal sonogram	Renal artery emboli
			Intrarenal abscess
			Perinephric abscess
Abdominal pain	Focal abdominal tenderness	Abdominal sonogram	**GI**
	Hepatomegaly	Abdominal CT	Liver abscesses
	Splenomegaly		Splenic abscesses
			Intestinal artery emboli (intestinal ischemia)
Rashes	Janeway lesions (painless hemorrhagic macules on hands and soles)	Skin biopsies (low yield for diagnosis)	**Skin, miscellaneous**
Focal painful lesions			Septic emboli
Visual complaints	Splinter hemorrhages (nail beds)		Immune complex vasculitis
	Subconjunctival hemorrhage		
	Petechiae		
	Osler's nodes (painful nodules)		
	Roth spots (funduscopic examination)		

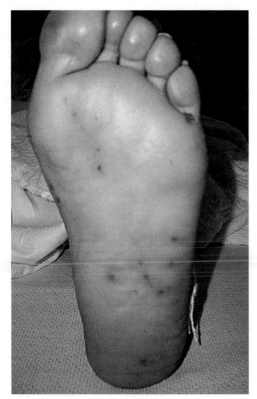

FIGURE 4–6 Osler's node causing pain within pulp of the big toe in a woman hospitalized with acute bacterial endocarditis. (Osler's nodes are painful: remember "O" for Ouch and Osler.) Note the multiple painless flat Janeway lesions over the sole of the foot. (Used with permission from David A. Kasper, DO, MBA. Originally published in: Chumley H. Bacterial endocarditis. In: Usatine RP, Smith MA, Mayeaux EJ Jr, Chumley H, Tysinger J [editors]. *The Color Atlas of Family Medicine*. New York, NY: McGraw-Hill; 2009:205–209.)

CHECKPOINT

5. Which patients are at highest risk for infective endocarditis?
6. What are the leading bacterial agents of infective endocarditis?
7. What features characterize infective endocarditis in intravenous drug users? In patients with prosthetic heart valves?
8. What hemodynamic features predispose to infective endocarditis?
9. What is the outcome of untreated bacterial endocarditis?
10. What are the risk factors for a fatal outcome? What are the most common causes of death in untreated infective endocarditis?

MENINGITIS

Clinical Presentation

Symptoms commonly associated with both bacterial and viral meningitis include acute onset of fever, headache, neck stiffness (**meningismus**), photophobia, and confusion. Bacterial meningitis causes significant morbidity (neurologic sequelae, particularly sensorineural hearing loss) and mortality and thus requires immediate antibiotic therapy. With rare exceptions, only supportive care with analgesics is necessary for viral meningitis.

Because the clinical presentations of bacterial and viral meningitis may be indistinguishable, laboratory studies of the cerebrospinal fluid are critical in differentiating these entities. **Cerebrospinal fluid leukocyte pleocytosis** (white blood cells in the cerebrospinal fluid) is the hallmark of meningitis. Bacterial meningitis is generally characterized by neutrophilic pleocytosis (predominance of polymorphonuclear neutrophils in the cerebrospinal fluid). Common causes of lymphocytic pleocytosis include viral infections (eg, enterovirus, West Nile virus), fungal infections (eg, cryptococcus in HIV-infected persons), and spirochetal infections (eg, neurosyphilis or Lyme neuroborreliosis). Noninfectious causes such as cancer, connective tissue diseases, and hypersensitivity reactions to drugs can also cause lymphocytic pleocytosis. The cerebrospinal fluid in bacterial meningitis is generally characterized by marked elevations in protein concentration, an extremely low glucose level, and, in the absence of previous antibiotic treatment, a positive Gram stain for bacteria. However, there is often significant overlap between the cerebrospinal fluid findings in bacterial and nonbacterial meningitis, and differentiating these entities at presentation is a significant clinical challenge.

Etiology

The microbiology of bacterial meningitis in the United States has changed dramatically following the introduction of the *Haemophilus influenzae* conjugate vaccine. The routine use of this vaccine in the pediatric population has essentially eliminated *H influenzae* as a cause of meningitis, resulting in a shift in median age among patients with bacterial meningitis from 9 months to 25 years.

Bacterial agents causing meningitis vary according to host age (Table 4–6). In infants younger than 3 months, *E coli*, *Listeria*, and group B streptococci are the most common causes of meningitis. For children 3 months to 18 years of age, *S pneumoniae* and *N meningitidis* are the most common causes, with *H influenzae* a concern among nonimmunized children. For adults aged 18–50 years, *S pneumoniae* and *N meningitidis* are the leading causes of meningitis, whereas the elderly are at risk for those pathogens as well as for *Listeria*. Additional bacteria must be considered for postneurosurgery patients (*S aureus, P aeruginosa*), patients with ventricular shunts (*S epidermidis, S aureus,* gram-negative bacilli), pregnant patients (*Listeria*), or neutropenic patients (gram-negative bacilli, including *P aeruginosa*). Subacute or chronic meningitides may be caused by *M tuberculosis*, fungi (eg, *Coccidioides immitis, Cryptococcus neoformans*), and spirochetes such as *Treponema pallidum* (the bacterium causing syphilis) or *Borrelia burgdorferi* (the bacterium causing Lyme disease). The diagnosis of meningitis caused by these organ-

TABLE 4–6 Common causes of bacterial meningitis in the United States by host age.

Pathogen	Age			
	< 3 Months	3 Months–18 Years	18–50 Years	> 50 Years
Group B streptococci	X			
E coli	X			
Listeria monocytogenes	X			X
N meningitidis		X	X	X
S pneumoniae		X	X	X
Aerobic gram-negative bacilli	X			X

isms may be delayed because many of these pathogens are difficult to culture and require special serologic or molecular diagnostic techniques.

Pathogenesis

The pathogenesis of bacterial meningitis involves a sequence of events in which virulent microorganisms overcome the host defense mechanisms (Table 4–7).

Most cases of bacterial meningitis begin with bacterial colonization of the nasopharynx (Figure 4–7, panel A). An exception is *Listeria,* which enters the bloodstream through ingestion of contaminated food. Pathogenic bacteria such as *S pneumoniae* and *N meningitidis* secrete an IgA protease that inactivates host antibody and facilitates mucosal attachment. Many of the causal pathogens also possess surface characteristics that enhance mucosal colonization. *N meningitidis* binds to nonciliated epithelial cells by finger-like projections known as **pili.**

Once the mucosal barrier is breached, bacteria gain access to the bloodstream, where they must overcome host defense mechanisms to survive and invade the CNS (Figure 4–7, panel B). The bacterial capsule, a feature common to *N meningitidis, H influenzae,* and *S pneumoniae,* is the most important virulence factor in this regard. Host defenses counteract the protective effects of the pneumococcal capsule by activat-

ing the alternative complement pathway, resulting in C3b activation, opsonization, phagocytosis, and intravascular clearance of the organism. This defense mechanism is impaired in patients who have undergone splenectomy, and such patients are predisposed to the development of overwhelming bacteremia and meningitis with encapsulated bacteria. Activation of the complement system membrane attack complex is an essential host defense mechanism against invasive disease by *N meningitidis,* and patients with deficiencies of the late complement components (C5–9) are at increased risk for meningococcal meningitis.

The mechanisms by which bacterial pathogens gain access to the CNS are largely unknown. Experimental studies suggest that receptors for bacterial pathogens are present on cells in the choroid plexus, which may facilitate movement of these pathogens into the subarachnoid space (Figure 4–7, panel C). Invasion of the spinal fluid by a meningeal pathogen results in increased permeability of the blood-brain barrier, with leakage of albumin into the subarachnoid space, where local host defense mechanisms are inadequate to control the infection. Normally, complement components are minimal or absent in the cerebrospinal fluid. Meningeal inflammation leads to increased, but still low, concentrations of complement, inadequate for opsonization, phagocytosis, and removal of encapsu-

TABLE 4–7 Pathogenetic sequence of bacterial neurotropism.

Neurotropic Stage	Host Defense	Strategy of Pathogen
1. Colonization or mucosal invasion	Secretory IgA	IgA protease secretion
	Ciliary activity	Ciliostasis
	Mucosal epithelium	Adhesive pili
2. Intravascular survival	Complement	Evasion of alternative pathway by polysaccharide capsule
3. Crossing of blood-brain barrier	Cerebral endothelium	Adhesive pili
4. Survival within CSF	Poor opsonic activity	Bacterial replication

Reproduced, with permission, from Quagliarello V, Scheld WM. Bacterial meningitis: Pathogenesis, pathophysiology, and progress. N Engl J Med. 1992;327:864.

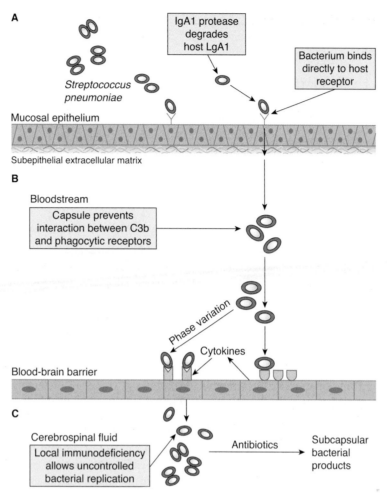

FIGURE 4–7 Pathogenic steps leading to pneumococcal meningitis. The pneumococcus adheres to and colonizes the nasopharynx. IgA1 protease protects the pneumococcus from host antibody (**A**). Once in the bloodstream, the bacterial capsule helps the pneumococcus to evade opsonization (**B**). The pneumococcus accesses the cerebrospinal fluid through receptors on the endothelial surface of the blood-brain barrier (**C**). (Redrawn, with permission, from Koedel U et al. Pathogenesis and pathophysiology of pneumococcal meningitis. Lancet Infect Dis. 2002;2:731.)

lated meningeal pathogens. Immunoglobulin concentrations are also low in the cerebrospinal fluid, with an average blood to cerebrospinal fluid IgG ratio of 800:1. Although the absolute quantity of immunoglobulin in the cerebrospinal fluid increases with infection, the ratio of immunoglobulin in the cerebrospinal fluid relative to that in the serum remains low.

The ability of meningeal pathogens to induce a marked subarachnoid space inflammatory response contributes to many of the pathophysiologic consequences of bacterial meningitis. Although the bacterial capsule is largely responsible for intravascular and cerebrospinal fluid survival of the pathogens, the subcapsular surface components (ie, the cell wall and lipopolysaccharide) of bacteria are more important determinants of meningeal inflammation. The major mediators of the inflammatory process are thought to be IL-1, IL-6, matrix metalloproteinases, and tumor necrosis factor (TNF). Within 1–3 hours after intracisternal inoculation of purified lipopolysaccharide in an animal model, there is a brisk release of TNF and IL-1 into the cerebrospinal fluid, preceding the development of inflammation. Indeed, direct inoculation of

TNF and IL-1 into the cerebrospinal fluid produces an inflammatory cascade identical to that seen with experimental bacterial infection.

Cytokine and proteolytic enzyme release leads to loss of membrane integrity, with resultant cellular swelling. The development of cerebral edema contributes to an increase in intracranial pressure, potentially resulting in life-threatening cerebral herniation (Figure 4–8). **Vasogenic cerebral edema** is principally caused by the increase in blood-brain barrier permeability. **Cytotoxic cerebral edema** results from swelling of the cellular elements of the brain because of toxic factors from bacteria or neutrophils. **Interstitial cerebral edema** reflects obstruction of flow of cerebrospinal fluid, as in hydrocephalus. The literature suggests that oxygen free radicals and nitric oxide may also be important mediators in cerebral edema. Other complications of meningitis include **cerebral vasculitis** with alterations in cerebral blood flow. The vasculitis leads to narrowing or thrombosis of cerebral blood vessels, resulting in ischemia and possible brain infarction.

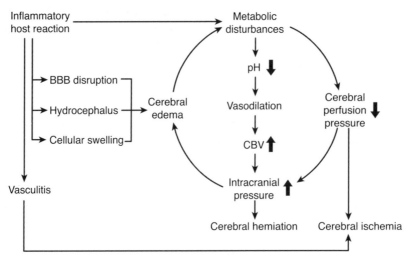

FIGURE 4–8 Pathophysiological alterations leading to neuronal injury during bacterial meningitis. BBB, blood-brain barrier; CBV, cerebral blood volume. (Redrawn, with permission, from Koedel U et al. Pathogenesis and pathophysiology of pneumococcal meningitis. Lancet Infect Dis. 2002;2:731.)

Understanding the pathophysiology of bacterial meningitis has therapeutic implications. Although bactericidal antibiotic therapy is critical for adequate treatment, rapid bacterial killing releases inflammatory bacterial fragments, potentially exacerbating inflammation and abnormalities of the cerebral microvasculature. In animal models, antibiotic therapy has been shown to cause rapid bacteriolysis and release of bacterial endotoxin, resulting in increased cerebrospinal fluid inflammation and cerebral edema.

The importance of the immune response in triggering cerebral edema has led researchers to study the role of adjuvant anti-inflammatory medications for bacterial meningitis. The use of corticosteroids has been shown to decrease the risk of sensorineural hearing loss among children with *H influenzae* meningitis and mortality among adults with pneumococcal meningitis, and these agents are routinely given at the time of initial antibiotic therapy.

Clinical Manifestations

Among patients who develop community-acquired bacterial meningitis, an antecedent upper respiratory tract infection is common. Patients with a history of head injury or neurosurgery, especially those with a persistent cerebrospinal fluid leak, are at particularly high risk for meningitis. Manifestations of meningitis in infants may be difficult to recognize and interpret; therefore, the physician must be alert to the possibility of meningitis in the evaluation of any febrile neonate.

Most patients with meningitis have a rapid onset of fever, headache, lethargy, and confusion. Fewer than half complain of neck stiffness, but nuchal rigidity is noted on physical examination in 30–70%. Other clues seen in a variable proportion of cases include altered mental status, nausea or vomiting, photophobia, **Kernig's sign** (resistance to passive extension of the flexed leg with the patient lying supine), and **Brudzinski's sign** (involuntary flexion of the hip and knee when the examiner passively flexes the patient's neck). More

than half of patients with meningococcemia develop a characteristic petechial or purpuric rash, predominantly on the extremities.

Although a change in mental status (lethargy, confusion) is common in bacterial meningitis, up to one third of patients present with normal mentation. From 10% to 30% of patients have cranial nerve dysfunction, focal neurologic signs, or seizures. Coma, papilledema, and Cushing's triad (bradycardia, respiratory depression, and hypertension) are ominous signs of impending **herniation** (brain displacement through the foramen magnum with brain stem compression), heralding imminent death.

Any patient suspected of having meningitis requires emergent lumbar puncture for Gram stain and culture of the cerebrospinal fluid, followed immediately by the administration of antibiotics and corticosteroids. Alternatively, if a focal neurologic process (eg, brain abscess) is suspected, antibiotics should be initiated immediately, followed by brain imaging (computed tomography or magnetic resonance imaging) and lumbar puncture performed only if there is no radiologic contraindication.

CHECKPOINT

11. What is the typical presentation of bacterial meningitis?
12. What are the major etiologic agents of meningitis, and how do they vary with age or other characteristics of the host?
13. What is the sequence of events in development of meningitis, and what features of particular organisms predispose to meningitis?
14. What are the diverse causes of cerebral edema in patients with meningitis?
15. Why is rapid bacteriolysis theoretically dangerous in meningitis?
16. What are the associated clinical manifestations of untreated bacterial meningitis?

PNEUMONIA

Clinical Presentation

The respiratory tract is the most common site of infection by pathogenic microorganisms. Pneumonia accounts for 1.2 million hospitalizations each year in the United States, with an estimated 58,000 deaths. Pneumonia, together with influenza, is the leading cause of death from an infectious disease in the United States.

Diagnosis and management of pneumonia require knowledge of host risk factors, potential infectious agents, and environmental exposures. Pneumonia is an infection of the lung tissue caused by a number of different bacteria, viruses, parasites, and fungi, resulting in inflammation of the lung parenchyma and accumulation of an inflammatory exudate in the airways. Infection typically begins in the alveoli, with secondary spread to the interstitium, resulting in consolidation and impaired gas exchange. Infection can also extend to the pleural space, causing **pleurisy** (inflammation of the pleura, characterized by pain on inspiration). The exudative response of the pleura to pneumonia is termed **parapneumonic effusion,** which itself can become infected and develop into frank pus (**empyema**).

Etiology

Despite technologic advances in diagnosis, a specific causative agent is not identified in as many as 50% of cases of community-acquired pneumonia. Even in cases in which a microbiologic diagnosis is made, there is usually a delay of several days before the pathogen can be identified and antibiotic susceptibility determined. Symptoms are nonspecific and do not reliably differentiate the various causes of pneumonia. Therefore, knowledge of the most common etiologic organisms is crucial in determining rational empiric antibiotic regimens. Bacterial causes of community pneumonia vary by comorbid disease and severity of pulmonary infection (Table 4–8).

S pneumoniae is the most common organism isolated in community-acquired pneumonia in both immunocompetent and immunocompromised individuals. Several additional organisms require special consideration in specific hosts or because of public health importance (Table 4–9). Understanding and identifying patient risk factors (eg, smoking, HIV infection) and host defense mechanisms (cough reflex, cell-mediated immunity) focuses attention on the most likely etiologic agents, guides empiric therapy, and suggests possible interventions to decrease further risk. For example, patients who have suffered strokes and have impaired ability to protect their airways are at risk for aspirating oropharyngeal secretions. Precautions such as avoiding thin liquids in these patients may decrease the risk of future lung infections. Likewise, an HIV-infected patient with a low CD4 lymphocyte count is at risk for pneumocystic pneumonia and should be given prophylactic antibiotics.

Pathogenesis

Although pneumonia is a relatively common disease, it occurs infrequently in immunocompetent individuals. This can be attributed to the effectiveness of host defenses, including anatomic barriers and cleansing mechanisms in the nasopharynx

TABLE 4–8 Common etiologic agents of community-acquired pneumonia as determined by severity of illness.

		Hospitalized	
Etiologic Agent	Outpatient	Mild to Moderate Infection (Not in ICU)	Severe Infection (Requiring ICU)
S pneumoniae	X	X	X
M pneumoniae	X	X	
C pneumoniae	X	X	
H influenzae	X	X	X
Respiratory viruses[1]	X	X	X
Legionella species		X	X
Enteric gram-negative bacilli		X	X
Anaerobes (aspiration)		X	X
S aureus			X
P aeruginosa			X

Adapted from Mandell LA, Wunderink RG, Anzuelo A, et al. Infectious Diseases Society of America/American Thoracic Society Consensus Guidelines on the Management of Community-Acquired Pneumonia in Adults. Clin Infect Dis. 2007;44:227–72.

[1]Influenza A and B, adenovirus, respiratory syncytial virus, and parainfluenza.

TABLE 4–9 Common risk factors and causes of pneumonia in specific adult hosts.

Risk Factor	Etiologic Agents		Pathogenetic Mechanism and Comments
	Acute Symptoms	**Subacute Chronic Symptoms**	
HIV infection	S pneumoniae	Fungi	Cell-mediated immune dysfunction
	H influenzae	M tuberculosis	Impaired humoral response
	P jirovecii		
	P aeruginosa		
Solid organ or bone marrow transplantation	Cytomegalovirus	Nocardia	Cell-mediated immune dysfunction
	Aspergillus species	Fungi	Neutropenia (bone marrow transplant)
	Legionella species	M tuberculosis	
	P jirovecii		
Chronic obstructive lung disease or smoking	S pneumoniae		Decreased mucociliary clearance
	H influenzae		
	Moraxella catarrhalis		
	P aeruginosa		
Structural lung disease (bronchiectasis)	P aeruginosa		
	Burkholderia cepacia		
	S aureus		
Alcoholism	K pneumoniae	Mixed anaerobic infection (lung abscess)	Aspiration of oropharyngeal contents
	Oral anaerobes		
Injection drug abuse	S aureus		Hematogenous spread
Environmental or animal exposure	Legionella species (infected water)	C immitis (Southwest USA)	Inhalation
	C psittaci (birds)	H capsulatum (east of Mississippi)	
	C burnetii (animals)	C neoformans (birds)	
	Hanta virus (rodents)		
Institutional exposure (hospital, nursing home, etc)	Gram-negative bacilli		Microaspirations
	P aeruginosa		Bypass of upper respiratory tract defense mechanisms (intubation)
	S aureus		
	Acinetobacter species		Hematogenous spread (intravenous catheters)
Postinfluenza	S aureus		Disruption of respiratory epithelium
	S pyogenes		Ciliary dysfunction
			Inhibition of PMNs

and upper airways and local humoral and cellular factors in the alveoli. Normal lungs are sterile below the first major bronchial divisions.

Pulmonary pathogens reach the lungs by one of four routes: (1) direct inhalation of infectious respiratory droplets, (2) aspiration of oropharyngeal contents, (3) direct spread along the mucosal membrane surface from the upper to the lower respiratory system, and (4) hematogenous spread. The pulmonary antimicrobial defense mechanisms are shown in Figure 4–9. Incoming air with suspended particulate matter is subjected to turbulence in the nasal passages and then to abrupt changes in direction as the airstream is diverted through the pharynx and along the branches of the tracheobronchial tree. Particles larger than 10 mm are trapped in the nose or pharynx; those with diameters of 2–9 mm are deposited on the mucociliary blanket; only smaller particles reach the alveoli. *M tuberculosis* and *Legionella pneumophila* are examples of bacteria that are deposited directly in the lower airways through inhalation of small airborne particles. Bacteria trapped in the upper airways can colonize the oropharynx and subsequently be transported into the lungs either by "microaspiration" or by overt aspiration through an open epiglottis (eg, in patients who lose consciousness after excessive alcohol intake).

The respiratory epithelium has special properties for fighting off infection. Epithelial cells are covered with beating cilia blanketed by a layer of mucus. Each cell has about 200 cilia that beat up to 500 times/min, moving the mucus layer upward toward the larynx. The mucus itself contains antimicrobial compounds such as lysozyme and secretory IgA antibodies.

Chronic cigarette smokers have decreased mucociliary clearance secondary to damage of cilia and must, therefore, rely more heavily on the cough reflex to clear aspirated material, excess secretions, and foreign bodies.

Bacteria that reach the terminal bronchioles, alveolar ducts, and alveoli are inactivated primarily by alveolar macrophages and neutrophils. Opsonization of the microorganism by complement and antibodies enhances phagocytosis by these cells.

Impairment at any level of host defenses increases the risk of developing pneumonia. Children with cystic fibrosis have defective ciliary activity and are prone to develop recurrent sinopulmonary infections, particularly with *S aureus* and *P aeruginosa*. Patients with neutropenia, whether acquired or congenital, are also susceptible to lung infections with gram-negative bacteria and fungi. Antigenic stimulation of T cells leads to the production of lymphokines that activate macrophages with enhanced bactericidal activity. HIV-infected patients have depleted CD4 T lymphocyte counts and are predisposed to a variety of bacterial (including mycobacterial) and fungal infections.

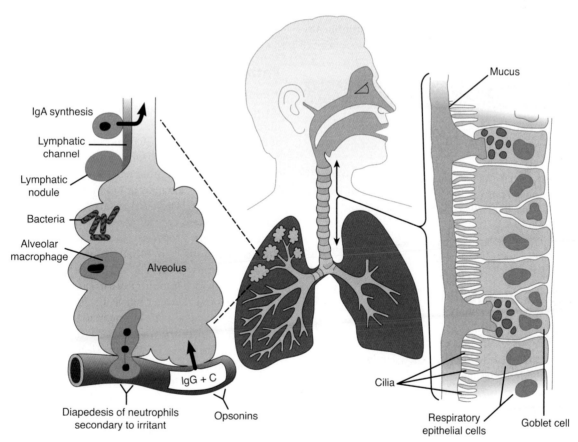

FIGURE 4–9 Pulmonary defense mechanisms. Abrupt changes in direction of airflow in the nasal passages can trap potential pathogens. The epiglottis and cough reflex prevent introduction of particulate matter in the lower airway. The ciliated respiratory epithelium propels the overlying mucous layer (right) upward toward the mouth. In the alveoli, cell-mediated immunity, humoral factors, and the inflammatory response defend against lower respiratory tract infections. (C, complement.) (Redrawn, with permission, from Storch GA. Respiratory system. In: *Mechanisms of Microbial Disease*, 4th ed. Schaechter M et al [editors]. Lippincott Williams & Wilkins, 2007.)

Clinical Manifestations

Most patients with pneumonia have fever, cough, tachypnea, tachycardia, and an infiltrate on chest x-ray film. Extrapulmonary manifestations that may provide clues to the etiologic agents include pharyngitis (*Chlamydia pneumoniae*), erythema nodosum rash (fungal and mycobacterial infections), and diarrhea (*Legionella*).

The following questions aid in guiding empiric therapy for a patient who presents with symptoms consistent with pneumonia: (1) Is this pneumonia community acquired or healthcare acquired (eg, hospital, nursing home)? (2) Is this patient immunocompromised (HIV infected, a transplant recipient)? (3) Is this patient an injection drug user? (4) Has this patient had a recent alteration in consciousness (suggestive of aspiration)? (5) Are the symptoms acute (days) or chronic (weeks to months)? (6) Has this patient lived in or traveled through geographic areas associated with specific endemic infections (histoplasmosis, coccidioidomycosis)? (7) Has this patient had recent zoonotic exposures associated with pulmonary infections (psittacosis, Q fever)? (8) Could this patient have a contagious infection of public health importance (tuberculosis)? (9) Could this patient's pulmonary infection be associated with a common source exposure (*Legionella* or influenza outbreak)?

CHECKPOINT

17. What are the important pathogens for patients with community-acquired pneumonia based on severity of illness and site of care?

18. What host features influence the likelihood of particular causes of pneumonia?

19. What are the four mechanisms by which pathogens reach the lungs?

20. What are the defenses of the respiratory epithelium against infection?

INFECTIOUS DIARRHEA

Clinical Presentation

Each year throughout the world more than 5 million people—most of them children younger than 1 year—die of acute infectious diarrhea (see also Chapter 13). Although death is a rare outcome of infectious diarrhea in the United States, morbidity is substantial. It is estimated that there are more than 200 million episodes each year, resulting in 1.8 million hospitalizations at a cost of $6 billion per year. The morbidity and mortality attributable to diarrhea are largely due to loss of intravascular volume and electrolytes, with resultant cardiovascular failure. For example, adults with cholera can excrete more than 1 L of fluid per hour. Contrast this with the normal volume of fluid lost daily in the stools (150 mL), and it is clear why massive fluid losses associated with infectious diarrhea can lead to dehydration, cardiovascular collapse, and death.

Gastrointestinal (GI) tract infections can present with primarily upper tract symptoms (nausea, vomiting, crampy epigastric pain), small intestine symptoms (profuse watery diarrhea), or large intestine symptoms (tenesmus, fecal urgency, bloody diarrhea). Sources of infection include person-to-person transmission (fecal-oral spread of *Shigella*), water-borne transmission (*Cryptosporidium*), food-borne transmission (*Salmonella* or *S aureus* food poisoning), and overgrowth after antibiotic administration (*Clostridium difficile*).

Etiology

A wide range of viruses, bacteria, fungi, and protozoa can infect the GI tract. However, in the majority of cases, symptoms are self-limited, and diagnostic evaluation is not performed. Patients presenting to medical attention are biased toward the subset with more severe symptoms (eg, high fevers or hypotension), immunocompromise (eg, HIV or neutropenia), or prolonged duration (eg, chronic diarrhea defined as lasting 14 days). An exception is large outbreaks of food-borne illness, in which epidemiologic investigations may detect patients with milder variants of disease.

Pathogenesis

A comprehensive approach to GI tract infections starts with the classic host-agent-environment interaction model. A number of host factors influence GI tract infections. Patients at extremes of age and with comorbid conditions (eg, HIV infection) are at higher risk for symptomatic infection. Medications that alter the GI microenvironment or destroy normal bacterial flora (eg, antacids or antibiotics) also predispose patients to infection. Microbial agents responsible for GI illness can be categorized according to type of organism (bacterial, viral, protozoal), propensity to attach to different anatomic sites (stomach, small bowel, colon), and pathogenesis (enterotoxigenic, cytotoxigenic, enteroinvasive). Environmental factors can be divided into three broad categories based on mode of transmission: (1) water borne, (2) food borne, and (3) person to person. Table 4–10 summarizes these relationships and provides a framework for assessing the pathogenesis of GI tract infections.

GI tract infections can involve the stomach, causing nausea and vomiting, or affect the small and large bowel, with diarrhea as the predominant symptom. The term "gastroenteritis" classically denotes infection of the stomach and proximal small bowel. Organisms causing this disorder include *Bacillus cereus, S aureus,* and a number of viruses (rotavirus, norovirus). *B cereus* and *S aureus* produce a preformed **neurotoxin** that, even in the absence of viable bacteria, is capable of causing disease, and these toxins represent major causes of food poisoning. Although the exact mechanisms are poorly understood, it is thought that neurotoxins act locally, through stimulation of the sympathetic nervous system with a resultant

TABLE 4–10 Approach to GI tract infections.

Paradigm	Categories	Epidemiology	Examples
Environment	Water borne	Fecal contamination of water supply	*Vibrio cholerae*
	Food borne	Contaminated food (bacteria or toxin)	*S aureus*
			Salmonella
	Person to person (fecal oral spread)	Child care centers	*Shigella*
			Rotavirus
Agent	Bacterial		*Campylobacter*
	Viral		Norovirus
	Parasitic		*Entamoeba histolytica*
Host	Age	Infants, elderly	Enterohemorrhagic *E coli*
	Comorbidity	HIV	*Cryptosporidium*
	Gastric acidity	Antacid use	*Salmonella*
	GI flora	Antibiotic use	*Clostridium difficile*
Site	Stomach	Gastroenteritis	*B cereus*
	Small intestine	Secretory diarrhea	*V cholerae*
	Large intestine	Inflammatory diarrhea	*Shigella*

increase in peristaltic activity, and centrally, through activation of emetic centers in the brain.

The spectrum of diarrheal infections is typified by the diverse clinical manifestations and mechanisms through which *E coli* can cause diarrhea. Colonization of the human GI tract by *E coli* is universal, typically occurring within hours after birth. However, when the host organism is exposed to pathogenic strains of *E coli* not normally present in the bowel flora, localized GI disease or even systemic illness may occur. There are five major classes of diarrheogenic *E coli*: enterotoxigenic (ETEC), enteropathogenic (EPEC), enterohemorrhagic (EHEC), enteroaggregative (EAEC), and enteroinvasive (EIEC) (Table 4–11). Features common to all pathogenic *E coli* are evasion of host defenses, colonization of intestinal mucosa, and multiplication with host cell injury. This organism, like all GI pathogens, must survive transit through the acidic gastric environment and be able to persist in the GI tract despite the mechanical force of peristalsis and competition for scarce nutrients from existing bacterial flora. Adherence can be nonspecific (at any part of the intestinal tract) or, more commonly, specific, with attachment occurring at well-defined anatomic areas.

TABLE 4–11 *Escherichia coli* in diarrheal disease.

Class	Susceptible Populations		Clinical Syndrome	Site	Toxins
	Developed Countries	Developing Countries			
ETEC	Returning travelers	Age < 5 years	Watery diarrhea	Small intestine	Heat-labile and heat-stable toxin
EIEC	Rare	All ages	Dysentery (bloody diarrhea, mucus, fever)	Large intestine > small intestine	*Shigella*-like enterotoxin
EHEC	Children, elderly	Rare	Hemorrhagic colitis; hemolytic uremic syndrome	Large intestine	Shiga toxins (Stx1 & Stx2)
EPEC	Rare	Age < 2 years	Watery diarrhea	Small intestine	Unknown
EAEC	Rare	Children	Persistent watery diarrhea	Small intestine	Enteroaggregative heat-stable enterotoxin

Once colonization and multiplication occur, the stage is set for host injury. Infectious diarrhea is clinically differentiated into secretory, inflammatory, and hemorrhagic types, with different pathophysiologic mechanisms accounting for these diverse presentations. **Secretory** (watery) diarrhea is caused by a number of bacteria (eg, *Vibrio cholerae*, ETEC, EAggEC), viruses (rotavirus, norovirus), and protozoa (*Giardia, Cryptosporidium*). These organisms attach superficially to enterocytes in the lumen of the small bowel. Stool examination is notable for the absence of fecal leukocytes, although in rare cases there is occult blood in the stools. Some of these pathogens elaborate **enterotoxins,** proteins that increase intestinal cyclic adenosine monophosphate (cAMP) production, leading to net fluid secretion. The classic example is cholera. The bacterium *V cholerae* produces cholera toxin, which causes prolonged activation of epithelial adenylyl cyclase in the small bowel, leading to secretion of massive amounts of fluid and electrolytes into the intestinal lumen (Figure 4–10). Clinically, the patient presents with copious diarrhea ("rice-water stools"), progressing to dehydration and vascular collapse without vigorous volume resuscitation. ETEC, a common cause of acute diarrheal illness in young children and the most common cause of diarrhea in travelers returning to the United States from developing countries, produces two enterotoxins. The heat-labile toxin (LT) activates adenylyl cyclase in a manner analogous to cholera toxin, whereas the heat-stable toxin (ST) activates guanylyl cyclase activity.

Inflammatory diarrhea is a result of bacterial invasion of the mucosal lumen, with resultant cell death. Patients with this syndrome are usually febrile, with complaints of crampy lower abdominal pain as well as diarrhea, which may contain visible mucous. The term **dysentery** is used when there are significant numbers of fecal leukocytes and gross blood. Pathogens associated with inflammatory diarrhea include EIEC, *Shigella, Salmonella, Campylobacter,* and *Entamoeba histolytica. Shigella,* the prototypical cause of bacillary dysentery, invades the enterocyte through formation of an endoplasmic vacuole, which is lysed intracellularly. Bacteria then proliferate in the cytoplasm and invade adjacent epithelial cells. Production of a **cytotoxin,** the Shiga toxin, leads to local cell destruction and death. EIEC resembles *Shigella* both clinically and with respect to the mechanism of invasion of the enterocyte wall; however, the specific cytotoxin associated with EIEC has not yet been identified.

Hemorrhagic diarrhea, a variant of inflammatory diarrhea, is primarily caused by EHEC. Infection with *E coli* O157:H7 has been associated with a number of deaths from the hemolytic-uremic syndrome, with several well-publicized outbreaks related to contaminated foods. EHEC causes a broad spectrum of clinical disease, with manifestations including (1) asymptomatic infection, (2) watery (nonbloody) diarrhea, (3) hemorrhagic colitis (bloody, noninflammatory diarrhea), and (4) hemolytic-uremic syndrome (an acute illness, primarily of children, characterized by anemia and renal failure). EHEC does not invade enterocytes; however, it does produce two Shiga-like toxins (Stx1 and Stx2) that closely resemble the Shiga toxin in structure and function. After binding of EHEC to the cell surface receptor, the A subunit of the Shiga toxin catalyzes the destructive cleavage of ribosomal RNA and halts protein synthesis, leading to cell death.

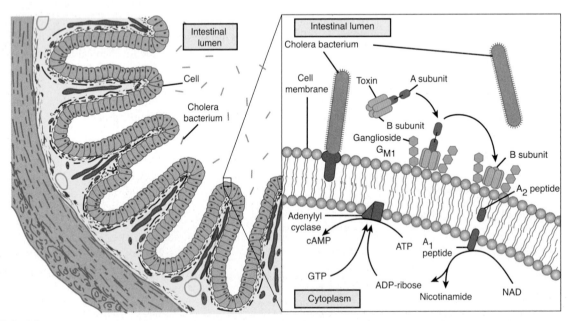

FIGURE 4–10 Pathogenesis of *Vibrio cholerae* and enterotoxigenic *E coli* (ETEC) in diarrheal disease. *V cholerae* and ETEC share similar pathogenetic mechanisms in causing diarrheal illness. The bacteria gain entry to the small intestinal lumen through ingestion of contaminated food (**left**). They elaborate an enterotoxin that is composed of one A subunit and five B subunits. The B subunits bind to the intestinal cell membrane and facilitate entry of part of the A subunit (**right**). Subsequently, this results in a prolonged activation of adenylyl cyclase and the formation of cyclic adenosine monophosphate (cAMP), which stimulates water and electrolyte secretion by intestinal endothelial cells. (Redrawn, with permission, from Vaughan M. Cholera and cell regulation. Hosp Pract. 1982;17(6):145–152.)

Clinical Manifestations

Clinical manifestations of GI infections vary depending on the on site of involvement (Table 4–10). For instance, in staphylococcal food poisoning, symptoms develop several hours after ingestion of food contaminated with neurotoxin-producing *S aureus*. The symptoms of staphylococcal food poisoning are profuse vomiting, nausea, and abdominal cramps. Diarrhea is variably present with agents causing gastroenteritis. Profuse watery (noninflammatory, nonbloody) diarrhea is associated with bacteria that have infected the small intestine and elaborated an enterotoxin (eg, *Clostridium perfringens, V cholerae*). In contrast, colitis-like symptoms (lower abdominal pain, tenesmus, fecal urgency) and an inflammatory or bloody diarrhea occur with bacteria that more commonly infect the large intestine. The incubation period is generally longer (> 3 days) for bacteria that localize to the large intestine, and colonic mucosal invasion can occur, causing fever, bacteremia, and systemic symptoms.

CHECKPOINT

21. How many individuals in the world die yearly of infectious diarrhea?
22. What are different modes of spread of infectious diarrhea? Give an example of each.
23. What are the different mechanisms by which infectious organisms cause diarrhea?

SEPSIS & SEPTIC SHOCK

Clinical Presentation

Sepsis is a leading cause of death in the United States, with more than 34,000 deaths occurring annually and an overall case fatality rate approaching 20%. The medical costs of sepsis in the United States exceed $17 billion annually. Rates of sepsis continue to rise secondary to medical advances such as the widespread use of indwelling intravascular catheters, increased implantation of prosthetic material (eg, cardiac valves and artificial joints), and administration of immunosuppressive drugs and chemotherapeutic agents. These interventions serve to increase the risk of infection and subsequent sepsis.

The study of sepsis has been facilitated by establishment of standardized case definitions (Table 4–12). The **systemic inflammatory response syndrome** (**SIRS**) is a nonspecific inflammatory state that may be seen with infection as well as with noninfectious states such as pancreatitis, pulmonary embolism, and myocardial infarction. Leukopenia and hypothermia, included in the SIRS case definition, are predictors of a poor prognosis when associated with sepsis. **Sepsis** is defined as the presence of SIRS associated with an infectious precipitant. **Severe sepsis** occurs when there is objective evidence of organ dysfunction (eg, renal failure, hepatic failure, altered mentation), usually associated with tissue hypoperfusion. The final stage of sepsis is **septic shock,** defined as

TABLE 4–12 Clinical definition of sepsis.

I. Systemic inflammatory response syndrome (SIRS)
Two or more of the following:
(1) Temperature of > 38 °C or < 36 °C
(2) Heart rate of > 90/min
(3) Respiratory rate of > 20/min or PaCO$_2$ < 32 mm Hg
(4) WBC count of > 12×10^9/L or < 4×10^9/L, or > 10% immature forms (bands)
II. Sepsis
SIRS plus evidence of infection
III. Severe sepsis
Sepsis plus organ dysfunction, hypotension, or hypoperfusion (including lactic acidosis, oliguria, acute alteration in mental status)
IV. Septic shock
Hypotension (despite fluid resuscitation) plus hypoperfusion abnormalities

hypotension (systolic blood pressure < 90 mm Hg or a 40 mm Hg decrease below the baseline systolic blood pressure) unresponsive to fluid resuscitation.

Etiology

Although evidence of infection is a diagnostic criterion for sepsis, only 28% of patients with sepsis have bacteremia, and slightly more than 10% will have **primary bacteremia,** defined as positive blood cultures without an obvious source of bacterial seeding. Common sites of infection among patients with sepsis syndrome (in decreasing order of frequency) include the respiratory tract, the genitourinary tract, abdominal sources (gall-bladder, colon), device-related infections, and wound or soft tissue infections.

The bacteriology of sepsis has evolved in the last decade. Gram-negative bacteria (*Enterobacteriaceae* and *Pseudomonas*), previously the most common cause of sepsis, have been surplanted by gram-positive organisms, which now cause more than 50% of cases. Staphylococci are the most common bacteria cultured from the bloodstream, presumably because of an increase in the prevalence of chronic indwelling venous access devices and implanted prosthetic material. For similar reasons, the incidence of fungal sepsis due to *Candida* species has risen dramatically in the last decade. Sepsis associated with *P aeruginosa, Candida,* or mixed (polymicrobial) organisms is an independent predictor of mortality.

Pathogenesis

The different stages of sepsis (SIRS to septic shock) represent a continuum, with patients often progressing from one stage to the next within days or even hours after admission. Sepsis generally starts with a localized infection. Bacteria may then invade the bloodstream directly (leading to bacteremia and positive blood cultures) or may proliferate locally and release toxins into the bloodstream. These toxins can arise from a structural component of the bacteria (eg, endotoxin) or may be exotoxins, which are proteins synthesized and released by the bacteria. **Endotoxin** is defined as the **lipopolysaccharide (LPS)** moiety contained in the outer membrane of gram-negative bacteria. Endotoxin is composed of an outer polysaccharide chain (the **O side chain**), which varies between species and is not toxic, and a highly conserved lipid portion (**lipid A**), which is embedded in the outer bacterial membrane. Injection of either purified endotoxin or lipid A is highly toxic in animal models, causing a syndrome analogous to septic shock in the absence of viable bacteria.

Until recently, sepsis was attributed solely to overstimulation of the host inflammatory response and uncontrolled release of inflammatory mediators. Although this undoubtedly occurs in a subset of patients, the failure of medical inter-

ventions aimed at blocking this response (eg, monoclonal antibodies directed against endotoxin, blockade of IL-1 and TNF, bradykinin antagonists, inhibition of cyclooxygenase with ibuprofen) suggests a more complex process. Studies have shown that, as sepsis persists, host immunosuppression plays a critical role. Specific stimuli such as organism, inoculum, and site of infection stimulate **CD4 T cells** to secrete cytokines with either inflammatory (type 1 helper T-cell) or anti-inflammatory (type 2 helper T-cell) properties (Figure 4–11). Among patients who die of sepsis, there is significant loss of cells essential for the adaptive immune response (B lymphocytes, CD4 T cells, dendritic cells). Genetically programmed cell death, termed **apoptosis,** is thought to play a key role in the decrease in these cell lines and downregulates the surviving immune cells. The clinical consequences of sepsis include hemodynamic changes (tachycardia, tachypnea), inappropriate vasodilation, and poor tissue perfusion, with resultant organ dysfunction (Figure 4–11).

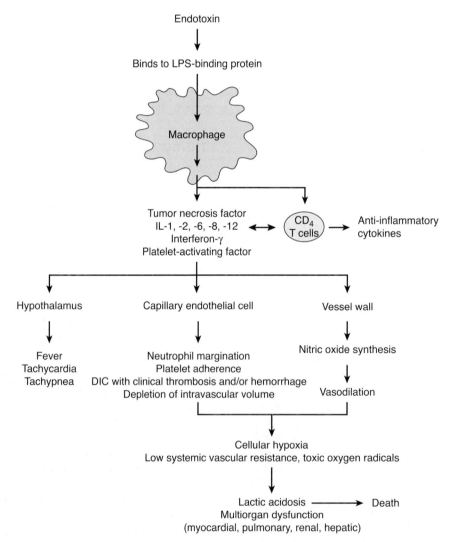

FIGURE 4–11 Pathogenic sequence of the events in septic shock. Activation of macrophages by endotoxin and other proteins leads to release of inflammatory mediators and immune modulation resulting in host tissue damage and, in some cases, death. (Redrawn, with permission, from Horn DL et al. What are the microbial components implicated in the pathogenesis of sepsis? Clin Infect Dis. 2000;31:852.)

A. Hemodynamic Alterations

All forms of shock result in inadequate tissue perfusion and subsequent cell dysfunction and death (see Chapter 11). In noninfectious forms (such as cardiogenic shock and hypovolemic shock), **systemic vascular resistance** is elevated as a compensatory mechanism to maintain blood pressure. In the hypoperfused tissues, there is enhanced extraction of oxygen from circulating red blood cells, leading to decreased pulmonary artery oxygenation. In contrast, early in septic shock there is hypovolemia from inappropriate arterial and venous dilation (low systemic vascular resistance) and leakage of plasma into the extravascular space. Even with correction of the hypovolemia, systemic vascular resistance remains low despite a compensatory increase in **cardiac output.** Inefficient oxygen extraction and tissue hypoperfusion result in an increased pulmonary artery oxygen content.

A hyperdynamic circulatory state, described as **distributive shock** to emphasize the maldistribution of blood flow to various tissues, is the common hemodynamic finding in sepsis. The release of vasoactive substances (including nitric oxide) results in loss of normal mechanisms of vascular autoregulation, producing imbalances in blood flow with regional shunting and relative hypoperfusion of some organs. Animal studies have documented predictable changes in organ blood flow, with a marked reduction in blood flow to the stomach, duodenum, small bowel, and pancreas; a moderate reduction in blood flow to the myocardium and the skeletal muscles; and relative preservation of perfusion to the kidneys and CNS.

Myocardial depression is a common finding in early septic shock. Initially, patients have low cardiac filling pressures and low cardiac output secondary to volume depletion and vasodilation. After fluid replacement, cardiac output is normal or increased but ventricular function is abnormal. From 24 to 48 hours after the onset of sepsis, left and right ventricular ejection fractions are reduced, and end-diastolic and end-systolic volumes are increased. This myocardial depression has been attributed to direct toxic effects of nitric oxide, TNF, and IL-1. Reduced ejection fraction and consequent myocardial depression are reversible in patients who survive the initial period of septic shock.

B. Vascular and Multiorgan Dysfunction

Most patients who die of septic shock have either refractory hypotension or multiple-organ failure. Refractory hypotension can occur from two mechanisms. First, some patients cannot sustain high cardiac output in response to the septic state and develop progressive high-output cardiac failure. Second, circulatory failure may be associated with severe vasodilation and hypotension refractory to intravenous fluid resuscitation and vasopressor therapy.

The development of multiple-organ failure represents the terminal phase of a hypermetabolic process that begins during the initial stages of shock. Organ failure results from microvascular injury induced by local and systemic inflammatory responses to infection. Maldistribution of blood flow is accentuated by impaired erythrocyte deformability, with microvascular obstruction. Aggregation of neutrophils and platelets may also reduce blood flow. Demargination of neutrophils from vascular endothelium results in further release of inflammatory mediators and subsequent migration of neutrophils into tissues. Components of the complement system are activated, attracting more neutrophils and releasing locally active substances such as prostaglandins and leukotrienes. The net result of all of these changes is microvascular collapse and, ultimately, organ failure.

The outcome of sepsis depends on the number of organs that fail: The mortality among patients with multiorgan failure (three or more organ systems) averages 70%. Respiratory failure develops in 18% of patients with sepsis. At the most severe end of the spectrum is **acute respiratory distress syndrome,** characterized by refractory hypoxia, decreased lung compliance, noncardiogenic pulmonary edema, and pulmonary hypertension. Renal failure, seen in 15% of cases, is usually a multifactorial process, with additive injury from intrarenal shunting, renal hypoperfusion, and administration of nephrotoxic agents (antibiotics and radiologic imaging dye). Other organs affected by sepsis include the CNS (altered mentation, coma) and the blood (disseminated intravascular coagulation).

Clinical Manifestations

The clinical manifestations of sepsis include those related to the systemic response to infections (tachycardia, tachypnea, alterations in temperature and leukocyte count) and those related to specific organ system dysfunction (cardiovascular, respiratory, renal, hepatic, and hematologic abnormalities). Sepsis sometimes begins with very subtle clues that can be easily confused with more common and less serious illnesses. Awareness of these early signs of sepsis can lead to early recognition and intervention. Nonspecific signs can include isolated tachypnea (without dyspnea), isolated tachycardia (with normal blood pressure), irritability or lethargy, and otherwise unexplained fever, rigors, or myalgias. Nonspecific laboratory abnormalities can include respiratory alkalosis, leukocytosis, and mild liver function abnormalities.

CHECKPOINT

24. What is the mortality rate of sepsis and septic shock in the United States?
25. What factors contribute to hospital-related sepsis?
26. Which organisms are most commonly associated with sepsis?
27. What is the role of the host immune system in the pathogenesis of sepsis?
28. What activates the immune response?
29. What are some distinctive hemodynamic features of septic shock versus noninfectious shock syndromes?

CASE STUDIES

Eva M. Aagaard, MD

(See Chapter 25, p. 676 for Answers)

CASE 11

A 55-year-old man who recently emigrated from China presents to the emergency department with fever. He states that he has had recurring fevers over the past 3 weeks, associated with chills, night sweats, and malaise. Today he developed new painful lesions on the pads of his fingers, prompting him to come to the emergency department. His medical history is remarkable for "being very sick as a child after a sore throat." He has recently had several teeth extracted for severe dental caries. He is taking no medications. On physical examination, he is febrile to 38.5 °C, blood pressure 120/80 mm Hg, heart rate 108 bpm, respiratory rate 16/min, with an oxygen saturation of 97% on room air. Skin examination is remarkable for painful nodules on the pads of several fingers and toes. He has multiple splinter hemorrhages in the nail beds and painless hemorrhagic macules on the palms of the hands. Ophthalmoscopic examination is remarkable for retinal hemorrhages. Chest examination is clear to auscultation and percussion. Cardiac examination is notable for a grade 3/6 holosystolic murmur heard loudest at the left lower sternal border, with radiation to the axilla. Abdominal and back examinations are unremarkable.

Questions

A. What is the likely diagnosis? What are some common predisposing factors to this disease? Which is most likely in this patient?
B. Which infectious agents are most likely to be involved?
C. What hemodynamic factors predispose to this disease? How do these factors contribute to the establishment of this disease and resistance to normal host immune responses?
D. What is the name given to the various lesions found on this man's hands and feet? What is the pathogenetic mechanism responsible for their formation?
E. What are some other common clinical manifestations of this disease? What are the most common causes of death in this disease? What factors are predictive of a fatal outcome?

CASE 12

A 25-year-old man presents to the emergency department with fever and in a confused, irrational state. He is accompanied by his wife, who provides the history. She states that he had been well until approximately 1 week ago, when he developed symptoms of upper respiratory tract infection that were slow to improve. On the morning of admission, he complained of progressive severe headache and nausea. He vomited once. He became progressively lethargic as the day progressed, and she brought him to the hospital. He has no other medical problems and takes no medications.

On examination, he is febrile to 39 °C, with a blood pressure of 95/60 mm Hg, heart rate of 100 bpm, and respiratory rate of 18/min. He is lethargic and confused, lying with his hand over his eyes. Funduscopic examination shows no papilledema. The neck is stiff, with a positive Brudzinski sign. Heart, lung, and abdominal examinations are unremarkable. Neurologic examination is limited by the patient's inability to cooperate but appears to be nonfocal. Kernig's sign (resistance to passive extension of the flexed leg with the patient lying supine) is negative.

Questions

A. What infectious diagnosis is suggested? What are the most likely etiologic agents in this patient? What would they be if he were a newborn? If he were a child?
B. What is the pathophysiologic sequence of events in the development of this disease? What features of the pathogens involved facilitate their ability to produce this disease?
C. What are the possible causes of cerebral edema in this patient?
D. What tests should be performed to confirm the diagnosis? What kinds of treatments should be started or considered? Why?

CASE 13

A 68-year-old man presents to the hospital emergency department with acute fever and persistent cough. He has had cough productive of green sputum for 3 days, associated with shortness of breath, left-sided pleuritic chest pain, fever, chills, and night sweats. His medical history is notable for chronic obstructive pulmonary disease, requiring intermittent steroid use. His medications include albuterol, ipratropium bromide, and corticosteroid inhalers. The patient lives at home and is active. On examination, he is febrile to 38 °C, with a blood pressure of 110/50 mm Hg, heart rate of 98 bpm, and respiratory rate of 20/min. Oxygen saturation is 92% on room air. He is a thin man in moderate respiratory distress, speaking in sentences of three or four words. Lung examination is notable for rales in the left lung base and left axilla and diffuse expiratory wheezes. The remainder of the examination is unremarkable. Chest x-ray film reveals a left lower lobe and lingular infiltrate. A diagnosis of pneumonia is made, and the patient is admitted to the hospital for administration of intravenous antibiotics.

Questions

A. On the basis of this patient's underlying condition and severity of illness, what are the likely pathogens involved in this case? How would your differential change if he required ICU admission?

B. What are the mechanisms by which pathogens reach the lungs?

C. What are the normal host defenses against pneumonia?

D. What are some common host risk factors for pneumonia? What are the pathogenetic mechanisms by which they increase the risk of pneumonia? Which of these risk factors are present in this patient?

CASE 14

A 21-year-old woman presents with the complaint of diarrhea. She returned from Mexico the day before her visit. The day before that, she had an acute onset of profuse watery diarrhea. She denies blood or mucus in the stools. She has had no associated fever, chills, nausea, or vomiting. She has no other medical problems and is taking no medications. Examination is remarkable for diffuse, mild abdominal tenderness to palpation without guarding or rebound tenderness. Stool is guaiac negative. Infectious diarrhea is suspected.

Questions

A. What are the different modes of spread of infectious diarrhea? Give an example of each.

B. What is the likely anatomic site of infection in this case? Why?

C. What is the most likely pathogen in this case? What is the pathogenetic mechanism by which it causes diarrhea?

CASE 15

A 65-year-old woman is admitted to the hospital with community-acquired pneumonia. She is treated with intravenous antibiotics and is given oxygen by nasal cannula. A Foley catheter is placed in her bladder. On the third hospital day she is switched to oral antibiotics in anticipation of discharge. On the evening of hospital day 3, she develops fever and tachycardia. Blood and urine cultures are ordered. The following morning, she is lethargic and difficult to arouse. Her temperature is 35 °C, blood pressure 85/40 mm Hg, heart rate 110 bpm, and respiratory rate 20/min. Oxygen saturation is 94% on room air. Head and neck examinations are unremarkable. Lung examination is unchanged from admission, with rales in the left base. Cardiac examination is notable for a rapid but regular rhythm, without murmurs, gallops, or rubs. Abdominal examination is normal. Extremities are warm. Neurologic examination is nonfocal. The patient is transferred to the ICU for management of presumed sepsis and given intravenous fluids and antibiotics. Blood and urine cultures are positive for gram-negative rods.

Questions

A. What factors contribute to hospital-related sepsis?

B. By what mechanism do gram-negative rods result in sepsis? What role does the immune response play in the pathogenesis of sepsis?

C. Describe the hemodynamic changes that result in septic shock?

D. By what mechanisms does sepsis result in multiorgan failure?

E. What factors predict a poor outcome in patients with sepsis?

REFERENCES

General

Finlay BB et al. Anti-immunology: Evasion of the host immune system by bacterial and viral pathogens. Cell. 2006 Feb 24;124(4):767–82. [PMID: 16497587]

Mandell GL et al. *Mandell, Douglas and Bennett's Principles and Practices of Infectious Diseases,* 6th ed. Elsevier Churchill Livingstone, 2005.

Pirofski LA et al. The damage-response framework of microbial pathogenesis and infectious diseases. Adv Exp Med Biol 2008;635:135–46. [PMID: 18841709]

Infective Endocarditis

Thiene G et al. Pathology and pathogenesis of infective endocarditis in native heart valves. Cardiovasc Pathol. 2006 Sep-Oct;15(5):256–63. [PMID: 16979032]

Tleyjeh I et al. A systematic review of population-based studies of infective endocarditis. Chest 2007 Sep;132(3):1025–35. [PMID: 17873196]

Wang A et al. International Collaboration on Endocarditis-Prospective Cohort Study Investigators. Contemporary clinical profile and outcome of prosthetic valve endocarditis. JAMA. 2007 Mar 28;297(12):1354–61. [PMID: 17392239]

Meningitis

Van de Beek D et al. Corticosteroids for acute bacterial meningitis. Cochrane Database Syst Rev. 2007 Jan 24;(1):CD004405. [PMID: 17253505]

Van de Beek D et al. Community-acquired bacterial meningitis in adults. N Engl J Med. 2006 Jan 5;354(1):44–53. [PMID: 16394301]

Van der Flier M et al. Reprogramming the host response in bacterial meningitis: how best to improve outcome? Clin Microbiol Rev. 2003 Jul;16(3):415–29. [PMID: 12857775]

Pneumonia

Kadioglu A et al. The role of *Streptococcus pneumoniae* virulence factors in host respiratory colonization and disease. Nat Rev Microbiol. 2008 Apr;6(4):288–301. [PMID: 18340341]

Mandell LA et al. Infectious Diseases Society of America/American Thoracic Society consensus guidelines on the management of community-acquired pneumonia in adults. Clin Infect Dis. 2007 Mar 1;44(Suppl 2):S27–72. [PMID: 17278083]

Infectious Diarrhea

Gascón J. Epidemiology, etiology, and pathophysiology of traveler's diarrhea. Digestion. 2006;73(Suppl 1):102–8. [PMID: 16498258]

Sepsis, Sepsis Syndrome, and Septic Shock

Rittirsch D et al. Harmful molecular mechanisms in sepsis. Nat Rev Immunol. 2008 Oct;8(10):776–87. [PMID: 18802444]

Rudiger A et al. Mechanisms of sepsis-induced cardiac dysfunction. Crit Care Med. 2007 Jun;35(6):1599–608. [PMID: 17452940]

Van der Poll T et al. Host-pathogen interactions in sepsis. Lancet Infect Dis. 2008 Jan;8(1):32–43. [PMID: 18063412]

Neoplasia

Mark M. Moasser, MD

Cell growth and maturation are normal events in organ development during embryogenesis, growth, and tissue repair and remodeling after injury. Disordered regulation of these processes can result in loss of control over cell growth, differentiation, and spatial confinement. Human neoplasia collectively represents a spectrum of diseases characterized by abnormal growth and invasion of cells. Although cancers are typically classified by their tissues of origin or anatomic location, many features are shared by all types. There is also considerable variation among patients with a given type of cancer in the nature of cellular alterations as well as the clinical presentation and course of disease. The recognition of overt malignancy by physical examination or imaging requires the presence in the body of about 1 billion malignant cells. A **preclinical phase** may sometimes be recognized. Preclinical signs may consist of, among others, polyps in the colon or dysplastic nevi on the skin—potential precursors of colon carcinoma and malignant melanoma, respectively. Such precursor lesions usually exhibit features of abnormal cell proliferation without the demonstration of invasiveness and may precede the development of an invasive malignancy by months to years, or may not progress to cancer within the individual's lifetime. More commonly, the preclinical phase goes undetected until invasive cancer, occasionally with regional or distant metastases, is already present. As is the case with other medical disorders, our understanding of the pathophysiology of neoplasia has been based on clinical and pathologic observations of large series of patients. More recently, cellular and molecular features of cancer cells have been described, and their relationships to certain neoplastic entities and clinical situations have extended our knowledge in this field.

CHECKPOINT

1. What is the preclinical phase of cancer?
2. How many malignant cells must be present before overt signs of cancer are evident?

THE MOLECULAR & BIOCHEMICAL BASIS OF NEOPLASIA

The process of neoplasia is a result of stepwise alterations in cellular function. These phenotypic changes confer proliferative, invasive, and metastatic potential that are the hallmarks of cancer. It is generally believed—although not conclusively proved—that genetic alterations underlie all cellular and biochemical aberrations responsible for the malignant phenotype. In addition to mutational changes that alter the genetic code, epigenetic changes also underlie cellular and biochemical aberrations that contribute to the malignant phenotype. Epigenetic phenomena influence gene expression and cell behavior, and although once acquired they are transmitted to daughter cells with cell division, they are not changes in the genetic code. An example of this is the silencing of certain genes by hypermethylation of DNA in the promoter region. An increasing number of genetic and cellular changes are being catalogued from the study of cancer cells, both in vivo, from primary tumors of patients, and in vitro, from established cancer cell lines grown in tissue culture. Some alterations are related to particular cellular phenotypes, such as a high proliferative rate or metastatic potential. Some of these changes are specific to a certain tumor type, whereas others are seen across different tumor types. In certain types of tumors, a particular genetic alteration is etiologically linked with, and is pathognomonic of, that cancer type and can play a significant role as a molecular marker of that disease and as a target for drug development. However, most types of cancers do not have unifying molecular characteristics. Although many of the most common types of cancers are categorized by their primary organ site, such as breast or prostate, this classification belies the heterogeneous nature of the cancers that can arise from that organ, and in actuality, what is currently called breast cancer is in fact a compilation of many diseases, previously difficult to categorize. Technological advances in high-throughput analysis of the entire cellular genome and of total cellular gene expression profiles have allowed the characterization of tumors by their molecular signatures. Ongoing studies are attempting to link molecular signatures with important predictive and prognostic clinical parameters. If confirmed, then their biologic relevance is established and in time molecular profiling will define a new system of classification of human tumor types.

Although the progressive phenotypic characteristics of neoplasia result predominantly through sequential molecular alterations and abnormal function of the proliferating tumor cells, it is now clear that at some level abnormal function of the host stromal cells is fundamentally involved in continued tumor progression. It is not clear whether the abnormal function of stromal cells in tumor progression is due to genetic changes in these host cells or whether it is through cell-to-cell communications established through juxtacrine signaling loops with tumor cells. Stromal cell abnormalities can be nonproliferative, such as secretion of requisite growth factors, or proliferative, such as an expansion of the blood vessel network to support the growth of enlarging tumors.

CHECKPOINT

3. What stepwise phenotype changes are the hallmarks of cancer?

GENETIC CHANGES IN NEOPLASIA

Maintaining genomic integrity is a fundamental cellular task. A complex cellular apparatus serves to recognize DNA damage or errors in replication, activate checkpoints to halt further cell replication, and implement corrective measures or signal suicidal cell death. One of the earliest phenomena observed in the course of tumor initiation is the development of defects in the genes involved in the machinery that guards the genome. This malfunction creates a degree of instability inherent in the genome that greatly increases the spontaneous rate at which genomic mutations or structural alterations occur and subsequently enables tumors to potentially acquire defects in an unlimited number of additional genes that may confer to them a growth advantage. Exposure to ionizing radiation and chemical carcinogens are environmental factors that can accelerate the accumulation of deleterious mutations. The cataloguing of these mutated genes has been a fundamental task of molecular oncology because it identifies genes whose functions are relevant to tumor

cells. Genes that confer a growth advantage to tumor cells through a loss-of-function alteration are named **tumor suppressor genes.** Genes that confer a growth advantage through a gain-of-function event are named **proto-oncogenes,** and their activated counterparts are named **oncogenes.** Tumor suppressor genes can be inactivated through **frame-shift mutation, deletion** of part or all of the gene, and gene silencing by way of **promoter methylation.** Proto-oncogenes can be activated through **mutation,** gene **amplification** and **overexpression, chromosomal translocation,** and possibly other mechanisms. Examples of oncogenes and tumor suppressor genes are listed in Tables 5–1 and 5–2. In general, during the gain-of-function alteration of a proto-oncogene, only one allele is mutated. In contrast, during the loss-of-function alteration of a tumor suppressor gene both alleles need to be inactivated. In certain cases, loss of one allele can result in reduction of gene expression. For some genes, this gene-dosage reduction is sufficient to permit tumorigenic growth.

In addition to being generated through the mutation of cellular proto-oncogenes, oncogenes can also be acquired through the introduction of foreign genomic material, typically transmitted by viruses. Although virally induced tumors are common in animals, only a few human tumors are directly caused by viral infection. Causative viruses and their associated malignancies are listed in Table 5–3. One such virus, human T-cell leukemia virus, is closely related to HIV and can cause a type of T-cell leukemia as a result of proteins encoded by the viral genome that are able to activate latent human genes. Human papillomavirus has long been linked epidemiologically to cervical cancer, and the serotypes most often linked have been found to encode proteins that can bind and inactivate host tumor suppressor gene products. In this situation, a causative gene is not necessarily introduced by the virus, but the viral genome is able to direct the inactivation of tumor suppressor gene products and thereby favor growth and proliferation as well as malignant potential. The ability of viruses to modulate the host cellular machinery—and in some cases retain altered mammalian genes that are oncogenic—is likely to have developed over the course of mammalian evolution, because an actively proliferating cell provides the optimal conditions for replication of virions and propagation of viral infections.

The diploid human genome naturally contains defective alleles of many genes, and although defective alleles are for the most part biologically silent, in the case of tumor suppressor genes, a defective allele can confer significant cancer risk to an individual and all family members harboring such an allele. The loss of function of a gene in adult tissues is statistically much more probable when only one functional allele exists in all cells from the beginning of life, and inherited susceptibility to cancer is almost always a result of germline passage of a defective tumor suppressor gene allele. Many of the identified tumor suppressor genes that are frequently inactivated in sporadic human tumors have also been

TABLE 5–1 **Representative oncogenes activated in human tumors.**

Oncogene	Cellular Function	Tumor Types Activated	Mechanism of Activation
EGFR/HER1	Growth factor receptor	Glioblastoma, lung and breast cancer	Mutation, amplification
HER2/Neu	Growth factor receptor	Breast, ovarian, gastric cancer	Amplification
PRAD1/Cyclin D1	Cell cycle regulator	Breast and esophageal cancer, lymphoma, parathyroid adenoma	Amplification, translocation
K-Ras, N-Ras, H-Ras	G protein, signal transduction	Multiple tumor types	Mutation
B-Raf	Signal transduction	Multiple tumor types, melanomas	Mutation
Src	Adhesion and cytoskeletal signaling, other functions	Colon, breast, lung cancer, sarcoma, melanoma	Unknown, rarely mutated
Myc	Transcription factor	Multiple tumor types	Amplification, mutation
Myb	Transcription factor	Leukemia	Amplification, overexpression
Fos	Transcription factor	Multiple tumor types	Overexpression
Int2/FGF3	Growth factor	Esophageal, gastric, head and neck cancers	Amplification
Fes/Fps	Signal transduction	Leukemia	Unknown
menin	Transcription factor	Pituitary, pancreas , parathyroid tumors	Mutation
Ret	Growth factor receptor	Parathyroid, medullary thyroid carcinoma, pheochromocytoma	Mutation

TABLE 5–2 **Representative tumor suppressor genes inactivated in human tumors or the human germline.**

Tumor Suppressor Gene	Cellular Function	Tumor Types Inactivated	Mechanism of Inactivation	Hereditary Syndromes with a Germline Inactivated Allele
p53	Cell cycle regulator	Multiple tumor types	Mutation	Li-Fraumeni
Rb	Cell cycle regulator	Retinoblastoma, small cell lung cancer, sarcoma	Deletion, mutation	Familial retinoblastoma
APC	Cell adhesion	Colon cancer	Deletion, mutation	Familial adenomatous polyposis
PTEN	Signal transduction, adhesion signaling	Glioblastomas, prostate cancer, breast cancer	Deletion, mutation	Cowden's
hMSH2	DNA mismatch repair	Colon cancer, endometrial cancer, melanoma	Mutation	Hereditary nonpolyposis colon cancer
hMLH1	DNA mismatch repair	Colon cancer, melanoma	Mutation	Hereditary nonpolyposis colon cancer
BRCA1	DNA ds-break repair	Breast and ovarian cancers	Mutation	Familial breast/ovarian
BRCA2	DNA ds-break repair	Breast and ovarian cancers	Mutation	Familial breast/ovarian
WT-1	Transcription factor	Wilms' tumor	Deletion, mutation	Childhood Wilms' tumor
NF-1	GTPase activator	Sarcoma, glioma	Deletion, mutation	Neurofibromatosis
NF-2	Cytoskeletal protein	Schwannoma	Mutation	Neurofibromatosis
VHL	Ubiquitin ligase	Kidney cancer, multiple tumor types	Mutation	Von Hippel-Lindau disease
p16/CDKN2	Cell cycle regulator	Melanoma, pancreatic and esophageal cancers	Mutation, deletion, methylation	Familial melanoma

TABLE 5–3 Oncogenic human viruses.

Virus Type	Virus Family	Associated Cancer Type
HTLV-I	Retrovirus (RNA virus)	T-cell leukemia/lymphoma
Hepatitis B	Hepadnavirus (hepatotropic DNA virus)	Hepatocellular carcinoma
Hepatitis C	Hepadnavirus	Hepatocellular carcinoma
Epstein-Barr	Herpesvirus (DNA virus)	Nasopharyngeal carcinoma
		Burkitt's lymphoma
		Immunoblastic lymphoma
		Hodgkin's disease
HHV-8 (KSHV)	Herpesvirus	Kaposi's sarcoma
		Body cavity lymphoma
HPV serotypes 16, 18, 33, 39	Papillomavirus (DNA virus)	Cervical carcinoma
		Anal carcinoma
HPV serotypes 5, 8, 17	Papillomavirus	Skin cancer

Key: HTLV, human T-cell leukemia-lymphoma virus; HHV-8, human herpesvirus-8; KSHV, Kaposi's sarcoma herpesvirus.

linked to specific hereditary cancer syndromes. In families with these syndromes, a defective allele of the responsible tumor suppressor gene is passed in the germline, and members who harbor this heterozygous genotype inherit a high risk for tumors in which the second allele has also been lost. An inherited mutation in one allele of the *p53* gene can cause the rare Li–Fraumeni syndrome, characterized by the early development of bone, breast, brain, and soft tissue tumors (sarcomas) along with other organ-specific tumors (such as adrenal cancer). Inherited mutations in single alleles of the *BRCA1* or *BRCA2* genes confer a high risk for breast or ovarian cancers. The hereditary cancer syndromes linked with many tumor suppressor genes are listed in Table 5–2. In contrast to single alleles of defective tumor suppressor genes, single alleles of mutationally activated oncogenes are not biologically silent and, if present in the germline, can have profound clinical manifestations, even embryonic demise. Because of this fact, inherited syndromes related to germline transmission of activated oncogenes are much more uncommon. A rare example, however, is the familial syndrome of **multiple endocrine neoplasia type II,** in which heterozygotes carrying an activated *RET* oncogene on chromosome 10 are at increased risk of developing two rare neural crest tumors: pheochromocytoma and medullary carcinoma of the thyroid, together with parathyroid tumors.

PROTO-ONCOGENES & TUMOR SUPPRESSOR GENES IN NORMAL PHYSIOLOGY & NEOPLASIA

Proteins encoded by proto-oncogenes and tumor suppressor genes perform diverse cellular functions. Not surprisingly, these include proteins that recognize and repair DNA damage, proteins that regulate the cell cycle, proteins that mediate growth factor signal transduction pathways and that regulate programmed cell death, and proteins involved in cell adhesion, proteolytic proteins, and transcription factors. The function of many proto-oncogenes and tumor suppressor genes remains unknown. Mutations that confer selective advantage to tumors are those that result in increased genomic instability, elimination of cell cycle checkpoints, inactivation of programmed cell death (apoptotic) pathways, increased growth factor signaling, decreased cell adhesion, and increased extracellular proteolysis. The expression and functions of many genes can be simultaneously affected through deregulation of transcription factors. With rapid advances in sequencing technologies and high-throughput capabilities to study normal and tumor genomes, aggressive efforts are in progress to identify all the tumor suppressor genes and proto-oncogenes in the human genome.

Tumor suppressor genes include proteins involved in DNA damage control, cell cycle control, programmed cell death, and cell adhesion. Examples include both the retinoblastoma protein and the **p16** cell cycle inhibitor, which function in regulation of the G1 checkpoint of the cell cycle. Loss of these genes can result in unchecked progression through the G1/S checkpoint. The *p53* tumor suppressor gene is a critical guardian of genomic integrity and serves to recognize DNA damage and consequently inhibit cell cycle progression and induce programmed cell death. Loss of *p53* can result in continued cell replication despite DNA damage and failure to activate programmed cell death. The fundamental importance of *p53* function and of genomic stability in the oncogenic process is underscored by the fact that *p53* mutations are the most common mutations in human cancers and are seen in more than half of all human tumors. The *PTEN* tumor suppressor gene is a phosphatase involved in the regulation of an important survival signaling pathway. Loss of *PTEN* function can result in unopposed survival signaling and failure to activate programmed cell death. **Cadherins** are proteins involved in cell–cell adhesion. Loss of cadherins can result in reduced cell adhesion, cell detachment, and metastasis. Table 5–2 presents a small list of examples of tumor suppressor genes. When fully identified, the entire list of human tumor suppressor genes will be much larger.

Proto-oncogenes include proteins involved in various steps of the extracellular growth factor signaling pathway from the membrane receptors to the membrane intermediates to the proteins mediating the cytoplasmic signaling cascades. The epidermal growth factor receptor (**EGFR**) binds a number of extracellular ligands and, in cooperation with its homolog,

HER2, signals proliferative and apoptotic pathways. Overactivity of EGFR or HER2 can lead to unregulated control of growth and apoptotic signaling. The gene for EGFR or HER1 is mutated or amplified in nearly half of all glioblastomas, is amplified in a fraction of breast cancers and other epithelial cancers, and is mutationally activated in a fraction of lung cancers. The *HER2* gene is amplified in 20% of breast cancers and confers a poorer prognosis. **Ras** is a membrane-bound signaling switch that functions immediately downstream of membrane receptors at a key branch point of cytoplasmic signaling. Mutational activation of Ras causes overactive cytoplasmic signaling and deregulation of proliferative and apoptotic pathways. Ras appears to be critically important in tumorigenesis because nearly one third of all human tumors harbor mutationally activated Ras. **Raf** is a serine-threonine kinase that functions downstream of Ras. Mutational activation of Raf similarly can lead to overactive signaling and deregulation of proliferative and apoptotic pathways and is commonly seen in many tumors. Table 5–1 presents a partial list of oncogenes identified in human malignancies, along with the tumor types in which they are commonly observed and the cellular function encoded by their proto-oncogene counterparts.

Another pathway frequently activated in many human cancers is the PI3 kinase signaling pathway. This pathway controls many cellular processes required for malignant transformation, particularly because it functions to allow the cell to deal with and respond to stress. Activation of this pathway allows cells to adapt to and survive in conditions of low oxygen, low nutrients, and other environmental stresses and signals processes leading to increased protein synthesis, increased energy production, use of alternative metabolic pathways, cell survival, and cell proliferation. This pathway can be activated by upstream signals or can be activated within the pathway by the mutational activation of PI3K or its downstream signal Akt or by mutational inactivation of its negative regulator PTEN.

It is now clear that the inactivation of a single tumor suppressor gene or the activation of a single oncogene is insufficient for the development of most types of human tumors. In fact, the process entails the sequential acquisition of a number of hits over a period of time leading to sequential cellular phenotypic changes from atypia to dysplasia to hyperplasia to in situ cancer to invasive and subsequently metastatic cancer. The largest body of evidence to support this theory has been generated from the molecular study of colon cancer and identifiable preneoplastic lesions, including adenomas and colonic polyps. In this model, the progressive development of neoplasia from premalignant to malignant to invasive lesions is associated with an increasing number of genetic abnormalities, including both oncogene activation and tumor suppressor gene inactivation. This theory is further supported by the identification of inherited abnormalities of several tumor suppressor genes, all associated with a strong familial tendency to develop colon cancer at a young age.

Some forms of human cancer appear to be more simplistic in evolution. A translocation of the long arm of chromosome 9 to the long arm of chromosome 22 leads to fusion of the *BCR* gene with the *c-Abl* gene and results in expression of the **BCR-Abl** oncoprotein seen in chronic myelogenous leukemia (CML). The expression of this oncogene in hematopoietic cells in animal models reproduces the disease. This oncogenic event is seen in virtually 100% of cases of this disease, and a treatment that inhibits the kinase activity of this oncoprotein produces remissions in nearly 100% of the patients. Thus, in contrast to the multistep process involved in most types of carcinogenesis, the steps necessary for the development of CML may be much simpler.

The identification of tumor suppressor genes and oncogenes as the fundamental enablers of tumorigenesis has led to the hypothesis that cancer can be successfully treated by treatments that counteract the biochemical sequelae of these molecular abnormalities. This has fueled attempts to develop therapeutic agents that can inhibit the function of activated oncoproteins or that can restore the function of inactivated tumor suppressor proteins.

HORMONES, GROWTH FACTORS, & OTHER CELLULAR GENES IN NEOPLASIA

Although structurally altered genes, classified as oncogenes or tumor suppressor genes, are key mediators of neoplasia, the role of unaltered genes is not to be dismissed and is likely equally important in carcinogenesis. Signaling proteins of all kinds may drive the oncogenic process through abnormal signaling: abnormal in time, duration, or intensity; abnormal tissue expression; or abnormal subcellular compartment localization. The regulation of growth in complex organisms requires specialized proteins for the normal growth, maturation, development, and function of cells and specialized tissue. The complexity of the human organism requires that these proteins be expressed at precisely coordinated points in space and time. An essential component of this regulation is the system of hormones, growth factors, and growth inhibitors. On binding to specific receptor proteins on the cell surface or in the cytoplasm, these factors lead to a complex set of signals that can result in a variety of cellular effects, including mitogenesis, growth inhibition, changes in cell cycle regulation, apoptosis, differentiation, and induction of a secondary set of genes. The actual end effects are dependent not only on the particular type of interacting factor and receptor but also on the cell type and milieu in which factor–receptor coupling occurs. This system allows for cell-to-cell interactions, whereby a factor secreted by one cell or tissue can enter the bloodstream and influence another set of distant cells (endocrine action) or act on adjacent cells (paracrine action). An autocrine action is also possible when a cell produces a factor that binds to a receptor on or in the same cell. Altered concentration of these growth factors as well as overexpression or mutations of the receptors can change the signaling behavior, contributing to a malignant phenotype. Only a subset of growth factor receptors are proto-oncogenes. However, many additional **growth factors** and **growth factor receptors** appear to be important in tumor growth and progression, although not classified as proto-oncogenes, because they serve tumorigenic causes without incurring mutations or without overexpression.

An important class of growth factor signaling molecules are the **growth factor receptor tyrosine kinases (RTKs)**. A number of tyrosine kinase receptor families exist, and in experimental models most are capable of transforming cells if activated or overexpressed. Although all of these abnormalities are not necessarily seen in naturally occurring human tumors, these experimental data highlight the potential inherent in these proteins and the important role they may be playing in tumor cells despite lacking the oncogene label. Members of the HER family of RTKs are commonly mutated or amplified in human tumors and exemplify the important role of RTKs in human neoplasia. In many other tumors, they likely play an important role despite having a normal sequence and expression level. For example, HER1 (also called EGFR) is not mutated or overexpressed in colon cancers, but it is sometimes activated by autocrine signaling in the cancer cells, and EGFR-targeted therapies are used to treat this type of cancer. The platelet-derived growth factor (PDGF) receptors, fibroblast growth factor receptors, vascular endothelial growth factor receptors, and insulin-like growth factor receptor are all families of RTKs that function similar to HER family RTKs. These receptors are, in general, not reported to be mutated or amplified in human tumors. However, there is increased expression in many tumors or aberrant expression in tumors from tissue types that ordinarily would not be expected to express that receptor. Alternatively, excessive production of receptor ligands is due to a variety of mechanisms (ie, loss of epigenetic silencing of the gene coding for the ligand or excessive gene transcription of the same gene). In experimental systems, each of these RTK systems has oncogenic potential, building a circumstantial case that they may be important players in human tumors.

Some growth factor signaling pathways function to inhibit cell growth and provide negative regulation in response to extracellular stimuli. Desensitization of cells to such growth inhibitors is common in tumors. An example of this is the **transforming growth factor-β (TGF-β)**. TGF-β has diverse biological effects. It potently inhibits cell proliferation but also stimulates the production and deposition of extracellular matrix (ECM) and adhesion factors. These functions are important in tissue remodeling during embryogenesis and wound repair. In some tumor types, the antiproliferative response to TGF-β is lost early on because of mutations in its downstream signaling components. However, continued secretion, and often oversecretion, of TGF-β by the tumor and stromal tissues leads to an increase in the production of ECM and adhesion factors and promotes the invasive and metastatic property of tumors.

Another important class of receptors is the large superfamily of **nuclear hormone receptors.** These include the cellular receptors for a variety of hormones, among them estrogen and progesterone, androgens, glucocorticoids, thyroid hormone, and retinoids. The actions of estrogen are

fundamentally important in the development of breast cancer. In women, oophorectomy early in life offers substantial protection against the development of breast cancer, and in animal models mammary carcinogenesis is significantly retarded in the absence of estrogen. Approximately half of all breast cancers are dependent on estrogen for proliferation. Although these data clearly implicate the estrogen signaling pathway in breast carcinogenesis, specific abnormalities of the **estrogen receptor** (**ER**) are not seen in breast cancers; therefore, the ER does not qualify as a tumor suppressor protein or an oncoprotein. It is possible that, although the loss of certain tumor suppressor genes or activation of certain oncogenes leads to the development of breast cancer, continued ER function is essential throughout this process and without ER function it cannot proceed. Alternatively, it is possible that abnormal ER signaling, perhaps as a result of altered cofactors, cross-talk, or phosphorylation status, drives breast carcinogenesis. Although the mechanism by which estrogen and its receptor drive breast cancers has not yet been determined, its fundamental role in this disease is well established. Furthermore, treatments that work through inhibiting the production of the active ligand or that inhibit the function of the ER are the most effective therapies for breast cancer yet developed and are highly active in the prevention and treatment of breast cancer. The **androgen receptor** (AR), similarly, plays a critical role in the development of prostate cancer, although occasional activating mutations of the AR have been reported in prostate cancers. On the contrary, the ability of retinoids (ligands for retinoic acid receptors) that are well known to participate in the differentiation of a variety of tissues during development to cause the differentiation of certain tumors in tissue culture models has been exploited as a treatment approach for acute promyelocytic leukemia (APL). APL is characterized by a t(15;17) chromosomal translocation resulting in the fusion of the *PML* gene with the **retinoic acid receptor-α (*RAR-α*)** gene. The resulting fusion protein blocks the differentiation of hematopoietic progenitor cells and eventually leads to the development of APL. This fusion protein is not by itself transforming in experimental models and cannot be categorized as a classic oncogene or tumor suppressor gene, but it is etiologically involved in the pathogenesis of APL. Because the fusion protein contains the ligand-binding domain of RAR-α, it remains sensitive to ligand and treatment of patients with the ligand all-*trans* retinoic acid results in differentiation of tumor cells and complete remission in most patients with this disease.

Other functional membrane proteins not related to growth can also be present on tumors cells. The MDR-1 gene product belongs to a class of ATP-dependent channel transporter proteins and is present on some normal epithelial cells. Its physiologic role may be to pump toxic molecules out of the cell, but in some tumor cells, its overexpression causes efflux of certain chemotherapeutic agents, leading to drug resistance. In some situations, its expression can be induced by long-term exposure to chemotherapy.

STROMAL, ADHESIVE, & PROTEOLYTIC PROTEINS

The preservation of tissue structure in multicellular organisms involves the orderly arrangement of cells within an architectural framework. This higher-level order is required to maintain tissue structure and organ function, and mechanisms are in place to enable remodeling during embryogenesis or during wound repair. A number of protein families serve to constitute the ECM, to embed cells within the ECM, to attach cells to each other, and to dissolve and reestablish the ECM when necessary. Abnormalities of these proteins frequently occur in later stages of tumorigenesis, account for the loss of architecture, and mediate the invasive and metastatic phenotype of tumor cells. Integrins are a large family of membrane proteins that bind ECM ligands, anchor cells to the ECM, and activate intracellular signaling pathways in response to ECM signals. Cells have the ability to express any of a large repertoire of integrin combinations and the specificity of integrin expression is not well understood. However, tumor cells can reshuffle their integrin expression profiles in favor of an invasive or metastatic phenotype. Cadherins are a family of membrane proteins that function in epithelial cell-to-cell adhesion. Loss of E-cadherin expression is seen in some human epithelial tumors leading to a more invasive phenotype. The expression and activity of many secreted and membrane-anchored proteases are increased in tumor cells. This includes the **matrix metalloprotease** family and the **serine protease** family of proteins. Increased protease activity leads to ECM degradation, triggering of the plasminogen activation cascade, and activation of transmembrane receptors through cleavage and shedding of their extracellular domains. Through abnormalities in deposition of ECM, of expression of cell adhesion proteins, and in activity of membrane and secreted proteases, cancer cells develop an invasive and ultimately a metastatic phenotype.

ALTERATIONS IN METABOLISM & OXYGENATION IN NEOPLASIA

In addition to abnormalities in cell proliferation and survival, signal transduction, adhesion, and migration, tumor cells have changes in metabolic pathways in order to meet their increased metabolic requirements. Oxygen pressure is reduced in tumor tissues, and tumor hypoxia signals changes in gene expression for adaptation to the hypoxic environment. Tumor cells secrete **angiogenic growth factors,** which signal the proliferation of vascular structures into tumor tissue for nutrition and oxygenation. The identification of tumor factors that signal pathologic neovascularization has been of particular interest because such factors could be targets for therapeutic drug development and produce treatments that inhibit tumor angiogenesis. The best studied proangiogenic factor is the **vascular endothelial growth factor** (**VEGF**), a mitogen to endothelial cells that is often se-

creted by tumor cells and activates the VEGF receptors in endothelial cells, leading to de novo vascularization. Although most cells may not ordinarily express VEGF, malignant transformation often results in the induction of VEGF expression by tumor cells, either directly through the effects of oncogenes or the loss of tumor suppressor genes or indirectly as a result of hypoxia and the induction of hypoxia-induced gene transcription. Other growth factors also have proangiogenic effects, including epidermal growth factor, fibroblast growth factor, PDGF, transforming growth factor-α, and others.

CELLULAR CHANGES IN NEOPLASIA

The molecular changes of neoplastic cells and their phenotypic behavior is a constantly evolving process. Every cell division can result in additional genomic abnormalities and a variety of phenotypic consequences. Certain genotypes result in proliferative, survival, or other biological attributes that favor its clonal expansion. Such neoplastic clones eventually overtake the tumor cell population and change its clinical behavior. This remodeling process occurs repeatedly with repeated cell division, recreating a process akin to evolution, albeit in a much faster timeframe. Attributes that are acquired early during the evolution of cancer include enhanced proliferation and survival. Changes that are acquired midpoint include the ability to overcome spacial limitations by invading surrounding tissues, the ability to survive under conditions of low oxygen and nutrients, and the ability to evade host immune defenses. Changes acquired later in the progression of neoplasia are the ability to travel to distant organs and the ability to resist anticancer treatments.

The changing nature of cancer with repeated cell proliferation cycles along constantly expanding cell lineages creates heterogeneity in the whole tumor cell population. Tumor cell heterogeneity is a common characteristic of many types of cancer. Although many or most of the cells that arise from cancer cell division themselves proceed to multiply, the changes with repeated cycles of cell division often lead to the loss of some of the more fundamental properties of the ancestral cancer cells. For example, many of the cells in a tumor are unable to give rise to a new tumor if isolated. In fact, only a small proportion of cancer cells appear to be capable of starting new colonies of cancer cells if isolated or if metastasized to a new site in the body. Such cells, named **cancer stem cells,** typically do not proliferate as fast but are capable of self-renewal and of generating daughter cells that can proliferate much faster and produce new tumors.

Current efforts explore the hypotheses that 1) defects in normal tissue stem cells within an organ give rise to cancer stem cells (see the Hematologic Malignancy section for a more detailed discussion) and 2) terminally differentiated cells (non-stem cells) usurp the machinery used by normal stem cells in the process of becoming cancer stem cells.

CLASSIFICATION OF NEOPLASIA

Neoplasia describes a large number of human diseases with extremely diverse characteristics. Therefore, the classification of neoplastic diseases into categories and subcategories is of great value in understanding them, diagnosing them, studying them, and developing treatments for them. Malignant transformation, by definition, results in abnormal cellular behavior. Tumor cells that have retained many of their specialized tissue functions and that are very similar appearing to their normal cellular counterparts are identified as well differentiated. Conversely, tumor cells that have lost much of their functions and that bear little similarity to their normal counterparts are identified as poorly differentiated. Poorly differentiated tumors are sometimes so abnormal that their cell or organ of origin cannot be recognized. However, although poorly differentiated tumor cells may have lost much of their specialized functions, their cellular ancestry can often still be recognized by more primitive characteristics.

The broadest classification of tumors relies on the most fundamental characterization of cell types based on their primitive embryologic origins. During early embryonic development, three cell lineages are established: ectoderm, endoderm, and mesoderm. All subsequent cells, including adult tumors, can be traced to one of these three cellular origins. As such, tumors are broadly classified into the categories of **carcinoma** if they originate from **ectodermal** or **endodermal** tissues or as **sarcomas** if they originate from **mesodermal** tissues. Even if completely unrecognizable by morphologic analysis, fundamental differences in the expression of certain proteins, especially intermediate filaments such as keratins and vimentin, will identify the lineage of origin.

Carcinomas are the most common cancer type and include all the common epithelial tissue cancers such as lung, colon, breast, and prostate cancers. **Sarcomas** arise from mesenchymal cell types, which are predominantly the connective tissues. Malignancies of blood cells, including leukemias and lymphomas, are technically a subtype of sarcomas because they are of mesenchymal origin. However, because of the highly specialized nature of hematologic cell types, they are generally grouped together and considered the entity of hematologic neoplasms, which includes leukemias and lymphomas. Further classification of carcinomas and sarcomas is based on the organ of origin. In the growing infant and child, mesenchymal tissues are very active in growth and remodeling, and mesenchymal tumors are common, including tumors of the muscle, cartilage, bone, and blood. In adults, the mesenchymal tissues are not very active, and epithelial tumors are by far the most common, including tumors of the lung, breast, prostate, and colon. Developments in gene expression profiling of tumors has enabled classification of tumors based on characteristic molecular portraits, and further work in this area may result in an entirely new classification of human tumors based on their gene expression profiles.

EPITHELIAL NEOPLASIA

Epithelial cells are in constant turnover, arising from a basal layer that continually generates new cells. The mature and functional layer of cells performs specialized tissue or organ functions, and with senescence it is eventually sloughed off. Proliferating epithelial cells normally observe anatomic boundaries such as the basement membrane that underlies the basal layer of cells in the epithelium. The potential to divide, migrate, and differentiate is tightly controlled. The stimulus to divide may be autonomous or exogenous as a response to factors from adjacent or distant cells. Inhibitory signals and factors may also be present and serve to function as negative regulators to check uncontrolled growth. The neoplastic phenotype of epithelial cells can be seen as a spectrum from **hyperplastic** to **preinvasive** to frankly **invasive** and **metastatic** neoplasia, as illustrated in Figure 5–1. Because of their embryonic origins, malignancies of epithelial origin are termed carcinomas. Hyperplasia can be a normal physiologic response in some situations, such as that which occurs in the lining of the uterus in response to estrogens before the ovulatory phase of the menstrual cycle. It may also be a pathologic finding and associated with a predisposition to progress to invasive carcinoma. In such instances of hyperplasia, there are usually accompanying disorders of maturation that may be recognizable by microscopic examination. These changes are termed **dysplasia, atypical hyperplasia,** or **metaplasia** depending on the type of epithelium in which they are observed. More aggressive proliferation without the ability to invade through the

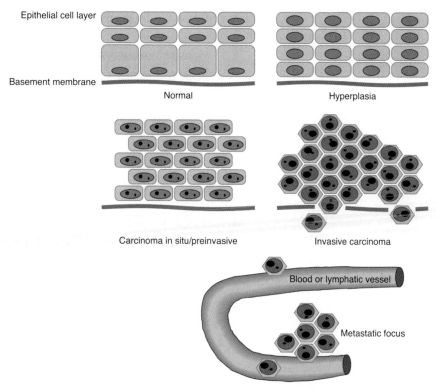

Epithelial cell layer

Basement membrane

Normal

Hyperplasia

Carcinoma in situ/preinvasive

Invasive carcinoma

Blood or lymphatic vessel

Metastatic focus

FIGURE 5–1 Schematic depiction of phenotypic transition of epithelial cells from hyperplasia to invasive carcinoma.

basement membrane is termed **preinvasive** carcinoma, or **carcinoma in situ.** Technically, these cells do not have the capacity to invade the basement membrane and metastasize, although they may over time progress to **invasive carcinoma.** The term "invasive carcinoma" implies that tissue boundaries, especially the basement membrane, have been breached. **Metastatic carcinoma** occurs via the lymphatic system to regional lymph nodes and via the bloodstream to distant organs and other tissues. This pattern of metastasis, however, is not unique to epithelial malignancies. Epithelial neoplasms in general have a variable propensity to spread to regional nodes and distant sites. It is assumed that the natural history of most tumors is to follow this pattern of spread over time. The specific genotypic and phenotypic changes necessary to accomplish this spread are not well understood; they may, in some cases, be shared across tumor types, and in other cases they are unique to a given neoplasia. Certain molecular characteristics have been linked to clinical characteristics, although the exact mode of action is not fully understood.

From a pathophysiologic standpoint, certain structural and functional characteristics must be acquired by malignant cells, as outlined in Table 5–4. An increase in growth rate through several mechanisms has been described for different tumor types. It is known that the proliferative fraction (the percentage of cells in S phase, or actively synthesizing DNA) is elevated, and more so in histologically and clinically aggres-

sive tumors. Changes in the tightly regulated cell cycle machinery have been observed, including abnormal levels of cyclins and other proteins that regulate cyclin-dependent kinases responsible for entry of the cell into S phase. Likewise, alterations of intermediate signaling proteins have been noted that couple external growth factor and hormonal stimuli to proliferation. The ability of cells to migrate and pass through cellular and ECM barriers can be enhanced in tumor cells. This can occur through the activation of proteolytic enzyme cascades from within the tumor cell or by the action of stromal cells that are directed to do so as a result of factors produced by nearby tumor cells. Through similar mechanisms, malignant cells can induce the formation of a microvasculature that is essential to support the continued growth of a tumor colony. Other functions necessary to breach the immune defenses and survive destruction by antitumor drugs can be mediated by the genetic program already possessed in latent form by tumor cells. Examples include modulation of antigens and alterations in drug metabolism or metabolic pathways that are targeted by certain drugs.

As described earlier, there is evidence that discrete phenotypic changes that arise from specific genetic alterations account for the progression from hyperplasia to metastatic neoplasia. Moreover, there is an interplay between these genetic changes and the inherent program of gene expression of a given epithelial type. Other highly regulated functions of

TABLE 5–4 Phenotypic changes in the progression of neoplasia.

1. Genomic instability

    Impaired DNA repair

    Aberrant cell cycle checkpoint control

2. Enhanced proliferation

    Autonomous growth

    Abnormalities of cell cycle control

    Exaggerated response to hormonal or growth factor stimuli

    Lack of response to growth inhibitors or cell contact inhibition

3. Evasion of immune system

    Antigen modulation and masking

    Elaboration of immune response antagonistic molecules

4. Invasion of tissue and stroma

    Attachment to extracellular matrix

    Secretion of proteolytic enzymes

    Recruitment of stromal cells to produce proteolytic enzymes

    Loss of cell cohesion

5. Ability to gain access to and egress from lymphatics and bloodstream

    Enhanced cell motility

    Recognition of endothelial protein sequences

    Cytoskeletal modifications

6. Establishment of metastatic foci

    Cell adhesion and attachment

    Tissue-specific tropism

7. Ability to recruit vascularization to support growth of primary or metastatic tumor

8. Drug resistance

    Altered drug metabolism and drug inactivation

    Increased synthesis of targeted enzymes

    Enhanced drug efflux

    Enhanced DNA damage repair

epithelial cells include active or passive transport of ions or molecules as well as synthesis and secretion of specific proteins. These functions may also be lost, altered, or even enhanced for specific tumor types and likewise can create specific pathophysiologic and clinical entities. Two epithelial neoplasms are discussed in further detail. Colon cancer is an example of an epithelial neoplasm for which precursor lesions have been well studied because we can seek out and biopsy such lesions by colonoscopy. Breast epithelial tissue is responsive to steroid hormones and growth factors that may play a role in the development and behavior of breast cancer.

CHECKPOINT

13. What factors determine the malignant potential of epithelial versus mesenchymal tumors?
14. What is the term applied to malignancies of epithelial origin?
15. What is the spectrum of characteristics of the neoplastic phenotype in epithelial cells?

1. Colon Carcinoma

The model of stepwise genetic alterations in cancer is best illustrated by observations made in colonic lesions representing different stages of progression to malignancy. Certain genetic alterations are found commonly in early-stage adenomas, whereas others tend to occur with significant frequency only after the development of invasive carcinoma. These changes are in keeping with the concept that serial phenotypic changes must occur in a cell for it to exhibit full malignant (invasive and metastatic) properties (Table 5–4). Two principal lines of evidence support the model of stepwise genetic alterations in colon cancer.

1. The rare familial syndromes associated with predisposition to colon cancer at an early age are now known to result from germline mutations. **Familial adenomatous polyposis** is the result of a mutation in the *APC* gene, which encodes a cell adhesion protein that has also been implicated in the control of β-catenin, a potent transcriptional activator. In the tumors that subsequently develop, the remaining allele has been lost. Similarly, **hereditary nonpolyposis colorectal cancer** is associated with germline mutations in DNA repair genes such as *hMSH2* and *hMLH1.* These genes can also be affected in sporadic cancers.

2. The carcinogenic effects of factors known to be linked to an increased risk of colon cancer constitute the second line of evidence for a genetic basis for colon cancer. Substances derived from bacterial colonic flora, ingested foods, or endogenous metabolites such as fecapentaenes, 3-ketosteroids, and benzo[α]pyrenes are mutagenic. Levels of these substances can be reduced by low-fat and high-fiber diets, and several epidemiologic studies confirm that such diets reduce the risk of colon cancer. Furthermore, because the risk of sporadic colon cancer in older individuals is mildly elevated in the presence of a positive family history, there may be other inherited genetic abnormalities that interact with environmental factors to cause colon cancer. The sequence of genetic changes may not need to be exact to lead to the development of an invasive cancer, although there is mounting

evidence that some genetic lesions tend to develop early, whereas others may develop late in the course of the natural disease. All phenotypic changes cannot be explained by a known genetic abnormality, nor do all identified genetic alterations have a known phenotypic result. However, the stepwise nature of genotypic and phenotypic abnormalities is well established.

The earliest molecular defect in the pathogenesis of colon cancer is the acquisition of somatic mutations in the *APC* gene in the normal colonic mucosa. This defect causes abnormal regulation of β-catenin, which leads to abnormal cell proliferation and the initial steps in tumor formation. Subsequent defects in the TGF-β signaling pathway inactivate this important growth inhibitory pathway and lead to further tumor mucosal proliferation and the development of small adenomas. Mutational activation of the *K-ras* gene leads to constitutive activation of an important proliferative signaling pathway, is common at these stages, and further increases the proliferative potential of the adenomatous tumor cells. Deletion or loss of expression of the *DCC* gene is common in the progression to invasive colon cancers. The *DCC* protein is a transmembrane protein of the immunoglobulin superfamily and may be a receptor for certain extracellular molecules that guide cell growth and or apoptosis. Mutational inactivation of *p53* is also a commonly observed step in the development of invasive colon cancer, seen in late adenomas and early invasive cancers, and leads to loss of an important cell cycle checkpoint and inability to activate the p53-dependent apoptotic pathways. Identification of genetic abnormalities in the progression of colon cancer to metastatic disease is currently under investigation.

In parallel to these sequential abnormalities in the regulation of cell proliferation, colon cancers also acquire defects in mechanisms that protect genomic stability. These generally involve mutations in mismatch repair genes or genes that prevent chromosomal instability. **Mismatch repair genes** are a family of genes that are involved in proofreading DNA during replication and include *MSH2, MLH1, PMS1,* and *PMS2.* Germline mutations in these genes cause the hereditary nonpolyposis colorectal cancer (HNPCC) syndrome. Nonhereditary colon cancers develop genomic instability through defects in the **chromosomal instability (CIN) genes.** Defects in these genes lead to the gain or loss of large segments or entire chromosomes during replication leading to aneuploidy.

The stepwise acquisition of genetic abnormalities described previously is associated with alterations in the phenotypic behavior of the colonic mucosa. The earliest change in the progression to colon cancer is the increase in cell number (hyperplasia) on the epithelial (luminal) surface. This produces an adenoma, which is characterized by gland-forming cells exhibiting increases in size and cell number but no invasion of surrounding structures (Figure 5–2). Presumably, these changes are due to enhanced proliferation and loss of cell cycle control but before acquisition of the capacity to invade ECM. Additional dysplastic changes such as loss of

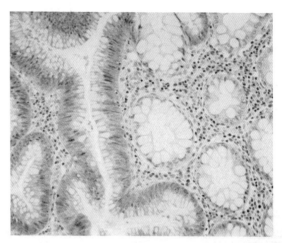

FIGURE 5–2 Edge of an adenomatous polyp, showing adenomatous change (**left**), compared with normal mucosal glands (**right**). Adenomatous change is characterized by increased size and stratification of nuclei and loss of cytoplasmic mucin. Note the arrangement of nuclei of the adenoma perpendicular to the basement membrane (polarity). (Reproduced, with permission, from Chandrasoma P, Taylor CE. *Concise Pathology*, 3rd ed. Originally published by Appleton & Lange. Copyright © 1998 by the McGraw-Hill Companies, Inc.)

mucin production and altered cell polarity may be present to a variable degree. Some adenomas may progress to carcinoma in situ and ultimately to invasive carcinoma. An early feature associated with disrupted architecture even before invasion occurs is the development of fragile new vessels or destruction of existing vessels that can cause microscopic bleeding. This can be tested for clinically as a fecal occult blood determination used for screening and early diagnosis of preinvasive and invasive colon cancer. It is not known whether all invasive colon cancers pass through a hyperplastic or preinvasive stage, and there is no information available for epithelial malignancies in general.

Further functional changes in the cell and surrounding tissue are also manifested in the preinvasive and invasive stages. Once the basement membrane is penetrated by invasive malignant cells, access can be gained to the regional lymphatics, and spread to regional pericolic lymph nodes can occur. Entry of cells into the bloodstream can lead to distant spread in a pattern that reflects venous drainage. Therefore, hematogenous spread from primary colon tumors to the liver is common, whereas rectal tumors usually disseminate to liver, lung, and bone. In addition to anatomic considerations, there may exist specific tropism of malignant cells mediated by surface proteins that cause the cells to preferentially home in on certain organs or sites.

Colonic epithelium is specialized to secrete mucus proteins and to absorb water and electrolytes (Chapter 13). The maintenance of a tight luminal barrier, intracellular charge differences, and the ability to exclude toxins are additional specialized functions. Some of these functions are maintained in the progression to neoplasia and may contribute to a specific phenotype of the malignant cell. One example is the expression of a transporter membrane protein, MDR-1, present on several types of epithelium, including the colon. MDR-1 is known to cause efflux of several compounds out of the cells, presumably as a protective mechanism to exclude toxins. In advanced colon cancer, this protein may contribute to the relative resistance of this and other tumor types to a variety of chemotherapeutic agents that are transported by MDR-1. In some cases, the activation of a latent gene encoding carcinoembryonic antigen (CEA) can result in measurable levels of the CEA protein in the serum of patients with localized or metastatic colon cancer as well as other adenocarcinomas.

CHECKPOINT

16. What are the two principal lines of evidence in favor of the model of stepwise genetic alterations in colon cancer?
17. What is an explanation for the frequent appearance of occult blood in stools of patients with even early colon carcinoma?
18. What are two genes whose products contribute to the classic phenotype of colon carcinomas?

2. Breast Carcinoma

The female breast is a specialized gland that undergoes repeated cycles of growth factor and hormone-induced changes that define the different stages of breast development (fetal, pubertal, menstrual, pregnancy-associated, and lactational growth together with postlactational involution). Deregulation in this complex biology leads to a diverse group of breast diseases inherently connected with growth factor or hormonal signaling. Factors associated with an increased risk of breast cancer development may provide clues to early driving forces. Prolonged usage of high doses of exogenous estrogen is a risk factor that implicates the estrogen signaling pathway. In contrast, reduced exposure to estrogen protects against the development of breast cancer. This has been demonstrated in ovariectomized animal models of breast carcinogenesis and is confirmed by clinical studies demonstrating that women who have undergone oophorectomy at a young age have a significant reduction in their lifetime risk of developing breast cancer. The clinical success of antiestrogen therapies provides proof of principle of the essential role of estrogen signaling in the pathogenesis of breast cancer. Agents that inhibit the production of estrogen or the ability of estrogen to activate the ER are highly effective in the treatment of patients with early or advanced breast cancer, are active in halting disease progression in patients with preinvasive breast cancers, and are also active in the primary prevention of breast cancer in women at risk. However, although the central role of estrogen signaling in the pathogenesis of breast cancer is now well established, the evidence to date does not etiologically implicate genetic abnormalities of the ER or its downstream targets in the development of breast cancer. It appears that ER signaling is a physiological pathway existing in breast epithelial cells whose continued signaling activity is favorable to, or perhaps even necessary for, the oncogenic process. Yet the estrogen signaling pathway is intact in only one half of patients diagnosed with breast cancer; the remaining half appear to have no expression of the ER or activity of the estrogen signaling pathway. This has led some investigators to believe that ER-negative breast cancer is a different disease with an alternative pathophysiology. Most likely, there are common early molecular steps in the development of ER-positive and ER-negative breast cancers; however, at an early or intermediate step, these pathways diverge, leading to the development of breast cancers with distinctly different phenotypes.

The specific signaling pathways that are pathologically or mutationally activated in the progression of breast epithelial cells to preinvasive and invasive cancer are yet undefined. However, the tyrosine kinase growth factor receptors of the human epidermal growth factor receptor (HER) family are prime candidates. Amplification of the *HER2* gene and overexpression of the HER2 protein are common in preinvasive and invasive breast cancers. Overexpression of the *HER1* gene, also called the EGFR, is also seen with less frequency. The HER3 protein is similarly overexpressed in a majority of breast cancers. Antibodies that target the HER2 receptor have activity in the treatment of breast cancer, further confirming the role of this receptor signaling pathway. The HER family receptors activate a number of downstream signaling pathways, including proliferative pathways, apoptotic pathways, and metabolic pathways. The PI3 kinase protein is frequently mutationally activated in breast cancers enhancing survival and stress response. Inactivating mutations of *p53* are also seen frequently in breast cancers and are associated with a worse prognosis.

The loss of genomic stability is also a common event in the pathogenesis of breast cancers. The group of genes involved in the DNA repair mechanism associated with breast cancers was identified in the hereditary breast and ovarian cancer syndromes. Five to 10% of breast cancer cases appear to be associated with an inherited predisposition and linked with predisposition to ovarian cancer. Familial clustering has long been noted in certain kindreds, and this led to the chromosomal localization of putative breast cancer susceptibility genes. This process is termed "linkage analysis," whereby the characteristic of developing breast cancer can be shown to segregate with certain markers of known chromosomal location. The identification of two discrete genes, **BRCA1** and **BRCA2,** then followed through the use of positional cloning, which describes a variety of strategies to pinpoint a gene over a large segment of the genome without knowledge of the gene's function but the presumption that mutations in this gene should be seen in susceptible individuals (eg, women with breast cancer in families with breast cancer clustering). Inherited mutations in the BRCA1 and BRCA2 genes appear to be associated with a likelihood of developing breast cancer over a lifetime of up to 80%. Mutations in these genes are also associated with a high incidence of ovarian cancer and can lead to increased incidences of prostate cancer, melanomas, and breast cancer in males. Both of these genes function as tumor suppressor genes such that breast tumors contain both the inherited abnormality in one allele as well as a somatic loss of the remaining allele. Although sporadic (nonfamilial) cases of breast cancer rarely contain *BRCA1* mutations, they may have reduced BRCA1 expression or may have abnormalities in other proteins that interact with BRCA1 to perform what appears to be a DNA repair function involving double-strand breaks in DNA. It is likely that other inherited genetic abnormalities will be identified that confer an increased risk of breast cancer. Generally, it will be more difficult to identify those that have only modest **penetrance** (ie, confer only a slight increase in breast cancer risk). Identifying mutations with high penetrance in individuals allows such individuals to take preventive measures. Identification of mutations with undefined penetrance or risk is less informative until future studies can better define their risk.

The scheme depicted in Figure 5–1 applies to progressive changes toward invasive breast carcinoma, and this full spectrum may be seen in patients who undergo biopsy to evaluate breast masses or mammographic abnormalities. Carcinoma in situ of the breast represents a preinvasive lesion in which enhanced proliferation and malignant cell morphology are observed but no invasion of the basement membrane can be demonstrated. Therefore, lymph nodal or distant metastases cannot occur at this stage, presumably because the invasive phenotype has not yet been acquired. Certain molecular abnormalities can be seen at this stage, including *HER2* oncogene amplification and *p53* tumor suppressor gene mutations, although the mechanisms through which these abnormalities operate are not well understood.

Cancer of the breast is almost always due to malignant transformation of the secretory epithelial cells. However, two distinct subtypes are recognized. Cancers arising from the collecting ducts are called ductal carcinomas, whereas those arising from the terminal lobules are called lobular carcinomas. **Ductal carcinomas** comprise the majority of breast cancers, and lobular carcinomas represent a minority. Both in situ and invasive breast cancers fall into these two common classifications. Ductal and lobular cancers have distinct morphologic characteristics as well as molecular features specific to each subtype. For example, **lobular carcinomas** have loss of the cell adhesion protein E-cadherin and typically grow in a more diffuse pattern with less formation of dense solid tumors. Consequently, lobular carcinomas are often more difficult to detect radiographically in their primary tumors and even in metastatic sites. Lobular cancers also have less frequent abnormalities of the p53 tumor suppressor protein and rarely have amplification of the *HER2* gene.

Progressive changes in epithelial cell morphology and behavior are seen in lesions that often predate the development of invasive breast cancer. Atypical ductal hyperplasia and atypical lobular hyperplasia are proliferative abnormalities of the breast epithelium, and their presence confers an increased risk of subsequent development of breast cancer. **Ductal carcinoma in situ** (DCIS) and **lobular carcinoma in situ** (LCIS) are noninvasive carcinomas that are more strongly associated with the concurrent or subsequent development of invasive breast cancer. Although these progressive cellular changes are well described in the progression to breast cancer, it is not clear that these are sequential steps that a clonal population of cells needs to undergo to evolve into invasive breast cancer. Alternatively, these may be various manifestations of a field defect in the breast epithelium, which leads cells to progress along any of several parallel oncogenic pathways. For example, the risk conferred by DCIS is not only of a subsequent invasive ductal cancer but also of an invasive lobular cancer, and the same is true for LCIS. In addition, although close to 50% of DCIS lesions have amplification and overexpression of *HER2*, only 20% of invasive cancers show this oncogenic molecular abnormality. It remains possible that invasive breast cancer and in situ breast cancer both arise from a common oncogenic pathway that ultimately diverges into separate in situ or invasive endpoints.

The hallmark of invasive breast cancer is the ability of the tumor cells to pass the basement membrane, invade the stroma, and gain access to lymphatic and vascular structures. The spread of tumor cells past the basement membrane to regional lymph nodes and to distant organs is the result of molecular events that are not yet well described. Cell surface proteins involved in adhesion and in degradation of ECM are likely involved. The phenotypic behavior of breast cancer among patients varies greatly, indicating the diverse nature of this disease. Some breast cancers metastasize with high frequency, whereas others rarely do so. Some breast cancers metastasize rapidly, whereas others do so after a long latent period. Some breast cancers preferentially metastasize to bone, whereas others prefer the liver or the lung as metastatic sites and yet others prefer the brain. Specific molecular features must underlie the diverse phenotypes of breast cancer, and indeed breast cancer is likely a compilation of many different disease subsets.

The development of techniques to simultaneously determine the expression of 10,000 or more genes is revolutionizing the way we classify cancers. New initiatives are underway that will likely reclassify breast cancers into disease subsets with specific prognostic and therapeutic implications. Early analysis of gene expression profiles of many patients has already identified distinct subsets labeled as a basal epithelial-like group, a luminal epithelial-like group, and a *HER2* overexpressing group. The basal group is characterized by low or absent expression of ER and other transcription factors, high expression of certain keratins, laminin, and certain integrins. The luminal group is characterized by the expression of a cluster of transcription factors that includes ER and has been further defined into luminal A, B, and C subgroups. The *HER2* overexpressing group is characterized by high expression of several genes in the *HER2* amplicon. These molecular portraits have biologic relevance because they are associated with distinct survival outcomes. Future molecular profiling studies may redefine this preliminary classification and may even classify breast cancers based on chemosensitivity profiles.

MESENCHYMAL, NEUROENDOCRINE, & GERM CELL NEOPLASIA

Mesenchymal, neuroendocrine, and germ cell neoplasms account for a large proportion of the tumors of childhood and young adulthood, ostensibly because these cells are actively dividing and more subject to mutational events. Table 5–5 is a representative list of mesenchymal, neuroendocrine, and germ cell tumors, as well as the embryologic cell groups from which they arise. Owing to the extensive migration and convolution of embryonic cell layers during early development, these tumor types may not evolve in specific anatomic sites. Neuroendo-crine tumors are derived from cells that migrate throughout the body and have developed specific enzymatic capabilities and accumulation of cytoplasmic proteins that serve a secretory function. As such, they are frequently identified by certain enzymatic markers, in particular, nonspecific esterase. Although they were all originally thought to arise from the neural crest, not all neuroendocrine tumors can be traced to the neural crest. Indeed tumors of this classification may not have a common embryonic ancestry. However, this tumor classification has been maintained because of their unique specialized secretory functions. Neuroendocrine tumors can secrete biologically active peptides and produce specific clinical syn-

TABLE 5–5 Neoplasia of mesenchymal, neuroendocrine, and germ cells.

Neoplasia Type	Embryonic Derivation	Neoplasia Type	Embryonic Derivation
Wilms' tumor	Metanephric blastema	Testicular, extragonadal germ cell tumors	
Neuroblastoma	Neuroblasts	Seminoma	
Retinoblastoma		Choriocarcinoma	
Ganglioneuroma		Embryonal carcinoma	
Neuroendocrine tumors	Neural crest	Endodermal sinus, yolk sac tumors	
Small cell carcinoma		Ovarian germ cell tumors	
Ewing's sarcoma		Sarcomas	Mesenchymal cell
Primitive neuroectodermal tumor		Rhabdomyosarcoma	Striated muscle
Malignant melanoma		Leiomyosarcoma	Smooth muscle
Pheochromocytoma		Liposarcoma	Adipocyte
Carcinoid		Osteosarcoma	Osteoblast
GI endocrine tumors		Chondrosarcoma	Chondrocyte
Insulinoma		Malignant fibrous histiocytoma	Fibroblast
Glucagonoma		Synovial sarcoma	Synovial cell
Somatostatinoma		Lymphangiosarcoma	Lymphatic endothelium
Gastrinoma		Hemangiosarcoma	Blood vessel endothelium
VIPoma		Kaposi's sarcoma	Endothelial cell + fibroblasts?
GRFoma		Hepatoblastoma	Mesenchymal cell + hepatocytes
Pituitary tumors		Mesothelioma	Mesothelial cell
Intracranial brain tumors		Schwannoma	Peripheral nerve sheath
Glioblastoma/astrocytoma	Glial precursors	Meningioma	Arachnoidal fibroblast
Ependymoma, oligodendroglioma, medulloblastoma		Adrenocortical carcinoma	Mesonephric mesenchyme
Germ cell tumors		Somatic (non-germ cell) testicular and ovarian cancers	Mesonephric mesenchyme
Teratoma (benign)	Germ cell		
Germinoma, dysgerminoma			

dromes because of their secretory activities. Germ cell tumors can arise within the testes or in extragonadal sites through which germ cells migrate during development. Mesenchymal cells, by virtue of their function, are distributed throughout the body, and mesenchymal tumors can arise at any anatomic site.

1. Carcinoid Tumors

Carcinoid tumors are one type of neuroendocrine tumor. They arise from neural crest tissue and, more specifically, from enterochromaffin cells, whose final resting place after embryonic migration is along the submucosal layer of the intestines and pulmonary bronchi. Reflecting this embryonic origin, carcinoid cells express the necessary enzymes to produce bioactive amines such as 5-hydroxytryptamine and other vasoactive serotonin metabolites as well as a variety of small peptide hormones. Cytoplasmic granules typical of neuroendocrine cells are also commonly seen. These features may also be shared by other tumors of neural crest origin. In contrast to epithelial neoplasms, morphologic changes observed with the light microscope do not distinguish between malignant and benign cells. The anatomic distribution of primary carcinoid tumors is consistent with embryonic development patterns, as listed in Table 5–6. Carcinoid tumors and other mesenchymal neoplasms have similar patterns of tissue invasion followed by local and distant spread to regional lymph nodes and distant organs. The characteristics of increased mitotic count (an indicator of rapid proliferation), nuclear pleomorphism, lymphatic and vascular invasion, and an undifferentiated growth pattern are associated with a higher rate of metastases and a less favorable clinical prognosis.

A frequent site of carcinoid metastasis is the liver. In this setting, especially with midgut carcinoid, there can be a constellation of symptoms (**carcinoid syndrome**) as a consequence of substances secreted into the blood (Table 5–7). These substances reflect the neuroendocrine origin of carcinoid and the latent machinery that can be activated inappropriately in the malignant state. Many of these peptides are vasoactive and can cause inter-

TABLE 5–7 Peptides secreted by carcinoid cells.

| Adrenocorticotropic hormone (ACTH) |
| Calcitonin |
| Gastrin |
| Glicentin |
| Glucagon |
| Growth hormone |
| Insulin |
| Melanocyte-stimulating hormone (β-MSH) |
| Motilin |
| Neuropeptide K |
| Neurotensin |
| Somatostatin |
| Pancreatic polypeptide |
| Substance K |
| Substance P |
| Vasoactive intestinal peptide |

mittent flushing as a result of vasodilation. Other symptoms often observed include secretory diarrhea, wheezing, and excessive salivation or lacrimation. Long-term tissue damage can also occur by exposure to these substances and their metabolites. Fibrosis of the pulmonary and tricuspid heart valves, mesenteric fibrosis, and hyperkeratosis of the skin have all been reported in patients with carcinoid syndrome. A urinary marker commonly used to aid in the diagnosis or to monitor patients being treated is a metabolite of serotonin, 5-hydroxyindoleacetic acid (**5-HIAA**), because the production of serotonin is also characteristic of carcinoid and other neuroendocrine tumors that are able to take up and decarboxylate amine precursors.

TABLE 5–6 Carcinoid tumor location by site of embryonic origin.

Foregut	Midgut	Hindgut
Esophagus	Jejunum	Rectum
Stomach	Ileum	
Duodenum	Appendix	
Pancreas	Colon	
Gallbladder and bile duct	Liver	
Ampulla of Vater	Ovary	
Larynx	Testes	
Bronchus	Cervix	
Thymus		

CHECKPOINT

19. What are some of the hormones and growth factors to which breast tissue respond?
20. What are some factors associated with increased risk of breast cancer?
21. What are the two main subtypes of breast cancer?
22. To what tissues do breast cancers tend to metastasize and why?
23. What products produced by carcinoid tumors reflect their embryonic origin?
24. What are some short-term symptoms and long-term complications precipitated by release of excessive amounts of these products?

2. Testicular Germ Cell Cancer

Testicular cancer arises chiefly from germ cells within the testes. Germ cells are the population of cells that give rise to spermatozoa through meiotic division and can, therefore, theoretically retain the ability to differentiate into any cell type. Some testicular neoplasms arise from remnant tissue outside the testes owing to the midline migration of germ cells that occurs during early embryogenesis. This is followed by the formation of the urogenital ridge and eventually by the aggregation of germ cells in the ovary or testes. As predicted by this pattern of migration, **extragonadal** testicular germ cell neoplasms are found in the midline axis of the lower cranium, mediastinum, or retroperitoneum. The pluripotent ability of the germ cell (ie, the ability of one cell to give rise to an entire organism) is most evident in benign germ cell tumors such as **mature teratomas.** These tumors often contain differentiated elements from all three germ cell layers, including teeth and hair in lesions termed **dermoid cysts.** Malignant teratomas can also exist as a spectrum bridging other germ cell layer-derived neoplasms such as sarcomas and epithelium-derived carcinomas. Malignant testicular cancers may coexist with benign mature teratomas, and the benign component sometimes becomes apparent only after the malignancy has been eradicated with chemotherapy.

Proteins expressed during embryonic or trophoblastic development such as alpha-fetoprotein and human chorionic gonadotropin can be secreted and measured in the serum. Testicular carcinoma follows a lymphatic and hematogenous pattern of spread to regional retroperitoneal nodes and distant organs such as lung, liver, bone, and brain. The exquisite sensitivity of even advanced testicular cancers to radiation and chemotherapy may be a result of the foreign nature of malignant germ cells when present in a mature organism. This foreign nature may create more specific activity of cytotoxic insults and stimulate a more vigorous immune rejection of tumor.

CHECKPOINT

25. From what cellular elements of the testes does testicular cancer generally arise?
26. What are some characteristic markers that may be monitored in testicular tumor progression?

3. Sarcomas

The sarcomas consist of a family of mesenchymal neoplasms whose morphologic appearance and anatomic distribution mirror the early mesenchymal elements from which they derive (Table 5–5). They arise in structures composed of the mesenchymal cell type or in locations where remnant cells eventually come to rest in the path of early tissue migration. Several of the less mature sarcomas that resemble more prim-

itive cells are seen in children, because this compartment of cells is usually dividing more rapidly. These sarcomas include rhabdomyosarcoma and osteosarcoma, which are less common in adults. The morphologic appearance of sarcomas does not involve perceptible architectural changes, because cell polarity and gland formation do not occur in normal mature mesenchymal cells such as muscle or cartilage. Nuclear pleomorphism and mitotic rate determine the grade of a tumor; a higher grade correlates with a higher propensity to invade local and distant structures and a poorer survival. Sarcomas also have a tendency to retain the cell appearance and repertoire of expressed proteins of the cell of origin. Bone matrix of calcium and phosphorus can form within osteosarcomas, and calcification of these tumors can be observed on radiography. There is less of a propensity for direct tissue invasion by sarcomas than by epithelial malignancies. However, tissue destruction can result when a sarcoma compresses but does not invade adjacent tissue, leading to the formation of a pseudocapsule. Sarcomas exhibit metastatic dissemination to regional lymph nodes and distant organs, especially the lungs. High-grade histologic features and anatomic location are factors influencing the likelihood and timing of metastases.

Various genetic abnormalities have been detected in sarcomas. Mutations in the *p53* tumor suppressor gene are the most commonly detected lesion, although such changes are also seen in epithelial neoplasms. The **NF1 tumor suppressor gene** was originally identified through a germline mutation of this gene in patients with type 1 neurofibromatosis. This inherited syndrome is characterized by café-au-lait hyperpigmented skin spots and multiple benign neurofibromas (benign tumors of Schwann cells) under the skin and throughout the body. These can degenerate into malignant **neurofibrosarcomas (malignant schwannoma).** *NF1* mutations have since been detected in sporadic sarcomas of different types. Defective or absent activity of the NF1 protein is known to cause enhanced activation of the G protein-signaling pathways. Given the complex set of cellular activities governed by G protein-mediated pathways, the mechanisms by which NF1 abnormalities contribute to the malignant phenotype are not fully understood.

CHECKPOINT

27. From what two kinds of locations do sarcomas arise?
28. What kinds of sarcomas are more common in children?
29. Are sarcomas more or less likely to directly invade tissues compared with epithelial malignancies?
30. To what sites do sarcomas commonly metastasize?
31. What is the most common genetic lesion in sarcomas?
32. What are the characteristics of type 1 neurofibromatosis, and what is a likely molecular basis for the development of neoplasia in this syndrome?

HEMATOLOGIC NEOPLASMS

Hematologic neoplasms are malignancies of cells derived from hematopoietic precursors. The true hematopoietic stem cell has the capacity for self-renewal and the ability to give rise to precursors (**colony-forming units**) that proliferate and terminally differentiate toward one of any lineage (Figure 5–3). Distinct hematologic neoplasms can arise from each of the mature cell types. Many of these arise in the bone marrow, circulate in the bloodstream, and can infiltrate certain organs and tissues. Others may form tumors in lymphoid tissue, particularly lymphomas, which arise from lymphoblasts. The lineage of a hematopoietic cell and the degree of differentiation along that lineage are associated with the cell surface expression of characteristic proteins, many of which are receptors, others are adhesion molecules and proteases, and some are of unknown function. These clusters of differentiation (CD) antigens have become essential diagnostic tools in the management of hematologic neoplasms, and some types of malignancies are defined by characteristic CD expression patterns.

The cellular ultrastructure and machinery of the malignant cell can somewhat resemble that of its cell of origin. A markedly enhanced proliferative rate and arrest of differentiation are the hallmarks of these neoplasms. Examination of the interphase nucleus of cells can sometimes reveal chromosomal abnormalities such as deletions (monosomy), duplications (trisomy), or balanced translocations. Certain types of hematologic neoplasms tend to have stereotypic chromosomal abnormalities. Given their clonal nature, these abnormalities will be evident on all malignant cells. In some cases of chromosomal translocation, a new fusion gene is formed and can result in production of a fusion protein possessing abnormal function compared with the original gene products (Table 5–8). This function usually involves loss of cell cycle control, abnormal signal transduction, or reprogrammed gene expression as a result of an aberrant transcription factor. In contrast to solid tumors, many hematologic malignancies are specifically linked to certain chromosomal translocations; therefore, karyotype studies are essential in the diagnosis of hematologic malignancies. On the other hand, solid tumors often contain a multitude of chromosomal abnormalities that are not disease specific or even reproducible. Other genetic changes described in hematologic malignancies include mutations or deletions of the *p53*, retinoblastoma (*Rb*), and Wilms' tumor (*WT1*) suppressor genes and activating mutations in the *N-ras* oncogene. Additional genetic changes can be detected in the clonal evolution of leukemias as disease progresses to a more aggressive form in the patient's course. This finding lends further support to the theory that neoplasia is the result of stepwise genetic alterations that correspond to the sequential acquisition of additional phenotypic changes that favor abnormal growth, invasion, and resistance to normal host defenses.

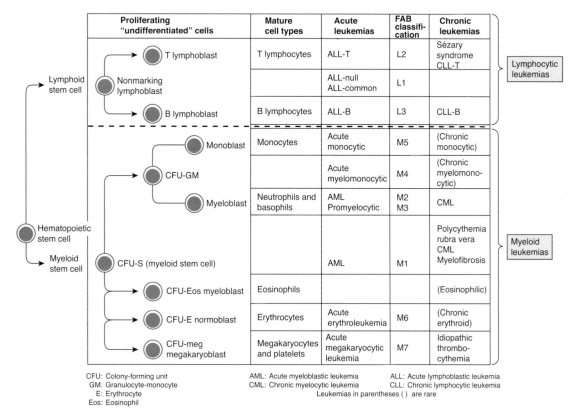

FIGURE 5–3 Classification of leukemias according to cell type and lineage. (Redrawn, with permission, from Chandrasoma P, Taylor CE. *Concise Pathology*, 3rd ed. Originally published by Appleton & Lange. Copyright © 1998 by the McGraw-Hill Companies, Inc.)

TABLE 5–8 Chromosomal translocations of hematologic neoplasms.

Neoplasm	Chromosomal Translocation	Fusion Gene Resulting from Translocation	Fusion Protein Function
Follicular lymphoma	t(14;18)	IgH-*bcl*-2	Inhibitor of apoptosis
Mantle cell lymphoma	t(11;14)	IgH-*bcl*-1	Cyclin
Follicular lymphoma	t(14;19)	IgH-*bcl*-3	Transcription repressor
Diffuse large cell lymphoma	t(3;14)	IgH/K/L-*bcl*-6	Transcription repressor
Burkitt's lymphoma	t(8;14)	IgH-*myc*	Transcription factor
Anaplastic large T-/null-cell lymphoma	t(2;5)	*NPM-ALK*	Tyrosine kinase
CML	t(9;22)	*bcr-abl*	Tyrosine kinase
AML M3	t(15;17)	*PML-RAR*	Transcription factor
AML	t(8;21)	*AML1*	Transcription factor
T-cell ALL	t(1;14)	*tal*-1-TCR	Transcription factor

Key: IgH, immunoglobulin heavy chain enhancer; TCR, T-cell receptor; RAR, retinoic acid receptor.

1. Lymphomas

Malignant lymphomas are a diverse group of cancers derived from the immune system, which result from neoplastic proliferation of B or T lymphocytes. These tumors may arise anywhere in the body, most commonly within lymph nodes but occasionally in other organs in which lymphoid elements reside. One subtype of lymphomas that are composed of mixtures of cell types with a unique biology is called Hodgkin's lymphomas, whereas all other types of lymphomas are referred to as non-Hodgkin's lymphomas.

Several factors are associated with the development of non-Hodgkin's lymphoma. These include congenital or acquired immunodeficiency states such as AIDS or iatrogenic immunosuppression used in organ transplantation. Viruses are associated with the pathogenesis of some types. For example, most cases of Burkitt's lymphoma that occur in Africa (endemic form) are associated with Epstein-Barr virus (EBV), whereas Burkitt's lymphoma occurring in temperate zones is associated with EBV in only 30% of cases. Human T-cell leukemia-lymphoma virus I (HTLV-I) plays a causative role in the genesis of adult T-cell leukemia-lymphoma, in which the malignant cells contain the integrated virus. Human herpesvirus-8 (HHV-8) has been associated with body cavity-based lymphoma, a rare B-cell lymphoma that occurs predominantly in patients with AIDS. Chronic immune stimulation may be a causal mechanism in the development of lymphomas as well. For example, chronic gastritis secondary to *Helicobacter pylori* infection may give rise to gastric mucosa-associated lymphoid tissue (MALT) lymphomas. Resolution of gastric MALT lymphoma may occur in the majority of patients with localized disease who are treated with antibiotics effective against *H pylori*.

The classification of lymphomas has evolved over several decades. The latest classification was devised by an international group of lymphoma specialists for the World Health Organization (Table 5–9). The new scheme characterizes non-Hodgkin's lymphomas according to the cell of origin using a combination of criteria: clinical and morphologic features, cytogenetics, and immunoreactivity with monoclonal antibodies that recognize B-cell and T-cell antigens, as well as genotypic determination of B-cell and T-cell receptor rearrangements. Most non-Hodgkin's lymphomas originate in B cells and express on their surface CD20, a B-cell marker. Their monoclonal origin can be inferred by characterization of the specific class of light chain that is expressed: Either kappa or lambda B-cell lymphomas are further classified as malignant expansions of cells from the germinal center, mantle zone, or marginal zone of normal lymph nodes.

Somatic gene rearrangements occur normally during B-cell and T-cell differentiation. The genes for variable and constant regions of the immunoglobulin heavy and light chains are discontinuous in the B-cell germline DNA but are combined by somatic rearrangement to produce a functional antibody molecule. The T-cell receptor gene is analogous to the immunoglobulin molecule in that discontinuous segments of this gene also undergo somatic rearrangement early in T-cell development. DNA hybridization by Southern blot analysis permits recognition of a band of electrophoretic mobility that serves as a fingerprint for a monoclonal population of lymphoma cells.

Most non-Hodgkin's lymphomas exhibit karyotypic abnormalities. The most prevalent translocations include t(8;14), t(14;18), and t(11;14) (Table 5–8). Each translocation involves the immunoglobulin heavy chain gene locus at chromosome 14q32 with an oncogene. Identification and cloning of the breakpoints have identified 8q24 as *c-myc*, 18q21 as *bcl-2*, and 11q13 as *bcl-1*. The proximity of these oncogenes to the immunoglobulin gene results in deregulation and increased expression of the oncogene product.

TABLE 5–9 World Health Organization classification of lymphoid neoplasms.

B-Cell Lymphomas	T-Cell and NK Cell Lymphomas
Precursor Cell Neoplasms	
B-cell lymphoblastic lymphoma	T-cell lymphoblastic lymphoma
Mature or Peripheral Lymphomas	
Lymphoplasmacytic lymphoma	Aggressive NK-cell leukemia
Splenic marginal zone B-cell lymphoma	Adult T-cell lymphoma/leukemia
Nodal marginal zone B-cell lymphoma	Extranodal NK/T-cell lymphoma
MALT lymphoma	Enteropathy-type T-cell lymphoma
Hairy cell leukemia	Hepatosplenic T-cell lymphoma
Follicular lymphoma	Primary subcutaneous T-cell lymphomas
Mantle-cell lymphoma	Mycosis fungoides
Diffuse large B-cell lymphoma	Anaplastic large-cell lymphoma
Mediastinal large B-cell lymphoma	Peripheral T-cell lymphoma
Burkitt's lymphoma	Angioimmunoblastic T-cell lymphoma
Hodgkin's lymphoma	
Classical: nodular sclerosis Hodgkin's	
Classical: lymphocyte-rich Hodgkin's	
Classical: mixed cellularity Hodgkin's	
Classical: lymphocyte depleted Hodgkin's	
Nonclassical: Nodular lymphocyte predominant Hodgkin's	

Representative subtypes of non-Hodgkin's lymphoma include the indolent lymphomas such as follicular lymphoma, marginal zone lymphomas, and the aggressive lymphomas such as mantle cell lymphoma, diffuse large-cell lymphoma, and Burkitt's lymphoma.

Follicular lymphomas are low-grade tumors that may be insidious in their presentation. The translocation t(14;18)(q32;q21) is found in more than 90% of follicular lymphomas. The mutation results in overexpression of the bcl-2 protein by these cells. The *bcl-2* is an oncogene that codes for a protein that blocks apoptosis when overexpressed. The absence of bcl-2 translocation as assessed by the highly sensitive polymerase chain reaction test may be a marker for complete remission status in patients whose lymphomas harbor this translocation. Spontaneous regression of lymph node size is common in patients with follicular lymphomas. However, this class of lymphoma is not curable with standard chemotherapy; although the patient with follicular lymphoma tends to have an indolent clinical course, transformation to a more aggressive grade of lymphoma occurs in 40–50% of patients by 10 years.

An important subtype of marginal zone lymphomas are the MALT lymphomas, which may originate in the stomach, lungs, skin, parotid gland, thyroid, breasts, and other extranodal sites, where they characteristically align themselves with epithelial cells. A close association has been established between gastric MALT lymphomas and *H pylori* infection.

Mantle cell lymphoma presents histologically as a monotonous population of small to medium-sized atypical lymphoid cells with a nodular or diffuse pattern that is composed of small lymphoid cells with irregular nuclear outlines. The diagnosis of mantle cell lymphoma is based on morphologic criteria with confirmation by monoclonal antibody staining against cyclin D1 (bcl-1). The t(11;14) translocation seen in the majority of cases of mantle cell lymphoma results in juxtaposition of the *PRAD1* gene on chromosome 11 with the immunoglobulin heavy chain gene on chromosome 14. This results in overexpression of the *PRAD1* gene product, cyclin D1. Cyclin D1 binds to and activates cyclin-dependent kinases, which are thought to facilitate cell cycle progression through the G1 phase of the cell cycle. This disease occurs more commonly among older males and presents with adenopathy and hepatosplenomegaly. Mantle cell lymphomas are significantly more resistant to treatment with combination chemotherapy than follicular lymphomas and are also incurable.

Diffuse large-cell lymphoma is the most prevalent subtype of non-Hodgkin's lymphoma. One third of presentations involve extranodal sites, particularly the head and neck, stomach, skin, bone, testis, and nervous system. Diffuse large B-cell lymphomas commonly harbor mutations or rearrangements of the *BCL6* gene.

Virtually all cases of Burkitt's lymphoma are associated with alterations of chromosome 8q24, resulting in overexpression of *c-myc*, an oncogene that encodes a transcriptional regulator of cell proliferation, differentiation, and apoptosis. Adults presenting with high tumor burdens and elevated serum lactate dehydrogenase have a poor prognosis. Disease with a large tumor burden may be associated with a hypermetabolic syndrome that is triggered by treatment as the tumor undergoes sudden lysis. This syndrome may lead to life-threatening hyperkalemia, hyperphosphatemia, hyperuricemia, and hypocalcemia.

Anaplastic large-cell lymphoma is characterized by the proliferation of highly atypical cells that express the CD30 antigen. These tumors usually express a T-cell phenotype and are associated with the chromosomal translocation t(2;5)(p23;q35), resulting in the nucleophosmin-anaplastic lymphoma kinase (NPM-ALK) fusion protein. Activation of the ALK receptor tyrosine kinase results in an unregulated mitogenic signal.

Another type of T-cell lymphoma is the adult T-cell leukemia-lymphoma, an aggressive disease associated with HTLV-I infection that is characterized by generalized adenopathy, polyclonal hypergammaglobulinemia, hypercalcemia, and lytic bone lesions.

Finally, Hodgkin's lymphoma is distinguished by the presence of the Reed–Sternberg giant cell of B-cell lineage, which is considered the malignant cell type in this neoplasm. The Reed–Sternberg cell constitutes only 1–10% of the total number of cells in pathologic specimens of this disease and is associated with an infiltrate of nonneoplastic inflammatory cells.

2. Acute & Chronic Myelogenous Leukemia

Acute myelogenous leukemia (AML), also termed acute nonlymphocytic leukemia (ANLL), is a rapidly progressive neoplasm derived from hematopoietic precursors, or myeloid stem cells, that give rise to granulocytes, monocytes, erythrocytes, and platelets. There is increasing evidence that genetic events occurring early in stem cell maturation can lead to leukemia. First, there is a lag time of 5–10 years to the development of leukemia after exposure to known causative agents such as chemotherapy, radiation, and certain solvents. Second, many cases of secondary leukemia evolve out of a prolonged "preleukemic phase" manifested as a **myelodysplastic syndrome** of hypoproduction with abnormal maturation without actual malignant behavior. Finally, examination of precursor cells at a stage earlier than the malignant expanded clone in a given type of leukemia can reveal genetic abnormalities such as monosomy or trisomy of different chromosomes. In keeping with the general molecular theme of neoplasia, additional genetic changes are seen in the malignant clone compared with the morphologically normal stem cell that developmentally precedes it.

Acute myelocytic leukemias are classified by morphology and cytochemical staining as shown in Table 5–10. **Auer rods** are crystalline cytoplasmic inclusion bodies characteristic of, though not uniformly seen in, all myeloid leukemias. In contrast to mature myeloid cells, leukemic cells have large immature nuclei with open chromatin and prominent nucleoli. The appearance of the individual types of AML mirrors the cell type from which they derive. M1 leukemias originate from early myeloid precursors with no apparent maturation toward any terminal myeloid cell type. This is apparent in the lack of granules or other features that mark more mature myeloid cells. M3 leukemias are a neoplasm of promyelocytes, precursors of granulocytes, and M3 cells exhibit abundant azurophilic granules that are typical of normal promyelocytes. M4 leukemias arise from myeloid precursors that can differentiate into granulocytes or monocytes, whereas M5 leukemias derive from precursors already committed to the monocyte lineage. Therefore, M4 and M5 cells both contain the characteristic folded nucleus and gray cytoplasm of monocytes, whereas M4 cells contain also granules of a granulocytic cytochemical staining pattern. M6 and M7 leukemias cannot be readily identified on morphologic grounds, but immunostaining for erythrocytic proteins is positive in M6 cells, and staining for platelet glycoproteins is apparent in M7 cells.

Chromosomal deletions, duplications, and balanced translocations had been noted on the leukemic cells of some patients before the introduction of molecular genetic techniques. Cloning of the regions where balanced translocations occur has, in some cases, revealed a preserved translocation site that reproducibly fuses one gene with another, resulting in the production of a new fusion protein. M3 leukemias show a very high frequency of the t(15;17) translocation that juxtaposes the PML gene with the *RAR-α* gene. *RAR-α* encodes a retinoic acid steroid hormone receptor, and PML encodes a transcription factor whose target genes are unknown. The fusion protein possesses novel biologic activity that presumably results in enhanced proliferation and a block of differentiation. Interestingly, retinoic acid can induce a temporary remission of M3 leukemia, supporting the importance of the *RAR-α*–PML fusion protein. Monosomy of chromosome 7 can be seen in leukemias arising out of the preleukemic syndrome of myelodysplasia or in de novo leukemias, and in both cases this finding is associated with a worse clinical prognosis. This monosomy as well as other serial cytogenetic changes can also be seen after relapse of treated leukemia, a situation characterized by a more aggressive course and resistance to therapy.

As hematopoietic neoplasms, acute leukemias involve the bone marrow and usually manifest abnormal circulating leukemic (blast) cells. Occasionally, extramedullary leukemic infiltrates known as **chloromas** can be seen in other organs and mucosal surfaces. A marked increase in the number of circulating blasts can sometimes cause vascular obstruction accompanied by hemorrhage and infarction in the cerebral and pulmonary vascular beds. This **leukostasis** results in symptoms such as strokes, retinal vein occlusion, and pulmonary infarction. In most cases of AML and other leukemias, peripheral blood counts of mature granulocytes, erythrocytes, and platelets are decreased. This is probably due to crowding of the bone marrow by blast cells as well as the elaboration of inhibitory substances by leukemic cells or alteration of the bone marrow stromal microenvironment and cytokine milieu necessary for normal hematopoiesis. Susceptibility to infections as a result of depressed granulocyte number and function and abnormal bleeding as a result of low platelet counts are common problems in patients initially presenting with leukemia.

TABLE 5–10 Classification of acute myelogenous leukemias (AML).

M1	Myeloblasts without differentiation
M2	Myeloblasts with some degree of differentiation
M3	Acute promyelocytic leukemia
M4	Acute myelomonocytic leukemia
M5	Acute monocytic leukemia
M6	Erythroleukemia
M7	Megakaryoblastic leukemia

Chronic myelogenous leukemia (CML) is an indolent leukemia manifested by an increased number of immature granulocytes in the marrow and peripheral circulation. One of the hallmarks of CML is the **Philadelphia chromosome,** a cytogenetic feature that is due to balanced translocation of chromosomes 9 and 22, resulting in a fusion gene, *bcr-abl,* that encodes a kinase that phosphorylates several key proteins involved in cell growth and apoptosis. The fusion gene can recreate a CML-like syndrome when introduced into mice. CML eventually transforms into acute leukemia (blast crisis), which is accompanied by further cytogenetic changes and a clinical course similar to that of acute leukemia. New classes of drugs that block the bcr-abl kinase by competing with the ATP-binding site, induce remissions in most patients in chronic phases of CML. Furthermore, resistance to these *bcr-abl* inhibitors can involve amplification of the bcr-abl breakpoint as well as the development (or clonal expansion) of mutations in the ATP-binding pocket of bcr-abl, which no longer allows binding of inhibitors.

SYSTEMIC EFFECTS OF NEOPLASIA

Many effects of malignancies are mediated not by the tumor cells themselves but by direct and indirect effects, as outlined in Tables 5–11 and 5–12. Direct effects (Table 5–11) include compression or invasion of vital structures such as blood and lymphatic vessels, nerves, spinal cord or brain, bone, airways, GI tract, and urinary tract. These may cause a typical pain pattern as well as dysfunction of the involved organ and obstruction of a conduit. On occasion, an inflammatory or desmoplastic host response rather than the tumor itself can result in the same effect.

Indirect effects (Table 5–12) are heterogeneous and poorly understood. Likewise, the onset and clinical course are unpredictable. When affecting distant targets uninvolved by tumor, they are collectively termed **paraneoplastic syndromes.** Some of these effects are stereotypic syndromes resulting from the elaboration of peptide hormones or cytokines with specific biologic activity, as shown in Table 5–12. The peptides secreted by a given neoplasm may reflect the tissue of origin or may be the result of activation of latent genes not normally expressed. Common examples of paraneoplastic phenomena include the syndrome of inappropriate antidiuretic hormone (SIADH), seen most often in small cell lung cancer. The result of ectopic ADH production is retention of free water and hyponatremia, which can result in altered sensorium, coma, and death. Another peptide secreted in cases of small cell lung cancer is ACTH, which can lead to Cushing's syndrome with excessive adrenocorticosteroids, skin fragility, central redistribution of body fat, proximal myopathy, and other features. Hypercalcemia can be seen in many types of malignancies, and its several causes include secretion of a parathyroid hormone–like peptide as a result of activation of the parathyroid hormone–related protein (PTHrP) gene, as well as the elaboration of local-acting cytokines that increase bone uptake in areas of tumor infiltration of bone.

In some malignancies such as carcinoid, several active peptides may act in concert to produce a constellation of symptoms and tissue effects. Cytokines such as the interleukins and tumor necrosis factor may be responsible for tumor-related fevers and weight loss. Some paraneoplastic syndromes are associated with the development of autoantibodies as a result of an immune response to tumor-associated antigens or an inappropriate production of antibody, as can be seen in lymphoid neoplasms. Finally, the nucleic acid, cytoplasmic, and membrane products of cell breakdown can result in electrolyte and other metabolic abnormalities as well as coagulopathic disorders, resulting in clotting or bleeding.

TABLE 5–11 Direct systemic effects of neoplasms.

Effect	Clinical Syndrome
Vessel compression	Edema, superior vena cava syndrome
Vessel invasion and erosion	Bleeding
Lymphatic invasion	Lymphedema
Nerve invasion	Pain, numbness, dysesthesia
Brain metastases	Weakness, numbness, headache, coordination and gait abnormalities, visual changes
Spinal cord compression	Pain, paralysis, incontinence
Bone invasion and destruction	Pain, fracture
Bowel obstruction and perforation	Nausea, vomiting, pain, ileus
Airway obstruction	Dyspnea, pneumonia, lung volume loss
Ureteral obstruction	Renal failure, urinary infection
Liver invasion and metastases	Hepatic insufficiency
Lung and pleural metastases	Dyspnea, chest pain
Bone marrow infiltration	Pancytopenia, infection, bleeding

CHECKPOINT

33. What are the hallmarks of hematologic malignancies?
34. What are some characteristics of low-grade lymphomas?
35. What are some characteristics of high-grade lymphomas?

TABLE 5–12 Indirect systemic effects of neoplasms.

Tumor Type	Cause of Indirect Effect	Clinical Syndrome
Effects of Hormone or Peptide Secretion		
Lung	ACTH	Cushing's syndrome
Lung, breast, kidney, others	PTH or PTH-related protein	Hypercalcemia
Lung	ADH, ANP	SIADH, hyponatremia
Germ cell, trophoblastic, hepatoblastoma	Gonadotropins (FSH, LH, βhCG)	Gynecomastia, precocious puberty
Lung, gastric	Growth hormone	Acromegaly
Carcinoid, neuroendocrine	Various vasoactive peptides	Flushing, wheezing, diarrhea
Sarcoma, mesothelioma, insulinoma	Insulin, insulin-like growth factor	Hypoglycemia
Cutaneous Effects		
GI	Unknown	Acanthosis nigricans (hyperkeratosis and hyperpigmentation in skin folds)
GI, lymphoma	Unknown	Leser-Trélat (large seborrheic) keratoses
Lymphoma, hepatoma, melanoma	Melanin deposits	Melanosis (skin darkening)
Lymphoma	Autoantibodies to subepidermal proteins	Skin bullae (blisters)
Myeloid leukemia	Neutrophilic skin infiltrates	Sweet's syndrome
Neurologic Effects		
Lung, prostate, colorectal, ovarian, cervical, others	Unknown	Subacute cerebellar degeneration
Lung, testicular, Hodgkin's disease	Unknown	Limbic encephalitis
Lung	Unknown	Dementia
Lung, others	Unknown	Amyotrophic lateral sclerosis
Lung, others	Unknown	Peripheral sensory or sensorimotor neuropathy
Lymphoma	Unknown, ?autoantibodies	Ascending radiculopathy (Guillain-Barré syndrome)
Lung, GI	Autoantibodies to voltage-gated Ca^{2+} channels	Eaton-Lambert (myasthenia-like) syndrome
Hematologic and Coagulopathic Effects		
Several	Unknown	Anemia
Adenocarcinomas (especially gastric)	Unknown	Microangiopathic hemolytic anemia
Several	Interleukin-1, -3 and hematopoietic growth factors	Granulocytosis
Hodgkin's, others	Eosinophilic hematopoietic growth factors	Eosinophilia
Several	Unknown	Thrombocytosis
Adenocarcinomas (especially pancreatic), others	Unknown, ?exposed phospholipids from cell membranes	Thrombosis
Adenocarcinoma (especially prostate)	Urokinase, other mediators of fibrinolysis	Disseminated intravascular coagulation

(continued)

TABLE 5–12 Indirect systemic effects of neoplasms. (Continued)

Tumor Type	Cause of Indirect Effect	Clinical Syndrome
	Metabolic Effects	
Various	Interleukin-1, tumor necrosis factor	Cachexia, anorexia
Lymphoma, others	Interleukins-1, -6	Fever
Hematologic neoplasms	Hypermetabolism/cell breakdown products	Hyperuricemia, hyperkalemia, hyperphosphatemia
Lymphoma, others	Tumor hypoxia	Lactic acidosis

Key: ACTH, adrenocorticotropic hormone; ADH, antidiuretic hormone (arginine vasopressin); ANP, atrial natriuretic protein; FSH, follicle-stimulating hormone; βhCG, human chorionic gonadotropin; LH, luteinizing hormone; PTH, parathyroid hormone; SIADH, syndrome of inappropriate secretion of antidiuretic hormone.

CASE STUDIES

Yeong Kwok, MD, & Eva M. Aagaard, MD

(See Chapter 25, p. 678 for Answers)

CASE 16

A 54-year-old man presents with several weeks of facial flushing and diarrhea. His symptoms began intermittently but are becoming more constant. A 24-hour urine collection reveals an elevated level of 5-hydroxyindoleacetic acid (5-HIAA), a metabolite of serotonin. An abdominal CT scan shows a 2-cm mesenteric mass in the ileum and likely metastatic tumors in the liver.

Questions

A. This patient has malignant carcinoid syndrome. From what type of tissue do carcinoid tumors arise, and how does this account for the body site where they first appear?

B. What accounts for the frequent association of systemic symptoms, the so-called carcinoid syndrome, with carcinoid tumors?

C. Why is the 24-hour urine collection for 5-HIAA useful in the diagnosis of carcinoid syndrome?

CASE 17

A 54-year-old man presents to the clinic for a routine checkup. He is well, with no physical complaints. The history is remarkable only for a father with colon cancer at age 55 years. Physical examination is normal. Cancer screening is discussed, and the patient is sent home with fecal occult blood testing supplies and scheduled for a colonoscopy. The fecal occult blood test results are positive. The colonoscopy reveals a villous adenoma as well as a 2-cm carcinoma.

Questions

A. How are the two lesions—adenoma and carcinoma—thought to be related?

B. What are the two principal lines of evidence in favor of such a model?

C. Describe the genetic alterations in the stepwise progression of colon cancer and the phenotypic changes associated with these alterations.

D. What is the explanation for the presence of occult blood in stools of patients with early colorectal cancer?

CASE 18

A 40-year-old woman presents for the evaluation of a left-sided breast lump. She does have a strongly positive family history, with her mother and one older sister both having had breast cancer. Physical examination is notable for a 2-cm lump in the left breast. A biopsy shows invasive ductal carcinoma. The tumor is positive for estrogen and HER2 receptors.

Questions

A. What genetic factors may have been involved in this patient's risk for developing breast cancer?

B. What are the two major subtypes of breast cancer?

C. How is our knowledge of the tumor receptors used in treatment of breast cancer?

D. Describe the distinction between invasive breast cancer and carcinoma in situ.

CASE 19

A 25-year-old man presents with a complaint of testicular enlargement. Examination reveals a hard nodule on the left testicle, 2 cm in diameter. Orchiectomy is diagnostic of testicular cancer.

Questions

A. From what cellular elements of the testes does testicular cancer generally arise? What is the normal development of these cells?

B. In addition to the testes, where else might testicular cancer arise? What is the explanation for this distribution?

C. What serum markers might be monitored to evaluate disease progression and response to therapy?

CASE 20

A 16-year-old previously healthy teenager presents with a 2-month history of pain and swelling of his knee. He thought it began after a soccer game, but it just has not gotten better. Physical examination shows marked swelling of the knee and the distal thigh. Radiographs show a 3-cm partially calcified mass in the distal femur, just above the knee joint. A biopsy reveals an osteosarcoma.

Questions

A. From which tissues do sarcomas arise?

B. Why are many sarcomas more common in children, adolescents, and young adults?

C. What accounts for the calcifications that can be seen in osteosarcomas?

CASE 21

A 28-year-old woman presents to her primary care physician with complaints of fatigue, intermittent fevers, and 5 pounds of weight loss over a 6-week period. Her medical history is remarkable for a renal transplantation at age 15 years performed for end-stage renal disease as a result of poststreptococcal glomerulonephritis. Physical examination reveals two enlarged, matted, nontender lymph nodes in the left anterior cervical chain; a firm, nontender 1.5-cm lymph node in the right groin; and an enlarged liver. Biopsy of the lymph nodes in the cervical region reveals follicular, cleaved-cell lymphoma.

Questions

A. One theory states that chronic immune stimulation or modulation may be an early step in lymphomagenesis. What observations support this view?

B. How would one classify her lymphoma? What are some characteristics of this grade of lymphoma?

C. From which cell line do follicular lymphomas originate? What are some of the common genetic mutations seen with this type of lymphoma? How might one of these mutations contribute to the formation of lymphoma?

D. What is the pathophysiologic mechanism causing this patient's fever and weight loss?

CASE 22

A 22-year-old woman presents with a 2-week history of fatigue, bleeding from her gums, and very heavy menstrual bleeding. Physical examination reveals a pale woman with an enlarged spleen and petechiae on her legs. A complete blood cell count shows a markedly elevated white cell count (WBC 178,000) with severe anemia (hemoglobin 7.8) and thrombocytopenia (platelet count 25,000). Blast cells (abnormally immature leukemic cells) comprise 30% of the total white cell count. A bone marrow biopsy is positive for AML of the M1 type.

Questions

A. How are leukemias classified in general, and more specifically how are AMLs classified?
B. What accounts for the patient's symptoms and physical findings? What other major symptoms or signs may be present?
C. What types of genetic abnormalities are responsible for the development of leukemias? How can this knowledge be used to treat some leukemias?

CASE 23

A 60-year-old man is brought to the emergency department by ambulance. He was in good health until yesterday when his wife noted that he seems somewhat confused. This morning she could not arouse him from sleep and called an ambulance. His past medical history is notable for a 40 pack-year history of smoking. On examination, he is noted to be responsive to painful stimuli, but not able to speak or follow commands. Chemistries are significant for severe hyponatremia (serum sodium 120 mEq/L). Chest x-ray film shows a 2-cm nodule in the right lung field suspicious for lung cancer. Biopsy confirms the diagnosis of small cell lung cancer.

Questions

A. What is a paraneoplastic syndrome? How does it exert its effects?
B. What is the likely mechanism for this patient's hyponatremia?
C. What other paraneoplastic syndromes can be seen in lung cancer?

REFERENCES

General

Bergers G et al. Tumorigenesis and the angiogenic switch. Nat Rev Cancer. 2003 Jun;3(6):401–10. [PMID: 12778130]

DeVita VT et al. *Cancer: Principles and Practice of Oncology*, 8th ed. Lippincott Williams & Wilkins, 2008.

Hanahan D et al. The hallmarks of cancer. Cell. 2000 Jan 7;100(1):57–70. [PMID: 10647931]

Hanash S. Integrated global profiling of cancer. Nat Rev Cancer. 2004 Aug;4(8):638–44. [PMID: 15286743]

Mendelsohn J et al. *The Molecular Basis of Cancer*, 3rd ed. WB Saunders, 2008.

Mueller MM et al. Friends or foes—Bipolar effects of the tumour stroma in cancer. Nat Rev Cancer. 2004 Nov;4(11):839–49. [PMID: 15516957]

Pardal R et al. Applying the principles of stem-cell biology to cancer. Nat Rev Cancer. 2003 Dec;3(12):895–902. [PMID: 14737120]

Colon Cancer

de la Chapelle A. Genetic predisposition to colorectal cancer. Nat Rev Cancer. 2004 Oct;4(10):769–80. [PMID: 15510158]

Lynch JP et al. The genetic pathogenesis of colorectal cancer. Hematol Oncol Clin North Am. 2002 Aug;16(4):775–810. [PMID: 12418049]

Narayan S et al. Role of APC and DNA mismatch repair genes in the development of colorectal cancers. Mol Cancer. 2003 Dec 12;2:41. [PMID: 14672538]

Breast Cancer

Fackenthal JD et al. Breast cancer risk associated with *BRCA1* and *BRCA2* in diverse populations. Nat Rev Cancer. 2007 Dec;7(12):937–48. [PMID: 18034184]

Martin M. Molecular biology of breast cancer. Clin Transl Oncol. 2006 Jan;8(1):7–14. [PMID: 16632434]

Stingl J et al. Molecular heterogeneity of breast carcinomas and the cancer stem cell hypothesis. Nat Rev Cancer. 2007 Oct;7(10):791–9. [PMID: 17851544]

Yager JD et al. Estrogen carcinogenesis in breast cancer. N Engl J Med. 2006 Jan 19;354(3):270–82. [PMID: 16421368]

Carcinoid

Oberg K. Carcinoid tumors: Molecular genetics, tumor biology, and update of diagnosis and treatment. Curr Opin Oncol. 2002 Jan;14(1):38–45. [PMID: 11790979]

Testicular Cancer

Horwich A et al. Testicular germ-cell cancer. Lancet. 2006 Mar 4;367(9512):754–65. [PMID: 16517276]

Sarcoma

Helman LJ et al. Mechanisms of sarcoma development. Nat Rev Cancer. 2003 Sep;3(9):685–94. [PMID: 12951587]

Lymphoma

Armitage JO et al. Lymphoma 2006: Classification and treatment. Oncology (Williston Park). 2006 Mar;20(3):231–9. [PMID: 16629256]

Bagg A. Role of molecular studies in the classification of lymphoma. Expert Rev Mol Diagn. 2004 Jan;4(1):83–97. [PMID: 14711352]

Isaacson PG et al. MALT lymphoma: From morphology to molecules. Nat Rev Cancer. 2004 Aug;4(8):644–53. [PMID: 15286744]

Jares P et al. Genetic and molecular pathogenesis of mantle cell lymphoma: perspectives for new targeted therapeutics. Nat Rev Cancer. 2007 Oct;7(10):750–62. [PMID: 17891190]

Küppers R. Mechanisms of B-cell lymphoma pathogenesis. Nat Rev Cancer. 2005 Apr;5(4):251–62. [PMID: 15803153]

Spagnolo DV et al. The role of molecular studies in lymphoma diagnosis: A review. Pathology. 2004 Feb;36(1):19–44. [PMID: 14757555]

Leukemia

Brunning RD. Classification of acute leukemias. Semin Diagn Pathol. 2003 Aug;20(3):142–53. [PMID: 14552428]

Goldman JM et al. Chronic myeloid leukemia—Advances in biology and new approaches to treatment. N Engl J Med. 2003 Oct 9;349(15):1451–64. [PMID: 14534339]

Paraneoplastic Syndromes

Albert ML et al. Paraneoplastic neurological degenerations: Keys to tumour immunity. Nat Rev Cancer. 2004 Jan;4(1):36–44. [PMID: 14708025]

Dalmau J et al. Paraneoplastic syndromes of the CNS. Lancet Neurol. 2008 Apr;7(4):327–40. [PMID: 18339348]

DeLellis RA et al. Chronic myeloid leukemia—Advances in biology and new approaches to treatment. Endocr Pathol. 2003 Winter; 14(4):303–17. [PMID: 14739488]

Blood Disorders

J. Ben Davoren, MD, PhD, & Sunny Wang, MD

NORMAL STRUCTURE & FUNCTION

Blood is an extremely complex fluid, composed of both formed elements (red cells, white cells, platelets) and plasma. Red blood cells (**erythrocytes**) are the most common formed elements, carrying oxygen to the cells of the body via their main component, **hemoglobin.** White blood cells are generally present at about 1/700th the number of erythrocytes and function as mediators of immune responses to infection or other stimuli of inflammation. Platelets are the formed elements that participate in coagulation. Plasma is largely water, electrolytes, and plasma proteins, all of which are very complex. The plasma proteins most important in blood clotting are the coagulation factors. Because blood circulates throughout the body, alterations in normal blood physiology—either formed elements or plasma proteins—may have widespread adverse consequences.

FORMED ELEMENTS OF BLOOD

Anatomy

A. Bone Marrow and Hematopoiesis

Although the mature formed elements of blood are quite different from each other in both structure and function, all of these cells develop from a common progenitor cell, or **stem cell,** population, which resides in the bone marrow. The developmental process is called **hematopoiesis** and represents an enormous metabolic task for the body. More than 100 billion cells are produced every day. This makes the bone marrow one of the most active organs in the body. In adults, most of the active marrow resides in the vertebrae, sternum, and ribs. In children, the marrow is more active in the long bones.

The process of differentiation from stem cell to mature erythrocyte, granulocyte, lymphocyte, monocyte, or platelet is shown in Figure 6–1. It is not clear exactly what early events

lead dividing stem cells down a particular path of development, but many different peptides, called **cytokines,** are clearly involved (Table 6–1); see also Chapter 3. Perhaps because mature white blood cells have a much shorter half-life in the circulation, white blood cell precursors usually outnumber red blood cell precursors by a ratio of 3:1 in the bone marrow.

The major hormone that stimulates the production of **erythrocytes** (**erythropoiesis**) is **erythropoietin.** This peptide is produced by the kidneys and regulates red blood cell production by a feedback system: When blood hemoglobin levels fall (**anemia**), oxygen delivery to the kidneys falls, and they produce more erythropoietin, causing the marrow to produce more red cells. When hemoglobin levels rise, the kidney produces less erythropoietin and the marrow fewer red cells.

For white blood cells, the situation is more complex. The most common cells are the **granulocytes,** so named because their cytoplasms are filled with granules. Of these, the neutrophils are the most prevalent and the most important cells in producing inflammation. Granulocyte production (**myelopoiesis**) can be affected by many cytokines at different stages of development. Figure 6–1 shows that interleukin-3 (IL-3), granulocyte colony-stimulating factor (G-CSF), and granulocyte-macrophage colony-stimulating factor (GM-CSF) are the most important. All three proteins have been purified, sequenced, and cloned. The latter two proteins are used therapeutically. Unlike G-CSF, GM-CSF also stimulates the maturation of a different white blood cell line, the **monocyte-macrophage line.** These cells are part of the immune system as well (eg, ingesting foreign bacteria) and can reside in skin and other tissues, not just blood. Their function, along with that of the B- and T-lymphocyte populations, is discussed more fully in Chapter 3.

Platelets are not cells but fragments of larger multinucleated cells in the marrow called **megakaryocytes.** Platelets are crucial to normal blood clotting. Platelet production is also stimulated by multiple cytokines but is dependent mainly on the action of

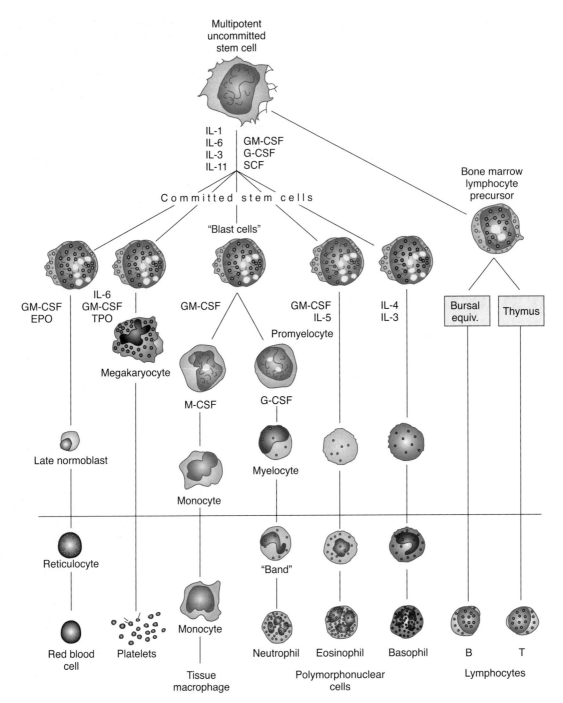

FIGURE 6–1 Hematopoiesis: development of the formed elements of blood from bone marrow stem cells. Cells below the horizontal line are found in normal peripheral blood. The principal cytokines that stimulate each cell lineage to differentiate are shown. (EPO, erythropoietin; TPO, thrombopoietin; CSF, colony-stimulating factor; G, granulocyte; M, macrophage; IL, interleukin; SCF, stem cell factor.) See Table 6–1 for details. (Redrawn, with permission, from Ganong WF. *Review of Medical Physiology,* 22nd ed. McGraw-Hill, 2005.)

IL-3, IL-6, and IL-11 and **thrombopoietin.** This peptide is produced by the liver, kidney, skeletal muscle, and marrow stroma. One model of **thrombopoiesis** proposes that the production of thrombopoietin occurs at a constant rate. However, the amount of this hormone free to interact with platelet precursors rises and falls, probably as a result of metabolism by the existing platelets in the blood. Therefore, a low platelet count stimulates thrombopoiesis. A second model proposes that low platelet lev-

els can induce increased production of thrombopoietin in marrow stromal cells, via various cytokines including platelet-derived growth factor (PDGF) and fibroblast growth factor (FGF). These two models are not necessarily mutually exclusive.

For all its complexity and metabolic activity, there is tremendous regulation of the marrow through the interaction of various cytokines. Normally, only the most mature elements in each cell lineage are released into the general circulation,

TABLE 6–1 **Cytokines that regulate hematopoiesis.**

Cytokine	Cell Lines Stimulated	Cytokine Source
IL-1	Erythrocyte	Multiple cell types
	Granulocyte	
	Megakaryocyte	
	Monocyte	
IL-3	Erythrocyte	T lymphocytes
	Granulocyte	
	Megakaryocyte	
	Monocyte	
IL-4	Basophil	T lymphocytes
IL-5	Eosinophil	T lymphocytes
IL-6	Erythrocyte	Endothelial cells
	Granulocyte	Fibroblasts
	Megakaryocyte	Macrophages
	Monocyte	
IL-11	Erythrocyte	Fibroblasts
	Granulocyte	Osteoblasts
	Megakaryocyte	
Erythropoietin	Erythrocyte	Kidney
		Kupffer cells of liver
SCF	Erythrocyte	Multiple cell types
	Granulocyte	
	Megakaryocyte	
	Monocyte	
G-CSF	Granulocyte	Endothelial cells
		Fibroblasts
		Monocytes
GM-CSF	Erythrocyte	Endothelial cells
	Granulocyte	Fibroblasts
	Megakaryocyte	Monocytes
		T lymphocytes
M-CSF	Monocyte	Endothelial cells
		Fibroblasts
		Monocytes
Thrombopoietin	Megakaryocyte	Liver, kidney

Key: IL, interleukin; CSF, colony-stimulating factor; G, granulocyte; M, macrophage; SCF, stem cell factor.

demonstrating this exquisite control over development. Complex negative-feedback mechanisms must be at work to maintain circulating quantities of each formed element at the consistent levels at which they are found.

Examination of the appropriateness of blood cell development is best undertaken with the microscope, using the **thin blood smear** (Figure 6–2). Modern technical equipment, which can optically sort cells by size and various optical reflective parameters, gives important information, especially about whether cell numbers are out of the normal ranges (Table 6–2). However, microscopic examination of the blood smear, usually using Wright's stain, gives additional information once an abnormality is detected and should always be done when a blood disorder is suspected on clinical grounds.

Physiology

A. Erythrocytes

Mature red blood cells are biconcave disk-shaped cells filled with hemoglobin, which function as the oxygen-carrying component of the blood. In contrast to most other cells, they

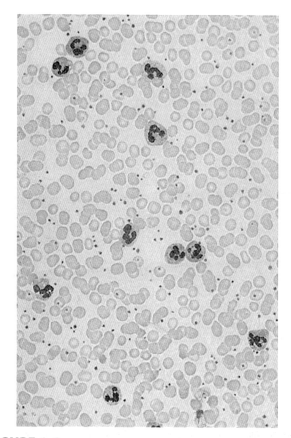

FIGURE 6–2 Normal thin blood smear, seen at low power (40×) with Wright's stain. Erythrocytes predominate and can be seen to be thin disks with central pallor (see text). Platelets are the numerous small, dark bodies. Larger cells with lobulated nuclei are mature neutrophils. Lymphocytes and monocytes are not present on this smear.

TABLE 6–2 Normal values obtained on automated blood count—formed elements of blood.

Element	Male Adult	Female Adult
Hemoglobin	14–18 g/dL	12–16 g/dL
Hematocrit (percentage of blood which is erythrocytes)	42–50%	37–47%
Red cell count	$4.6–6 \times 10^6/\mu L$	$4.2–5.4 \times 10^6/\mu L$
Mean corpuscular volume (MCV)	80–100 fL	80–100 fL
White blood cell (total) count	4000–11,000/μL	4000–11,000/μL
Neutrophils	2500–7500/μL	2500–7500/μL
Lymphocytes	1500–3500/μL	1500–3500/μL
Monocytes	200–800/μL	200–800/μL
Eosinophils	60–600/μL	60–600/μL
Basophils	< 100/μL	< 100/μL
Platelets	150,000–400,000/μL	150,000–400,000/μL

do not have nuclei at maturity; their nuclei are extruded during the final phase of erythrocyte development. The presence of erythrocytes with nuclei in the peripheral blood smear suggests an underlying disease state. Normal red cells are about 8 μm in diameter, a size that is larger than the smallest capillaries. However, their biconcave shape gives them enough flexibility to slip through small capillaries and deliver oxygen to the tissues. Once extruded from the bone marrow, individual erythrocytes function for about 120 days before they are removed from the circulation by the spleen.

In a typical blood smear (stained with Wright's stain), erythrocytes dominate the microscopic field, and their biconcave disk shape resembles that of a doughnut. There is a thicker outer rim that appears red owing to the hemoglobin present and an area of central pallor where the disk is thinnest. Young erythrocytes (reticulocytes) appear bluer (basophilic) because they still contain some ribosomes and mitochondria for a few days after the nuclei are extruded.

Hemoglobin is the most important substance in the erythrocyte. This protein is actually a tetramer, made of two α-protein subunits and two β-protein subunits (in normal adult hemoglobin, called hemoglobin A). Each α- or β-subunit contains the actual oxygen-binding portion of the complex, **heme.** Heme is a compound whose centrally important atom is iron; it is this atom that actually binds oxygen in the lungs and subsequently releases it in the tissues of the body. A low level of hemoglobin in the blood, from a variety of causes (see later discussion), is **anemia,** the most common general blood disorder.

B. Granulocytes: Neutrophils, Eosinophils, and Basophils

The granulocytes are the most common white blood cells; of these, neutrophils are most abundant, followed by eosinophils and basophils (Table 6–2). Developmentally, all three types are similar: As they mature, their nuclei become more convoluted and multilobed, and each develops a cytoplasm filled with granules. These granules contain a variety of enzymes, prostaglandins, and mediators of inflammation, with specific factors dependent on the cell type. Early progenitor cells for each type of granulocyte ("blasts") are indistinguishable on microscopic examination of the bone marrow, but under the influence of different cytokines, they become morphologically distinct cell types.

Basophils contain very dark blue or purple granules when stained with either Giemsa's or Wright's stain. Basophil granules are large and usually obscure the nucleus because of their density. Normally, basophils function in hypersensitivity reactions (as described in Chapter 3). However, their numbers can be increased in diseases not associated with hypersensitivity, such as chronic myelogenous leukemia.

Eosinophils contain large, strikingly "eosinophilic" granules (staining red with Wright's or Giemsa's stain). Eosinophil nuclei are usually bilobed. Normally, eosinophils function as part of the inflammatory response to parasites too large to be engulfed by individual immune cells. They are also involved in some allergic reactions.

Neutrophils contain granules that are "neutrophilic" (ie, neither eosinophilic nor basophilic). Although they predominate in the blood, their major function is actually in the tissues; they must leave the blood by inserting themselves between the endothelial cells of the vasculature to reach sites of injury or infection. Their granules contain highly active enzymes such as **myeloperoxidase,** which, along with the free radical oxygen ions produced by membrane enzymes such as nicotinamide adenine dinucleotide phosphate (NADPH) **oxidase,** kill bacteria that neutrophils ingest via endocytosis or phagocytosis. They are the "first line of defense" against bacterial pathogens, and low numbers of them (leukopenia) lead directly to a high incidence of significant bacterial infections (see later discussion). Of all the cells produced by the bone marrow, the neutrophils comprise the greatest fraction. Their life span in blood, only 8 hours, is much shorter than that of any other cell type. Evidence of their importance and their short survival is commonly manifested, because examination of the blood smear under the microscope in a patient with an active infection may show not only increased numbers of mature, multilobed neutrophils (neutrophilia) but also increased numbers of less mature cells. These less mature cells, released from a large storage pool in the bone marrow, are called **bands** and have a characteristic horseshoe-shaped nucleus that is not yet fully lobulated. The phenomenon of finding these cells in the peripheral blood is called a **left shift** of the granulocyte lineage.

C. Other White Blood Cells: Monocytes and Lymphocytes

Both monocytes and lymphocytes arise from the common stem cell. It is the widespread **pluripotential** ability of stem cells to differentiate into these cells in addition to the granulocytes, erythrocytes, and platelets that makes bone marrow transplantation a therapeutic option for immune system disorders and malignancies. Monocytes have a very long life span, probably several months, but spend only about 3 days in the circulation. They mostly reside in tissues and act there as immune cells that engulf (**phagocytose**) bacteria and subsequently can "present" components of these bacteria to lymphocytes in a way that further amplifies and refines the immune response (Chapter 3). On blood smear evaluation, monocytes are the largest cells seen, with irregular but not multilobed nuclei and pale blue cytoplasm, often with prominent vacuoles.

Lymphocyte precursors leave the marrow early and require extramedullary (outside of the marrow) maturation to become normally functioning immune cells in either the blood or the lymphatic system (Figure 6–3). Their crucial roles in recognizing "self" versus "nonself" and in modulating virtually all aspects of the immune response are described in Chapter 3. On microscopic examination of the blood smear, lymphocytes are small cells, slightly larger than an erythrocyte, with dark nuclei essentially filling the entire cell; only a thin rim of light blue cytoplasm is normally seen. Granules are sparse or absent.

D. Platelets

Platelets are the smallest formed elements in the blood. They are fragments of larger, multinucleated cells, which are the largest discrete constituents of the bone marrow (**megakaryocytes**), but platelets have no nuclei of their own. Most platelets remain in the circulation, but a substantial minority are trapped in the spleen; this phenomenon becomes important in a variety of immune-mediated decreases in platelet count (**thrombocytopenia;** see later discussion). In the setting of a normal platelet count, they have a circulatory half-life of about 10 days. In cases of thrombocytopenia, their half-life decreases, as they are consumed in the routine maintenance of vascular integrity.

Platelets are integral components of the coagulation system. Their membranes provide an important source of phospholipids, which are required for the function of the coagulation system proteins (Figure 6–4), and contain important receptors that allow attachment to endothelial cells (**platelet adhesion**) so that a **platelet plug** can be formed in response to blood vessel injury. This prevents further blood loss after trauma and limits the coagulation response to the site of injury rather than letting coagulation proceed inappropriately.

The cytoplasm is also important for platelet function, particularly the intracellular **dense granules** and **alpha granules.** The phenomenon of platelet activation is also called "degranulation" and can be initiated by exposure of platelets to the activated blood coagulation factor **thrombin,** adenosine 5′-diphosphate (ADP), or collagen. This last reaction is probably the most important, occurring when collagen, normally in the basement membrane below the endothelial cells, is exposed to the blood after injury. Platelet activation can also be induced by exposure to **platelet-activating factor** (**PAF**), a neutrophil-derived phospholipid cytokine.

During platelet activation, the dense and alpha granules release further activators of platelet activity, such as ADP, and platelet factor 4, which can also bind to endothelial cells. It is important because it binds to the most commonly used therapeutic anticoagulant, heparin (see later discussion). The last step in platelet activity is platelet aggregation, where platelets stick to each other, firming up the platelet plug. On examination of the blood smear, platelets are small, irregularly shaped blue or purple granular bodies. In conditions in which platelet numbers are rising as a result of increased marrow activity, more immature platelets can be identified by their larger size.

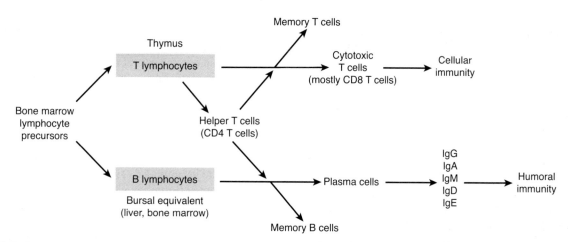

FIGURE 6–3 Development of the immune system from the common bone marrow stem cell. (Redrawn, with permission, from Ganong WF. *Review of Medical Physiology*, 22nd ed. McGraw-Hill, 2005.)

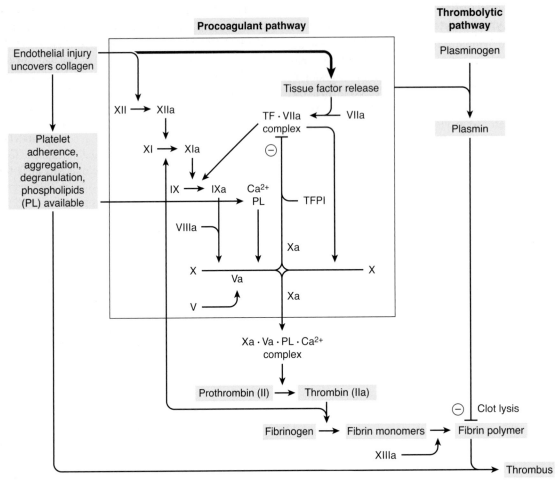

FIGURE 6–4 Coagulation and thrombolytic systems, showing balanced activity between them.

COAGULATION FACTORS & THE COAGULATION CASCADE

Anatomy

The coagulation system is remarkably complex in both structure and function. Many proteins are involved, produced by different cell types of the body, with both inactive and active forms regulated in a fine balance. The coagulation system provides for immediate activation when there is blood loss that needs to be stemmed but also confines its activity to the site of blood loss. Otherwise, coagulation might occur throughout the entire circulatory system, which would be incompatible with life.

There are two major components of the coagulation system: platelets (discussed previously) and the coagulation factors, which are plasma proteins. The end result of coagulation factor activity is quite simple: the formation of a complex of cross-linked **fibrin** molecules and platelets that terminate hemorrhage after injury. However, the sophisticated **coagulation cascade** provides several points of control over this event (Figure 6–4).

The coagulation factors do not generally circulate in active forms. Most of them are enzymes (serine proteases) and remain dormant until they are needed. This is accomplished by having other enzymes (the other proteases in the cascade) available that can cleave the inactive factors into active ones. Presumably, the many interactions in the cascade allow a small increase in the activity of two key early enzymes, factors VII and XI, to be amplified. This results in a timely change in the availability of thrombin, which cleaves fibrinogen, leaving fibrin to form the clot. All of the factors have roman numerals, and the inactive forms are written without annotation (eg, factor II, also known as prothrombin). The activated forms of the factors are signified by the letter "a" (eg, factor IIa, also known as thrombin).

Most of the coagulation factors are made by the liver, but factor XIII derives from platelets and factor VIII is made by endothelial cells. Factors II, VII, IX, and X are particularly important factors (Table 6–3) because they are all dependent on the liver enzyme γ-carboxylase. Gammacarboxylase is dependent on vitamin K, and the oral anticoagulant **warfarin** acts by interfering with vitamin K activity. Two of the anticoagulant proteins, protein S and protein C (see later discussion), are also vitamin K dependent.

Physiology

The coagulation cascade, diagrammed in Figure 6–4, is a highly complex, regulated interaction of proteins. The critical step for the entire process, around which the procoagulant and anticoagulant balance is centered, is the activation of factor X to factor Xa. Factor Xa forms a complex with factor Va and calcium, and it is here also that the phospholipids (PLs) from platelet membranes come into play, helping to ensure that coagulation is proceeding in the appropriate place in the circulation where a

TABLE 6–3 Coagulation factors of plasma.

Name	Production Source
Procoagulant factors	
Factor I (fibrinogen)	Liver
Factor II (prothrombin)	Liver
Factor III (tissue thromboplastin)	Tissue
Factor IV (calcium)	...
Factor V (proaccelerin)	Liver
Factor VI (obsolete = factor Va)	...
Factor VII (proconvertin)	Liver
Factor VIII (antihemophilic factor)	Endothelial cells
Factor IX (Christmas factor)	Liver
Factor X (Stuart-Prower factor)	Liver
Factor XI (plasma thromboplastin antecedent)	Liver
Factor XII (Hageman factor)	Liver
Factor XIII (fibrin-stabilizing factor)	Platelets
Anticoagulant factors	
Antithrombin	Liver
Protein C	Liver
Protein S	Liver
Plasminogen	Liver
Tissue factor pathway inhibitor	Endothelial cells

clot is necessary, namely, at the platelet plug. This Xa-Va-Ca^{2+}-PL complex, prothrombinase, converts prothrombin to thrombin and can convert multiple molecules per complex. It is not the result of simple binding but rather of proteolytic cleavage of prothrombin, and the complex is free to act on other prothrombin molecules nearby. This mechanism provides more amplification of a system built on multiple levels of amplification.

Thrombin is also a serine protease. It cleaves the ubiquitous plasma protein fibrinogen into fibrin monomers, which are small insoluble proteins and polymerize with each other to form the complex **fibrin.** This conglomerate can subsequently be solidified by chemical cross-links catalyzed by factor XIIIa, which is formed from factor XIII by the proteolytic activity of thrombin.

The tight control of factor X activity begins as soon as coagulation begins. Tissue factor, also called **thromboplastin,** is a lipid-rich protein material released on tissue injury. It directly activates factor VII and, complexed with factor VIIa, subsequently activates both factor IX and factor X. Factor Xa, however, binds to another plasma (and lipid-bound) protein called tissue factor pathway inhibitor (TFPI). TFPI not only inhibits the further activity of factor Xa itself, but the combination of factor Xa and TFPI greatly inhibits factor VIIa. Downstream prothrombinase activity can only be sustained if the initial injury continues to generate enough factor IXa (and VIIIa) to activate more factor X. The alternative pathway to production of IXa is the conversion of factor XI to XIa, the result of activation of protease factor XII by high-molecular-weight kininogen (the precursor of the vasoactive peptide bradykinin) and kallikrein (an enzyme) in the presence of collagen. Exposed collagen is usually a result of vascular injury and leads to platelet adhesion and aggregation (see prior discussion). Factor XI may also be activated by thrombin in a different positive feedback step.

Factor IXa requires one more collaborator to activate factor X: factor VIII, normally complexed to **von Willebrand factor (vWF),** the protein that allows platelets to adhere to endothelial cells. Factor VIII is activated by its release from vWF. Factors VIIIa and IXa, in the presence of phospholipids (again, usually from platelets) and calcium, together activate factor X.

Two complex anticoagulant systems also help control coagulation. The first is the **thrombolytic system,** which is principally involved in dissolving clots that have already formed. In this system, **plasmin,** a serum protease, cleaves fibrin, resulting in breakup of the clot and creating fibrin degradation products that inhibit thrombin. Completing this feedback loop, plasmin is formed from its own inactive precursor protein, **plasminogen,** by thrombin. Plasminogen can also be cleaved by **tissue plasminogen activator (t-PA)** to form plasmin; t-PA and related proteins are now used clinically, injected intravenously or intra-arterially, to break up clots that form in coronary arteries, to treat heart attacks, and in cerebral arteries, to treat strokes.

The second anticoagulant system is characterized by a group of inhibitors of the coagulation factors. They are composed of antithrombin, protein S, and protein C (see later discussion). Antithrombin is a protease inhibitor and physically blocks the action of the serine proteases in the cascade. Its activity is enhanced up to 2000-fold by heparin. Protein C, activated by thrombin, cleaves factor Va into an inactive form so that the prothrombinase complex cannot cleave prothrombin into thrombin. Protein C requires protein S as a cofactor. This complex also inactivates factor VIIIa.

LABORATORY TESTING OF THE COAGULATION PROCESS

Assays are available for determining both the absolute level and the activity of each of the coagulation factors, but in practice there are two common in vitro tests of coagulation function, both reported as "seconds required to form a clot": the prothrombin time (PT) and the activated partial thromboplastin time (aPTT). The tests are designed in such a way that the results will be prolonged out of the normal range in different pathologic states, but significant alterations in the coagulation pathway inevitably lead to changes in both tests because of the multiple interactions of the involved factors.

PT is the test used clinically to monitor the effects of warfarin. Because all vitamin K–dependent factor levels are lowered by warfarin, eventually the aPTT will also become abnormal with high enough doses; but factor VII has the shortest half-life of those factors, so its levels fall first. Because of its critical role in clotting, thrombin is the principal factor whose activity must be reduced to achieve and maintain therapeutic anticoagulation. The aPTT is prolonged most easily when there are reduced levels of factor VIII or factor IX activity, regardless of whether these factors are present at low concentrations or are present at normal concentrations but are being actively inhibited by other molecules. The aPTT is also very sensitive to the presence of heparin bound to antithrombin and is used to monitor the anticoagulant effects of unfractionated heparin. Low-molecular-weight heparins (a specific purified subset of unfractionated heparin) in combination with antithrombin preferentially inhibit factor Xa. In the doses of low-molecular-weight heparins usually given for prevention or treatment of thrombosis, the aPTT will not be prolonged (at least not into the usual "therapeutic range" for unfractionated heparin) despite good evidence of anticoagulation efficacy if factor Xa activity is measured directly.

CHECKPOINT

4. Name the vitamin K–dependent clotting factors and the organ in which they are synthesized.
5. The extrinsic and intrinsic coagulation pathways converge with the activation of which clotting factor?
6. Describe the two anticoagulant systems that participate in clotting homeostasis.

OVERVIEW OF BLOOD DISORDERS

FORMED ELEMENT DISORDERS

Disorders of red cells, white cells, and platelets are separated for discussion because one or the other is found to be the most abnormal during laboratory testing. However, because of the clonal nature of hematopoiesis, many disorders affect all the formed elements of the blood. This is perhaps best demonstrated in the "blast crisis" phase of chronic myelogenous leukemia, in which the majority of both myeloid and lymphoid cells in the blood may be shown to express an identical gene rearrangement, called *bcr-abl* or Philadelphia chromosome, that has arisen in a single abnormal progenitor cell.

1. Red Cell Disorders

There are many red cell abnormalities, but the principal ones are a variety of anemias. **Anemia** is defined as an abnormally low hemoglobin concentration in the blood. There are several methods of classification, but the prevailing systems are based on red cell size and shape.

In normal persons, erythrocytes are of uniform size and shape, and the automated blood count shows a mean corpuscular volume (MCV) near 90 fL, which is the estimated volume of a single cell. Automated systems usually report abnormalities of red cells as changes in hemoglobin concentration, red cell number, and MCV. Small cells (with low MCVs) are termed **microcytic,** and cells larger than normal are termed **macrocytic.** The relative nonuniformity of cell shapes (**poikilocytosis**) or sizes (**anisocytosis**) can further aid in subclassifying erythrocyte disorders.

The morphologic classification of anemias is set forth in Table 6–4 and Figure 6–5. In general, the microcytic anemias are due to abnormalities in hemoglobin production, either in number of hemoglobin molecules per cell or in type of hemoglobin molecules (**hemoglobinopathies**). **Iron deficiency anemia** resulting from chronic blood loss and the **thalassemias** are examples of microcytic anemia.

The macrocytic anemias reflect either abnormal nuclear maturation or a higher fraction of young, large red cells (reticulocytes). When the nuclei of maturing red cells appear too young and large for the amount of hemoglobin in the cytoplasm, the macrocytic anemia is termed **megaloblastic.** These anemias are most often due either to vitamin deficiencies (vitamin B_{12} or folic acid) or drugs that interfere with DNA synthesis. Abnormal nuclear maturation can also be due to clonal proliferation in the bone marrow, producing preleukemic states termed the **myelodysplastic syndromes.**

TABLE 6–4 Morphologic classification and common causes of anemia.

Type	MCV	Common Causes
Macrocytic	Increased	Folic acid deficiency
		Vitamin B$_{12}$ deficiency
		Liver disease
		Alcohol
		Hypothyroidism
		Drugs (sulfonamides, zidovudine, antineoplastic agents)
		Myelodysplastic syndromes
Microcytic	Decreased	Iron deficiency
		Thalassemias
Normocytic	Normal	Aplastic anemia
		Anemia of chronic disease
		Chronic renal failure
		Hemolytic anemia
		Spherocytosis

The normocytic anemias can be due to multiple causes: decreased numbers of red cell precursors in the marrow (primary failure called aplastic anemia, replacement of marrow elements with cancer, certain viral infections, or autoimmune inhibition called **pure red cell aplasia**), low levels of erythropoietin (resulting from chronic renal failure), or chronic inflammatory diseases that affect the availability of iron in the marrow. Other normocytic anemias can be secondary to decreased life span of the cells that are produced. Examples of this phenomenon are acute blood loss; **autoimmune hemolytic anemias,** in which antibodies or complement bind to red cells and cause their destruction; **sickle cell anemia,** in which the abnormal hemoglobin polymerizes and obliterates the usual resilience of the red cell, and **hereditary spherocytosis** or **hereditary elliptocytosis,** in which defects in the erythrocyte membrane affect their ability to squeeze through the capillary microcirculation.

Anemias are very common. In contrast, an elevated hemoglobin concentration, termed **erythrocytosis,** is uncommon. Elevations in hemoglobin concentration can occur as a secondary phenomenon because of increased erythropoietin levels, such as that found in smokers or people who live at high altitudes (whose low blood oxygen levels stimulate erythropoietin production). Some tumors, especially renal tumors, can also make erythropoietin. Primary **polycythemia** is an abnormality of the bone marrow itself. This myeloproliferative syndrome leads to an increased red cell mass and consequent low erythropoietin levels by the negative-feedback mechanism discussed previously.

2. White Blood Cell Disorders

Abnormalities in white cell numbers occur commonly (Table 6–5), whereas abnormalities of function are rare. Neoplastic transformation in the form of leukemia (granulocytes and monocytes) or lymphoma (lymphocytes) is fairly common. The leukemias are discussed in Chapter 5.

Changes in neutrophil count are the most common white cell abnormality detected on the automated blood count. Increased numbers of neutrophils (**leukocytosis**) suggest acute or chronic infection or inflammation but can be a sign of many conditions. These include stress, because adrenal corticosteroids cause **demargination** of neutrophils from blood vessel walls.

Decreased numbers of neutrophils (**neutropenia**) can be seen in overwhelming infection and benign diseases such as **cyclic neutropenia** (see later discussion) but can also be seen when the bone marrow is infiltrated with tumor or involved by the myelodysplastic syndromes. Many drugs can also directly suppress marrow production, and because neutrophils have the shortest half-life in the blood of any cell produced by the marrow, their numbers may fall quickly.

Lymphocyte numbers can vary substantially (Table 6–6). Lymphocyte counts are classically elevated in viral infections, such as infectious mononucleosis. However, persistent elevations suggest malignancies, particularly **chronic lymphocytic leukemia,** which may not cause any symptoms and be incidentally discovered on a routine blood count.

Decreased lymphocyte counts (**lymphopenia**) are a common complication of corticosteroid therapy but are most worrisome for immunodeficiency states; HIV directly infects lymphocytes, and the likelihood of opportunistic infections increases as lymphocyte counts fall, resulting in AIDS.

3. Platelet Disorders

Abnormalities in platelet number are fairly common, particularly low counts (**thrombocytopenia**). Causes are listed in Table 6–7. Decreased production of platelets occurs when the marrow is affected by a variety of diseases or when thrombopoietin production by the liver is impaired, as in cirrhosis. Increased destruction of platelets is much more prevalent. There are three general mechanisms. Because a significant number of platelets normally reside in the spleen, any increase in spleen size or activity (**hypersplenism**) leads to lower platelet counts. Platelet consumption because of ongoing clotting will also lower counts. Most commonly, however, there is immune-mediated consumption caused by either drugs or autoantibodies. The latter are usually directed against the platelet membrane antigen gpIIb/IIIa.

Functional platelet disorders are common, especially the acquired disorders resulting from uremia (renal failure) or aspirin, which inhibits the platelet enzyme cyclooxygenase and decreases platelet aggregability. Inherited abnormalities are unusual with the exception of **von Willebrand's disease,** which results from either quantitative or qualitative defect of

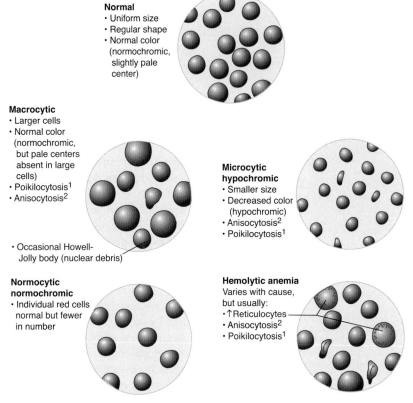

Normal
- Uniform size
- Regular shape
- Normal color (normochromic, slightly pale center)

Macrocytic
- Larger cells
- Normal color (normochromic, but pale centers absent in large cells)
- Poikilocytosis[1]
- Anisocytosis[2]

- Occasional Howell-Jolly body (nuclear debris)

Microcytic hypochromic
- Smaller size
- Decreased color (hypochromic)
- Anisocytosis[2]
- Poikilocytosis[1]

Normocytic normochromic
- Individual red cells normal but fewer in number

Hemolytic anemia
Varies with cause, but usually:
- ↑Reticulocytes
- Anisocytosis[2]
- Poikilocytosis[1]

FIGURE 6–5 Thin blood smear appearance of erythrocytes in the different morphologic types of anemias. (1, Poikilocytosis [variation in shape]; 2, anisocytosis [variation in size].)   (Redrawn, with permission, from Chandrasoma P, Taylor CR. *Concise Pathology*, 3rd ed. Originally published by Appleton & Lange. Copyright © 1998 by the McGraw-Hill Companies, Inc.)

TABLE 6–5 Causes of abnormal neutrophil counts.

Neutrophilia	Neutropenia
Increased marrow activity	*Decreased marrow activity*
Bacterial infections	Drugs (antineoplastic agents, antibiotics, gold, certain diuretics, anti-thyroid agents, antihistamines, antipsychotics)
Acute inflammation	Radiation exposure
Leukemia and myeloproliferative disorders	Megaloblastic anemia
Release from marrow pool	Cyclic neutropenia
Stress (catecholamines)	Kostmann's (infantile) neutropenia
Corticosteroids	Aplastic anemias
Endotoxin exposure	Myelodysplastic syndromes
Demargination into blood	Marrow replacement by tumor
Bacterial infections	*Decreased neutrophil survival*
Hypoxemia	Sepsis
Stress (catecholamines)	Viral or rickettsial infection
Corticosteroids	Immune destruction associated with drugs
Exercise	Immune destruction associated with autoantibodies (systemic lupus erythematosus, Felty's syndrome)
	Hypersplenism

TABLE 6–6 Causes of abnormal lymphocyte counts.

Lymphocytosis
Medium to large, atypical lymphocytes predominant
Viral infections (mononucleosis, mumps, measles, hepatitis, rubella)
Active immune responses, particularly in children
Toxoplasmosis
Lymphoma with circulating cells
Chronic lymphocytic leukemia
Small, mature lymphocytes predominant
Chronic infections (tuberculosis)
Autoimmune diseases (myasthenia gravis)
Metabolic diseases (Addison's disease)
Lymphoma with circulating cells
Chronic lymphocytic leukemia
Immature cells predominant
Acute lymphocytic leukemia
Lymphoblastic lymphoma
Lymphopenia
Immunodeficiency states (AIDS)
Corticosteroid therapy
Toxic drugs
Cushing's syndrome

TABLE 6–7 Causes of platelet abnormalities.

Thrombocytosis
Myeloproliferative disorders, especially essential thrombocythemia
Postsplenectomy
Reactive (postsurgical, posthemorrhage, anemias)
Inflammatory disorders
Malignancies
Thrombocytopenia
Decreased production
Aplastic anemia
Marrow infiltration
Vitamin B_{12} and folate deficiencies
Radiation or chemotherapy
Hereditary
Infection (HIV, parvovirus, CMV)
Cirrhosis (low thrombopoietin levels)
Decreased survival
Immune mediated (idiopathic, systemic lupus erythematosus, drug induced, neonatal from maternal IgG)
Hypersplenism
Disseminated intravascular coagulation
Thrombotic thrombocytopenic purpura, hemolytic uremic syndrome
Prosthetic valves
Qualitative platelet disorders
Inherited
Bernard-Soulier syndrome (adhesion defect)
Glanzmann's thrombasthenia (aggregation defect)
Storage pool disease (granule defect)
Von Willebrand's disease
Wiskott-Aldrich syndrome
Acquired
Uremia
Dysproteinemias
Chronic liver disease
Drug induced (especially aspirin)

von Willebrand factor, the carrier protein for factor VIII. This factor also acts as a bridge between platelets and the endothelium and thus is crucial for formation of the platelet plug in the coagulation cascade.

Elevations in the platelet count above normal (**thrombocytosis**) are relatively common and are especially apt to occur in recovery from iron deficiency anemia upon iron repletion. In the myeloproliferative disorders, such as polycythemia, platelet counts are often high. In **essential thrombocythemia**, platelet counts may be higher than 1,000,000/µL.

COAGULATION FACTOR DISORDERS

The most important coagulation factor disorders are quantitative rather than qualitative and usually hereditary rather than acquired (Table 6–8). Exceptions to this rule are **acquired factor inhibitors**, which are antibodies that bind to one of the coagulation factors, most often factor VIII. These may or may not cause clinical bleeding problems, but they can be extremely difficult to

TABLE 6–8 Coagulation factor deficiencies.

Factor	Disease	Inheritance Pattern	Frequency	Disease Severity
Fibrinogen	Afibrinogenemia	Autosomal recessive	Rare	Variable
	Dysfibrinogenemia	Autosomal dominant	Rare	Variable
Factor V	Parahemophilia	Autosomal recessive	Very rare	Moderate to severe
Factor VII		Autosomal recessive	Very rare	Moderate to severe
Factor VIII	Hemophilia A	X-linked recessive	Common	Mild to severe
vWF	von Willebrand's disease	Autosomal dominant	Common	Mild to moderate
Factor IX	Hemophilia B	X-linked recessive	Uncommon	Mild to severe
Factor X		Autosomal recessive	Rare	Variable
Factor XI	Rosenthal's syndrome	Autosomal recessive	Uncommon	Mild
Factor XII	Hageman trait	Autosomal recessive or dominant	Rare	Asymptomatic
Factor XIII		Autosomal recessive	Rare	Severe

treat. The quantitative disorders that most commonly cause bleeding are **hemophilia A** (deficiency of factor VIII) and **hemophilia B** (deficiency of factor IX). Both are X chromosome-linked recessive traits, and affected males have very low levels of factor VIII or IX. It is not clear why all affected males do not have complete absence of factor VIII or IX activity. Hemophilia A is more common, with a prevalence of 1:10,000 males worldwide. Both disorders lead to spontaneous and excessive post-traumatic bleeding, particularly into joints and muscles. Females with the trait have 50% of the normal amount of either factor and tend not to have any bleeding problems; in general, one needs only half of the normal quantities of most coagulation factors to clot normally. The aPTT test is usually designed to become abnormal when factor VIII or IX activities fall below 50% of normal.

Vitamin K deficiency also leads to quantitative declines in the levels of factors II, VII, IX, and X and proteins C and S; prolongation of the prothrombin time may result.

Quantitative inherited abnormalities of the anticoagulation systems also occur. Protein S deficiency, protein C deficiency, and antithrombin deficiency all occur and lead to abnormal clotting problems, as discussed in the next section.

Finally, the condition of **consumptive coagulopathy** or **disseminated intravascular coagulation** (**DIC**) needs to be included. This condition is generally due to overwhelming infection, specific leukemias or lymphomas, or massive hemorrhage. In DIC, the coagulation factors become depleted. Often there is simultaneous activation of the fibrinolytic system as well, and uncontrolled bleeding may occur throughout the entire circulatory system. PT and aPTT are usually both abnormal.

CHECKPOINT

7. Define anemia and suggest three causes each for macrocytic and microcytic anemia.
8. What are some categories of explanations for a white blood cell number that is substantially increased or decreased compared with the normal range?
9. What are the three general mechanisms of thrombocytopenia?
10. What is the nature of the defects in hemophilia A and B?

PATHOPHYSIOLOGY OF SELECTED BLOOD DISORDERS

RED CELL DISORDERS

1. Iron Deficiency Anemia

Etiology

Iron deficiency anemia is the most common form of anemia. Although in many developing countries dietary deficiency of iron can occur, in developed nations the main cause is loss of iron, almost always through blood loss from the GI or genitourinary tracts.

Because of recurrent menstrual blood loss, premenopausal women represent the population with the highest incidence of iron deficiency. The incidence in this group is even higher because of iron losses during pregnancy, because the developing fetus efficiently extracts maternal iron for use in its own hematopoiesis. In men or in postmenopausal women with iron deficiency, GI bleeding is usually the cause. Blood loss in this case may be due to relatively benign disorders, such as peptic ulcer, arteriovenous malformations, or angiodysplasia (small vascular abnormalities along the intestinal walls). More serious causes are inflammatory bowel disease or malignancy. Endoscopic investigation to exclude malignancy is mandatory in patients without a known cause of iron deficiency.

There are other less common causes of iron deficiency, but almost all are related to blood loss: Bleeding disorders, hemoptysis, and hemoglobinuria are the chief possibilities.

Pathogenesis

Body iron stores are generally sufficient to last several years, but there is a constant loss of iron in completely healthy persons, such that iron balance depends on adequate intake and absorption. Dietary iron is primarily absorbed in the duodenum. Absorption is increased in the setting of anemia, hypoxia, and systemic iron deficiency. Iron is also recycled from senescent erythrocytes via macrophage phagocytosis and lysis. The export of iron to plasma from these cellular sites is regulated by **hepcidin,** a 25-amino acid peptide produced by the liver. Hepcidin binds to ferroportin, a transmembrane protein, inducing its internalization and lysosomal degradation. When iron stores are low, hepcidin production is reduced and ferroportin molecules are expressed on the basolateral membrane of enterocytes, where they transfer iron from the cytoplasm of enterocytes to plasma **transferrin.** Conversely, when iron stores are adequate or elevated, hepcidin production is increased, resulting in the internalization of ferroportin and reduced export of iron into plasma. In inflammatory states, hepcidin production is increased, leading to the internalization of **ferroportin** on macrophages and the trapping of recycled iron within macrophage stores.

Iron is stored in most body cells as **ferritin,** a combination of iron and the protein apoferritin. It is also stored as **hemosiderin,** which is ferritin partly stripped of the apoferritin protein shell. Iron is transported in blood bound to its carrier protein transferrin. Because of the complex interactions between these molecules, a simple measurement of serum iron rarely reflects body iron stores (see later discussion).

Iron is found predominantly in hemoglobin and is present also in **myoglobin,** the oxygen-storing protein of skeletal muscle. The main role for iron is as the ion in the center of the body's oxygen-carrying molecule, **heme.** Held stably in the ferrous form by the other atoms in heme, iron reversibly binds oxygen. Each protein subunit of hemoglobin contains one heme molecule; because hemoglobin exists as a tetramer, four iron molecules are needed in each hemoglobin unit. When there is iron deficiency, the final step in heme synthesis is interrupted (Figure 6–6). In this step, ferrous iron is inserted into protoporphyrin IX by the enzyme ferrochelatase; when heme synthesis is interrupted, there is inadequate heme production. Globin biosynthesis is inhibited by heme deficiency through a **heme-regulated translational inhibitor (HRI).** Elevated HRI activity (a result of heme deficiency) inhibits a key transcription initiation factor for heme synthesis, eIF2. Thus, less heme and fewer globin chains are available in each red cell precursor. This directly causes anemia, a decrease in the hemoglobin concentration of the blood.

As noted, heme is also the oxygen acceptor in myoglobin; therefore, iron deficiency will also lead to decreased myoglobin production. Other proteins also are dependent on iron; most of these are enzymes. Many use iron in the heme molecule, but some use elemental iron. Although the exact implications of iron deficiency on their activity is not known, these enzymes are crucial to metabolism, energy production, DNA synthesis, and even brain function.

Pathology

As iron stores are depleted, the peripheral blood smear pattern evolves. In early iron deficiency, the hemoglobin level of the blood falls but individual erythrocytes appear normal. In response to a falling oxygen level, erythropoietin levels rise and stimulate the marrow, but the hemoglobin level cannot rise in response because of the iron deficiency. Other hormones are presumably also stimulated, however, and the resulting "revved-up" marrow usually causes an elevated blood platelet count. An elevated white cell count is less common. Reticulocytes are notably absent.

Eventually, the hemoglobin concentration of individual cells falls, leading to the classic picture of microcytic, hypochromic erythrocytes (Figure 6–5). This is most commonly found as an abnormally low MCV of red cells on the automated hemogram. There is also substantial anisocytosis and poikilocytosis, seen on the peripheral smear, and **target cells** may be seen. The target shape occurs because there is a relative excess of red cell membrane compared with the amount of hemoglobin within the cell, so that the membrane bunches up in the center.

Laboratory results are often confusing. A low serum ferritin level is diagnostic of iron deficiency, but even in obvious cases, levels can be normal; ferritin levels rise in acute or chronic inflammation or significant illnesses, which can themselves be the cause of iron (blood) loss. Serum iron levels fall in many illnesses, and levels of its serum carrier, transferrin, fluctuate as well, so neither of them is a consistent indicator of iron deficiency, nor is their ratio, the transferrin saturation. If ferritin levels are not diagnostic, clinical practice now focuses on measuring soluble transferrin receptor (sTfR) in the serum. Transferrin receptors (TfRs) are membrane glycoproteins that facilitate iron transport from plasma transferrin into body cells. Erythroid precursors increase their expression of membrane TfR in the setting of iron deficiency but not anemia of chronic disease. Some membrane TfR is released into the serum as sTfR. The amount of sTfR in the serum reflects the amount of membrane TfR. A high ratio of sTfR to ferritin predicts iron deficiency when ferritin is not diagnostically low.

Other than observing a hematologic response to empiric iron supplementation, bone marrow biopsy can be used to confirm a diagnosis of iron deficiency. Iron is normally found

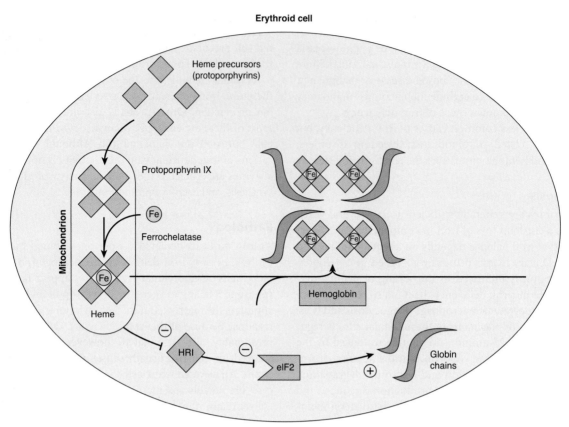

FIGURE 6–6 Heme synthesis, emphasizing the role of iron and the insertion of heme into individual globin chains to make hemoglobin, and the role of the heme-regulated translational inhibitor (HRI) of globin synthesis. Normal concentrations of heme keep the activity of HRI low, preserving normal globin synthesis.

in the macrophages of the marrow, where it supplies erythrocyte precursors; intracellular hemosiderin is easily visualized with Prussian blue stain. These macrophages do not stain at all if there is iron deficiency.

Clinical Manifestations

All anemias lead to classic symptoms of decreased oxygen-carrying capacity (ie, fatigue, weakness, and shortness of breath, particularly dyspnea on exertion), and iron deficiency is no exception. Decreased oxygen-carrying capacity leads to decreased oxygen delivery to metabolically active tissues, which nonetheless must have oxygen; this leads directly to fatigue. The compensatory mechanisms of the body lead to additional symptoms and signs of anemia. Some patients appear pale not only because there is less hemoglobin per unit of blood (oxygenated hemoglobin is red and gives color to the skin) but also because superficial skin blood vessels constrict, diverting blood to more vital structures. Patients may also respond to the anemia with tachycardia. This increased cardiac output is appropriate because one way to increase oxygen delivery to the tissues is to increase the number of times each hemoglobin molecule is oxygenated in the lungs every hour. This tachycardia may cause benign cardiac murmurs due to the increased blood flow.

Abnormalities of the GI tract occur because iron is also needed for proliferating cells. **Glossitis,** where the normal tongue papillae are absent, can occur, as can gastric atrophy with **achlorhydria** (absence of stomach acid). The achlorhydria may compound the iron deficiency because iron is best absorbed in an acidic environment, but this complication is quite unusual.

In children, there may be significant developmental problems, both physical and mental. Iron-deficient children, mostly in developing regions, perform poorly on tests of cognition compared with iron-replete children. Iron therapy can reverse these findings if started early enough in childhood. The exact mechanism of cognitive loss in iron deficiency is not known. Another unexplained but often observed phenomenon in severe iron deficiency is **pica,** a craving for nonnutritive substances such as clay or dirt.

Many patients have no specific symptoms or findings at all, and their iron deficiency is discovered because of anemia noted on a blood count obtained for another purpose. It is of interest that mild anemias (hemoglobins of 11–12 g/dL) may be tolerated very well because they develop slowly. In addition to the physiologic compensatory mechanisms discussed previously (increased cardiac output, diversion of blood flow from less metabolically active areas), there is a biochemical adaptation as well. The ability to transfer oxygen from hemoglobin to cells is partly dependent on a small molecule in erythrocytes called **2,3-biphosphoglycerate (2,3-BPG)**. In high concentrations, the ability to unload oxygen in the tissues is increased. Chronic anemia leads to elevated 2,3-BPG concentrations in erythrocytes.

Other patients who do not present with symptoms directly related to the anemia present instead with symptoms or signs related directly to blood loss. Because the most common site of unexpected (nonmenstrual) blood loss is the GI tract, patients often have visible changes in the stool. There may be gross blood (**hematochezia**), which is more common with bleeding sites near the rectum, or black, tarry, metabolized blood (**melena**) from more proximal sites. Significant blood loss from the urinary tract is very uncommon.

CHECKPOINT

11. What is the most common form of anemia and its most likely cause in a premenopausal woman? In a man?
12. Why is the serum ferritin level often not a good indicator of whether anemia is due to iron deficiency?
13. What are some disorders associated with iron deficiency anemia?
14. What are the physiologic adaptations to slowly developing iron deficiency anemia?

2. Pernicious Anemia

Etiology

Pernicious anemia is a megaloblastic anemia in which there is abnormal erythrocyte nuclear maturation. Unlike in many other types of anemia such as that resulting from iron deficiency, hemoglobin synthesis is normal. Pernicious anemia is the end result of a cascade of events that are autoimmune in origin. The ultimate effect is a loss of adequate stores of vitamin B_{12} (cobalamin), which is a cofactor involved in DNA synthesis. Rapidly proliferating cells are those most often affected, predominantly bone marrow cells and those of the GI epithelium. The nervous system is also affected, demonstrating that this is a systemic disease. Anemia is merely the most common manifestation.

Besides pernicious anemia, cobalamin deficiency can also be due to bacterial overgrowth in the intestine (because bacteria compete with the host for cobalamin), intestinal malabsorption of vitamin B_{12} involving the terminal ileum (such as in Crohn's disease), surgical removal of the antrum of the stomach (gastrectomy), and, rarely, dietary deficiency, which occurs only in strict vegetarians. In the diet, cobalamin is found only in animal products.

Pernicious anemia is most common in older patients of Scandinavian descent but is found in a wide variety of ethnic groups. In the United States, black females are one of the most common groups. Pernicious anemia accounts for only a small percentage of patients with anemia, however.

Pathogenesis

The initial events in the pathogenetic cascade begin in the stomach (Figure 6–7). The gastric parietal cells are initially affected by an autoimmune phenomenon that leads to two discrete effects: loss of gastric acid (**achlorhydria**) and loss of **intrinsic factor.** Pernicious anemia interferes with both the initial availability and the absorption of vitamin B_{12}: Stomach acid is required for the release of cobalamin from foodstuffs, and intrinsic factor is a glycoprotein that binds cobalamin and is required for the effective absorption of cobalamin in the terminal ileum. Both stomach acid and intrinsic factor are made exclusively by parietal cells.

Evidence for the autoimmune destruction of parietal cells is strong: Patients with pernicious anemia have atrophy of the gastric mucosa, and pathologic specimens show infiltrating lymphocytes, which are predominantly antibody-producing B cells. In addition, 90% or more of patients have antibodies in their serum directed against parietal cell membrane proteins. The major protein antigen appears to be H^+-K^+ ATPase, the **proton pump,** which is responsible for the production of stomach acid. Cytotoxic T cells whose receptors recognize H^+-K^+ ATPase may also contribute to the gastric atrophy. More than half of patients also have antibodies to intrinsic factor itself or the intrinsic factor-cobalamin complex. Furthermore, patients with pernicious anemia have a higher incidence of other autoimmune diseases, such as Graves' disease. Lastly, corticosteroid therapy, used as first-line therapy for many autoimmune disorders, may reverse the pathologic findings in pernicious anemia. Despite this evidence, the exact mechanism of the inciting event remains unknown.

Complete vitamin B_{12} deficiency develops slowly, even after total achlorhydria and loss of intrinsic factor occur. Liver stores of vitamin B_{12} are adequate for several years. However, the lack of this vitamin eventually leads to alterations in DNA synthesis and in the nervous system, altered myelin synthesis.

In DNA synthesis, cobalamin, along with folic acid, is crucial as a cofactor in the synthesis of deoxythymidine from deoxyuridine (Figure 6–8). Cobalamin accepts a methyl group from methyltetrahydrofolate, which leads to the formation of two important intracellular compounds. The first is methylcobalamin, which is required for the production of the amino acid methionine from homocysteine. The second is reduced tetrahydrofolate, which is required as the single-carbon donor in purine synthesis. Thus, cobalamin deficiency depletes stores of reduced tetrahydrofolate and impairs DNA synthesis because of lowered purine production. In cobalamin deficiency, other reduced folates may substitute for tetrahydrofolate (and may explain why pharmacologic doses of folic acid can partially reverse the megaloblastic blood cell changes, but not the neurologic changes, seen in pernicious anemia). However, methyltetrahydrofolate, normally the methyl donor to cobalamin, accumulates. This folate cannot be retained intracellularly because it cannot be **polyglutamated;** the addition of multiple glutamate residues leads to a charged compound that does not freely diffuse out of the cell. Therefore, there is

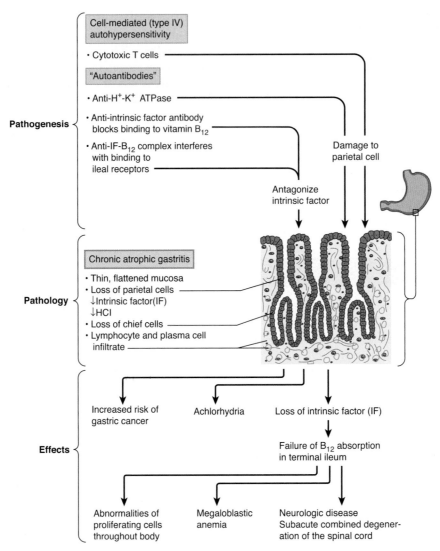

FIGURE 6–7 Pathogenesis and effects of pernicious anemia (autoimmune atrophic gastritis). (Redrawn, with permission, from Chandrasoma P, Taylor CR. *Concise Pathology*, 3rd ed. Originally published by Appleton & Lange. Copyright © 1998 by the McGraw-Hill Companies, Inc.)

relative folate deficiency in pernicious anemia as well. In addition, methionine may serve as a principal donor of methyl groups to these other "substituting" reduced folates; because methionine cannot be produced in cobalamin deficiency, this compounds the problems in purine synthesis.

The exact mechanism of the neurologic consequences of pernicious anemia, with **demyelination** (loss of the myelin sheaths around nerves), is not known. Defects in the methionine synthase pathway have been suggested but not proven experimentally. Instead, observations in cobalamin-deficient gastrectomized rats implicate an imbalance of cytokines and growth factors as a potential mediator of nerve damage. The synthesis of the cytokine **tumor necrosis factor (TNF)** is regulated by S-adenosyl-methione, a product of methionine. Deficiency of methionine may indirectly lead to neuropathy via unregulated production of TNF, a myelinolytic cytokine, among other mechanisms.

The production of succinyl-coenzyme A (CoA) is also dependent on the presence of cobalamin. It is not clear whether a decrease in the production of succinyl-CoA, which may affect fatty acid synthesis, is also involved in the demyelinating disease.

Pathology

The gastric disorders associated with pernicious anemia are dominated by the picture of **chronic atrophic gastritis** (Figure 6–7). The normally tall columnar epithelium is replaced by a very thin mucosa, and there is obvious infiltration of plasma cells and lymphocytes. Pernicious anemia also increases the risk for gastric adenocarcinoma. Thus, pathologic examination may also reveal cancer.

The peripheral blood smear picture (Figure 6–5) varies, depending on the length of time the patient has been cobalamin deficient. In early stages, the patient may have mild macrocytic anemia, and large ovoid erythrocytes (**macro-**

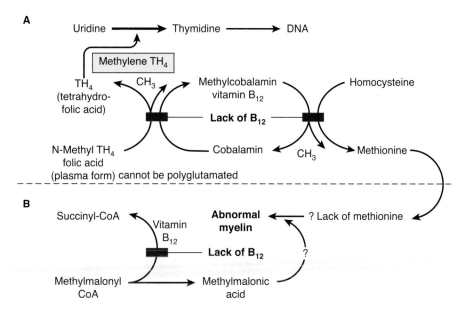

FIGURE 6–8 Role of cobalamin (vitamin B_{12}) and folic acid in nucleic acid and myelin metabolism. Lack of either cobalamin or folic acid retards DNA synthesis (**A**) and lack of cobalamin leads to loss of folic acid, which cannot be held intracellularly unless polyglutamated. Lack of cobalamin also leads to abnormal myelin synthesis, probably via a deficiency in methionine production (**B**). (Redrawn, with permission, from Chandrasoma P, Taylor CR. *Concise Pathology*, 3rd ed. Originally published by Appleton & Lange. Copyright © 1998 by the McGraw-Hill Companies, Inc.)

ovalocytes) are commonly seen. In full-blown megaloblastic anemia, however, there are abnormalities in all cell lines. The classic picture reveals significant anisocytosis and poikilocytosis of the red cell line, and there are hypersegmented neutrophils, revealing the nuclear dysgenesis from abnormal DNA synthesis (Figure 6–9). In severe cases of pernicious anemia, the red and white cell series are easily mistaken for acute leukemia because the cells look so atypical.

The bone marrow, however, is less suggestive of acute leukemia, and megaloblastic changes—nuclei that are too large and immature in cells with mature, hemoglobin-filled cytoplasm—are seen at each stage of erythrocyte development. These cells are not seen in the peripheral blood because the abnormal erythrocytes generally are destroyed in the marrow (**intramedullary hemolysis**) by unexplained processes. This compounds the anemia. Megaloblastic changes can be seen in the marrow even in the absence of obvious changes on the peripheral blood smear.

Spinal cord abnormalities consist of demyelination of the posterolateral spinal columns, called **subacute combined degeneration.** Peripheral nerves may also show demyelination. Demyelination eventually results in neuronal cell death, which is also obvious on pathologic examination. Because neurons do not divide, new neurons cannot replace the dead ones.

Laboratory findings include elevated lactate dehydrogenase (LDH) and, sometimes, indirect bilirubin consistent with the hemolysis occurring in the bone marrow. LDH is directly released from lysed red cells, and free hemoglobin is metabolized to bilirubin. Serum vitamin B_{12} levels are usually low, revealing the deficient state. Antibodies to intrinsic factor are usually detectable. Serum elevations of both methylmalonic

acid (MMA) and homocysteine together (see Figure 6–8) are highly predictive of B_{12} deficiency. The Schilling test, which assesses the oral absorption of vitamin B_{12} with and without added intrinsic factor, is no longer used, because of lack of availability of radioactively labeled vitamin B_{12}. Typically, the approach is to first measure serum B_{12} and, if equivocal, to obtain serum levels of MMA and homocysteine.

Clinical Manifestations

The clinical presentation consists of one or more symptoms related to the underlying deficiency. Anemia is the most commonly encountered abnormality and is often very severe; hemoglobin levels of 4 g/dL (less than a third of normal) can be seen. This degree of anemia is rare with other causes, such as iron deficiency. Typical symptoms are fatigue, dyspnea, or dizziness, because a decreased red cell mass equals decreased oxygen-carrying capacity of the blood. High-output congestive heart failure is relatively common, with tachycardia and signs of left ventricular failure (Chapter 10). Because oxygen demands are constant (or rise with exercise) and oxygen-carrying capacity is falling, the only way to maintain tissue oxygenation in anemia is to increase cardiac output (ie, the number of times per minute each red cell is fully oxygenated by the lungs). Eventually, however, the left ventricle fails.

However, symptoms may be mild because the anemia develops slowly as a result of the extensive liver storage of vitamin B_{12}. Patients with anemia usually adapt over time to slow changes in oxygen-carrying capacity. The same changes in 2,3-BPG that encourage oxygen delivery to the tissues from the hemoglobin in red cells in other anemias occur in vitamin B_{12} deficiency.

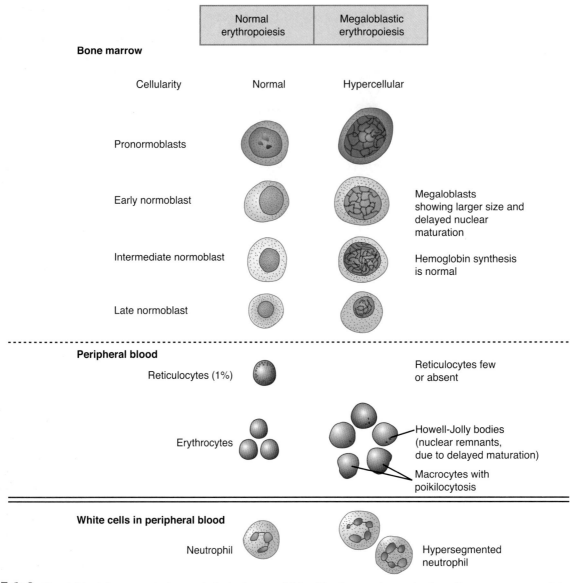

	Normal erythropoiesis	Megaloblastic erythropoiesis
Bone marrow		
Cellularity	Normal	Hypercellular
Pronormoblasts		
Early normoblast		Megaloblasts showing larger size and delayed nuclear maturation
Intermediate normoblast		Hemoglobin synthesis is normal
Late normoblast		
Peripheral blood		
Reticulocytes (1%)		Reticulocytes few or absent
Erythrocytes		Howell-Jolly bodies (nuclear remnants, due to delayed maturation) Macrocytes with poikilocytosis
White cells in peripheral blood		
Neutrophil		Hypersegmented neutrophil

FIGURE 6–9 Megaloblastic hematopoiesis: morphologic changes visible with microscopic examination of bone marrow or peripheral blood. (Redrawn, with permission, from Chandrasoma P, Taylor CR. *Concise Pathology*, 3rd ed. Originally published by Appleton & Lange. Copyright © 1998 by the McGraw-Hill Companies, Inc.)

GI symptoms are less prevalent and include malabsorption, muscle wasting (unusual), diarrhea (more common), and **glossitis** (most common). In glossitis, the normal tongue papillae are absent regardless of whether the tongue is painful, red, and "beefy" or pale and smooth.

Neurologic symptoms are least likely to improve with cobalamin replacement therapy. As with other neuropathies involving loss of myelin from large peripheral sensory nerves, numbness and tingling (**paresthesias**) occur frequently and are the most common symptoms. Demyelination and neuronal cell death in the posterolateral "long tracts" of the spinal cord interfere with delivery of positional information to the brainstem, cerebellum, and sensory cortex. Patients, therefore, complain of loss of balance and coordination. Examination reveals impaired **proprioception** (position sense) and vibration sense. True dementia may also occur when demyelination involves the brain. Importantly but somewhat unexpectedly, neurologic symptoms may occur in the absence of any changes in the peripheral blood smear suggestive of pernicious anemia.

CHECKPOINT

15. Name two crucial cofactors in DNA synthesis whose deficiency results in pernicious anemia. In what specific biochemical pathways do they participate?

16. Why neurologic defects are observed in prolonged pernicious anemia?

17. Why symptoms of pernicious anemia are usually relatively mild?

18. Are changes in the peripheral blood smear necessary for neurologic effects of vitamin B_{12} deficiency?

WHITE CELL DISORDERS

1. Malignant Disorders

The most important leukocyte abnormalities are the malignant disorders leukemia and lymphoma. They are discussed in Chapter 5.

2. Cyclic Neutropenia

Absolute neutropenia, characterized by neutrophil counts less than 1500–2000/µL (> 2 SD below the mean in normals) is a commonly encountered problem in medicine and can be due to a large number of disease entities (Table 6–5). Cyclic neutropenia, however, is rare. It is of interest because it provides insight into normal neutrophil production and function. It is characterized by a lifetime history of neutrophil counts that decrease to zero or near zero for 3–5 days at a time every 3 weeks and then rebound. Interestingly, the peripheral blood neutrophil counts and monocyte counts oscillate in opposite phases on this 3-week cycle.

Etiology

Classic, childhood-onset cyclic neutropenia results from mutations in the gene, *ELA2*, which encodes for a single enzyme, neutrophil elastase (NE). NE is found in the primary azurophilic granules of neutrophils and monocytes. There are approximately 100 cases in the literature, most of which are consistent with an autosomal dominant inheritance. However, sporadic adult cases also occur, and these are associated with neutrophil elastase mutations. There does not seem to be a racial predilection or gender bias in incidence.

Pathogenesis

The neutrophil count in blood is stable in normal individuals, reflecting the fact that there is a large storage pool of granulocytes in the marrow. The marrow reserve exceeds the circulating pool of neutrophils by 5- to 10-fold. This large pool is necessary because it takes nearly 2 weeks for the full development of a neutrophil from an early stem cell within the bone marrow, yet the average life span of a mature neutrophil in blood is less than 12 hours.

In cyclic neutropenia, the storage pool is not adequate. Daily measurements of neutrophil counts in the blood reveal striking variations in their number. Studies of neutrophil kinetics in affected patients reveal that the defect is in abnormal production, rather than abnormal disposition of neutrophils. Neutrophil production occurs in discrete waves even in normal individuals. As neutrophils differentiate from an early progenitor cell, they produce neutrophil elastase, which is thought to inhibit the differentiation of myeloblasts in a negative feedback loop. This results in an oscillatory wave with peaks and troughs of neutrophil production. As neutrophil numbers increase in the marrow, a peak is obtained where enough neutrophil elastase causes a drop in neutrophil differ-

entiation. Then, as the number of neutrophils drops again to a nadir, the production of neutrophil elastase also declines, allowing the number of neutrophils to climb once again. In cyclic neutropenia, it is hypothesized that the mutant neutrophil elastase may have an excessive inhibitory effect, causing prolonged trough periods and inadequate storage pools to maintain a normal peripheral neutrophil count. However, once they are extruded from the marrow, the neutrophils appear to have a normal life span (Figure 6–10).

The myeloid progenitor for neutrophil can also produce monocytes. Therefore, during neutrophil nadirs, the myeloid progenitor cell can preferentially differentiate to the monocyte lineage, giving the opposing oscillatory waves of neutrophils and monocytes seen in these patients (see Figure 6–11).

The waves are remarkably constant in their periodicity. Almost every patient has a cycle between 19 and 22 days, and each patient's cycle length is constant during his or her lifetime. Neutrophils and monocytes are not the only marrow elements that cycle. Platelet and reticulocyte counts also cycle with the same cycle length, but, in contrast to the blood neutrophil count, clinically significant decreases are not observed. This is presumably because the blood life spans of these elements are so much longer than the life span of neutrophils. Because multiple cell lines are seen to cycle, it is believed that neutrophil elastase mutations accelerate the process of **apoptosis** (programmed cell death) in early progenitor cells, as well, unless they are "rescued" by G-CSF.

Clinically, administration of pharmacologic doses of G-CSF (filgrastim) to affected individuals has three interesting effects that partially overcome the condition. First, although cycling continues, mean neutrophil counts increase at each point in the cycle, such that patients are rarely neutropenic. Second, cycling periodicity decreases immediately from 21 days to 14 days. Third, other cell line fluctuations change in parallel; their cycle periodicity also decreases to 14 days, suggesting that an early progenitor cell is indeed at the center of this illness. However, the fact that cycling does not disappear demonstrates that there are other abnormalities yet to be discovered. It also suggests that there may be an inherent cycling of all stem cells in normal individuals that is modulated by multiple cytokines in the marrow.

Pathology

The pathologic features of cyclic neutropenia are seen mostly in the laboratory. The peripheral blood smear appears normal except for the paucity of neutrophils—mature or immature—during the nadirs of each cycle. Individual neutrophils appear normal. The bone marrow, however, shows striking differences depending on the day of the cycle on which it is examined. During the nadir of each cycle, there are increased numbers of early myeloid precursors such as promyelocytes and myelocytes, and mature neutrophils are rare. This picture is similar to that seen in acute leukemia, but 10 days later, as circulating neutrophil counts are rising, an entirely normal-appearing marrow is typical.

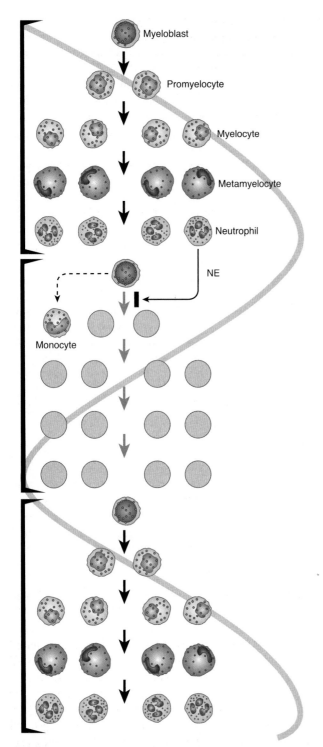

FIGURE 6–10 Feedback loop hypothesis to explain hematopoietic cycling. Neutrophil elastase (NE) is postulated to inhibit further differentiation by a myeloblast. Blue sinewave denotes neutrophil count oscillations. In this model, NE is produced by the terminally differentiating cohort of neutrophils and ultimately feeds back to inhibit further production of neutrophils, which results in loss of the inhibitory cycle—at least for a while, until production of the neutrophils resumes, followed again by the inhibitory action of NE in a cyclic manner. (Redrawn from: Horwitz MS et al. Neutrophil elastase in cyclic and severe congenital neutropenia. *Blood.* 2007 Mar 1;109(5):1817–24. Copyright American Society of Hematology.)

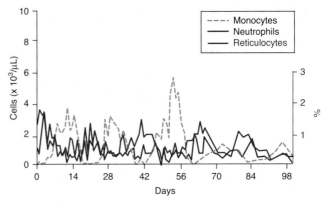

FIGURE 6–11 Regular cyclic variation of monocytes, reticulocytes, and neutrophils in a patient with cyclic neutropenia. Note that monocytes and reticulocytes tend to rise when the neutrophils fall. (Redrawn, with permission, from Dale D, Hammond WP. Cyclic neutropenia: A clinical review. Blood Rev. 1988;2:178.)

Clinical Manifestations

In general, neutropenia from any cause places patients at risk for severe bacterial infections, generally from enteric organisms, because of the alteration in host defenses in the gastrointestinal tract. This is especially true when the neutropenia is due to administration of chemotherapeutic agents, because chemotherapy also affects the lining of the GI tract. Neutrophils, with their ability to engulf bacteria and deliver toxic enzymes and oxidizing free radicals to sites of infection, normally serve as the first line of host defenses against the bacteria that inhabit the gut. Such patients are also at risk for fungal infections if the neutropenia lasts more than several days; this is because it takes longer for fungi to reproduce and invade the bloodstream. Untreated infections of either type can be rapidly fatal, particularly if the neutrophil count is less than about 250/μL.

In cyclic neutropenia, then, recurrent infections are to be expected, and deaths from infections with intestinal organisms have been reported. Each cycle is characterized by malaise and fever coincident with the time neutrophil counts are falling. Cervical lymphadenopathy is almost always present as are oral ulcers. These symptoms usually last for about 5 days and then subside until the next cycle.

When infections occur, the site is usually predictable. Skin infections, specifically small superficial pyogenic abscesses (**furunculosis**) or bacterial invasion of the dermis or epidermis (**cellulitis**), are the most common and respond to antibiotic therapy with few sequelae. The next most common infection site is usually the gums, and chronic gingivitis is evident in about half of patients. It is also the most noticeably improved problem when patients receive therapy with filgrastim. Other infections are unusual, but any neutropenic patient is at risk for infection from organisms that reside in the GI system. In the few patients who have required abdominal surgery during their neutropenia, ulcers similar to those seen in the mouth have been noted; this destruction of the normal mucosal barrier presumably eases entry of intestinal bacteria into the bloodstream. Because the period of greatest susceptibility to infection is only a few days in each cycle, most patients grow and develop normally.

CHECKPOINT

19. How long does it take for a neutrophil to develop from a stem cell in the bone marrow? Once fully mature, what is its life span?
20. At what level of neutropenia does the incidence of infection dramatically increase?
21. What are the most common sites and types of infections observed in neutropenic patients?
22. What is the probable underlying abnormality in cyclic neutropenia?

PLATELET DISORDERS

1. Drug-Associated Immune Thrombocytopenia

Etiology

Thrombocytopenia, defined as the occurrence of platelet levels below the normal laboratory range, is a commonly encountered abnormality. Although there are many causes (Table 6–7), the possibility of a drug-induced immune thrombocytopenia should always be considered.

Many drugs have been associated with this phenomenon, and the most common ones are listed in Table 6–9. In practice, the association between a given drug and thrombocytopenia is usually made clinically rather than with specific tests. Thrombocytopenia usually occurs at least 5–7 days after exposure to the drug, if given for the first time. The suspect drug is stopped and platelet counts rebound within a few days. Rechallenge with the drug, which is rarely done, almost always reproduces the thrombocytopenia.

Heparin is the most important cause of thrombocytopenia because of its frequent use in hospitalized patients; its use also carries the potential to cause a life-threatening thrombotic syndrome. The pathophysiology of the thrombocytopenia caused by heparin is also the most completely described.

Pathogenesis

Although the phenomenon of drug-induced thrombocytopenia has been known for decades to be immune in nature, the specific mechanisms have long been controversial. The association of antibodies with platelets leads to their destruction via the spleen. The spleen acts as the major "blood filter" and recognizes platelets bound to antibodies as abnormal and thus removes them. Spleen removal also occurs in autoimmune (idiopathic) thrombocytopenia, which is relatively common and difficult to distinguish clinically from drug-induced thrombocytopenia.

TABLE 6–9 Common drugs that may cause thrombocytopenia.

Abciximab	Heparin
Acetaminophen	Hydrochlorothiazide
Acetazolamide	Indinavir
Allopurinol	Interferon alfa
Amiodarone	Iodinated contrast agents
Amphotericin B	Methyldopa
Aspirin	Nonsteroidal antiinflammatory drugs
Atorvastatin	Ondansetron
Captopril	Penicillins
Carbamazepine	Pentoxifylline
Cephalosporins	Phenothiazines
Chlorothiazide	Phenytoin
Chlorthalidone	Prednisone
Cimetidine	Procainamide
Clopidrogel	Quinidine
Cocaine	Quinine
Danazol	Ranitidine
Digoxin	Rifampin
Ethanol	Sulfonamides (antibiotics and hypoglycemics)
Famotidine	
Fluconazole	Ticlopidine
Furosemide	Valproic acid
Gold salts	Vancomycin

There are various mechanisms underlying drug-induced immune thrombocytopenia. Quinine- or NSAID-induced thrombocytopenia involves the tight binding of antibody to normal platelets only in the presence of the sensitizing drug. The antibody usually targets epitopes on the glycoprotein IIb/IIIa or Ib/IX complexes, the major platelet receptors for fibrinogen and von Willebrand factor, respectively. Penicillin and cephalosporin antibiotics are believed to lead to platelet destruction via hapten-dependent antibodies. The drug acts as a hapten, a small molecule that only elicits an immunologic response when it is bound to a large carrier molecule or protein. Some drugs (gold salts, procainamide, and possibly sulfonamides) can induce autoantibodies that are capable of binding to and destroying platelets even in the absence of the sensitizing drug.

For heparin, there is clear evidence of binding to a platelet protein, platelet factor 4 (PF4). PF4 resides in the alpha granules of platelets and is released when they are activated. It binds back onto the platelet surface through a specific PF4 receptor molecule, further increasing platelet activation. It also binds with high affinity to heparin and to heparin-like glycosaminoglycan molecules present on the vascular endothelium. This non–immune-based adhesion to PF4 can lead to mild thrombocytopenia via promotion of platelet binding to fibrinogen and subsequent aggregation, known as **heparin-induced thrombocytopenia (HIT) type I**. This can happen in 30% of patients exposed to heparins without clinical sequelae. However, the combination of heparin with PF4 can also act as an antigenic stimulus that provokes the production of immunoglobulin G (IgG) directed against the combination. This immunologic response is known as **heparin-induced thrombocytopenia (HIT) type II**. These antibodies can occur in 17% of patients treated with unfractionated heparin and 8% of those treated with low-molecular-weight heparins. About 20% of these patients with heparin-PF4 antibodies will develop a serious clinical syndrome, which paradoxically involves both thrombocytopenia 5–10 days after drug exposure and a prothrombotic state via increased platelet activation.

Thrombocytopenia occurs in HIT type II after a series of steps. First, PF4 is released from platelets either by heparin itself or by other stimuli. Heparin then binds to PF4, forming an antigenic complex that results in the production of IgG antibodies that can bind directly to this compound. The new complex of IgG-heparin-PF4 binds to platelets through the platelet Fc receptor, via its IgG end. Platelets bound with this antibody complex are then destroyed by the spleen.

Despite the resulting thrombocytopenia, HIT type II leads to a prothrombotic state via the additional binding of the heparin-PF4 portion to the PF4 receptor on platelets, promoting platelet cross-linking, activation, and aggregation (Figure 6–12).

Because each end of this IgG-heparin-PF4 molecule can bind to a platelet, it is possible that platelets can become cross-linked by a single molecule. Many platelets could actually interact in this fashion, leading to further platelet aggregation and activation. Clinically, this decreases the numbers of circulating platelets, but it may also lead to creation of a thrombus at the site of activation. Thus, despite the fact that heparin is the most commonly used anticoagulant, in this case it may

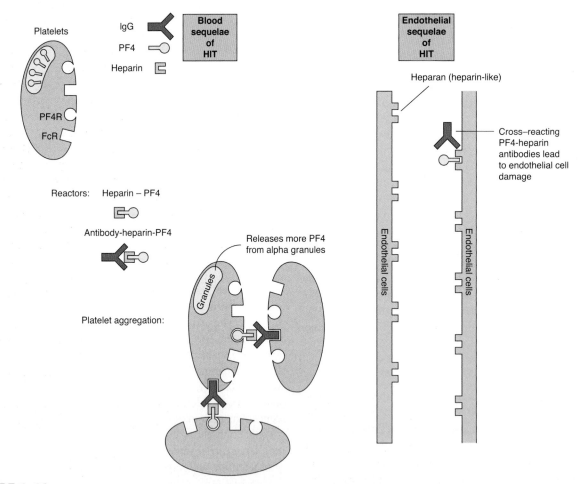

FIGURE 6–12 Pathogenesis of heparin-induced thrombocytopenia (HIT). IgG is the autoantibody against the heparin-PF4 complex. Platelets can bind to each other and become activated via either the IgG-Fc receptor interaction or the PF4-PF4 receptor interaction or both. Aggregation and thrombus formation may thus occur. Furthermore, IgG may bind to endothelial cell bound heparan-PF4 construct and cause vascular damage, which may also provoke thrombus formation.

actually provoke coagulation. Furthermore, the activation of platelets via this mechanism leads to increased amounts of circulating PF4, which can bind to more heparin and continue the cycle. The excess PF4 can also bind to the endothelial surface via the heparin-like glycosaminoglycans described earlier. It is thus possible that the antibodies to the heparin-PF4 construct could bind to the endothelial cells as well, which may lead to endothelial cell injury, further increasing the risk of local thrombosis by generating tissue factor and ultimately thrombin. Lastly, there is some evidence that macrophages may release tissue factor in response to these antibodies, further stimulating the coagulation cascade.

Pathology

The peripheral blood smear is not strikingly abnormal unless platelet counts are less than about 75,000/μL, and then it is usually abnormal only because relatively few platelets are seen. Platelet morphology, however, is usually normal, although large platelets can be seen. These large platelets are less mature and are a bone marrow compensation for a low peripheral platelet count, with platelet production from megakaryocytes being increased. Although drugs—heparin in particular—may cause platelet aggregation in vivo and in vitro, this is usually not apparent on review of the blood smear.

The bone marrow usually appears normal, although the megakaryocyte number may be relatively increased, presumably reflecting an attempt to increase the number of platelets (megakaryocyte fragments) in the circulation. In a few cases of immune-mediated thrombocytopenia, however, there may be decreased numbers of megakaryocytes. There are many hypotheses as to why this may occur, but it most likely means that the antigenic combination of drug-platelet protein is also occurring on megakaryocytes, so that they as well as the platelets in the peripheral circulation are being immunologically destroyed. This destruction would not involve the spleen, of course, but would require antibody-dependent cell killing.

In patients who develop heparin-induced thrombocytopenia and thrombosis, thrombi are seen that are relatively rich in platelets when compared with "typical" thrombi seen in other situations. They are described as "white clots." The thrombi may be either arterial or venous.

Clinical Manifestations

Despite that the platelet count in immune-mediated thrombocytopenia can be extremely low (< 10,000/μL, compared with a normal value of over 150,000/μL), significant bleeding is unusual. More often there is easy bruising with minimal trauma. With platelet counts of less than about 5000/μL, pinpoint hemorrhages (**petechiae**) may spontaneously occur in the skin or mucous membranes. These are self-limited because the plasma coagulation factors are still intact, and only a small number of aggregated platelets are needed to provide adequate phospholipid for the clotting cascade.

The relationship between the likelihood of bleeding and the platelet count is not linear. The **bleeding time** test used clinically to evaluate platelet function does not even begin to be abnormally prolonged until the platelet count is less than 90,000/μL. Spontaneous bleeding is unlikely until platelet counts are less than 20,000/μL but is still uncommon until counts are less than about 5000/μL. This assumes that patients do not have other abnormalities of hemostasis, which is not always true. For example, aspirin inhibits platelet aggregation and increases the likelihood of bleeding. When bleeding from thrombocytopenia does occur, it is most often mucosal or superficial in the skin. This is most commonly seen as a nosebleed (epistaxis), but bleeding of the gums, GI tract, or bladder mucosa may be seen.

As mentioned, however, when immune thrombocytopenia occurs as a result of heparin, paradoxical clotting may occur instead of bleeding. This may cause a very confusing picture, because the heparin may have been given therapeutically for another thrombosis; it may be difficult to determine whether the new thrombosis is an extension of the initial clot or a new one referable to the heparin. However, the occurrence of the simultaneous thrombocytopenia provides a clue.

When heparin-induced thrombocytopenia and thrombosis do occur, the clinical manifestation of the new thrombosis will depend on the site of the thrombus. Most studies of this disorder suggest that when thrombosis occurs, it is at the site of previous vascular injury or abnormality. Thus, in patients with atherosclerotic vascular disease, arterial thromboses are much more common than venous clots. Patients have the rapid onset of severe pain, usually in an extremity, with a cool, pale limb. Pulses are absent. This can be life threatening or at least extremity threatening because oxygen flow to the affected area is cut off, and emergency clot removal or vascular bypass surgery may be necessary. Venous clots also occur in a manner similar to typical venous clots (see later discussion). In addition to stopping heparin, patients with type II HIT need anticoagulation to prevent and treat thrombosis formation. Direct thrombin inhibitors, (argatroban, lepirudin, or bivalirudin) provide a direct means of blocking the effects of thrombin, a primary mediator of the coagulation cascade.

CHECKPOINT

23. What is the most common category of cause of thrombocytopenia?
24. Name the antibodies to which platelet protein are implicated in the pathogenesis of heparin-induced thrombocytopenia?
25. By what mechanism can heparin-induced thrombocytopenia actually increase clot formation?
26. Why is major bleeding unusual in drug-induced thrombocytopenia?

COAGULATION DISORDERS

1. Inherited Hypercoagulable States

Etiology

The formation of blood clots in otherwise normal vessels is distinctly abnormal because the coagulation system in mammalian species is both positively and negatively balanced by so many factors. Nonetheless, there are a number of diseases that result in abnormal clotting (**thrombosis**). Abnormal clotting states may be either primary, in that the abnormalities are due to genetic predispositions involving the coagulation factors themselves, or secondary (ie, acquired) because of changes in coagulation factors, blood vessels, or blood flow.

As first noted by the pathologist Virchow more than 150 years ago, there are three possible contributors to formation of an abnormal clot (thrombus): decreased blood flow, vessel injury or inflammation, and changes in the intrinsic properties of the blood. Persistent physiologic changes in any of these three factors (Virchow's triad) are referred to as the "hypercoagulable states."

The primary, or inherited, hypercoagulable states are all autosomal dominant genetic defects. This means that carriers (heterozygotes) are affected. Except for hyperprothrombinemia, all lead to only moderate (50%) decreases in the levels of the relevant factors. Despite the relatively modest fall, affected individuals are predisposed to abnormal thrombosis. These disorders are relatively rare in the general population, but they do account for a significant percentage of young patients who come to medical attention with thromboses. The specific states to be discussed are activated protein C resistance (the most commonly encountered abnormality), protein C deficiency, protein S deficiency, antithrombin deficiency, and the prothrombin 20210 AG abnormality. Hyperhomocystinemia, an inborn error of metabolism, is also an inherited hypercoagulable state, but because it does not involve the coagulation cascade, it is not further discussed here.

Pathogenesis

In the coagulation cascade, activated factor V (Va) plays a pivotal role (Figure 6–13). It is required for significant activation of factor X (to Xa), which is the central control factor involved in the entire cascade. Factor Va thus makes an excellent negative control point, so that once clot formation has begun, it does not go on unchecked.

Protein C is the major inhibitor of factor Va. Although it is an anticoagulation factor, its production is contingent on vitamin K-dependent γ-carboxylation, just like the coagulation factors II, VII, IX, and X. Protein C, when activated by the presence of clotting that generates thrombin, cleaves factor Va into an inactive form, and activation of factor X is thus slowed. By itself, however, protein C only weakly influences factor Va; its negative effect on factor Va is enhanced by a protein cofactor, protein S.

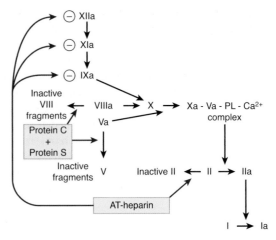

FIGURE 6–13 Central role of factor V in the control of the coagulation cascade. The action of each of the negative control factors: protein S, protein C, and antithrombin, is shown in color.

Factor V does not provide the only negative control point, however. Protein C also inhibits activated factor VIIIa. Factors II, IX, X, XI, and XII (the serine proteases) are inhibited by a different molecule, antithrombin (AT). The action of AT itself is also regulated and is highly dependent on the binding of an accelerator, heparin, or similar molecules that are present in abundance along the endothelial cells that line the vasculature. Evidence suggests that AT may also inhibit the factor VII–tissue factor complex.

The fact that deficiencies of protein S, protein C, and antithrombin activity cause clinically significant thrombosis demonstrates an important concept: It is the lack of adequate anticoagulant activity rather than the overproduction of procoagulant activity that characterizes most of the hypercoagulable states.

A. Activated Protein C Resistance—Activated protein C resistance is the most common inherited hypercoagulable state, with as many as 2–5% of the general population heterozygous for the abnormality. Up to 25% of patients who have venous thrombosis without an inciting event are found to have activated protein C resistance in a large patient series. Most of the cases are due to a single DNA base pair mutation in the factor V gene, where guanine (G) is replaced by adenine (A). This single base change leads to substitution of the amino acid glutamine for arginine at position 506, and the altered factor V is referred to as "factor V Leiden," named for the town in the Netherlands where it was discovered. This amino acid change alters the three-dimensional conformation of the cleavage site within factor Va, where activated protein C normally binds to inactivate it. Thus, factor Va molecules can continue to enhance factor Xa's conversion of prothrombin to thrombin (factor IIa), and coagulation is not inhibited.

B. Protein C Deficiency—Protein C deficiency is common; up to 1 of every 200 individuals in the population is a heterozygote. Yet thrombosis is uncommon among these individuals. The families that are thrombosis prone are thought to carry additional genetic factors, in addition to protein C deficiency, that increase their risk for thrombosis.

As noted earlier, protein C inactivates factors Va and VIIIa but requires protein S for its own action. Protein C is also dependent on the presence of platelet phospholipid and calcium. In protein C deficiency, there is less inhibition of the prothrombinase complex, leading to relatively unrestricted clot formation. Normally, some of the thrombin generated in the cascade binds to an endothelial cell protein, thrombomodulin, and this complex activates protein C in the first place. This "negative feedback loop" is thus lost in protein C deficiency.

Protein C deficiency is not all one disease, however, unlike the factor V Leiden abnormality discussed previously. Type I deficiency refers to individuals with decreased levels of protein C. Type II deficiency denotes cases with normal protein C levels but low protein C activity.

C. Protein S Deficiency—Protein S deficiency is also an uncommon heterogeneous disorder. Type I protein S deficiency refers to cases with low free and total protein S levels. Type II deficiency, which is the least encountered, refers to an abnormal functioning protein S. Type III deficiency refers to only low levels of free protein S. In the coagulation cascade, when factors Va and Xa are complexed together, the inactivation site on factor Va is "hidden" from protein C. Protein S, not a protease itself, exposes this site so that protein C can cleave Va. Because protein S is so crucial, deficiency of protein S also leads to the unregulated procoagulant action of factor Xa.

D. Antithrombin Deficiency—Antithrombin (AT) deficiency is less common than any of the previously discussed disorders, with approximately 1 in 2000 cases in the general population. AT binds to and inhibits not just thrombin (whence its name) but also the activated forms of factors IX, X, XI, and XII and perhaps the factor VII–tissue factor complex as well. Unlike protein C's proteolytic cleavage of factor Va, AT binds to each factor, directly blocking their activity; it is not an enzyme. This action is accelerated—up to 2000 times—in a reversible manner by the anticoagulant molecule heparin, which binds to AT via its pentasaccharide sequence. The anticoagulant fondaparinux is a synthetic version of this five-saccharide sequence, and thus, it can also bind to AT. In AT deficiency, then, multiple coagulation steps are unbalanced, and the coagulation cascade may proceed unrestrained. More than 100 different AT mutations have been reported. Type I molecular defects involve a parallel decrease in antigen and activity, while Type II defects involve a dysfunctional molecule that has decreased activity, but normal or near-normal antigen levels.

E. Hyperprothrombinemia—A mutation in the untranslated region of the prothrombin gene (a single base pair mutation, called 20210 AG) is associated with elevated plasma prothrombin levels and an increased risk of thrombosis. Presum-ably, this leads to excess thrombin generation when the prothrombinase complex is activated. This is probably the second most common hereditary hypercoagulable state after factor V Leiden. It is the first hereditary thrombophilia associated with overproduction of procoagulant factors.

Pathology

The pathologic features of thrombi in hypercoagulable states are indistinguishable from those of genetically normal individuals on a gross anatomic or microscopic basis, except that there is a greater likelihood in hypercoagulable states of having a clot in unusual sites. (See Clinical Manifestations section.)

Most of the pathologic features of the hereditary hypercoagulable states consist of laboratory abnormalities, and findings depend on which laboratory tests are requested. In the evaluation of patients suspected of having a hereditary hypercoagulable state, there are two basic types of laboratory abnormalities. The first type is quantitative: Specific immunologic assays can define the relative amount of protein C, protein S, antithrombin, or fibrinogen present in a given patient's serum, but they do not evaluate the function of any of these molecules. The second type is qualitative: The assays for protein C or protein S activity (rather than amount) measure the ability (or inability) of the patient's protein C or S to prolong a clotting time in vitro. Activated protein C resistance can be evaluated with a different clotting assay, but generally the presence of the specific mutation in factor V Leiden is assessed by the polymerase chain reaction, because the full sequence of the molecule is known. The polymerase chain reaction is also used for detecting the 20210 AG prothrombin abnormality. Prothrombin levels can also be measured and are consistently in the highest quartile of prothrombin levels found.

Clinical Manifestations

Most thromboembolic events encountered in clinical practice are secondary, not primary. Patients have blood clots usually in the deep veins of the legs for two reasons: (1) because of sluggish blood flow (in high-capacity, low-flow veins) compared with other sites, particularly when inactive (bedridden after surgery or as a result of illness); and (2) because the extremities are more likely to sustain injury than the trunk. Trauma causes blood vessel compression or injury; thus, two elements of Virchow's triad are more readily observed in the legs than elsewhere.

These venous clots in the legs (commonly referred to as deep venous thromboses [DVTs]) usually present with pain, swelling, and redness below the level of the thrombus, with normal arterial pulses and distal extremity perfusion. Because blood return to the central circulation is blocked in these high-capacity vessels, superficial collateral veins just under the skin may be prominent and engorged. The swelling is mechanical, because normal arterial blood flow continues to the extremity while venous return is compromised, leading to engorgement. Pain occurs primarily as a result of the swelling alone but can also occur from lactic acid buildup in the muscles of the legs. This happens when the pressure in the legs increases to the point that it compromises arterial blood flow and adequate oxygen delivery to those muscles.

Pulmonary emboli, the major source of morbidity and mortality after DVT of the lower extremity, typically present with acute-onset shortness of breath, hypoxemia, and a history suggesting an initial DVT that has now broken off and migrated through the right side of the heart to the pulmonary arterial system. The presence of the clot blocks blood flow from the heart to a portion of lung; thus, the blood returning from the lung to the heart is not fully oxygenated. The degree of hypoxemia depends on how much of the blood flow is blocked and whether the patient has any underlying lung disease.

The clinical presentations of all of the hypercoagulable states are similar, but there are some interesting differences. DVTs tend to occur (whether there is a hypercoagulable state or not) in patients with a history of trauma, pregnancy, oral contraceptive use, or immobility but rarely in adolescents or young adults. The inherited hypercoagulable states are suspected in patients who present with a thromboembolic event, usually because they are young or have recurrent clots. Events that occur without any specific risks, of course, are particularly suspect. Because of the dominant pattern of inheritance, suspicion is aroused when other family members have had clotting problems, and this underscores the importance of taking a family history.

Despite the distinct coagulation abnormalities, most thromboses still occur in usual sites (ie, the deep veins of the legs with or without pulmonary embolism). Other unusual sites, however, are much more likely than in patients without underlying coagulation disorders, such as the sagittal sinus of the skull or the mesenteric veins in the abdomen. The propensity for clotting notwithstanding, arterial thromboses are extremely rare.

Interestingly, not all patients—probably not even a majority—with an inherited hypercoagulable state develop symptomatic thromboses; this is particularly true for heterozygotes. Each disorder is slightly different, presumably because of the redundancy of the factors in the coagulation cascade, and the penetrance of each state varies in individual patients because of factors we do not yet understand. For this reason, many patients come to medical attention with a clot in a "usual" spot with a "typical" risk factor: sustaining an injury, having an extremity immobilized, having surgery, or being pregnant.

Homozygous protein C or protein S deficiencies have the highest likelihood of causing illness. Both conditions usually result in thrombosis, which is fatal in early life (neonatal purpura fulminans), although some patients may not present until their teens even with these profound defects. Heterozygotes for protein C deficiency are actually unlikely to develop a thrombosis over their lifetimes, although they are about six times more likely to do so than members of the general population. A similar propensity is true for the heterozygous protein S state.

Antithrombin deficiency is another significant defect in terms of the likelihood of developing thrombosis. These patients have a lifetime 10-fold increased risk for thrombosis.

The situation is complex in the case of activated protein C resistance. Proteins C and S can still cleave factor VIIIa and the factor V abnormality is a relative rather than an absolute insensitivity to activated protein C. There is still negative control of the clotting cascade at the factor X step by tissue factor pathway inhibitor (TFPI) as well.

Heterozygotes for activated protein C resistance probably represent more than one third of all patients with familial thromboses. An individual's risk of developing a clot, however, is lower than with protein S or protein C deficiency. Heterozygosity for factor V Leiden results in a lifelong 5-fold increased risk for venous thrombosis.

Even homozygous factor V Leiden does not inevitably cause thrombosis. Families in which homozygous females have had repeated pregnancies without difficulty have been carefully described. This is somewhat surprising because pregnancy, a hypercoagulable state itself, leads to decreases in protein S concentration, which would be expected to amplify the resistance to protein C. Nevertheless, case-control studies suggest at least a 30-fold increased risk of thrombosis versus the general population for homozygotes for factor V Leiden.

Persons with the prothrombin 20210 AG mutation are nearly all heterozygotes, with about a threefold higher risk of thrombosis than the general population.

CHECKPOINT

27. What constitutes Virchow's triad of factors predisposing to formation of intravascular clots?
28. Deficiencies in what proteins can result in clinically significant thromboses?
29. What is the basis for activated protein C resistance?

CASE STUDIES

Eva M. Aagaard, MD, & Yeong Kwok, MD

(See Chapter 25, p. 681 for Answers)

CASE 24

A 65-year-old previously well man presents to the clinic with complaints of fatigue of 3-months' duration. Questioning reveals diffuse weakness and feeling winded when walking uphill or climbing more than one flight of stairs. All of the symptoms have slowly worsened over time. There are no other complaints, and the review of systems is otherwise negative. The patient has no significant medical history, social history, or family history. On physical examination, he appears somewhat pale, with normal vital signs. The physical examination is unremarkable except for his rectal examination, which reveals brown, guaiac-positive stool (suggests the presence of blood in the stool). A blood test reveals anemia.

Questions

A. What is the most likely form of anemia in this man? What is the probable underlying cause?

B. What is the mechanism by which this disorder results in anemia?

C. What might one expect to see in the peripheral blood smear?

D. What other tests might be ordered to confirm the diagnosis?

E. What is the pathophysiologic mechanism of this patient's fatigue, weakness, and shortness of breath? Why is he pale?

CASE 25

A 58-year-old black woman presents to the emergency department with complaints of progressive fatigue and weakness for the past 6 months. She is short of breath after walking several blocks. On review of systems, she mentions mild diarrhea. She has noted intermittent numbness and tingling of her lower extremities and a loss of balance while walking. She denies other neurologic or cardiac symptoms and has no history of black or bloody stools or other blood loss. On physical examination she is tachycardiac to 110 bpm; other vital signs are within normal limits. Head and neck examination is notable for pale conjunctivas and a beefy red tongue with loss of papillae. Cardiac examination shows a rapid regular rhythm with a grade 2/6 systolic murmur at the left sternal border. Lung, abdominal, and rectal examination findings are normal. Neurologic examination reveals decreased sensation to light touch and vibration in the lower extremities. The hematology consultant on call is asked to see this patient because of a low hematocrit level.

Questions

A. What vitamin deficiency is the probable cause of this woman's anemia? How does this result in anemia?

B. What might one expect the peripheral blood smear to look like? What other blood tests may be ordered, and what results are anticipated? What test might differentiate the various causes of this vitamin deficiency?

C. Workup reveals pernicious anemia. What is the pathogenesis of this disease? What is the evidence to support an autoimmune origin?

D. What is the pathophysiologic mechanism of this woman's symptoms of tachycardia, paresthesias, and impaired proprioception?

CASE 26

A 6-year-old boy presents to the pediatric emergency department. His mother states that he has had 3 days of general malaise and fevers to 38.5 °C. He has no other localizing symptoms. Medical history is remarkable for multiple febrile illnesses. His mother says, "It seems like he gets sick every month." Physical examination is notable for cervical lymphadenopathy and oral ulcers. Blood tests reveal a neutrophil count of 200/μL. The patient is admitted to the hospital. Blood, urine, and cerebrospinal fluid cultures are negative, and over 48 hours, his neutrophil counts return to normal. He is then discharged.

Questions

A. What is the likely pathogenesis of cyclic neutropenia? What evidence supports this theory?

B. What aspects of this case presentation support the diagnosis of cyclic neutropenia? What is the expected clinical course?

C. Assuming that the diagnosis of cyclic neutropenia is correct, what would one expect the peripheral blood smear to look like? What would the bone marrow examination results be at this second admission? What would they be in 2 weeks?

CASE 27

A 36-year-old man was admitted to hospital after sustaining multiple fractures to the lower extremities by jumping from a three-story building in a suicide attempt. His fractures required surgical repair. He has no significant medical history. Current medications include morphine for pain and subcutaneous heparin for prophylaxis against deep venous thrombosis. Consultation with a hematologist is requested because of a dropping platelet count. On physical examination, the patient has multiple bruises, and his lower extremities are casted bilaterally. Examination is otherwise normal. Laboratory tests from the last several days reveal a platelet count that has dropped from 170,000/μL on admission to 30,000/μL 5 days later.

Questions

A. What is the most likely cause of this man's thrombocytopenia?

B. By what mechanisms does heparin sometimes cause thrombocytopenia?

C. What are the possible clinical consequences of this patient's thrombocytopenia?

CASE 28

A 23-year-old woman presents to the emergency department with a chief complaint of acute onset of shortness of breath. It is associated with right-sided chest pain, which increases with inspiration. She denies fever, chills, cough, or other respiratory symptoms. She has had no lower extremity swelling. She has not been ill, bedridden, or immobile for prolonged periods. Her medical history is notable for an episode about 2 years ago of deep venous thrombosis in the right lower extremity while taking oral contraceptives. She has been otherwise healthy and is currently taking no medications. The family history is notable for a father who died of a pulmonary embolism. On physical examination she appears anxious and in mild respiratory distress. She is tachycardiac to 110 bpm, with a respiratory rate of 20/min. She has no fever, and blood pressure is stable. The remainder of the physical examination is normal. Chest x-ray film is normal. Ventilation-perfusion scan reveals a high probability of pulmonary embolus. Given her history of deep vein thrombosis, a hypercoagulable state is suspected.

Questions

A. What constitutes Virchow's triad of predisposing factors for venous thrombosis? Which components of the triad may be present in this patient?

B. What are some causes of inherited hypercoagulable states specifically associated with the coagulation cascade? How do they result in hypercoagulability?

C. How might this woman be evaluated for the presence of an inherited hypercoagulable state?

REFERENCES
General Hematology

Beutler E et al. *Williams Hematology,* 7th ed. McGraw-Hill, 2006.

Colman RW et al. *Hemostasis and Thrombosis: Basic Principles and Clinical Practice,* 4th ed. Lippincott Williams & Wilkins, 2000.

Hoffman R et al. *Hematology: Basic Principles and Practice,* 4th ed. Churchill Livingstone, 2004.

Iron-Deficiency Anemia

Beutler E et al. Iron deficiency and overload. Hematol Am Soc Hematol Educ Program. 2003:40–61. [PMID: 14633776]

Brugnara C. Iron deficiency and erythropoiesis: New diagnostic approaches. Clin Chem. 2003 Oct;49(10):1573–8. [PMID: 14500582]

Cook JD et al: The quantitative assessment of body iron. Blood 2003;101(9):3359. [PMID: 12521995]

Ganz T: Hepcidin and its role in regulating systemic iron metabolism. Hematol Am Soc Hematol Educ Program. 2006:29–35, 507. [PMID: 17124036]

Wish JB. Assessing iron status: beyond serum ferritin and transferrin saturation. Clin J Am Soc Nephrol. 2006 Sep;1(Suppl 1):S4–8. [PMID: 17699374]

Pernicious Anemia

Andrès E et al. Vitamin B_{12} (cobalamin) deficiency in elderly patients. CMAJ 2004 Aug 3;171(3):251–9. [PMID: 15289425]

Carmel R et al. Update on cobalamin, folate, and homocysteine. Hematol Am Soc Hematol Educ Program. 2003:62–81. [PMID: 14633777]

Hvas AM et al. Diagnosis and treatment of vitamin B_{12} deficiency— An update. Haematologica. 2006 Nov;91(11):1506–12. [PMID: 17043022]

Solomon LR. Disorders of cobalamin (vitamin B_{12}) metabolism: Emerging concepts in pathophysiology, diagnosis and treatment. Blood Rev. 2007 May;21(3):113–30. [PMID: 16814909]

Cyclic Neutropenia

Berliner N. Lessons from congenital neutropenia: 50 years of progress in understanding myelopoiesis. Blood. 2008 Jun 15;111(12):5427–32. [PMID: 18544696]

Dale DC et al. Cyclic neutropenia. Semin Hematol. 2002 Apr;39(2):89–94. [PMID: 11957190]

Grenda DS et al. Mutations of the *ELA2* gene found in patients with severe congenital neutropenia induce the unfolded protein response and cellular apoptosis. Blood. 2007 Dec 15;110(13): 4179–87. [PMID: 17761833]

Horwitz MS et al. Neutrophil elastase in cyclic and severe congenital neutropenia. Blood. 2007 Mar 1;109(5):1817–24. [PMID: 17053055]

Drug-Induced Thrombocytopenia

Aster RH et al. Drug-induced immune thrombocytopenia. N Engl J Med. 2007 Aug 9;357(6):580–7. [PMID: 17687133]

Baldwin ZK et al. Contemporary standards for the diagnosis and treatment of heparin-induced thrombocytopenia (HIT). Surgery. 2008 Mar;143(3):305–12. [PMID: 18291250]

Davoren A et al. Heparin-induced thrombocytopenia and thrombosis. Am J Hematol. 2006 Jan;81(1):36–44. [PMID: 16369980]

Kravitz MS et al. Thrombocytopenic conditions–autoimmunity and hypercoagulability: Commonalities and differences in ITP, TTP, HIT, and APS. Am J Hematol. 2005 Nov;80(3):232–42. [PMID: 16247748]

Menajovsky LB. Heparin-induced thrombocytopenia: Clinical manifestations and management strategies. Am J Med. 2005 Aug;118(Suppl 8A):21S–30S. [PMID: 16125511]

Hypercoagulable States

Abildgaard U. Antithrombin—Early prophecies and present challenges. Thromb Haemost. 2007 Jul;98(1):97–104. [PMID: 17597998]

Dahlbäck B. Advances in understanding pathogenic mechanisms of thrombophilic disorders. Blood. 2008 Jul 1;112(1):19–27. [PMID: 18574041]

Segers K et al. Coagulation factor V and thrombophilia: Background and mechanisms. Thromb Haemost. 2007 Sep;98(3):530–42. [PMID: 17849041]

Nervous System Disorders

7

Catherine Lomen-Hoerth, MD, PhD, & Robert O. Messing, MD

The major functions of the nervous system are to detect, analyze, and transmit information. Information is gathered by sensory systems, integrated by the brain, and used to generate signals to motor and autonomic pathways for control of movement and of visceral and endocrine functions. These actions are controlled by neurons, which are interconnected to form signaling networks that comprise motor and sensory systems. In addition to neurons, the nervous system contains neuroglial cells that serve a variety of immunologic and support functions and modulate the activity of neurons. Understanding the pathophysiology of nervous system disease requires knowledge of neural and glial cell biology and the anatomy of neural networks. The first part of this chapter reviews several basic aspects of histology, cellular physiology, and anatomy of the nervous system.

Understanding the causes of neurologic diseases requires knowledge of molecular and biochemical mechanisms. Discoveries in the fields of molecular biology and genetics have made available important information about the mechanisms of several disease states. Several neurologic disorders in which some of the molecular mechanisms of pathogenesis are known are discussed later in this chapter including motor neuron disease, Parkinson's disease, myasthenia gravis, epilepsy, Alzheimer's disease, and stroke. Exciting advances in our understanding and overlap of these diseases are leading to new therapeutic targets and the hope of better treating these devastating diseases.

NORMAL STRUCTURE & FUNCTION OF THE NERVOUS SYSTEM

HISTOLOGY & CELL BIOLOGY

Neurons

The major function of neurons is to receive, integrate, and transmit information to other cells. Neurons consist of three parts: **dendrites,** which are elongated processes that receive information from the environment or from other neurons; the **cell body,** which contains the nucleus; and the **axon,** which may be up to 1 m long and conducts impulses to muscles, glands, or other neurons (Figure 7–1). Most neurons are multipolar, containing one axon and several dendrites. Bipolar neurons have one dendrite and one axon and are found in the cochlear and vestibular ganglia, retina, and olfactory mucosa. Spinal sensory ganglia contain pseudounipolar neurons that have a single process that emanates from the cell body and divides into two branches, one extending to the spinal cord and the other extending to the periphery. Axons and dendrites usually branch extensively at their ends. Dendritic branching can be very complex, with the result that a single neuron may receive thousands of inputs. Axon branching allows several target cells to simultaneously receive a message from one neuron. Each branch of the axon terminates on the next cell at a **synapse,** which is a structure specialized for information transfer from the axon to muscle, to glands, or to another neuron. Synapses between neurons most often occur between axons and dendrites but may occur between an axon and a cell body, between two axons, or between two dendrites.

Signals are propagated electrically along axons. Like other cells, neurons maintain cell size and osmolarity primarily through the action of Na^+-K^+ ATPase, which actively pumps Na^+ out of cells in exchange for K^+. This results in the formation of concentration gradients for Na^+ and K^+ across the cell membrane. The membrane is practically impermeable to Na^+, but the presence of K^+ leak channels permits the flow of K^+ out of cells. This produces a difference in electrical charge across the membrane that counters transport of K^+ from the cell. The flow of ions continues until the opposing electrical

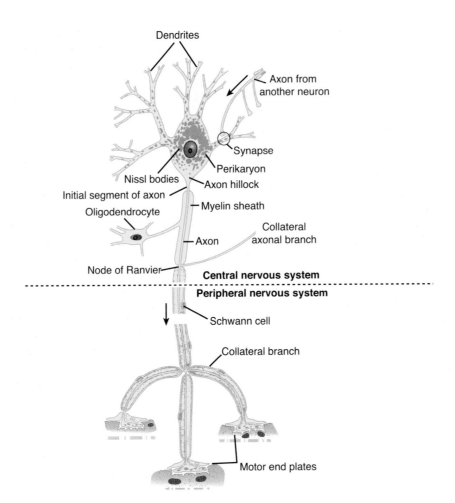

FIGURE 7–1   Schematic drawing of a Nissl-stained motor neuron. The myelin sheath is produced by oligodendrocytes in the central nervous system and by Schwann cells in the peripheral nervous system. Note the three motor end plates, which transmit the nerve impulse to striated skeletal muscle fibers. (Redrawn, with permission, from Junqueira LC, Carneiro J: *Basic Histology*, 10th ed. McGraw-Hill, 2003.)

force reaches a value that balances the diffusional force and the membrane reaches the **equilibrium potential** for K$^+$ (E$_K$). E$_K$ is calculated by the Nernst equation:

$$E_K = 2.3 \frac{RT}{F} \log \frac{[K^+]_o}{[K^+]_i}$$

where

R = gas constant (2 kcal mol^{-1} °K^{-1})

T = absolute temperature (°K)

F = Faraday's constant (2.3 × 10^4 kcal V^{-1} mol^{-1})

[K$^+$]$_o$ = concentration of K$^+$ outside the cell

[K$^+$]$_i$ = concentration of K$^+$ inside the cell

In most neurons, the resting membrane potential (E$_m$) is 50–100 mV and lies close to E$_K$ since the leak of K$^+$ is the major determinant of the charge difference across the membrane.

The membrane potential may be altered by increasing the permeability of the membrane to another ion, which drives the resting membrane potential toward the equilibrium potential for that ion. Neurons are highly specialized to use rapid changes

in membrane potential to generate electrical signals. This is accomplished by **ligand-gated** and **voltage-gated ion channels** that allow the passage of Na$^+$, K$^+$, Ca^{2+}, or Cl$^-$ ions in response to electrical or chemical stimuli. These channels are composed of protein complexes embedded in the lipid membrane to form aqueous pores to the inside of the cell. In general, channels are selective for a particular species of ion. An array of charged amino acids within voltage-dependent channels detects changes in voltage and induces a conformational change in the channel to alter ion permeability. Binding sites for **neurotransmitters** such as glutamate, γ-aminobutyric acid (GABA), glycine, and acetylcholine exist on ligand-gated channels and, when occupied, induce a conformational change to open the channel.

Electrical signals are propagated in neurons because a voltage change across the membrane in one part of a neuron is propagated to other parts. Passive spread of a voltage disturbance weakens with increasing distance from the source unless energy-dependent processes amplify the signal. Passive spread of electrical signals works well over short distances and is a major mechanism of signal propagation in dendrites. However, long-distance communication down axons to nerve terminals requires amplification. This is accomplished through the generation of self-propagating waves of excitation known as **action potentials.**

An action potential arises primarily from voltage-dependent changes in membrane permeability to Na^+ and K^+ (Figure 7–2). If a depolarizing stimulus raises the membrane potential to about –45 mV, voltage-gated Na^+ channels open, allowing influx of Na^+ and further depolarization toward E_{Na} (± 50 mV). Nearby areas of membrane are depolarized to the threshold for Na^+ channel activation, propagating a wave of depolarization from the initial site. The resting potential is restored quickly by a combination of events. First, Na^+ channels close rapidly and remain in an inactive state until the membrane potential returns to negative levels for several milliseconds. Voltage-dependent K^+ channels open as the membrane potential peaks, speeding the efflux of K^+ from cells and driving the membrane potential back to E_K. K^+ channels are also inactivated, but more slowly than Na^+ channels, and this may transiently hyperpolarize cells. Plasma membrane ion exchangers and ion pumps then counteract the ion fluxes and eventually restore the resting state.

Neurons transmit signals chemically to other cells at synapses (Figure 7–3). Presynaptic and postsynaptic cells are electrically isolated from each other and separated by a narrow synaptic cleft. Signaling across the cleft occurs through the release of neurotransmitters from the terminal of the presynaptic neuron. Most neurotransmitters are stored in membrane-bound synaptic vesicles and are released into the synaptic cleft by Ca^{2+}-dependent exocytosis. Depolarization of the nerve terminal opens voltage-gated Ca^{2+} channels, stimulating Ca^{2+} influx and neurotransmitter release. Neurotransmitters diffuse across the cleft and bind to receptors on ligand-gated ion channels concentrated at the postsynaptic membrane. This produces local permeability changes, altering the membrane potential of the postsynaptic cell. If the response is depolarizing, an action potential may be generated if there are enough voltage-gated Na^+ channels nearby and the membrane potential has been raised to the threshold for their activation. Receptor-gated ion channels are highly selective for a particular neurotransmitter and for the type of ions they pass, which determines whether they generate excitatory or inhibitory responses. In general, **excitatory neurotransmitters,** such as glutamate, open cation channels that allow influx of Na^+ or Ca^{2+} and generate a depolarizing **excitatory postsynaptic potential. Inhibitory neurotransmitters** such as GABA and glycine open Cl^- channels and generate an **inhibitory postsynaptic potential,** keeping the postsynaptic membrane near E_{Cl} (= –70 mV). Termination of

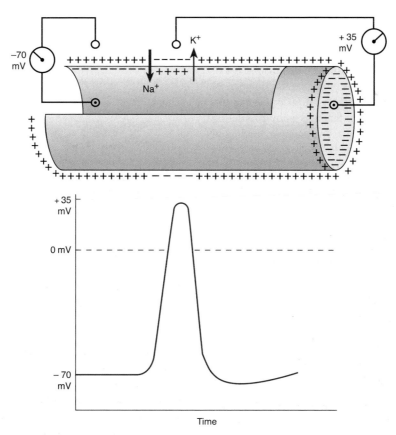

FIGURE 7–2 Conduction of the nerve impulse through an unmyelinated nerve fiber. In the resting axon, there is a difference of 70 mV between the interior of the axon and the outer surface of its membrane (resting potential). During the impulse passage, more Na^+ (thick arrow) passes into the axon interior than the amount of K^+ (thin arrow) that migrates in the opposite direction. In consequence, the membrane polarity changes (the membrane becomes relatively positive on its inner surface), and the resting potential is replaced by an action potential (+35 mV here). (Redrawn, with permission, from Junqueira LC, Carneiro J. *Basic Histology,* 10th ed. McGraw-Hill, 2003.)

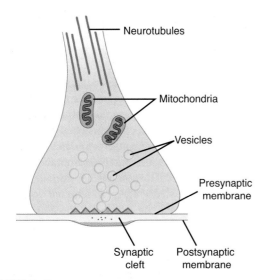

FIGURE 7–3 Schematic drawing of a synaptic terminal. Vesicles pass through the presynaptic membrane and release a transmitter substance into the synaptic cleft. (Redrawn, with permission, from Waxman SG. *Clinical Neuroanatomy*, 25th ed. McGraw-Hill, 2003.)

the signal is achieved by removal of the neurotransmitter from the synaptic cleft. Acetylcholine is hydrolyzed by acetylcholinesterase at the postsynaptic membrane. Other neurotransmitters such as glutamate are removed by specific membrane transporters on nerve terminals or glial cells.

Not all neurotransmitter receptors are ion channels. Many receptors are coupled to cellular enzymes that regulate levels of **intracellular second messengers** to modulate the function of ion channels and many other cell proteins. A major mechanism by which messengers regulate ion channels is by promoting **phosphorylation** of channel subunits. For example, binding of the neurotransmitter norepinephrine to β-adrenergic receptors activates the enzyme **adenylyl cyclase** and stimulates the production of cyclic adenosine monophosphate (**cAMP**). The cAMP, in turn, activates a cAMP-dependent protein kinase that can phosphorylate voltage-gated calcium channels. In many cases, this increases the duration of time the channel remains open once it is activated, resulting in increased Ca^{2+} influx through the channel. Other neurotransmitter receptors, such as $α_1$-adrenergic, muscarinic cholinergic, or metabotropic glutamate receptors, are coupled to the enzyme **phospholipase C,** which catalyzes the hydrolysis of the membrane lipid phosphatidylinositol-4,5-bisphosphate. Binding of neurotransmitter to the receptor activates phospholipase C to produce two second messengers: **1,2-diacylglycerol** and **inositol-1,4,5-trisphosphate.** Diacylglycerol activates several enzymes of the protein kinase C family, some of which phosphorylate ion channels and either enhance or suppress their function. Inositol-1,4,5-trisphosphate binds an intracellular receptor that is itself a calcium ionophore, allowing release of calcium from intracellular stores into the cytosol. This calcium signal activates several calcium-dependent enzymes, including phosphatases and kinases that can alter the phosphorylation state and function of several ion channels and other cell proteins.

Astrocytes

Astrocytes serve a variety of metabolic, immunologic, structural, and nutritional support functions required for normal function of neurons. They possess numerous processes that radiate from the cell body, surrounding blood vessels and covering the surfaces of the brain and spinal cord (Figure 7–4). Astrocytes express voltage- and ligand-gated ion channels and regulate K^+ and Ca^{2+} concentrations within the interstitial space. Many synapses are invested with astrocytic processes, and this allows astrocytes to modulate neurotransmission by regulating extracellular concentrations of these cations. Astrocytes provide structural and trophic support for neurons through the production of extracellular matrix molecules such as laminin and through release of growth factors such as nerve growth factor, fibroblast growth factors, and brain-derived neurotrophic factor. End-feet of astrocytic processes at blood vessels provide sites for release of cytokines and chemoattractants during CNS injury. Astrocytes respond to brain injury by

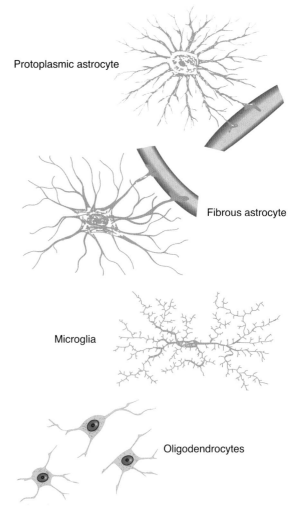

FIGURE 7–4 Drawings of neuroglial cells as seen in slides stained by metallic impregnation. Observe that only astrocytes exhibit vascular end-feet, which cover the walls of blood capillaries. (Redrawn, with permission, from Junqueira LC, Carneiro J. *Basic Histology*, 10th ed. McGraw-Hill, 2003.)

increasing in size—and in some cases in number—through a process called **reactive astrocytosis.** This phenotypic change is characterized by an increase in cells expressing glial-fibrillary acidic protein and by synthesis and release of cytokines that regulate inflammatory responses and entry of hematogenous cells into the CNS. Astrocytes play an important role also in terminating neuronal responses to glutamate, the most abundant excitatory neurotransmitter in the brain. In cell cultures, neurons die in the presence of high levels of glutamate unless astrocytes are present. Glutamate transporters present on astrocyte cell membranes remove glutamate from the synapse. Astrocytes also contain glutamine synthase, which converts glutamate to glutamine, detoxifying the CNS of both glutamate and ammonia.

Oligodendrocytes & Schwann Cells

Plasma membranes of oligodendrocytes in the CNS and Schwann cells in the peripheral nervous system envelop axons. For many axons, the membranes of these glial cells are wrapped layer on layer around the axon, forming a myelin sheath (Figure 7–5). Gaps form between myelin sheaths from neighboring glia and produce **nodes of Ranvier** where a small portion of the axon is exposed to the interstitial space and where voltage-dependent Na$^+$ channels are clustered in the axonal membrane. Between the nodes, myelin insulates the axon from the extracellular space, allowing efficient spread of depolarization from one node to another. This allows action potentials to propagate rapidly by jumping from node to node in a process called **saltatory conduction.**

Microglia

Although peripheral blood lymphocytes and monocytes enter from the circulation and patrol the CNS, microglia, which reside in the CNS, function as the main immune effector cells. They appear to be derived from bone marrow precursors of macrophage-monocyte lineage and invade the CNS during the perinatal period. Microglia cells are activated by brain injury, infection, or neuronal degeneration. Activation is characterized by proliferation, migration into damaged tissue, increased or de novo expression of surface receptors, includ-

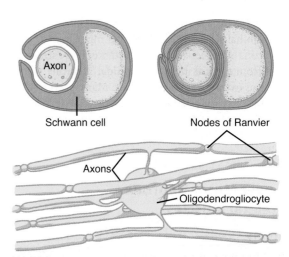

FIGURE 7–5 Myelination of axons. **Top left:** Unmyelinated axon. **Top right:** Myelinated axon. Note that the cell membrane of the Schwann cell has wrapped itself around the axon. **Bottom:** Myelination of several axons in the CNS by an oligodendrogliocyte. (Redrawn, with permission, from Ganong WF. *Review of Medical Physiology*, 22nd ed. McGraw-Hill, 2005.)

ing CD45 (leukocyte common antigen), MHC class I and class II and immunoglobulin Fc receptors, and secretion of several cytokines, reactive oxygen intermediates, and proteinases. This response functions to remove dead tissue and destroy invading organisms but may contribute to CNS damage, particularly in certain CNS inflammatory and degenerative diseases.

CHECKPOINT

1. What are the primary functions of neurons, astrocytes, and microglia?
2. What role does myelin play in axonal conduction?
3. What is responsible for the resting membrane potential and for the generation of action potentials?
4. What are some of the major neurotransmitters in the nervous system, and what effects do they produce when they bind to their receptors?

FUNCTIONAL NEUROANATOMY

To understand neuroanatomy, it is useful to study structures as parts of functional systems.

MOTOR SYSTEM

Large **alpha motor neurons** of the spinal cord ventral horns and brainstem motor nuclei (facial nucleus, trigeminal motor nucleus, nucleus ambiguus, hypoglossal nucleus) extend axons into spinal and cranial nerves to innervate skeletal muscles. Damage to these **lower motor neurons** results in loss of all voluntary and reflex movement because they comprise the output of the motor system. Neurons in the precentral gyrus and neighboring cortical regions (**upper motor neurons**) send axons to synapse with lower motor neurons. Axons from these upper motor neurons comprise the **corticospinal** and **corticobulbar tracts.** The motor cortex and spinal cord are connected with other deep cerebral and brainstem motor nuclei, including the caudate nucleus, putamen, globus pallidus, red nuclei, subthalamic nuclei, substantia nigra, reticular nuclei, and neurons of the cerebellum. Neurons in these structures are distinct from cortical motor (**pyramidal**) neurons and are referred to as **extrapyramidal** neurons. Many parts of the cerebral cortex are connected by fiber tracts to the primary motor cortex. These connections are important for complex patterns of movement and for coordinating motor responses to sensory stimuli.

1. Lower Motor Neurons & Skeletal Muscles

Anatomy

Each alpha motor neuron axon contacts up to about 200 muscle fibers, and together they constitute the **motor unit** (Figure 7–6). Axons of the motor neurons intermingle to form spinal ventral roots, plexuses, and peripheral nerves. Muscles are innervated from specific segments of the spinal cord, and each muscle is supplied by at least two roots. Motor fibers are rearranged in the plexuses so that most muscles are supplied by one peripheral nerve. Thus, the distribution of muscle weakness differs in spinal root and peripheral nerve lesions.

Physiology

The lower motor neurons are the final common pathway for all voluntary movement. Therefore, damage to lower motor neurons or their axons causes flaccid weakness of innervated muscles. In addition, muscle tone or resistance to passive movement is reduced, and deep tendon reflexes are impaired or lost. Tendon reflexes and muscle tone depend on the activity of alpha motor neurons (Figure 7–7), specialized sensory receptors known as muscle spindles, and smaller **gamma motor neurons** whose axons innervate the spindles. Some gamma motor neurons are active at rest, making the spindle fibers taut

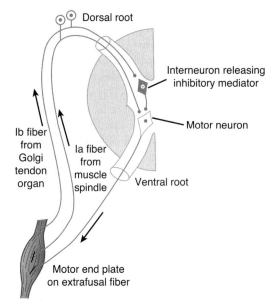

FIGURE 7–7 Diagram illustrating the pathways responsible for the stretch reflex and the inverse stretch reflex. Stretch stimulates the muscle spindle, and impulses pass up the Ia fiber to excite the motor neuron. It also stimulates the Golgi tendon organ, and impulses passing up the Ib fiber activate the interneuron to release the inhibitory mediator glycine. With strong stretch, the resulting hyperpolarization of the motor neuron is so great that it stops discharging. (Redrawn, with permission, from Ganong, WF. *Review of Medical Physiology*, 22nd ed. McGraw-Hill, 2005.)

and sensitive to stretch. Tapping on the tendon stretches the spindles, which causes them to send impulses that activate alpha motor neurons. These in turn fire, producing the brief muscle contraction observed during the **myotactic stretch reflex.** Alpha motor neurons of antagonist muscles are simultaneously inhibited. Both alpha and gamma motor neurons are influenced by descending fiber systems, and their state of activity determines the level of tone and activity of the stretch reflex.

Each point of contact between nerve terminal and skeletal muscle forms a specialized synapse known as a **neuromuscular junction** composed of the presynaptic motor nerve terminal and a postsynaptic motor end plate (Figure 7–8). Presynaptic terminals store synaptic vesicles that contain the neurotransmitter acetylcholine. The amount of neurotransmitter within a vesicle constitutes a quantum of neurotransmitter. Action potentials depolarize the motor nerve terminal, opening voltage-gated calcium channels and stimulating calcium-dependent release of neurotransmitter from the terminal. Released acetylcholine traverses the synaptic cleft to the postsynaptic (end plate) membrane, where it binds to nicotinic cholinergic receptors. These receptors are ligand-gated cation channels, and, on binding to acetylcholine, they allow entry of extracellular sodium into the motor end plate. This depolarizes the motor end plate, which in turn depolarizes the muscle fiber. After activation, cholinergic receptors are rapidly inactivated, reducing sodium entry. They remain inactive until acetylcholine dissociates from the receptor. This is facilitated by the enzyme acetylcholinesterase, which hydrolyzes acetylcholine and is present in the postsynaptic zone.

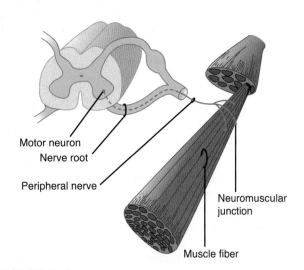

Motor neuron
Nerve root
Peripheral nerve
Neuromuscular junction
Muscle fiber

FIGURE 7–6 Anatomic components of the motor unit. (Redrawn, with permission, from Greenberg DA, Aminoff MJ, Simon RP. *Clinical Neurology*, 5th ed. McGraw-Hill, 2002.)

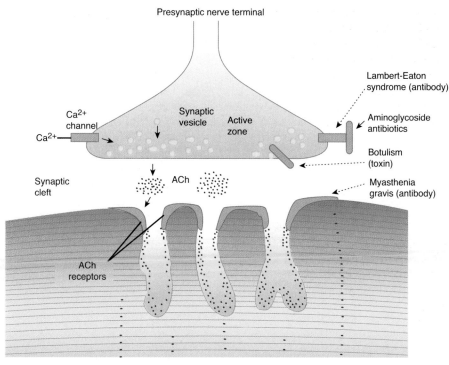

Presynaptic nerve terminal

Lambert-Eaton
syndrome (antibody)

Aminoglycoside
antibiotics

Botulism
(toxin)

Myasthenia
gravis (antibody)

Ca²⁺
channel

Ca²⁺

Synaptic
vesicle

Active
zone

Synaptic
cleft

ACh

ACh
receptors

Postsynaptic muscle membrane

FIGURE 7–8 Sites of involvement in disorders of neuromuscular transmission. **Left:** Normal transmission involves depolarization-induced influx of calcium (Ca²⁺) through voltage-gated channels. This stimulates release of acetylcholine (ACh) from synaptic vesicles at the active zone and into the synaptic cleft. ACh binds to ACh receptors and depolarizes the postsynaptic muscle membrane. **Right:** Disorders of neuromuscular transmission result from blockage of Ca²⁺ channels (Lambert-Eaton syndrome or aminoglycoside antibiotics), impairment of Ca²⁺-mediated ACh release (botulinum toxin), or antibody-induced internalization and degradation of ACh receptors (myasthenia gravis). (Redrawn, with permission, from Greenberg DA, Aminoff MJ, Simon RP. *Clinical Neurology,* 5th ed. McGraw-Hill, 2002.)

Neuromuscular transmission may be disturbed in several ways (Figure 7–8). In the **Lambert-Eaton myasthenic syndrome,** antibodies to calcium channels inhibit calcium entry into the nerve terminal and reduce neurotransmitter release. In these cases, repetitive nerve stimulation facilitates accumulation of calcium in the nerve terminal and increases acetylcholine release. Clinically, limb muscles are weak, but if contraction is maintained, power increases. Electrophysiologically, there is an increase in the amplitude of the muscle response to repetitive nerve stimulation. **Aminoglycoside antibiotics** also impair calcium channel function and cause a similar syndrome. Proteolytic toxins produced by *Clostridium botulinum* cleave specific presynaptic proteins, preventing neurotransmitter release at both neuromuscular and parasympathetic cholinergic synapses. As a result, patients with **botulism** develop weakness, blurred vision, diplopia, ptosis, and large unreactive pupils. In **myasthenia gravis,** autoantibodies to the nicotinic acetylcholine receptor (AChR) block neurotransmission by inhibiting receptor function and activating complement-mediated lysis of the postsynaptic membrane. Myasthenia gravis is discussed in greater detail later in this chapter.

Motor nerves exert trophic influences on the muscles they innervate. Denervated muscles undergo marked atrophy, losing more than half of their original bulk in 2–3 months. Nerve fibers are also required for organization of the muscle end plate

and for the clustering of cholinergic receptors to that region. Receptors in denervated fibers fail to cluster and become spread across the muscle membrane. Muscle fibers within a denervated motor unit may then discharge spontaneously, giving rise to a visible twitch (**fasciculation**) within a portion of a muscle. Individual fibers may also contract spontaneously, giving rise to **fibrillations,** which are not visible to the examiner but can be detected by electromyography. Fibrillations usually appear 7–21 days after damage to lower motor neurons or their axons.

CHECKPOINT

5. From where do lower motor neurons emanate, and to where do they send axons?
6. Describe four mechanisms that can disturb the function of the neuromuscular junction.

2. Upper Motor Neurons

Anatomy

The motor cortex is the region from which movements can be elicited by electrical stimuli (Figure 7–9). This includes the primary motor area (Brodmann area 4), premotor cortex (area

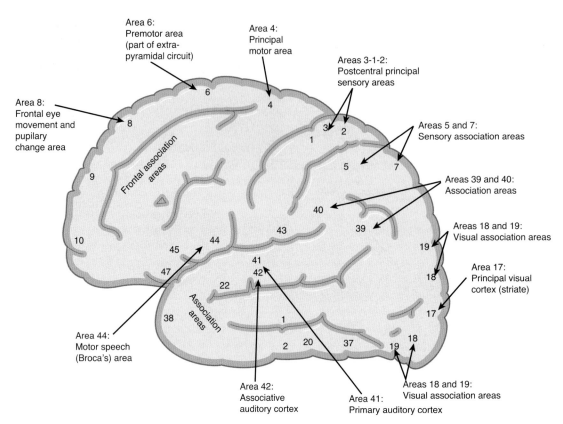

FIGURE 7–9 Lateral aspect of the cerebrum. The cortical areas are shown according to Brodmann, with functional localizations. (Redrawn, with permission, from Waxman SG. *Neuroanatomy with Clinical Correlations,* 25th ed. McGraw-Hill, 2003.)

6), supplementary motor cortex (medial portions of 6), and primary sensory cortex (areas 3, 1, and 2). In the motor cortex, groups of neurons are organized in vertical columns, and discrete groups control contraction of individual muscles. Planned movements and those guided by sensory, visual, or auditory stimuli are preceded by discharges from prefrontal, somatosensory, visual, or auditory cortices, which are then followed by motor cortex pyramidal cell discharges that occur several milliseconds before the onset of movement.

Cortical motor neurons contribute axons that converge in the corona radiata and descend in the posterior limb of the internal capsule, cerebral peduncles, ventral pons, and medulla. These fibers constitute the **corticospinal** and **corticobulbar tracts** and together are known as upper motor neuron fibers (Figure 7–10). As they descend through the diencephalon and brainstem, fibers separate to innervate extrapyramidal and cranial nerve motor nuclei. The lower brainstem motor neurons receive input from crossed and uncrossed corticobulbar fibers, although neurons that innervate lower facial muscles receive primarily crossed fibers.

In the ventral medulla, the remaining corticospinal fibers course in a tract that is pyramidal in shape in cross section— thus, the name **pyramidal tract.** At the lower end of the medulla, most fibers decussate, although the proportion of crossed and uncrossed fibers varies somewhat between individuals. The bulk of these fibers descend as the lateral corticospinal tract of the spinal cord.

Different groups of neurons in the cortex control muscle groups of the contralateral face, arm, and leg. Neurons near the ventral end of the central sulcus control muscles of the face, whereas neurons on the medial surface of the hemisphere control leg muscles (Figure 7–10). Because the movements of the face, tongue, and hand are complex in humans, a large share of the motor cortex is devoted to their control. A somatotopic organization is also apparent in the lateral corticospinal tract of the cervical cord, where fibers to motor neurons that control leg muscles lie laterally and fibers to cervical motor neurons lie medially.

Physiology

Upper motor neurons are the final common pathway between cortical and subcortical structures, such as the basal ganglia, in the planning, initiation, sequencing, and modulation of all voluntary movement. Much has been learned about the normal function of upper motor neurons through the study of animals and humans with focal brain lesions. Upper motor neuron pathways can be interrupted in the cortex, subcortical white matter, internal capsule, brainstem, or spinal cord. Unilateral upper motor neuron lesions spare muscles innervated by lower motor neurons that receive bilateral cortical input, such as muscles of the eyes, jaw, upper face, pharynx, larynx, neck, thorax, and abdomen. Unlike paralysis resulting from lower motor neuron lesions, paralysis from upper motor neuron lesions is rarely

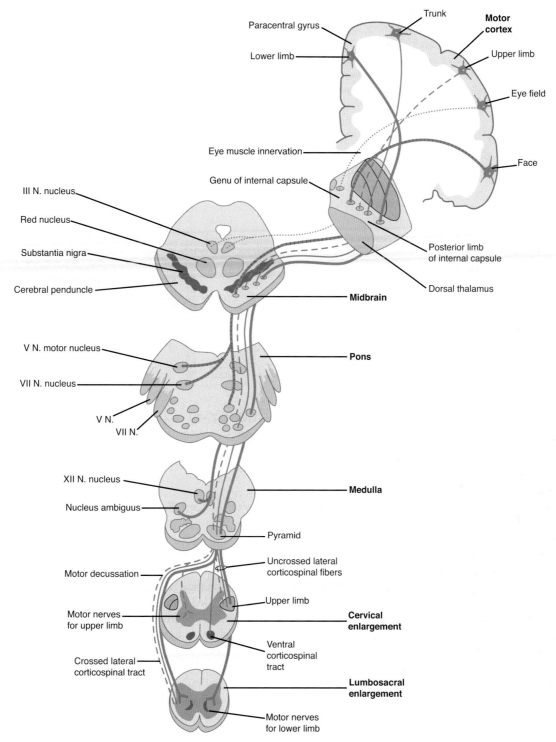

FIGURE 7–10 Schematic illustration of upper motor neuron pathways. (Redrawn, with permission, from Adams M, Victor RD. *Principles of Neurology*, 8th ed. McGraw-Hill, 2005.)

complete for a prolonged period of time. Acute lesions, particularly of the spinal cord, often cause flaccid paralysis and absence of spinal reflexes at all segments below the lesion. With spinal cord lesions, this state is known as **spinal shock.** After a few days to weeks, a state known as **spasticity** appears, characterized by increased tone and hyperactive stretch reflexes. A similar but less striking sequence of events can occur with acute cerebral lesions.

Upper motor neuron lesions cause a characteristic pattern of limb weakness and change in tone. Antigravity muscles of the limbs become more active relative to other muscles. The arms tend to assume a flexed, pronated posture, and the legs become extended. In contrast, muscles that move the limbs out of this posture (extensors of the arms and flexors of the legs) are preferentially weakened. Tone is increased in antigravity muscles (flexors of the arms and extensors of the legs), and if these muscles are stretched rapidly, they respond with an abrupt catch, followed by a rapid increase and then a decline in resistance as passive movement continues. This sequence constitutes the **"clasp knife"** phenomenon. **Clonus**—a series of involuntary muscle contractions in response to passive stretch—may be present, especially with spinal cord lesions.

Pure pyramidal tract lesions in animals cause temporary weakness without spasticity. In humans, lesions of the cerebral peduncles also cause mild paralysis without spasticity. It appears that control of tone is mediated by other tracts, particularly corticorubrospinal and corticoreticulospinal pathways. This may explain why the degrees of weakness and spasticity often do not correspond in patients with upper motor neuron lesions.

The distribution of paralysis resulting from upper motor neuron lesions varies with the location of the lesion. Lesions above the pons impair movements of the contralateral lower face, arm, and leg. Lesions below the pons spare the face. Lesions of the internal capsule often impair movements of the contralateral face, arm, and leg equally, because motor fibers are packed closely together in this region. In contrast, lesions of the cortex or subcortical white matter tend to differentially affect the limbs and face because the motor fibers are spread over a larger area of brain. Bilateral cerebral lesions cause weakness and spasticity of cranial, trunk, and limb muscles, which leads to dysarthria, dysphonia, dysphagia, bifacial paresis, and sometimes reflexive crying and laughing (**pseudobulbar palsy**).

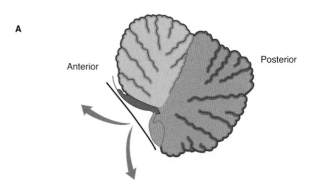

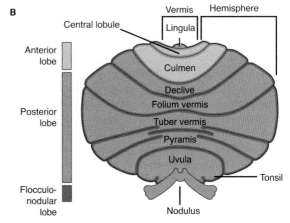

FIGURE 7–11 Anatomic divisions of the cerebellum in midsagittal view: (**A**) unfolded (arrows) and (**B**) viewed from behind. (Redrawn, with permission, from Greenberg DA, Aminoff MJ, Simon RP. *Clinical Neurology*, 5th ed. McGraw-Hill, 2002.)

CHECKPOINT

7. Define the motor cortex and describe its organization.
8. Fibers from which nuclei and in which tracts constitute upper motor neurons? What is their path?
9. Describe the somatotopic organization of motor neurons in the cortex.
10. What are the characteristics of weakness and tone in upper motor neuron lesions?
11. How is the distribution of paralysis and spasticity affected by the location of an upper motor neuron lesion?

3. Cerebellum

Anatomy

The cerebellar cortex can be divided into three anatomic regions (Figure 7–11B). The **flocculonodular lobe,** composed of the flocculus and the nodulus of the vermis, has connections to vestibular nuclei and is important for the control of posture and eye movement. The **anterior lobe** (Figure 7–11A) lies rostral to the primary fissure and includes the remainder of the vermis. It receives proprioceptive input from muscles and ten-

dons via the dorsal and ventral spinocerebellar tracts and influences posture, muscle tone, and gait. The **posterior lobe,** which comprises the remainder of the cerebellar hemispheres, receives major input from the cerebral cortex via the pontine nuclei and middle cerebellar peduncles and is important for the coordination and planning of voluntary skilled movements initiated from the cerebral cortex.

Efferent fibers from these lobes project to deep cerebellar nuclei, which in turn project to the cerebrum and brainstem through two main pathways (Figure 7–12). The fastigial nucleus receives input from the vermis and sends fibers to bilateral vestibular nuclei and reticular nuclei of the pons and medulla via the inferior cerebellar peduncles. Other regions of the cerebellar cortex send fibers to the **dentate, emboliform, and globose nuclei,** whose efferents form the superior cerebellar peduncles, enter the upper pons, decussate completely in the lower midbrain, and travel to the contralateral red nucleus. At the red nucleus, some fibers terminate, whereas others ascend to the ventrolateral nucleus of the thalamus, whence thalamic neurons send ascending efferent fibers to the motor cortex of the same side. A smaller group of fibers descend after decussation in the midbrain and terminate in reticular nuclei of the lower brainstem. Thus, the cerebellum controls movement through connections with cerebral motor cortex and brainstem nuclei.

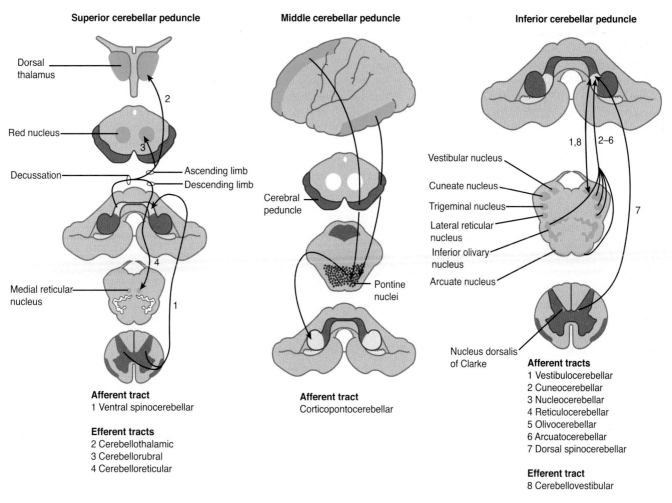

FIGURE 7–12 Cerebellar connections in the superior, middle, and inferior cerebellar peduncles. The peduncles are indicated by gray shading and the areas to and from which they project by blue shading. (Redrawn, with permission, from Greenberg DA, Aminoff MJ, Simon RP. *Clinical Neurology,* 5th ed. McGraw-Hill, 2002.)

Physiology

The cerebellum is responsible for the coordination of muscle groups, control of stance and gait, and regulation of muscle tone. Rather than causing paralysis, damage to the cerebellum interferes with the performance of motor tasks. The major manifestation of cerebellar disease is **ataxia,** in which simple movements are delayed in onset and their rates of acceleration and deceleration are decreased, resulting in **intention tremor** and **dysmetria** ("overshooting"). Lesions of the cerebellar hemispheres affect the limbs, producing limb ataxia, whereas midline lesions affect axial muscles, causing truncal and gait ataxia and disorders of eye movement. Cerebellar lesions are often associated with **hypotonia** as a result of depression of activity of alpha and gamma motor neurons. If a lesion of the cerebellum or cerebellar peduncles is unilateral, the signs of limb ataxia appear on the same side as the lesion. However, if the lesion lies beyond the decussation of efferent cerebellar fibers in the midbrain, the clinical signs are on the side opposite the lesion.

CHECKPOINT

12. What is the overall role of the cerebellum?

13. What are the anatomic regions of the cerebellum, what do they control, and through which other regions of the brain do they make connections?

14. What are the consequences of damage to the cerebellum, and what symptoms and signs are seen in patients with cerebellar lesions?

15. Below what point do unilateral cerebellar lesions manifest on the opposite side?

4. Basal Ganglia

Anatomy

Several subcortical, thalamic, and brainstem nuclei are critical for regulating voluntary movement and maintaining posture. These include the basal ganglia (ie, the caudate nucleus and putamen [corpus striatum]), globus pallidus, substantia nigra, and subthalamic nuclei. They also include the red nuclei and the mesencephalic reticular nuclei. The major pathways that involve the basal ganglia form three neuronal circuits (Figure 7–13). The first is the cortical-basal ganglionic-thalamic-cortical loop. Inputs mainly from premotor, primary motor, and primary sensory cortices (areas 1, 2, 3, 4, and 6) project to the corpus striatum, which sends fibers to the medial and lateral portions of the globus pallidus. Fibers from the globus pallidus form the ansa and fasciculus lenticularis, which sweep through the internal capsule and project onto ventral and intralaminar thalamic nuclei. Axons from these nuclei project to the premotor and primary motor cortices (areas 4 and 6), completing the loop. In the second loop, the substantia nigra sends dopaminergic fibers to the corpus striatum, which has reciprocal connections with the substantia nigra. The substantia nigra also projects to the ventromedial thalamus. The third loop is composed of reciprocal connections between the globus pallidus and the subthalamic nucleus. The subthalamic nucleus also sends efferents to the substantia nigra and corpus striatum.

Physiology

Basal ganglia circuits regulate the initiation, amplitude, and speed of movements. Diseases of the basal ganglia cause abnormalities of movement and are collectively known as **movement disorders.** They are characterized by motor deficits (bradykinesia, akinesia, loss of postural reflexes) or abnormal activation of the motor system, resulting in rigidity, tremor, and involuntary movements (chorea, athetosis, ballismus, and dystonia).

Several neurotransmitters are found within the basal ganglia, but their role in disease states is only partly understood. **Acetylcholine** is present in high concentrations within the corpus striatum, where it is synthesized and released by large Golgi type 2 neurons (Figure 7–14). Acetylcholine acts as an excitatory transmitter at medium-sized spiny striatal neurons that synthesize and release the inhibitory neurotransmitter γ-aminobutyric acid (**GABA**) and project to the globus pallidus. **Dopamine** is synthesized by neurons of the substantia nigra, whose axons form the nigrostriatal pathway that terminates in the corpus striatum. Dopamine released by these fibers inhibits striatal GABAergic neurons. In Parkinson's disease, degeneration of nigral neurons leads to loss of dopaminergic inhibition and a relative excess of cholinergic activity. This increases GABAergic output from the striatum and contributes to the paucity of movement that is a cardinal manifestation of the disease. Anticholinergics and dopamine agonists tend to restore the normal balance of striatal cholinergic and dopaminergic inputs and are effective in treatment. The pathogenesis of Parkinson's disease is discussed later in this chapter.

Huntington's disease is inherited as an autosomal dominant disorder. When disease onset occurs later in life, patients develop involuntary, rapid, jerky movements (**chorea**) and slow writhing movements of the proximal limbs and trunk (**athetosis**). When disease onset occurs earlier in life, patients develop signs of parkinsonism with tremor (cogwheeling) and stiffness. The spiny GABAergic neurons of the striatum preferentially degenerate, resulting in a net decrease in GABAergic output from the striatum. This contributes to the development of chorea and athetosis. Dopamine antagonists, which block inhibition of remaining striatal neurons by dopa-

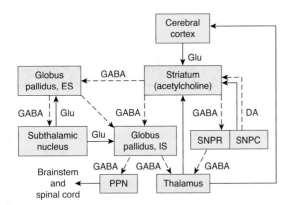

FIGURE 7–13 Diagrammatic representation of the principal connections of the basal ganglia. Solid lines indicate excitatory pathways; dashed lines indicate inhibitory pathways. The transmitters are indicated in the pathways, where they are known. Glu, glutamate; DA, dopamine. Acetylcholine is the transmitter produced by interneurons in the striatum (ie, the putamen and the caudate nucleus, which have similar connections). SNPR, substantia nigra, pars reticulata; SNPC, substantia nigra, pars compacta; ES, external segment; IS, internal segment. The subthalamic nucleus also projects to the pars compacta of the substantia nigra; this pathway has been omitted for clarity. (Redrawn, with permission, from Ganong WF. *Review of Medical Physiology,* 22nd ed. McGraw-Hill, 2005.)

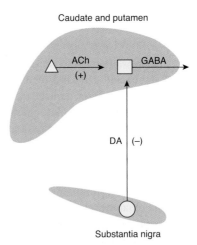

FIGURE 7–14 Simplified neurochemical anatomy of the basal ganglia. Dopamine (DA) neurons exert a net inhibitory effect and acetylcholine (ACh) neurons a net excitatory effect on the GABAergic output from the striatum. In Parkinson's disease, DA neurons degenerate. The net effect is to increase GABAergic output from the striatum. (Redrawn, with permission, from Greenberg DA, Aminoff MJ, Simon RP. *Clinical Neurology,* 5th ed. McGraw-Hill, 2002.)

minergic striatal fibers, reduce the involuntary movements. Neurons in deep layers of the cerebral cortex also degenerate early in the disease, and later this extends to other brain regions, including the hippocampus and hypothalamus. Thus, the disease is characterized by cognitive defects and psychiatric disturbances in addition to the movement disorder.

The gene for the disease is located on chromosome 4p and encodes for a 3144-amino acid protein, **huntingtin,** which is widely expressed and interacts with several proteins involved in intracellular trafficking and endocytosis, gene transcription, and intracellular signaling. The protein contains a trinucleotide (CAG) repeat of 11–34 copies that encodes a polyglutamine domain and is expanded in patients with the disease. Deletion of the gene in mice causes embryonic death, whereas heterozygous animals are healthy. Transgenic mice with an expanded repeat develop a neurodegenerative disorder, suggesting that the disease results from the toxic effect of a gain of function mutation.

The mechanisms by which mutant huntingtin causes disease are not certain. The mutant protein is degraded, and the resulting fragments that contain the glutamine repeats form aggregates, which are deposited in nuclear and cytoplasmic inclusions. These fragments may bind abnormally to other proteins and interfere with normal protein processing or disrupt mitochondrial function. Nuclear fragments may interfere with nuclear functions such as gene expression. For example, in the cerebral cortex, mutant huntingtin reduces the production of brain-derived neurotrophic factor by suppressing its transcription. In addition, normal huntingtin is protective for cortical and striatal neurons and blocks the processing of procaspase 9, thereby reducing **apoptosis** (programmed cell death). Therefore, both loss of neurotrophic support and enhanced caspase activity could promote striatal cell loss in Huntington's disease.

CHECKPOINT

16. Which are the component nuclei of the basal ganglia, and what is their functional role?

17. What are the clinical consequences of lesions in the basal ganglia?

18. What are some of the neurotransmitters within the basal ganglia, and what is their role in disorders of basal ganglia function?

SOMATOSENSORY SYSTEM

Somatosensory pathways confer information about touch, pressure, temperature, pain, vibration, and the position and movement of body parts. This information is relayed to thalamic nuclei and integrated in the sensory cortex of the parietal lobes to provide conscious awareness of sensation. Information is also relayed to cortical motor neurons to adjust fine movements and maintain posture. Some ascending sensory fibers, particularly pain fibers, enter the midbrain and project to the amygdala and limbic cortex, where they contribute to emotional responses to pain. In the spinal cord, painful stimuli activate local pathways that induce the firing of lower motor neurons and cause a reflex withdrawal. Thus, somatosensory pathways provide tactile information, guide movement, and serve protective functions.

Anatomy

A variety of specialized end organs and free nerve endings transduce sensory stimuli into neural signals and initiate the firing of sensory nerve fibers. Fibers that mediate cutaneous sensation from the trunk and limbs travel in sensory or mixed sensorimotor nerves to the spinal cord (Figure 7–15). Cutaneous sensory nerves contain small myelinated Aδ fibers that transmit information about pain and temperature, larger myelinated fibers that mediate touch and pressure sensation, and more numerous unmyelinated pain and autonomic C fibers. Myelinated proprioceptive fibers and afferent and efferent muscle spindle fibers are carried in the larger sensorimotor nerves. The cell bodies of the sensory neurons are in the dorsal root ganglia, and their central projections enter the spinal cord via the dorsal spinal roots. Innervation of the skin, muscles, and surrounding connective tissue is segmental, and each root innervates a region of skin known as a **dermatome** (Figure 7–16). Cell bodies of the sensory neurons that innervate the face reside in the trigeminal ganglion and send their central projections in the trigeminal nerve to the brainstem. The trigeminal innervation of the face is subdivided into three regions, each innervated by one of the three divisions of the trigeminal nerve.

The dorsal roots enter the dorsal horn of the spinal cord (Figure 7–15). Large myelinated fibers divide into ascending and descending branches and either synapse with dorsal gray neurons within a few cord segments or travel in the **dorsal columns,** terminating in the gracile or cuneate nuclei of the lower medulla on the same side. Secondary neurons of the dorsal horn also send axons up the dorsal columns. Fibers in the dorsal columns are displaced medially as new fibers are added, so that in the cervical cord, leg fibers are located medially and arm fibers laterally (Figure 7–15). The gracile and cuneate nuclei send fibers that cross the midline in the medulla and ascend to the thalamus as the **medial lemniscus** (Figure 7–17). The dorsal column-lemniscal system carries information about pressure, limb position, vibration, direction of movement, recognition of texture and shape, and two-point discrimination.

Thinly myelinated and unmyelinated fibers enter the lateral portion of the dorsal horn and synapse with dorsal spinal neurons within one or two segments. The majority of secondary fibers from these cells cross in the anterior spinal commissure and ascend in the anterolateral spinal cord as the **lateral spinothalamic tracts.** Crossing fibers are added to the inner side of the tract, so that in the cervical cord the leg fibers are located superficially and arm fibers are deeper. These fibers carry information about pain, temperature, and touch sensation.

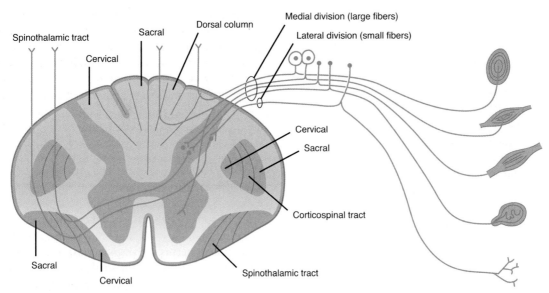

FIGURE 7–15 Schematic illustration of a spinal cord segment with its dorsal root, ganglion cells, and sensory organs. Sensory organs shown (from top to bottom) are the pacinian corpuscle, muscle spindle, tendon organ, encapsulated ending, and free nerve endings. The somatotopic arrangement of fibers in the dorsal columns, spinothalamic tract, and corticospinal tract is also shown. (Redrawn, with permission, from Waxman SG. *Neuroanatomy with Clinical Correlations,* 25th ed. McGraw-Hill, 2003.)

Sensation from the face is carried by trigeminal sensory fibers that enter the pons and descend to the medulla and upper cervical cord (Figure 7–18). Fibers carrying information about pain and temperature sensation terminate in the **nucleus of the spinal tract of cranial nerve V,** which is continuous with the dorsal horn of the cervical cord. Touch, pres-

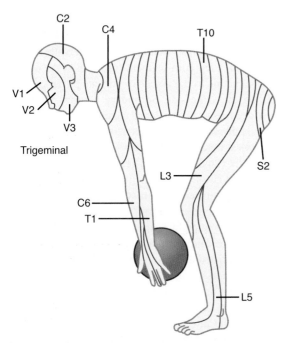

FIGURE 7–16 Segmental distribution of the body viewed in the approximate quadruped position, including sensory distribution of the trigeminal (V) cranial nerve. (Redrawn, with permission, from Waxman SG. *Neuroanatomy with Clinical Correlations,* 25th ed. McGraw-Hill, 2003.)

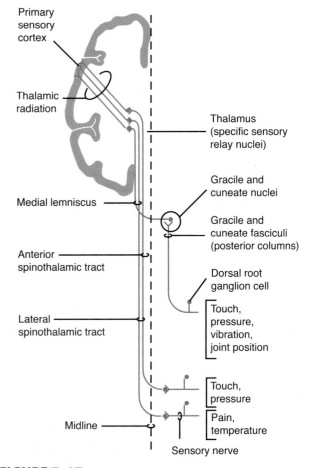

FIGURE 7–17 Sensory pathways conveying touch, pressure, vibration, joint position, pain, and temperature sensation. (Redrawn, with permission, from Greenberg DA, Aminoff MJ, Simon RP. *Clinical Neurology,* 5th ed. McGraw-Hill, 2002.)

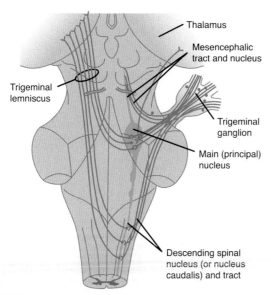

FIGURE 7–18 Schematic drawing of the trigeminal system. (Redrawn, with permission, from Waxman SG. *Neuroanatomy with Clinical Correlations*, 25th ed. McGraw-Hill, 2003.)

sure, and postural information is conveyed by fibers that terminate in the **main sensory** and **mesencephalic nuclei of the trigeminal nerve.** Axons arising from trigeminal nuclei cross the midline and ascend as the **trigeminal lemniscus** just medial to the spinothalamic tract. Fibers from the spinothalamic tract, medial lemniscus, and trigeminal lemniscus merge in the midbrain and terminate along with sensory fibers ascending from the spinal cord in the posterior thalamic nuclei, mainly in the nucleus ventralis posterolateralis. These thalamic nuclei project to the primary somatosensory cortex (Brodmann areas 3, 1, and 2) and to a second somatosensory area on the upper bank of the sylvian fissure (lateral cerebral sulcus). The primary somatosensory region is organized somatotopically like the primary motor cortex.

Physiology

A. Pain

Free nerve endings of unmyelinated C fibers and small-diameter myelinated Aδ fibers in the skin convey sensory information in response to chemical, thermal, and mechanical stimuli. Intense stimulation of these nerve endings evokes the sensation of pain. In contrast to skin, most deep tissues are relatively insensitive to chemical or noxious stimuli. However, inflammatory conditions can sensitize sensory afferents from deep tissues to evoke pain on mechanical stimulation. This sensitization appears to be mediated by bradykinin, prostaglandins, and leukotrienes released during the inflammatory response. Information from primary afferent fibers is relayed via sensory ganglia to the dorsal horn of the spinal cord and then to the contralateral spinothalamic tract, which connects to thalamic neurons that project to the somatosensory cortex.

Damage to these pathways produces a deficit in pain and temperature discrimination and may also produce abnormal painful sensations (**dysesthesias**) usually in the area of sensory loss. Such pain is termed **neuropathic pain** and often has a strange burning, tingling, or electric shocklike quality. It may arise from several mechanisms. Damaged peripheral nerve fibers become highly mechanosensitive and may fire spontaneously without known stimulation. They also develop sensitivity to norepinephrine released from sympathetic postganglionic neurons. Electrical impulses may spread abnormally from one fiber to another (**ephaptic conduction**), enhancing the spontaneous firing of multiple fibers. Neuropeptides released by injured nerves may recruit an inflammatory reaction that stimulates pain. In the dorsal horn, denervated spinal neurons may become spontaneously active. In the brain and spinal cord, synaptic reorganization occurs in response to injury and may lower the threshold for pain. In addition, inhibition of pathways that modulate transmission of sensory information in the spinal cord and brainstem may promote neuropathic pain.

Pain-modulating circuits exert a major influence on the perceived intensity of pain. One such pathway (Figure 7–19) is composed of cells in the periaqueductal gray matter of the midbrain that receive afferents from frontal cortex and hypothalamus and project to rostroventral medullary neurons. These in turn project in the dorsolateral white matter of the spinal cord and terminate on dorsal horn neurons. Additional

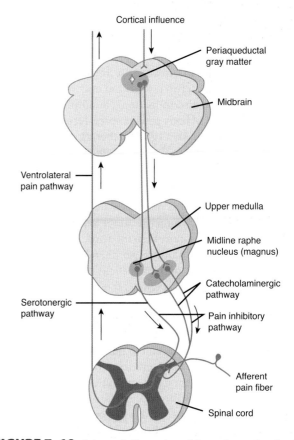

FIGURE 7–19 Schematic illustration of the pathways involved in pain control. (Courtesy A Basbaum.)

descending pathways arise from other brainstem nuclei (locus ceruleus, dorsal raphe nucleus, and nucleus reticularis gigantocellularis). Major neurotransmitters utilized by these systems include endorphins, serotonin, and norepinephrine, providing the rationale for the use of opioids, serotonin agonists, and serotonin and norepinephrine reuptake inhibitors in the treatment of pain.

B. Proprioception and Vibratory Sense

Receptors in the muscles, tendons, and joints provide information about deep pressure and the position and movement of body parts. This allows one to determine an object's size, weight, shape, and texture. Information is relayed to the spinal cord via large Aα and Aβ myelinated fibers and to the thalamus by the dorsal column-lemniscal system. Detecting vibration requires sensing touch and rapid changes in deep pressure. This depends on multiple cutaneous and deep sensory fibers and is impaired by lesions of multiple peripheral nerves, the dorsal columns, medial lemniscus, or thalamus but rarely by lesions of single nerves. Vibratory sense is often impaired together with proprioception.

C. Discriminative Sensation

Primary sensory cortex provides awareness of somatosensory information and the ability to make sensory discriminations. Touch, pain, temperature, and vibration sense are considered the primary modalities of sensation and are relatively preserved in patients with damage to sensory cortex or its projections from the thalamus. In contrast, complex tasks that require integration of multiple somatosensory stimuli and of somatosensory stimuli with auditory or visual information are impaired. These include the ability to distinguish two points from one when touched on the skin (**two-point discrimination**), localize tactile stimuli, perceive the position of body parts in space, recognize letters or numbers drawn on the skin (**graphesthesia**), and identify objects by their shape, size, and texture (**stereognosis**).

D. Anatomy of Sensory Loss

The patterns of sensory loss often indicate the level of nervous system involvement. Symmetric distal sensory loss in the limbs, affecting the legs more than the arms, usually signifies a generalized disorder of multiple peripheral nerves (**polyneuropathy**). Sensory symptoms and deficits may be restricted to the distribution of a single peripheral nerve (**mononeuropathy**) or two or more peripheral nerves (**mononeuropathy multiplex**). Symptoms limited to a dermatome indicate a spinal root lesion (**radiculopathy**).

In the spinal cord, segregation of fiber tracts and the somatotopic arrangement of fibers give rise to distinct patterns of sensory loss. Loss of pain and temperature sensation on one side of the body and of proprioception on the opposite side occurs with lesions that involve one half of the cord on the side of the proprioceptive deficit (**Brown-Séquard syndrome;** Figure 7–20). Compression of the upper spinal cord causes loss of pain, temperature, and touch sensation first in the legs,

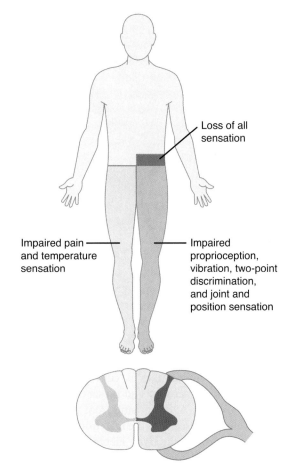

FIGURE 7–20 Brown-Séquard syndrome with lesion at left tenth thoracic level (motor deficits not shown). (Redrawn, with permission, from Waxman SG. *Neuroanatomy with Clinical Correlations,* 25th ed. McGraw-Hill, 2003.)

because the leg spinothalamic fibers are most superficial. More severe cord compression compromises fibers from the trunk. In patients with spinal cord compression, the lesion is often above the highest dermatome involved in the deficit. Thus, radiographic studies should be tailored to visualize the cord at and above the level of the sensory deficit detected on examination. Intrinsic cord lesions that involve the central portions of the cord often impair pain and temperature sensation at the level of the lesion because the fibers crossing the anterior commissure and entering the spinothalamic tracts are most centrally situated. Thus, enlargement of the central cervical canal in **syringomyelia** typically causes loss of pain and temperature sensation across the shoulders and upper arms (Figure 7–21).

Brainstem lesions involving the spinothalamic tract cause loss of pain and temperature sensation on the opposite side of the body. In the medulla, such lesions can involve the neighboring spinal trigeminal nucleus, resulting in a "crossed" sensory deficit involving the ipsilateral face and contralateral limbs. Above the medulla, the spinothalamic and trigeminothalamic tracts lie close together, and lesions there cause contralateral sensory loss of the face and limbs. In the midbrain and thalamus, medial lemniscal fibers run together with pain and temperature fibers, and lesions are more likely to

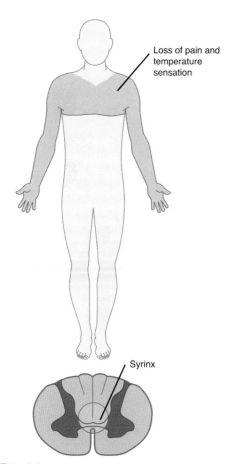

FIGURE 7–21 Syringomyelia (the presence of a cavity in the spinal cord resulting from breakdown of gliomatous new formations, presenting clinically with pain and paresthesias followed by muscular atrophy of the hands) involving the cervicothoracic portion of the cord. (Redrawn, with permission, from Waxman SG. *Neuroanatomy with Clinical Correlations,* 25th ed. McGraw-Hill, 2003.)

impair all primary sensation contralateral to the lesion. Because sensory fibers converge at the thalamus, lesions there tend to cause fairly equal loss of pain, temperature, and proprioceptive sensation on the contralateral half of the face and body. Lesions of the sensory cortex in the parietal lobe impair discriminative sensation on the opposite side of the body, whereas detection of the primary modalities of sensation may remain relatively intact.

CHECKPOINT

19. What fibers carry pain, and how are they segregated from fibers that carry proprioception information in the spinal cord?
20. What are the differences in characteristics of sensory loss at different levels of the nervous system?
21. What is the function of the sensory cortex in the parietal lobe, and what are the clinical features of damage to this region?

VISION & CONTROL OF EYE MOVEMENTS

The visual system provides our most important source of sensory information about the environment. The visual system and pathways for the control of eye movements are among the best characterized pathways in the nervous system. Familiarity with these neuroanatomic features is often extremely valuable in localization of neurologic disease.

Anatomy

The cornea and lens of the eye refract and focus images on the photosensitive posterior portion of the retina. The posterior retina contains two classes of specialized photoreceptor cells, **rods** and **cones,** which transduce photons into electrical signals. At the retina, the image is reversed in the horizontal and vertical planes so that the inferior visual field falls on the superior portions of the retina and the lateral field is detected by the nasal half of the retina.

Fibers from the nasal half of the retina traverse the medial portion of the optic nerve and cross to the other side at the **optic chiasm** (Figure 7–22). Each **optic tract** contains fibers from the same half of the visual field of both eyes. The optic tracts terminate in the **lateral geniculate nuclei** of the thalamus. Lateral geniculate neurons send fibers to the primary visual cortex in the occipital lobe (area 17, **calcarine cortex;** see Figure 7–9). These fibers form the **optic radiations,** which extend through the white matter of the temporal lobes and the inferior portion of the parietal lobes.

Eye movements are produced by the extraocular muscles, which function in pairs to move the eyes along three axes (Figure 7–23). These muscles are innervated by the **oculomotor** (III), **trochlear** (IV), and **abducens** (VI) nerves. The oculomotor nerve innervates the ipsilateral **medial, superior,** and **inferior rectus muscles** and the **inferior oblique muscles.** It also supplies the ipsilateral levator palpebrae, which elevates the eyelid. The oculomotor nerve also carries parasympathetic fibers that mediate pupillary constriction (see later discussion). Trochlear nerve fibers decussate before leaving the brainstem, and each trochlear nerve supplies the contralateral **superior oblique muscle.** The abducens nerve innervates the **lateral rectus muscle** of the same side.

Cortical and brainstem gaze centers innervate the extraocular motor nuclei and provide for supranuclear control of gaze. A **vertical gaze center** is located in the midbrain tegmentum, and **lateral gaze centers** are present in the pontine paramedian reticular formation. Each lateral gaze center sends fibers to the neighboring ipsilateral abducens nucleus and, via the **medial longitudinal fasciculus,** to the contralateral oculomotor nucleus. Therefore, activation of the right lateral gaze center stimulates conjugate deviation of the eyes to the right. Rapid **saccadic eye movements** are initiated by the **frontal eye fields** in the premotor cortex that stimulate conjugate movement of the eyes to the opposite side. Slower eye movements involved in pursuit of moving objects are controlled by parieto-occipital gaze centers, which stimulate conjugate gaze

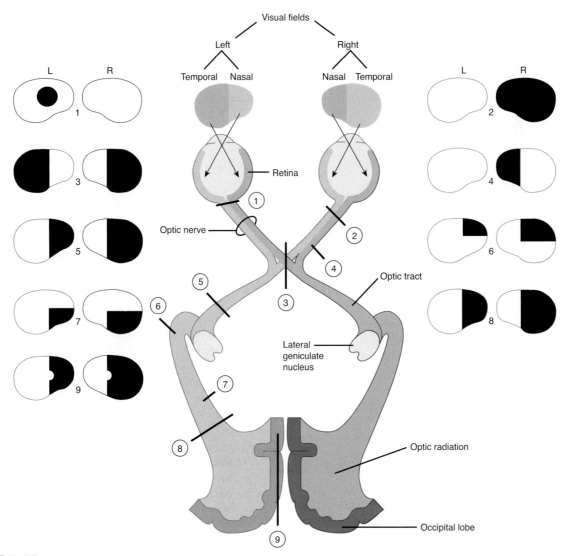

FIGURE 7–22 Common visual field defects and their anatomic bases. (1) Central scotoma caused by inflammation of the left optic disk (optic neuritis) or optic nerve (retrobulbar neuritis). (2) Total blindness of the right eye from a complete lesion of the right optic nerve. (3) Bitemporal hemianopia caused by pressure exerted on the optic chiasm by a pituitary tumor. (4) Right nasal hemianopia caused by a perichiasmal lesion (eg, calcified internal carotid artery). (5) Right homonymous hemianopia from a lesion of the left optic tract. (6) Right homonymous superior quadrantanopia caused by partial involvement of the optic radiation by a lesion in the left temporal lobe (Meyer's loop). (7) Right homonymous inferior quadrantanopia caused by partial involvement of the optic radiation by a lesion in the left parietal lobe. (8) Right homonymous hemianopia from a complete lesion of the left optic radiation. A similar defect may also result from lesion. (9) Right homonymous hemianopia (with macular sparing) resulting from posterior cerebral artery occlusion. (Redrawn, with permission, from Greenberg DA, Aminoff MJ, Simon RP. *Clinical Neurology,* 5th ed. McGraw-Hill, 2002.)

to the side of the gaze center. These cortical areas control eye movements through their connections with the brainstem gaze centers.

The size of the pupils is determined by the balance between parasympathetic and sympathetic discharge to the pupillary muscles. The parasympathetic oculomotor **nuclei of Edinger-Westphal** send fibers in the oculomotor nerves that synapse in the ciliary ganglia within the orbits and innervate the pupillary constrictor muscles.

The motor portion of pupillary dilation is controlled by a three-neuron system (Figure 7–24). It is composed of axons from neurons in the posterolateral hypothalamus that descend through the lateral brainstem tegmentum and the intermediolateral column of the cervical spinal cord to the level of T1. There they terminate on preganglionic sympathetic neurons within the lateral gray matter of the thoracic cord. These neurons send axons that synapse with postganglionic neurons in the superior cervical ganglion. Postganglionic neurons send fibers that travel with the internal carotid artery and the first division of the trigeminal nerve to innervate the iris. The fibers also innervate the tarsal muscles of the eyelids. Damage to these pathways causes **Horner's syndrome,** which consists of miosis, ptosis, and sometimes impaired sweating ipsilateral to the lesion.

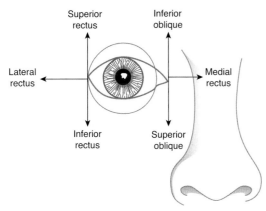

FIGURE 7–23 Extraocular muscles subserving the six cardinal positions of gaze. The eye is adducted by the medial rectus and abducted by the lateral rectus. The adducted eye is elevated by the inferior oblique and depressed by the superior oblique; the abducted eye is elevated by the superior rectus and depressed by the inferior rectus. (Redrawn, with permission, from Greenberg DA, Aminoff MJ, Simon RP. *Clinical Neurology*, 5th ed. McGraw-Hill, 2002.)

Physiology

A. Vision

The rods are sensitive to low levels of light and are most numerous in the peripheral regions of the retina. In retinitis pigmentosa, there is degeneration of the retina that begins in the periphery. Poor twilight vision is thus an early symptom of this disorder. Cones are responsible for perception of stimuli in bright light and for discrimination of color. They are concentrated in the macular region, which is crucial for visual acuity. In disorders of the retina or optic nerve that impair acuity, diminished color discrimination is often an early sign.

Visual processing begins in the retina, where information gathered from rods and cones is modified by interactions among bipolar, amacrine, and horizontal cells. Amacrine and bipolar cells send their output to ganglion cells, whose axons comprise the optic nerve. Photoreceptors convey information about the absolute level of illumination. Retinal processing renders ganglion cells sensitive to simultaneous differences in contrast for detection of edges of objects.

Ganglion cell axons terminate in a highly ordered fashion in well-defined layers of the lateral geniculate nuclei. Because of the separation of fibers in the optic chiasm, the receptive fields of cells in the lateral geniculate lie in the contralateral visual field. Geniculate neurons are arranged in six layers, and ganglion cell axons from each eye terminate in separate layers. Cells in different layers are in register, so that the receptive fields of cells in the same part of each layer are in corresponding regions of the two retinas. A greater proportion of cells are devoted to the macular region of both retinas. This reflects use of the central retina for high acuity and color vision. Some visual processing occurs in the geniculate, particularly for contrast and edge perception and detection of movement.

In the primary visual cortex, visual fields from the eyes are also represented in a topographic projection. Cortical neu-

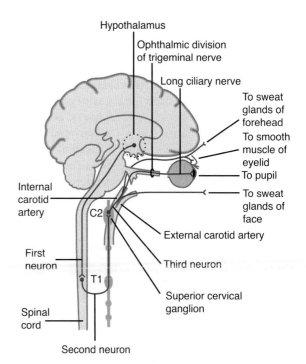

FIGURE 7–24 Oculosympathetic pathways. This three-neuron pathway projects from the hypothalamus to the intermediolateral column of the spinal cord, then to the superior cervical (sympathetic) ganglion, and finally to the pupil, the smooth muscle of the eyelids, and the sweat glands of the forehead and face. Interruption of these pathways results in Horner's syndrome. (Redrawn, with permission, from Greenberg DA, Aminoff MJ, Simon RP. *Clinical Neurology*, 5th ed. McGraw-Hill, 2002.)

rons are functionally organized in columns perpendicular to the cortical surface. Geniculate fibers terminate within layer IV of the visual cortex, and cells within a column above and below layer IV show the same eye preference and similar receptive fields. Narrow alternating columns of cells supplied by one eye or the other lie next to each other (**ocular dominance columns**). A tremendous amount of visual processing occurs in primary visual cortex, including the synthesis of complex receptive fields and determination of axis orientation, position, and color. The retina is not simply represented as a map on the cortex; rather, each area of the retina is represented in multiple columns and analyzed with respect to position, color, and orientation of objects. As in the geniculate, a major portion of the primary visual cortex is devoted to analysis of information derived from the macular regions of both retinas. Cortical areas 18 and 19 (and many other areas) provide higher levels of visual processing.

The anatomic organization of the visual system is useful for localizing neurologic disease (Figure 7–22). Lesions of the retina or optic nerves (**prechiasmal lesions**) impair vision from the ipsilateral eye. Lesions that compress the central portion of the chiasm, such as pituitary tumors, disrupt crossing fibers from the nasal halves of both retinas, causing **bitemporal hemianopia**. Lesions involving structures behind the chiasm (**retrochiasmal lesions**) cause visual loss in the contralateral field of both eyes. Lesions that completely destroy the optic tract, lateral geniculate nucleus, or optic radiations on one side produce a contralateral **homonymous hemianopia.** Selective destruction of temporal lobe optic radiations causes **superior quadrantanopia,** and lesions of the parietal optic radiations cause **inferior quadrantanopia.** The posterior portions of the optic radiations and the calcarine cortex are supplied mainly by the posterior cerebral artery, although the macular region of the visual cortex receives some collateral supply from the middle cerebral artery. Therefore, a lesion of primary visual cortex generally causes contralateral homonymous hemianopia, but if it is due to posterior cerebral artery occlusion it may spare macular vision.

B. Eye Movements

Conjugate eye movements are regulated by proprioceptive information from neck structures and information about head movement and position from the vestibular system. This information is used to maintain fixation on a stationary point when moving the head. In a comatose patient, the integrity of these oculovestibular and oculocephalic pathways can be assessed by the "doll's eye" maneuver. This is elicited by briskly turning the head, which normally results in conjugate movement of the eyes in the opposite direction in a comatose patient. Irrigation of the ear with 10–20 mL of cold water reduces the activity of the labyrinth on that side and elicits jerk nystagmus, with the fast component away from the irrigated ear in a conscious individual. In coma, the fast saccadic component is lost, and the vestibular influence on eye movements dominates. Cold-water irrigation then results in deviation of the eyes toward the irrigated ear. These caloric responses are lost with midbrain or pontine lesions, with damage to the labyrinths, or with drugs that inhibit vestibular function.

C. Pupillary Function

The size of the pupils is controlled by the amount of ambient light sensed by the retina (Figure 7–25). Fibers from each retina terminate within midbrain pretectal nuclei that send fibers to both Edinger-Westphal nuclei. The fibers mediate pupillary constriction in bright light. In dim light, this reflex is inhibited and the influence of sympathetic fibers predominates, causing pupillary dilatation. The pupillary constrictor fibers release acetylcholine, which activates muscarinic AChRs and thus stimulates contraction of the pupillary sphincter muscle of the iris. Sympathetic pupillary fibers release norepinephrine, which activates α_1-adrenergic receptors, causing contraction of the radial muscle of the iris. Drugs that inhibit muscarinic receptors, such as atropine, or that stimulate α_1-adrenergic receptors, such as epinephrine, dilate the pupils, whereas drugs that stimulate muscarinic receptors or block α_1-adrenergic receptors cause pupillary constriction.

CHECKPOINT

22. What is the pathway of fibers from the retina to the visual cortex?
23. What is the innervation of the extraocular muscles?
24. Describe how lesions in various parts of the visual pathways produce characteristic visual field defects.

HEARING & BALANCE

Anatomy

Structures of the middle ear serve to amplify and transmit sounds to the cochlea, where specialized sensory cells (hair cells) are organized to detect ranges in amplitude and frequency of sound. The semicircular canals contain specialized hair cells that detect movement of endolymphatic fluid contained within the canals. Similar hair cells in the saccule and utricle detect movement of the otolithic membrane, which is composed of calcium carbonate crystals embedded in a matrix. The semicircular canal hair cells detect angular acceleration, whereas the hair cells of the utricle and saccule detect linear acceleration. Axons from auditory and vestibular neurons comprise the eighth cranial nerve, which traverses the petrous bone, is joined by the facial nerve, and enters the posterior fossa through the auditory canal. Auditory fibers terminate in the cochlear nuclei of the pons, and vestibular fibers terminate in the vestibular nuclear complex.

Cochlear neurons send fibers bilaterally to a network of auditory nuclei in the midbrain, and impulses are finally relayed through the medial geniculate thalamic nuclei to the

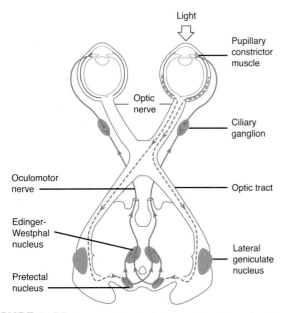

FIGURE 7–25 Anatomic basis of the pupillary light reflex. The afferent visual pathways from the retina to the pretectal nuclei of the midbrain are represented by dashed lines, the efferent pupilloconstrictor pathways from the midbrain to the retinas by solid lines. Note that illumination of one eye results in bilateral pupillary constriction. (Redrawn, with permission, from Greenberg DA, Aminoff MJ, Simon RP. *Clinical Neurology,* 5th ed. McGraw-Hill, 2002.)

auditory cortex in the superior temporal gyri. Vestibular nuclei have connections with the cerebellum, red nuclei, brainstem gaze centers, and brainstem reticular formation. The vestibular nuclei exert considerable control over posture through descending vestibulospinal, rubrospinal, and reticulospinal pathways.

Physiology

A. Hearing

There are three types of hearing loss: (1) **conductive deafness,** which is due to diseases of the external or middle ear that impair conduction and amplification of sound from the air to the cochlea; (2) **sensorineural deafness,** resulting from diseases of the cochlea or eighth cranial nerve; and (3) **central deafness,** resulting from diseases affecting the cochlear nuclei or auditory pathways in the CNS. Because of the redundancy of central pathways, almost all cases of hearing loss are due to conductive or sensorineural deafness. Besides hearing loss, auditory diseases may cause **tinnitus,** the subjective sensation of noise in the ear. Tinnitus resulting from disorders of the cochlea or eighth cranial nerve sounds like a constant nonmusical tone and may be described as ringing, whistling, hissing, humming, or roaring. Transient episodes of tinnitus occur in most individuals and are not associated with disease. When persistent, tinnitus is often associated with hearing loss.

Conductive and sensorineural deafness may be distinguished by examining hearing with a vibrating 512-Hz tuning fork. In the **Rinne test,** the tuning fork is held on the mastoid process behind the ear and then is placed at the auditory meatus. If the sound is louder at the meatus, the test is positive. Normally the test is positive because sound transmitted through air is amplified by middle-ear structures. In sensorineural deafness, although sound perception is reduced, the Rinne test is still positive because middle-ear structures are intact. In conductive deafness, sounds are heard less well through air and the test is negative. In the **Weber test,** the tuning fork is applied to the forehead at the midline. In conductive deafness, the sound is heard best in the abnormal ear, whereas with sensorineural deafness the sound is heard best in the normal ear. **Audiometry** can distinguish types of hearing loss. In general, sensorineural deafness causes greater loss of high-pitched sounds, whereas conductive deafness causes more loss of low-pitched sounds.

B. Vestibular Function

In contrast to hearing, vestibular function is commonly disturbed by small brainstem lesions. The vestibular nuclei occupy a large portion of the lateral brainstem, extending from medulla to midbrain. Although there are extensive bilateral connections between vestibular nuclei and other motor pathways, these connections are not redundant but are highly lateralized and act in concert to control posture, balance, and conjugate eye movement.

Patients with diseases of the vestibular system complain of disequilibrium and dizziness. Cerebellar disease also causes disequilibrium, but this is often described as a problem with coordination rather than a feeling of dizziness in the head. Interpretation of the complaint of dizziness can often be difficult. Many patients use the term loosely to describe sensations of light-headedness, weakness, or malaise. Directed questioning is often required to establish whether there is truly an abnormal sensation of movement (**vertigo**).

Vertigo may be due to disease of the labyrinth or vestibular nerve (peripheral vertigo) or to dysfunction of brainstem and CNS pathways (central vertigo). In general, peripheral vertigo is more severe and associated with nausea and vomiting, especially if the onset is acute. Diseases of the semicircular canal neurons or their fibers frequently cause rotational vertigo, whereas diseases involving the utricle or saccule cause sensations of tilting or listing, as on a boat. Traumatic and ischemic lesions may cause associated hearing loss. Dysfunction of one labyrinth often causes horizontal and rotatory **jerk nystagmus.** The slow phase of the nystagmus is caused by the unopposed action of the normal labyrinth, which drives the eyes to the side of the lesion. The fast-jerk phase is due to a rapid saccade, which maintains fixation.

Vertigo resulting from lesions of the CNS is usually less severe than peripheral vertigo and is often associated with other findings of brainstem dysfunction. In addition, nystagmus associated with central lesions may be present in vertical or multiple directions of gaze. Common causes of central vertigo include brainstem ischemia, brainstem tumors, and multiple sclerosis.

CONSCIOUSNESS, AROUSAL, & COGNITION

Anatomy

Consciousness is awareness of self and the environment. It has two aspects: **arousal,** which is the state of wakefulness, and **cognition,** which is the sum of mental activities. This distinction is useful because neurologic disorders can affect arousal and cognition differently. Arousal is generated by activity of the ascending reticular activating system (Figure 7–26), which is composed of neurons within the central mesencephalic brainstem, the lateral hypothalamus, and the medial, intralaminar, and reticular nuclei of the thalamus. Widespread projections from these nuclei synapse on distal dendritic fields of large pyramidal neurons in the cerebral cortex and generate an arousal response. Cognition is the chief function of the cerebral cortex, particularly of prefrontal cortex and cortical association areas of the occipital, temporal, and parietal lobes. Some specialized mental functions are localized to specific cortical regions. Several subcortical nuclei in the basal ganglia and thalamus are intimately linked with cortical association areas, and damage to these nuclei or their interconnections with cortex may give rise to cognitive deficits similar to those observed with cortical lesions.

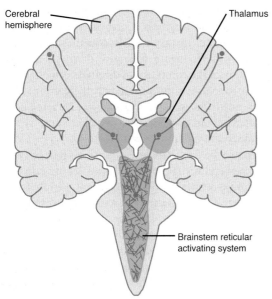

FIGURE 7–26 Brainstem reticular activating system and its ascending projections to the thalamus and cerebral hemispheres. (Redrawn, with permission, from Greenberg DA, Aminoff MJ, Simon RP. *Clinical Neurology*, 5th ed. McGraw-Hill, 2002.)

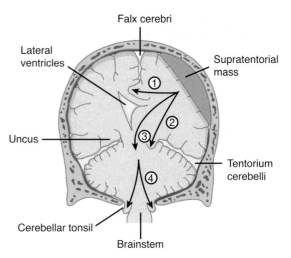

FIGURE 7–27 Anatomic basis of herniation syndromes. An expanding supratentorial mass lesion may cause brain tissue to be displaced into an adjacent intracranial compartment, resulting in (1) cingulate herniation under the falx cerebri, (2) downward transtentorial (central) herniation, (3) uncal herniation over the edge of the tentorium, or (4) cerebellar tonsillar herniation into the foramen magnum. Coma and ultimately death result when (2), (3), or (4) produces brainstem compression. (Redrawn, with permission, from Greenberg DA, Aminoff MJ, Simon RP. *Clinical Neurology*, 5th ed. McGraw-Hill, 2002.)

Physiology

A. Arousal

The reticular activating system is excited by a wide variety of stimuli, especially somatosensory stimuli. It is most compact in the midbrain and can be damaged by central midbrain lesions, resulting in failure of arousal, or **coma.** Higher nuclei and projections are less localized, and lesions rostrad to the midbrain, therefore, must be bilateral to cause coma.

Less severe dysfunction causes **confusional states** in which consciousness is clouded and the patient is sleepy, inattentive, and disoriented. Alertness is reduced, and the patient appears drowsy or falls asleep easily without frequent stimulation. More awake patients perceive stimuli slowly but are distractible, assigning important and irrelevant stimuli equal value. Perceptions may be distorted, leading to **hallucinations,** and the patient may be unable to organize and interpret a complex set of stimuli. The inability to perceive properly interferes with learning and memory and with problem solving. Thoughts become disorganized and tangential, and the confused patient may maintain false beliefs even in the face of evidence of their falsity (**delusions**). In some cases, the confusional state presents as **delirium,** which is characterized by heightened alertness, disordered perception, agitation, delusions, hallucinations, convulsions, and autonomic hyperactivity (sweating, tachycardia, hypertension).

Coma may result from structural or metabolic causes. Some structural lesions of the cerebral hemispheres, such as hemorrhages, large areas of ischemic infarction, abscesses, or tumors can expand over minutes or a few hours and cause brain tissue to herniate into the posterior fossa (Figure 7–27). If lateral within the temporal lobe, the expanding mass may drive the uncus of the temporal lobe into the ambient cistern surrounding the midbrain, compressing the ipsilateral third cranial nerve (**uncal herniation**). This causes pupillary dilation and impaired function of eye muscles innervated by that nerve. Continued pressure distorts the midbrain, and the patient lapses into coma with posturing of the limbs. With continued herniation, pontine function is impaired, causing loss of oculovestibular responses. Eventually, medullary function is lost and breathing ceases. Hemispheric lesions closer to the midline compress the thalamic reticular formation structures and can cause coma before eye findings develop (**central herniation**). With continued pressure, midbrain function is affected, causing the pupils to dilate and the limbs to posture. With progressive herniation, pontine vestibular and then medullary respiratory functions are lost.

Several nonstructural disorders that diffusely disturb brain function can produce a confusional state or, if severe, coma (Table 7–1). Most of these disorders are acute, and many, particularly those caused by drugs and metabolic toxins, are reversible. Clues to the cause of these "metabolic" encephalopathies are provided by general physical examination, drug screens, and certain blood studies. When these disorders cause coma, pupillary light responses are usually preserved despite impaired oculovestibular or respiratory function. This finding is of great help in distinguishing metabolic from structural causes of coma.

Neurons in the dorsal midbrain and especially nuclei within the pontine reticular formation are important for **sleep.** Thus, lesions involving the pons may preserve consciousness but disturb sleep. In contrast, diffuse lesions of the

TABLE 7–1 Nonstructural causes of confusional states and coma.

Drugs (sedative-hypnotics, ethanol, opioids)
Global cerebral ischemia
Hepatic encephalopathy
Hypercalcemia
Hyperosmolar states
Hyperthermia
Hypoglycemia
Hyponatremia
Hypoxia
Hypothyroidism
Meningitis and encephalitis
Seizure or prolonged postictal state
Subarachnoid hemorrhage
Thyrotoxicosis
Uremia
Wernicke's encephalopathy

neocortex, such as those resulting from global cerebral ischemia, may preserve the reticular activating system and brainstem sleep centers, resulting in a patient with preserved sleep-wake cycles who cannot interact in any meaningful way with the environment (coma vigil or apallic state).

B. Cognition

Several disorders disturb cognition rather than the level of consciousness. Specific cortical regions generally mediate different cognitive functions, although there is considerable overlap and interconnection between cortical and subcortical structures in all mental tasks. When several of these abilities are impaired, the patient is said to suffer from **dementia.** Dementia is discussed in more detail later in this chapter.

The prefrontal cortex (Figure 7–9) generally refers to areas 9, 10, 11, 12, 45, 46, and 47 of Brodmann on the superior and lateral surfaces of the frontal lobes and the anterior cingulate, parolfactory, and orbitofrontal cortex inferiorly and mesially. These regions are essential for orderly planning and sequencing of complex behaviors, attending to several stimuli or ideas simultaneously, concentrating and flexibly altering the focus of concentration, grasping the context and meaning of information, and controlling impulses, emotions, and thought sequences. Damage to the frontal lobes or connections to the caudate and dorsal medial nuclei of the thalamus causes the **frontal lobe syndrome.** Patients may suffer dramatic alterations in personality and behavior, whereas most sensorimo-

tor functions remain intact. Some patients become vulgar in speech, slovenly, grandiose, and irascible, whereas others lose interest, spontaneity, curiosity, and initiative. The affect may become apathetic and blunted (**abulia**). Some patients lose the capacity for creativity and abstract reasoning and the ability to solve problems while becoming excessively concrete in their thinking. Often they are distractible and unable to focus attention when presented with multiple stimuli. The most dramatic manifestations are seen after bilateral frontal lobe damage; unilateral damage can lead to subtle alterations in behavior that may be difficult to detect. Involvement of premotor areas may lead to incontinence, inability to perform learned motor tasks (**apraxia**), variable increases in muscle tone (**paratonia**), and appearance of primitive grasp and oral reflexes (sucking, snouting, and rooting).

In about 90% of people, **language** is a function of the left hemisphere. Whereas 99% of right-handed people are left hemisphere dominant, about 40% of left-handed people are right hemisphere dominant for language. In most left-handed people, hemispheric dominance for language is incomplete, and damage to the dominant hemisphere tends to disturb language less severely than in right-handed individuals. The cortical regions most critical for language include Broca's area (area 44), Wernicke's area (area 22), the primary auditory cortex (areas 41 and 42), and neighboring frontal and temporoparietal association areas (Figure 7–9). Injury to these areas or their connections to other cortical regions result in **aphasia.** Lesions in the frontal speech areas cause nonfluent, dysarthric, halting speech, whereas lesions of the temporal speech area cause fluent speech that contains many errors or may be totally devoid of understandable words. Patients with damage to temporal speech areas also lack comprehension of spoken words. Isolation of the temporal speech area from the occipital lobes causes an inability to read (**alexia**). Portions of the parietal lobe adjacent to the temporal lobe are important for retrieval of previously learned words, and damage here may result in **anomia.** The inferior parietal region is important for the translation of linguistic messages generated in the temporal language areas into visual symbols. Damage to this region may result in an inability to write (**agraphia**).

Memory requires that information be registered by the primary somatosensory, auditory, or visual cortex. Posterior cortical areas involved in comprehension of language are needed for immediate processing of spoken or written events and recalling them immediately. The hippocampi and their connections to the dorsal medial nuclei of the thalamus and the mamillary nuclei of the hypothalamus constitute a limbic system network crucial for learning and processing of events for long-term storage. When these areas are damaged, the patient is unable to learn new material or retrieve memories from the recent past. The most severe symptoms occur with bilateral lesions; unilateral disease causes more subtle learning deficits. Memories that remain with a person for years are considered remote memories and are stored in corresponding association cortex areas (eg, visual cortex for scenes). Remote memories remain intact in patients with damage to limbic structures required for learning. However, they may be lost by damage to cortical association areas. Understanding the mechanisms by which recent memories are transferred from the limbic memory network to association cortex for long-term storage is a major goal of current research.

The parietal association cortex is the region principally involved in visuomotor integration of constructional tasks. The visual cortex is required for observation, whereas the auditory cortex and the temporal language cortex are necessary for drawing objects on command. The inferior parietal cortex (areas 39 and 40) integrates visual and auditory information, and the output from this region is translated into motor patterns by motor cortex. Thus, lesions to the parietal lobes commonly cause constructional impairment. Damage to either hemisphere may result in constructional errors. Drawings may show rotation of objects, disorientation of objects on the background, fragmentation of design, inability to draw angles properly, or omission of parts of a figure presented for copying. It is often difficult to determine which side is damaged, although if language is preserved a nondominant parietal deficit is more likely.

Calculation ability, abstract reasoning, problem solving, and several other aspects of intelligence are difficult to localize because they require integration of several cortical regions. They are frequently disturbed by diseases that cause widespread cortical dysfunction, such as those that cause dementia.

CHECKPOINT

25. What is the network of neurons that maintain normal arousal and consciousness?
26. What are the symptoms and signs of cerebral herniation caused by focal brain lesions?
27. Which cognitive functions are controlled by the frontal lobes and by the parietal association cortex?
28. What regions of the cortex are important for language and memory?

PATHOPHYSIOLOGY OF SELECTED NEUROLOGIC DISORDERS

Nervous system disease may be caused by a wide variety of degenerative, metabolic, structural, neoplastic, or inflammatory conditions that affect neurons, glia, or both. The resultant dysfunction is expressed by either neuronal hyperactivity, as seen during seizures, or decreased activity of neurons, as observed after a stroke. The specific functional abnormalities observed depend on the network of neurons affected. For example, because amyotrophic lateral sclerosis is a disorder of upper and lower motor neurons, neurologic deficits are limited to the motor system. In Parkinson's disease, dopaminergic neurons of the substantia nigra degenerate, causing symptoms of extrapyramidal motor system dysfunction. In patients with ischemic stroke, the particular constellation of deficits is determined by the vascular territory affected. Therefore, an understanding of the pathophysiology of neurologic disease requires an analysis of events occurring at both the cellular level and the level of neural networks.

MOTOR NEURON DISEASE

Clinical Presentation

Motor neuron diseases predominantly affect the anterior horn cells of the spinal cord and are characterized by wasting and weakness of skeletal muscles. Spontaneous discharges of degenerating motor nerve fibers occur, giving rise to muscle twitches known as **fasciculations** (see prior discussion). Electromyography characteristically shows features of denervation, including increased numbers of spontaneous discharges (**fibrillations**) in resting muscle and a reduction in the number of motor units detected during voluntary contraction. Sprouting of remaining healthy motor fibers may occur, leading to the appearance of large, polyphasic motor unit potentials (reinnervation).

The **spinal muscular atrophies** (**SMAs**) are a heterogeneous group of genetic diseases characterized by selective degeneration of lower motor neurons. The most common form is autosomal recessive with childhood onset and has a frequency of between 1:6,000 and 1:10,000. Childhood SMA has been divided into three types depending on age of onset and clinical progression. SMA I is infantile spinal muscular atrophy (**Werdnig-Hoffman disease**), a disorder that manifests usually within the first 3 months of life. Infants with this condition have difficulty sucking, swallowing, and breathing. Atrophy and fasciculations are found in the tongue and limb muscles. SMA I is rapidly progressive, leading to death from respiratory complications usually by age 3. SMA II begins in the latter half of the first year of life. It progresses more slowly than the infantile form, and patients may survive into adulthood. SMA III (**Kugelberg-Welander disease**) is a juvenile form that develops after age 2. Patients develop weakness of proximal limb muscles with relative sparing of bulbar muscles. The pattern of weakness can falsely suggest a myopathy such as limb-girdle dystrophy rather than a motor neuron disease. The course is gradually progressive, leading to disability in adulthood. All three forms of SMA are due to deletions or mutations in the survival motor neuron 1 (*SMN1*) gene on chromosome 5q13. The SMN gene product is expressed in all tissues and appears to be involved in RNA metabolism. Loss of SMN function promotes apoptosis of lower motor neurons.

It is not yet known why motor neurons are selectively affected. Recent clinical trials are aimed at adjusting the levels of the SMN protein to try to modulate disease progression using drugs such as hydroxyurea and valproic acid.

In adults, motor neuron disease usually begins between the ages of 20 and 80 years, with an average age at onset of 56 years. It is commonly sporadic but is familial in up to 10% of cases. Several varieties have been described, depending on relative involvement of upper or lower motor neurons and bulbar or spinal anterior horn cells. For example, X-linked spinobulbar atrophy is an X-linked recessive disorder that typically manifests clinically in the fourth or fifth decade and is associated with an expanded CAG repeat in the androgen receptor gene. As with other genetic disorders associated with triplet repeat expansions, the neurodegeneration is associated with neuronal inclusions. Testosterone promotes the development of inclusions, and women homozygous for the mutation develop only mild symptoms. Moreover, female mice carrying the mutation show motor impairment after testosterone administration, whereas castration reduces impairment in male mice. These findings have led to testing of gonadotropin-releasing hormone antagonists, which reduce testosterone release from the testes, as treatments for the disease.

The most common form of motor neuron disease in adults is **amyotrophic lateral sclerosis (ALS)**, in which mixed upper and lower motor neuron deficits are found in limb and bulbar muscles. In 80% of patients, the initial symptoms are due to weakness of limb muscles. Complaints are often bilateral but asymmetric. Involvement of bulbar muscles causes difficulty with swallowing, chewing, speaking, breathing, and coughing.

Neurologic examination reveals a mixture of upper and lower motor neuron signs. There is usually no involvement of extraocular muscles or sphincters. The disease is progressive and generally fatal within 3–5 years, with death usually resulting from pulmonary infection and respiratory failure.

Pathology & Pathogenesis

In ALS, there is selective degeneration of motor neurons in the primary motor cortex and the anterolateral horns of the spinal cord. Many affected neurons show cytoskeletal disease with accumulations of intermediate filaments in the cell body and in axons. There is only a subtle glial cell response and little evidence of inflammation. The cause is unknown, but biochemical and genetic studies have provided several clues.

A. Glutamate Signaling and RNA Processing

Glutamate (Figure 7–28) is the most abundant excitatory neurotransmitter in the CNS. Glutamate activates a large family of receptors that either open cation channels (ionotropic receptors) or activate phospholipase C (metabotropic receptors), which catalyzes the formation of the second messenger, inositol-1,4,5-trisphosphate (IP_3). Influx of Na^+ and Ca^{2+} through glutamate-gated cation channels depolarizes cells, whereas IP_3 stimulates release of Ca^{2+} from intracellular storage sites. The net effect of these events is to generate an excitatory postsynaptic potential and raise the concentration of free intracellular Ca^{2+} in the cytosol of the postsynaptic neuron. This Ca^{2+} signal activates calcium-sensitive enzymes and is quickly terminated

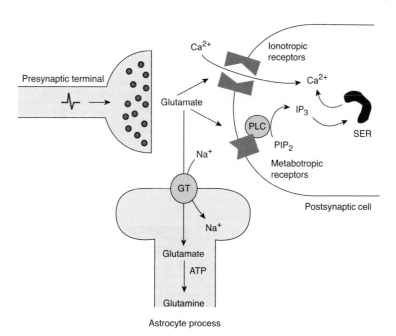

FIGURE 7–28 Glutamatergic neurotransmission. Depolarization stimulates release of glutamate from presynaptic terminals into the synaptic cleft, where it binds to ionotropic or metabotropic glutamate receptors, stimulating Ca^{2+} influx and activation of phospholipase C (PLC). PLC catalyzes hydrolysis of phosphatidylinositol-4,5-bisphosphate (PIP_2) to produce inositol-1,4,5-trisphosphate (IP_3), which causes release of Ca^{2+} from storage sites in smooth endoplasmic reticulum (SER). Synaptic actions of glutamate are terminated mainly by uptake through Na^+-dependent glutamate transporters (GT) on glia. In astrocytes, glutamate is converted into glutamine by glutamine synthetase.

by removal of glutamate from the synapse and by mechanisms for calcium sequestration and extrusion in the postsynaptic cell. Breakdown of normal mechanisms for terminating the excitatory signal leads to sustained elevations of intracellular Ca^{2+} that cause cell death.

Glutamate is removed from synapses by transport proteins on surrounding astrocytes and nerve terminals. In astrocytes, it is metabolized to glutamine and can be shuttled back to neurons for reconversion into glutamate. In 60% of patients with sporadic ALS, there is a large decrease in glutamate transport activity in the motor cortex and spinal cord but not in other regions of the CNS. This has been associated with a loss of the astrocytic glutamate transporter protein excitatory amino acid transporter 2 (EAAT2), perhaps resulting from a defect in splicing of its messenger RNA. In cultured spinal cord slices, pharmacologic inhibition of glutamate transport induces motor neuron degeneration. Thus, selective loss of a glutamate transporter may cause excitotoxicity in ALS by increasing extracellular levels of glutamate.

A second alteration in glutamate signaling has been found recently in spinal motor neurons from five patients with ALS. RNA editing is a process whereby gene-specified codons are altered by RNA-dependent deaminases. In GluR2 receptor subunits, this process is virtually 100% efficient, resulting in conversion of a glutamine to arginine in the second transmembrane domain of this subunit, which markedly reduces the calcium permeability of a major subclass of glutamate receptors. Editing efficiency was reduced in more than 50% of neurons from the patients with ALS. Because transgenic mice that express GluR2 made artificially more permeable to calcium develop a motor neuron disease late in life, it is possible that defective editing of GluR2 contributes to ALS pathogenesis. These findings suggest that sporadic ALS may be caused by a defect in RNA metabolism.

B. Free Radicals

About 10% of ALS cases are familial and 20% of these familial cases are due to missense mutations in the **cytosolic copper-zinc superoxide dismutase (*SOD1*)** gene on the long arm of chromosome 21. SOD1 catalyzes the formation of hydrogen peroxide from superoxide anion. Hydrogen peroxide is then detoxified by catalase or glutathione peroxidase to form water. Not all mutations reduce *SOD1* activity, and the disorder is typically inherited as an autosomal dominant trait, suggesting that familial ALS results from a gain rather than a loss of function. This is supported by the finding that transgenic mice expressing mutant *SOD1* develop motor neuron disease analogous to human familial ALS, whereas mice lacking SOD1 do not develop motor neuron disease. One hypothesis suggests that the mutant enzyme has an altered substrate specificity catalyzing the reduction of hydrogen peroxide to yield hydroxyl radicals and utilizing peroxynitrite to produce nitration of tyrosine residues in proteins. This is consistent with elevated levels of carbonyl proteins in the brain and elevated levels of free nitrotyrosine

in the spinal cord of ALS patients. EAAT2 may also be inactivated by mutant SOD1, thereby promoting excitotoxicity. Some mutations also promote the formation of SOD aggregates, which may be neurotoxic.

C. Cytoskeletal Proteins

Motor neurons tend to be very large, with extremely long axons, and cytoskeletal proteins that maintain axonal structure may be critical targets for motor neuron injury. A role for neurofilament dysfunction in ALS is supported by the finding that neurofilamentous inclusions in cell bodies and proximal axons are an early feature of ALS pathology. In addition, mutations in the heavy chain neurofilament subunit (NF-H) have been detected in some patients with sporadic ALS, suggesting that NF-H variants may be a risk factor for ALS. Peripherin is another intermediate filament protein found with neurofilaments in neuronal inclusions in ALS and in mice with *SOD1* mutations. Peripherin expression is increased in response to cell injury, and overexpression of peripherin causes a late-onset motor neuron disease in mice. Inclusions containing peripherin and neurofilaments may interfere with axonal transport, resulting in failure to maintain axonal structure and transport of macromolecules such as neurotrophic factors required for motor neuron survival.

D. TDP-43

An exciting recent discovery of the protein transactive response DNA-binding protein 43 (TDP 43) may offer new clues to the etiology of this disorder. This newly discovered protein is the major component of the ubiquitinated, tau-negative, inclusions that are the pathological hallmark of sporadic and familial ALS and frontotemporal dementia (FTD). It is also found in some cases of Alzheimer's disease and Parkinson's disease. Mutations in this gene, which is located on chromosome 1, co-segregate with disease in familial forms of ALS and FTD and are not found in *SOD1* familial ALS. FTD and ALS overlap in approximately 15–25% of cases and these disorders are starting to be referred to as "TDP-43 proteinopathies." Several other genes and gene regions have been identified to cause both FTD and ALS such as *TARDBP* on chromosome 1p36.2, *MAPT* on chromosome *7q21*, and *DCTN1* on chromosome 2p13.

CHECKPOINT

29. What are the clinical features of motor neuron disease?
30. What gene is responsible for some cases of familial ALS, and what is a postulated molecular mechanism by which the mutation causes disease?
31. What two other mechanisms may play a role in motor neuron degeneration?

PARKINSON'S DISEASE

Clinical Presentation

Parkinsonism is a clinical syndrome of rigidity, bradykinesia, tremor, and postural instability. Most cases are due to Parkinson's disease, an idiopathic disorder with a prevalence of about 1–2 per 1000. In the first half of the last century, parkinsonism was a common sequela of von Economo's encephalitis. Parkinsonism can also result from exposure to certain toxins such as manganese, carbon disulfide, 1-methyl-4-phenyl-1,2,3,6-tetrahydropyridine (MPTP), and carbon monoxide. Several drugs, particularly butyrophenones, phenothiazines, metoclopramide, reserpine, and tetrabenazine, can cause reversible parkinsonism. Parkinsonism may also result from repeated head trauma or may be a feature of several basal ganglia diseases, including Wilson's disease, some cases of early onset Huntington's disease, Shy-Drager syndrome, striatonigral degeneration, and progressive supranuclear palsy. In these disorders, other symptoms and signs are present along with parkinsonism.

Pathology & Pathogenesis

In Parkinson's disease, there is selective degeneration of monoamine-containing cell populations in the brainstem and basal ganglia, particularly of pigmented dopaminergic neurons of the substantia nigra. In addition, scattered neurons in basal ganglia, brainstem, spinal cord, and sympathetic ganglia contain eosinophilic, cytoplasmic inclusion bodies (**Lewy bodies**). These contain filamentous aggregates of α-synuclein, along with parkin, synphilin, neurofilaments, and synaptic vesicle proteins.

Important clues about the pathogenesis of Parkinson's disease have been discovered through study of the potent neurotoxin MPTP. MPTP is a by-product of synthesis of a synthetic opioid derivative of meperidine. Illicit use of opioid preparations heavily contaminated with MPTP led to several cases of parkinsonism in the early 1980s. MPTP selectively injures dopaminergic neurons in the brain and produces a clinical syndrome very similar to Parkinson's disease.

MPTP enters the brain (Figure 7–29) and is converted by monoamine oxidase B present in glia and serotonergic nerve terminals to N-methyl-4-phenyldihydropyridine (MPDP$^+$), which diffuses across glial membranes and then undergoes nonenzymatic oxidation and reduction to the active metabolite N-methyl-4-phenylpyridinium (MPP$^+$). Plasma membrane transporters that normally act to terminate the action of monoamines by removing them from synapses take up MPP$^+$. Internalized MPP$^+$ inhibits oxidative phosphorylation by interacting with complex I of the mitochondrial electron transport chain. This inhibits ATP production and reduces metabolism of molecular oxygen, allowing for increased formation of peroxide, hydroxyl radicals, and superoxide radicals that react with lipids, proteins, and nucleic acids that cause cell injury. In support of a role for mitochondrial dys-

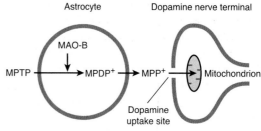

FIGURE 7–29 Proposed mechanism of MPTP-induced parkinsonism. MPTP enters brain astrocytes and is converted to MPDP$^+$ through the action of monoamine oxidase type B (MAO-B). MPDP$^+$ is then metabolized extracellularly to MPP$^+$, which is taken up through dopamine uptake sites on dopamine nerve terminals and concentrated in mitochondria. The resulting disturbance of mitochondrial function can lead to neuronal death. (Redrawn, with permission, from Greenberg DA, Aminoff MJ, Simon RP. *Clinical Neurology,* 5th ed. McGraw-Hill, 2002.)

function and oxidative damage in the pathogenesis of Parkinson's disease is evidence that the insecticide rotenone, which inhibits mitochondrial complex I, produces parkinsonism in animals with degeneration of nigrostriatal dopaminergic neurons and cytoplasmic inclusions that resemble Lewy bodies. Exposure to paraquat, a common herbicide that is structurally similar to MPP$^+$ and also inhibits complex I, can lead to selective degeneration of dopaminergic neurons and aggregation of α-synuclein. Furthermore, impaired complex I activity has been observed in cell lines derived from Parkinson's disease patients, and one genetic variant of NADH dehydrogenase 3 in complex I is associated with a reduced risk of the disease among Caucasians. Thus, alterations in mitochondrial complex I activity appear to play an important role in the pathogenesis of Parkinson's disease.

The reasons why dopaminergic neurons appear selectively vulnerable to complex I inhibition are not clear. Although controversial, some evidence suggests that dopamine can promote neurotoxicity. Addition of exogenous dopamine is toxic to neurons in culture. Dopamine undergoes autooxidation to generate superoxide radicals or is metabolized by monoamine oxidase to generate hydrogen peroxide. Superoxide dismutase catalyzes the conversion of superoxide to H_2O_2, which is converted by glutathione peroxidase and catalase to water. However, H_2O_2 can also react with ferrous iron to form highly reactive hydroxyl radicals. Thus, dopamine within dopaminergic neurons may provide a source of reactive oxygen species, which, when coupled with reduced complex I function, may promote cell death.

Approximately 5% of Parkinson's disease cases are familial. Genetic studies have identified causative mutations in five genes that provide important information about molecular pathways involved in the disease. These genes include the genes for α-synuclein (*PARK1*), parkin (*PARK2*), DJ-1 (*PARK7*), ubiquitin-C-hydrolase-L1 (*PARK5*), PTEN (phosphatase and tensin homolog deleted on chromosome 10)-induced kinase 1 (*PINK1*), and leucine-rich repeat kinase 2 (*LRRK2*).

Mutations in the gene for α-synuclein on chromosome 4q21-23 cause autosomal dominant Parkinson's disease. Alpha-synuclein is found in nerve terminals in close proximity to synaptic vesicles. Its normal function is not known. Overexpression of nonmutant human α-synuclein in transgenic mice results in formation of Lewy bodies, reduced dopaminergic terminals in the striatum, and impaired motor performance. Genomic triplication of α-synuclein leading to overexpression has been documented in a human family with autosomal dominant Parkinson's disease. This suggests that it is the production of neuronal inclusions containing α-synuclein rather than a change in α-synuclein function that contributes to degeneration of dopaminergic neurons. Interestingly, mice lacking α-synuclein are resistant to the toxic effects of the complex I inhibitor MPTP, suggesting that mitochondrial dysfunction generates an environment that favors α-synuclein aggregation and neurodegeneration.

Misfolded, damaged, or unassembled proteins are generally degraded by a process involving covalent attachment of ubiquitin. Ubiquitin is a 76-residue protein that marks proteins for processing by a proteolytic complex (**proteasome**). A missense mutation in one component of the ubiquitin-proteasome system, ubiquitin carboxyl terminal hydrolase L1, has been found in one family with autosomal dominant Parkinson's disease. Mutations in *parkin* on chromosome 6q25 have been identified in cases of autosomal recessive juvenile parkinsonism. *Parkin* is a ubiquitin E3 ligase that catalyzes the addition of ubiquitin to specific proteins to target them for degradation. Known mutations cause loss of function, which presumably leads to a disturbance in protein degradation. However, most patients with *parkin* mutations lack Lewy bodies, suggesting that other mechanisms, such as increased oxidative stress, cause neurodegeneration in these patients. In support of this mechanism is the finding that *Drosophila* mutants that lack *parkin* show mitochondrial pathology.

The most common known genetic form of Parkinson's disease was recently discovered. In 4% of familial cases of Parkinson's disease and 1% of sporadic cases, *LRRK2* mutations are the cause. It is most common in patients from the Middle East and southern Europe. Interestingly, the penetrance is not complete and the risk of obtaining the disease when the mutation is present greatly increases between the ages of 69 and 79 years. This form of Parkinson's disease tends to be more benign than idiopathic Parkinson's disease.

CHECKPOINT

32. What are the clinical features of parkinsonism?

33. What are some of the causes of this syndrome?

34. What are two major mechanisms proposed to explain the pathophysiology of Parkinson's disease?

MYASTHENIA GRAVIS

Clinical Presentation

Myasthenia gravis is an autoimmune disorder of neuromuscular transmission. The major clinical features are fluctuating fatigue and weakness that improve after a period of rest and after administration of acetylcholinesterase inhibitors. Muscles with small motor units, such as ocular muscles, are most often affected. Oropharyngeal muscles, flexors and extensors of the neck, proximal limb muscles, and the erector spinae muscles are involved less often. In severe cases, all muscles are weak, including the diaphragm and intercostal muscles, and death may result from respiratory failure.

About 5% of patients have coexistent hyperthyroidism. Rheumatoid arthritis, systemic lupus erythematosus, and polymyositis are also more common in patients with myasthenia gravis than in the general population, and up to 30% of patients have a maternal relative with an autoimmune disorder. These associations suggest that patients with myasthenia gravis share a genetic predisposition to autoimmune disease.

Pathology & Pathogenesis

The major structural abnormality in myasthenia gravis is a simplification of the postsynaptic region of the neuromuscular synapse. The muscle end plate shows sparse, shallow, and abnormally wide or absent synaptic clefts. In contrast, the number and size of the presynaptic vesicles are normal. Scattered collections of lymphocytes, some within the vicinity of motor end plates, may be present. IgG and the C3 component of complement are present at the postsynaptic membrane.

Electrophysiologic studies indicate that the postsynaptic membrane has a decreased response to applied acetylcholine. Studies with iodine-125–labeled α-bungarotoxin, which binds with high affinity to muscle nicotinic AChRs, show a 70–90% decrease in the number of receptors per end plate in affected muscles. Circulating antibodies to the receptor are present in 90% of patients, and the disorder may be passively transferred to animals by administration of IgG from affected patients. Moreover, immunization with AChR protein from muscle can produce myasthenia in experimental animals. The antibodies block acetylcholine binding and receptor activation (Figure 7–30). In addition, the antibodies cross-link receptor molecules, increasing receptor internalization and degradation. Bound antibody also activates complement-mediated destruction of the postsynaptic region, resulting in simplification of the end plate. Many patients who lack antibodies to the AChR have autoantibodies instead against the muscle-specific receptor tyrosine kinase (MuSK), which is an important mediator of acetylcholine receptor clustering at the end plate. These antibodies inhibit clustering of receptors in muscle cell culture.

During repetitive stimulation of a motor nerve, the number of quanta released from the nerve terminal declines with successive stimuli. Normally, this causes no clinical impairment

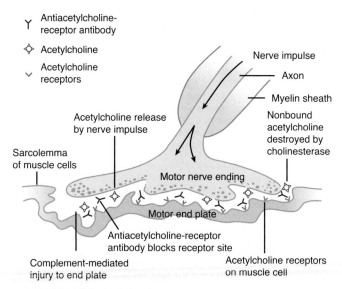

FIGURE 7–30 Pathogenesis of myasthenia gravis. Acetylcholine released at the nerve ending by the nerve impulse normally binds with acetylcholine receptors. This evokes the action potential in the muscle. In myasthenia gravis, antiacetylcholine receptor antibody binds to the acetylcholine receptor and inhibits the action of acetylcholine. Bound antibody evokes immune-mediated destruction of the end plate. (Redrawn, with permission, from Chandrasoma P, Taylor CE. *Concise Pathology,* 3rd ed. Originally published by Appleton & Lange. Copyright © 1998 by the McGraw-Hill Companies, Inc.)

because a sufficient number of AChR channels are opened by the reduced level of neurotransmitter. However, in myasthenia gravis, where there is a deficiency in the number of functional receptors, neuromuscular transmission fails at lower levels of quantal release. Electrophysiologically, this is measured as a decremental decline in the compound muscle action potential during repetitive stimulation of a motor nerve. Clinically, this is manifested by muscle fatigue with sustained or repeated activity.

Treatment has reduced the mortality rate from approximately 30% to 5% in generalized myasthenia gravis. The two basic strategies for treatment that stem from knowledge of the pathogenesis are to increase the amount of acetylcholine at the neuromuscular junction and to inhibit immune-mediated destruction of AChRs.

By preventing metabolism of acetylcholine, cholinesterase inhibitors can compensate for the normal decline in released neurotransmitter during repeated stimulation. Therapy with cholinesterase inhibitors can also cause a paradoxical increase in weakness known as a **cholinergic crisis.** This is due to an excess of acetylcholine. At the molecular level, binding of acetylcholine first opens nicotinic cation channels, but with continued exposure to the agonist the channels desensitize and shut down again. The desensitized channels recover their sensitivity to acetylcholine only after the neurotransmitter is removed. Removal of acetylcholine is impaired when cholinesterase activity is inhibited. This can result in depolarization block of neurotransmission similar to the effect of the depo-

larizing paralytic agent succinylcholine or organophosphate insecticides and nerve gases that markedly inhibit acetylcholinesterase. Therefore, the dose of cholinesterase inhibitors must be carefully regulated to reduce myasthenia but avoid a cholinergic crisis.

Plasmapheresis, corticosteroids, and immunosuppressant drugs are effective in reducing levels of autoantibody to AChRs and suppressing disease. The thymus is thought to play an important role in the pathogenesis of the disease by supplying helper T cells sensitized against thymic proteins that cross-react with AChRs. In most patients with myasthenia gravis, the thymus is hyperplastic, and 10–15% have thymomas. Thymectomy is indicated if a thymoma is suspected. In patients with generalized myasthenia without thymoma, thymectomy induces remission in 35% and improves symptoms in another 45% of patients.

For patients with AChR antibody–negative myasthenia gravis who test positive for the MuSK antibody, the clinical features and treatment are different. Patients tend to be younger women with bulbar weakness, and muscle atrophy is often seen, particularly in the tongue, making the diagnosis more difficult. Results of repetitive stimulation studies and single-fiber EMG studies in the limbs are often normal, necessitating facial studies to make a diagnosis. Cholinesterase inhibitors often make these patients worse, but plasma exchange is very effective, as is less conventional immunosuppressive therapy. Thymectomy is not clearly beneficial in this population.

CHECKPOINT

35. What is the clinical presentation of myasthenia gravis?
36. What causes this disorder?
37. What is the pathophysiology of symptoms in myasthenia gravis?

EPILEPSY

Clinical Presentation

Seizures are paroxysmal disturbances in cerebral function caused by an abnormal synchronous discharge of cortical neurons. The epilepsies are a group of disorders characterized by recurrent seizures. Approximately 0.6% of people in the United States suffer from recurrent seizures, and idiopathic epilepsy accounts for more than 75% of all seizure disorders. In some forms of idiopathic epilepsy, a genetic basis is apparent. Other forms are secondary to brain injury from stroke, trauma, a mass lesion, or infection. About two thirds of new cases arise in children, and most of these cases are idiopathic or caused by trauma. In contrast, seizures or epilepsy with onset in adult life is more often due to underlying brain lesions or metabolic causes.

Seizures are classified by behavioral and electrophysiologic data (Table 7–2). **Generalized tonic-clonic seizures** are attacks characterized by sudden loss of consciousness followed rapidly by tonic contraction of muscles, causing limb extension and arching of the back. The tonic phase lasts 10–30 seconds and is followed by a clonic phase of limb jerking. The jerking builds in frequency to a peak after 15–30 seconds and then slows gradually over another 15–30 seconds. Thereafter, the patient remains unconscious for several minutes. As consciousness is regained, there is a period of postictal confusion lasting several minutes. In patients with recurrent seizures or an underlying structural or metabolic abnormality, confusion may persist for a few hours. Focal abnormalities may be present on neurologic examination during the postictal period. Such findings suggest a focal brain lesion requiring further laboratory and radiologic study.

Typical **absence seizures** begin in childhood and usually remit by adulthood. Seizures are characterized by brief lapses in consciousness lasting several seconds without loss of posture. These spells may be associated with eyelid blinking, slight head movement, or brief jerks of limb muscles. Immediately after the seizure, the patient is fully alert. The spells may occur several times through the day and impair school performance. The electroencephalogram (EEG) shows characteristic runs of spikes and waves at a rate of three per second, particularly after hyperventilation (Figure 7–31). The disorder is transmitted as an autosomal dominant trait with incomplete penetrance.

Some forms of epilepsy cause seizures with only a tonic or clonic phase. In others, the seizure is manifested by sudden loss of muscle tone (atonic seizures). In myoclonic epilepsy, sudden, brief contractions of muscles occur. Myoclonic seizures are found in certain neurodegenerative diseases or after diffuse brain injury, as occurs during global cerebral ischemia.

Partial seizures are caused by focal brain disease. Therefore, in general, patients with simple or complex partial seizures should be investigated for underlying brain lesions. **Simple partial seizures** begin with motor, sensory, visual, psychic, or

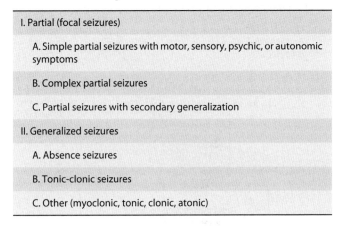

TABLE 7–2 Simplified classification of seizures.

I. Partial (focal seizures)
A. Simple partial seizures with motor, sensory, psychic, or autonomic symptoms
B. Complex partial seizures
C. Partial seizures with secondary generalization
II. Generalized seizures
A. Absence seizures
B. Tonic-clonic seizures
C. Other (myoclonic, tonic, clonic, atonic)

autonomic phenomena depending on the location of the seizure focus. Consciousness is preserved unless the seizure discharge spreads to other areas, producing a tonic-clonic seizure (**secondary generalization**). **Complex partial seizures** are characterized by the sudden onset of impaired consciousness with stereotyped, coordinated, involuntary movements (**automatisms**). Immediately before impairment of consciousness, there may be an aura consisting of unusual abdominal sensations, olfactory or sensory hallucinations, unexplained fear, or illusions of familiarity (déjà vu). Seizures usually last for 2–5 minutes and are followed by postictal confusion. Secondary generalization may occur. The seizure focus usually lies in the temporal or frontal lobe.

Pathogenesis

Normal neuronal activity occurs in a nonsynchronized manner, with groups of neurons inhibited and excited sequentially during the transfer of information between different brain areas. Seizures occur when neurons are activated synchronously. The kind of seizure depends on the location of the abnormal activity and the pattern of spread to different parts of the brain.

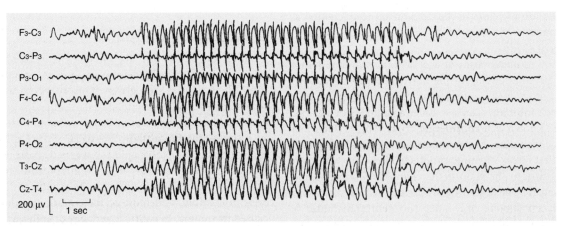

FIGURE 7–31 EEG of a patient with typical absence (petit mal) seizures, showing a burst of generalized 3-Hz spike-and-wave activity (center of record) that is bilaterally symmetric and bisynchronous. Odd-numbered leads indicate electrode placements over the left side of the head; even numbers, those over the right side. (Redrawn, with permission, from Greenberg DA, Aminoff MJ, Simon RP. *Clinical Neurology,* 5th ed. McGraw-Hill, 2002.)

Interictal spike discharges are often observed on EEG recordings from epileptic patients. These are due to synchronous depolarization of a group of neurons in an abnormally excitable area of brain. Experimentally, this is known as the **paroxysmal depolarizing shift** and is followed by a hyperpolarizing afterpotential that is the cellular correlate of the slow wave that follows spike discharges on the EEG. The shift is produced by depolarizing currents generated at excitatory synapses and by subsequent influx of sodium or calcium through voltage-gated channels.

Normally, discharging excitatory neurons activate nearby inhibitory interneurons that suppress the activity of the discharging cell and its neighbors. Most inhibitory synapses utilize the neurotransmitter GABA. Voltage-gated and calcium-dependent potassium currents are also activated in the discharging neuron to suppress excitability. In addition, adenosine generated from adenosine triphosphate (ATP) released during excitation further suppresses neuronal excitation by binding to adenosine receptors present on nearby neurons. Disruption of these inhibitory mechanisms by alterations in ion channels, or by injury to inhibitory neurons and synapses, may allow for the development of a seizure focus. In addition, groups of neurons may become synchronized if local excitatory circuits are enhanced by reorganization of neural networks after brain injury.

Spread of a local discharge occurs by a combination of mechanisms. During the paroxysmal depolarizing shift, extracellular potassium accumulates, depolarizing nearby neurons. Increased frequency of discharges enhances calcium influx into nerve terminals, increasing neurotransmitter release at excitatory synapses by a process known as **posttetanic potentiation.** This involves increased calcium influx through voltage-gated channels and through the N-methyl-D-aspartate (NMDA) subtype of glutamate receptor-gated ion channels. NMDA receptor-gated channels preferentially pass calcium ions but are relatively quiescent during normal synaptic transmission because they are blocked by magnesium ions. Magnesium block is relieved by depolarization. In contrast, the effect of inhibitory synaptic neurotransmission appears to decrease with high-frequency stimulation. This may be partly due to rapid desensitization of GABA receptors at high concentrations of released GABA. The net effect of these changes is to recruit neighboring neurons into a synchronous discharge and cause a seizure.

In secondary epilepsy, loss of inhibitory circuits and sprouting of fibers from excitatory neurons appear to be important for the generation of a seizure focus. In several of the idiopathic epilepsies, genetic studies have identified mutations in ion channels. For example, benign familial neonatal convulsions have been linked to mutations in two homologous voltage-gated K$^+$ channels: KCNQ2 encoded by a gene on chromosome 20q13.3 and KCNQ3 encoded by a gene on chromosome 8q24. Two forms of generalized epilepsy associated with febrile seizures have been linked to mutations in voltage-gated Na$^+$ channel subunits. Another rare condition, autosomal dominant nocturnal frontal lobe epilepsy, is associated with mutations on chromosome 20q13.2 in the gene for the α4 subunit of neuronal nicotinic cholinergic receptors.

Animal models have provided clues to the pathogenesis of absence seizures. Absence seizures arise from synchronous thalamic discharges that are mediated by activation of low-threshold calcium currents (T or "transient" currents) in thalamic neurons. The anticonvulsant ethosuximide blocks T channels and suppresses absence seizures in humans. T channels are more likely to be activated after hyperpolarization of the cell membrane. Activation of GABA$_B$ receptors hyperpolarizes thalamic neurons and facilitates T-channel activation. Lethargic (lh/lh) mice demonstrate frequent absence spells accompanied by 5- to 6-Hz spike-wave discharges on the EEG and respond to drugs used in human absence epilepsy. A single mutation in a gene on chromosome 2 results in this autosomal recessive disorder. There is an increase in the number of GABA$_B$ receptors in the cerebral cortex in these mice, and the GABA$_B$ agonist baclofen worsens the seizures, whereas antagonists alleviate them. This suggests that abnormal regulation of GABA$_B$ receptor function or expression may be important in the pathogenesis of absence seizures. This is supported by the finding that γ-hydroxybutyrate, which causes behavioral and electroencephalographic alterations similar to those seen during absence attacks, activates GABA$_B$ receptors and that GABA$_B$ agonists increase and GABA$_B$ antagonists reduce spike-wave discharges in rats genetically susceptible to absence seizures (GAERS rats).

The main targets for currently available anticonvulsants are (1) voltage-gated ion channels that are involved in the generation of action potentials and in neurotransmitter release and (2) ligand-gated channels that modulate synaptic excitation and inhibition. Many agents act by more than one mechanism. Several anticonvulsants and some of their presumed mechanisms of action are listed in Table 7–3.

CHECKPOINT

38. What is the clinical presentation of the major types of seizures?

39. What are some disorders that lead to secondary epilepsy and what changes in brain structure lead to secondary epilepsy?

40. What kinds of mutations have been associated with idiopathic epilepsies?

DEMENTIA & ALZHEIMER'S DISEASE

1. Clinical Features of Dementia

Dementia is an acquired decline in intellectual function resulting in loss of social independence. There is impairment of memory and at least one other area of cortical function, such as language, calculation, spatial orientation, decision making,

TABLE 7–3 Known mechanisms of action of some anticonvulsant drugs.

Drug	Main Indications	Mechanisms of Action
Phenytoin	Generalized tonic-clonic and partial seizures	Inhibition of voltage-gated sodium and calcium channels
Carbamazepine	Generalized tonic-clonic and partial seizures	Inhibition of voltage-gated sodium and calcium channels
Phenobarbital	Generalized tonic-clonic and partial seizures	Enhancement of GABA$_A$ receptor function
Valproate	Generalized tonic-clonic, absence, myoclonic, and partial seizures	Increases levels of GABA by inhibiting succinic semialdehyde dehydrogenase
Ethosuximide	Absence seizures	Inhibition of low-threshold (T-type) voltage-gated calcium channels
Felbamate	Generalized tonic-clonic and partial seizures	Antagonist of NMDA subtype of glutamate receptors; enhances action of GABA at GABA$_A$ receptors
Lamotrigine	Generalized tonic-clonic and partial seizures	Inhibition of voltage-gated sodium channels
Vigabatrin	Partial and secondarily generalized seizures	Increases GABA levels by inhibiting GABA transaminase
Tiagabine	Partial seizures	Increased GABA levels by inhibiting GAB$_A$ reuptake

judgment, and abstract reasoning. In contrast to patients with confusional states, symptoms progress over months to years, and alertness is preserved until the very late stages of disease. Dementia affects 5–20% of persons over age 65, and, although not part of normal aging, its incidence increases with age. The most common causes, which are listed in Table 7–4, account for almost 90% of cases. Treatable causes are important to rec-

TABLE 7–4 Major causes of dementia.

Alzheimer's disease (> 50% of cases)
Multiple cerebral infarcts
Dementia with Lewy bodies
Alcoholism
Normal pressure hydrocephalus
Primary or metastatic CNS neoplasms
Frontotemporal dementia
Parkinson's disease
Huntington's disease
Pick's disease
Prion diseases (eg, Creutzfeldt-Jakob disease)
Neurosyphilis
HIV infection
Hypothyroidism
Deficiency of vitamins B$_{12}$, B$_6$, B$_1$, or niacin
Chronic meningitis
Subdural hematoma

ognize and include hypothyroidism, vitamin B$_{12}$ deficiency, neurosyphilis, brain tumor, normal pressure (communicating) hydrocephalus, and chronic subdural hematoma. In addition, although not curable, dementia associated with HIV infection may be slowed by antiretroviral treatment. About 10–15% of patients referred for evaluation of dementia suffer from depression (**"pseudodementia"**), which may also respond to treatment.

Cerebrovascular disease is the second most common cause of dementia (after Alzheimer's disease). Dementia results from either multiple infarctions in the territory of major cerebral vessels (**multi-infarct dementia**) or from subcortical infarctions in the distributions of deep penetrating arterioles (**lacunar state, Binswanger's disease, subcortical arteriosclerotic encephalopathy**). There is usually a history of stepwise progression of neurologic deficits, focal signs on neurologic examination, and multiple infarctions on brain imaging studies. Patients generally have a history of hypertension or other risk factors for atherosclerosis.

Chronic drug intoxication is often listed as a cause of dementia but actually produces a confusional state. The existence of alcohol-induced dementia is controversial. Although animal and cell culture studies provide evidence for a direct neurotoxic effect of alcohol, dementia in alcoholic patients also results from associated nutritional deficiency, from recurrent head trauma, and (rarely) from acquired hepatocerebral degeneration, a complication of chronic hepatic insufficiency caused by alcoholic cirrhosis.

2. Alzheimer's Disease

Clinical Features

Alzheimer's disease is the most common cause of dementia and accounts for more than 50% of cases. It is a slowly progressive disorder that runs a course of 5–10 years and typically begins with impairment of learning and recent memory. Anomia, aphasia, and acalculia eventually develop, causing loss of employment and inability to manage finances. Spatial disorientation causes patients to become lost easily, and apraxias lead to difficulty with cooking, cleaning, and self-care. A frontal lobe gait disorder may appear, with short, shuffling steps, flexed posture, difficulty turning, and a tendency to fall backward (**retropulsion**) similar to that seen in Parkinson's disease. In later stages, social graces are lost, and psychiatric symptoms such as paranoia, hallucinations, and delusions may appear. Terminally ill patients are bedridden, mute, and incontinent.

Pathology

The pathology of Alzheimer's disease is characterized by extracellular neuritic plaques in the cerebral cortex and in walls of meningeal and cerebral blood vessels (Figure 7–32). These plaques contain a dense core of amyloid material surrounded by dystrophic neurites (axons, dendrites), reactive astrocytes, and microglia. Other structural changes include the formation of intraneuronal neurofibrillary tangles, neuronal and synaptic loss, reactive astrocytosis, and microglial proliferation. Controversy exists as to which features are most related to the pathogenesis of the disease. Formation of neuritic plaques is particularly characteristic for Alzheimer's disease, but there is little evidence that the course or onset of disease correlates with plaque number. Neurofibrillary tangles are paired helical filaments composed of a hyperphosphorylated form of the microtubule protein tau. They are not specific for Alzheimer's disease and occur in several other neurodegenerative disorders. In general, all pathologic changes are most prominent in the hippocampus, entorhinal cortex, association cortex, and basal forebrain. This accounts for the early symptoms of memory loss and disturbance of higher cortical functions, with preservation of primary sensory and motor function until later in the course.

Amyloid plaques

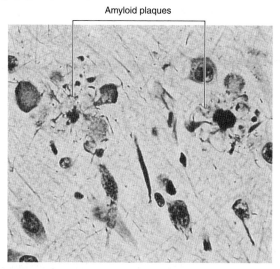

FIGURE 7–32 Amyloid plaques in cerebral cortex in Alzheimer's disease.

Pathophysiology

A. Amyloid β-Peptide—The major protein in neuritic plaques is **amyloid β-peptide** (Aβ), which is proteolytically derived from a membrane protein, the β-**amyloid precursor protein** (**APP**) encoded by a gene on chromosome 21q21.3-22.05. APP interacts with extracellular matrix and supports the growth of neurites in neuronal cultures. Genetic evidence implicates Aβ in the pathogenesis of Alzheimer's disease. Almost all patients with trisomy 21 (Down syndrome) develop pathologic changes indistinguishable from those seen in Alzheimer's disease, suggesting that having an increased copy of the *APP* gene increases the metabolism of APP to Aβ. About 10% of cases of Alzheimer's disease are familial, with early onset (before age 65 years) and autosomal dominant inheritance. In approximately 5% of these families, Alzheimer's disease is strongly linked to missense mutations immediately flanking the Aβ sequence in the *APP* gene. Transgenic mice expressing human APP with these mutations show elevated levels of Aβ, behavioral abnormalities, and neuritic plaques. The APP mutations result in either increased production of all forms of Aβ or mainly in the long 42-amino-acid form, $A\beta_{42}$, which self-aggregates and promotes plaque formation. Aβ is toxic to cultured neurons and stimulates production of cytokines from microglial cells. Aβ also triggers the release of glutamate from glial cells and may injure neurons through excitotoxicity. This evidence links increased production of Aβ, particularly $A\beta_{42}$, to Alzheimer's disease and suggests that Aβ causes the neurodegeneration. Transgenic mice that express mutant forms of familial human APP develop synaptic dysfunction before plaque deposition, indicating that diffusible forms of Aβ are neurotoxic. This may explain why plaque number and disease severity correlate poorly.

B. Presenilins—The enzymatic pathways that regulate Aβ formation are critical areas of current research that may lead to new treatments. Some clues have come from analysis of additional families with Alzheimer's disease. APP is cleaved at the amino terminal of the Aβ sequence by the membrane-anchored protease BACE, or beta-amyloid precursor protein cleaving enzyme, which is also known as beta-secretase. This cleavage generates a 99-amino-acid carboxyl terminal fragment. A second enzymatic activity termed γ-secretase cleaves this fragment to yield Aβ. Almost 70% of familial cases of Alzheimer's disease have been linked to missense mutations in the gene *PS-1/S182*, which encodes a seven-trans-membrane protein (**presenilin 1**) on chromosome 14q24.3. Another 20% of cases have been linked to mutations in another gene, *STM2* (**presenilin 2**), on chromosome 1q31-42. The proteins encoded by these genes are 67% identical in amino acid sequence and presumably have similar functions. Current evidence indicates that the presenilins are subunits of γ-secretase, because mutant mice lacking either presenilin show reduced γ-secretase function, and mutations designed to inhibit the predicted aspartyl protease function of presenilins eliminate γ-secretase activity. Mutant variants of presenilins associated with familial Alzheimer's disease increase the production of $A\beta_{42}$. This suggests that these mutations produce Alzheimer's disease by selectively altering γ-secretase activity to favor production of the longer, amyloid-producing form of A. In addition, γ-secretase is important for processing Notch proteins and other substrates critical for neuronal function, and mice deficient in presenilins show deficiencies in spatial memory and synaptic plasticity. Thus, γ-secretase deficiency may contribute to neurodegeneration in patients with presenilin mutations.

C. Apolipoprotein E—The majority of patients with Alzheimer's disease are older than 60 years, and in about 50% of these patients the e4 isoform of **apolipoprotein E (apoE4)** has been identified as a risk factor. ApoE is a 34-kDa protein that mediates the binding of lipoproteins to the low-density lipoprotein (LDL) receptor and the LDL receptor-related protein (LRP). It is synthesized and secreted by astrocytes and macrophages and is thought to be important for mobilizing lipids during normal development of the nervous system and during regeneration of peripheral nerves after injury. There are three major isoforms (apoE2, apoE3, and apoE4), which arise from different alleles (e2, e3, and e4) of a single gene on chromosome 19q13.2. The e3 allele is the most common, accounting for about 75% of all alleles, whereas e2 and e4 account for roughly 10% and 15%, respectively. The e4 allele is associated with increased risk and earlier onset of both familial and sporadic late-onset Alzheimer's disease. In contrast, inheritance of e2 is associated with decreased risk and later onset. It is important to note that Alzheimer's disease develops in the absence of e4 and also that many persons with e4 escape disease. Therefore, genotyping is not currently recommended as a useful genetic test.

The mechanism by which apoE alleles alter disease risk is not certain. In cultured neurons, apoE3 increases neurite outgrowth in the presence of very low-density lipoproteins, whereas apoE4 inhibits outgrowth. Alzheimer patients who are homozygous for the e4 allele have larger and denser senile plaques than patients homozygous for the e3 allele. ApoE is found in neuritic plaques, and apoE4 binds Aβ more readily than does apoE3. Therefore, apoE4 may facilitate plaque formation or reduce the clearance of Aβ from brain tissue. In addition, apoE enters neurons and binds the microtubule-associated protein tau, which is the major constituent of neurofibrillary tangles. ApoE3 binds tau much more avidly than apoE4. Binding of apoE3 to tau may prevent the formation of neurofibrillary tangles and support normal microtubule assembly required for neurite outgrowth.

CHECKPOINT

41. What are the treatable causes of dementia?
42. What are the clinical features of Alzheimer's disease?
43. In which proteins are there mutations associated with familial forms of Alzheimer's disease?
44. What is the association between apolipoprotein E and Alzheimer's disease?

STROKE

Clinical Presentation

Stroke is a clinical syndrome characterized by the sudden onset of a focal neurologic deficit that persists for at least 24 hours and is due to an abnormality of the cerebral circulation. It is the third leading cause of death in the United States. The incidence of stroke increases with age and is higher in men than in women. Significant risk factors include hypertension, hypercholesterolemia, diabetes, smoking, heavy alcohol consumption, and oral contraceptive use.

Pathophysiology

A. Vascular Supply

The focal symptoms and signs that result from stroke correlate with the area of brain supplied by the affected blood vessel. Strokes may be classified into two major categories based on pathogenesis: ischemic stroke and hemorrhage (Table 7–5). In ischemic stroke, vascular occlusion interrupts blood flow to a specific brain region, producing a fairly characteristic pattern of neurologic deficits resulting from loss of functions controlled by that region. The pattern of deficits resulting from hemorrhage is less predictable because it depends on the location of the bleed and also on factors that affect the function of brain regions distant from the hemorrhage (eg, increased intracranial pressure, brain edema, compression of neighboring brain tissue, and rupture of blood into ventricles or subarachnoid space).

TABLE 7–5 Classification of stroke.

Ischemic stroke
Thrombotic occlusion
Large vessels (major cerebral arteries)
Small vessels (lacunar stroke)
Venous occlusion
Embolic
Artery to artery
Cardioembolic
Hemorrhage
Intraparenchymal hemorrhage
Subarachnoid hemorrhage
Subdural hemorrhage
Epidural hemorrhage
Hemorrhagic ischemic infarction

B. Ischemic Stroke

Ischemic strokes result from thrombotic or embolic occlusion of cerebral vessels. Neurologic deficits caused by occlusion of large arteries (Figure 7–33) result from focal ischemia to the area of brain supplied by the affected vessel (Figure 7–34) and produce recognizable clinical syndromes (Table 7–6). Not all signs are present in every patient, because the extent of the deficit depends on the presence of collateral blood flow, individual variations in vascular anatomy, blood pressure, and exact location of the occlusion. Thrombosis usually involves the internal carotid, middle cerebral, or basilar arteries. Symptoms typically evolve over several minutes and may be preceded by brief episodes of reversible focal deficits known as **transient ischemic attacks.** Emboli from the heart, aortic arch, or carotid arteries usually occlude the middle cerebral artery, because it carries more than 80% of blood flow to the cerebral hemisphere. Emboli that travel in the vertebral and basilar arteries commonly lodge at the apex of the basilar artery or in one or both posterior cerebral arteries.

Ischemic strokes involving occlusion of small arteries occur at select locations, where perfusion depends on small vessels that are end arteries. Most result from a degenerative change in the vessel, described pathologically as **lipohyalinosis,** that is caused by chronic hypertension and predisposes to occlu-

sion. The most common vessels involved are the lenticulostriate arteries, which arise from the proximal middle cerebral artery and perfuse the basal ganglia and internal capsule. Also commonly affected are small branches of the basilar and posterior cerebral arteries that penetrate the brainstem and thalamus. Occlusion of these vessels causes small areas of tissue damage known as **lacunar infarctions.** These typically occur in the putamen, caudate, thalamus, pons, and internal capsule and less commonly in subcortical white matter and cerebellum. Lacunar infarctions produce several fairly stereotyped clinical syndromes. The two most common are pure motor stroke and pure sensory stroke. In pure motor stroke, the infarction is usually within the internal capsule or pons contralateral to the weak side. In pure sensory stroke, the infarction is usually in the contralateral thalamus.

Several vascular, cardiac, and hematologic disorders can cause focal cerebral ischemia (Table 7–7). The most common is **atherosclerosis** of the large arteries of the neck and base of the brain (Figure 7–35). Atherosclerosis is thought to arise from injury to vascular endothelial cells by mechanical, biochemical, or inflammatory insults (see Chapter 11). Endothelial injury stimulates attachment of circulating monocytes and lymphocytes that migrate into the vessel wall and stimulate proliferation of smooth muscle cells and fibroblasts. This

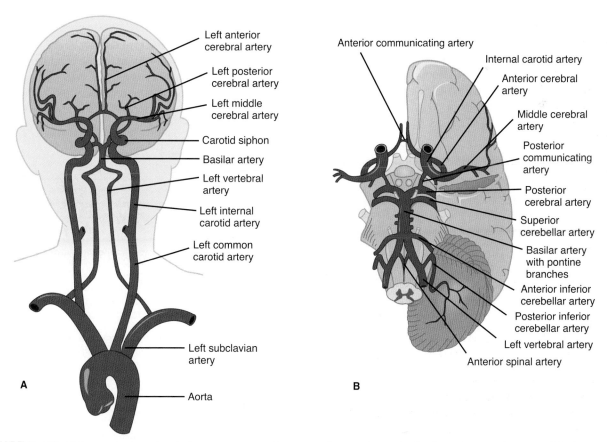

FIGURE 7–33 Major cerebral arteries. **A:** Anterior view. **B:** Inferior view showing the circle of Willis and principal arteries of the brainstem.
(Redrawn, with permission, from Waxman SG. *Neuroanatomy with Clinical Correlations,* 25th ed. McGraw-Hill, 2003.)

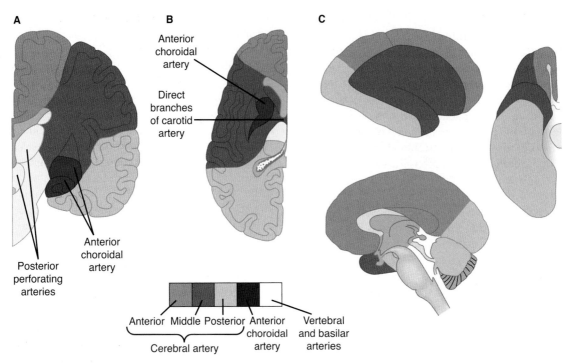

FIGURE 7–34 Vascular territories of the major cerebral arteries. **A:** Coronal section through the cerebrum. **B:** Horizontal section through the cerebrum. **C:** Vascular supply to the cerebral cortex.   (Redrawn, with permission, from Chusid JG. *Correlative Neuroanatomy and Functional Neurology,* 19th ed. Originally published by Appleton & Lange. Copyright © 1985 by the McGraw-Hill Companies, Inc.)

leads to the formation of a fibrous plaque. Damaged endothelial cells also provide a nidus for aggregation and activation of platelets. Activated platelets secrete growth factors that encourage further proliferation of smooth muscle and fibroblasts. The plaque may eventually enlarge to occlude the vessel or may rupture, releasing emboli.

C. Hemorrhage

Epidural and **subdural hematomas** typically occur as sequelae of head injury. Epidural hematomas arise from damage to an artery, typically the middle meningeal artery, which can be ruptured by a blow to the temporal bone. Blood dissects the dura from the skull and compresses the hemisphere lying be-

TABLE 7–6 Vascular territories and clinical features in ischemic stroke.

Artery	Territory	Symptoms and Signs
Anterior cerebral	Medial frontal and parietal cortex, anterior corpus callosum	Paresis and sensory loss of contralateral leg and foot
Middle cerebral	Lateral frontal, parietal, occipital, and temporal cortex and adjacent white matter, caudate, putamen, internal capsule	Aphasia (dominant hemisphere), neglect (nondominant hemisphere), contralateral hemisensory loss, homonymous hemianopia, hemiparesis
Vertebral (posterior inferior cerebellar)	Medulla, lower cerebellum	Ipsilateral cerebellar ataxia, Horner's syndrome, crossed sensory loss, nystagmus, vertigo, hiccup, dysarthria, dysphagia
Basilar (including anterior inferior cerebellar, superior cerebellar)	Lower midbrain, pons, upper and mid cerebellum	Nystagmus, vertigo, diplopia, skew deviation, gaze palsies, hemi- or crossed sensory loss, dysarthria, hemi- or quadriparesis, ipsilateral cerebellar ataxia, Horner's syndrome, coma
Posterior cerebral	Distal territory: medial occipital and temporal cortex and underlying white matter, posterior corpus callosum	Contralateral homonymous hemianopia, dyslexia without agraphia, visual hallucinations and distortions, memory defect, cortical blindness (bilateral occlusion)
	Proximal territory: upper midbrain, thalamus	Sensory loss, ataxia, third nerve palsy, contralateral hemiparesis, vertical gaze palsy, skew deviation, hemiballismus, choreoathetosis, impaired consciousness

TABLE 7–7 Conditions associated with focal cerebral ischemia.

Vascular disorders
Atherosclerosis
Fibromuscular dysplasia
Vasculitis
Systemic (polyarteritis nodosa, lupus, giant cell, Wegner's, Takayasu's)
Primary CNS
Meningitis (syphilis, tuberculosis, fungal, bacterial, herpes zoster)
Drug induced (cocaine, amphetamines)
Carotid or vertebral artery dissection
Lacunar infarction
Migraine
Multiple progressive intracranial occlusions (moyamoya syndrome)
Venous or sinus thrombosis
Cardiac disorders
Mural thrombus
Rheumatic heart disease
Arrhythmias
Endocarditis
Mitral valve prolapse
Paradoxic embolus
Atrial myxoma
Prosthetic heart valves
Hematologic disorders
Thrombocytosis
Polycythemia
Sickle cell disease
Leukocytosis
Hypercoagulable states (homocysteinemia, protein S deficiency, antiphospholipid syndrome, sickle cell disease)

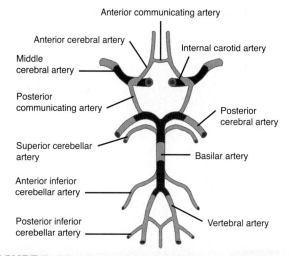

FIGURE 7–35 Sites of predilection (dark red areas) for atherosclerosis in the intracranial arterial circulation. (Redrawn, with permission, from Greenberg DA, Aminoff MJ, Simon RP. *Clinical Neurology*, 5th ed. McGraw-Hill, 2002.)

Subarachnoid hemorrhage may occur from head trauma, extension of blood from another compartment into the subarachnoid space, or rupture of an arterial aneurysm. Cerebral dysfunction occurs because of increased intracranial pressure and from poorly understood toxic effects of subarachnoid blood on brain tissue and cerebral vessels. The most common cause of spontaneous (nontraumatic) subarachnoid hemorrhage is rupture of a **berry aneurysm,** which is thought to arise from a congenital weakness in the walls of large vessels at the base of the brain. The aneurysms become symptomatic in adulthood, usually after the third decade. Rupture suddenly elevates intracranial pressure, which can interrupt cerebral blood flow and cause a generalized concussive injury. This results in loss of consciousness in about half of patients. With very large hemorrhages, global cerebral ischemia can cause severe brain damage and prolonged coma. Focal ischemia may later result from vasospasm of arteries at or near the site of rupture. Recurrence of hemorrhage within the first few days is a common and often fatal complication.

Intraparenchymal hemorrhage may result from acute elevations in blood pressure or from a variety of disorders that weaken vessels. The resultant hematoma causes a focal neurologic deficit by compressing adjacent structures. In addition, metabolic effects of extravasated blood disturb the function of surrounding brain tissue, and nearby vessels are compressed, causing local ischemia. Chronic hypertension is the most common predisposing factor. In hypertensive patients, small **Charcot-Bouchard aneurysms** appear in the walls of small penetrating arteries and are thought to be the major sites of rupture. Most vulnerable are the small vessels that are also involved in lacunar infarction. Hypertensive hemorrhages occur mainly in the basal ganglia, thalamus (Figure 7–36), pons, and cerebellum and less commonly in subcortical white matter. Other causes of intraparenchymal hemorrhage include **vascular malformations,** which contain abnormally fragile

low. Initial loss of consciousness from the injury is due to concussion and may be transient. Neurologic symptoms then return a few hours later as the hematoma exerts a mass effect that may be severe enough to cause brain herniation (Figure 7–27). Subdural hematomas usually arise from venous blood that leaks from torn cortical veins bridging the subdural space. These may be ruptured by relatively minor trauma, particularly in the elderly. The blood is under low pressure, and symptoms resulting from mass effect may not appear for several days.

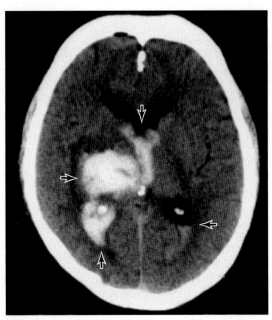

FIGURE 7–36 CT scan in hypertensive intracerebral hemorrhage. Blood is seen as a high-density signal at the site of hemorrhage in the thalamus (left arrow) and its extension into the third ventricle (top arrow) and the occipital horns of the ipsilateral (bottom arrow) and contralateral (right arrow) lateral ventricles. (Reproduced, with permission, from Greenberg DA, Aminoff MJ, Simon RP. *Clinical Neurology,* 5th ed. McGraw-Hill, 2002.)

vessels susceptible to rupture at normal arterial pressures, and certain **brain tumors,** such as glioblastoma multiforme, which induce proliferation of fragile vessels within the tumor. Certain **platelet** and **coagulation disorders** may predispose to intracerebral hemorrhage by inhibiting coagulation. **Cocaine** and **amphetamines** cause rapid elevation of blood pressure and are common causes of intraparenchymal hemorrhage in young adults. Hemorrhage may be related to spontaneous bleeding from the acute elevation in blood pressure, rupture of an occult vascular abnormality, or drug-induced vasculitis. **Cerebral amyloid angiopathy** is a disorder that occurs mainly in the elderly and may be associated with Alzheimer's disease. Deposition of amyloid weakens the walls of small cortical vessels and causes lobar hemorrhage, often at several sites.

D. Excitotoxicity

Most efforts to intervene in stroke have focused on the vasculature. In ischemic stroke, these efforts include restoring circulation through surgical endarterectomy and reducing thrombosis with anticoagulant, antiplatelet, and thrombolytic drugs. A complementary approach is to attempt to reduce the vulnerability of brain tissue to ischemic damage. This is based on observations that CNS glutamate homeostasis is markedly altered during ischemia, leading to increased and toxic levels of extra-cellular glutamate.

Neurons deep within an ischemic focus die from energy deprivation. However, at the edge of the ischemic region, neurons appear to die because of excessive stimulation of glutamate receptors (Figure 7–37). As noted, glutamate is

released at excitatory synapses, and glutamate levels in the extracellular space are normally tightly regulated by sodium-dependent reuptake systems in neurons and glia. In glia, glutamate is further detoxified by conversion to glutamine via the ATP-dependent enzyme glutamine synthetase. Glutamine is then released by glia and taken up by neurons, where it is repackaged into synaptic vesicles for subsequent release. Ischemia deprives the brain of oxygen and glucose, and the resultant disruption in cellular metabolism depletes neurons and glia of energy reserves required to maintain normal transmembrane ion gradients. This leads to accumulation of intracellular Na^+ and collapse of the transmembrane Na^+ gradient, which in turn inhibits glutamate uptake. Declining energy reserves also reduce conversion of glutamate to glutamine in glia. Both events promote accumulation of extracellular glutamate, which stimulates glutamate receptors on surrounding neurons, causing entry of Ca^{2+} and Na^+. The influx of cations depolarizes these neurons, stimulating additional Ca^{2+} influx through voltage-gated channels.

Ischemia also disrupts K^+ homeostasis, leading to an increase in the concentration of extracellular K^+ ($[K^+]_o$). Neuronal activity can rapidly increase $[K^+]_o$, and one major function of glial cells is to keep $[K^+]_o$ at about 3 mmol/L to help neurons maintain their resting membrane potential. Two energy-dependent transporters are particularly important for removal of extracellular K^+ by glia: a Na^+-K^+ ATPase and an anion transporter that cotransports K^+ and Na^+ with Cl. In ischemia, these energy-dependent mechanisms fail, and K^+ released into the extracellular space can no longer be taken up by glia. This depolarizes neurons because the gradient of K^+ across neuronal membranes determines the level of the resting membrane potential. Depolarization activates release of neurotransmitters, increasing accumulation of glutamate at excitatory synapses and in the extracellular space.

The net effect of these events is a tremendous influx of Na^+ and Ca^{2+} into neurons through glutamate- and voltage-gated ion channels. The resultant overload in intracellular Ca^{2+} appears to be especially toxic and may exceed the ability of the neuron to extrude or sequester the cation. This results in sustained activation of a variety of calcium-sensitive enzymes, including proteases, phospholipases, and endonucleases, leading to cell death. In support of an excitotoxic mechanism of cell death in stroke are animal studies that demonstrate a reduction in the size of ischemic lesions after treatment with glutamate receptor antagonists.

CHECKPOINT

45. What are the differences between the clinical presentation of stroke resulting from ischemia and stroke caused by spontaneous hemorrhage?

46. What are the most common causes of stroke?

47. What role does glutamate play in neuronal injury during ischemia?

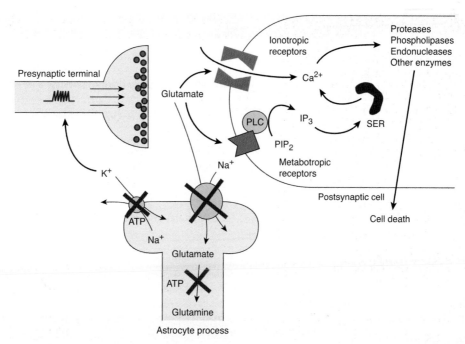

FIGURE 7–37 Excitotoxicity in neuronal ischemia. Depletion of energy supplies inhibits Na$^+$-K$^+$ ATPase, leading to accumulation of extracellular K$^+$ and a decline in extracellular Na$^+$. The rise in extracellular K$^+$ depolarizes nerve terminals, causing release of glutamate. The reduction in extracellular Na$^+$ reduces Na$^+$-dependent glutamate uptake, potentiating synaptic effects of released glutamate. This generates a sustained increase in intracellular Ca^{2+} in the postsynaptic cell, leading to cell death. Bold "X" denotes inhibition of Na$^+$-K$^+$ ATPase (**left**), glutamate transporters (**right**), and glutamine synthetase. Other abbreviations are defined in the legend to Figure 7–28.

CASE STUDIES

Eva M. Aagaard, MD, & Yeong Kwok, MD

(See Chapter 25, p. 684 for Answers)

CASE 29

A 63-year-old man comes to the clinic with a several-month history of difficulty with his gait and coordination. He finds walking difficult and has almost fallen on a number of occasions, especially when trying to change directions. He has also found that using his hands is difficult, and other people have noticed that his hands shake. Physical examination is notable for a resting tremor in the hands that disappears with intentional movement. He has a shuffling gait with difficulty turning. There is so-called cogwheeling rigidity in his arms, a jerky sensation with passive flexion and extension of the arms.

Questions

A. What is the likely diagnosis? What clinical factors make this diagnosis likely?

B. What are the underlying pathologic changes responsible for the clinical presentation?

C. What are some possible molecular mechanisms responsible for the pathologic changes?

CASE 30

A 35-year-old woman presents to the clinic with a chief complaint of double vision. She reports intermittent and progressively worsening double vision for approximately 2 months, rarely at first but now every day. She works as a computer programmer, and the symptoms increase the longer she stares at the computer screen. She has also noted a drooping of her eyelids, which seems to worsen with prolonged working at the screen. Both symptoms subside with rest. She is generally fatigued but has noted no other weakness or neurologic symptoms. Her medical history is unremarkable. Physical examination is notable only for the neurologic findings. Cranial nerve examination discloses impaired lateral movement of the right eye and bilateral ptosis, which worsen with repetitive eye movements. Motor, sensory, and reflex examinations are otherwise unremarkable.

Questions

A. What is the likely diagnosis? What is the pathogenesis of this disease?

B. What other neurologic manifestations might one expect to see?

C. What is the mechanism by which this patient's ocular muscle weakness increases with prolonged activity?

D. What associated conditions should be investigated in this patient?

E. What treatments should be considered?

CASE 31

A 73-year-old man is brought in by his wife with concerns about his worsening memory. He is a retired engineer who has recently been getting lost in the neighborhood where he has lived for 30 years. He has been found wandering and has often been brought home by neighbors. When asked about this, he becomes upset and defensive and states that he was just trying to get some exercise. He has also had trouble dressing himself and balancing his checkbook. A physical examination is unremarkable, except that he scores 12 points out of 30 on the Mini-Mental Status Examination, a test of cognitive function. A metabolic workup is normal. A computed tomography scan of the head shows generalized brain atrophy, though perhaps only what would be expected for his age. He is diagnosed with dementia, likely from Alzheimer's disease.

Questions

A. If a brain biopsy is done, what is likely to be found?

B. Where in the brain are the changes most prominent, and how does that explain the progression of symptoms?

C. What is the role of the amyloid peptide in Alzheimer's disease?

D. Is there a role for genetic testing to determine risk for development of Alzheimer's disease at this time?

CASE 32

A middle-aged man is transported to the emergency department unconscious and accompanied by a nurse from the medical floor. The nurse states that the patient was in line in front of her in the hospital cafeteria when he suddenly fell to the floor. He then had a "generalized tonic-clonic seizure." She called for assistance and accompanied him to the emergency department. No other historical information is available. On physical examination, the patient is confused and unresponsive to commands. He is breathing adequately and has oxygen in place via nasal prongs. His vital signs are as follows: temperature, 38 °C; blood pressure, 170/90 mm Hg; heart rate, 105 bpm; respiratory rate, 18/min. Oxygen saturation is 99% on 2 L of oxygen. Neurologic examination is notable for reactive pupils of 3 mm, intact gag reflex, decreased movement of the left side of the body, and Babinski reflexes bilaterally. Examination is otherwise unremarkable.

Questions

A. Describe what is meant by a generalized tonic-clonic seizure.

B. What are some of the underlying causes of seizure disorders? Which cause might you be most concerned about in this patient?

C. What is the likely pathophysiology of seizures in this patient?

CASE 33

A 72-year-old man presents to the emergency department with acute onset of right-sided weakness. The patient was eating breakfast when he suddenly lost strength in the right side of his body such that he was unable to move his right arm or leg. He also noted a loss of sensation in the right arm and leg and difficulty speaking. His wife called 911, and he was brought to the emergency department. His medical history is remarkable for long-standing hypertension, hypercholesterolemia, and recently diagnosed coronary artery disease. On physical examination, his blood pressure is 190/100 mm Hg. Neurologic examination is notable for right facial droop and a dense right hemiparesis. The Babinski reflex is present on the right. CT scan of the brain shows no evidence of hemorrhage. He is admitted to the neurologic ICU.

Questions

A. What is the diagnosis? Which artery or vascular territory is apt to be involved?

B. What are some risk factors for this condition?

C. What are the possible mechanisms by which this man developed these focal neurologic deficits? Which are most likely in this patient? Why?

D. What underlying disorder may be responsible? How does it result in stroke?

REFERENCES

General

Hille B. *Ion Channels of Excitable Membranes,* 3rd ed. Sinauer, 2001.

Kandel ER, Schwartz JH, Tessel TM (editors). *Principles of Neural Science,* 4th ed. McGraw-Hill, 2000.

Rosenberg RN et al (editors). *The Molecular and Genetic Basis of Neurological Disease,* 2nd ed. Butterworth-Heinemann, 1997.

Victor M, Ropper AH, Adams RD. *Principles of Neurology,* 7th ed. McGraw-Hill, 2000.

Functional Neuroanatomy

Greenberg DA et al. *Clinical Neurology,* 5th ed. McGraw Hill, 2002.

Haerer A. *De Jong's The Neurologic Exam,* 5th ed. Lippincott Williams & Wilkins, 1992.

Parent A. *Carpenter's Human Neuroanatomy,* 9th ed. Williams & Wilkins, 1996.

Patten J. *Neurological Differential Diagnosis,* 2nd ed. Springer, 1996.

Motor Neuron Disease

Julien J-P. Amyotrophic lateral sclerosis: Unfolding the toxicity of the misfolded. Cell. 2001 Feb 23;104(4):581–91. [PMID: 11239414]

Kawahara Y et al. Glutamate receptors: RNA editing and death of motor neurons. Nature. 2004 Feb 26;427(6977):801. [PMID: 14985749]

Rowland LP et al. Amyotrophic later sclerosis. N Engl J Med. 2001 May 31;344(22):1688–700. [PMID: 11386269]

Van Deerlin VM et al. *TARDBP* mutations in amyotrophic lateral sclerosis with TDP-43 neuropathology: A genetic and histopathological analysis. Lancet Neurol. 2008 May;7(5):409–16. [PMID: 18396105]

Parkinson's Disease

Dawson TM et al. Molecular pathways of neurodegeneration in Parkinson's disease. Science. 2003 Oct 31;302(5646):819–22. [PMID: 14593166]

Goedert M. Alpha-synuclein and neurodegenerative diseases. Nat Rev Neurosci. 2001 Jul;2(7):492–501. [PMID: 11433374]

Le W et al. Mutant genes responsible for Parkinson's disease. Curr Opin Pharmacol. 2004 Feb;4(1):79–84. [PMID: 15018843]

Marras C et al. Changing concepts in Parkinson disease: Moving beyond the decade of the brain. Neurology. 2008 May 20;70(21):1996–2003. [PMID: 18490620]

Myasthenia Gravis

De Baets M et al. The role of autoantibodies in myasthenia gravis. J Neurol Sci. 2002 Oct 15;202(1-2):5–11. [PMID: 12220686]

McConville J et al. Diseases of the neuromuscular junction. Curr Opin Pharmacol. 2002 Jun;2(3):296–301–301. [PMID: 12020474]

Vincent A et al. Myasthenia gravis seronegative for acetylcholine receptor antibodies. Ann N Y Acad Sci. 2008;1132:84–92. [PMID: 18567857]

Epilepsy

Avoli M et al. Generalized epileptic disorders: An update. Epilepsia. 2001 Apr;42(4):445–57. [PMID: 11440339]

Epilepsia 2001;42:445.French JA et al. Clinical practice. Initial management of epilepsy. N Engl J Med. 2008 Jul 10;359(2):166–76. [PMID: 18614784]

Steinlein OK. Genetic mechanisms that underlie epilepsy. Nat Rev Neurosci. 2004 May;5(5):4008. [PMID: 15100722]

Dementia & Alzheimer's Disease

Bossy-Wetzel E et al. Molecular pathways to neurodegeneration. Nat Med. 2004 Jul;10(Suppl):S2–9. [PMID: 15272266]

Marjaux E et al. Presenilins in memory, Alzheimer's disease, and therapy. Neuron. 2004 Apr 22;42(2):189–92. [PMID: 15091335]

Ross CA et al. Protein aggregation and neurodegenerative disease. Nat Med. 2004 Jul;10(Suppl):S10–7. [PMID: 15272267]

Selkoe DJ. Alzheimer's disease: Genes, proteins, and therapy. Physiol Rev. 2001 Apr;81(2):741–66. [PMID: 11274343]

Stroke

Arundine M et al. Molecular mechanisms of glutamate-dependent neurodegeneration in ischemia and traumatic brain injury. Cell Mol Life Sci. 2004 Mar;61(6):657–68. [PMID: 15052409]

Mohr JP et al. *Stroke: Pathophysiology, Diagnosis, and Management,* 4th ed. Churchill Livingstone, 2004.

C H A P T E R

Diseases of the Skin

8

Timothy H. McCalmont, MD

NORMAL SKIN

The skin is the most accessible organ of the human body. Its most basic function is simply a protective one. As a barrier, the skin holds off desiccation and disease by keeping moisture in and pathogens out. Nevertheless, characterization of the skin as mere "plastic wrap" is a gross underestimation of the anatomic and physiologic complexity of this vital structure.

Unlike parenchymal organs, end-organ dysfunction or failure is not a prerequisite for the diagnosis of a skin disease, because all skin diseases can be observed clinically irrespective of their functional effects. Among the spectacular array of neoplastic, inflammatory, infectious, and genetic cutaneous disorders, some elicit only trivial aberrations in skin structure or function, whereas others lead to profound and morbid consequences.

ANATOMY

The integumentary system consists of a layer of tissue, 1–4 mm thick, that covers all exposed surfaces of the body. The skin merges uninterruptedly with the structurally similar envelope of the mucous membranes, but skin is distinct from mucosa in that it contains adnexal structures such as the eccrine units that exude sweat and the folliculosebaceous units that produce hairs and oils. There is considerable variation in skin thickness and composition, depending on the requirements of a particular body site. For example, the thinnest skin overlies the eyelids, where delicacy and mobility are essential. The thickest skin is present on the upper trunk, where sturdiness exceeds mobility in importance. The surfaces of the palms and soles are characterized by a high density of eccrine sweat units, reflecting the importance of this region in regulation of temperature; an absence of hairs, which would interfere with sensation; and accentuation of the cornified layer (see later discussion), contributing to the tackiness needed to handle objects deftly. The size of the structures between sites can also vary greatly,

best illustrated by the contrast between large terminal hair follicles found on the scalp, bearded areas, and genital skin and the small vellus hair follicles found at most other sites.

HISTOLOGY

Using a light microscope, two important skin layers are easily identifiable: a stratified squamous epithelium, the **epidermis;** and a layer of connective tissue, the **dermis.** The subjacent adipose tissue is considered as a third layer by some and is referred to as the **subcutis.**

The epidermis consists of keratinocytes arrayed in four distinct substrata: the basal, spinous, granular, and cornified layers (Figure 8–1). Basal keratinocytes include the proliferative pool of keratinocytes. These cells divide, giving rise to progeny that are displaced toward the skin surface. As the keratinocytes move outwardly, they progressively flatten and accumulate keratin filaments within their cytoplasm. Individual keratinocytes are tightly bound together by intracellular junctions called desmosomes (Figure 8–2). The desmosomal junctions appear as delicate "spines" between cells in conventional microscopic sections and are most conspicuous in the epidermal spinous layer (Figure 8–3). Keratin filaments are linked intracellularly and are also attached to the desmosomes, forming a network that is vital to structural integrity.

Melanocytes and Langerhans' cells are dendritic cells that are intercalated among the keratinocytes of the epidermis. Melanocytes, which are positioned in the basal layer, synthesize a reddish-brown biochrome, melanin, and dispense it to numerous adjacent keratinocytes through their dendrites (Figure 8–4). This distribution system permits melanin to provide a dispersed screen against the potentially harmful ultraviolet rays of the sun. Langerhans' cells share a similar arborized morphology but are positioned in the midspinous layer. Langerhans' cells are bone marrow-derived antigen-presenting cells (see also Chapter 3).

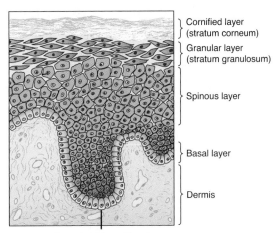

FIGURE 8–1 Although the epidermis biologically displays a gradient of differentiation, four distinct layers are recognized on the basis of microscopic appearance. Cuboidal germinative keratinocytes serve as a foundation in the basal layer; cells with ample cytoplasm and prominent desmosomes constitute the spinous layer; cells with cytoplasmic granularity resulting from an accumulation of keratin complexes and other structural proteins are found in the granular layer; and anucleate, flattened keratinocytes comprise the tough, membrane-like cornified layer. (Redrawn, with permission, from Orkin M, Maibach HI, Dahl MV [editors]. *Dermatology.* Originally published by Appleton & Lange. Copyright © 1991 by the McGraw-Hill Companies, Inc.)

The epidermal-dermal junction, or basement membrane zone, is a structure that welds the epidermis to the dermis and contributes to the skin barrier. The juncture of the epidermis and dermis is arrayed in an undulating fashion to increase the surface area of binding between the two structures and to resist shearing forces. The downward projections of the epidermis are referred to as **rete ridges,** and the upward projections of the superficial dermis are called **dermal papillae** (Figure 8–5). Although the basement membrane comprises a thin eosinophilic (pink) band beneath the basal cells in conventional microscopical sections, it has a sophisticated multilayered structure that reaches from the hemidesmosomes of

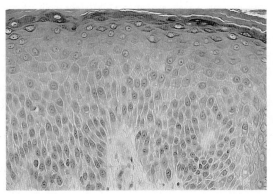

FIGURE 8–3 With conventional light microscopy, the numerous desmosomes of the spinous layer appear as delicate attachments ("spines") between individual keratinocytes.

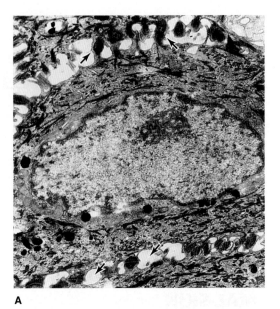

A

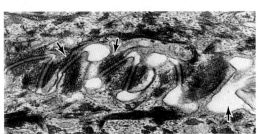

B

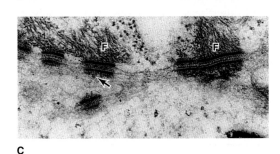

C

FIGURE 8–2 In an ultrastructural view of a human keratinocyte (**A**), numerous desmosomes (**B**) appear as plaques that tightly bind two cell membranes together. With very high magnification (**C**), the attachment of cytoplasmic keratin filaments (**F**) to the desmosomes can be appreciated. (Reproduced, with permission, from Junqueira LO, Carneiro J, *Basic Histology,* 10th ed. McGraw-Hill, 2003.)

the basal keratinocytes to the collagen bundles of the superficial dermis (Figure 8–6). The lamina densa and lamina lucida are two of the layers of the basement membrane zone and are so named because of their electron-dense and electron-lucid appearance when viewed ultrastructurally.

The dermis consists of a connective tissue gel composed largely of proteins and mucopolysaccharides (so-called ground substance). This matrix serves as the scaffolding that supports the complex neurovascular networks, which course through the skin, and also supports the eccrine (sweat gland) and follic-

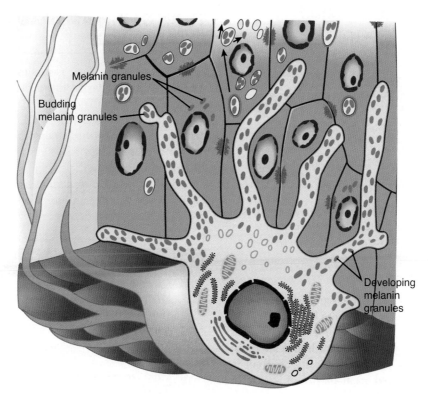

Melanin granules

Budding melanin granules

Developing melanin granules

FIGURE 8–4 The human melanocyte displays a branching morphology, and the dendrites of the cell maintain contact with 35–40 adjacent keratinocytes in a multicellular structure termed the epidermal melanin unit. The function of the unit is the effective dispersion of melanin pigment, packaged in organelles known as melanosomes, across a broad surface area. (Redrawn, with permission, from Junqueira LO, Carneiro J. *Basic Histology,* 10th ed. McGraw-Hill, 2003.)

ular (hair) adnexal structures. The vast majority of the fibrous structural proteins of the dermis are composed of collagen types I and III, and a network of elastic microfibrils is also woven throughout the full dermal thickness. Fibrocytes, the synthetic units of the structural proteins, are ubiquitous, and there are also mast cells and dendritic immune cells arrayed throughout the dermis. A discussion of the fine structure of the dermis—the dermal vascular and neural networks and the adnexal structures—is beyond the scope of this chapter.

OVERVIEW OF SKIN DISEASES

In the broadest and simplest sense, there are two types of skin diseases: growths and rashes. A skin growth is a cyst, a malformation, or a benign or malignant neoplasm, something that presents clinically as a bump on the skin. A rash is, with rare exception, a nonneoplastic skin disease; it is more precisely referred to as an inflammatory skin condition or a **dermatitis.** The pathophysiologic aspects of the huge number of described growths and rashes exceed the scope of this chapter, and our discussion will focus on nine prototypical rashes.

TYPES OF SKIN LESIONS

Physicians interested in the skin learned decades ago that the accurate diagnosis and classification of the many patterns of dermatitis were dependent on a standardized nomenclature for the description and documentation of rashes. When used in association with a few well-chosen adjectives, the terms used to describe the prototypical types of inflammatory skin lesions (so-called primary lesions) permit vivid description of a rash. To illustrate the importance of terminology, imagine trying to describe a patient's condition over the telephone to another physician. Talking about a red raised rash may truthfully describe the eruption in some sense, but the mental image evoked could be any one of dozens of skin diseases. The only way to accurately characterize an eruption is by the use of precisely defined terms.

The most important types of primary lesions include macules and patches, papules and plaques, vesicles and bullae, pustules, and nodules. The terms **macule** and **patch** denote flat areas of discoloration without any discernible change in texture. Macules are 1 cm or less in diameter, whereas patches

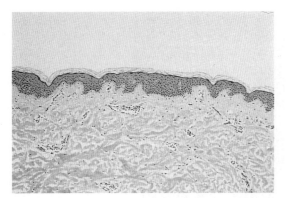

FIGURE 8–5 The undulating configuration of the epidermal-dermal junction consists of downward extensions of the epidermis, known as rete ridges, and upward extensions of the dermis, known as dermal papillae.

exceed 1 cm in size. **Papules** and **plaques** are elevated, palpable skin lesions in which the breadth of the lesion exceeds its thickness. A papule is small, 1 cm or less in diameter, whereas a plaque exceeds 1 cm in size. **Vesicles** and **bullae** are fluid-filled spaces within the skin. Vesicles are less than 1 cm in diameter, whereas bullae exceed 1 cm in size. A vesicle or bulla containing purulent fluid is known as a **pustule**. A **nodule** is a solid, rounded skin lesion in which diameter and thickness are roughly equal.

TYPES OF INFLAMMATORY SKIN DISEASES

Different inflammatory processes involve different structures within the skin and display different microscopic patterns. Experience has shown that pattern analysis can serve as a useful means of diagnosis and classification. Pattern analysis is dependent on accurate recognition of the distribution of inflammation within the skin as well as recognition of the specific structures affected by the inflammatory reaction. There are nine distinct patterns of dermatitis (Table 8–1; Figure 8–7). Eight of these patterns and some of the diseases that produce them are discussed in detail next.

CHECKPOINT

1. What are the two most basic barrier functions of skin?
2. How is skin distinct from mucosa? Why are these terms important?
3. What are the main primary lesions? Why are these terms important?
4. What are the main patterns of inflammatory skin disease?
5. What is the value of knowing the microscopic pattern of inflammation of a skin lesion? What additional information is needed for this information to be most useful?

PATHOPHYSIOLOGY OF SELECTED SKIN DISEASES

PSORIASIFORM DERMATITIS: PSORIASIS

Clinical Presentation

Psoriasis is a common chronic, persistent or relapsing, scaling skin condition. Individual lesions are distinctive in their classic form: sharply marginated and erythematous and surmounted by silvery scales (Figure 8–8). Most patients with

psoriasis have a limited number of fixed plaques, but there is great variation in clinical presentation.

Epidemiology & Etiology

Psoriasis affects between 1% and 2% of individuals of both sexes in most ethnic groups. The most common age at onset is the third decade, but psoriasis can develop soon after birth, and psoriasis of new onset has been documented in a centenarian.

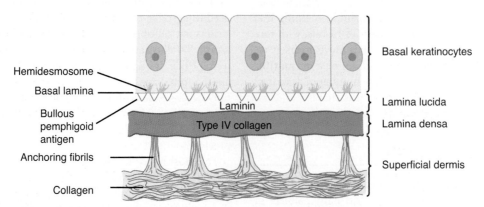

FIGURE 8–6 Schematic diagram of the basement membrane zone of human epidermis. (Redrawn, with permission, from Orkin M, Maibach HI, Dahl MV [editors]. *Dermatology.* Originally published by Appleton & Lange. Copyright © 1991 by the McGraw-Hill Companies, Inc.)

TABLE 8–1 Patterns of inflammatory skin disease.

Pattern	Description	Prototypes
Perivascular dermatitis	Perivascular inflammatory infiltrate without significant involvement of the epidermis	Urticaria (hives)
Spongiotic dermatitis	Inflammatory infiltrate associated with intercellular epidermal edema (spongiosis)	Allergic contact dermatitis (poison oak dermatitis)
Psoriasiform dermatitis	Inflammatory infiltrate associated with epidermal thickening as a result of elongation of rete ridges	Psoriasis
Interface dermatitis	Cytotoxic inflammatory reaction with prominent changes in the lower epidermis, characterized by vacuolization of keratinocytes	Erythema multiforme Lichen planus
Vesiculobullous dermatitis	Inflammatory reaction associated with intraepidermal or subepidermal cleavage	Bullous pemphigoid
Vasculitis	Inflammatory reaction focused on the walls of cutaneous vessels	Leukocytoclastic vasculitis
Folliculitis	Inflammatory reaction directed against folliculo-sebaceous units	Acne folliculitis
Nodular dermatitis	Inflammatory reaction with a nodular or diffuse dermal infiltrate in the absence of significant epidermal changes	Cutaneous sarcoidosis
Panniculitis	Inflammatory reaction involving the subcutaneous fat	Erythema nodosum

Several lines of evidence have established that genetic factors contribute to the development of psoriasis. There is a high rate of concordance for psoriasis in monozygotic twins and an increased incidence in relatives of affected individuals. The gene products of specific class I alleles of the major histocompatibility complex (MHC) are overexpressed in patients with psoriasis. Psoriasis is not merely a genetic disorder, however, because some susceptible individuals never develop characteristic lesions. In other predisposed individuals, a number of environmental factors, including infection and physical injury, can serve as triggers for the development of psoriasis (Table 8–2).

Histopathology & Pathogenesis

Psoriasis is the prototypical form of psoriasiform dermatitis, a pattern of inflammatory skin disease in which the epidermis is thickened as a result of elongation of rete ridges (Figures 8–7 and 8–9). In psoriatic lesions, epidermal thickening reflects excessive epidermopoiesis (epidermal proliferation). The increase in epidermopoiesis is reflected in shortening of the duration of the keratinocyte cell cycle and doubling of the proliferative cell population. Because of these alterations, lesional skin contains up to 30 times as many keratinocytes per unit area as normal skin. Evidence of excessive proliferation is also manifest microscopically as numerous intraepidermal mitotic figures.

During normal keratinocyte maturation, nuclei are eliminated as cells enter the cornified layer and condense to form a semipermeable envelope. In psoriasis, the truncation of the cell cycle leads to an accumulation of cells within the cornified layer with retained nuclei, a pattern known as parakeratosis. As parakeratotic cells accumulate, neutrophils migrate to the cornified layer. Histopathologically, the silvery scale of psoriatic plaques consists of a thick layer of parakeratotic keratinocytes with numerous intercalated neutrophils. At times, the number of neutrophils in the stratum corneum is so great that lesions assume a pustular appearance.

Psoriasis also induces endothelial cell hyperproliferation that yields pronounced dilation, tortuosity, and increased permeability of capillaries in the superficial dermis (Figure 8–10). The vascular alterations contribute to the bright erythema seen clinically. The capillary changes are most pronounced at the advancing margins of psoriatic plaques.

After years of study, a large number of immunologic abnormalities have been documented in psoriatic skin, but a precise sequence of events that eventuates in epidermal hyperproliferation has not been established. The association between psoriasis and specific MHC class I molecules implicates CD8 lymphocytes because the complex of MHC class I protein and antigen is established as the ligand of the T-cell receptor of CD8 cells (see also Chapter 3). Overexpression of a large number of cytokines has also been reported. Interleukin-2 (IL-2) overexpression is a common if not fundamental aberration, reflected in the observation that systemic IL-2 therapy for metastatic malignancy may precipitate severe exacerbations of psoriasis in predisposed individuals.

Clinical Manifestations

The cardinal features of the plaques of psoriasis include sharp margination, bright erythema, and nonconfluent whitish or silvery scales. Lesions can occur at any site, but the scalp, the

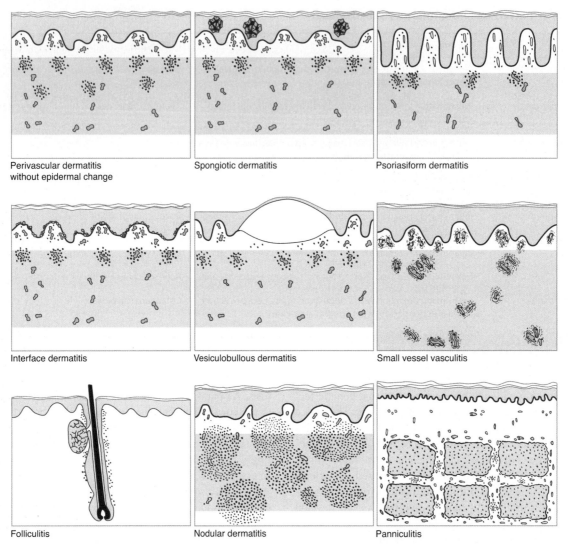

Perivascular dermatitis
without epidermal change

Spongiotic dermatitis

Psoriasiform dermatitis

Interface dermatitis

Vesiculobullous dermatitis

Small vessel vasculitis

Folliculitis

Nodular dermatitis

Panniculitis

FIGURE 8–7 Nine patterns of inflammatory skin disease. (See also Table 8–1.)

extensor surfaces of the extremities, and the flexural surfaces are often involved. Psoriasis commonly affects the nail bed and matrix, yielding pitted or markedly thickened dystrophic nails. Mucosal surfaces are spared.

The only extracutaneous manifestation of psoriasis is psoriatic arthritis, a deforming, asymmetric, oligoarticular arthritis that can involve small or large joints. The distal interphalangeal joints of the fingers and toes are characteristically involved. Psoriatic arthritis is classified as one of the seronegative spondyloarthropathies, distinguishable from rheumatoid arthritis by a lack of circulating autoantibodies (so-called rheumatoid factors) or circulating immune complexes and by linkage with specific MHC class I alleles, including HLA-B27.

There are many variants of psoriasis, all of which are histopathologically similar but which differ greatly in clinical distribution (Table 8–3).

CHECKPOINT

6. What evidence supports a genetic role in the development of psoriasis? An environmental role?

7. Which cell types hyperproliferate in psoriasis?

8. What immunologic defects have been identified in psoriasis?

INTERFACE DERMATITIS: LICHEN PLANUS

Clinical Presentation

Lichen planus is a distinctive itchy eruption that usually presents with numerous small papules. Individual lesions have angulate borders, flat tops, and a violaceous hue, attributes

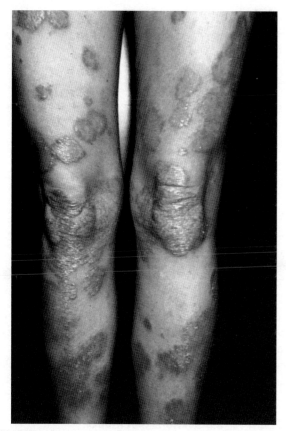

FIGURE 8–8 Classic plaque-type psoriasis (psoriasis vulgaris) consisting of sharply marginated scaling plaques accentuated over the extensor aspects of the extremities. (Reproduced, with permission, from Orkin M, Maibach HI, Dahl MV [editors]. *Dermatology*. Appleton & Lange, 1991.)

TABLE 8–2 Factors that induce or exacerbate psoriasis.

Physical factors
Trauma (so-called Koebner phenomenon)
Abrasions
Contusions
Lacerations
Burns
Sunburn[1]
Bites
Surgical incisions
Cold weather
Infections
Viral bronchitis
Streptococcal pharyngitis
Human immunodeficiency virus (HIV) infection
Medications or medication-related
Antimalarial agents
Lithium
β-Adrenergic blocking agents
Corticosteroid withdrawal

[1]Ultraviolet (UV) light in modest doses inhibits psoriasis and has been utilized as effective therapy for decades. UV light only exacerbates psoriasis when presented in toxic doses (sunburn).

that form the basis of their alliterative description as pruritic polygonal purple papules (Figure 8–11). The individual papules of lichen planus sometimes coalesce to form larger plaques. Minute whitish streaks, barely visible to the naked eye and known as Wickham's striae, are characteristically found on the surfaces of lesions.

Epidemiology & Etiology

Lichen planus generally develops in adulthood and affects women slightly more commonly than men. Although the factors that trigger lichen planus remain obscure in many pa-

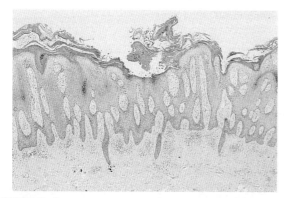

FIGURE 8–9 Histopathologic features of psoriasis at low magnification. The rete ridges are strikingly and evenly elongated, and the overlying cornified layer contains cells with retained nuclei (parakeratosis), a pattern that reflects the increased epidermal turnover.

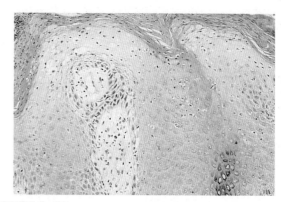

FIGURE 8–10 In a psoriatic plaque at high magnification, dilated capillaries are evident in an edematous portion of the superficial dermis.

TABLE 8–3 **Variants of psoriasis.**

Variant	Cutaneous Findings and Distribution	Other Features
Plaque-type psoriasis (psoriasis vulgaris)	Large stationary plaques with prominent scales, commonly involving the scalp and the extensor surfaces of the extremities	
Guttate psoriasis	Scaling papules or small plaques, usually 0.5–1.5 cm in diameter, scattered on the trunk and proximal extremities	Lesions often induced or exacerbated by streptococcal pharyngitis
Erythrodermic psoriasis	Generalized erythematous plaques involving the face, trunk, and extremities, with only slight scaling	
Pustular psoriasis, generalized	Generalized eruption of sterile pustules involving erythematous skin of the trunk and extremities, often with sparing of the face	Associated with fever; may occur in pregnancy
Pustular psoriasis, localized	Scaling erythematous plaques, studded with pustules, involving the palms, soles, and nails	
Inverse psoriasis	Slightly scaling, erythematous plaques involving the axillary and inguinal regions, with sparing of areas usually involved in plaque-type disease	

tients, it is clear that the rash represents a cell-mediated immune reaction that directly or indirectly damages basal keratinocytes of the epidermis. Observations that suggest a cell-mediated mechanism include the occurrence of lichen planus–like eruptions as a manifestation of graft-versus-host disease after bone marrow transplantation and the development of a lichen planus–like eruption in mice after injection of sensitized, autoreactive T cells. Although most lichen planus is idiopathic, drugs are one established cause of lichen planus or lichen planus–like reactions. Therapeutic gold and antimalarial agents are the medications most closely linked to the development of lichenoid eruptions, but a long list of other agents has accumulated (Table 8–4).

Histopathology & Pathogenesis

Lichen planus is a form of lichenoid interface dermatitis, a type of inflammatory skin disease in which a dense infiltrate of lymphocytes occupies the papillary dermis and the superficial dermis immediately subjacent to the epidermis, in association with vacuolization of the lower epidermis (Figure 8–12). The papil-

lary dermal infiltrate is composed largely, if not entirely, of T lymphocytes. Some of the T cells are also found within the epidermis, where adjacent vacuolated, injured keratinocytes are found. Dense eosinophilic (pink) globules, known as **colloid bodies,** are also identifiable within the epidermis and the infil-

TABLE 8–4 **Medications that induce lichenoid (lichen planus–like) reactions.**

Therapeutic gold
Antimalarial agents
Quinacrine
Quinidine
Quinine
Chloroquine
Penicillamine
Thiazide diuretics
β-Blocking agents
Antibiotics
Tetracycline
Streptomycin
Dapsone
Isoniazid
Anticonvulsants
Carbamazepine
Phenytoin
Nonsteroidal anti-inflammatory drugs

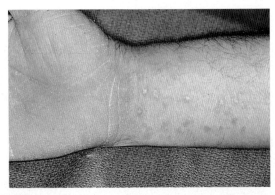

FIGURE 8–11 Pruritic polygonal flat-topped papules of lichen planus are present in a common location, the flexor surface of the wrist.

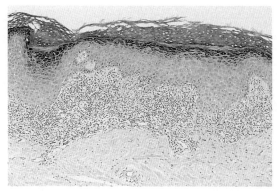

FIGURE 8–12 Histopathologic features of lichen planus at low magnification. There is a bandlike infiltrate of lymphocytes that impinges on the epidermal-dermal junction, and some keratinocytes adjacent to the infiltrate show cytoplasmic vacuolization.

trate (Figure 8–13). Colloid bodies represent condensed, anucleate keratinocytes that have succumbed to the inflammatory reaction. Although the keratinocytes bear the brunt of the lymphocyte attack, melanocytes may be coincidentally destroyed in the reaction as "innocent bystanders." Free melanin pigment is released as melanocytes are damaged, and the pigment is phagocytosed by dermal macrophages known as melanophages.

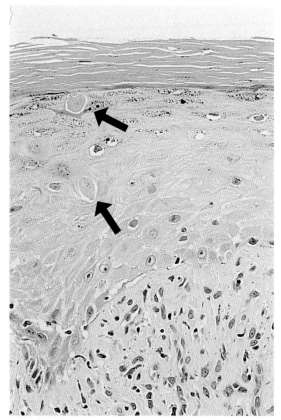

FIGURE 8–13 Necrotic keratinocytes (so-called colloid bodies) in a lesion of lichen planus appear as rounded globules (arrow) along the epidermal-dermal junction. Necrotic cells are also evident in the upper epidermis.

In incipient lesions of lichen planus, CD4 helper T lymphocytes predominate, and some of the cells have been found in proximity to macrophages and Langerhans' cells (see also Chapter 3). In contrast, CD8 cytotoxic T cells comprise the bulk of the infiltrate in mature lesions. This shift in infiltrating T-cell composition is thought to reflect the afferent and efferent aspects of lesional development. In the afferent phase, causative antigens are processed and presented to helper T cells, probably in the context of specific HLA determinants. The stimulated CD4 lymphocytes then elaborate specific cytokines that lead to the recruitment of cytotoxic lymphocytes. Cell-mediated cytotoxicity and cytokines such as interferon-γ and tumor necrosis factor (TNF) are then thought to contribute to the vacuolization and necrosis of keratinocytes as a secondary event.

The clinical appearance of lichen planus lesions reflects several synchronous alterations in the skin. The dense array of lymphocytes in the superficial dermis yields the elevated, flat-topped appearance of each papule or plaque. The chronic inflammatory reaction induces accentuation of the cornified layer (hyperkeratosis) of the epidermis, which contributes to the superficial whitish coloration perceived as Wickham's striae. Although the many melanophages that accumulate in the papillary dermis hold a brownish black pigment, the fact that the pigmented cells are embedded in a colloidal matrix such as the skin permits extensive scattering of light, a phenomenon known as the Tyndall effect. Thus, the human eye interprets a lesion of lichen planus as dusky or violaceous despite the fact that the pigment that serves as the basis for the coloration is melanin.

Clinical Manifestations

Lichen planus affects both skin and mucous membranes. Papules are generally distributed bilaterally and symmetrically. The sites most commonly involved include the flexor surfaces of the extremities, the genital skin, and the mucous membranes. Rarely, lichen planus may involve the mucosa of internal organs, such as the esophagus. Cutaneous lesions are virtually never seen on the palms, soles, or face.

In general, lichen planus variants can be grouped into three categories.

A. Lichen Planus Papules Arrayed in an Unusual Configuration

In these variants, typical individual papules of lichen planus are grouped in a distinctive larger pattern. In annular lichen planus, small lichenoid papules coalesce to form a larger ring. Linear and zosteriform patterns of lichen planus have also been observed. When lichen planus presents in an unusual configuration, it is prone to be underdiagnosed or misdiagnosed.

B. Lichen Planus Papules Arrayed at Distinctive Sites

Although most lichen planus is widespread, at times papules are restricted to a specific body site, such as the mouth (oral lichen planus) or genitalia. Nearly 25% of all lichen planus patients have disease limited to the mucous membranes.

C. Lichen Planus Papules with Unusual Clinical Morphology

Some examples of lichen planus defy clinical recognition because the appearance of the individual lesions is atypical. Erosive, vesiculobullous, atrophic, and hypertrophic lesions can be seen. In **erosive lichen planus,** the interface reaction that is directed against the epidermis is so profound that the entire epidermis becomes necrotic and ulceration ensues. The closely related entity **vesiculobullous lichen planus** is also characterized by an intense interface reaction that yields necrosis of the epidermal junctional zone across a broad front. As a result of basal layer necrosis, the epidermis becomes detached from its dermal attachments and a blister develops. In **atrophic lichen planus,** the rate of destruction of keratinocytes by the lichenoid interface reaction exceeds the rate of epidermal regeneration, and the epidermis becomes attenuated as a result. In contrast, in **hypertrophic lichen planus,** the rate of epidermal regeneration triggered by the interface reaction exceeds the rate of destruction, and thick, verrucous, hyperkeratotic lesions develop. All of these variants are histopathologically similar with the exception of the foci of ulceration seen in erosive lichen planus.

CHECKPOINT

9. What skin cells are damaged by cell-mediated immune reactions in lichen planus?
10. Which drugs have been most commonly implicated in licheniform eruptions?
11. What synchronous alterations in the skin are reflected in the clinical appearance of lichen planus?

INTERFACE DERMATITIS: ERYTHEMA MULTIFORME

Clinical Presentation

Erythema multiforme is an acute cutaneous eruption that presents with a wide spectrum of clinical severity. The eruption is commonly brief and self-limited, but repetitive or generalized attacks can be disabling or even life threatening. As the name implies, variation in lesional morphology can be seen, but most patients present with a monomorphous pattern in a given bout. The prototypical lesion is a red macule or thin papule that expands centrifugally and develops a dusky or necrotic center, creating a target-like pattern (Figure 8–14).

Epidemiology & Etiology

Erythema multiforme is an uncommon but distinctive skin disease that afflicts men and women in nearly equal numbers. The peak incidence is in the second to fourth decades of life, and onset during infancy or early childhood is a rarity. Like li-

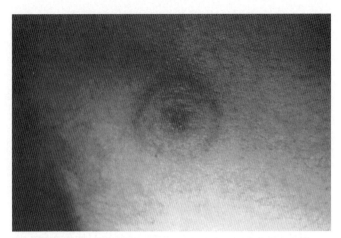

FIGURE 8–14 A target lesion—a characteristic pattern seen in erythema multiforme—consists of a papule or plaque with a central zone of epidermal necrosis surrounded by a rim of erythema. (Reproduced, with permission, from Jordon RE [editor]. *Immunologic Diseases of the Skin.* Originally published by Appleton & Lange. Copyright © 1991 by the McGraw-Hill Companies, Inc.)

chen planus, erythema multiforme represents a cell-mediated immune reaction that eventuates in necrosis of epidermal keratinocytes. Herpes simplex viral infection and reactions to medications have been established as the most common causes of erythema multiforme. Other cases are idiopathic.

Histopathology & Pathogenesis

Erythema multiforme is a prototypical form of vacuolar interface dermatitis. In contrast to lichen planus, which typically presents with a dense obscuring lichenoid infiltrate within the superficial dermis, in erythema multiforme the inflammatory infiltrate is sparse. Thus, the vacuolated keratinocytes that are widely distributed within the epidermal basal layer are conspicuous in the face of a sparse infiltrate, and the damaged keratinocytes serve as the basis for the name of this pattern of inflammatory skin disease.

The dermal infiltrate in erythema multiforme is composed of a mixture of CD4 and CD8 T lymphocytes. CD8 cytotoxic cells are also found within the epidermis, in proximity to vacuolated and necrotic keratinocytes. Keratinocytes that are killed in the course of the inflammatory reaction become anucleate and are manifest microscopically as round, dense, eosinophilic bodies similar to the colloid bodies of lichen planus (Figure 8–15).

Although lichen planus and erythema multiforme are clinically, microscopically, and etiologically distinct, both appear to share a common pathogenetic pathway in which specific inciting agents recruit effector lymphocytes into the epidermis and papillary dermis. After this recruitment, keratinocytes are injured and killed by the combined negative influences of cytotoxicity and cytokines, such as interferon-γ and TNF.

Many cases of so-called erythema multiforme minor are triggered by herpes simplex viral infection. A relationship between erythema multiforme and herpetic infection had

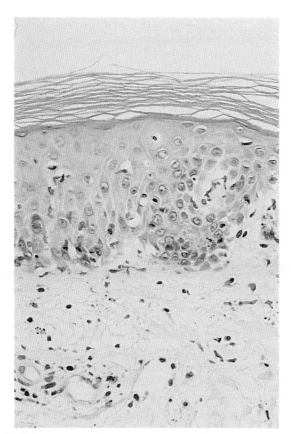

FIGURE 8–15 Histopathologic features of erythema multiforme, a type of vacuolar interface dermatitis. There is a modest infiltrate of lymphocytes in the vicinity of the epidermal-dermal junction where vacuolated and necrotic keratinocytes are conspicuous.

long been suspected based on the documentation of preceding herpes simplex lesions in patients with erythema multiforme. The relationship was strengthened after antiherpetic drug therapy, in the form of oral acyclovir, was shown to suppress the development of erythema multiforme lesions in some individuals. Molecular studies have substantiated the relationship by confirming the presence of herpes simplex DNA within skin from erythema multiforme lesions. Herpesvirus DNA is also demonstrable within peripheral blood lymphocytes and within lesional skin after resolution but not within nonlesional skin. These findings suggest that viral DNA is disseminated from the primary infection in the peripheral blood and becomes integrated into the skin at specific target sites. The herpetic genomic fragments then contribute to the development of a cytotoxic effector response in their chosen target tissue, the skin.

The target-like clinical appearance of many erythema multiforme lesions reflects zonal differences in the intensity of the inflammatory reaction and its deleterious effects. At the periphery of an erythema multiforme lesion, only sparse inflammation, slight edema, and subtle vacuolization of the epidermis are apparent in the outer erythematous halo. In contrast, the dusky "bull's eye" often shows pronounced epidermal vacuolization, with areas of near-complete epidermal necrosis.

Clinical Manifestations

Erythema multiforme is generally limited to the skin and mucous membranes. The lesions develop rapidly in crops and are initially distributed on acral surfaces, although proximal spread to the trunk and face occurs not uncommonly. Mucosal erosions and ulcers are seen in roughly 25% of cases, and mucositis can be the sole presenting feature of the disease. Although erythema multiforme is an epithelial disorder, nonspecific constitutional symptoms such as malaise can also occur.

Although the spectrum of erythema multiforme exists as a continuum, a given patient is usually classified as having minor or major disease. The disorder is referred to as **erythema multiforme minor** when there are scattered lesions confined to the skin or when skin lesions are observed in association with limited mucosal involvement. A diagnosis of **erythema multiforme major** is based on the presence of prominent involvement of at least two of three mucosal sites: oral, anogenital, or conjunctival. Many examples of erythema multiforme major also display severe, widespread cutaneous involvement. Erythema multiforme major encompasses **Stevens-Johnson syndrome,** a term that connotes profound mucosal involvement with or without cutaneous lesions, as well as toxic **epidermal necrolysis.** In the latter, which most commonly represents an idiosyncratic reaction to a medication, vast regions of the skin and mucosa undergo extensive necrosis (Figure 8–16) with secondary vesiculation. Pathologically, toxic epidermal necrolysis is similar to a severe burn in that the integrity of a patient's skin fails completely, with a resulting increased risk for infectious and metabolic sequelae.

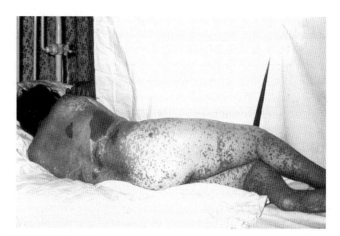

FIGURE 8–16 Toxic epidermal necrolysis is a form of erythema multiforme that usually represents an adverse reaction to a medication. Generalized maculopapular erythema of the trunk and extremities is followed by extensive desquamation, as illustrated on this patient's back, resulting from epidermal necrosis. Patients are often admitted to a burn unit for acute care. (Reproduced, with permission, from Lyell A. Toxic epidermal necrolysis: The scalded skin syndrome: a reappraisal. Br J Dermatol. 1979;100(1):69–86.)

VESICULOBULLOUS DERMATITIS: BULLOUS PEMPHIGOID

Clinical Presentation

Bullous pemphigoid is a blistering disease in which tense fluid-filled spaces develop within erythematous, inflamed skin. The blisters in bullous pemphigoid develop because of detachment of the epidermis from the dermis (subepidermal vesiculation) as the result of a specific inflammatory reaction directed against structural proteins. The term "pemphigoid" reflects the clinical similarity of bullous pemphigoid to pemphigus, another form of blistering skin disease that is characterized by intraepidermal rather than subepidermal vesiculation. The distinction between bullous pemphigoid and pemphigus is an important one, because bullous pemphigoid has a more favorable prognosis.

Epidemiology & Etiology

Bullous pemphigoid is generally a disorder of the elderly. There are rare reports of bullous pemphigoid in children and young adults, but the vast majority of patients are older than 60 years. There is no sex predilection.

It has been known for years that immunoglobulins and complement are deposited along the epidermal-dermal junction in bullous pemphigoid. The deposited antibodies are specific for antigens within the basement membrane zone, and bullous pemphigoid thus represents a form of autoimmune skin disease. The specific factors that induce autoantibody production have not been identified.

Histopathology & Pathogenesis

Microscopically, biopsies from fully developed bullous pemphigoid lesions show a subepidermal cleft containing lymphocytes, eosinophils, and neutrophils as well as eosinophilic (pink) material that represents extravasated macromolecules such as fibrin (Figure 8–17). An inflammatory infiltrate of eosinophils, neutrophils, and lymphocytes is also evident in the dermis beneath the cleft. These findings represent the aftermath of an inflammatory reaction centered on the basement membrane zone.

Insights into this reaction can be obtained from direct immunofluorescence microscopy, in which fluorochrome-labeled anti-immunoglobulin G (IgG), anti-IgA, anti-IgM, and anti-

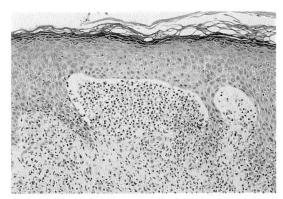

FIGURE 8–17 Histopathologic features of bullous pemphigoid. There is a subepidermal cleft that contains numerous eosinophils and lymphocytes, and a similar infiltrate is present in the superficial dermis. Ultrastructurally, the separation is within the lamina lucida of the basement membrane zone, at the level of the bullous pemphigoid antigen (see Figure 8–6).

complement antibodies are incubated with lesional skin. Using an ultraviolet microscope to localize the fluorochrome, tagged antibodies that are specific for IgG and complement component C3 are found in a linear distribution along the epidermal-dermal junction (Figure 8–18). Circulating IgG that binds to the basement membrane zone of human epidermis is also identifiable in bullous pemphigoid patients. These antibodies are capable of complement fixation, and pathogenicity has been confirmed by injection into laboratory animals, in whom the antibodies bind to the junctional zone and induce blisters.

Characterization of the antigen bound by these autoantibodies has yielded a 230-kDa protein within the lamina lucida. The protein, known as the "bullous pemphigoid antigen," has been localized to the hemidesmosomal complex of the epidermal basal cell (Figure 8–6). Its exact structural or functional role has not been established.

Based on these findings, blister formation is believed to begin with the binding of IgG to the bullous pemphigoid antigen with subsequent activation of the classic complement cascade (Chapter 3). Complement fragments induce mast cell degranulation and attract neutrophils. The presence of eosinophils in the infiltrate of bullous pemphigoid is probably a reflection of mast cell degranulation, because mast cell granules contain eosinophil chemotactic factors. Numerous enzymes are released by granulocytes and mast cells during the reaction, and enzymatic digestion is thought to be the primary mechanism behind the separation of the epidermis from the dermis. It is also possible that the bullous pemphigoid antigen plays a vital structural role that is compromised by autoantibody binding, leading to cleavage.

Clinical Manifestations

Patients with bullous pemphigoid present with large, tense blisters on an erythematous base (Figure 8–19). Lesions are most commonly distributed on the extremities and lower

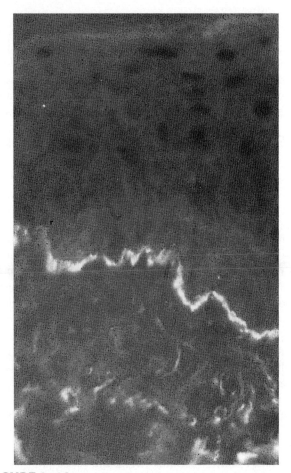

FIGURE 8–18 Direct immunofluorescence findings in lesional skin from a bullous pemphigoid patient. When fluorochrome-stained sections are viewed through an ultraviolet microscope, a bright linear band, signifying deposition of immunoglobulin G, is evident along the epidermal-dermal junction. (Reproduced, with permission, from Jordon RE [editor]. *Immunologic Diseases of the Skin*. Originally published by Appleton & Lange. Copyright © 1991 by the McGraw-Hill Companies, Inc.)

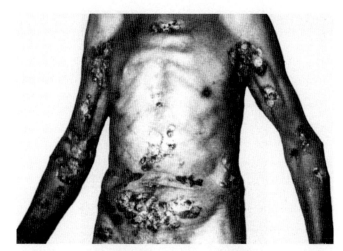

FIGURE 8–19 Large tense bullae on erythematous bases are distributed over the lower trunk and proximal extremities of this elderly man with bullous pemphigoid. (Reproduced, with permission, from Jordon RE [editor]. *Immunologic Diseases of the Skin*. Originally published by Appleton & Lange. Copyright © 1991 by the McGraw-Hill Companies, Inc.)

Bullous pemphigoid is a disease of the skin and mucous membranes only, and systemic involvement has never been documented. Some patients with bullous pemphigoid have developed skin lesions synchronously with a diagnosis of malignancy, but careful studies with age-matched controls have not demonstrated an increased incidence of bullous pemphigoid in cancer patients.

CHECKPOINT

15. How do pemphigus and pemphigoid differ and why is the distinction important?
16. How does Ig binding to the bullous pemphigoid antigen cause blistering in lesions of bullous pemphigoid?
17. Is there a connection between bullous pemphigoid and cancer?

VASCULITIS: LEUKOCYTOCLASTIC VASCULITIS

Clinical Presentation

Leukocytoclastic vasculitis is an inflammatory disorder affecting small blood vessels of the skin that typically presents as an eruption of reddish or violaceous papules, a pattern known as **palpable purpura** (Figure 8–20). The lesions develop in crops, and individual papules persist for a few days or weeks and generally less than a month. Although each individual lesion is transient, the duration of the eruption can vary from weeks to months, and in exceptional cases crops can develop over a period of years.

trunk, but blisters can develop at any site. Most patients experience considerable pruritus in association with their blisters, possibly triggered by the many eosinophils in the dermal infiltrate. Mucous membrane lesions develop in up to one third of patients and are usually clinically innocuous, in contrast to the variants of erythema multiforme.

Some patients with bullous pemphigoid present with itchy, erythematous plaques, with no blistering for an extended period of time, but blisters eventually develop in most patients. This pattern is known as preeruptive or urticarial bullous pemphigoid. Immunofluorescence and histopathologic examination of biopsies from such patients reveals junctional deposition of autoantibodies and complement in association with an eosinophil-rich infiltrate, implying that the inflammatory reaction is identical to that of conventional bullous pemphigoid. The explanation for the delayed blistering seen in these patients is not presently known.

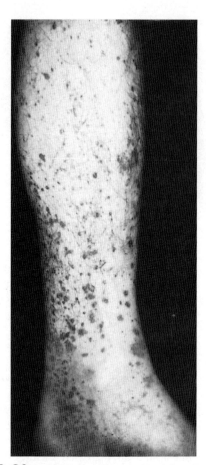

FIGURE 8–20 Purpuric papules are scattered on the lower extremity in leukocytoclastic vasculitis. (Reproduced, with permission, from Jordon RE [editor]. *Immunologic Diseases of the Skin*. Originally published by Appleton & Lange. Copyright © 1991 by the McGraw-Hill Companies, Inc.)

Epidemiology & Etiology

Leukocytoclastic vasculitis can develop at any age, and the incidence is equal in both sexes. The most common precipitants include infections and medications. Bacterial, mycobacterial, and viral infections can all trigger bouts, but poststreptococcal and poststaphylococcal eruptions are most common.

A wide variety of drugs have been established as leukocytoclastic vasculitis elicitors, including antibiotics, thiazide diuretics, and nonsteroidal anti-inflammatory agents. Among antibiotics, penicillin derivatives are the foremost offenders.

Histopathology & Pathogenesis

The name of this disorder conveys its chief pathological attributes, namely an inflammatory reaction involving blood vessels in association with an accumulation of necrotic nuclear (leukocytoclastic) debris. The key steps that contribute to this pattern include the accumulation of triggering molecules within the walls of small blood vessels, subsequent stimulation of the complement cascade with the elaboration of chemoattractants, and entry of neutrophils with oxidative enzyme release, eventuating in cellular destruction and nuclear fragmentation.

The molecules that trigger leukocytoclastic vasculitis are immune complexes, consisting of antibodies bound to exogenous antigens that are usually derived from microbial proteins or medications. Circulating immune complexes have been documented by laboratory assays of serum from patients with active leukocytoclastic vasculitis, and the presence of circulating complexes can also be deduced based on the finding of low serum complement levels during exacerbations. The exact factors that lead to preferential deposition of immune complexes within small cutaneous vessels (venules) remain unknown, but the fact that venules exhibit relatively high permeability in the face of a relatively low flow rate is probably contributory. The deposited complexes are detectable within vessel walls by direct immunofluorescence testing (Figure 8–21).

After becoming trapped in tissue, immune complexes activate the complement cascade, and localized production of chemotactic fragments (such as C5a) and vasoactive molecules ensues (Chapter 3). Chemoattractants draw neutrophils out of vascular lumens and into vascular walls, where release of neutrophilic enzymes results in destruction of the immune complexes, the neutrophils, and the vessel. Microscopically, this stage is characterized by an infiltrate of neutrophils, neutrophilic nuclear dust, and protein (fibrin) in the vessel wall, a pattern that has historically been called "fibrinoid necrosis" (Figure 8–22). Throughout the inflammatory reaction, the integrity of the channel is progressively compromised. As cellular interstices widen, erythrocytes and fibrin exude through the vessel wall and enter the surrounding dermis.

Leukocytoclastic vasculitis lesions are raised and papular because lesional skin is altered and expanded by an intense vasocentric infiltrate containing numerous neutrophils. The erythematous or purpuric quality of leukocytoclastic vasculitis is attributable to the numerous extravasated erythrocytes that accumulate in the dermis of fully developed lesions. In patients with repetitive or persistent leukocytoclastic vasculitis, extravasated erythrocyte debris is metabolized into hemosiderin, which accumulates within macrophages (siderophages) in the deep dermis. The dermal hemosiderin can contribute to a dusky, violaceous clinical appearance, clinically similar to but pathologically distinct from the pigmentary changes seen in lichen planus. After resolution of the eruption, the hyperpigmentation resolves slowly over a period of weeks to months as the hemosiderin is resorbed.

Clinical Manifestations

Lesions of leukocytoclastic vasculitis can develop at any site but are usually distributed on the lower extremities or in dependent areas. Although purpuric lesions comprise the most common clinical pattern, a variety of other morphologic patterns, including vesicopustules, necrotic papules, and ulcers, can develop. These patterns often reflect secondary ischemic changes that are superimposed on the primary vasculitic papule. Vesicopustules develop after ischemic necrosis of the epidermis results in subepidermal separation or after massive dermal accumulation of neutrophils secondary to immune

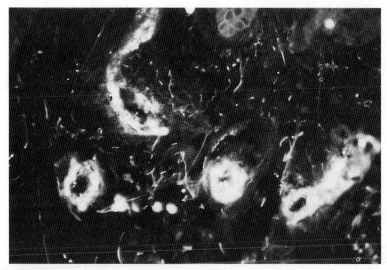

FIGURE 8–21 Direct immunofluorescence microscopy localizes complement component C3 within the walls of small cutaneous vessels. The complement fragments are present after activation of the complement cascade by immune complexes. Immunoglobulin deposition within vessel walls is detectable by the same method. (Reproduced, with permission, from Jordon RE [editor]. *Immunologic Diseases of the Skin*. Originally published by Appleton & Lange. Copyright © 1991 by the McGraw-Hill Companies, Inc.)

complex deposition. Necrotic papules, eschars, and ulcers are end-stage lesions that develop after total necrosis of the epidermis and superficial dermis. In essence, these lesions represent vasculitic infarcts.

Leukocytoclastic vasculitis is not merely a dermatitis but often part of a systemic vasculitis involving small vessels. In such cases, the vascular eruption is accompanied by arthralgias, myalgias, and malaise. Arthralgias and myalgias are probably attributable to vasculitic changes in small vessels in joint capsules and soft tissue. Vasculitic involvement of the kidneys, liver, and GI tract can also occur. Such involvement of abdominal organ systems often presents clinically as abdominal pain. Laboratory studies are important to evaluate possible renal or hepatic impairment.

CHECKPOINT

18. Why are leukocytoclastic vasculitis lesions papular?
19. What are the most common precipitants of leukocytoclastic vasculitis?
20. When leukocytoclastic vasculitis is part of a systemic vasculitis, what additional symptoms are typically observed?

SPONGIOTIC DERMATITIS: ALLERGIC CONTACT DERMATITIS

Clinical Presentation

Allergic contact dermatitis is an eruption, usually pruritic, caused by a specific immune-mediated reaction to a substance that has touched the skin. The acute phase is characterized by

erythematous papules, vesicles, and bullae confined to the area of primary contact of the "allergen" (Figure 8–23). Often the blisters break down and result in weeping and formation of a yellowish crust.

Epidemiology & Etiology

Reliable data on the incidence of allergic contact dermatitis are impossible to gather because of the vast number of people affected, including those with mild disease who do not come to medical attention. However, the disorder has been estimated to cost millions annually in occupation-related direct medical costs and lost productivity.

The factors that determine which individuals will react to which substances are not known, although HLA types are thought to play a role. Some animal models of allergic contact dermatitis demonstrate autosomal inheritance patterns.

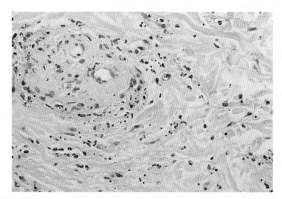

FIGURE 8–22 Histopathologic features of leukocytoclastic vasculitis, a form of small-vessel vasculitis. Neutrophils, neutrophilic nuclear debris, and amorphous protein deposits are present within the expanded wall of a cutaneous venule.

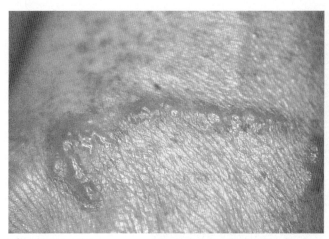

FIGURE 8–23 Allergic contact dermatitis resulting from poison ivy. Confluent, linear, eruptive vesicles with surrounding erythema. (Reproduced, with permission, from Hurwitz RM, Hood AF. *Pathology of the Skin: Atlas of Clinical-Pathological Correlation.* Appleton & Lange, 1998.)

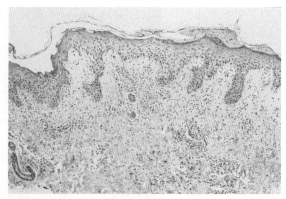

FIGURE 8–25 Histopathologic features of allergic contact dermatitis, a type of acute spongiotic dermatitis. There is a perivascular and interstitial infiltrate of inflammatory cells. The paleness of the papillary dermis is due to edema. Note the scale-crust of serum and inflammatory cells overlying the epidermis.

Histopathology & Pathogenesis

As the term "spongiotic dermatitis" implies, spongiosis is the pathologic hallmark of this category of skin disease. The term "spongiosis" refers to edema of the epidermis, which separates keratinocytes from one another. Microscopically, edema makes visible the normally indiscernible "spines," or desmosomes, which interconnect the keratinocytes (Figures 8–7 and 8–24). Spongiosis may be slight and barely perceptible microscopically or so massive that it is evident clinically as a blister. Spongiotic dermatitis is accompanied by a variable amount of perivascular inflammation that may be around the superficial vascular plexus or the superficial and deep vascular plexuses or perivascular and interstitial in distribution (Figure 8–25). The infiltrate is typically composed of lymphocytes, but eosinophils are often concurrently present in significant numbers in spongiotic dermatitis.

The series of events leading to the development of allergic contact dermatitis has been and continues to be intensively studied, because the mechanism of development of contact hypersensitivity in the skin is analogous to cell-mediated rejection of organs used for transplantation. Delayed-type (type IV) hypersensitivity reactions consist of two phases: induction (sensitization) and elicitation. In the induction phase, the allergen that has come into contact with an individual who is naive to that allergen binds to an endogenous protein and alters it to make it appear foreign. This protein-allergen complex is then intercepted by the immunosurveillance cells of the skin: the Langerhans' cells. Langerhans' cells are bone marrow–derived dendritic cells that reside in the epidermis and form a network at the interface of the immune system with the environment. They engulf the complex, partially degrade ("process") it, migrate to the lymph nodes, and present antigenic fragments on the cell surface in conjunction with an MHC-II molecule. The Langerhans' cells with antigen–MHC-II complexes on the surface contact naive T cells possessing T-cell receptors that specifically recognize the MHC-II–allergen complex. The binding of the T-cell receptors to the MHC-II–allergen complex in the context of important costimulatory molecules on the surface of the Langerhans' cells stimulates clonal expansion of reactive T cells. This process progresses over a period of days. If the allergen exposure is transient, the first exposure often does not result in a reaction at the exposure site. However, a contingent of "armed and ready" memory T cells is now policing the skin, waiting for the allergen to reappear. The individual is said to be sensitized.

The elicitation phase begins once the sensitized individual encounters the antigen again. Memory T cells from the prior exposure have been policing the skin constantly. The Langerhans' cells again process antigen and migrate to lymph nodes, but presentation and T-cell proliferation also occur at the site of contact with the allergen. Nonspecific T cells in the vicinity are recruited and stimulated by the inflammatory cytokines released by the specifically reactive T cells, and an amplification loop ensues, eventuating in clinically recognizable dermatitis. This complex series of events takes time to develop,

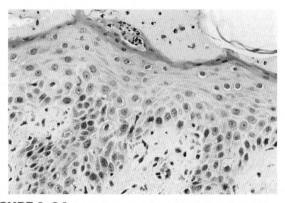

FIGURE 8–24 Allergic contact dermatitis. Intercellular edema has made the "spines" (desmosomes) between keratinocytes visible.

resulting in the 24- to 48-hour delay between reexposure and eruption. Many individuals have experienced this delay in their own personal experience with poison ivy or poison oak. The onset of these disorders never occurs while the yardwork is being completed or during the hike but always a day or two later.

Delayed-type hypersensitivity serves the organism's need for defense against noxious invaders such as viruses; responding T cells recognize virally infected cells and selectively kill them. The development of contact allergy represents an aberrance of this protective mechanism, and the allergen invokes a somewhat nonselective onslaught of T cells that damage the epidermis and result in spongiotic dermatitis histopathologically and a pruritic erythematous blistering eruption clinically.

Clinical Manifestations

Few skin diseases are as well embedded in the lay lexicon as poison ivy and poison oak, which are among the most common causes of allergic contact dermatitis. For those who have been unfortunate enough to experience a full-blown case of poison ivy or oak (so-called *Rhus* dermatitis, after the genus of plant involved), the salient features of the eruption are well known, manifest as an extremely pruritic erythematous eruption on areas of skin exposed directly to the allergenic plant leaves. The eruption consists of erythematous papules, papulovesicles, vesicles, or bullae, often in a linear pattern where the offending leaf was drawn across the skin. Linear streaks, although characteristic, are not always noted because the eruption will assume the pattern of the exposure: A hand covered in allergen that then touches the face may result in a rash in a nonlinear configuration.

A common misconception regarding *Rhus* dermatitis is that blister fluid from broken blisters (or even touching the blistered area) causes the eruption to spread. In fact, once the eruption has developed, the allergen has been irreversibly bound to other proteins or has been so degraded that it cannot be transferred to other sites. Apparent spread of the eruption to other sites can be accounted for by several possible scenarios. First, the *Rhus* allergen is tremendously stable and can persist on unwashed clothing and remain capable of inducing allergic contact dermatitis for up to 1 year. Inadvertent contact with contaminated clothes or other surfaces may induce new areas of dermatitis that are often thought to represent spread and not additional contact. (Washing the skin with soap and water soon after contact with the offending sap will usually abort development of the eruption.) Second, intense allergic contact dermatitis can induce an eruption on skin that was never contacted by allergen. This poorly understood phenomenon is termed "autosensitization." The autosensitization eruption consists of erythematous papules or papulovesicles that are often confined to the hands and feet but may be generalized. The pattern of individual lesions is not linear or geometric, as it is at the original site of allergic contact dermatitis.

Importantly, *Rhus* is but one cause of allergic contact dermatitis. The list of known antigens numbers in the thousands, and there are countless ways for these substances to come into contact with the skin. Often an unnatural geometric pattern of an eruption is the clue to an "outside-in" disease, caused by a contactant. Importantly, a contact eruption does not develop immediately on contact but only after a delay of 24–48 hours. This sometimes makes identification of the offending agent difficult as the connection between exposure and eruption is obscured by the time delay. Patch testing is a useful clinical technique for helping to pinpoint a possible cause when an unknown contactant is suspected as the origin of a persistent or recurrent eruption. In patch testing, a panel of small amounts of standardized antigens are applied in an array to unaffected skin (typically on the back) and left in place for 48 hours. The patches are then removed and the skin is inspected for development of erythema or vesiculation; wherever a reaction is present, the substance that induced the reaction is noted. Readings are performed again at 96 hours to detect long-delayed reactions. To be useful clinically, positive patch test reactions must be correlated with the pattern of the original eruption and the overall clinical context.

CHECKPOINT

21. What is spongiosis?
22. What are the two phases of development of allergic contact dramatized? What steps are involved in each?
23. What is the role of patch testing in patients with suspected allergic contact dermatitis?

PANNICULITIS: ERYTHEMA NODOSUM

Clinical Presentation

Panniculitis is an inflammatory process that occurs in the fat of the subcutis. Erythema nodosum is the most common form of panniculitis, presenting most often with tender red nodules on the anterior lower legs (Figure 8–26). The number of lesions is variable, but typically a dozen or more lesions may be present at onset.

Because the infiltrate in panniculitis occurs deeply in the skin, demarcation of individual lesions is often indistinct. Fever and constitutional symptoms—in particular arthralgias—may accompany the onset of erythema nodosum. The duration of the eruption is typically a few weeks to a few months.

Epidemiology & Etiology

Erythema nodosum is a common condition, although precise data regarding its prevalence are not available. Women seem especially susceptible to its development, and there is an adult female–male predominance of 3:1. This is not true in child-

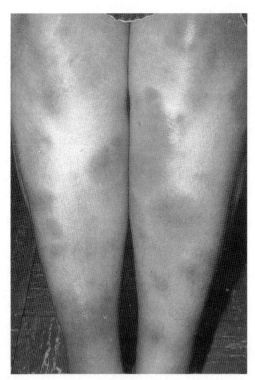

FIGURE 8–26 Erythema nodosum on the lower legs of a woman. The lesions are firm, painful, red or red-brown plaques and nodules. Lesion borders are indistinct. (Reproduced, with permission, from Hurwitz RM, Hood AF. *Pathology of the Skin: Atlas of Clinical-Pathological Correlation.* Originally published by Appleton & Lange. Copyright © 1998 by the McGraw-Hill Companies, Inc.)

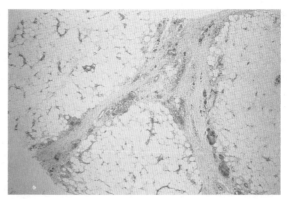

FIGURE 8–27 Histopathologic features of erythema nodosum, a form of septal panniculitis. The septa are thickened and inflamed. There is little inflammation of the fat lobules.

finding of considerable diagnostic value (Figure 8–28). The septa are thickened and may become fibrotic depending on the density of the infiltrate and the duration of the reaction. Even though the infiltrate is largely confined to subcutaneous septa, there is commonly an element of fat necrosis at the edges of the subcutaneous lobules in erythema nodosum. Evidence of fat necrosis may be seen in the form of an infiltrate of foamy (lipid-laden) macrophages at the periphery of subcutaneous lobules or in the form of small stellate clefts within multinucleate macrophages, indicating an element of lipomembranous fat necrosis.

The favored hypothesis regarding the mechanism of development of erythema nodosum is that of a delayed-type hypersensitivity reaction occurring in the septal fat. Immune complex deposition has not been found in the lesions. It is not yet known why systemic hypersensitivity is localized to the fat in such microscopically distinctive fashion.

Clinical Manifestations

As mentioned, erythema nodosum presents as tender, deep-seated, red to red-brown nodules. As the lesions age, they evolve to more "bruise-like" patches or thin plaques. Erythema

hood cases, in which boys and girls are equally affected. Erythema nodosum represents a final common pathway of inflammation that may develop in response to any one of a number of general causes, including infection, medication, hormones (including pregnancy), and inflammatory disease. Streptococcal pharyngitis, sulfonamide-containing drugs, estrogen-containing oral contraceptives, and inflammatory bowel disease are well-known inducers of the disorder.

Histopathology & Pathogenesis

Panniculitis can be separated into two broad categories based on the distribution of inflammation: mostly septal panniculitis and mostly lobular panniculitis (Figure 8–7). The septa are the fibrous divisions between fat compartments and contain the neurovascular bundles. The lobules are the conglomerations of adipocytes demarcated by septa. The modifier "mostly" is meant to convey that the inflammatory process is not strictly confined to a single compartment but, in fact, will frequently spill over from one to the other. An important step in making a specific histopathologic diagnosis is deciding where the majority of the inflammatory response is located.

In the case of erythema nodosum, the inflammatory response occurs in the septal compartment and consists of lymphocytes, histiocytes, and granulocytes (neutrophils and eosinophils) (Figure 8–27). Multinucleated histiocytes within the septa are a

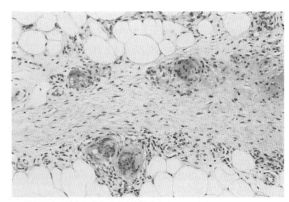

FIGURE 8–28 Erythema nodosum. There are multiple large multinucleated giant cells in this septum. Note the prominent fibrous background with increased cellularity.

nodosum tends to occur on the anterior shins but may involve the thighs, the extensor forearms, and, rarely, the trunk. Because the lesions represent a hypersensitivity response to some inciting stimulus, they may persist or continue to develop in crops for as long as the stimulus is present. In the case of streptococci-associated erythema nodosum, the lesions will probably resolve within a few weeks after successful antibiotic treatment of the primary infection. A prolonged course of erythema nodosum should prompt a search for persistent infection and possible other causes. Erythema nodosum may also be the presenting sign of sarcoidosis (see following discussion).

CHECKPOINT

24. What are the two general categories of panniculitis?
25. Which category of panniculitis does erythema nodosum fit into? What are the features of erythema nodosum clinically? Histopathologically?
26. What are some common precipitators of erythema nodosum?

NODULAR DERMATITIS: SARCOIDOSIS

Clinical Presentation

Sarcoidosis is an enigmatic systemic disease with a hugely variable clinical spectrum ranging from mild asymptomatic skin papules to life-threatening lung disease. Lesions are often red-brown dermal papules or nodules that may occur anywhere on the cutaneous surface but have a special predilection for the face (Figure 8–29). Similar nodular granulomas can occur in the pulmonary tree and other viscera.

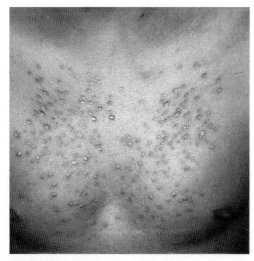

FIGURE 8–29 Reddish-brown papules on the chest typical of sarcoidosis. (Reproduced, with permission, from Hurwitz RM, Hood AF. *Pathology of the Skin: Atlas of Clinical-Pathological Correlation.* Originally published by Appleton & Lange. Copyright © 1998 by the McGraw-Hill Companies, Inc.)

Epidemiology & Etiology

Sarcoidosis can affect patients of any age or ethnic background but does occur more frequently in young adults and, in the United States, is more common in people of black African descent. Among this population, estimates of disease incidence range from 35.5 to 64 cases per 100,000 compared with 10–14 cases per 100,000 in whites. In Europe, Irish and Scandinavian populations are at increased risk.

Numerous causes of sarcoidosis have been proposed, including infectious agents. Among these, *Mycobacterium* species (especially *M tuberculosis*) have been favored suspects, although investigation has yielded contradictory results. Other proposed etiologic agents include *Histoplasma*, viruses, and minute systematized foreign particles (which may incite a reactive process in susceptible individuals), although no solid evidence supporting these suspected causes exists. One report found polarizable foreign material in diseased skin of patients with sarcoidosis, but the authors emphasized that this finding probably reflects the propensity of sarcoidal lesions to develop around a nidus of foreign material in affected patients and does not imply that sarcoidosis is directly caused by foreign detritus. The extent to which genetic heritage determines the susceptibility of an individual to sarcoidosis is not clear, although a higher than expected incidence of sarcoidosis among siblings of affected patients is suggestive of a genetic role.

Histopathology & Pathogenesis

Sarcoidosis is manifest microscopically as collections of tissue macrophages (ie, histiocytes), known as granulomas, situated within the dermis (Figures 8–30 and 8–31). Unlike tuberculoid granulomas of tuberculosis, sarcoidal granulomas are noncaseating and do not show central coagulation necrosis. Multinucleated histiocytes formed by the fusion of individual cells are a common finding (Figure 8–32). The characteristic microscopical appearance of sarcoidal granulomas is of small numbers of lymphocytes around the granulomas ("naked granulomas"). This appearance contrasts with the dense lymphocytic infiltrate that blankets the granulomas in many other granulomatous disorders, including tuberculosis. Sarcoidal granulomas can occupy almost the entire dermis in affected skin or may occur only in relatively small foci that are widely spaced. Histochemical stains for infectious organisms are generally negative.

Just as the cause of sarcoidosis remains unknown, the mechanisms of granuloma formation in sarcoidosis are not completely understood. In general, certain antigenic stimuli elicit a T-cell reaction (see prior discussion regarding pathogenesis of allergic contact dermatitis). Antigens presented in the proper context induce the responding T cells to release various cytokines. The specific cytokines **monocyte chemotactic factor** and **migration inhibitory factor,** along with a host of others, recruit macrophages to the site and direct the cells to remain there. Even though lymphocytes are a small

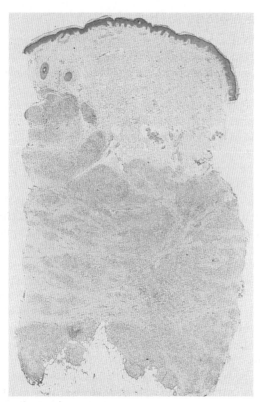

FIGURE 8–30 Histopathologic features of sarcoidosis, a nodular dermatitis. Note the dense infiltrate of inflammatory cells throughout most of the dermis.

component of sarcoidal granulomas microscopically, they are believed to be crucial to the pathogenesis of the disease.

Studies of the organization of sarcoidal granulomas suggest a pattern of lymphocyte arrangement similar to that of tuberculoid leprosy, a condition in which a potent immune response keeps the *M leprae* organisms in relative check. In these conditions, the lymphocytes present within the centers of the granulomas are CD4 positive, whereas CD8-positive cells are arranged at the periphery. This structure may allow the CD4 helper cells to direct the immune response to center around an offending antigen while the CD8 suppressor cells

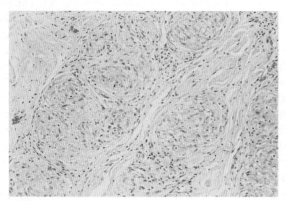

FIGURE 8–31 Sarcoidosis. Pale-staining histiocytes form nodular aggregates among the collagen of the dermis.

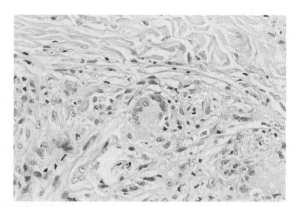

FIGURE 8–32 Sarcoidosis. Multinucleated giant cells such as the one seen here in the center of the field are common in sarcoidal granulomas.

limit the extent of the response. Granulomas are not organized in this fashion in lepromatous leprosy, and the lack of an effective suppressive reaction permits uncontrolled proliferation of *M leprae* bacilli.

Clinical Manifestations

The clinical picture in sarcoidosis is quite broad. The spectrum of symptoms in an individual patient depends on which tissues are involved and to what extent. There are several prototypical presentations. One consists of bilateral pulmonary hilar lymphadenopathy (resulting from sarcoidal granulomas in perihilar lymph nodes) and acute erythema nodosum, a combination known as Löfgren's syndrome. Fever, arthralgias, uveitis, and lung parenchymal involvement are common in Löfgren's syndrome. Another variant of sarcoidosis involves the nose, with beadlike papules at the rims of the nares. This presentation is known as lupus pernio, a term of some antiquity that still enjoys widespread use in dermatology. More recently, the designation "nasal rim sarcoidosis" has been proposed for this variant. This cutaneous finding usually indicates significant involvement of the tracheobronchial tree or lung parenchyma.

Skin disease occurs in systemic sarcoidosis in only one third of cases, although about 80% of patients with sarcoidosis of the skin have concurrent systemic disease. The lungs are commonly involved, and the possibility of lung involvement should always be investigated in any case of sarcoidosis. The spectrum of lesions of sarcoidosis in the skin includes skin-colored to red-brown papules, plaques, and nodules, hair loss (alopecia) on the scalp or other sites, pigmentary alteration, ulcers, and numerous other patterns mimicking many other diseases. New dermal papules or nodules arising within tattoos that have been present even for many years are a well-recognized phenomenon in sarcoidosis. This should not be surprising because tattoo pigment is a foreign body that is phagocytosed by tissue macrophages and probably serves as a nidus for the development of lesions of sarcoidosis.

Diagnosing sarcoidosis may be difficult. It is often a diagnosis of exclusion. Only when the clinical spectrum is consistent with sarcoidosis and standard investigations have failed to uncover a clear origin (infectious or otherwise) can a diagnosis of sarcoidosis be issued with confidence. Helpful studies include chest x-ray films and bone films with findings suggestive of sarcoidosis or a biopsy of skin or other involved tissue showing the noncaseating granulomas characteristic of the disease.

CHECKPOINT

27. Who gets sarcoidosis? How common is it?
28. What pattern of inflammatory skin disease does sarcoidosis exhibit?
29. How does the pathology of skin lesions of sarcoidosis correspond to clinical lesions?

FOLLICULITIS & PERIFOLLICULITIS: ACNE

Clinical Presentation

Acne most commonly presents as follicle-based comedones, inflammatory papules, or pustules on the face, neck, chest, and back (Figures 8–33 and 8–34). Teenagers are stereotypically afflicted, but neonatal acne and adult acne are common also. Disfiguring nodulocystic acne with resulting severe scarring does not occur before puberty.

Epidemiology

Acne vulgaris is so common that it is said by some authors to affect practically everyone at some point in their lives. The peak incidence is at 18 years of age, although significant numbers of adults up to age 40 years are affected.

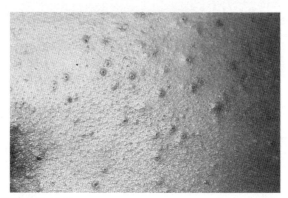

FIGURE 8–33 Acne vulgaris. There are numerous papules with central black plugs termed open comedones or "blackheads." (Reproduced, with permission, from Hurwitz RM, Hood AF. *Pathology of the Skin: Atlas of Clinical-Pathological Correlation*. Originally published by Appleton & Lange. Copyright © 1998 by the McGraw-Hill Companies, Inc.)

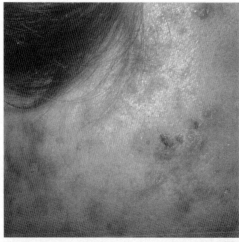

FIGURE 8–34 Acne vulgaris. The red papules and crusts with occasional scars are typical of inflammatory acne. (Reproduced, with permission, from Hurwitz RM, Hood AF. *Pathology of the Skin: Atlas of Clinical-Pathological Correlation*. Originally published by Appleton & Lange. Copyright © 1998 by the McGraw-Hill Companies, Inc.)

Histopathology & Pathogenesis

Histopathologically, comedonal acne is manifest as a widened follicle with a dense keratin plug within its infundibulum. If the follicular orifice is patulous, the acne lesion is said to be an open comedone. If the orifice is normal and the follicle is expanded below the skin surface, the lesion is termed a closed comedone. Secondary inflammatory changes occur commonly within plugged follicular units. Neutrophils may accompany the keratinous plug with the follicular canal, creating a pustular lesion. Inflammatory acne lesions are a consequence of follicles that have ruptured with resultant spillage of keratinous debris into the perifollicular dermis, evoking a dense inflammatory reaction with a mixture of neutrophils, lymphocytes, and histiocytes (Figure 8–35).

Understanding of the evolution of acne lesions has led to therapies that are effective for the vast majority of cases. There are four essential components to the development of acne lesions: (1) plugging of the folliculosebaceous unit; (2) sebum production; (3) overgrowth of the bacterium *Propionibacterium acnes* within the plugged follicle; and (4) a secondary inflammatory response. The formation of keratin plugs within follicles is a complex process that is thought to be genetically controlled on a cellular level. Keratinocytes become sticky and fail to slough appropriately, yielding follicular plugging. Contrary to a commonly held belief, being "dirty" does not cause acne, and vigorous or frequent cleansing does not improve the condition. However, some exogenous substances such as oily cosmetics or petrolatum-based hair care products may promote comedone formation and thus exacerbate acne.

Plugged follicles alone would never become more than comedones, however, if it were not for sebum production and *P acnes* overgrowth. *P acnes* is a commensal organism of the

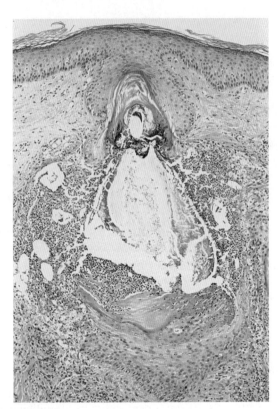

FIGURE 8–35 Histopathologic features of acne. There is a follicle with a central keratin plug. The follicle walls have ruptured and numerous neutrophils fill the dermis around the follicle. This lesion would correspond to an erythematous papule seen in inflammatory acne (see Figure 8–33).

skin. However, with ample sebum as a food source within the well-protected environment of a plugged follicle, *P acnes* overgrowth occurs. The sebum becomes broken down to constituent lipids and free fatty acids. The failure of keratinous debris and sebum to exit the follicle freely expands the follicular canal. The bacteria release factors chemotactic for neutrophils, and their infiltration of the follicle results in pustule formation. Neutrophilic enzymes weaken the follicle wall and follicular rupture occurs, releasing large amounts of inflammatory reactants into the dermis. Lymphocytes, macrophages, and more neutrophils respond, and the comedonal lesion is transformed into an inflamed papule, pustule, or nodule of acne. Follicular rupture and an intense secondary inflammatory reaction may eventuate with profound scarring in some hosts.

Clinical Manifestations

The spectrum of acne severity is quite broad. In the neonate, maternal androgens stimulate enlargement of and sebum overproduction from sebaceous glands. The presence of sebum promotes *P acnes* overgrowth, and acne ensues until the maternal androgens have cleared and the sebaceous glands atrophy to a normal neonatal size. Significant sebum production does not begin again until puberty. Under the stimulation of androgens at puberty, sebaceous glands enlarge once again and produce sebum in the sebaceous areas of the body, namely the face, neck, chest, and back (the same areas affected most by acne). Onset may be gradual or rapid, and severity may range from primarily comedonal to inflammatory papules and pustules to highly inflammatory, painful nodules. Severe scarring variants may be explosive in onset and present with systemic symptoms of fever and arthralgias.

Acne may present as a component of a syndrome, as in polycystic ovary disease (ie, Stein-Leventhal syndrome) or so-called SAPHO syndrome (*s*ynovitis, *a*cne, *p*almoplantar pustulosis, *h*yperostosis, and *o*steitis). At least in Stein-Leventhal syndrome, there may be hormonal influences that predispose to the acne lesion development. Acne treatments are often multifaceted and address restoring normal keratinization and desquamation to follicular keratinocytes via topical or systemic vitamin A analogs (ie, retinoids), controlling *P acnes* and inflammation with antibiotics (such as topical benzoyl peroxide or oral erythromycin or tetracycline), and decreasing sebum production with retinoids or antiandrogen medications such as spironolactone. On a practical note, patients are usually instructed to avoid excessive face washing because it is not helpful in ameliorating acne and may cause secondary irritation, making topical treatments less tolerable. Gently washing the face once a day with a mild facial cleanser or mild soap is all that is required. Patients are also advised to use nongreasy cosmetics, usually those labeled as noncomedogenic, as well as hair care products without petrolatum.

CHECKPOINT

30. Why do some infants develop acne? What factors explain its spontaneous resolution?
31. What is the pathophysiology of lesion development in acne?
32. What are some broad treatment categories for acne, and which aspect of acne pathogenesis does each address?

CASE STUDIES

Eva M. Aagaard, MD, & Yeong Kwok, MD

(See Chapter 25, p. 686 for Answers)

CASE 34

A 25-year-old woman presents with a complaint of rash that has developed over the last several weeks and seems to be progressing. On examination, she is noted to have several plaquelike lesions over the extensor surfaces of both upper and lower extremities as well as similar lesions on her scalp. The plaques are erythematous, with silvery scales, and are sharply marginated.

Questions

A. What is the likely diagnosis? Is this skin disease genetic, environmental, or both? Based on what evidence?

B. What are the pathophysiologic mechanisms behind the development of the plaques, scale, and erythema characteristic of this disorder?

C. What immunologic defects have been implicated in patients with this skin disease?

CASE 35

A 35-year-old woman who recently returned from Africa presents to the clinic with complaints of a rash. During her trip, she developed an itchy rash on both arms. She has an unremarkable medical history. Medications recently taken include chloroquine for malaria prophylaxis. Examination discloses multiple small violaceous papules on the flexor surfaces of the arms. The lesions have angular borders and flat tops. Some of the lesions have minute white streaks on the surface, barely visible to the naked eye.

Questions

A. What is the likely diagnosis? What is the possible underlying cause?

B. What is the pathophysiologic mechanism by which these skin lesions are formed?

C. What histopathologic changes in the skin are responsible for the appearance of these lesions as violaceous papules with minute white striae?

CASE 36

A 27-year-old woman presents to the urgent care clinic complaining of a red, itchy rash developing suddenly the day before on her arms and legs and spreading to the trunk. She denies ulcers in the mouth or genital area. Her medical history is unremarkable except for occasional episodes of genital herpes. The most recent outbreak was approximately 2 weeks ago. She generally takes oral acyclovir on such occasions, but her prescription has run out and so she did not take any with her last bout. On physical examination, she has multiple erythematous papules over the arms, legs, and trunk. Many of the papules have a central area of duskiness or clearing, such that the lesions resemble targets. There is no evidence of mucosal involvement.

Questions

A. What is the likely diagnosis?

B. What is the pathophysiologic mechanism by which these skin lesions are formed? In what ways is this disease similar to and different from lichen planus?

C. What factors may have triggered this rash? What evidence supports this link?

D. What is responsible for the target-like appearance of these lesions, and what does the histopathology show?

CASE 37

A 65-year-old man presents to the dermatology clinic with a complaint of blisters developing on his abdomen and extremities over the last week. The lesions consisted initially of red patches followed by blister formation. They are pruritic but not painful. The patient has no other complaints and denies mucous membrane involvement. Examination shows only multiple large, tense blisters with an erythematous base over the lower trunk and extremities. The clinical picture is felt to be most consistent with bullous pemphigoid.

Questions

A. What is the major differential diagnosis for multiple bullae? How do these diseases differ, and why is the distinction important?

B. What is the most likely diagnosis, and what would one expect histologic examination to show?

C. What would one expect to find on direct immunofluorescence microscopy?

D. What is the presumed mechanism by which blister formation occurs in bullous pemphigoid?

CASE 38

A 60-year-old man presents to the clinic with complaints of a recurring rash. He states that for the last 2–3 months he has had several episodes of a painless, nonpruritic rash over his distal lower extremities. The lesions are described as purple and raised. His medical history is remarkable for hepatitis C—with no history of cirrhosis—and peripheral neuropathy. The patient has recently been treated for otitis media with amoxicillin. He has taken no other medications. Physical examination is notable only for multiple reddish-purple papules over the distal lower extremities (palpable purpura). The underlying skin is hyperpigmented. Biopsy reveals neutrophils, neutrophilic debris, and amorphous protein deposits involving the small blood vessels, consistent with fibrinoid necrosis.

Questions

A. What is the likely dermatologic diagnosis? What are some possible precipitants of that disease in this patient?

B. What is the underlying pathogenetic mechanism by which the lesions are formed?

C. What histologic characteristics are responsible for the appearance of the lesions as papular and purpuric?

D. What additional symptoms should this patient be asked about? Should any laboratory tests be ordered?

CASE 39

A 30-year-old woman presents to the clinic complaining that she has "an itchy rash all over the place." She noticed that her legs became red, itchy, and blistered about 2 days after she had been hiking in a heavily wooded area. She says that scratching broke the blisters and afterward the rash became much worse and spread all over. She is convinced that the rash could not be poison ivy because once before she was exposed to that plant and did not develop a rash. On examination there are erythematous vesicles and bullae in linear streaks on both of her legs. Some areas are weepy, with a yellowish crust. There are ill-defined erythematous plaques studded with papulovesicles on the trunk and arms.

Questions

A. What is the likely diagnosis? What feature on the physical examination is the cardinal sign?

B. What made the eruption spread?

C. How do you explain the diagnosis to the patient in light of the fact that she did not develop a rash after known exposure to poison ivy in the past? Why didn't the rash appear until 2 days after the apparent exposure?

CASE 40

A 45-year-old-woman presents to clinic with a rash on her legs for 2 months. She notes that the rash started soon after babysitting her niece, who had "strep throat." She initially had a sore throat herself, but it stopped hurting after she took 2 days worth of antibiotics she had left over from a previous prescription. On examination, on the anterior lower legs, she has several scattered ill-defined erythematous nodules, which are tender to palpation.

Questions

A. What is the likely diagnosis? What is the probable cause? What might explain why the eruption has persisted?

B. What are some other common causes of this condition?

C. What is the pathophysiologic mechanism of skin lesion formation?

D. What are the histopathologic findings of this disease?

CASE 41

A 52-year-old African American man presents to the clinic with a rash that has been worsening for several months. Review of systems is notable for a chronic cough. Examination reveals multiple red-brown dermis-based papules on the trunk, arms, and face. Several lesions are clustered near the nares. The exam is otherwise unremarkable.

Questions

A. What is the likely diagnosis? What information is necessary to confirm the diagnosis?

B. What organ system (in addition to the skin) is at risk for disease involvement based on the clinical examination?

C. What are the histopathologic features of this disease?

D. How does it present clinically?

CASE 42

A 15-year-old girl presents to the clinic complaining of "pimples" for 6 months. She has been using an over-the-counter face wash four times a day to keep the oil and dirt off, but it has not helped. Examination reveals several dozen erythematous papules and pustules over the forehead and central face with scattered open and closed comedones. A diagnosis of moderate inflammatory acne is entertained.

Questions

A. Why has her meticulous cleansing practice not helped her condition? What advice do you give her regarding facial cleansing?

B. What is the life cycle of an inflammatory papule of acne?

C. What are some general categories of acne treatment, and what component of lesion development does each address?

REFERENCES

General

Ackerman AB, Ragaz A. *The Lives of Lesions: Chronology in Dermatopathology.* Masson, 1984.

Bolognia J et al (editors). *Dermatology,* 2nd ed. Mosby, 2008.

James W et al. *Andrews' Diseases of the Skin,* 10th ed. Elsevier, 2005.

Psoriasis

Fitch E et al. Pathophysiology of psoriasis: Recent advances on IL-23 and Th17 cytokines. Curr Rheumatol Rep. 2007 Dec;9(6):461–7. [PMID: 18177599]

Ghoreschi K et al. Immunopathogenesis and role of T cells in psoriasis. Clin Dermatol. 2007 Nov-Dec;25(6):574–80. [PMID: 18021895]

Griffiths CE et al. Pathogenesis and clinical features of psoriasis. Lancet. 2007 Jul 21;370(9583):263-71. [PMID: 17658397]

MacDonald A et al. Psoriasis: Advances in pathophysiology and management. Postgrad Med J. 2007 Nov;83(985):690–7. [PMID: 17989268]

Myers WA et al. Psoriasis and psoriatic arthritis: Clinical features and disease mechanisms. Clin Dermatol. 2006 Sep-Oct;24(5):438–47. [PMID: 16966023]

Naldi L et al. The clinical spectrum of psoriasis. Clin Dermatol. 2007 Nov-Dec;25(6):510–8. [PMID: 18021886]

Nickoloff BJ et al. The cytokine and chemokine network in psoriasis. Clin Dermatol. 2007 Nov-Dec;25(6):568–73. [PMID: 18021894]

Lichen Planus

Ismail SB et al. Oral lichen planus and lichenoid reactions: Etio-patho-genesis, diagnosis, management and malignant transform-ation. J Oral Sci. 2007 Jun;49(2):89–106. [PMID: 17634721]

Mithani SK et al. Molecular genetics of premalignant oral lesions. Oral Dis. 2007 Mar;13(2):126–33. [PMID: 17305612]

Parodi A et al. Prevalence of stratified epithelium-specific antinuclear antibodies in 138 patients with lichen planus. J Am Acad Dermatol. 2007 Jun;56(6):974–8. [PMID: 17270314]

Scully C et al. Oral mucosal disease: lichen planus. Br J Oral Maxillo-fac Surg. 2008 Jan;46(1):15–21. [PMID: 17822813]

Wenzel J et al. Type I interferon-associated cytotoxic inflammation in lichen planus. J Cutan Pathol. 2006 Oct;33(10):672–8. [PMID: 17026519]

Erythema Multiforme

Caproni M et al. Expression of cytokines and chemokine receptors in the cutaneous lesions of erythema multiforme and Stevens-Johnson syndrome/toxic epidermal necrolysis. Br J Dermatol. 2006 Oct;155(4):722–8. [PMID: 16965421]

French LE. Toxic epidermal necrolysis and Stevens Johnson syn-drome: Our current understanding. Allergol Int. 2006 Mar;55(1):9–16. [PMID: 17075281]

Khalili B et al. Pathogenesis and recent therapeutic trends in Stevens-Johnson syndrome and toxic epidermal necrolysis. Ann Allergy Asthma Immunol. 2006 Sep;97(3):272–80. [PMID: 17042130]

Lamoreux MR et al. Erythema multiforme. Am Fam Physician. 2006 Dec 1;74(11):1883–8. [PMID: 17168345]

Scully C et al. Oral mucosal diseases: erythema multiforme. Br J Oral Maxillofac Surg. 2008 Mar;46(2):90–5. [PMID: 17767983]

Bullous Pemphigoid

Di Zenzo G et al. Bullous pemphigoid: physiopathology, clinical fea-tures and management. Adv Dermatol. 2007;23:257–88. [PMID: 18159905]

Kasperkiewicz M et al. The pathophysiology of bullous pemphigoid. Clin Rev Allergy Immunol. 2007 Oct;33(1-2):67–77. [PMID: 18094948]

Leukocytoclastic Vasculitis

Claudy A. Pathogenesis of leukocytoclastic vasculitis. Eur J Derma-tol. 1998 Mar;8(2):75–9. [PMID: 9649707]

Crowson AN et al. Cutaneous vasculitis: A review. J Cutan Pathol. 2003 Mar;30(3):161–73. [PMID: 12641775]

Grunwald MH et al. Leukocytoclastic vasculitis: Correlation between different histologic stages and direct immunofluores-cence results. Int J Dermatol. 1997 May;36(5):349–52. [PMID: 9199981]

Sais G et al. Adhesion molecule expression and endothelial cell activa-tion in cutaneous leukocytoclastic vasculitis. An immuno-histologic and clinical study in 42 patients. Arch Dermatol. 1997 Apr;133(4):443–50. [PMID: 9126007]

Sais G et al. Prognostic factors in leukocytoclastic vasculitis: A clini-copathologic study of 160 patients. Arch Dermatol. 1998 Mar;134(3):309–15. [PMID: 9521029]

Tai YJ et al. Retrospective analysis of adult patients with cutaneous leukocytoclastic vasculitis. Australas J Dermatol. 2006 May;47(2):92–6. [PMID: 16637802]

Allergic Contact Dermatitis

Fyhrquist-Vanni N et al. Contact dermatitis. Dermatol Clin. 2007 Oct;25(4):613–23. [PMID: 17903620]

Lepoittevin JP et al (editors). *Allergic Contact Dermatitis: The Molec-ular Basis*. Springer, 1998.

Saint-Mezard P et al. The role of CD4+ and CD8+ T cells in contact hypersensitivity and allergic contact dermatitis. Eur J Dermatol. 2004 May-Jun;14(3):131–8. [PMID: 15246935]

Erythema Nodosum

Mert A et al. Erythema nodosum: An experience of 10 years. Scand J Infect Dis. 2004;36(6-7):424–7. [PMID: 15307561]

Requena L et al. Erythema nodosum. Semin Cutan Med Surg. 2007 Jun;26(2):114–25. [PMID: 17544964]

Schwartz RA et al. Erythema nodosum: A sign of systemic disease. Am Fam Physician. 2007 Mar 1;75(5):695–700. [PMID: 17375516]

Sarcoidosis

Marchell RM et al. Chronic cutaneous lesions of sarcoidosis. Clin Dermatol. 2007 May-Jun;25(3):295–302. [PMID: 17560307]

Tchernev G. Cutaneous sarcoidosis: The "great imitator": etio-patho-genesis, morphology, differential diagnosis, and clinical manage-ment. Am J Clin Dermatol. 2006;7(6):375–82. [PMID: 17173472]

Acne

Ayer J et al. Acne: More than skin deep. Postgrad Med J. 2006 Aug;82(970):500–6. [PMID: 16891439]

Harper JC et al. Pathogenesis of acne: Recent research advances. Adv Dermatol. 2003;19:1–10. [PMID: 14626815]

McInturff JE et al. The role of toll-like receptors in the pathophysiol-ogy of acne. Semin Cutan Med Surg. 2005 Jun;24(2):73–8. [PMID: 16092794]

Pawin H et al. Physiopathology of acne vulgaris: Recent data, new understanding of the treatments. Eur J Dermatol. 2004 Jan-Feb;14(1):4–12. [PMID: 14965788]

Webster GF. The pathophysiology of acne. Cutis. 2005 Aug;76(2 Suppl):4–7. [PMID: 16164150]

Pulmonary Disease

Thomas J. Prendergast, MD, Stephen J. Ruoss, MD, & Eric J. Seeley, MD

The principal physiologic role of the lungs is to make oxygen available to tissues for metabolism and to remove the main byproduct of that metabolism, carbon dioxide. The lungs perform this function by moving inspired air into close proximity to the pulmonary capillary bed to enable gas exchange by simple diffusion. This is accomplished at a minimal workload, is regulated efficiently over a wide range of metabolic demand, and takes place with close matching of ventilation to lung perfusion. The extensive surface area of the respiratory system must also be protected from a broad variety of infectious or noxious environmental insults.

Humans possess a complex and efficient respiratory system that satisfies these diverse requirements. When injury to components of the respiratory system occurs, the integrated function of the whole is disrupted. The consequences can be profound. Airway injury or dysfunction results in obstructive lung diseases, including bronchitis and asthma, whereas parenchymal lung injury can produce restrictive lung disease or pulmonary vascular disease. To understand the clinical presentations of lung disease, it is necessary first to understand the anatomic and functional organization of the lungs that determines normal function.

CHECKPOINT

1. What are the two principal physiologic roles of the lungs?
2. What are the requirements for successful lung function?

NORMAL STRUCTURE & FUNCTION OF THE LUNGS

ANATOMY

The mature respiratory system consists of visceral pleura-covered lungs contained by the chest wall and diaphragm, the latter serving under normal conditions as the principal bellows muscle for ventilation. The lungs are divided into lobes, each demarcated by intervening visceral pleura. Each lung possesses an upper and lower lobe; the middle lobe and lingula are the third lobes in the right and left lungs, respectively. At end expiration, most of the volume of the lungs is air (Table 9–1), whereas almost half of the mass of the lungs is accounted for by blood volume. It is a testament to the delicate structure of the gas-exchanging region of the lungs that alveolar tissue has a total weight of only 250 g but a total surface area of 75 m^2.

Connective tissue fibers and surfactant serve to maintain the anatomic integrity of this large and complex surface area. The connective tissue fibers are highly organized collagen and elastic structures. They radiate into the lungs, dividing segments, investing airways and vessels, and supporting alveolar walls with a very elastic and delicate fibrous network. The multidirectional elastic support provided by this network allows the lung, from alveoli to conducting airways, to support itself and retain airway patency despite large changes in volume.

Surfactant is a complex material produced by type II alveolar cells and composed of multiple phospholipids and specific associated proteins. The presence of surfactant covering the alveolar epithelial surface produces a marked reduction of surface tension, allowing expansion of alveoli with a transpulmonary distending pressure of less than 5 cm H_2O. In the absence of this surface-active layer, increasing surface tension associated with a reduction of alveolar volume during expiration would collapse alveoli. The distending pressure required to reexpand these alveoli would be greater than normal ventilatory effort could produce. The physiologic function of surfactant thus enhances the anatomic stability of the lungs.

TABLE 9–1 Components of normal human lung.

Component	Volume (mL) or Mass (g)	Thickness (μm)
Gas (functional residual capacity)	2400	
Tissue	900	
Blood	400	
Lung	500	
Support structures	250	
Alveolar walls	250–300	
Epithelium	60–80	0.18
Endothelium	50–70	0.10
Interstitium	100–185	0.22

Reproduced, with permission, from Murray JF, Nadel JA. *Textbook of Respiratory Medicine,* 4th ed. Copyright Elsevier/Saunders, 2005.

Airway & Epithelial Anatomy

Further anatomic division of the lungs is based primarily on the separation of the tracheobronchial tree into **conducting airways,** which provide for movement of air from the external environment to areas of gas exchange, and **terminal respiratory units,** or **acini,** the airways and associated alveolar structures participating directly in gas exchange (Figure 9–1). The proximal conducting airways are lined by ciliated pseudostratified columnar epithelial cells, are supported by a cartilaginous skeleton in their walls, and contain secretory glands in the epithelial wall. The ciliated epithelium has a uniform orientation of cilia that beat in unison toward the pharynx. This ciliary action, together with the mucus layer produced by submucosal mucous secretory glands, provides a mechanism for the continuous transport of contaminating or excess material out of the lungs. Circumferential airway smooth muscle is also present but, as with secretory glands, is reduced and then lost as the airways branch farther into the lung and diminish in caliber. The smallest conducting airways are nonrespiratory **bronchioles.** They are characterized by a loss of smooth muscle and cartilage but retention of a cuboidal epithelium that may be ciliated and which is not a site of gas exchange. The lobes of the lung are divided into less distinct lobules, defined as collections of terminal respiratory units incompletely bounded by connective tissue septa. Terminal respiratory units are the final physiologic and anatomic unit of the lung, with walls of thin alveolar epithelial cells that provide gas exchange with the alveolar capillary bed.

The principal site of resistance to airflow in the lungs is in medium-sized bronchi (Figure 9–2). This seems counterintuitive because one would expect smaller caliber airways to be the major site of resistance. Repetitive branching of the small airways leads to a profound increase in cross-sectional area

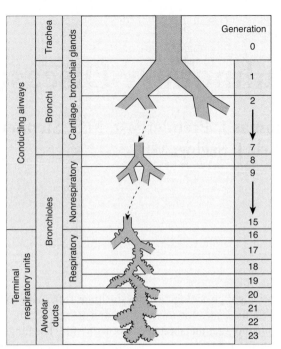

FIGURE 9–1 Subdivision of conducting airways and terminal respiratory units. This schematic illustration demonstrates the subdivisions of both the conducting airways and the respiratory airways. Successive branching produces increasing generations of airways, beginning with the trachea. Note that gas-exchanging segments of the lung are encountered only after extensive branching, with concomitant decrease in airway caliber and increase in total cross-sectional area (see Figures 9–2 and 9–3). (Redrawn, with permission, from Weibel ER. *Morphometry of the Human Lung.* Springer, 1963.)

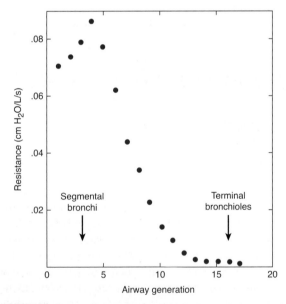

FIGURE 9–2 Location of the principal site of airflow resistance. The second- through fifth-generation airways include the segmental bronchi and larger bronchioles. They present the greatest resistance to airflow in normal individuals. The smaller airways contribute relatively little despite their smaller caliber because of the enormous number arranged in parallel. Compare with Figure 9–3. (Redrawn, with permission, from West JB. *Respiratory Physiology: The Essentials,* 4th ed. Williams & Wilkins, 1990.)

that does not normally contribute significantly to airway resistance (Figure 9–3). Under pathologic conditions such as asthma, in which smaller bronchi and bronchioles become narrowed, airway resistance can increase dramatically.

The pulmonary arterial system runs in close association with the branching bronchial tree throughout the lungs (Figure 9–4). Control of arterial flow and bronchial caliber is tightly regulated and this anatomic arrangement provides the ideal setting for the continuous matching of ventilation and perfusion to different lung segments.

Pulmonary Nervous System

The lungs are richly innervated with neural fibers from parasympathetic (vagal), sympathetic, and the so-called nonadrenergic, noncholinergic (NANC) systems. Efferent fibers include the following: (1) parasympathetic fibers, with muscarinic cholinergic efferents that mediate bronchoconstriction, pulmonary vasodilation, and mucous gland secretion; (2) sympathetic fibers, whose stimulation produces bronchial smooth muscle relaxation, pulmonary vasoconstriction, and inhibition of secretory gland activity; and (3) the NANC system, with multiple transmitters implicated, including adenosine triphosphate (ATP), nitric oxide (NO), and peptide neurotransmitters such as substance P and vasoactive intestinal peptide (VIP). The NANC system participates in inhibitory events, including bronchodilation, and may function as the predominant reciprocal balance to the excitatory cholinergic system.

Pulmonary afferents consist principally of the vagal sensory fibers. These include the following:

1. Fibers from bronchopulmonary stretch receptors, located in the trachea and proximal bronchi. Stimulation of these fibers by lung inflation results in bronchodilation and an increased heart rate.
2. Fibers from irritant receptors, which are also found in proximal airways. Stimulation of these fibers by diverse nonspecific stimuli elicits efferent responses, including cough, bronchoconstriction, and mucus secretion.
3. C fibers, or fibers from juxtacapillary (J) receptors, are unmyelinated fibers ending in lung parenchyma and bronchial walls and respond to mechanical and chemical stimuli. The reflex responses associated with stimulation of C fibers include a rapid shallow breathing pattern, mucus secretion, cough, and heart rate slowing with inspiration.

Vascular & Lymphatic Anatomy

The pulmonary vascular system has two main components: the pulmonary vessels and the bronchial vessels (Figure 9–4). Pulmonary arteries are smooth muscle-invested vessels running with the bronchial tree and providing perfusion to lung parenchyma. They are very sensitive to the alveolar PO_2, with a prominent hypoxic vasoconstrictor response. This provides a sensitive mechanism for matching alveolar perfusion with ventilation. Pulmonary veins, in turn, drain alveolar lung parenchyma, taking a course in the intralobular septa distinct from the pulmonary bronchovascular bundle. Bronchial vessels arise from the systemic circulation to supply blood to nearly all the intrapulmonary structures except the parenchyma, including the bronchial tree, pulmonary nervous system and lymphatics, and connective tissue septa. Bronchial arteries anastomose with capillaries of the pulmonary circulation but normally contribute only 1–2% of total pulmonary circulation. This flow can increase dramatically in the setting of chronic inflammation and may be a major source of hemoptysis.

Pulmonary lymphatics develop along with the airway and vascular systems of the lung. Lymphatics are found in connective tissue spaces of the visceral pleura, the peribronchovascular sheath, and interlobular septa. Lymphatics are found as far distally as the terminal respiratory bronchioles but do not enter the connective tissue space of the alveolar walls (Figure 9–4). Thus, fluid that finds its way into the alveolar interstitium must move the short distance to the region of terminal bronchioles to gain access to draining lymphatics. Both visceral and parietal pleura contain associated lymphatics. These vessels—in particular, the lymphatics associated with the parietal pleura—are responsible for the rapid clearance of fluid from the pleural space.

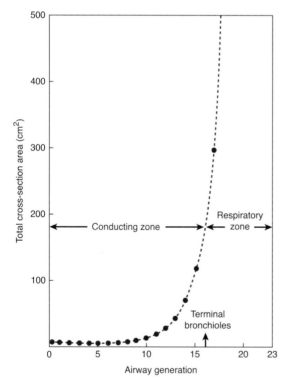

FIGURE 9–3 Airway generation and total airway cross-sectional area. Note the extremely rapid increase in total cross-sectional area in the respiratory zone (compare with Figure 9–1) and the fall in resistance as a consequence of the increase in cross-sectional area increase (compare with Figure 9–2). As a result, the forward velocity of gas during inspiration becomes very low at the level of the respiratory bronchioles, and gas diffusion becomes the chief mode of ventilation. (Redrawn, with permission, from West JB. *Respiratory Physiology: The Essentials,* 4th ed. Williams & Wilkins, 1990.)

LUNG VOLUMES, CAPACITIES, AND THE NORMAL SPIROGRAM

The volume of gas in the lungs is divided into volumes and capacities as shown in the bars to the left of the figure below. Lung volumes are primary: They do not overlap each other. **Tidal volume (V_T)** is the amount of gas inhaled and exhaled with each resting breath. A normal tidal volume in a 70-kg person is approximately 350–400 mL. **Residual volume (RV)** is the amount of gas remaining in the lungs at the end of a maximal exhalation. Lung capacities are composed of two or more lung volumes. The **vital capacity (VC)** is the total amount of gas that can be exhaled after a maximal inhalation. The vital capacity and the residual volume together constitute the **total lung capacity (TLC)**, or the total amount of gas in the lungs at the end of a maximal inhalation. The **functional residual capacity (FRC)** is the amount of gas in the lungs at the end of a resting tidal breath. (**IC, inspiratory capacity; IRV, inspiratory reserve volume; ERV, expiratory reserve volume.**)

The spirogram at the right in the figure is drawn in real time. The first tidal breath shown takes 5 seconds, indicating a respiratory rate of 12 breaths/min. The **forced vital capacity (FVC)** maneuver begins with an inhalation from FRC to TLC (lasting about 1 second) followed by a forceful exhalation from TLC to RV (lasting about 5 seconds). The amount of gas exhaled during the first second of this maneuver is the **forced expiratory volume in 1 second (FEV$_1$)**. Normal subjects expel approximately 80% of the FVC in the first second. The **ratio of the FEV$_1$ to FVC** (referred to as the FEV$_1$%) is diminished in patients with obstructive lung disease and increased in patients with restrictive lung disease.

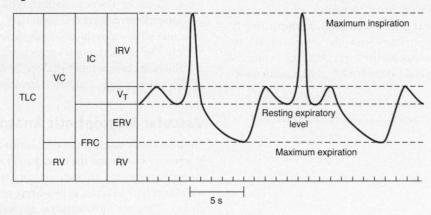

(Redrawn, with permission, from Staub NC. *Basic Respiratory Physiology*. Churchill Livingstone, 1991.)

Immune Structure & Function

Of all the body's organs, the lungs have a unique exposure to environmental insults. Nonexertional ventilation in an adult totals about 6000 L of air per day, an amount that is increased substantially with activity. This exposure to an open, nonsterile environment imposes an ongoing risk of toxic, infectious, or inflammatory insults. Furthermore, the pulmonary circulation contains the only capillary bed in the body through which the entire circulating blood volume must flow in each cardiac cycle. As a consequence, the lung is an obligatory vascular sieve and functions as a principal site of defense against hematogenous spread of infection or other noxious influences. Protection of the lungs from environmental and infectious injury involves a set of complex responses capable of providing a timely and successful defense against attack via the airways or the vascular bed. As outlined in Table 9–2, it is convenient for discussion purposes to separate these responses into two major categories—nonspecific physical and chemical protections and specific immune structures and actions—all functioning in such a way to prevent injury to or microbial invasion of the very large epithelial and vascular area of the lung.

CHECKPOINT

3. What are the roles of the connective tissue and surfactant systems in lung function?

4. What is the role of ciliary action of the respiratory epithelium?

5. Why are medium-sized bronchi rather than small airways the major site of resistance to airflow in the lungs?

6. What are the physiologic functions of the efferent parasympathetic, sympathetic, and NANC neural systems of the lung?

7. What are the categories of afferent vagal sensory receptors?

8. What are the different roles of the pulmonary and bronchial arteries?

9. What sensitive mechanism do the pulmonary arteries have for matching alveolar perfusion with ventilation?

10. What are the components of the nonspecific defense system of the lungs?

11. What are the humoral and cellular components of the specific immune defense system of the lungs?

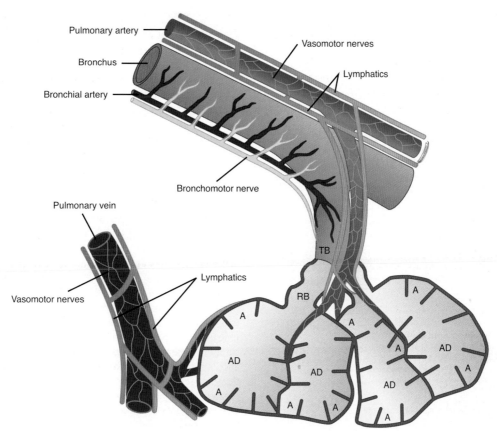

FIGURE 9–4 Airway, vascular, and lymphatic anatomy of the lung. This schematic diagram demonstrates the general anatomic relationships of the airways and terminal respiratory units with the vascular and lymphatic systems of the lung. Important points are as follows: (1) The pulmonary arterial system runs adjacent to the bronchial tree, while the draining pulmonary veins are found distant from the airways; (2) the bronchial wall blood supply is provided by bronchial arteries, branches of systemic arterial origin; (3) lymphatics are found adjacent to both the arterial and venous systems and are very abundant in the lung; and (4) lymphatics are found as far distally as the terminal respiratory bronchioles, but they do not penetrate to the alveolar wall. (A, alveolus; AD, alveolar duct; RB, respiratory bronchiole; TB, terminal bronchiole.) (Redrawn, with permission, from Staub NC. The physiology of pulmonary edema. Hum Pathol. 1970;1:419.)

PHYSIOLOGY

At rest, the lungs take 4 L/min of air and 5 L/min of blood, direct them within 0.2 μm of each other, and then return both to their respective pools. With maximal exercise, flow may increase to 100 L/min of ventilation and 25 L/min of cardiac output. The lungs thereby perform their primary physiologic function of making oxygen available to the tissues for metabolism and removing the major byproduct of that metabolism, carbon dioxide. The lungs perform this task largely free of conscious control, all the while maintaining $PaCO_2$ within 5% tolerance. It is a magnificent feat of evolutionary plumbing and neurochemical control.

Static Properties: Compliance & Elastic Recoil

The lung maintains its extremely thin parenchyma over an enormous surface area by means of an intricate supporting architecture of collagen and elastin fibers. Anatomically, as well as physiologically and functionally, the lung is an elastic organ.

The lungs inflate and deflate in response to changes in volume of the semirigid thoracic cage in which they are suspended. An analogy would be to inflate a blacksmith's bellows by pulling the handles apart, thus increasing the volume of the bellows, lowering pressure, and causing inflow of air. Air enters the lungs when the pressure in the pleural space is reduced by the expansion of the chest wall. The volume of air entering the lungs depends on the change in pleural pressure and the **compliance** of the respiratory system. Compliance is an intrinsic elastic property that relates a change in volume to a change in pressure. The compliance of both the chest wall and the lungs contribute to the compliance of the respiratory system (Figure 9–5). The compliance of the chest wall does not change significantly with thoracic volume, at least within the physiologic range. The compliance of the lungs varies inversely with lung volume. At functional residual capacity (FRC), the lungs are normally very compliant, approximately 200 mL/cm H_2. Thus, a reduction of 5 cm H_2O pressure in the pleural space will draw a breath of 1 L.

The tendency of a deformable body to return to its baseline shape is its **elastic recoil.** The elastic recoil of the chest wall is determined by the shape and structure of the thoracic cage.

TABLE 9–2 Lung defenses.

I. Nonspecific defenses
1. Clearance
a. Cough
b. Mucociliary escalator
2. Secretions
a. Tracheobronchial (mucus)
b. Alveolar (surfactant)
c. Cellular components (including lysozyme, complement, surfactant proteins, defensins)
3. Cellular defenses
a. Nonphagocytic
Conducting airway epithelium
Terminal respiratory epithelium
b. Phagocytic
Blood phagocytes (monocytes)
Tissue phagocytes (alveolar macrophages)
4. Biochemical defenses
a. Proteinase inhibitors (α_1-protease inhibitor, secretory leukoprotease inhibitor)
b. Antioxidants (eg, transferrin, lactoferrin, glutathione, albumin)
II. Specific immunologic defenses
1. Antibody mediated (B-lymphocyte–dependent immunologic responses)
a. Secretory immunoglobulin (IgA)
b. Serum immunoglobulins
2. Antigen presentation to lymphocytes
a. Macrophages and monocytes
b. Dendritic cells
c. Epithelial cells
3. Cell mediated (T-lymphocyte–dependent) immunologic responses
a. Cytokine mediated
b. Direct cellular cytotoxicity
4. Nonlymphocyte cellular immune responses
a. Mast cell dependent
b. Eosinophil dependent

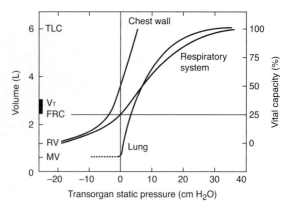

FIGURE 9–5 Interaction of the pressure-volume properties of the lungs and the chest wall. Resting lung volume (functional residual capacity [FRC]) represents the equilibrium point where the elastic recoil of the lung (tendency to collapse inward) and the chest wall (tendency to spring outward) are exactly balanced. Other lung volumes can also be defined by reference to this diagram. Total lung capacity (TLC) is the point where the inspiratory muscles cannot generate sufficient force to overcome the elastic recoil of the lungs and chest wall. Residual volume (RV) is the point where the expiratory muscles cannot generate sufficient force to overcome the elastic recoil of the chest wall. Compliance is calculated by taking the slope of these pressure-volume relationships at a specific volume. Note that the compliance of the lungs is greater at low lung volumes but falls considerably above two thirds of vital capacity. (Modified from Staub NC. *Basic Respiratory Physiology*. Churchill Livingstone, 1991.)

Two components contribute to lung elastic recoil. The first is tissue elasticity; the second is related to the forces needed to change the shape of the air-liquid interface of the alveolus (Figure 9–6). Expanding the lungs requires overcoming local surface forces that are directly proportionate to the local **surface tension.** Surface tension is a physical property that reflects the greater attraction between molecules of a liquid rather than between molecules of that liquid and adjacent gas. At the air-liquid interface of the lung, molecules of water at the interface are more strongly attracted to each other than they are to the air above. This creates a net force drawing water molecules together in the plane of the interface. If the interface is stretched over a curved surface, that force acts to collapse the curve. The law of Laplace quantifies this force: The pressure needed to keep open the curve (in this case represented by a sphere) is directly proportionate to the surface tension at the interface and inversely proportionate to the radius of the sphere (Figure 9–7).

Surfactant is a mixture of phospholipid (predominantly dipalmitoylphosphatidylcholine [DPPC]) and specific surfactant proteins. These hydrophobic molecules displace water molecules from the air-liquid interface, thereby reducing surface tension. This reduction has three physiologic implications: First, it reduces the elastic recoil pressure of the lungs, thereby reducing the pressure needed to inflate them. This results in reduced work of breathing. Second, it allows surface forces to vary with alveolar surface area, thereby promoting

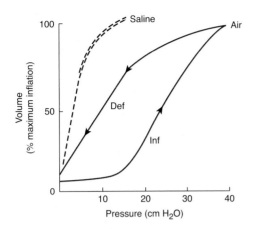

FIGURE 9–6 Effect of surface forces on lung compliance: a simple experiment demonstrating the effect of surface tension at the air-liquid interface of excised cat lungs. When inflated with saline, there are no surface forces to overcome and the lungs are both more compliant and show no difference (hysteresis) between the inflation and deflation curves. When inflated with air, the pressure required to distend the lung is greater at every volume. The difference between the two represents the contribution of surface forces. There is also a pronounced hysteresis that reflects surfactant recruited into the alveolar liquid during inflation (Inf), where it further reduces surface forces during deflation (Def). (Redrawn, with permission, from Morgan TE. Pulmonary surfactant. N Engl J Med. 1971;284:1185.)

alveolar stability and protecting against atelectasis (Figure 9–7). Third, it limits the reduction of hydrostatic pressure in the pericapillary interstitium caused by surface tension. This reduces the forces promoting transudation of fluid and the tendency to accumulate interstitial edema.

Pathologic states may result from changes in lung elastic recoil related to an increase in compliance (emphysema), a decrease in compliance (pulmonary fibrosis; Figure 9–8), or a disruption of surfactant with an increase in surface forces (infant respiratory distress syndrome [IRDS]).

Dynamic Properties: Flow & Resistance

Inflation of the lungs must overcome three opposing forces: elastic recoil, including surface forces; inertia of the respiratory system; and resistance to airflow. Because inertia is negligible, the work of breathing can be divided into work to overcome elastic forces and work to overcome flow resistance.

Resistance to flow depends on the nature of the flow. Under conditions of **laminar** or **streamlined flow,** resistance is described by Poiseuille's equation: Resistance is directly proportionate to the length of the airway and the viscosity of the gas and inversely proportionate to the fourth power of the radius. A reduction by one half of airway radius leads to a 16-fold increase in airway resistance. Airway caliber is, therefore, the principal determinant of airway resistance under laminar flow conditions. Under conditions of **turbulent flow,** the driving pressure needed to achieve a given flow rate is proportionate to the square of the flow rate. Turbulent flow is also dependent on gas density and not on gas viscosity.

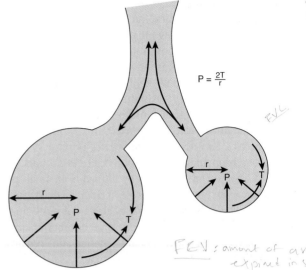

FIGURE 9–7 The importance of surface tension. If two connected alveoli have the same surface tension, then the smaller the radius, the greater the pressure tending to collapse the sphere. This could lead to alveolar instability, with smaller units emptying into larger ones. Alveoli typically do not have the same surface tension because surface forces vary according to surface area as a result of the presence of surfactant. Because the relative concentration of surfactant in the surface layer of the sphere increases as the radius of the sphere falls, the effect of surfactant is increased at low lung volumes. This tends to counterbalance the increase in pressure needed to keep alveoli open at diminished lung volume and adds stability to alveoli, which might otherwise tend to collapse into one another. Surfactant thus protects against regional collapse of lung units, a condition known as atelectasis, in addition to its other functions. (r, radius of alveolus; T, surface tension; P, gas pressure.)

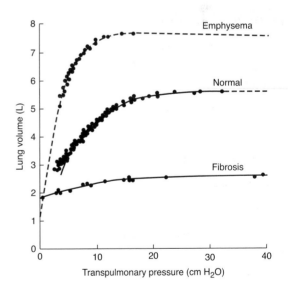

FIGURE 9–8 Static expiratory pressure-volume curves in normal subjects and patients with emphysema and pulmonary fibrosis. The underlying physiologic abnormality in emphysema is a dramatic increase in lung compliance. Such patients tend to breathe at very high lung volumes. Patients with pulmonary fibrosis have very noncompliant lungs and breathe at low lung volumes. (Redrawn, with permission, from Pride NB, Macklem PT. Lung mechanics in disease. In: Vol III, Part 2, of *Handbook of Physiology.* Section 3. Respiratory System. Fishman AP [editor]. American Physiological Society, 1986.)

Most of the resistance to normal breathing arises in the medium-sized bronchi and not in the smaller bronchioles (Figure 9–2). There are two main reasons for this counterintuitive finding. First, airflow in the normal lung is not laminar but turbulent, at least from the mouth to the small peripheral airways. Thus, where flow is highest (in the segmental and subsegmental bronchi), resistance is dependent chiefly on flow rates. There is a transition to laminar flow approaching the terminal bronchioles as a consequence of increased cross-sectional area and decreased flow rates (Figure 9–3). In the respiratory bronchioles and alveoli, there is no bulk flow of gas, and gas movement occurs by diffusion. In small peripheral airways, airway caliber is the principal determinant of resistance. The caliber of peripheral airways is quite small, but repetitive branching creates a very large number of small airways arranged in parallel. Their resistance adds reciprocally, making their contribution to total airway resistance minor under normal conditions.

Airway resistance is determined by several factors. Many disease states affect bronchial smooth muscle tone and cause **bronchoconstriction,** producing an abnormal narrowing of the airways. Airways may also be narrowed by hypertrophy (chronic bronchitis) or infiltration (sarcoidosis) of the airway mucosa. Physiologically, the radial traction of the lung interstitium supports the airways and increases their caliber as lung volume increases. Conversely, as lung volume decreases, airway caliber also decreases and resistance to airflow increases. Patients with airflow obstruction often breathe at large lung volumes in an effort to maximize elastic lung recoil; this supports a larger airway caliber and thus minimizes resistance.

Analysis in terms of laminar and turbulent flow assumes that the airways are rigid tubes. In fact, they are highly compressible. The compressibility of the airways underlies the important phenomenon of **effort-independent flow.** It is an old clinical observation that airflow rates during expiration can be increased with effort only up to a certain point. Beyond that point, further increases in effort do not increase flow rates. The explanation for this phenomenon relies on the concept of an **equal pressure point.**

Pleural pressure is generally negative (subatmospheric) throughout quiet breathing. The peribronchiolar pressure that surrounds the conducting airways reflects pleural pressure. Hence, during quiet breathing, the airways are surrounded by negative pressure that helps to keep them open. Pleural and peribronchiolar pressure may become positive during forced expiration. In this case, the airways are surrounded by positive pressure. The equal pressure point occurs where the pressure inside the airway equals the surrounding peribronchiolar pressure, leading to instability and potential airway collapse (Figure 9–9).

The equal pressure point is not an anatomic site but a functional result that helps to clarify different mechanisms of airflow obstruction. Because the pressure driving expiratory airflow is lung elastic recoil pressure, a reduction in recoil pressure will lead to cessation of flow at higher lung volumes. Patients with emphysema lose lung elastic recoil and may

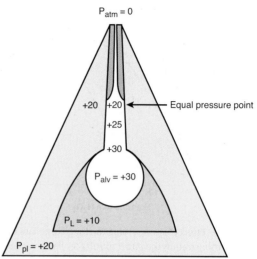

FIGURE 9–9 The concept of the equal pressure point. For air to flow through a tube, there must be a pressure difference between the two ends. In the case of forced expiration with an open glottis, this driving pressure is the difference between alveolar pressure (the sum of pleural pressure and lung elastic recoil pressure) and atmospheric pressure (assumed to be zero). Frictional resistance causes a fall in this driving pressure along the length of the conducting airways. At some point, the driving pressure may equal the surrounding peribronchial pressure; in this event, the net transmural pressure is zero. This defines the equal pressure point. Downstream (toward the mouth) from the equal pressure point, pressure outside the airway is greater than the driving pressure inside the airway. This net negative pressure tends to collapse the airway, resulting in dynamic compression. The more forcefully one expires, the more the pressure surrounding collapsible airways increases. Flow becomes effort independent. (P_{pl}, pleural pressure; P_L, lung elastic recoil pressure; P_{alv}, alveolar pressure; P_{atm}, atmospheric pressure.)

have severely impaired expiratory flow even with airways of normal caliber. Conversely, an increase in recoil pressure will oppose dynamic compression. Patients with pulmonary fibrosis may have abnormally high flow rates despite severely reduced lung volumes. The presence of airway disease augments the drop in pressure along the airways and may generate an equal pressure point at high lung volumes.

The Work of Breathing

The amount of energy needed to maintain the respiratory muscles during quiet breathing is small, approximately 2% of basal oxygen consumption. Increasing ventilation in normal humans consumes relatively little oxygen until ventilation approaches 70 L/min. In patients with lung disease, the energy requirements are greater at rest and increase dramatically with exercise. Patients with emphysema may not be able to increase their ventilation by more than a factor of 2 because the oxygen cost of breathing exceeds the additional oxygen made available to the body.

A constant minute ventilation can be achieved through multiple combinations of respiratory rate and tidal volume. The two components of the work of breathing—elastic forces and resistance to airflow—are affected in opposite ways by changes in frequency and depth of breathing. Elastic resistance is minimized by rapid, shallow breathing; resistive forces are minimized by slow, large tidal volume breathing. Figure 9–10 shows how these two components can be summed to provide a total work of breathing for different frequencies at a constant minute ventilation. The setpoint for respiration is that point at which the total work of breathing is minimized. In normal humans, this occurs at a frequency of approximately 15 breaths/min. In different diseases, this pattern is altered to compensate for the underlying physiologic abnormality.

Distribution of Ventilation & Perfusion

Inhaled air is not distributed equally to all regions of the lung. In the healthy individual, this is due principally to the fractal geometry of repetitive branching of airways and vessels and the effects of gravity on pleural pressure. Pleural pressure varies from the top to the bottom of the lung by approximately 0.25 cm H_2O/cm. It is more negative at the apex and more positive at the base. The effect is shifted to an anteroposterior distribution in the supine position and is greatly diminished (although not abolished) at zero gravity.

Regional ventilation is dependent on regional pleural pressure (Figure 9–11). More negative pleural pressure at the lung apex causes greater expansion of the apical alveoli. Given the shape of the lung's pressure-volume curve, lung compliance is greater at low lung volumes, and ventilation is preferentially distributed to the lower lobes at FRC.

Pulmonary blood flow is a low-pressure system that functions in a gravitational field across 30 vertical centimeters. The distribution of blood flow to the lungs is not uniform under resting conditions. In the upright position, there is a nearly linear increase in blood flow from the top to the bottom of the lung. The details of distribution are portrayed in Figure 9–12.

Multiple factors besides gravity regulate blood flow. The most important is **hypoxic pulmonary vasoconstriction.** The smooth muscle cells of the pulmonary arterioles are sensitive to alveolar PO_2 (much more so than to arterial PO_2). As alveolar PO_2 falls, there is arteriolar constriction, an increase in local resistance to flow, and redistribution of flow to regions of higher alveolar PO_2. This is an extremely effective mechanism when regionalized. It can greatly diminish local blood flow without a significant increase in mean pulmonary arterial pressure when it affects less than 20% of the pulmonary circulation. Global alveolar hypoxia results in pulmonary hypertension.

Matching of Ventilation to Perfusion

The functional role of the lungs is to place ambient air in close proximity to circulating blood to permit gas exchange by simple diffusion. To accomplish this, air and blood flow must be directed to the same place at the same time. In other words, ventilation and perfusion must be matched. A failure to match ventilation to perfusion, or $\dot{V}/\dot{Q}$ **mismatch**, lies behind most abnormalities in O_2 and CO_2 exchange.

In the normal individual, a typical resting minute ventilation is 6 L/min. Approximately one third of this amount fills the conducting airways and constitutes dead space or wasted ventilation. Resting alveolar ventilation is, therefore, approximately 4 L/min, whereas pulmonary artery blood flow is 5 L/min. This yields an overall ratio of ventilation to perfusion of 0.8. As noted previously, neither ventilation nor perfusion is homogeneously distributed. Both are preferentially distributed to dependent regions at rest, although the increase in gravity-dependent flow is more marked with perfusion than with ventilation. Hence, the ratio of ventilation to perfusion is highest at the apex and lowest at the base (Figure 9–13).

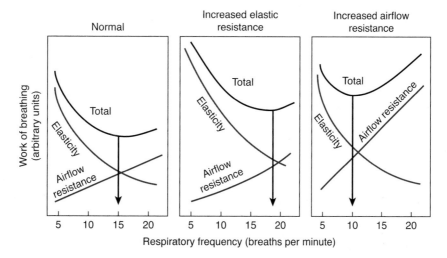

FIGURE 9–10 Minimizing the work of breathing. These diagrams divide the total work of breathing at the same minute ventilation into elastic and resistive components. In disease states that increase elastic forces (eg, pulmonary fibrosis), total work is minimized by rapid, shallow breathing; with increased airflow resistance (eg, chronic bronchitis), total work is minimized by slow deep breathing. (Redrawn, with permission, from Nunn JF. *Nunn's Respiratory Physiology,* 4th ed. Butterworth-Heinemann, 1993.)

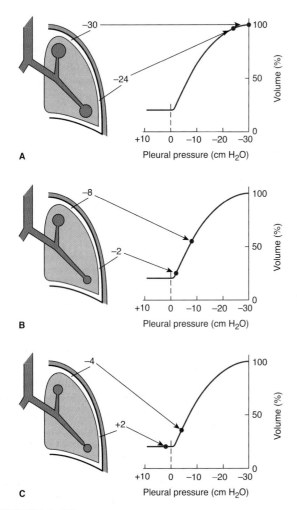

FIGURE 9–11 Distribution of ventilation at different lung volumes. The effect of gravity and the weight of the lung cause pleural pressure to become more negative toward the apex of the lung. The effect of this change in pressure is to increase the expansion of apical alveoli. **A:** Total lung capacity. At high lung volumes, the compliance curve of the lung is flat; alveoli are almost equally expanded because pressure differences cause small changes in lung volume. **B:** Functional residual capacity. During quiet breathing, the lower lobes are on the steep part of the pressure-volume curve. This increased compliance at lower volumes is why ventilation at FRC is preferentially distributed to the lower lobes. **C:** Residual volume. Below functional residual capacity (FRC), there may be dependent lung units that are exposed to positive pleural pressures. These units may collapse, leading to areas of lung that are perfused but not ventilated. (Reprinted, with permission, from Hinshaw HC, Murray JF. *Diseases of the Chest*, 4th. Philadelphia, WB Saunders, 1979.)

Alterations in the distribution of ventilation to perfusion ratios are extremely important and underlie the functional impairment in many disease states. The distribution may favor high $\dot{V}/\dot{Q}$ ratios, with the limiting case being alveolar dead space (ventilation without perfusion, or $\dot{V}/\dot{Q} = \infty$); or it may favor low $\dot{V}/\dot{Q}$ ratios, with the limiting case being a shunt (perfusion without ventilation, or $\dot{V}/\dot{Q} = 0$). These two shifts affect respiratory function differently.

Approximately one third of resting minute ventilation in normal individuals goes to fill the main conducting airways. This is the **anatomic dead space;** it represents ventilation to areas that do not participate in gas exchange. If gas-exchanging regions of the lung are ventilated but not perfused, as may occur in pulmonary embolism or various forms of pulmonary vascular disease, these regions also fail to function in gas exchange. They are referred to as **alveolar dead space, or wasted ventilation** (Figure 9–14, lower panel). Functionally, some percentage of the work of breathing then supports ventilation that does not participate in gas exchange, thus reducing the overall efficiency of ventilation. In the absence of respiratory compensation, an increase in alveolar dead space will cause disturbances in both arterial PO_2 and arterial PCO_2: PaO_2 will fall and $PaCO_2$ will rise. However, because the respiratory control center is exquisitely sensitive to small changes in $PaCO_2$, the most common response to an increase in wasted ventilation is an increase in total minute ventilation that maintains $PaCO_2$ nearly constant. PaO_2 is normal or may be reduced if the fraction of wasted ventilation is large. The A-a ΔPO_2 is increased (as is discussed below in the Distribution of Ventilation & Perfusion section).

A shunt occurs when ventilation is eliminated but perfusion continues, as might happen with atelectatic lung or in areas of lung consolidation (alveoli filled with fluid or infected debris) (Figure 9–14, mid panel). Such a right-to-left shunt permits mixed venous blood to pass to the systemic arterial circulation without coming in contact with alveolar gas. This typically causes a fall in both PO_2 and PCO_2. The reason can be seen in the diagram: The remaining respiratory unit is overventilated relative to its blood flow (large arrow).

The hyperventilation of some lung regions can compensate for a shunt through other regions but only for a possible rise in PCO_2 and not for the fall in PO_2. The reason is straightforward: The CO_2 content of blood is linearly related and inversely proportionate to alveolar ventilation. Increased ventilation to one respiratory unit can reduce the CO_2 content of blood leaving that unit. The CO_2 content of the mixture is the mean of the two units. Because the PCO_2 is directly proportionate to the CO_2 content, the reduced CO_2 content of the hyperventilated units compensates for lack of ventilation to the dead space.

The O_2 content of blood is not linearly related to alveolar ventilation (Figure 9–15). The sigmoid shape of the hemoglobin-oxygen dissociation curve indicates that blood is nearly maximally saturated with oxygen at basal ventilation. Increasing ventilation to one respiratory unit does not significantly increase the O_2 content of blood leaving that unit. The O_2 content of blood leaving a low $\dot{V}/\dot{Q}$ area is the mean of normal blood oxygen content and desaturated, shunted blood. The reduced oxygen content of the mixture tends to lie on the steep portion of the hemoglobin-oxygen dissociation curve. The result is that modest falls in oxygen content lead to large falls in the PO_2.

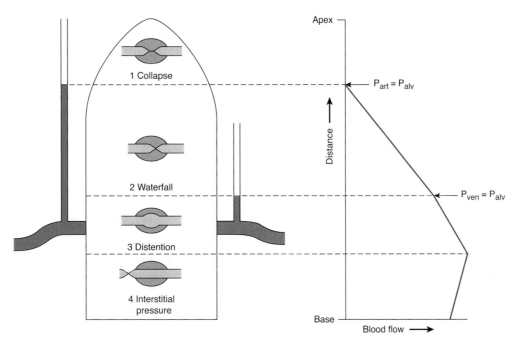

FIGURE 9–12 Effect of changing hydrostatic pressure on the distribution of pulmonary blood flow. Capillary blood flow in different regions of the lung is governed by three pressures: pulmonary arterial pressure, pulmonary venous pressure, and alveolar pressure. Pulmonary arterial pressure must be greater than pulmonary venous pressure to maintain forward perfusion; there are, therefore, three potential arrangements of these variables. **Zone 1:** $P_{alv} > P_{art} > P_{ven}$. There is no capillary perfusion in areas where alveolar pressure is greater than the capillary perfusion pressure. Because alveolar pressure is normally zero, this only occurs where mean pulmonary arterial pressure is less than the vertical distance from the pulmonary artery. **Zone 2:** $P_{art} > P_{alv} > P_{ven}$. Pulmonary arterial pressure exceeds alveolar pressure, but alveolar pressure exceeds pulmonary venous pressure. The driving pressure along the capillary is dissipated by resistance to flow until the transmural pressure is negative and compression occurs. This zone of collapse then regulates flow, which is intermittent and dependent on fluctuating pulmonary venous pressures. **Zone 3:** $P_{art} > P_{ven} > P_{alv}$. Flow is independent of alveolar pressure because the pulmonary venous pressure exceeds atmospheric pressure. **Zone 4:** Zone of extra-alveolar compression. In dependent lung regions, lung interstitial pressure may exceed pulmonary arterial pressure. In this event, capillary flow is determined by compression of extra-alveolar vessels. The right side of the diagram shows a near-continuous distribution of blood flow from the top of the lung to the bottom, demonstrating that in the normal lung there are no discrete zones. The normal human lung at FRC spans 30 vertical centimeters, half of which distance is above the pulmonary artery and left atrium; and representative pulmonary arterial pressures are 33/11 cm H_2O with a mean of 19 cm H_2O. There is, therefore, no physiologic zone 1 in upright humans except perhaps in late diastole. Left atrial pressure averages 11 cm H_2O and is sufficient to create zone 3 conditions two thirds of the distance from the heart to the apex. However, in patients undergoing positive-pressure mechanical ventilation, alveolar pressure is not atmospheric. Under conditions of positive end-expiratory pressure (PEEP), P_{alv} may be as high as 15–20 cm H_2O. This potentially shifts the entire distribution of pulmonary blood flow. (Adapted and reprinted with permission, from Hughes JM et al: Effect of lung volume on the distribution of pulmonary blood flow in man. Respir Physiol. 1968;4(1):58–72.)

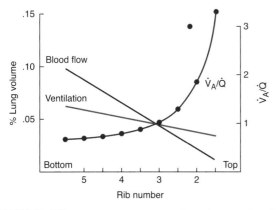

FIGURE 9–13 Changing distribution of ventilation and perfusion down the upright lung. The two straight lines reflect the progressive increases in ventilation and perfusion. The slope is steeper for perfusion. The ratio of ventilation to perfusion is, therefore, lowest at the base and highest at the apex. (Redrawn, with permission, from West JB. *Ventilation/blood flow and gas exchange,* 5th ed. Oxford Blackwell, 1990.)

Ventilation/perfusion mismatching commonly occurs between the extremes of shunts and wasted ventilation. The effect on arterial blood gases of shifts in the distribution of $\dot{V}/\dot{Q}$ ratios can be predicted from the discussion of the limiting cases (Figure 9–16). At the top of Figure 9–16 is a respiratory unit where on one side (B) ventilation has been reduced but perfusion maintained. This defines an area of low $\dot{V}/\dot{Q}$ ratio. The effect on lung function can be understood by dividing it into an area with a normal $\dot{V}/\dot{Q}$ ratio (A) and an area of shunted blood (C). The physiologic effect of low $\dot{V}/\dot{Q}$ areas is similar to the effect of shunts: hypoxemia without hypercapnia. The difference between them can also be seen in this schematic. Shunted blood comes into no contact with inspired air; therefore, no amount of additional oxygen supplied to the inspired air will reverse the fall in systemic arterial PO_2. A low $\dot{V}/\dot{Q}$ area does come in contact with inspired air and can be reversed with increased inspired oxygen. A true shunt is the limiting case of a low $\dot{V}/\dot{Q}$ area where the ratio is zero.

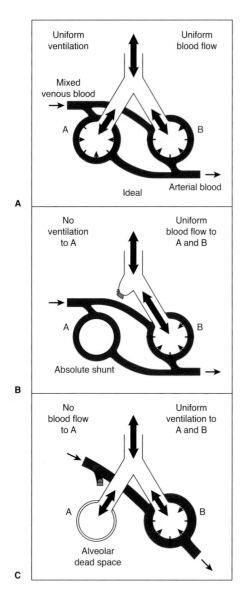

FIGURE 9–14 Three models of the relationship of ventilation to perfusion. In this schematic representation, the circles represent respiratory units, with tubes depicting the conducting airways. The colored channels represent the pulmonary blood flow, which enters the capillary bed as mixed venous blood (blue) and leaves it as arterialized blood (red). Large arrows show distribution of inspired gas; small arrows show diffusion of O_2 and CO_2. In the idealized case (A), the PO_2 and PCO_2 leaving both units are identical. See B and C. See text for details. (Redrawn, with permission, from Comroe J. *Physiology of Respiration,* 2nd ed. Year Book, 1974.)

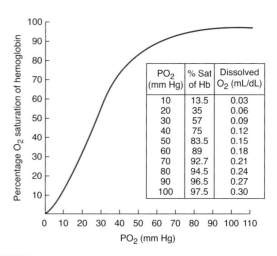

FIGURE 9–15 Oxygen-hemoglobin dissociation curve. pH 7.40, temperature 38 °C. (Data from Severinghaus JW. J Appl Physiol. 1966;21: 1108.)

effect of high $\dot{V}/\dot{Q}$ areas is to increase respiration to maintain $PaCO_2$. This may be done unconsciously. It becomes a clinical problem when the individual cannot maintain an increased minute ventilation.

Arterial blood gases detect major disturbances in respiratory function. One attempt to assess more subtle abnormalities of gas exchange is to calculate the difference between the alveolar and arterial PO_2. This is referred to as the A-a ΔPO_2 or A-a DO_2. The alveolar-capillary membrane permits full equilibration of alveolar and end-capillary oxygen tension under normal $\dot{V}/\dot{Q}$ matching. There is nonetheless a small A-a ΔPO_2 in normal individuals as a result of right-to-left shunting through the bronchial veins and the thebesian veins of the left heart. This accounts for approximately 2% of resting cardiac output and leads to an A-a ΔPO_2 of 5–8 mm Hg in healthy young adults. Normal values increase with age, presumably as a result of closure of dependent airways with consequent shift toward low $\dot{V}/\dot{Q}$ ratios. Further increases in the A-a ΔPO_2 reflect areas of low $\dot{V}/\dot{Q}$ ratio, including shunting. Increasing the fractional inspired concentration of oxygen (FiO_2) also increases this value: A normal A-a ΔPO_2 breathing 100% oxygen is approximately 100 mm Hg.

Control of Breathing

The lungs inflate and deflate passively in response to changes in pleural pressure. Therefore, control over respiration lies in control of the striated muscles—chiefly the diaphragm but also the intercostals and abdominal wall—that change pleural pressure.

These muscles are under both automatic and voluntary control. The rhythm of spontaneous breathing originates in the brainstem, specifically in several groups of interconnected neurons in the medulla. Research into the generation of the respiratory rhythm has identified that it originates in the neurons in the pre-Bötzinger complex. Respiratory neurons are either inspiratory or expiratory and may fire early, late, or in

At the bottom of Figure 9–16 is a respiratory unit where on one side blood flow has been decreased (B) but ventilation maintained. This defines an area of high $\dot{V}/\dot{Q}$ ratio. The effect on lung function can be understood by dividing the unit into an area with a normal $\dot{V}/\dot{Q}$ ratio (A) and (this time) an area of wasted ventilation (C). As expected, the effect of high $\dot{V}/\dot{Q}$ ratios is to increase the amount of ventilation necessary to maintain a normal arterial PCO_2. Because the respiratory control system is very sensitive to small changes in $PaCO_2$ and the lungs have enormous excess capacity, the physiologic

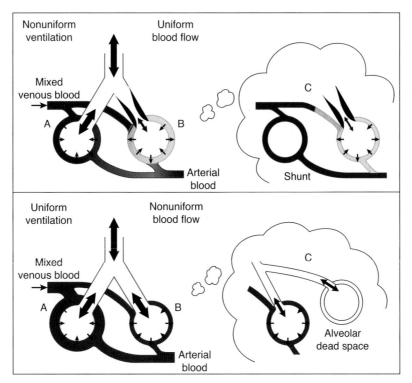

FIGURE 9–16 Ventilation/perfusion mismatching. (Blue, deoxygenated; red, oxygenated.) See text for details. (Redrawn, with permission, from Comroe J. *Physiology of Respiration*, 2nd ed. Year Book, 1974.)

an accelerating fashion during the respiratory cycle. Their integrated output is an efferent signal via the phrenic nerve (diaphragm) and spinal nerves (intercostals and abdominal wall) to generate rhythmic contraction and relaxation of the respiratory musculature. The result is spontaneous breathing without conscious input. However, by attending to breathing, the reader may hold his or her breath. Eating, speaking, singing, swimming, and defecating all depend on voluntary control over automatic breathing.

A. Sensory Input

The frequency, depth, and timing of spontaneous breathing are modified by information provided to the respiratory center from both chemical and mechanical sensors (Figure 9–17).

There are chemoreceptors in the peripheral vasculature and in the brainstem. The peripheral chemoreceptors are the carotid bodies, located at the bifurcation of the common carotid arteries and the aortic bodies near the arch of the aorta. The carotid bodies are particularly important in humans. They function as sensors of arterial oxygenation. There is a graded increase in firing of the carotid body in response to a fall in the PaO_2. This response is most marked below 60 mm Hg. An increase in the $PaCO_2$ or a fall in arterial pH potentiates the response of the carotid body to decreases in the PaO_2.

In humans, the carotid bodies are solely responsible for the increased ventilation seen in response to hypoxia. Bilateral carotid body resection, which has been performed to treat disabling dyspnea and may happen as an unintended conse-

quence of carotid thromboendarterectomy, results in a complete loss of this hypoxic ventilatory drive. The response to an increase in $PaCO_2$ remains intact. Central chemoreceptors

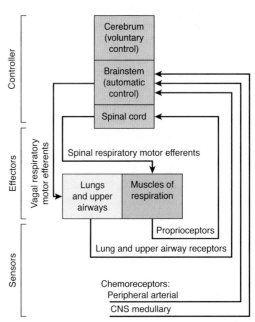

FIGURE 9–17 Schematic representation of the respiratory control system. The interrelationships among the CNS controller, effectors, and sensors are shown as are the connections among these components. (Redrawn, with permission, from Berger AJ et al. Regulation of respiration. N Engl J Med 1977;297:92, 138, 194.)

mediate the response to changes in $PaCO_2$. There is growing evidence that these chemoreceptors are widely dispersed throughout the brainstem. They are separate from the neurons that generate the respiratory rhythm. The increased ventilatory response to elevation in $PaCO_2$ is mediated through changes in chemoreceptor pH. The blood-brain barrier permits free diffusion of CO_2 but not hydrogen ions. CO_2 is hydrated to carbonic acid, which ionizes and lowers brain pH. Central chemoreceptors probably respond to these changes in intracellular hydrogen ion concentration.

There are a variety of pulmonary stretch receptors located in airway smooth muscle and mucosa whose afferent fibers are carried in the vagus nerve. They discharge in response to lung distention. Increasing lung volume decreases the rate of respiration by increasing expiratory time. This is known as the Hering-Breuer reflex. There are unmyelinated C fibers located near the pulmonary capillaries (hence juxtacapillary [J] receptors). These fibers are quiet during normal breathing but can be directly stimulated by intravenous administration of irritant chemicals such as capsaicin. They appear to stimulate the increased respiratory drive in interstitial edema and pulmonary fibrosis. Skeletal movement transmitted by proprioceptors in joints, muscles, and tendons causes an increase in respiration and may have some role in the increased ventilation of exercise. Finally, there are muscle spindle receptors in the diaphragm and intercostals that provide feedback on muscle force. They may be involved in the sensation of dyspnea when the work of breathing is disproportionate to ventilation.

B. Integrated Responses

Under normal conditions in healthy people, the hydrogen ion concentration in the region of the central chemoreceptors determines the drive to breathe. Changes in chemoreceptor pH are largely determined by the $PaCO_2$. The PaO_2 is not an important part of the baseline respiratory drive under normal conditions.

Breathing is stimulated by a fall in the PaO_2, a rise in the $PaCO_2$, or an increase in the hydrogen ion concentration of arterial blood (fall in arterial pH).

Ventilation increases approximately 2–3 L/min for every 1 mm Hg rise in $PaCO_2$. This response (Figure 9–18) occurs first through sensitization of the carotid body receptor. The carotid body will increase its firing in response to an increased $PaCO_2$ even in the absence of changes in the PaO_2. This accounts for approximately 15% of the ventilatory response to hypercapnia. The majority of the response is mediated through pH changes in the region of the central chemoreceptors. Changes in arterial pH are additive to changes in $PaCO_2$. CO_2 response curves under conditions of metabolic acidosis have an identical slope but are shifted to the left. The ventilatory response to an increased $PaCO_2$ falls with age, sleep, and aerobic conditioning and with increased work of breathing.

The individual response to hypoxemia is extremely variable. Normally, there is little increase in ventilation until the PaO_2 falls below 50–60 mm Hg. At this point, there is a rapid increase in ventilation that reaches its maximum at approxi-

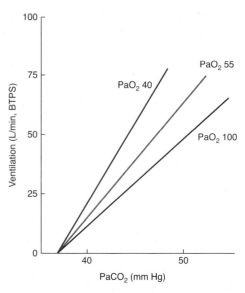

FIGURE 9–18   Ventilatory response to CO_2. The curves represent changes in minute ventilation plotted against changes in inspired PCO_2 at different values of alveolar PO_2. There is a linear increase in ventilation with increasing PCO_2. The rate of increase is greater at lower PO_2 values, but the curves begin from a common point where ventilation should cease in response to lowered PCO_2. In awake humans, arousal maintains ventilation even when the PCO_2 falls below this level; when lightly anesthetized, apnea does occur. In the case of metabolic acidosis, this x-intercept is shifted to the left but the slope of the lines remains virtually unchanged. This indicates that the effects of metabolic acidosis are separate from and additive to the effects of respiratory acidosis. (BTPS, body temperature and pressure, saturated with water vapor.)   (Redrawn, with permission, from Ganong WF. *Review of Medical Physiology*, 22nd ed. McGraw-Hill, 2005.)

mately 32 mm Hg. Below this level, further decreases in PaO_2 lead to depression of ventilation. The response to hypoxia is affected by the $PaCO_2$. An increase in the alveolar PCO_2 will shift the isocapnic O_2 response curve upward and to the right (Figure 9–19).

A fall in arterial hydrogen ion concentration increases minute ventilation. This response results chiefly from stimulation of the carotid bodies and is independent of changes in $PaCO_2$. There is a response to severe metabolic acidosis in the absence of carotid bodies. It is assumed that this response is mediated by central chemoreceptors; it may represent breakdown of the blood-brain barrier.

C. Special Situations

1. **Chronic hypercapnia**—In patients with chronic hypercapnia, brain pH is returned toward normal by compensatory changes in bicarbonate levels. This makes the central chemoreceptors less sensitive to further changes in arterial $PaCO_2$. In this instance, a patient's minute ventilation may depend on tonic stimuli from the carotid bodies. If such a patient were given high concentrations of inspired oxygen, it could reduce carotid body output and lead to a fall in minute ventilation. In rare cases, this can be extreme enough to cause a rapid rise in $PaCO_2$ and coma.

2. **Chronic hypoxia**—Long-term residence at high altitude—or sleep apnea with repeated episodes of severe oxygen desaturation—may blunt the hypoxic ventilatory response. In such individuals, the development of lung disease and hypercapnia may ablate endogenous stimuli to breathing. This pattern is seen in patients with obesity-hypoventilation syndrome.

3. **Exercise**—Exercise may increase minute ventilation up to 25 times the resting level. Strenuous but submaximal exercise in a healthy individual typically causes no change or only a slight rise in PaO_2 as a result of increased pulmonary blood flow and better matching of ventilation and perfusion, with no change or a slight fall in $PaCO_2$. Changes in arterial oxygenation are, therefore, not a factor behind the increased ventilatory response to exercise. The reason for the increased ventilatory response is not known with certainty. Two contributing factors are the increased production of carbon dioxide and increased afferent discharge from joint and muscle proprioceptors.

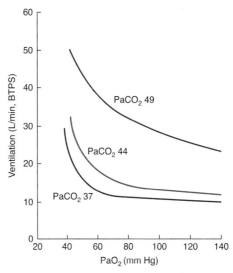

FIGURE 9–19 Isocapnic ventilatory response to hypoxia. These curves represent changes in minute ventilation plotted against changes in alveolar PO_2 when the alveolar PCO_2 is held constant at 37, 44, or 49 mm Hg. When the PCO_2 is in the normal range (37–44 mm Hg), there is little increase in ventilation until the PO_2 is reduced to between 50 and 60 mm Hg. This response is not linear, as is the response to an increased PCO_2, but resembles a rectangular hyperbola asymptotic to infinite ventilation (at a PO_2 in the low 30s) and ventilation without tonic stimulation from the carotid bodies (which occurs above a PO_2 of 500 mm Hg). Not shown is the fall in minute ventilation that occurs with extreme hypoxia (PO_2 values below 30 mm Hg) as a result of depression of the respiratory center. (Redrawn, with permission, from Ganong WF. Review of *Medical Physiology,* 22nd ed. McGraw-Hill, 2005.)

CHECKPOINT

12. What are the components of lung elastic recoil? What is the role of surfactant?

13. What three opposing forces must be overcome normally to inflate the lungs?

14. What are four factors affecting airway resistance?

15. What are the components of the work of breathing?

16. What factors regulate ventilation, and what factors regulate perfusion?

17. How are ventilation and perfusion normally matched?

18. What are the effects of changing CO_2 and O_2 levels on respiratory control?

PATHOPHYSIOLOGY OF SELECTED LUNG DISEASES

OBSTRUCTIVE LUNG DISEASES: ASTHMA & CHRONIC OBSTRUCTIVE PULMONARY DISEASE (COPD)

The fundamental physiologic problem in obstructive diseases is increased resistance to airflow as a result of caliber reduction of conducting airways. This increased resistance can be caused by processes (1) within the lumen, (2) in the airway wall, or (3) in the supporting structures surrounding the airway. Examples of luminal obstruction include the increased secretions seen in asthma and chronic bronchitis. Airway wall thickening and airway narrowing can result from the inflammation seen in both asthma and chronic bronchitis or from the bronchial smooth muscle contraction in asthma. Emphysema is the classic example of obstruction caused by loss of surrounding supporting structure, with expiratory airway collapse resulting from the destruction of lung elastic tis-

sue. Although the causes and clinical presentations of these diseases are distinct, the common elements of their physiology are instructive.

1. Asthma

Clinical Presentation

Asthma is a disease of airway inflammation and airflow obstruction characterized by the presence of intermittent symptoms, including wheezing, chest tightness, shortness of breath (dyspnea), and cough together with demonstrable bronchial hyperresponsiveness. Exposure to defined allergens or to various nonspecific stimuli initiates a cascade of cellular activation events in the airways, resulting in both acute and chronic inflammatory processes mediated by a complex and integrated assortment of locally released cytokines and other mediators. Release of mediators can alter airway smooth muscle tone and responsiveness, produce mucus hypersecretion, and damage airway epithelium. These pathologic events result in chronically abnormal airway architecture and function.

Inherent in the definition of asthma is the possibility of considerable variation in the magnitude and manifestations of the disease within and between individuals over time. For example, whereas many asthmatic patients have infrequent and mild symptoms, others may have persistent or prolonged symptoms of great severity. Similarly, initiating or exacerbating stimuli may be quite different between individual patients.

Etiology & Epidemiology

Asthma is the most common chronic pulmonary disease, affecting as many as one third of adolescents in some countries. The highest prevalence rates are reported in Australia and New Zealand; in the United States, the prevalence is 4–8%. Asthma is more common in children and occurs more frequently in boys than in girls. Data pertaining to deaths from asthma are incomplete and somewhat variable but suggest a trend toward increased hospitalization and mortality rates in recent decades, despite greater availability of effective pharmacologic treatment. A number of explanations have been offered, including the deleterious side effects of medications and increasing exposure to indoor and industrial pollution.

Atopy, or the production of immunoglobulin E (IgE) antibodies in response to exposure to allergens, is common in asthmatics and plays a role in evolution of the disease. Asthma has conventionally been divided into extrinsic and intrinsic asthma depending on the presence or absence, respectively, of accompanying atopy. There are some characteristic differences between the two groups. For example, intrinsic asthma is characterized by a later age at onset, a lack of apparent allergic sensitization by testing, and a tendency toward greater disease severity. However, the two types share the pathologic features of airway inflammation, hyperresponsiveness, and obstruction, so the distinction has not proved useful clinically.

The fundamental abnormality in asthma is increased reactivity of airways to stimuli. As outlined in Table 9–3, there are many known provocative agents for asthma. These can be broadly categorized as (1) physiologic or pharmacologic mediators of asthmatic airway responses, (2) allergens that can induce airway inflammation and reactivity in sensitized individuals, and (3) exogenous physicochemical agents or stimuli that produce airway hyperreactivity. Some of these provocative agents will produce responses in asthmatics only (eg, exercise, adenosine), whereas others produce characteristically magnified responses in asthmatics that can be used to distinguish them from normals under controlled testing conditions (eg, histamine, methacholine; see later discussion).

Asthmatics typically have early and late responses to provocative stimuli. In the early asthmatic response, there is an onset of airway narrowing within 10–15 minutes after exposure and improvement by 60 minutes. This can sometimes be

TABLE 9–3 Asthma: Provocative factors.

Physiologic and pharmacologic mediators of normal smooth muscle contraction
Histamine
Methacholine
Adenosine triphosphate
Physicochemical agents
Exercise; hyperventilation with cold, dry air
Air pollutants
Sulfur dioxide
Nitrogen dioxide
Viral respiratory infections (eg, influenza A)
Ingestants
Propranolol
Aspirin; NSAIDs
Allergens
Low-molecular-weight chemicals (eg, penicillin, isocyanates, anhydrides, chromate)
Complex organic molecules (eg, animal danders, dust mites, enzymes, wood dusts)

followed by a late asthmatic response, which appears 4–8 hours after an initial stimulus. Although the mechanisms producing these two responses are different, they are part of a common process of airway inflammation.

Pathogenesis

There is no known single mechanism that serves to explain the occurrence of asthma in all individuals. There are, however, common events that characterize the pathologic processes that produce asthma. It is important to recognize the central role of airway inflammation in the evolution of asthma.

The earliest events in asthmatic airway responses are the activation of local inflammatory cells, principally mast cells and eosinophils. This can occur by specific IgE-dependent mechanisms or indirectly via other processes (eg, osmotic stimuli or chemical irritant exposure). Acute-acting mediators, including leukotrienes, prostaglandins, and histamine, rapidly induce smooth muscle contraction, mucus hypersecretion, and vasodilation with endothelial leakage and local edema formation. Epithelial cells appear also to be involved in this process, releasing leukotrienes and prostaglandins as well as inflammatory cytokines on activation. Some of these preformed and rapidly acting mediators possess chemotactic activity, recruiting additional inflammatory cells such as eosinophils and neutrophils to airway mucosa.

A critical process that accompanies these acute events is the recruitment, multiplication, and activation of immune inflammatory cells through the actions of a network of locally released cytokines and chemokines. Cytokines and chemokines participate in a complex and prolonged series of events that result in perpetuation of local airway inflammation and hyperresponsiveness (Table 9–4). These events include promoting growth of mast cells and eosinophils, influx and proliferation of T lymphocytes, and differentiation of B lymphocytes to IgE- and IgA-producing plasma cells. An important component of this process now appears to be the differentiation and activation of helper T lymphocytes of the T_H2 phenotype. These T_H2 lymphocytes, through their production of cytokines, including IL-3, IL-4, IL-5, IL-6, IL-9, IL-10, and IL-13, promote activation of mast cells, eosinophils, and other effector cells and drive IgE production by B cells, all of which are pathologic components of the asthma phenotype. Thus, through their specific mediators, these multiple cells participate in the many proinflammatory processes that are active in the airways of asthmatics. Among these are injury to epithelial cells and denudation of the airway, greater exposure of afferent sensory nerves, and consequent neurally mediated smooth muscle hyperresponsiveness; the upregulation of IgE-mediated mast cell and eosinophil activation and mediator release, including acute and long-acting mediators; and submucosal gland hypersecretion with increased mucus volume. Concurrently, the production of

growth factors such as TGF-β, TGF-α, and fibroblast growth factor (FGF) by epithelial cells as well as macrophages and other inflammatory cells drives the process of tissue remodeling and submucosal airway fibrosis. This submucosal fibrosis can result in the fixed airway obstruction that may accompany the chronic airway inflammation in asthma.

Pathology

The histopathologic features of asthma reflect the cellular processes at play. Airway mucosa is thickened, edematous, and infiltrated with inflammatory cells, principally lymphocytes, eosinophils, and mast cells. Hypertrophied and contracted airway smooth muscle is seen. Bronchial and bronchiolar epithelial cells are frequently damaged, in part by eosinophil products such as major basic protein and eosinophil chemotactic protein, which are cytotoxic for epithelium. Epithelial injury and death leave portions of the airway lumen denuded, exposing autonomic and probably noncholinergic, nonadrenergic afferents that can mediate airway hyperreactivity. Secretory gland hyperplasia and mucus hypersecretion are seen, with mucus plugging of airways a prominent finding in severe asthma. Even in mildly involved asthmatic airways, inflammatory cells are found in increased numbers in the mucosa and submucosa, and subepithelial myofibroblasts are noted to proliferate and produce increased interstitial collagen; this may explain the component of relatively fixed airway obstruction seen in some asthmatics. The pathologic findings seen in severe fatal asthma parallel the pathologic events described previously but reflect the greater magnitude of the insult. More severe airway epithelial injury and loss are noted, often with severe and complete obstruction of the airway lumen by mucus plugs.

Pathophysiology

Local cellular events in the airways have important effects on lung function. As a consequence of airway inflammation and smooth muscle hyperresponsiveness, the airways are narrowed, resulting in an increase in airway resistance (recall that Raw ∝ $1/\text{radius}^4$). Thus, where under normal physiologic circumstances the small-caliber peripheral airways do not contribute significantly to airflow resistance, in asthma, as these airways narrow, they contribute substantially to airflow obstruction. Mucus hypersecretion and additional bronchoconstrictor stimuli may exacerbate obstructive lung physiology. Bronchial neural function also appears to play a role in the evolution of asthma, although this is probably of secondary importance. Cough and reflex bronchoconstriction mediated by vagal efferents follows stimulation of bronchial irritant receptors. Peptide neurotransmitters may also play a role. The proinflammatory neuropeptide substance P can be released from unmyelinated afferent fibers in the airways and can induce smooth muscle contraction and mediator release from mast cells. Vasoactive intestinal peptide (VIP) is the peptide neurotransmitter of some airway nonadrenergic, noncholinergic neurons and functions as a bronchodilator; interruption of its action by cleavage of VIP can promote bronchoconstriction.

TABLE 9–4 Asthma: Cellular inflammatory events.

Epithelial cell activation or injury
Cytokine (IL-8) and chemokine release, with neutrophil chemotaxis or activation
Antigen presentation to lymphocytes
Secretory epithelial cell hyperplasia and hypersecretion
Epithelial death; increased magnitude of airway sensory neural reflexes
Lymphocyte activation
Antigen exposure with lymphocyte proliferation
Increased cytokine and chemokine expression; activation of additional effector cells (dendritic cells, mast cells, eosinophils, macrophages)
Activation of B cells; increased IgE synthesis
Augmented lymphocyte activation by local cytokines
Mast cell and eosinophil activation
Eosinophil release of cytotoxic and acute proinflammatory mediators
IgE-mediated mast cell activation, with acute mediator release (eg, histamine, leukotrienes, platelets activating factor)
New expression of multiple cytokines by mast cells, with multiple effector cell activation, as with lymphocytes

Airway obstruction occurs diffusely, although not homogeneously, throughout the lungs. As a result, ventilation of respiratory units becomes nonuniform and the matching of ventilation to perfusion is altered. Areas of both abnormally low and abnormally high $\dot{V}/\dot{Q}$ ratios exist, with the low $\dot{V}/\dot{Q}$ ratio regions contributing to hypoxemia. Pure shunt is unusual in asthma even though mucus plugging is a common finding, particularly in severe, fatal asthma. Arterial CO_2 tension is usually normal to low, given the increased ventilation seen with asthma exacerbations. Even mild hypercapnia should be viewed as an ominous sign during a severe asthma attack, indicating progressive airway obstruction, muscle fatigue, and falling alveolar ventilation.

Clinical Manifestations

The manifestations of asthma are readily explained by the presence of airway inflammation and obstruction.

A. Symptoms and Signs—The variability of symptoms and signs is an indication of the tremendous range of disease severity, from mild and intermittent disease to chronic, severe, and sometimes fatal asthma.

1. **Cough**—Cough results from the combination of airway narrowing, mucus hypersecretion, and the neural afferent hyperresponsiveness seen with airway inflammation. It can also be a consequence of nonspecific inflammation after superimposed infections, particularly viral, in asthmatic patients. By virtue of the compressive narrowing and high velocity of airflow in central airways, cough provides sufficient shear and propulsive force to clear collected mucus and retained particles from narrowed airways.

2. **Wheezing**—Smooth muscle contraction, together with mucus hypersecretion and retention, results in airway caliber reduction and prolonged turbulent airflow, producing auscultatory and audible wheezing. The intensity of wheezing does not correlate well with the severity of airway narrowing; as an example, with extreme airway obstruction, airflow may be so reduced that wheezing is barely detectable if at all.

3. **Dyspnea and chest tightness**—The sensations of dyspnea and chest tightness are the result of a number of concerted physiologic changes. The greater muscular effort required to overcome increased airway resistance is detected by spindle stretch receptors, principally of intercostal muscles and the chest wall. Hyperinflation from airway obstruction results in thoracic distention. Lung compliance falls, and the work of breathing increases, also detected by chest wall sensory nerves and manifested as chest tightness and dyspnea. As obstruction worsens, increased $\dot{V}/\dot{Q}$ mismatching produces hypoxemia. Rising arterial CO_2 tension and, later, evolving arterial hypoxemia (each alone or together as synergistic stimuli) will stimulate respiratory drive through the peripheral and central chemoreceptors. This stimulus in the setting of respiratory muscle fatigue produces progressive dyspnea.

4. **Tachypnea and tachycardia**—Tachypnea and tachycardia may be absent in mild disease but are virtually universal in acute exacerbations.

5. **Pulsus paradoxus**—Pulsus paradoxus is a fall of more than 10 mm Hg in systolic arterial pressure during inspiration. It appears to occur as a consequence of lung hyperinflation, with compromise of left ventricular filling, together with augmented venous return to the right ventricle during more vigorous inspiration in severe obstruction. With increased right ventricular end-diastolic volume during inspiration, the intraventricular septum is moved to the left, compromising left ventricular filling and output. The consequence of this decreased output is a decrease in systolic pressure during inspiration, or pulsus paradoxus.

6. **Hypoxemia**—The presence of increasing $\dot{V}/\dot{Q}$ mismatching with airway obstruction produces areas of low $\dot{V}/\dot{Q}$ ratios, resulting in hypoxemia. Shunt is unusual in asthma.

7. **Hypercapnia and respiratory acidosis**—In mild to moderate asthma, ventilation is normal or increased, and the arterial PCO_2 is either normal or decreased. In severe attacks, airway obstruction persists or increases and respiratory muscle fatigue supervenes, with the evolution of alveolar hypoventilation and increasing hypercapnia and respiratory acidosis. It is important to note that this can occur in the face of continued tachypnea, which is not equivalent to alveolar hyperventilation.

8. **Obstructive defects by pulmonary function testing**—Patients with mild asthma may have entirely normal pulmonary function between exacerbations. During active asthma attacks, all indices of expiratory airflow are reduced, including FEV_1, FEV_1/FVC ($FEV_1\%$), and peak expiratory flow rate (Figure 9–20). FVC is often also

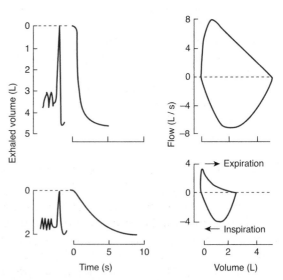

FIGURE 9–20 Obstructive ventilatory defect. Spirograms and flow-volume curves are shown for a normal patient (top panels) and a patient with an obstructive ventilatory defect (bottom panels). (Redrawn, with permission, from Murray JF, Nadel JA. *Textbook of Respiratory Medicine*, 4th ed. Copyright Elsevier/Saunders, 2005.)

reduced as a result of premature airway closure before full expiration. Administration of a bronchodilator results in the improvement of airflow obstruction. As a consequence of the airflow obstruction, incomplete emptying of lung units at end expiration results in acute and chronic hyperinflation; total lung capacity (TLC), functional residual capacity (FRC), and residual volume (RV) can be increased. Pulmonary diffusing capacity for carbon monoxide (DLCO) is often increased as a consequence of the increased lung (and lung capillary blood) volume.

9. **Bronchial hyperresponsiveness**—Bronchial provocation testing reveals nonspecific hyperresponsiveness in virtually all asthmatics, including those with mild disease and normal routine pulmonary function testing. Bronchial hyperresponsiveness is defined as either (1) a 20% decrease in FEV_1 in response to a provoking factor that, at the same intensity, causes less than a 5% change in a normal individual; or (2) a 20% increase in the FEV_1 in response to an inhaled bronchodilating drug. Methacholine and histamine are the agents for which standardized provocation testing has been established. Other agents have been used to establish specific exposure sensitivities; examples include sulfur dioxide and toluene diisocyanate.

CHECKPOINT

19. What is the fundamental physiologic problem in obstructive lung disease? Give an example of each of its three principal sources.
20. What are the pathologic events that contribute to chronically abnormal airway architecture in asthma?
21. What are the three categories of provocative agents that can trigger asthma?
22. Which acute-acting mediators contribute to asthmatic airway responses?
23. What are some histopathologic features of asthma?
24. Name three reasons for increased airway resistance in asthma.
25. Why is arterial PCO_2 usually low in asthma exacerbations?
26. What are some of the common symptoms and signs of acute asthma?

2. COPD: Chronic Bronchitis & Emphysema

"Chronic obstructive pulmonary disease" is an intentionally imprecise term used to denote a process characterized by the presence of chronic bronchitis or emphysema that may lead to the development of airway obstruction. The obstruction may be partially reversible. Although chronic bronchitis and emphysema are often regarded as independent processes, they share some common etiologic factors and are frequently encountered together in the same patient. It is for the purpose of including both under the same broad category that the definition remains imprecise: It reflects what we currently know about the evolution of these diseases.

Clinical Presentation

A. Chronic Bronchitis—Chronic bronchitis is defined by a clinical history of productive cough for 3 months of the year for 2 consecutive years. Dyspnea and airway obstruction, often with an element of reversibility, are intermittently to continuously present. Cigarette smoking is by far the leading cause, although other inhaled irritants may produce the same process. The predominant pathologic event is an inflammatory process in the airways, with mucosal thickening and mucus hypersecretion, resulting in diffuse airflow obstruction.

B. Emphysema—Pulmonary emphysema is a condition marked by irreversible enlargement of the airspaces distal to the terminal bronchioles, accompanied by destruction of their walls without obvious fibrosis. In contrast to chronic bronchitis, the primary pathologic defect in emphysema is not in the airways but rather in the respiratory unit walls, where the loss of elastic tissue results in a loss of appropriate recoil tension to support distal airways during expiration. Progressive dyspnea and nonreversible obstruction accompany the airspace destruction without significant productive cough. Furthermore, the loss of alveolar surface area and the accompanying capillary bed for gas exchange contribute to the progressive hypoxia and dyspnea. Pathologic and etiologic distinctions can be made among various patterns of emphysema, but the clinical presentations of all are similar.

Etiology & Epidemiology

Because of the overlap of these two diseases in individuals and the common causes encountered in both, epidemiologic data generally consider both diseases together under the rubric of COPD. COPD affects more than 10 million persons in the United States; chronic bronchitis is the diagnosis in approximately 75% of cases and emphysema in the remainder. The incidence, prevalence, and mortality rates of COPD increase with age and are higher in men, whites, and persons of lower socioeconomic status. Cigarette smoking remains the principal cause of disease in up to 90% of patients with chronic bronchitis and emphysema. However, only 15–20% of smokers develop COPD. The reasons for differences in disease susceptibility are unknown but may include genetic factors. The most important identified single risk factor for the evolution of COPD—other than cigarette smoking—is deficiency of α_1-protease inhibitor. Its absence can lead to early onset of severe emphysema. Alpha$_1$-protease inhibitor is a circulating protein capable of inhibiting several types of proteases, including neutrophil elastase, which is implicated in the genesis of emphysema (see Pathophysiology section later). Autosomal dominant mutations, especially in northern Europeans, produce abnormally low serum and tissue levels of this inhibitor, altering the balance of connective tissue synthesis and proteolysis. A homozygous mutation (the ZZ genotype) results in inhibitor levels 10–15% of normal. The risk of emphysema, particularly in smokers who carry this mutation, is dramatically increased.

Population-based studies suggest that chronic dust (including silica and cotton) or chemical fume exposure can lead to COPD, but the contribution of these factors appears to be minor compared with tobacco use.

A. Chronic Bronchitis—A number of pathologic airway changes are seen in chronic bronchitis, although none are uniquely characteristic of this disease. The clinical features of chronic bronchitis can be attributed to chronic airway injury and narrowing. The principal pathologic features are inflammation of airways, particularly small airways, and hypertrophy of large airway mucous glands, with increased mucus secretion and accompanying mucus obstruction of airways (Figure 9–21). The airway mucosa is variably infiltrated with inflammatory cells, including polymorphonuclear leukocytes and lymphocytes. Mucosal inflammation can substantially narrow the bronchial lumen. As a consequence of the chronic inflammation, the normal ciliated pseudostratified columnar epithelium is frequently replaced by patchy squamous metaplasia. In the absence of normal ciliated bronchial epithelium, mucociliary clearance function is severely diminished or completely abolished. Hypertrophy and hyperplasia of submucosal glands are prominent features, with the glands often making up more than 50% of the bronchial wall thickness. Mucus hypersecretion accompanies mucous gland hyperplasia, contributing to luminal narrowing. Bronchial smooth muscle hypertrophy is common, and hyperresponsiveness to nonspecific bronchoconstrictor stimuli (including histamine and methacholine) can be seen. Bronchioles are often infiltrated with inflammatory cells and are distorted, with associated peribronchial fibrosis. Mucus impaction and luminal obstruction of smaller airways are often seen. In the absence of any superimposed process, such as pneumonia, the gas-exchanging lung parenchyma, composed of terminal respiratory units, is largely undamaged. The result of these combined changes is chronic airway obstruction and impaired clearance of airway secretions.

The nonuniform airway obstruction of chronic bronchitis has substantial effects on ventilation and gas exchange. Obstruction with prolonged expiratory time produces hyperinflation. Altered ventilation/perfusion relationships include areas of high and low $\dot{V}/\dot{Q}$ ratios. The latter is largely responsible for the more significant resting hypoxemia seen in chronic bronchitis compared with emphysema. True shunt (perfusion with no ventilation) is unusual in chronic bronchitis.

B. Emphysema—The principal pathologic event in emphysema is thought to be a continuing destructive process resulting from an imbalance of local oxidant injury and proteolytic (particularly elastolytic) activity caused by a deficiency of protease inhibitors (Figure 9–22). Oxidants, whether endogenous (superoxide anion) or exogenous (eg, cigarette smoke), can inhibit the normal protective function of protease inhibitors, allowing progressive tissue destruction.

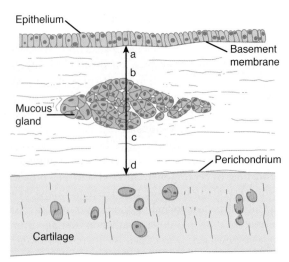

FIGURE 9–21 Bronchial wall anatomy. Structure of a normal bronchial wall. In chronic bronchitis, the thickness of the mucous glands increases and can be expressed as the ratio of (b–c)/(a–d); this is known as the Reid index. (Redrawn, with permission, from Thurlbeck WM. Chronic airflow obstruction in lung disease. In: *Major Problems in Pathology*. Bennington JL [editor]. Saunders, 1976.)

In contrast to chronic bronchitis, which is a disease of the airways, emphysema is a disease of the surrounding lung parenchyma. The physiologic consequences result from three important changes: 1) destruction of terminal respiratory units, 2) loss of alveolar capillary bed, and 3) loss of the supporting structures of the lung, including elastic connective tissue. The loss of elastic connective tissue produces a lung with diminished elastic recoil and increased compliance. In the absence of normal elastic recoil, the normal support of noncartilaginous airways is lost. Premature expiratory collapse of airways ensues, with characteristic obstructive symptoms and physiologic findings.

The pathologic picture of emphysema is one of progressive destruction of terminal respiratory units or lung parenchyma distal to terminal bronchioles. Airway inflammatory changes are minimal if present, although some mucous gland hyperplasia can be seen in large conducting airways. The interstitium of respiratory units harbors some inflammatory cells, but the chief finding is a loss of alveolar walls and enlargement of airspaces. Alveolar capillaries are also lost, which can result in decreased diffusing capacity and progressive hypoxemia, particularly with exercise.

Alveolar destruction is not uniform in all cases of emphysema. Anatomic variants have been described on the basis of the pattern of destruction of the terminal respiratory unit (or acinus, as it is also known). In centriacinar emphysema, destruction is focused in the center of the terminal respiratory unit, with the respiratory bronchioles and alveolar ducts relatively spared. This pattern is most frequently associated with prolonged smoking. Panacinar emphysema involves destruction of the terminal respiratory unit globally, with diffuse airspace distention. This pattern is typically, although not uniquely, seen in α_1-protease inhibitor deficiency. It is impor-

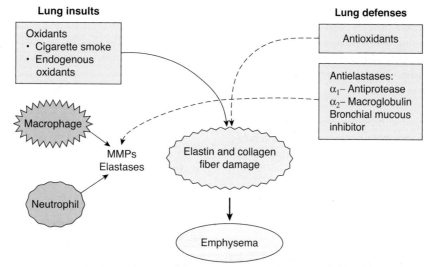

FIGURE 9–22 Schema of elastase-antielastase hypothesis of emphysema. Activation is represented by solid lines, inhibition by dashed lines. The lung is protected from elastolytic damage by α_1-protease inhibitor and α_2 macroglobulin. Bronchial mucus inhibitor protects the airways. Elastase is derived primarily from neutrophils, but macrophages secrete an elastase-like metalloprotease and may ingest and later release neutrophil elastase. Oxidants derived from neutrophils and macrophages or from cigarette smoke may inactivate α_1-protease inhibitor and may interfere with lung matrix repair. Endogenous antioxidants such as superoxide dismutase, glutathione, and catalase protect the lung against oxidant injury.

tant to note that the distinction between these two patterns is largely pathologic; there is no significant difference in the clinical presentation. An additional emphysema pattern of clinical importance is bullous emphysema. Bullae are large confluent airspaces formed by greater local destruction or progressive distention of lung units. They are important because of the compressive effect they can have on surrounding lung and the large physiologic dead space associated with these structures.

Clinical Manifestations

A. Chronic Bronchitis—The clinical manifestations of chronic bronchitis are principally the result of the obstructive and inflammatory airway process.

1. **Productive cough**—Cough is productive of thick, often purulent sputum owing to the ongoing local inflammation and the high likelihood of bacterial colonization and infection. Sputum viscosity is increased largely as a result of the presence of free DNA (of high molecular weight and highly viscous) from lysed cells. With increased inflammation and mucosal injury, hemoptysis can occur but is usually scant. Cough, which is very effective in clearing normal airways, is much less effective because of the narrow airway caliber and the greater volume and viscosity of secretions.

2. **Wheezing**—Persistent airway narrowing and mucus obstruction can produce localized or more diffuse wheezing. This may be responsive to bronchodilators, representing a reversible component to the obstruction.

3. **Inspiratory and expiratory coarse crackles**—Increased mucus production, together with defective mucociliary escalator function, leaves excessive secretions in the airways, even with the increased coughing. These are heard prominently in larger airways during tidal breathing or with cough.

4. **Cardiac examination**—Tachycardia is common, especially with exacerbations of bronchitis or with hypoxemia. If hypoxemia is significant and chronic, pulmonary hypertension can result; cardiac examination reveals a prominent pulmonary valve closing sound (P_2) or elevated jugular venous pressure and peripheral edema because of right heart failure.

5. **Imaging**—Typical chest radiographic findings include increased lung volumes with relatively depressed diaphragms consistent with hyperinflation. Prominent parallel linear densities ("tram track lines") of thickened bronchial walls are common. Cardiac size may be increased, suggesting right heart volume overload. Prominent pulmonary arteries are common and are consistent with pulmonary hypertension.

6. **Pulmonary function tests**—Diffuse airway obstruction is demonstrated on pulmonary function testing as a global reduction in expiratory flows and volumes. FEV_1, FVC, and the FEV_1/FVC ($FEV_1\%$) ratio are all reduced. The expiratory flow-volume curve shows substantial limitation of flow (Figure 9–20). Some patients may respond to bronchodilators. Measurement of lung volumes reveals an increase in the RV and FRC, reflecting air trapped in the lung as a result of diffuse airway obstruction and early airway closure at higher lung volumes. DLCO is normal, reflecting a preserved alveolar capillary bed.

7. **Arterial blood gases**—Ventilation/perfusion mismatching is common in chronic bronchitis. The A-a ΔPO_2 is increased and hypoxemia is common mainly because of significant areas of low $\dot{V}/\dot{Q}$ ratios (physiologic shunt); hypoxemia at rest tends to be more profound than in emphysema. With increasing obstruction, increasing

PCO_2 (hypercapnia) and respiratory acidosis, with compensatory metabolic alkalosis, are seen.

8. **Polycythemia**—Chronic hypoxemia is associated with a variable erythropoietin-mediated increase in hematocrit. With more severe and prolonged hypoxia, the hematocrit may increase to well over 50%.

B. Emphysema—Emphysema presents as a noninflammatory disease manifested by dyspnea, progressive nonreversible airway obstruction, and abnormalities of gas exchange, particularly with exercise.

1. **Breath sounds**—Breath sounds in emphysema are typically decreased in intensity, reflecting decreased airflow, prolonged expiratory time, and prominent lung hyperinflation. Wheezes, when present, are of diminished intensity. Airway sounds, including crackles and rhonchi, are unusual in the absence of superimposed processes such as infection.

2. **Cardiac examination**—Tachycardia may be present as in chronic bronchitis, especially with exacerbations or hypoxemia. Pulmonary hypertension is a common consequence of pulmonary vascular obliteration and concomitant hypoxemia. Cardiac examination may reveal prominent pulmonary valve closure (increased P_2, pulmonary component of the second heart sound) or elevated jugular venous pressure and the peripheral edema resulting from right heart failure.

3. **Imaging**—Hyperinflation is common, with flattened hemidiaphragms and an increased anteroposterior chest diameter. Parenchymal destruction produces attenuated lung peripheral vascular markings, often with proximal pulmonary artery dilation as a result of secondary pulmonary hypertension. Cystic or bullous changes may also be seen.

4. **Pulmonary function tests**—Lung parenchymal destruction and the loss of lung elastic recoil are the fundamental causes of the observed abnormalities of pulmonary function. The loss of elastic recoil in lung tissue supporting the airways results in increased dynamic compression of airways (Figure 9–9), especially during forced expiration; all flow rates are reduced. With premature airway collapse, FEV_1, FVC, and the FEV_1/FVC (FEV_1% ratio) are all reduced. As with chronic bronchitis and asthma, the expiratory flow-volume curve shows substantial limitation in flow (Figure 9–20). Expiratory time prolongation, early airway closure caused by loss of elastic recoil, and consequent air trapping produce increases in the RV and FRC. TLC is increased, although often a substantial amount of this increase comes from gas trapped in poorly or noncommunicating lung units, including bullae. The DLCO is generally decreased in proportion to the extent of emphysema, reflecting the progressive loss of alveoli and their capillary beds.

5. **Arterial blood gases**—Emphysema is a disease of alveolar wall destruction. The loss of the alveolar capillaries creates areas of high ventilation relative to perfusion.

Typically, patients with emphysema will adapt to high $\dot{V}/\dot{Q}$ ratios by increasing their minute ventilation. They may maintain nearly normal PO_2 and PCO_2 levels despite advanced disease. Examination of arterial blood gases invariably reveals an increase in the A-a ΔPO_2. With greater disease severity and further loss of capillary perfusion, the DLCO falls, leading to exercise-related and, ultimately, resting arterial hemoglobin desaturation. Hypercapnia, respiratory acidosis, and a compensatory metabolic alkalosis are common in severe disease.

6. **Polycythemia**—As in chronic bronchitis, chronic hypoxemia is frequently associated with an elevated hematocrit.

CHECKPOINT

27. What is the leading cause of chronic bronchitis?
28. Describe the pathophysiologic changes in emphysema versus chronic bronchitis.
29. Mutations of which protein are strongly correlated with an increased risk of emphysema?
30. Name eight symptoms and signs of chronic bronchitis.
31. Name six symptoms and signs of emphysema.

RESTRICTIVE LUNG DISEASE: IDIOPATHIC PULMONARY FIBROSIS

The term "diffuse parenchymal lung disease" denotes a broad collection of pulmonary processes, some of unknown cause, whose common feature is the infiltration of inflammatory cells and fluid and scarring of lung parenchyma (Figure 9–23). The common consequence of these diverse pathologic processes is widespread lung fibrosis, producing increased lung elastic recoil and decreased lung compliance, which we know as restrictive lung disease.

Diffuse parenchymal lung disease is often referred to as interstitial lung disease, but the modifier "interstitial" is an inadequate characterization of the pathophysiologic process. The lung interstitium is the anatomic space bounded by the basement membranes of epithelium and endothelium and normally contains mesenchymal cells (eg, fibroblasts), extracellular matrix molecules (eg, collagen, elastin, and proteoglycans), and a few tissue leukocytes, including mast cells and lymphocytes. So-called interstitial lung diseases are not typically restricted to the anatomic interstitium but also involve inflammation of the alveolar epithelium and conducting airway mucosa. The resulting fibrosis is generally present throughout the lung parenchyma, with global effects on lung structure and function.

The pathologic processes and physiologic consequences seen in idiopathic pulmonary fibrosis are typical of other causes of diffuse parenchymal lung disease, particularly in their advanced stages. For that reason, idiopathic pulmonary fibrosis is discussed as an example.

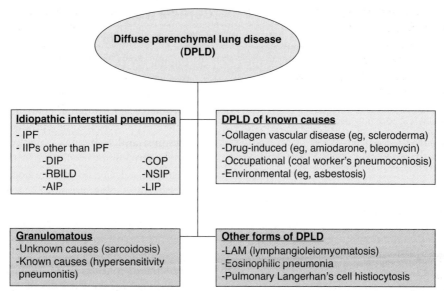

FIGURE 9–23 Categories of diffuse parenchymal lung disease that often lead to restrictive lung disease. In the absence of underlying malignancy or history of chemical or radiation therapy, diffuse parenchymal lung disease can be broadly grouped into the clinical categories shown. DIP, diffuse interstitial pneumonia, RBILD, respiratory bronchiolitis-associated interstitial lung disease, AIP, acute idiopathic pneumonia, COP, cryptogenic organizing pneumonia, NSIP, nonspecific interstitial pneumonia, LIP, lymphocytic interstitial pneumonia.

Clinical Presentation

Idiopathic pulmonary fibrosis, previously known as interstitial pulmonary fibrosis or cryptogenic fibrosing alveolitis, is an uncommon disease of unknown etiology. It is marked by chronic inflammation of alveolar walls, resulting in diffuse and progressive fibrosis and destruction of normal lung architecture. This process produces not only a restrictive defect, with altered ventilation and increased work of breathing, but destructive and obliterative vascular injury that can severely impair normal pulmonary perfusion and gas exchange.

The usual presentation of idiopathic pulmonary fibrosis is with the insidious onset of progressive dyspnea, generally accompanied by a dry and persistent hacking cough. Fever and chest pain are generally absent. With disease progression, dyspnea often worsens and occurs even at rest. Digital cyanosis and clubbing are commonly seen. In the later stages of the disease, increasing pulmonary hypertension can lead to right heart failure and peripheral edema.

Etiology & Epidemiology

Idiopathic pulmonary fibrosis typically presents in the fifth to seventh decades of life, with a slight male predominance. There is no known causative agent. Many environmental exposures and specific systemic diseases can produce a clinical pattern similar if not identical to that seen in idiopathic pulmonary fibrosis. It is important to consider alternative causes when evaluating a patient with diffuse parenchymal lung disease because this may alter the evaluation or the treatment options. A familial form of pulmonary fibrosis has been described but is uncommon; typical cases do not appear to have a genetic basis.

Pathophysiology

The primary insult that leads to the fibrotic response is unknown. Even in diffuse parenchymal diseases of known cause, such as hypersensitivity lung disease or asbestosis, the specific events in disease initiation are not clearly established. There is, however, a common series of cellular events that mediate and regulate the inflammatory process and fibrotic response in idiopathic pulmonary fibrosis as well as in other diffuse parenchymal lung diseases. This set of events, outlined in Table 9–5, includes (1) initial tissue injury; (2) vascular injury and activation, with increased permeability, exudation of plasma proteins into the extravascular space, and variable thrombosis and thrombolysis; (3) epithelial injury and activation, with loss of barrier integrity and release of proinflammatory mediators; (4) increased leukocyte adherence to activated endothelium, with transit of activated leukocytes into the interstitium; and (5) continued injury and repair processes characterized by alterations in cell populations and increased matrix production.

An extensive and complex array of effector and target cells and their specific products are thought to mediate the inflammatory and fibrotic events in idiopathic pulmonary fibrosis.

The initial pathophysiologic event in idiopathic pulmonary fibrosis is injury and activation of alveolar epithelium and endothelium. Type I epithelial cells are lost and replaced by proliferating type II cells. Airway epithelial cells participate in cytokine-mediated recruitment and activation of inflammatory cells, including neutrophils and lymphocytes. Recruitment and activation of both neutrophils and lymphocytes are also mediated by the injury and activation of vascular endothelium; this occurs through the coordinated action of multiple cytokines and the display of a specific repertoire of cellular adhesion molecules both on endothelial cells and on specific

TABLE 9–5 Cellular events involved in lung injury and fibrosis.

Tissue injury
Vascular endothelium activation and permeability changes, with thrombosis and thrombolysis
Epithelial injury and activation
Leukocyte influx, activation, and proliferation
Further tissue injury, remodeling, and fibrosis:
Perpetuation of tissue inflammation
Incomplete or delayed resolution of interstitial thrombosis
Fibroblast proliferation and matrix molecule production or deposition
Epithelial proliferation and re-population

leukocytes. Fibroblasts are also activated by these local proinflammatory cytokines, with proliferation in the interstitium, submucosa, and alveolar lumen. Fibroblasts serve a dual role, magnifying local inflammatory events through their release of cytokines while producing the matrix molecules, including collagen, involved in tissue fibrosis. The perpetuation of this pattern of fibroblast activation and proliferation—and increased tissue matrix deposition—occurs under the influence of inflammatory cells. These include not only lymphocytes, alveolar macrophages, and neutrophils but also resident mast cells and eosinophils, which are variably increased in number.

The histologic findings predict the physiologic abnormalities associated with diffuse parenchymal lung disease. The process of lung injury and scarring is not uniform or synchronous. The disease is typically a nonhomogeneous process, with areas of intense injury and fibrosis often intermixed with relatively spared lung. In the early stages of disease, infiltration of alveolar structures by leukocytes accompanies patchy type II epithelial hyperplasia in alveoli. Destruction of normal alveolar epithelium also causes significant change in the production and turnover of surfactant, with an increase in the alveolar surface tension in affected lung units. This is followed by increasing tissue leukocytosis, fibroblast proliferation, and increasing scar formation. Lymphocytes—predominantly T cells—and mast cells are found in markedly increased numbers in alveolar interstitium and submucosal regions. Collagen and elastin deposition are markedly increased. Later in the course of the disease, progressive alveolar destruction is seen, with large areas of fibrosis and residual airspaces lined by cuboidal epithelium; this appears on radiographs as honeycombing. With this alveolar destruction, the accompanying vascular bed is obliterated, also in a patchy pattern.

This pattern of lung injury produces an altered physiology that includes increased elastic recoil and poor lung compliance, altered gas exchange, and pulmonary vascular abnormalities.

Clinical Manifestations

A. Symptoms and Signs

1. **Cough**—With the bronchial and bronchiolar distortion that accompanies fibrotic damage to terminal respiratory units, chronic irritation of airways occurs, producing a chronic cough. Although epithelial cells may be injured, mucus hypersecretion and a productive cough are not seen.
2. **Dyspnea and tachypnea**—Multiple factors contribute to dyspnea in pulmonary fibrosis. With fibrosis of lung parenchyma as well as a decrease in normal surfactant effects, a greater distending pressure is required for inspiration. Increased stimuli from C fibers in fibrotic alveolar walls or stretch receptors in the chest wall may sense the increased force necessary to inflate the less compliant lungs. The diminished capillary bed and thickened alveolar-capillary membrane contribute to limitation of diffusion and increasing hypoxia with exercise. In severe disease, altered gas exchange with $\dot{V}/\dot{Q}$ mismatching can produce hypoxia even at rest. Tachypnea is the consequence of hypoxia and the apparent increased drive from lung sensory receptor stimuli. A rapid and shallow breathing pattern reduces ventilatory work in the face of increased lung elastic recoil.
3. **Inspiratory crackles**—Diffuse fine, dry inspiratory crackles are common and reflect the successive opening on inspiration of respiratory units that are collapsed owing to the fibrosis and the loss of normal surfactant.
4. **Digital clubbing**—Clubbing of the fingers and toes is a common finding, but the cause is unknown. There is no established link with any specific physiologic variable, including hypoxemia.
5. **Cardiac examination**—As with hypoxemia from other causes, cardiac examination can reveal evidence of pulmonary hypertension with prominent pulmonary valve closure sound (P_2). This can be accompanied by right heart overload or decompensation, with elevated jugular venous pressure, the murmur of tricuspid regurgitation, or a right-sided third heart sound (S_3).

B. Imaging

The characteristic radiographic findings include small lung volumes, with increased densities more prominent in the lung periphery. Fibrosis surrounding expanded small airspaces is seen as honeycombing. With pulmonary hypertension, central pulmonary arteries are enlarged, while the peripheral vascular destruction produces rapid attenuation of vessels out from the hilar regions.

C. Pulmonary Function Tests

Lung fibrosis typically produces a restrictive ventilatory pattern, with reductions in TLC, FEV_1, and FVC, while maintaining a preserved or even increased ratio of FEV_1/FVC ($FEV_1\%$) (Figure 9–24). The increased elastic recoil produces normal to increased expiratory flow rates when adjusted for lung volume. The DLCO in lung fibrosis is progressively reduced as a function of the fibrotic obliteration of lung capillaries.

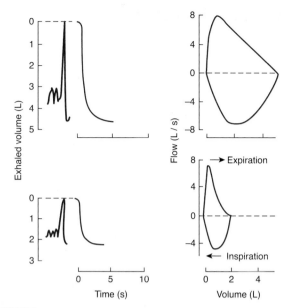

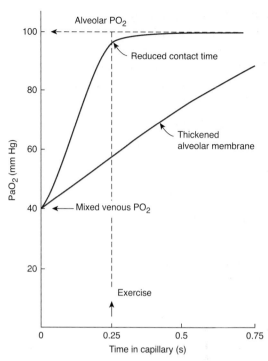

FIGURE 9–24 Restrictive ventilatory defect. Spirograms and flow-volume curves are shown for a normal patient (**top panels**) and a patient with a restrictive ventilatory defect (**bottom panels**). Compare with Figure 9–20. (Redrawn, with permission, from Murray JF, Nadel JA. *Textbook of Respiratory Medicine,* 4th ed. Copyright Elsevier/Saunders, 2005.)

FIGURE 9–25 Change in PaO_2 along the pulmonary capillary. The typical transit time at rest for an erythrocyte through an alveolar capillary is 0.75 seconds. In the normal lung, the partial pressure difference and rate of diffusion of O_2 across the alveolar-capillary barrier assure complete saturation of hemoglobin in 0.25 seconds. Thus, even with the shorter capillary transit time of exercise, the normal lung allows for essentially complete saturation of hemoglobin in the alveolar capillary. If the alveolar-capillary barrier is thickened, as is the case in lung fibrosis, diffusion rates are diminished and alveolar-capillary blood may not be fully saturated with O_2 even at rest. Obviously, greater desaturation of arterial blood can occur with progressive exercise. (Redrawn, with permission, from West JB. *Pulmonary Pathophysiology: The Essentials,* 6th ed. Philadelphia: Lippincott Williams & Wilkins, 2003.)

D. Arterial Blood Gases

Hypoxemia is common in pulmonary fibrosis and results from an increased physiologic dead space and relatively fixed minute ventilation. This leads to an increase in both high and low $\dot{V}/\dot{Q}$ mismatching areas. Diffusion impairment worsens with the severity of fibrosis; this is a common and significant contributor to exercise-induced desaturation but less frequently causes resting hypoxia except in severe disease (Figure 9–25). The increased cardiac output during exercise reduces the transit time for blood through alveolar capillary beds, increasing the limitation in oxygen loading of hemoglobin. Arterial PCO_2 is also reduced as a consequence of increased ventilation under the stimuli of hypoxia and lung fibrosis. Only in the later stages of disease or during exercise, when the increased lung elastic recoil and work of breathing prevent appropriate ventilation, does the $PaCO_2$ rise above normal. Hypercapnia is a grave sign, implying an inability to maintain adequate alveolar ventilation as a result of elevated VD/VT or excess work of breathing.

CHECKPOINT

32. How does interstitial lung disease affect lung function?
33. Name five events in the pathophysiology of idiopathic pulmonary fibrosis.
34. Name eight symptoms and signs of idiopathic pulmonary fibrosis.

PULMONARY EDEMA

Clinical Presentation

Pulmonary edema is the accumulation of excess fluid in the extravascular space of the lungs. This accumulation may occur slowly, as in a patient with occult renal failure, or with dramatic suddenness, as in a patient with left ventricular failure after an acute myocardial infarction. Pulmonary edema most commonly presents with dyspnea. Dyspnea is breathing perceived by a patient as both uncomfortable or anxiety-provoking and disproportionate to the level of activity. The patient at first notices dyspnea only with exertion but may progress to experience dyspnea at rest. In severe cases, pulmonary edema may be accompanied by edema fluid in the sputum and can cause acute respiratory failure.

Etiology

Pulmonary edema is a common problem associated with a variety of medical conditions (Table 9–6). In light of these multiple causes, it is helpful to think about pulmonary edema in terms of underlying physiologic principles.

Pathophysiology

All blood vessels leak. In the adult human, leakage from the pulmonary circulation represents less than 0.01% of pulmonary blood flow, or a baseline filtration of approximately 15 mL/h. Two thirds of this flow occurs across the pulmonary capillary endothelium into the pericapillary interstitial space (Figure 9–26). This is one of two extravascular spaces in the lung—the interstitial space and the airspaces—that contain the alveoli and connecting airways. These two spaces are protected by different barriers. The pulmonary capillary endothelium limits extravasation into the interstitial space while the alveolar epithelium lines the airspaces and protects them against the free movement of fluid. Edema fluid does not readily enter the alveolar space because the alveolar epithelium is nearly impermeable to the passage of protein. This protein barrier creates a powerful osmotic gradient that favors accumulation of fluid in the interstitium.

The amount of fluid that crosses the pulmonary capillary endothelium is determined by the surface area of the capillary bed, the permeability of the vessel wall, and the net pressure driving it across that wall (transmural or driving pressure). The transmural pressure represents the balance between the net hydrostatic forces that tend to move fluid out of the capillary and the net colloid osmotic forces that tend to keep it in. The Starling equation $Jv \approx ([Pc - Pi] - \sigma[\pi c - \pi i])$ illustrates this relationship mathematically, where Jv is the net fluid movement in or out of the lungs, Pc is the capillary hydrostatic pressure, Pi is the interstitial hydrostatic pressure, σ is the reflection coefficient, and πc and πi are the capillary and interstitial hydrostatic pressures. An imbalance in one or more of these four factors—capillary endothelial permeability, alveolar epithelial permeability, hydrostatic pressure, and colloid osmotic pressure—lies behind nearly all clinical presentations of pulmonary edema.

In the shorthand of clinical practice, these four factors are grouped into two types of pulmonary edema: cardiogenic, referring to edema resulting from a net increase in transmural pressure (hydrostatic or osmotic); and noncardiogenic, referring to edema resulting from increased permeability. The former is primarily a mechanical process, the latter primarily an inflammatory one. However, these two types of pulmonary edema are not exclusive but closely linked: Pulmonary edema occurs when the transmural pressure is excessive for a given capillary permeability. For instance, in the presence of damaged capillary endothelium, small increases in otherwise normal transmural pressure may cause large increases in edema formation. Similarly, if the alveolar epithelial barrier is damaged, even the baseline filtration across an intact endothelium may cause alveolar flooding.

TABLE 9–6 Causes of pulmonary edema.

Increased pulmonary capillary transmural pressure
Increased left atrial pressure
Left ventricular failure, acute or chronic
Mitral valve stenosis
Pulmonary venous hypertension
Pulmonary veno-occlusive disease
Increased capillary blood volume
Iatrogenic volume expansion
Chronic renal failure
Reduction of interstitial pressure
Rapid reexpansion of collapsed lung
Decreased plasma colloid osmotic pressure
Hypoalbuminemia: nephrotic syndrome, hepatic failure
Increased pulmonary capillary endothelial permeability
Circulating toxins: bacteremia, acute pancreatitis
Infectious pneumonia
Disseminated intravascular coagulation
Nonthoracic trauma accompanied by hypotension ("shock lung")
High-altitude pulmonary edema
Following cardiopulmonary bypass
Increased alveolar epithelial permeability
Inhaled toxins: oxygen, phosgene, chlorine, smoke
Aspiration of acidic gastric contents
Drowning and near-drowning
Depletion of surfactant through high tidal volume positive-pressure mechanical ventilation
Reduced lymphatic clearance
Lung resection (lobectomy) with regional lymph node sampling
Lymphangitic spread of carcinoma
Following lung transplant
Mechanism uncertain
Neurogenic pulmonary edema
Narcotic overdose
Multiple transfusions

Several mechanisms aid in the clearance of ultrafiltrate and protect against its accumulation as pulmonary edema. Although there are no lymphatics in the alveolar septa, there

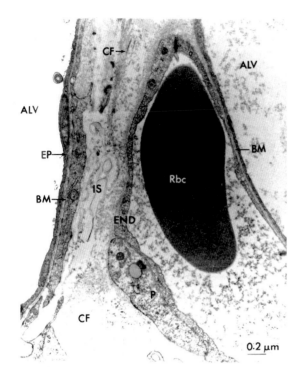

FIGURE 9–26 Interstitial pulmonary edema. Electron micrograph showing the alveolar septum and a pulmonary capillary in cross section. On the right, the basement membrane of the alveolar epithelium and the capillary endothelium are fused. This barrier is, therefore, thin (0.2 μm), which optimizes gas exchange and inhibits accumulation of edema fluid. On the other side, the interstitial space contains connective tissue that is in continuity with the loose connective tissue of the perivascular and peribronchial interstitium. Edema fluid first accumulates in this pericapillary space. The continuity of the interstitial spaces provides a pathway for movement of edema fluid centrally away from areas of gas exchange. (ALV, alveolus; EP, epithelial cell; BM, basement membrane; IS, interstitial space; Rbc, red blood cell; CF, pericapillary fluid; END, endothelial cell.) (Reproduced, with permission, from Fishman AP. Pulmonary edema. Circulation. 1972;46:390.)

are "juxta-alveolar" lymphatics in the pericapillary space that normally clear all the ultrafiltrate. The pericapillary interstitium is contiguous with the perivascular and peribronchial interstitium. The interstitial pressure there is negative relative to the pericapillary interstitium, so edema fluid tracks centrally, away from the airspaces. In effect, the perivascular and peribronchiolar interstitium acts as a sump for edema fluid. It can accommodate approximately 500 mL with only a small rise in interstitial hydrostatic pressure. Because this edema fluid is protein depleted relative to blood, there is an osmotic balance that favors resorption from the interstitium into the bloodstream. This is the major source of resorption of fluid from these collection areas. The perivascular and peribronchiolar interstitium is also contiguous with the interlobular septa and the visceral pleura. In the event of pulmonary edema, there is increased interstitial flow into the pleural space where parietal pleural lymphatics are very efficient at clearance. Pleural effusions seen in patients with increased pulmonary venous pressure represent another reservoir for

edema fluid, one that may compromise respiratory function less than would having the same fluid in the lung parenchyma. Finally, there is evidence that edema fluid may track along the interstitium into the mediastinum where it is taken up by lymphatics.

At some undefined critical level after the perivascular and peribronchiolar interstitium have been filled, increased interstitial hydrostatic pressure causes edema fluid to enter the alveolar space (Figure 9–27). The pathway into the alveolar space remains unknown.

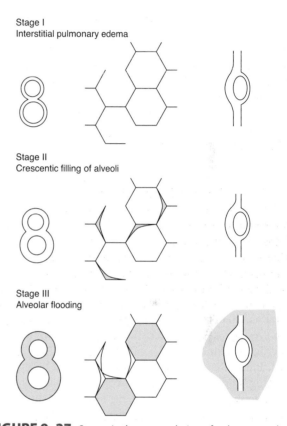

FIGURE 9–27 Stages in the accumulation of pulmonary edema fluid. The three columns represent three anatomic views of the progressive accumulation of pulmonary edema fluid. From left to right, the columns represent a cross section of the bronchovascular bundle showing the loose connective tissue surrounding the pulmonary artery and bronchial wall, a cross section of alveoli fixed in inflation, and the pulmonary capillary in cross section. The first stage is eccentric accumulation of fluid in the pericapillary interstitial space. The limitation of edema fluid to one side of the pulmonary capillary maintains gas transfer better than symmetric accumulation. When formation of edema fluid exceeds lymphatic removal, it distends the peribronchovascular interstitium. At this stage, there is no alveolar flooding, but there is some crescentic filling of alveoli. The third stage is alveolar flooding. Note that each individual alveolus is either totally flooded or has minimal crescentic filling. This pattern probably occurs because alveolar edema interferes with surfactant and, above some threshold, there is an increase in surface forces that greatly increases the transmural pressure and causes flooding. (Redrawn, with permission, from Nunn JF. *Nunn's Applied Respiratory Physiology*, 6th ed. Copyright Elsevier/Butterworth-Heinemann, 2005.)

In the case of cardiogenic pulmonary edema, increased transmural pressure may result from increased pulmonary venous pressure (causing increased capillary hydrostatic pressure), increased alveolar surface tension (thereby lowering interstitial hydrostatic pressure), or decreased capillary colloid osmotic pressure. When the rate of ultrafiltration rises beyond the capacity of the pericapillary lymphatics to remove it, interstitial fluid accumulates. If the rate of formation continues to exceed lymphatic clearance, alveolar flooding results. Because it is an ultrafiltrate of plasma, the edema fluid of cardiogenic pulmonary edema initially has a low protein content, generally less than 60% of the patient's plasma protein content.

Noncardiogenic (increased permeability) pulmonary edema is sometimes referred to clinically as acute respiratory distress syndrome (ARDS). Alveolar fluid accumulates as a result of loss of integrity of the alveolar epithelium, allowing solutes and large molecules such as albumin to enter the alveolar space. These changes may result from direct injury to the alveolar epithelium by inhaled toxins or pulmonary infection, or they may occur after primary injury to the capillary endothelium by circulating toxins as in sepsis or pancreatitis. This is in contrast to cardiogenic pulmonary edema, in which both the alveolar epithelium and the capillary endothelium are usually intact. Owing to the disrupted epithelial barrier, edema fluid in increased permeability edema has a high protein content, generally more than 70% of the plasma protein content. The list of potential causes of injury is broad and is associated with a diverse group of clinical entities (Table 9–6). So many different problems are grouped together in this syndrome because they share injury to the alveolar epithelium and damage to pulmonary surfactant, which results in characteristic changes in pulmonary mechanics and function.

With inhalation injury, such as that produced by mustard gas during World War I, there is direct chemical injury to the alveolar epithelium that disrupts this normally tight cellular barrier. The presence of high-protein fluid in the alveolus, particularly the presence of fibrinogen and fibrin degradation products, inactivates pulmonary surfactant, causing large increases in surface tension. This results in a fall in pulmonary compliance and alveolar instability, leading to areas of atelectasis. Increased surface tension decreases the interstitial hydrostatic pressure and favors further fluid movement into the alveolus. A damaged surfactant monolayer may increase susceptibility to infection as well.

Circulating factors may act directly on the capillary endothelium or may affect it through various immunologic mediators. A common instance is gram-negative bacteremia. Bacterial endotoxin does not cause endothelial damage directly; it causes neutrophils and macrophages to adhere to endothelial surfaces and release a variety of inflammatory mediators such as leukotrienes, thromboxanes, and prostaglandins as well as oxygen radicals that cause oxidant injury. Both macrophages and neutrophils may release proteolytic enzymes that cause further

damage. Alveolar macrophages may also be stimulated. Vasoactive substances may cause intense pulmonary vasoconstriction, leading to capillary failure.

The pathology of increased permeability pulmonary edema reflects these changes. The lungs appear grossly edematous and heavy. The surface appears violaceous, and hemorrhagic fluid exudes from the cut pleural surface. Microscopically, there is cellular infiltration of the interalveolar septa and the interstitium by inflammatory cells and erythrocytes. Type I pneumocytes are damaged, leaving a denuded alveolar barrier. Hyaline membranes form in the absence of alveolar epithelium. These are sheets of pink proteinaceous material composed of plasma proteins, fibrin, and coagulated cellular debris. Fibrosis occurs in some cases. However, complete recovery with regeneration from the type II pneumocytes of the alveolar epithelium may also occur.

Clinical Manifestations

Cardiogenic and noncardiogenic pulmonary edema both result in increased extravascular lung water, and both may result in respiratory failure. Given the differences in pathophysiology, it is not surprising that the clinical manifestations are very different in the two syndromes.

A. Increased Transmural Pressure Pulmonary Edema (Cardiogenic Pulmonary Edema)

Early increases in pulmonary venous pressure may be asymptomatic. The patient may notice only mild exertional dyspnea or a nonproductive cough stimulated by activation of irritant receptors coupled with C fibers. Orthopnea and paroxysmal nocturnal dyspnea occur when recumbency causes redistribution of blood or edema fluid, usually pooled in the lower extremities, into the venous circulation, thereby increasing thoracic blood volume and pulmonary venous pressures.

Clinical signs begin with the accumulation of interstitial fluid. Physical examination may reveal a third heart sound, but there is a paucity of lung findings in purely interstitial edema. The earliest sign is frequently a chest radiograph showing an increase in the caliber of the upper lobe vessels ("pulmonary vascular redistribution") and fluid accumulating in the perivascular and peribronchial spaces ("cuffing"). It may also show Kerley B lines, which represent fluid in the interlobular septa. Pulmonary compliance falls, and the patient begins to breathe more rapidly and shallowly to minimize the increased elastic work of breathing. As alveolar flooding begins, there are further decreases in lung volume and pulmonary compliance. With some alveoli filled with fluid, there is an increase in the fraction of the lung that is perfused but poorly ventilated. This shift toward low $\dot{V}/\dot{Q}$ ratios causes an increase in A-a ΔPO_2, if not frank hypoxemia. Supplemental oxygen corrects the hypoxemia. The $PaCO_2$ is normal or low, reflecting the increased drive to breathe. The patient may become sweaty and cyanotic. The sputum may show edema fluid that is pink from capillary hemorrhage and frothy from protein. Auscultation reveals inspiratory crackles chiefly at the bases, where the hydrostatic pressure is greatest, but potentially throughout both lungs. Rhonchi and wheezing ("cardiac asthma") may occur. The radiograph shows areas of alveolar flooding.

B. Increased Permeability Pulmonary Edema (Noncardiogenic Pulmonary Edema)

The most common form of increased-permeability pulmonary edema is ARDS. ARDS is the final common pathway of a number of different serious medical conditions, all of which lead to increased pulmonary capillary leak. The range of clinical presentations includes all the diagnoses in the adult ICU, including sepsis, aspiration of gastric contents, pneumonia, and pancreatitis. Nevertheless, there are clinical observations that mirror the pathophysiology.

After the initial insult (eg, an episode of high-grade bacteremia), there is generally a period of stability, reflecting the time it takes for various immunologic mediators to damage the pulmonary capillary integrity. Surfactant is inactivated, leading to a significant increase in surface forces and markedly reduced pulmonary compliance. For the first 24–48 hours after the insult, the patient may experience increased work of breathing, manifested by dyspnea and tachypnea but without abnormalities in the chest radiograph. At this early stage, the increased A-a ΔPO_2 reflects alveolar edema and $\dot{V}/\dot{Q}$ mismatching and is corrected by increased FiO_2 and increased minute ventilation. Pathologically, there is alveolar edema, hemorrhage, and atelectasis. The clinical picture may improve, or there may be a further fall in compliance and disruption of pulmonary capillaries, leading to areas of true shunting and refractory hypoxemia. The combination of increased work of breathing and progressive hypoxemia usually requires mechanical ventilation. Alveolar filling with inflammatory fluid leads to decreased efficacy of surfactant and increased atelectasis. This process, which leads to decreased lung compliance (ie, stiffer lungs), is heterogenous and may increase ventilation/perfusion imbalance. The high pressures required to ventilate these patients may overdistend normal alveoli and reduce blood flow to areas of adequate ventilation. Hypoxemia can be profound, and hypercapnia due to increasing dead space ventilation may ensue. Radiographically, there may be diffuse alveolar infiltrates or "whiteout" of the lungs, representing diffuse confluent alveolar filling. Pathologically, diffuse alveolar damage (DAD) is seen, characterized by inflammatory cells and the formation of hyaline membranes. The mortality rate is 30–40%. Most patients die from some complication of their presenting illness, not from refractory hypoxemia. Of those who survive, most will recover near-normal lung function, but their recovery may be prolonged to 6 or even 12 months. A significant number will develop new reactive airway disease or pulmonary fibrosis.

CHECKPOINT

35. What four factors are involved in the production of pulmonary edema? How are they affected in cardiogenic versus noncardiogenic causes of pulmonary edema?

36. What are the common causes of noncardiogenic pulmonary edema?

37. Is lung damage from increased permeability pulmonary edema reversible? If so, how?

38. What are the two major reasons that mechanical ventilation is often required in severe pulmonary edema?

PULMONARY EMBOLISM

Clinical Presentation

The English word "embolus" derives from a Greek word meaning "plug" or "stopper." A pulmonary embolus consists of material that gains access to the venous system and then to the pulmonary circulation. Eventually, it reaches a vessel whose caliber is too small to permit free passage, and there it forms a plug, occluding the lumen and obstructing perfusion. There are many types of pulmonary emboli. The most common is pulmonary thromboembolism, which occurs when venous thrombi, chiefly from the lower extremities, migrate to the pulmonary circulation (Table 9–7).

A normal function of the pulmonary microcirculation is to remove venous emboli. The lungs possess both excess functional capacity and a redundant vascular supply, making them a superb filter for preventing small thrombi and platelet aggregates from gaining access to the systemic circulation. However, large thromboemboli, or an accumulation of smaller ones, can cause substantial impairment of cardiac and respiratory function and death.

TABLE 9–7 Types of pulmonary emboli.

Material	Clinical Setting
Air	Cardiac surgery, neurosurgery, improper manipulation of central venous catheters
Amniotic fluid	Active labor
Fat	Long bone fracture, liposuction
Foreign body	Pieces of intravenous devices, talc
Oil	Lymphangiography
Parasite eggs	Schistosomiasis
Septic emboli	Endocarditis, thrombophlebitis
Thrombus	Deep venous thrombosis
Tumor	Renal cell carcinoma with invasion of vena cava

Pulmonary thromboemboli are common and cause significant morbidity. They are found at autopsy in 25–50% of hospitalized patients and are considered a major contributing cause of death in a third of those. However, the diagnosis is made antemortem in only 10–20% of cases.

Etiology & Epidemiology

Pulmonary embolism and deep venous thrombosis represent a continuum of a single disease that has been coined venous thromboembolic disease, or VTE. Thromboemboli almost never originate in the pulmonary circulation; they arrive there by traveling through the venous circulation.

More than 95% of pulmonary thromboemboli arise from thrombi in the deep veins of the lower extremity: the popliteal, femoral, and iliac veins. Venous thrombosis below the popliteal veins or occurring in the superficial veins of the leg is clinically common but not a risk factor for pulmonary thromboembolism because thrombi in these locations rarely migrate to the pulmonary circulation without first extending above the knee. Since fewer than 20% of calf thrombi will extend into the popliteal veins, isolated calf thrombi may be observed with serial tests to exclude extension into the deep system and do not necessarily require anticoagulation. Venous thromboses occasionally occur in the upper extremities or in the right side of the heart; this happens most commonly in the presence of intravenous catheters or cardiac pacing wires and may be of increasing clinical importance as the use of long-term intravenous catheters increases.

Risk factors for pulmonary thromboembolism are, therefore, the risk factors for the development of venous thrombosis in the deep veins of the legs (deep venous thrombosis) (Table 9–8). The German pathologist Rudolf Virchow stated these risk factors in 1856: venous stasis, injury to the vascular wall, and increased activation of the clotting system. His observations are still valid today.

The most prevalent risk factor in hospitalized patients is stasis from immobilization, especially in those undergoing surgical procedures. The incidence of calf vein thrombosis in patients who do not receive heparin prophylaxis after total knee replacement is reported to be as high as 84%; it is more than 50% after hip surgery or prostatectomy. The risk of fatal pulmonary thromboembolism in these patients may be as high as 5%. Physicians caring for these patients must, therefore, be aware of the magnitude of the risk and institute appropriate prophylactic therapy (Tables 9–8 and 9–9).

Malignancy and tissue damage at surgery are the two most common causes of increased activation of the coagulation system. Abnormalities in the vessel wall contribute little to venous as opposed to arterial thrombosis. However, prior thrombosis can damage venous valves and lead to venous incompetence, which promotes stasis.

Advances now permit identification of genetic disorders in up to one third of unselected patients with venous thrombosis and in more than half of patients with familial thrombosis

TABLE 9–8 Risk factors for venous thrombosis.

Increased venous stasis
Bed rest
Immobilization, especially after orthopedic surgery
Low cardiac output states
Pregnancy
Obesity
Hyperviscosity
Local vascular damage, especially prior thrombosis with incompetent valves
Central venous catheters
Increasing age
Increased coagulability
Tissue injury: surgery, trauma, myocardial infarction
Malignancy
Presence of a lupus anticoagulant
Nephrotic syndrome
Oral contraceptive use, especially estrogen administration
Genetic coagulation disorders: resistance to activated protein C (factor V Leiden); prothrombin 20210A mutation; hyperhomocysteinemia; thermolabile variant of methylenetetrahydrofolate reductase (MTHFR); deficiency of antithrombin III, protein C or its cofactor, protein S, or of plasminogen; dysfunctional fibrinogen; antiphospholipid antibody syndrome

(Table 9–8). It is now clear that these genetic variants may interact with other factors (eg, oral contraceptive use, dietary deficiencies) to increase thrombosis risk.

Pathophysiology

Venous thrombi are composed of a friable mass of fibrin, with many erythrocytes and a few leukocytes and platelets randomly enmeshed in the matrix. When a venous thrombus travels to the pulmonary circulation, it causes a broad array of pathophysiologic changes (Table 9–10).

A. Hemodynamic Changes

Every patient with a pulmonary embolus has some degree of mechanical obstruction. The effect of mechanical obstruction depends on the proportion of the pulmonary circulation obstructed and the presence or absence of preexisting cardiopulmonary disease. In patients without preexisting cardiopulmonary disease, pulmonary arterial pressure increases in proportion to the fraction of the pulmonary circulation occluded by emboli. If that fraction is greater than about one third, pulmonary artery pressures will rise out of the normal range

TABLE 9–9 Risk of postoperative deep venous thrombosis or pulmonary embolus in patients who do not receive anticoagulant prophylaxis.

Risk Category	Incidence of Calf Deep Venous Thrombosis	Incidence of Proximal Deep Venous Thrombosis	Incidence of Fatal Pulmonary Embolus
High risk	40–80%	10–20%	1–5%
1. Age > 40			
2. Anesthesia > 30 min			
3. At least one of the following:			
a. Orthopedic surgery			
b. Pelvic or abdominal cancer surgery			
c. History of deep venous thrombosis or pulmonary embolus			
d. Hereditary coagulopathy			
Moderate risk	10–40%	2–10%	0.1–0.7%
1. Age > 40			
2. Anesthesia > 30 min			
3. At least one of the following secondary risk factors:			
a. Immobilization			
b. Obesity			
c. Malignancy			
d. Estrogen use			
e. Varicose veins			
f. Paralysis			
Low risk	< 10%	< 1%	< 0.01%
1. Any age			
2. Anesthesia < 30 min			
3. No secondary risk factors			

Modified and reproduced, with permission, from Merli G. Update: Deep vein thrombosis and pulmonary embolism prophylaxis in orthopedic surgery. Med Clin North Am. 1993;77:397.

and cause right ventricular strain. The pulmonary circulation can adapt to increased flow, but this depends on (1) recruitment of underperfused capillaries, which may not be available because of obstruction, and (2) relaxation of central vessels, which does not occur instantaneously. In patients with preexisting cardiopulmonary disease, increases in pulmonary artery pressures do not correlate with extent of embolization. In these studies, there were relatively few patients with both preexisting cardiopulmonary disease and extensive arterial occlusion. A correlation may be obscured by the possibility that massive emboli may either kill patients with preexisting cardiopulmonary disease or perhaps make them too unstable for angiography.

The most devastating and feared complication of acute pulmonary thromboembolism is sudden occlusion of the pulmo-nary outflow tract, reducing cardiac output to zero and causing immediate cardiovascular collapse and death. Large emboli that do not completely occlude vessels, particularly in patients with compromised cardiac function, may cause an acute increase in pulmonary vascular resistance. This leads to acute right ventricular strain and a fatal fall in cardiac output. Such dramatic presentations occur in less than 5% of cases and are essentially untreatable. They serve to highlight the importance of primary prevention of venous thrombosis.

B. Changes in Ventilation/Perfusion Relationships

Pulmonary thromboembolism reduces or eliminates perfusion distal to the site of the occlusion. The immediate effect is to increase the proportion of lung segments with high $\dot{V}/\dot{Q}$ ratios. If

TABLE 9–10 Pathophysiologic changes in pulmonary embolism.

Pulmonary Physiology	Change with Pulmonary Thromboembolism	Mechanism of Observed Change
Hemodynamics	Increased pulmonary vascular resistance	Vascular obstruction
		Vasoconstriction mediated by thromboxane A2 and serotonin
Gas exchange	Decreased pO$_2$ (hypoxemia)	Increased perfusion of lung units with low $\dot{V}/\dot{Q}$ ratios
		Decreased cardiac output with decrease in mixed venous PO$_2$
		Right-to-left shunting
	Increased alveolar dead space	Vascular obstruction
		Increased perfusion of lung units with high $\dot{V}/\dot{Q}$ ratios
Work of breathing	Decreased lung compliance	Loss of surfactant causing alvelolar edema and hemorrhage
	Increased airway resistance	Reflex bronchoconstriction
Ventilatory control	Increased respiratory rate (hyperventilation)	Reflex stimulation of irritant receptors

there is complete obstruction to flow, then the $\dot{V}/\dot{Q}$ ratio reaches infinity. This represents alveolar dead space. An increase in dead space ventilation impairs the excretion of carbon dioxide. This tendency is generally compensated by hyperventilation. After several hours, hypoperfusion interferes with production of surfactant by alveolar type II cells. Surfactant is depleted, resulting in alveolar edema, alveolar collapse, and areas of atelectasis. Edema and collapse may result in lung units with little or no ventilation. If there is perfusion to these segments, there will be an increase in lung units with low $\dot{V}/\dot{Q}$ ratios or areas of true shunting, both of which will contribute to arterial hypoxemia.

C. Hypoxemia

Mild to moderate hypoxemia with a low PaCO$_2$ is the most common finding in acute pulmonary thromboembolism. Mild hypoxemia may be obscured by the tendency to rely on oximetry alone, because more than half of patients will have oxygen saturations (SaO$_2$) above 90% (Figure 9–28). Historically, the A-a ΔPO$_2$ was thought to be a more sensitive indica-

tor of pulmonary embolism because it compensates for the presence of hypocapnia and the amount of inspired FiO$_2$. However, the recent Prospective Investigation of Pulmonary Embolism Diagnosis II (PIOPED II) study has called this thinking into question. An A-a ΔPO$_2$ less than 20, which is normal or near normal depending on patient age, was found in one third of patients with an acute PE identified by CT scanning (Figure 9–28).

There is no one mechanism that will fully account for hypoxemia. Two causes have been mentioned previously. An increase in lung units with low $\dot{V}/\dot{Q}$ ratios impairs oxygen delivery. In patients whose underlying disease makes them unable to increase their minute ventilation, an increase in lung units with high $\dot{V}/\dot{Q}$ ratios can also result in hypoxemia. In some patients with preexisting impaired cardiac function or with large emboli that cause acute right ventricular strain, cardiac output may fall, with a resultant fall in the mixed venous oxygen concentration. This is an important cause of hypoxemia in seriously ill patients. Finally, there may be true right-to-left shunts. Such

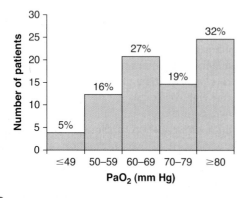

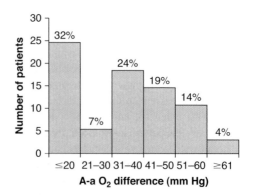

FIGURE 9–28 Arterial PO$_2$ and A-a O$_2$ difference in 74 patients with PE from the PIOPED II study. Blood gases were drawn while patients were breathing room air. (Reproduced, with permission, from Stein PD et al. Clinical characteristics of patients with acute pulmonary embolism: data from PIOPED II. Am J Med. 2007; 120:871.)

shunts have been described in a small percentage of patients with severe hypoxemia in the setting of an acute pulmonary thromboembolism. It is presumed that these represent pulmonary artery to pulmonary venous shunting, or perhaps opening of a foramen ovale, but their exact location is unknown.

Obstruction of small pulmonary arterial branches that act as end arteries leads to pulmonary infarction in about 10% of cases. It is generally associated with some concomitant abnormality of the bronchial circulation such as is seen in patients with left ventricular failure and chronically elevated left atrial pressures.

Clinical Manifestations

A. Symptoms and Signs

The classic triad of a sudden onset of dyspnea, pleuritic chest pain, and hemoptysis occurs in a minority of cases. In a recent large study of patients with PE, dyspnea was present in 73% of cases and pleuritic chest pain was present 44% of the time. Dyspnea probably results from reflex bronchoconstriction as well as increased pulmonary artery pressure, loss of pulmonary compliance, and stimulation of C fibers. In patients with large emboli, there may be an element of acute right heart strain. Pleuritic chest pain is much more common than pulmonary infarction; one group has suggested that the pain is caused by areas of pulmonary hemorrhage. Hemoptysis is seen with pulmonary infarction but may also result from transmission of systemic arterial pressures to the microvasculature via bronchopulmonary anastomoses, with subsequent capillary disruption. It may reflect hemorrhagic pulmonary edema from surfactant depletion or neutrophil-associated capillary injury. Syncope may signal a massive embolus.

The most compelling physical finding is not in the chest but the leg: a swollen, tender, warm and reddened calf that provides evidence for deep venous thrombosis. The absence of such evidence does not exclude the diagnosis, because the clinical examination is insensitive, and the absence of signs may indicate that the entire thrombus has embolized. Auscultatory chest findings are common but nonspecific. Atelectasis may lead to inspiratory crackles; infarction may cause a focal pleural friction rub; and the release of mediators may cause wheezing. In large embolization, one may find signs of acute right ventricular strain such as a right ventricular lift and accentuation of the pulmonary component of the second heart sound.

B. Electrocardiography

Less than 25% of cardiograms are normal in the setting of acute pulmonary thromboembolism. However, the findings are usually nonspecific. The most common abnormalities are sinus tachycardia, T-wave inversion in the precordial leads, and nonspecific ST- and T-wave changes. The classic finding of an acute right ventricular strain pattern on ECG—a deep S wave in lead I and both a Q wave and an inverted T wave in lead III ($S_1Q_3T_3$)—was observed in 11% of patients in the Urokinase Pulmonary Embolism Trial.

C. Laboratory Findings

An increase in the A-a ΔPO_2 is seen in more than two thirds of cases, and hypoxemia is a common yet nonspecific finding. Measurement of the degradation product of cross-linked fibrin, D-dimers, can be used to exclude the diagnosis of PE in patients deemed to have a low pretest probability of PE based on clinical criteria. Depending on the specific assay and patient population, the D-dimer has a high sensitivity (85–99%) and moderate to high specificity (40–93%). Most studies suggest that D-dimer cannot be used to exclude PE in a patient with an intermediate or a high pretest probability for PE.

Brain natriuretic peptide (BNP), an indicator of ventricular stretch, and cardiac troponins, which indicate cardiac myocyte death, are commonly measured in patients with PE. Due to low sensitivity and specificity, these markers cannot be used to diagnose PE. However, an elevation of BNP or troponins in the setting of known PE has been shown to correlate with the presence of right ventricular overload and greater risk of adverse outcomes, including respiratory failure and death.

D. Imaging

The chest radiograph was normal in only 12% of patients with confirmed pulmonary thromboembolism in the PIOPED study. The most common findings were atelectasis, parenchymal infiltrates, and pleural effusions. However, the prevalence of these findings was the same in hospitalized patients without suspected pulmonary thromboembolism. Local oligemia (Westermark's sign) or pleura-based areas of increased opacity that represent intraparenchymal hemorrhage (Hampton's hump) are rare. The chest radiograph is necessary to exclude other common lung diseases and to permit interpretation of the ventilation/perfusion scan, but it does not itself establish the diagnosis. Paradoxically, it may be most helpful when normal in the setting of acute severe hypoxemia.

E. Ventilation/Perfusion Scanning

A perfusion scan is obtained by injecting microaggregated albumin with a particle size of 50–100 μm into the venous system and allowing the particles to embolize to the pulmonary capillary bed (approximate diameter 10 μm). The substance is labeled with a gamma-emitting isotope of technetium (Tc-99m pertechnetate) that permits imaging of the distribution of pulmonary blood flow. A ventilation scan is performed by having the patient breathe xenon (Xe-133) or a radioactive aerosol and doing sequential scans during inhalation and exhalation. A normal perfusion scan excludes clinically significant pulmonary thromboembolism. A segmental or larger perfusion defect in a radiographically normal area that shows normal ventilation is diagnostic. This is referred to as a "mismatched" defect and is highly specific (97%) for pulmonary thromboembolism.

Only a minority of ventilation/perfusion scans reveal clearly diagnostic findings, however. The PIOPED study demonstrated that nondiagnostic ventilation/perfusion scans can

TABLE 9–11   Positive and negative predictive values of CT angiography for acute pulmonary embolism (PE).

	Clinical Probability[1] (%)					
	High		Intermediate		Low	
CT Scan Results	PE+/No. of Patients	%	PE+/No. of Patients	%	PE+/No. of Patients	%
CT+ (likelihood PE present)	22/23	96	93/101	92	22/38	58
CT– (likelihood PE absent)	9/15	60	121/136	89	158/164	96

Data from Multidetector computed tomography for acute pulmonary embolism. N Engl J Med. 2006;354(12):2317–2327.

[1]Clinical probability based on the Wells score: less than 2.0, low probability; 2.0–6.0, moderate probability; more than 6.0, high probability.

stratify a patient's risk of pulmonary thromboembolism. Furthermore, within the categories of high-, medium-, and low-probability studies, the clinician's pretest assessment of the probability of pulmonary thromboembolism can further stratify patients.

F. Computed Tomography and Pulmonary Angiography

Computed tomography scanning with intravenous contrast (CT pulmonary angiography) has widely supplanted $\dot{V}/\dot{Q}$ scanning as the initial test of choice to diagnose PE. The diagnostic strength of this imaging modality lies in its high negative predictive value and its ability to indentify other conditions that cause dyspnea and chest pain (eg, aortic dissection and pneumonia). Multiple trials have shown a high sensitivity and specificity of this imaging technique, although the diagnostic utilities are in part dependent on patient selection and the experience of the interpreting radiologist. The PIOPED II trial evaluated CT angiography for the diagnosis of PE and found a sensitivity of 83% and specificity 96% (Table 9–11). Several other studies indicate that the risk of PE after a negative CT scan in patients with a low or intermediate clinical probability of PE is less than 2%. Consistent with the first PIOPED trial comparing $\dot{V}/\dot{Q}$ scanning and traditional pulmonary angiography, pretest probability based on clinical risk scores must be taken into account when interpreting CT pulmonary angiography. If the results are discordant, further testing, such as $\dot{V}/\dot{Q}$ scanning or lower extremity Doppler ultrasonography, must be considered.

G. Resolution

The variability among patients is so great that generalizations are hard to make. The largest number of patients monitored serially with quantitative assessments was in the Urokinase Pulmonary Embolism Trial. In that study, serial perfusion scans showed substantial resolution of perfusion defects at 9–14 days (Table 9–12). More recent studies, some involving quantitative angiography, have tended to support the time course of these findings.

In a few patients, pulmonary emboli do not resolve completely but become organized and incorporated into the pulmonary arterial wall as an epithelialized fibrous mass, producing what is termed chronic pulmonary thromboembolism. This entity presents with stenosis of the central pulmonary arteries with associated pulmonary hypertension and right ventricular failure (cor pulmonale). Treatment is surgical.

TABLE 9–12   Resolution of heparin-treated pulmonary thromboembolism assessed by serial perfusion scanning.

Time after Event	Number of Patients	Resolution (%±SD)
24 h	70	7±28
2 days	65	16±30
3 days	65	21±30
5 days	69	32±31
7 days	67	42±32
14 days	62	56±30
3 months	60	75±26
6 months	55	77±25
12 months	50	77±23

From The Urokinase Pulmonary Embolism Trial. Circulation. 1973;47(suppl 2):1.

CHECKPOINT

39. Where do 95% of pulmonary thromboemboli originate?
40. What are the risk factors for pulmonary thromboemboli?
41. What hemodynamic changes are brought about by significant pulmonary thromboemboli?
42. What changes in ventilation/perfusion relationships are brought about by significant pulmonary thromboemboli?
43. Suggest some possible explanations for hypoxemia in pulmonary thromboembolism.
44. What are the clinical manifestations of pulmonary thromboembolism?

CASE STUDIES

Eva M. Aagaard, MD, & Yeong Kwok, MD

(See Chapter 25, p. 690 for Answers)

CASE 43

A 25-year-old previously well woman presents to your office with complaints of episodic shortness of breath and chest tightness. She has had the symptoms on and off for about 2 years but states that they have worsened lately, occurring two or three times a month. She notes that the symptoms are worse during the spring months. She has no exercise-induced or nocturnal symptoms. The family history is notable for a father with asthma. She is single and works as a secretary in a high-tech firm. She lives with a roommate, who moved in approximately 2 months ago. The roommate has a cat. The patient smokes occasionally when out with friends, drinks socially, and has no history of drug use. Examination is notable for mild end-expiratory wheezing. The history and physical examination are consistent with a diagnosis of asthma. Pulmonary function tests are ordered to confirm the diagnosis.

Questions

A. What are the three categories of provocative agents that can trigger asthma? What are some possible triggers in this patient?

B. Describe the early events responsible for the pathogenesis of asthma. How does this result in chronic airway inflammation and airway hyperresponsiveness?

C. What pathogenetic mechanisms are responsible for this patient's symptoms of wheezing, shortness of breath, and chest tightness?

D. What might you expect the results of her pulmonary function tests to be? Why?

CASE 44

A 68-year-old man presents to the clinic with a complaint of shortness of breath. He states that he has become progressively more short of breath for the last 2 months, such that he is now short of breath with walking one block. In addition, he has noted a nonproductive cough. He denies fever, chills, night sweats, chest pain, orthopnea, or paroxysmal nocturnal dyspnea. He has noted no lower extremity edema. The medical history is unremarkable. Physical examination is remarkable for a respiratory rate of 19/min and fine dry inspiratory crackles heard throughout both lung fields. Digital clubbing is present. A diagnosis of idiopathic pulmonary fibrosis is made.

Questions

A. What are the cellular events involved in lung injury and fibrosis in idiopathic pulmonary fibrosis?

B. What pathophysiologic mechanisms are responsible for this patient's symptoms of dyspnea and cough? What pathogenetic mechanisms are responsible for his physical findings of tachypnea, inspiratory crackles, and digital clubbing?

C. What might you expect the chest x-ray film to show? The pulmonary function tests?

CASE 45

A 72-year-old man presents to the emergency department complaining of severe shortness of breath. He has long-standing poorly controlled hypertension and history of coronary artery disease and two myocardial infarctions. About 1 week before admission, he had an episode of substernal chest pain lasting approximately 30 minutes. Since then he has noted progressive shortness of breath to the point that he is now dyspneic on minimal exertion such as walking across the room. He notes a new onset of shortness of breath while lying down. He is only comfortable when propped up by three pillows. He is occasionally awakened from sleep acutely short of breath. On examination he is afebrile, with a blood pressure of 160/100 mm Hg, heart rate of 108/min, respiratory rate of 22/min, and oxygen saturation of 88% on room air. He is pale, cool, and diaphoretic. Jugular venous pressure is 10 cm H_2O. Chest auscultation reveals rales in both lungs to the mid lung fields. Cardiac examination is tachycardiac, with an audible S3 and S4. No murmurs or rubs are heard. Extremities are without edema. The ECG shows left ventricular hypertrophy and Q waves in the anterior and lateral leads, consistent with this patient's history of hypertension and myocardial infarction. Chest x-ray film reveals bilateral fluffy infiltrates consistent with pulmonary edema. He is admitted to the ICU with a diagnosis of congestive heart failure and possible myocardial infarction.

Questions

A. What are the four factors that account for almost all cases of pulmonary edema? Which are probably responsible for this patient's pulmonary edema?

B. How does poor cardiac function cause pulmonary edema?

CASE 46

A 57-year-old man undergoes total knee replacement for severe degenerative joint disease. Four days after surgery, he develops an acute onset of shortness of breath and right-sided pleuritic chest pain. He is now in moderate respiratory distress with a respiratory rate of 28/min, heart rate of 120 bpm, and blood pressure of 110/70 mm Hg. Oxygen saturation is 90% on room air. Lung examination is normal. Cardiac examination reveals tachycardia but is otherwise unremarkable. The right lower extremity is postsurgical, healing well, with 2+ pitting edema, calf tenderness, erythema, and warmth; the left leg is normal. He has a positive Homan's sign on the right. Acute pulmonary embolism is suspected.

Questions

A. Where did the pulmonary embolism probably arise from?

B. What are this patient's risk factors for thromboembolism?

C. What are the hemodynamic changes seen in acute pulmonary embolism?

D. What changes might be expected in ventilation/perfusion relationships? What might you expect this patient's A-a ΔPO_2 to be?

CASE 47

A 46-year-old man presents to the hospital with a 5-day history of worsening cough, high fever, and shortness of breath. On physical examination, he is noted to be tachypneic (respiratory rate of 30 breaths/min), hypoxic with a low oxygen saturation (89%), and febrile (39°C). Chest x-ray film reveals infiltrates in both lower lobes. A complete blood count reveals a high white blood cell count. He is admitted to the hospital. Despite treatment with oxygen and antibiotics, he becomes more hypoxic and requires endotracheal intubation and mechanical ventilation. Blood cultures grow *Streptococcus pneumoniae*. Despite mechanical ventilation using high oxygen concentrations, his arterial blood oxygen level remains low. His chest x-ray film shows progression of infiltrates throughout both lung fields. He is diagnosed with acute respiratory distress syndrome (ARDS).

Questions

A. What are the main pathophysiologic factors in ARDS that cause accumulation of extravascular fluid in the lungs?

B. What are the common causes of ARDS?

C. What accounts for the severe hypoxia often found in ARDS, despite the use of mechanical ventilation and high concentrations of oxygen?

REFERENCES

General

Crystal RG et al: *The Lung: Scientific Foundations,* 2nd ed. Lippincott-Raven, 1997.

Hlastala MP et al: *Physiology of Respiration,* 2nd ed. Oxford University Press, 2001.

Lumb AB et al: *Nunn's Applied Respiratory Physiology,* 5th ed. Butterworth-Heinemann, 1999.

Murray JF: *The Normal Lung,* 2nd ed. WB Saunders, 1986.

Murray JF et al: *Textbook of Respiratory Medicine,* 4th ed. WB Saunders, 2005.

West JB: *Pulmonary Pathophysiology: The Essentials,* 6th ed. Lippincott Williams & Wilkins, 2003.

West JB: *Respiratory Physiology: The Essentials,* 7th ed. Lippincott Williams & Wilkins, 2004.

Physiology and Pathophysiology

Booth S et al: The use of oxygen in the palliation of breathlessness. A report of the expert working group of the Scientific Committee of the Association of Palliative Medicine. Respir Med. 2004;98(1):66. [PMID: 14959816]

Laghi F et al: Disorders of the respiratory muscles. Am J Respir Crit Care Med. 2003;168(1):10. [PMID: 12826594]

Leach RM et al: Oxygen transport–2. Tissue hypoxia. BMJ. 1998;317(7169):1370. [PMID: 9812940]

Treacher DF et al: Oxygen transport–1. Basic principles. BMJ. 1998;317(7168):1302. [PMID: 9804723]

Weisman IM et al: ATS/ACCP Statement on cardiopulmonary exercise testing. Am J Respir Crit Care Med. 2003;167(2):211. [PMID: 12524257]

West JB: The physiologic basis of high-altitude diseases. Ann Intern Med. 2004;141(10):789. [PMID: 15545679]

West JB: Understanding pulmonary gas exchange: Ventilation-perfusion relationships. J Appl Physiol. 2004;97(5):1603. [PMID: 15475551]

Obstructive Lung Disease

Barnes PJ. New concepts in chronic obstructive pulmonary disease. Annu Rev Med. 2003;54:113–29. [PMID: 12359824]

Effros RM et al. Asthma: New developments concerning immune mechanisms, diagnosis and treatment. Curr Opin Pulm Med. 2007 Jan;13(1):37–43. [PMID: 17133123]

Mannino DM et al. The epidemiology and economics of chronic obstructive pulmonary disease. Proc Am Thorac Soc. 2007 Oct 1;4(7):502–6. [PMID: 17878461]

Orozco-Levi M. Structure and function of the respiratory muscles in patients with COPD: Impairment or adaptation? Eur Respir J Suppl. 2003 Nov;46:41s–51s. [PMID: 14621106]

Rodrigo GJ et al. Acute asthma in adults: A review. Chest. 2004 Mar;125(3):1081–102. [PMID: 15006973]

Sciurba FC. Physiologic similarities and differences between COPD and asthma. Chest. 2004 Aug;126(2 Suppl):117S–24S. [PMID: 15302772]

Sutherland ER et al. Management of chronic obstructive pulmonary disease. N Engl J Med. 2004 Jun 24;350(26):2689–97. [PMID: 15215485]

Wedzicha JA et al. COPD exacerbations: Defining their cause and prevention. Lancet. 2007 Sep 1;370(9589):786–96. [PMID: 17765528]

Restrictive Lung Disease

Kaminski N. Microarray analysis of idiopathic pulmonary fibrosis. Am J Respir Cell Mol Biol. 2003 Sep;29(3 Suppl):S32–6. [PMID: 14503551]

Martinez FJ et al. Pulmonary function testing in idiopathic interstitial pneumonias. Proc Am Thorac Soc. 2006 Jun;3(4):315–21. [PMID: 16738195]

Noble PW. Idiopathic pulmonary fibrosis. New insights into classification and pathogenesis usher in a new era therapeutic approaches. Am J Respir Cell Mol Biol. 2003 Sep;29(3 Suppl):S27–31. [PMID: 14503550]

Thannickal VJ et al. Mechanisms of pulmonary fibrosis. Annu Rev Med. 2004;55:395–417. [PMID: 14746528]

Pulmonary Edema

Ketai LH et al. A new view of pulmonary edema and acute respiratory distress syndrome. J Thorac Imaging. 1998 Jul;13(3):147–71. [PMID: 9671417]

Ware LB et al. Acute pulmonary edema. N Engl J Med. 2005 Dec 29;353(26):2788–96. [PMID: 16382065]

Acute Respiratory Failure and ARDS

Gattinoni L et al. Lung recruitment in patients with the acute respiratory distress syndrome. N Engl J Med. 2006 Apr 27;354(17):1775–86. [PMID: 16641394]

Hess DR. The evidence for noninvasive positive-pressure ventilation in the care of patients in acute respiratory failure: A systematic review of the literature. Respir Care. 2004 Jul;49(7):810–29. [PMID: 15222912]

Malhotra A. Low-tidal-volume ventilation in the acute respiratory distress syndrome. N Engl J Med. 2007 Sep 13;357(11):1113–20. [PMID: 17855672]

Petrucci N et al. Ventilation with smaller tidal volumes: A quantitative systematic review of randomized controlled trials. Anesth Analg. 2004 Jul;99(1):193–200. [PMID: 15281529]

Ventilation with lower tidal volumes as compared with traditional tidal volumes for acute lung injury and the acute respiratory distress syndrome. The Acute Respiratory Distress Syndrome Network. N Engl J Med. 2000 May 4;342(18):1301–8. [PMID: 10793162]

Pulmonary Embolism

Eliott CG. Pulmonary physiology during pulmonary embolism. Chest. 1992 Apr;101(4 Suppl):163S–71S. [PMID: 1555481]

Fedullo PF et al: Clinical practice. The evaluation of suspected pulmonary embolism. N Engl J Med. 2003 Sep 25;349(13):1247–56. [PMID: 14507950]

Stein PD et al. Challenges in the diagnosis acute pulmonary embolism. Am J Med. 2008 Jul;121(7):565–71. [PMID: 18589050]

Stein PD et al. Clinical characteristics of patients with acute pulmonary embolism: Data from PIOPED II. Am J Med. 2007 Oct;120(10):871–9. [PMID: 17904458]

Stein PD et al. D-dimer for the exclusion of acute venous thrombosis and pulmonary embolism: A systematic review. Ann Intern Med. 2004 Apr 20;140(8):589–602. [PMID: 15096330]

Stein PD et al. Multidetector computed tomography for acute pulmonary embolism. N Engl J Med. 2006 Jun 1;354(22):2317–27. [PMID: 16738268]

Tapson VF. Acute pulmonary embolism. N Engl J Med. 2008 Mar 6;358(10):1037–52. [PMID: 18322285]

The PIOPED Investigators. Value of the ventilation/perfusion scan in acute pulmonary embolism. Results of the prospective investigation of pulmonary embolism diagnosis (PIOPED). JAMA. 1990 May 23–30;263(20):2753–9. [PMID: 2332918]

Cardiovascular Disorders: Heart Disease

Fred M. Kusumoto, MD

Diseases of the cardiovascular system frequently confront the physician involved in the day-to-day care of patients. Knowledge of the underlying pathophysiologic processes associated with diseases of the heart and blood vessels provides a critical framework for patient management. This chapter deals with diseases of the heart and the next one with diseases of the blood vessels. Normal cardiac structure and function are summarized here, and pathophysiologic mechanisms for commonly encountered cardiac problems are then discussed, with emphasis on arrhythmias, congestive heart failure, valvular heart disease, coronary artery disease, and pericardial disease.

NORMAL STRUCTURE & FUNCTION OF THE HEART

ANATOMY

The heart is a complex organ whose primary function is to pump blood through the pulmonary and systemic circulations. It is composed of four muscular chambers: the main pumping chambers, the left and right ventricles, and the left and right atria, which act like "priming pumps" responsible for the final 20–30% of ventricular filling (Figure 10–1A). Peripheral venous return from the inferior and superior venae cavae fills the right atrium and ventricle (through the open tricuspid valve) (Figure 10–1B). With atrial contraction, additional blood flows through the tricuspid valve and completes the filling of the right ventricle. Unoxygenated blood is then pumped to the pulmonary artery and lung by the right ventricle through the pulmonary valve (Figure 10–1C). Oxygenated blood returns from the lung to the left atrium via four pulmonary veins (Figure 10–1D). Sequential left atrial and ventricular contraction pumps blood back to the peripheral tissues. The mitral valve separates the left atrium and ventricle, and the aortic valve separates the left ventricle from the aorta (Figures 10–1D and 10–1E).

The heart lies free in the pericardial sac, attached to mediastinal structures only at the great vessels. During embryologic development, the heart invaginates into the pericardial sac like a fist pushing into a partially inflated balloon. The pericardial sac is composed of a serous inner layer (visceral pericardium) directly apposed to the myocardium and a fibrous outer layer called the parietal pericardium. Under normal conditions, approximately 40–50 mL of clear fluid, which probably is an ultrafiltrate of plasma, fills the space between the layers of the pericardial sac.

The left main and right coronary arteries arise from the root of the aorta and provide the principal blood supply to the heart (Figure 10–2). The large left main coronary artery usually branches into the left anterior descending artery and the circumflex coronary artery. The left anterior descending coronary artery gives off diagonal and septal branches that supply blood to the anterior wall and septum of the heart, respectively. The circumflex coronary artery continues around the heart in the left atrioventricular groove and gives off large obtuse marginal arteries that supply blood to the left ventricular free wall. The right coronary artery travels in the right atrioventricular groove and supplies blood to the right ventricle via acute marginal branches. The posterior descending artery, which supplies blood to the posterior and inferior walls of the left ventricle, arises from the right coronary artery in 80% of people (right-dominant circulation) and from the circumflex artery in the remainder (left-dominant circulation).

Contraction of the heart chambers is coordinated by several regions in the heart that are composed of myocytes with specialized automaticity (pacemaker) and conduction properties

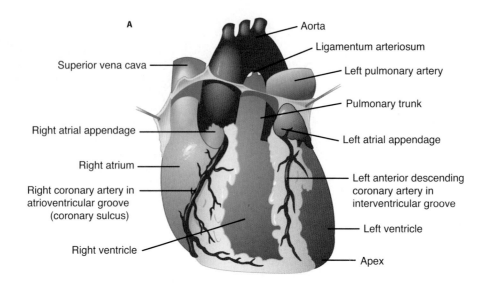

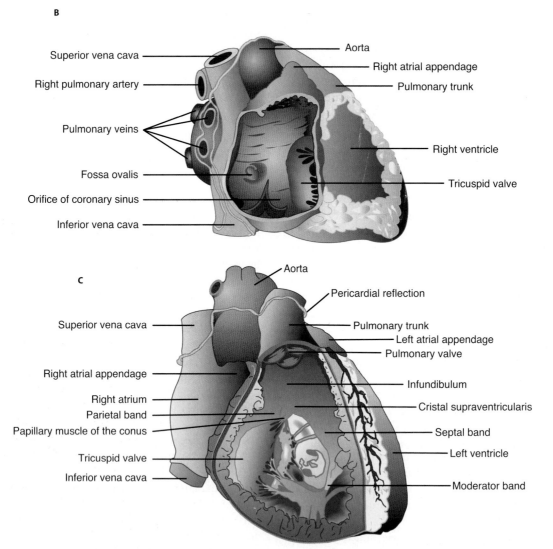

FIGURE 10–1 Anatomy of the heart. **A:** Anterior view of the heart. **B:** View of the right heart with the right atrial wall reflected to show the right atrium. **C:** Anterior view of the heart with the anterior wall removed to show the right ventricular cavity. (Redrawn, with permission, from Cheitlin MD, Sokolow M, McIlroy MB. *Clinical Cardiology,* 6th ed. Originally published by Appleton & Lange. Copyright © 1993 by the McGraw-Hill Companies, Inc.) (*continued*)

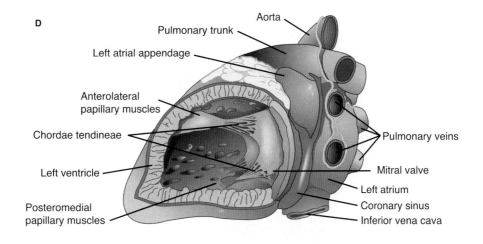

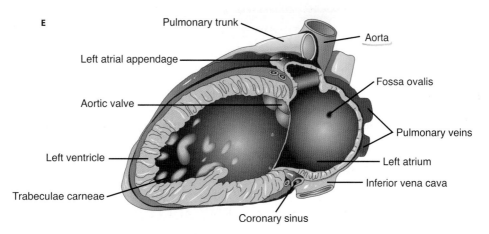

FIGURE 10–1 (*Continued*) Anatomy of the heart. **D:** View of the left heart with the left ventricular wall turned back to show the mitral valve. **E:** View of the left heart from the left side with the left ventricular free wall and mitral valve cut away to reveal the aortic valve. (Redrawn, with permission, from Cheitlin MD, Sokolow M, McIlroy MB. *Clinical Cardiology*, 6th ed. Originally published by Appleton & Lange. Copyright © 1993 by the McGraw-Hill Companies, Inc.)

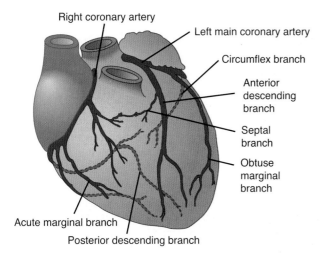

FIGURE 10–2 Coronary arteries and their principal branches in humans. (Redrawn, with permission, from Ross G. The cardiovascular system. In: *Essentials of Human Physiology*. Ross G [editor]. Copyright © 1978 by Year Book Medical Publishers, Inc., Chicago.)

(Figure 10–3). Cells in the sinoatrial (SA) node and the atrioventricular (AV) node have fast pacemaker rates (SA node: 60–100 beats/min; AV node: 40–70 beats/min), and the His bundle and Purkinje fibers are characterized by rapid rates of conduction. Because it has the fastest intrinsic pacemaker rhythm, the SA node is usually the site of initiation of the cardiac electrical impulse during a normal heartbeat. The impulse then rapidly depolarizes both the left and right atria as it travels to the AV node. Conduction velocity slows from 1 m/s in atrial tissue to 0.05 m/s in nodal tissue. After the delay in the AV node, the impulse moves rapidly down the His bundle (1 m/s) and Purkinje fibers (4 m/s) to simultaneously depolarize the right and left ventricles. The atria and ventricles are separated by a fibrous framework that is electrically inert, so that under normal conditions the AV node and the contiguous His bundle form the only electrical connection between the atria and ventricles. This arrangement allows the atria and ventricles to beat in a synchronized fashion and minimizes the chance of electrical feedback between the chambers.

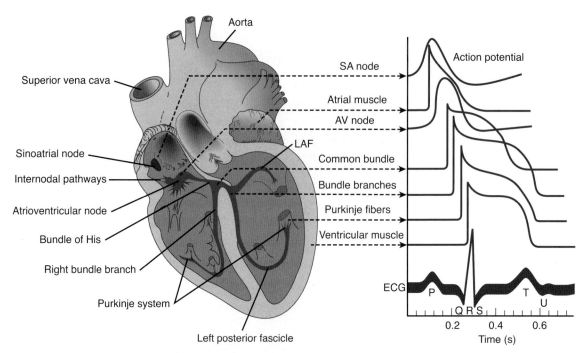

FIGURE 10–3 Conducting system of the heart. Typical transmembrane action potentials for the SA and AV nodes, other parts of the conduction system, and the atrial and ventricular muscles are shown along with the correlation to the extracellularly recorded electrical activity (ie, the electrocardiogram [ECG]). The action potentials and ECG are plotted on the same time axis but with different zero points on the vertical scale. The PR interval is measured from the beginning of the P wave to the beginning of the QRS. (LAF, left anterior fascicle.) (Redrawn, with permission, from Ganong WF. *Review of Medical Physiology*, 22nd ed. McGraw-Hill, 2005.)

The electrical activity of the heart can be measured from the body surface at standardized positions by electrocardiography. On the electrocardiogram (ECG), the P wave represents depolarization of atrial tissue; the electrocardiographic wave (QRS) interval, ventricular depolarization; and the T wave, ventricular repolarization (Figure 10–3). Because normal ventricular depolarization occurs almost simultaneously in the right and left ventricles—usually within 60–100 ms—the QRS complex is narrow. Although the electrical activity of the small specialized conduction tissues cannot be measured directly from the surface, the interval between the P wave and the start of the QRS complex (PR interval) represents primarily the conduction time of the AV node and His bundle.

HISTOLOGY

Ventricular myocytes are normally 50–100 mm long and 10–25 mm wide. Atrial and nodal myocytes are smaller, whereas myocytes of the Purkinje system are larger in both dimensions. Myocytes are filled with hundreds of parallel striated bundles termed myofibrils. Myofibrils are composed of repeating units, termed sarcomeres, that form the major contractile unit of the myocyte (Figure 10–4). Sarcomeres are complex structures composed of the contractile proteins, myosin, and actin, which are connected by cross-bridges, and a regulatory protein complex, tropomyosin. (See Cellular Physiology section later.)

PHYSIOLOGY

Physiology of the Whole Heart

Because the ventricles are the primary physiologic pumps of the heart, analysis has focused on these chambers, particularly the left ventricle. Function of intact ventricles is traditionally studied by evaluating pressure-time and pressure-volume relationships.

In **pressure-time analysis** (Figure 10–5), pressures in the chambers of the heart and the great vessels are measured during the cardiac cycle and plotted as a function of time. At the beginning of the cardiac cycle, the left atrium contracts, forcing additional blood into the left ventricle and giving rise to an *a* wave on the left atrial pressure tracing. At end diastole, the mitral valve closes, producing the first heart sound (S_1), and a brief period of isovolumic contraction follows during which both the aortic and the mitral valve are closed but the left ventricle is actively contracting. When intraventricular pressure rises to the level of aortic pressure, the aortic valve opens and blood flows into the aorta. Beyond this point, the aorta and left ventricle form a contiguous chamber with equal pressures, but left ventricular volume decreases as blood is expelled. Left ventricular contraction stops and ventricular relaxation begins, and end systole is reached when intraventricular pressure falls below aortic pressure. The aortic valve then closes, and the second heart sound (S_2) is heard. Throughout systole, blood has slowly accumulated in the left atrium (because the mitral

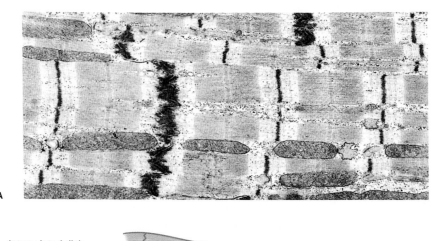

A

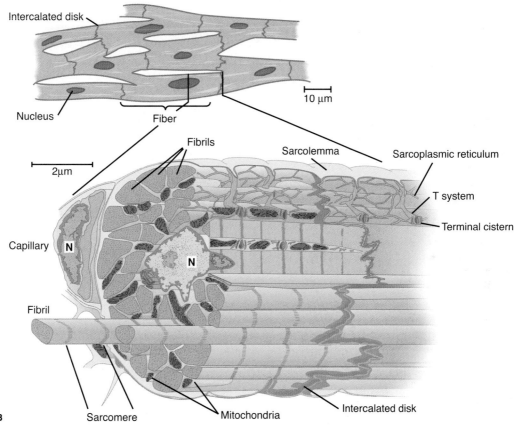

B

FIGURE 10–4 **A:** Electron photomicrograph of cardiac muscle. The fuzzy thick lines are intercalated disks (× 12,000). (Reproduced, with permission, from Bloom W, Fawcett DW. *A Textbook of Histology,* 10th ed. Saunders, 1975.) **B:** Diagram of cardiac muscle as seen under the light microscope (**top**) and the electron microscope (**bottom**). (N, nucleus.) (Redrawn, with permission, from Braunwald E, Ross J, Sonnenblick EH. Mechanisms of contraction of the normal and failing heart. N Engl J Med. 1967;277:794.)

valve is closed), giving rise to the *v* wave on the left atrial pressure tracing. During the first phase of diastole—isovolumic relaxation—no change in ventricular volume occurs, but continued relaxation of the ventricle leads to an exponential fall in left ventricular pressure. Left ventricular filling begins when left ventricular pressure falls below left atrial pressure and the mitral valve opens. Ventricular relaxation is a relatively long process that begins before the aortic valve closes and extends past mitral valve opening. The rate and extent of ventricular

relaxation depend on multiple factors: heart rate, wall thickness, chamber volume and shape, aortic pressure, sympathetic tone, and presence or absence of myocardial ischemia. Once the mitral valve opens, there is an initial period of rapid filling of the ventricle that contributes 70–80% of blood volume to the ventricle and occurs largely because of the atrioventricular pressure gradient. By mid-diastole, flow into the left ventricle has slowed, and the cardiac cycle begins again with the next atrial contraction. Right ventricular pressure-time analysis is

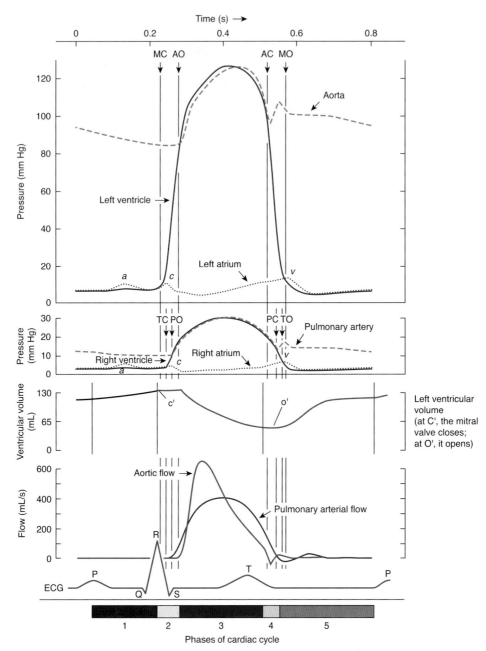

FIGURE 10–5 Diagram of events in the cardiac cycle. From top downward: pressure (in millimeters of mercury) in aorta, left ventricle, left atrium, pulmonary artery, right ventricle, right atrium; blood flow (mL/s) in ascending aorta and pulmonary artery; ECG. Abscissa, time in seconds. (Valvular opening and closing are indicated by AO and AC, respectively, for the aortic valve; MO and MC for the mitral valve; PO and PC for the pulmonary valve; TO and TC for the tricuspid valve.) Events of the cardiac cycle at a heart rate of 75 beats/min. The phases of the cardiac cycle identified by the numbers at the bottom are as follows: 1, atrial systole; 2, isovolumetric ventricular contraction; 3, ventricular ejection; 4, isovolumetric ventricular relaxation; 5, ventricular filling. Note that late in systole aortic pressure actually exceeds left ventricular pressure. However, the momentum of the blood keeps it flowing out of the ventricle for a short period. The pressure relationships in the right ventricle and pulmonary artery are similar. (Redrawn, with permission, from Milnor WR. The circulation. In: *Medical Physiology*, 2 vols. Mountcastle VB [editor]. Mosby, 1980.)

similar but with lower pressures because the impedance to flow in the pulmonary vascular system is much lower than in the systemic circulation.

In **pressure-volume analysis** (Figure 10–6), pressure during the cardiac cycle is plotted as a function of volume rather than time. During diastole, as ventricular volume increases

during both the initial rapid filling period and atrial contraction, ventricular pressure increases (curve **da**). The shape and position of this curve, the **diastolic pressure-volume relationship,** are dependent on relaxation properties of the ventricle, the elastic recoil of the ventricle, and the distensibility of the ventricle. The curve shifts to the left

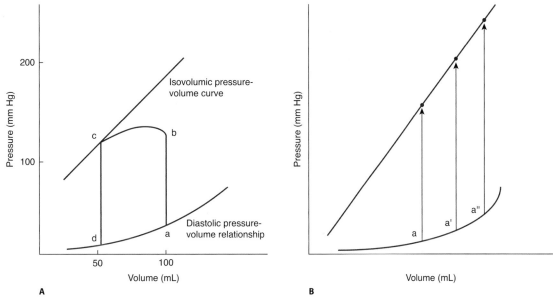

FIGURE 10–6 **A:** Pressure-volume loop for the left ventricle. During diastole the left ventricle fills and pressure increases along the diastolic pressure-volume curve from **d** to **a.** Line **ab** represents isometric contraction, and **bc** the ejection phase of systole. The aortic valve closes at point **c,** and pressure drops along **cd** (isovolumic relaxation), until the mitral valve opens at point **d** and the cycle repeats. The distance from **b** to **c** represents the stroke volume ejected by that beat. Point **a** represents end-diastole and point **c,** end-systole. **B:** If the left ventricle is filled by varying amounts **a, a', a''** and allowed to undergo isovolumic contraction, a relatively linear relationship, the isovolumic pressure-volume relation, can be defined.

(higher pressure for a given volume) if relaxation of the ventricle is decreased, the ventricle loses elastic recoil, or the ventricle becomes stiffer. At the beginning of systole, active ventricular contraction begins and volume remains unchanged (isovolumic contraction period) (**ab**). When left ventricular pressure reaches aortic pressure, the aortic valve opens, and ventricular volume decreases as the ventricle expels its blood (curve **bc**). At end systole (**c**), the aortic valve closes and isovolumic relaxation begins (**cd**). When the mitral valve opens, the ventricle begins filling for the next cardiac cycle, repeating the entire process. The area encompassed by this loop represents the amount of work done by the ventricle during a cardiac cycle. The position of point **c** is dependent on the **isovolumic systolic pressure-volume curve.** If the ventricle is filled with variable amounts of blood (preloads) and allowed to contract but the aortic valve is prevented from opening, a relatively linear relationship exists, termed the isovolumic systolic pressure-volume curve (Figure 10–6B). The slope and position of this line describe the inherent contractile state of the ventricle. If contractility is increased by catecholamines or other positive inotropes, the line will shift to the left.

Pressure-volume relationships help illustrate the effects of different stresses on cardiac output. Cardiac output of the ventricle is the product of the **heart rate** and the volume of blood pumped with each beat (**stroke volume**). The width of the pressure-volume loop is the difference between end-diastolic volume and end-systolic volume, or the stroke volume (Figure 10–6). The stroke volume is dependent on three parameters: contractility, afterload, and preload (Figure 10–7). Changing

the contractile state of the heart will change the width of the pressure-volume loop by changing the position of the isovolumic systolic pressure curve. The impedance against which the heart must work is termed **afterload;** increased afterload (aortic pressure for the left ventricle) will cause a decrease in stroke volume. **Preload** is the amount of filling of the ventricle at end-diastole. Up to a point, the more a myocyte or ventricular chamber is stretched, the more it will contract (**Frank-Starling relationship**), so that increased preload will lead to an increase in stroke volume.

Pressure-time and pressure-volume relationships are critical for understanding the pathophysiologic mechanisms of diseases that affect the entire ventricular chamber function, such as heart failure and valvular abnormalities.

Cellular Physiology

A. Ventricular and Atrial Myocytes

The cellular mechanism of myocyte contraction after electrical stimulation is too complex to be fully addressed in this section, but excellent discussions of electromechanical coupling can be found. Briefly, when the myocyte is stimulated, sodium channels on the cell surface membrane (sarcolemma) open, and sodium ions (Na^+) flow down their electrochemical gradient into the cell. This sudden inward surge of ions is responsible for the sharp upstroke of the myocyte action potential (phase 0) (Figure 10–8). A plateau phase follows during which the cell membrane potential remains relatively unchanged owing to the inward flow of calcium ions (Ca^{2+}) and the outward flow of potassium ions (K^+) through several different

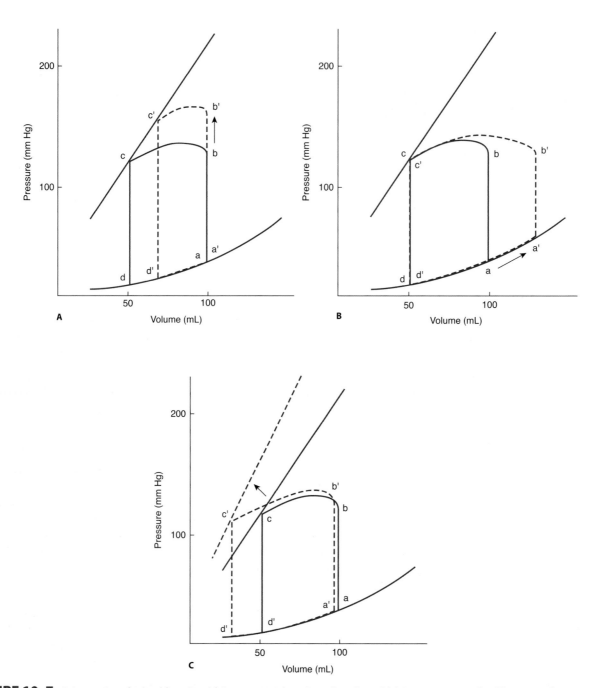

FIGURE 10–7 **A:** Increasing afterload from **b** to **b'** decreases stroke volume from **bc** to **b'c'**. **B:** Increasing preload from **a** to **a'** increases stroke volume from **bc** to **b'c'**, but at the expense of increased end-diastolic pressure. **C:** Increasing contractile state shifts the isovolumic pressure-volume relationship leftward, increasing stroke volume from **bc** to **b'c'**.

specialized potassium channels. Repolarization occurs because of continued outward flow of K^+ after inward flux of Ca^{2+} has stopped.

Within the cell, the change in membrane potential from the sudden influx of Na^+ and the subsequent increase in intracellular Ca^{2+} causes the sarcoplasmic reticulum to release large numbers of calcium ions via specialized Ca^{2+} release channels. The exact signaling mechanism is not known. Once in the cytoplasm, however, Ca^{2+} released from the sarcoplasmic reticulum binds with the regulatory proteins troponin and tropomyosin. Myosin and actin are then allowed to interact and the cross-bridges between them bend, giving rise to contraction (Figure 10–9). The process of relaxation is poorly understood also but appears to involve return of Ca^{2+} to the sarcoplasmic reticulum via two transmembrane sarcoplasmic reticulum-embedded proteins: Ca^{2+}-ATPase and phospholamban. Reuptake of Ca^{2+} is an active process that requires adenosine triphosphate (ATP).

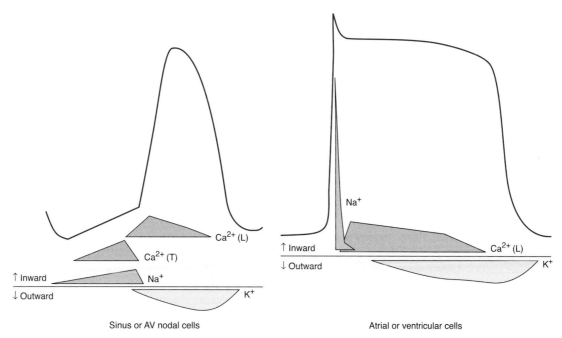

Sinus or AV nodal cells   *Atrial or ventricular cells*

FIGURE 10–8 Changes in ionic conductances responsible for generating action potentials for ventricular or atrial tissue (right) and a sinus or AV node cell (left). In nodal cells rapid Na^+ channels are absent, so that the action potential upstroke is much slower. Diastolic depolarization observed in nodal cells is due to decreased K^+ efflux and slow Na^+ and Ca^{2+} influx. Ca^{2+} (T): influx via Ca^{2+} (T) channels; Ca^{2+} (L): influx via Ca^{2+} (L) channels.

B. Pacemaker Cells

The action potential of pacemaker cells is different from that described for ventricular and atrial myocytes (Figure 10–8). Fast sodium channels are absent, so that rapid phase 0 depolarization is not observed in SA nodal and AV nodal cells. In addition, these cells are characterized by increased automaticity from a relatively rapid spontaneous phase 4 depolarization. A combination of reduced outward flow of K^+ and inward flow of Na^+ and Ca^{2+} via specialized channels appears to be responsible for this dynamic change in membrane potential. Myofibrils are sparse, although present, in the specialized pacemaker cells.

CHECKPOINT

1. What are the differences in pacemaker and conduction properties in different regions of the heart, and why do these differences explain the observation that cardiac electrical impulses normally arise in the SA node?
2. Describe pressure-time analysis through the cardiac cycle.
3. Describe pressure-volume analysis through the cardiac cycle.
4. What are preload and afterload?
5. Briefly describe the molecular mechanism of electromechanical coupling in cardiac myocyte contraction.

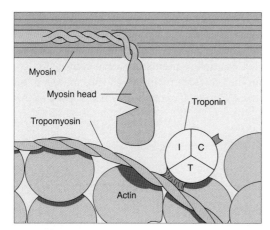
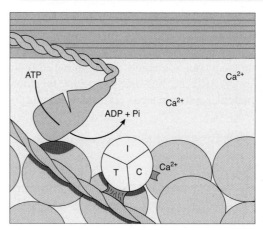

FIGURE 10–9 Initiation of muscle contraction by Ca^{2+}. When Ca^{2+} binds to troponin C, tropomyosin is displaced laterally, exposing the binding site for myosin on actin (dark area). Hydrolysis of ATP then changes the conformation of the myosin head and fosters its binding to the exposed site. For simplicity, only one of the two heads of the myosin-II molecule is shown. (Redrawn, with permission, from Ganong WF. *Review of Medical Physiology*, 22nd ed. McGraw-Hill, 2005.)

PATHOPHYSIOLOGY OF SELECTED CARDIOVASCULAR DISORDERS

ARRHYTHMIAS

At rest, the heart is normally activated at a rate of 50–100 beats/min. Abnormal rhythms of the heart (arrhythmias) can be classified as either too slow (bradycardias) or too fast (tachycardias).

Bradycardia

Bradycardia can arise from two basic mechanisms. First, reduced automaticity of the sinus node can result in slow heart rates or pauses. As shown in Figure 10–10, if sinus node pacemaker activity ceases, the heart will usually be activated at a slower rate by other cardiac tissues with pacemaker activity. Reduced sinus node automaticity can occur during periods of increased vagal tone (sleep, carotid sinus massage, "common faint"), with increasing age and secondary to drugs (beta-blockers, calcium channel blockers).

Second, slow heart rates can occur if the cardiac impulse is prevented from activating the ventricles normally because of blocked conduction (Figure 10–11). Because the fibrous valvular annulus is electrically inert, the AV node and His bundle normally form the only electrically active connection between the atria and the ventricles. Although this arrangement is useful for preventing feedback between the two chambers, it also makes the AV node and His bundle vulnerable sites for blocked conduction between the atria and ventricles. Although block can be observed in either the left or right bundle branches, bradycardia does not necessarily occur, because the ventricles can still be activated by the contralateral bundle. Atrioventricular block has been classified as first degree when there is an abnormally long atrioventricular conduction time (PR interval > 0.22 s) but activation of the atria and ventricles still demonstrates 1:1 association. In second-degree atrioventricular block, some but not all atrial impulses are conducted to the ventricles. Finally, in third-degree block, there is no association between atrial and ventricular activity. Atrioventricular block can occur with increasing age, with increased vagal input, and as a side effect of certain drugs. Atrioventricular block can sometimes be observed also in congenital disorders such as muscular dystrophy, tuberous sclerosis, and maternal systemic lupus erythematosus and in acquired disorders such as sarcoidosis, gout, Lyme disease, systemic lupus erythematosus, ankylosing spondylitis, and coronary artery disease.

Bradycardia resulting from either decreased automaticity or blocked conduction calls for evaluation to detect reversible causes. However, implantation of a permanent pacemaker is often required.

Tachycardia

Tachycardias can arise from three basic cellular mechanisms (Figure 10–12). First, increased automaticity resulting from more rapid phase 4 depolarization can cause rapid heart rate. Second, if repolarization is delayed (longer plateau period), spontaneous depolarizations (caused by reactivation of sodium or calcium channels) can sometimes occur in phase 3 or phase 4 of the action potential. These depolarizations are called triggered activity because they are dependent on the existence of a preceding action potential. If these depolarizations reach threshold, tachycardia can occur in certain pathologic conditions. Third, and most commonly, tachycardias can arise from a reentrant circuit. Any condition that gives rise to parallel but electrically separate regions with different conduction velocities (such as the border zone of a myocardial infarction or an accessory atrioventricular connection) can serve as the substrate for a reentrant circuit.

The best studied example of reentrant tachyarrhythmias is Wolff-Parkinson-White syndrome (Figure 10–13). As mentioned, the AV node normally forms the only electrical connection between the atria and the ventricles. Perhaps because of incomplete formation of the annulus, an accessory atrioventricular connection is found in approximately 1 in 1000 persons. This accessory pathway is usually composed of normal atrial or ventricular tissue. Because part of the ventricle is "pre-excited" over the accessory pathway rather than via the AV node, the surface ECG shows a short PR interval and a relatively wide QRS with a slurred upstroke, termed a **delta wave.** Because the atria and ventricles are linked by two parallel connections, reentrant tachycardias are readily initiated. For example, a premature atrial contraction could be blocked in the accessory pathway but still conduct to the ventricles via the AV node. If enough time has elapsed so that the accessory

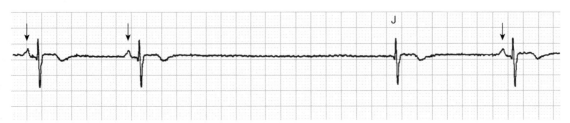

FIGURE 10–10 Rhythm strip showing bradycardia resulting from sinus node pause. Atrial activity **(arrows)** suddenly ceases, and after approximately 3 s a junctional escape beat is observed (J).

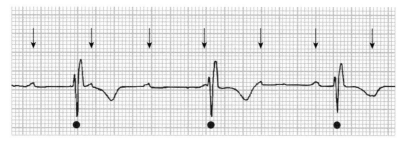

FIGURE 10–11 Rhythm strip demonstrating third-degree (complete) heart block with no association between atrial activity **(arrows)** and ventricular activity **(dots).**

pathway has recovered excitability, the cardiac impulse can travel in retrograde fashion to the atria over the accessory pathway and initiate a reentrant tachycardia.

The best example of tachycardias from triggered activity is the long QT syndrome. More than 40 years ago, investigators described several clusters of patients with a congenital syndrome associated with a long QT interval and ventricular arrhythmias. Data have shown that the long QT interval can be due to several specific ion channel defects. For example, reduced function of potassium channels leads to a prolonged plateau period (Figure 10–14). The prolonged plateau phase in ventricular tissue leads to a prolonged QT interval. These patients are prone to triggered activity because of reactivation of sodium and calcium channels (early after depolarizations). Triggered activity in the ventricles can lead to life-threatening ventricular arrhythmias.

Regardless of the mechanism, the approach to immediate clinical management of tachycardias depends on whether the QRS complex is narrow or wide. If the QRS complex is narrow, depolarization of the ventricles must be occurring normally over the specialized conduction tissues of the heart, and the arrhythmia must be originating at or above the AV node (supraventricular) (Figure 10–15).

A wide QRS complex suggests that ventricular activation is not occurring normally over the specialized conduction tissues of the heart. The tachycardia either is arising from ventricular tissue or is a supraventricular tachycardia with aberrant conduction over the His-Purkinje system or an accessory pathway. Criteria have been developed for distinguishing between ventricular and supraventricular tachycardia with aberrance.

CONGESTIVE HEART FAILURE

Inadequate pump function of the heart, which leads to congestion resulting from fluid in the lungs and peripheral tissues, is a common end result of many cardiac disease processes. Congestive heart failure (CHF) is present in approximately 3 million people in the United States; more than 400,000 new cases are reported annually. The clinical presentation is highly variable; for an individual patient, symptoms and signs depend on how quickly heart failure develops and whether it involves the left, right, or both ventricles.

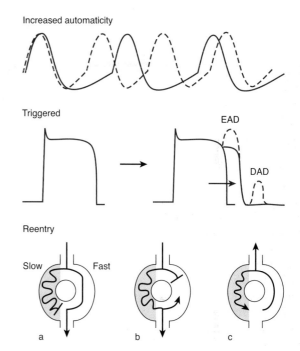

FIGURE 10–12 Tachyarrhythmias can arise from three different mechanisms. First, increased automaticity from more rapid phase 4 depolarization can cause arrhythmias. Second, in certain conditions, spontaneous depolarizations during phase 3 (early afterdepolarizations; EAD) or phase 4 (late afterdepolarizations; DAD) can repetitively reach threshold and cause tachycardia. This appears to be the mechanism of the polymorphic ventricular tachycardia (torsades de pointes) observed in some patients taking procainamide or quinidine and the arrhythmias associated with digoxin toxicity. Third, the most common mechanism for tachyarrhythmia is reentry. In reentry, two parallel pathways with different conduction properties exist (perhaps at the border zone of a myocardial infarction or a region of myocardial ischemia). The electrical impulse normally travels down the fast pathway and the slow pathway (shaded region), but at the point where the two pathways converge the impulse traveling down the slow pathway is blocked since the tissue is refractory from the recent depolarization via the fast pathway (a). However, when a premature beat reaches the circuit, block can occur in the fast pathway, and the impulse will travel down the slow pathway (shaded region) (b). After traveling through the slow pathway the impulse can then enter the fast pathway in retrograde fashion (which because of the delay has recovered excitability), and then reenter the slow pathway to start a continuous loop of activation, or reentrant circuit (c).

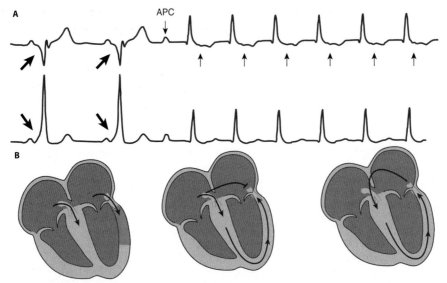

FIGURE 10–13 Reentrant tachyarrhythmia resulting from Wolff-Parkinson-White syndrome. **A:** First two beats demonstrate sinus rhythm with preexcitation of the ventricles over an accessory pathway. The large arrows show the delta wave. An atrial premature contraction (APC) blocks in the accessory pathway, which leads to normalization of the QRS, and the atria are activated in retrograde fashion via the accessory pathway (small arrows) and supraventricular tachycardia ensues. **B:** The left panel schematically depicts the first two beats of the rhythm strip. The QRS is wide owing to activation of the ventricles over both the AV node and the accessory pathway. The middle panel depicts the atrial premature contraction, which is blocked in the accessory pathway but conducts over the AV node. In the right panel, the atria are activated in retrograde fashion over the accessory pathway, and a reentrant circuit is initiated.

1. Left Ventricular Failure

Clinical Presentation

Patients with left ventricular failure most commonly present with a sensation of breathlessness (dyspnea), particularly when lying down (orthopnea) or at night (paroxysmal noc-

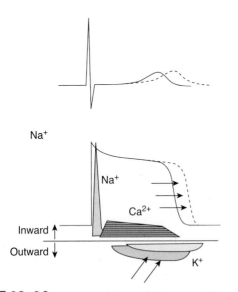

FIGURE 10–14 In certain patients with the long QT syndrome, potassium channel function is reduced (diagonal arrows), which leads to prolongation of the action potential of ventricular myocytes and prolongation of the QT interval. In some cases, reactivation of sodium and calcium channels can lead to triggered activity that can initiate life-threatening ventricular arrhythmias.

turnal dyspnea). In addition, the patient may complain of blood-tinged sputum (hemoptysis) and occasionally chest pain. Fatigue, nocturia, and confusion can also be caused by heart failure.

On physical examination, the patient usually has elevated respiratory and heart rates. The skin may be pale, cold, and sweaty. In severe heart failure, palpation of the peripheral pulse may reveal alternating strong and weak beats (pulsus alternans). Auscultation of the lungs reveals abnormal sounds, called rales, that have been described as "crackling leaves." In addition, the bases of the lung fields may be dull to percussion. On cardiac examination, the apical impulse is often displaced laterally and sustained. Third and fourth heart sounds can be heard on auscultation of the heart. Because many patients with left ventricular failure also have accompanying failure of the right ventricle, signs of right ventricular failure may also be present (see next section).

Etiology

Heart failure is a pathophysiologic complex associated with dysfunction of the heart and is a common end point for many diseases of the cardiovascular system. There are many possible causes (Table 10–1), and the specific reason for heart failure in a given patient must always be sought. In general, heart failure can be caused by (1) inappropriate workloads placed on the heart, such as volume overload or pressure overload; (2) restricted filling of the heart; (3) myocyte loss; or (4) decreased myocyte contractility. Any one of these causes can initiate an evolving sequence of events that are described next.

Atrial fibrillation   Atrial flutter

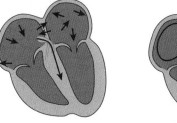

AV nodal
reentrant tachycardia

Atrioventricular
reentrant tachycardia

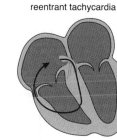

Atrial tachycardia

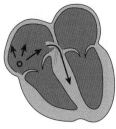

FIGURE 10–15 In supraventricular tachycardia, the QRS is narrow because the ventricles are depolarized over the normal specialized conduction tissues (light blue region). Five possible arrhythmias are commonly encountered. First, in atrial fibrillation, multiple microreentrant circuits can lead to chaotic activation of the atrium. Because impulses are reaching the AV node at irregular intervals, ventricular depolarization is irregular. Second, in atrial flutter, a macroreentrant circuit, traveling up the interatrial septum and down the lateral walls, can activate the atria in a regular fashion at approximately 300 beats/min. The AV node can conduct only every other or every third beat, so that the ventricles are depolarized at 150 or 100 beats/min. In AV nodal reentrant tachycardia, slow and fast pathways exist in the region of the AV node and a microreentrant circuit can be formed. Fourth, in atrioventricular reentry, an abnormal connection between the atrium and ventricle exists so that a macroreentrant circuit can be formed with the AV node forming the slow pathway, and the abnormal atrioventricular connection, the fast pathway. Finally, in atrial tachycardia an abnormal focus of atrial activity as a result of either reentry, triggered activity, or abnormal automaticity can activate the atria in a regular fashion.

Pathophysiology

The pathophysiology of heart failure is complex and must be understood at multiple levels. Traditionally, research has focused on the hemodynamic changes of the failing heart, considering the heart as an isolated organ. However, studies of the failing heart have emphasized the importance of understanding changes at the cellular level and the neurohormonal interactions between the heart and other organs of the body (Table 10–2).

TABLE 10–1 Causes of left ventricular failure.

Volume overload
Regurgitant valves (mitral or aortic)
High-output states: anemia, hyperthyroidism
Pressure overload
Systemic hypertension
Outflow obstruction: aortic stenosis, asymmetric septal hypertrophy
Loss of muscle
Myocardial infarction from coronary artery disease
Connective tissue disease: systemic lupus erythematosus
Loss of contractility
Poisons: alcohol, cobalt, doxorubicin
Infections: viral, bacterial
Genetic mutations of cellular architecture or sarcomere proteins
Restricted filling
Mitral stenosis
Pericardial disease: constrictive pericarditis and pericardial tamponade
Infiltrative diseases: amyloidosis

TABLE 10–2 Pathophysiologic changes associated with heart failure.

Hemodynamic changes
Decreased output (systolic dysfunction)
Decreased filling (diastolic dysfunction)
Neurohormonal changes
Sympathetic system activation
Renin-angiotensin system activation
Vasopressin release
Cytokine release
Cellular changes
Inefficient intracellular Ca^{2+} handling
Adrenergic desensitization
Myocyte hypertrophy
Reexpression of fetal phenotype proteins
Cell death (apoptosis)
Fibrosis

A. Hemodynamic Changes—From a hemodynamic standpoint, heart failure can arise from worsening systolic or diastolic function or, more frequently, a combination of both. In **systolic dysfunction,** the isovolumic systolic pressure curve of the pressure-volume relationship is shifted downward (Figure 10–16A). This reduces the stroke volume of the heart with a concomitant decrease in cardiac output. To maintain cardiac output, the heart can respond with three compensatory mechanisms: First, increased return of blood to the heart (preload) can lead to increased contraction of sarcomeres (Frank-Starling relationship). In the pressure-volume relationship, the heart

operates at **a′** instead of **a**, and stroke volume increases, but at the cost of increased end-diastolic pressure (Figure 10–16D). Second, increased release of catecholamines can increase cardiac output by both increasing the heart rate and shifting the systolic isovolumetric curve to the left (Figure 10–16C). Finally, cardiac muscle can hypertrophy and ventricular volume can increase, which shifts the diastolic curve to the right (Figure 10–16B). Although each of these compensatory mechanisms can temporarily maintain cardiac output, each is limited in its ability to do so, and if the underlying reason for systolic dysfunction remains untreated, the heart ultimately fails.

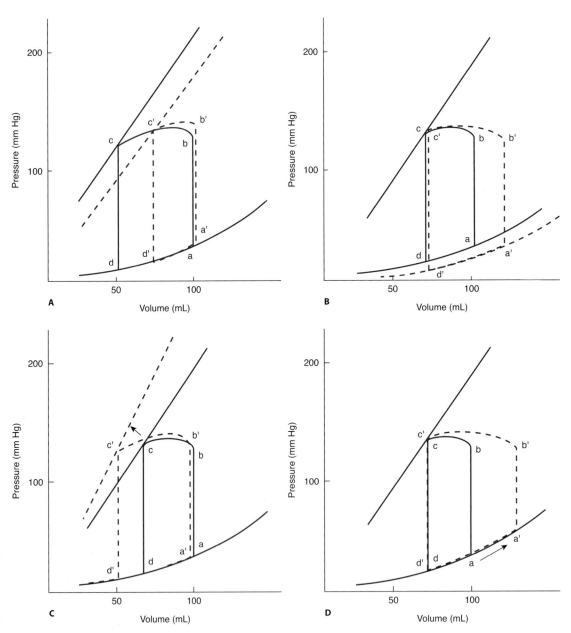

FIGURE 10–16   **A:** Systolic dysfunction is represented by shifting of the isovolumic pressure-volume curve to the right (dashed line), thus decreasing stroke volume. The ventricle can compensate by (**B**) shifting the diastolic pressure-volume relationship rightward (dashed line) by increasing left ventricular volume or elasticity, (**C**) increasing contractile state (dashed line) by activation of circulating catecholamines, and (**D**) increasing filling or preload (**a** to **a′**).

In **diastolic dysfunction,** the position of the systolic iso-volumic curve remains unchanged (contractility of the myocytes is preserved). However, the diastolic pressure-volume curve is shifted to the left, with an accompanying increase in left ventricular end-diastolic pressure and symptoms of congestive heart failure (Figure 10–17). Diastolic dysfunction can be present in any disease that causes decreased relaxation, decreased elastic recoil, or increased stiffness of the ventricle. Hypertension, which often leads to increases in left ventricular wall thickness, can cause diastolic dysfunction by changing all three parameters. Lack of sufficient blood to myocytes (ischemia) can also cause diastolic dysfunction by decreasing relaxation. If ischemia is severe, as in myocardial infarction, irreversible damage to the myocytes can occur, with replacement of contractile cells by fibrosis, which will lead to systolic dysfunction. In most patients, a combination of systolic and diastolic dysfunction is responsible for the symptoms of heart failure.

B. Neurohumoral Changes

—After an injury to the heart (Table 10–1), increased secretion of endogenous neurohormones and cytokines is observed. Initially, increased activity of the adrenergic system and the renin-angiotensin system provides a compensatory response that maintains perfusion of vital organs. However, over time these changes can lead to progressive deterioration of cardiac function.

Increased sympathetic activity occurs early in the development of heart failure. Elevated plasma norepinephrine levels cause increased cardiac contractility and an increased heart rate that initially help maintain cardiac output. However, continued increases lead to increased preload (as a result of venous vasoconstriction) and afterload (from arterial vasoconstriction), which can worsen heart failure. In addition, sympathetic hyperactivity causes deleterious cellular changes, which are discussed in the next section.

Reduced renal blood pressure stimulates the release of renin and increases the production of angiotensin II. Both angiotensin II and sympathetic activation cause efferent glomerular arteriolar vasoconstriction, which helps maintain the glomerular filtration rate despite a reduced cardiac output. Angiotensin II stimulates aldosterone synthesis, which leads to sodium resorption and potassium excretion by the kidneys. However, a vicious circle is initiated as continued hyperactivity of the renin-angiotensin system leads to severe vasoconstriction, increased afterload, and further reduction in cardiac output and glomerular filtration rate.

Heart failure is associated with increased release of vasopressin from the posterior pituitary gland. Vasopressin is another powerful vasoconstrictor that also promotes reabsorption of water in the renal tubules.

Heart failure is associated with the release of cytokines and other circulating peptides. Cytokines are a heterogeneous family of proteins that are secreted by macrophages, lymphocytes, monocytes, and endothelial cells in response to injury. The **interleukins (ILs)** and **tumor necrosis factor** (TNF) are the two major groups of cytokines that may have an important pathophysiologic role in heart failure. Upregulation of the gene responsible for TNF with an accompanying increase in circulating plasma levels of TNF has been found in patients with heart failure. TNF appears to have an important role in the cycle of myocyte hypertrophy and cell death (apoptosis) described in the next section. Preliminary in vitro data suggest that IL-1 may accelerate myocyte hypertrophy. Another peptide important for mediating some of the pathophysiologic effects observed in heart failure is the potent vasoconstrictor **endothelin,** which is released from endothelial cells. Preliminary data have suggested that excessive endothelin release may be responsible for hypertension in the pulmonary arteries observed in patients with left ventricular heart failure. Endothelin is also associated with myocyte growth and deposition of collagen in the interstitial matrix.

C. Cellular Changes

—Pathophysiologic changes at the cellular level are very complex and include changes in Ca^{2+} handling, adrenergic receptors, contractile apparatus, and myocyte structure.

In heart failure, both delivery of Ca^{2+} to the contractile apparatus and reuptake of Ca^{2+} by the sarcoplasmic reticulum are slowed. Decreased levels of messenger ribonucleic acid (mRNA) for the specialized Ca^{2+} release channels have been reported by some investigators. Similarly, myocytes from failing hearts have reduced levels of mRNA for the two sarcoplasmic reticulum proteins phospholamban and Ca^{2+}-ATPase.

Two major classes of adrenergic receptors are found in the human heart. Alpha$_1$-adrenergic receptors are important for induction of myocardial hypertrophy; levels of $\alpha 1$ receptors are slightly increased in heart failure. Heart failure is associ-

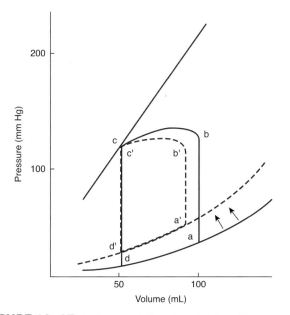

FIGURE 10–17 In diastolic dysfunction, the diastolic pressure-volume relation is shifted upward and to the left (dashed line), which leads to an elevated left ventricular end-diastolic pressure **a'** and reduced stroke volume.

ated with significant β-adrenergic receptor desensitization as a result of chronic sympathetic activation. This effect is mediated by downregulation of $β_1$-adrenergic receptors, downstream uncoupling of the signal transduction pathway, and upregulation of inhibitory G proteins. All of these changes lead to a further reduction in myocyte contractility.

Cardiac myocytes cannot proliferate once they have matured to their adult form. However, there is a constant turnover of the contractile proteins that make up the sarcomere. In response to the hemodynamic stresses associated with heart failure, angiotensin II, TNF, norepinephrine, and other molecules induce protein synthesis via intranuclear mediators of gene activity such as c-*fos*, c-*jun*, and c-*myc*. This causes myocyte hypertrophy with an increase in sarcomere numbers and a reexpression of fetal and neonatal forms of myosin and troponin. Reexpression of fetal contractile proteins causes the development of large myocytes that do not contract normally and have decreased ATPase activity.

The heart enlarges in response to continued hemodynamic stress. Changes in myocardial size and shape associated with heart failure are collectively referred to as left ventricular remodeling. Several tissue changes appear to mediate this process. First, heart failure is associated with myocyte loss via a process called apoptosis (programmed cell death). Unlike the process of necrosis, apoptotic cells initially demonstrate decreased cell volume without disruption of the cell membrane. However, as the apoptotic process continues, the myocyte ultimately dies, and "holes" are left in the myocardium. Loss of myocytes places increased stress on the remaining myocytes. The process of apoptosis is accelerated by the proliferative signals that stimulate myocyte hypertrophy such as TNF. Although apoptosis is a normal process that is essential in organs made up of proliferating cells, in the heart apoptosis initiates a vicious circle whereby cell death causes increased stress that leads to hypertrophy and further acceleration of apoptosis.

A second tissue change observed in heart failure is an increased amount of fibrous tissue in the interstitial spaces of the heart. Collagen deposition is due to activation of fibroblasts and myocyte death. Endothelin release leads to interstitial collagen deposition. The increase in connective tissue increases chamber stiffness and shifts the diastolic pressure-volume curve to the left.

Finally, heart failure is associated with gradual dilation of the ventricle. Myocyte "slippage" as a result of activation of collagenases that disrupt the collagen network may be responsible for this process.

Clinical Manifestations

A. Symptoms

1. **Shortness of breath, orthopnea, paroxysmal nocturnal dyspnea**—Although many details of the physiologic mechanisms for the sensation of breathlessness are unclear, the inciting event probably is a rise in pulmonary capillary pressures as a consequence of elevated left ventricular and atrial pressures. The rise in pulmonary capillary pressure relative to plasma oncotic pressure causes fluid to move into the interstitial spaces of the lung (pulmonary edema), which can be seen on chest x-ray film (Figure 10–18). Interstitial edema probably stimulates juxtacapillary J receptors, which in turn causes reflex shallow and rapid breathing. Replacement of air in the lungs by blood or interstitial fluid can cause a reduction of vital capacity, restrictive physiology, and air trapping as a result of closure of small airways. The work of breathing increases as the patient tries to distend stiff lungs, which can lead to respiratory muscle fatigue and the sensation of dyspnea. Alterations in the distribution of ventilation and perfusion result in relative ventilation-perfusion mismatch, with consequent widening of the alveolar-arterial O_2 gradient, hypoxemia, and increased dead space. Edema of the bronchial walls can lead to small airway obstruction and produce wheezing ("cardiac asthma"). Shortness of breath occurs in the recumbent position (orthopnea) because of reduced blood pooling in the extremities and abdomen, and, because the patient is operating on the steep portion of the diastolic pressure-volume curve, any increase in blood return leads to marked elevations in ventricular pressures. Patients usually learn to minimize orthopnea by sleeping with the upper body propped up by two or more pillows. Sudden onset of severe respiratory distress at night—paroxysmal nocturnal dyspnea—probably occurs because of the reduced adrenergic support of ventricular function that occurs with sleep, the increase in blood return as described previously, and normal nocturnal depression of the respiratory center.

2. **Fatigue, confusion**—Fatigue probably arises because of inability of the heart to supply appropriate amounts of blood to skeletal muscles. Confusion may arise in advanced heart failure because of underperfusion of the cerebrum.

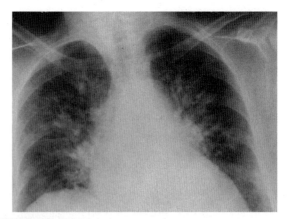

FIGURE 10–18 Posteroanterior chest x-ray film in a man with acute pulmonary edema resulting from left ventricular failure. Note the bat's wing density, cardiac enlargement, increased size of upper lobe vessels, and pulmonary venous congestion. (Reproduced, with permission, from Cheitlin MD, Sokolow M, McIlroy MB. *Clinical Cardiology*, 6th ed. Originally published by Appleton & Lange. Copyright © 1993 by the McGraw-Hill Companies, Inc.)

3. **Nocturia**—Heart failure can lead to reduced renal perfusion during the day while the patient is upright, which normalizes only at night while the patient is supine, with consequent diuresis.

4. **Chest pain**—If the cause of failure is coronary artery disease, patients may have chest pain secondary to ischemia (angina pectoris). In addition, even without ischemia, acute heart failure can cause chest pain by unknown mechanisms.

B. Physical Examination

1. **Rales, pleural effusion**—Increased fluid in the alveolar spaces from the mechanisms described previously can be heard as rales. Increased capillary pressures can also cause fluid accumulation in the pleural spaces.

2. **Displaced and sustained apical impulse**—In most people, contraction of the heart can be appreciated by careful palpation of the chest wall (apical impulse). The normal apical impulse is felt in the midclavicular line in the fourth or fifth intercostal space and is palpable only during the first part of systole. When the apical impulse can be felt during the latter part of systole, it is sustained. Sustained impulses suggest that increases in left ventricular volume or mass are present. In addition, when left ventricular volume is increased as a compensatory mechanism of heart failure, the apical impulse is displaced laterally.

3. **Third heart sound (S_3)**—The third heart sound is a low-pitched sound that is heard during rapid filling of the ventricle in early diastole (Figure 10–19A). The exact mechanism responsible for the genesis of the third heart sound is not known, but the sound appears to result either from the sudden deceleration of blood as the elastic limits of the ventricular chamber are reached or from the actual impact of the ventricular wall against the chest wall. Although a third heart sound is normal in children and young adults, it is rarely heard in healthy adults older than 40 years. In these individuals, the presence of a third heart sound is almost pathognomonic of ventricular failure. The increased end-systolic volumes and pressures characteristic of the failing heart are probably responsible for the prominent third heart sound. When it arises because of left ventricular failure, the third heart sound is usually heard best at the apex. It can be present in patients with either diastolic or systolic dysfunction.

4. **Fourth heart sound (S_4)**—Normally, sounds arising from atrial contraction are not heard. However, if there is increased stiffness of the ventricle, a low-pitched sound at end-diastole that occurs concomitantly with atrial contraction can sometimes be heard (Figure 10–19B). As with the third heart sound, the exact mechanism for the genesis of the fourth heart sound is not known. However, it probably arises from the sudden deceleration of blood in a non-compliant ventricle or from the sudden impact of a stiff ventricle against the chest wall. It is best heard laterally over the apex at the point of maximal impulse, particularly when the patient is partially rolled over onto the left side. The fourth heart sound is commonly heard in any patient with heart failure resulting from diastolic dysfunction.

5. **Pale, cold, and sweaty skin**—Patients with severe heart failure often have peripheral vasoconstriction, which maintains blood flow to the central organs and head. In some cases, the skin appears dusky because of reduced oxygen content in venous blood as a result of increased oxygen extraction from peripheral tissues that are receiving low blood flow. Sweating occurs because body heat cannot be dissipated through the constricted vascular bed of the skin.

2. Right Ventricular Failure

Clinical Presentation

Symptoms of right ventricular failure include shortness of breath, pedal edema, and abdominal pain.

The findings on physical examination are similar to those of left ventricular failure but in different positions, because the right ventricle is anatomically anterior and to the right of the left ventricle (Figure 10–1). Patients with right ventricular failure may have a third heart sound heard best at the sternal border or a sustained systolic heave of the sternum. Inspection of the neck reveals elevated jugular venous pressures. Because the most common cause of right ventricular failure is left ventricular failure, signs of left ventricular failure are often also present.

Etiology

Right ventricular failure can be due to several causes. As mentioned, left ventricular failure can cause right ventricular failure because of the increased afterload placed on the right ventricle. Increased afterload can also be present from abnormalities of the pulmonary arteries or capillaries. For example, increased flow from a congenital shunt can cause reactive pulmonary artery constriction, increased right ventricular afterload, and, ultimately, right ventricular failure. Right ventricular failure can occur as a sequela of pulmonary disease (cor pulmonale) because of destruction of the pulmonary capillary bed or hypoxia-induced vasoconstriction of the pulmonary arterioles. Right ventricular failure can also be caused by right ventricular ischemia, usually in the setting of an inferior wall myocardial infarction (Table 10–3).

Pathophysiology

The pathophysiology of right ventricular failure is similar to that described for the left ventricle. Both systolic and diastolic abnormalities of the right ventricle can be present and usually occur because of inappropriate loads placed on the ventricle or primary loss of myocyte contractility.

Patients with isolated right ventricular failure (pulmonary hypertension, cor pulmonale) can have a mechanical reason for left ventricular failure. The interventricular septum is usually bowed toward the thinner walled and lower pressure right

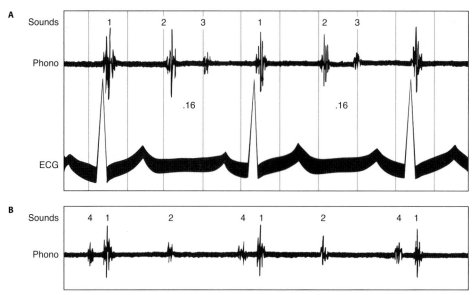

FIGURE 10–19 **A:** Phonocardiogram showing typical third heart sound (S$_3$). It follows the second sound (S$_2$) by 0.16 s. (Courtesy Roche Laboratories Division of Hoffman-La Roche, Inc.) **B:** Phonocardiogram showing a fourth heart sound (S$_4$) and its relation to first sound (S$_1$).

ventricle. When right ventricular pressure increases relative to the left, the interventricular septum can bow to the left and prevent efficient filling of the left ventricle, which may lead to pulmonary congestion. Rarely, the bowing can be so severe that left ventricular outflow can be partially obstructed. This phenomenon is termed a "reversed Bernheim effect."

Clinical Manifestations

A. Shortness of Breath—If there is left ventricular failure, patients may be short of breath because of pulmonary edema as discussed previously. In patients with right-sided failure resulting from pulmonary disease, shortness of breath may be a manifestation of the underlying disease (eg, pulmonary embolus, chronic obstructive pulmonary disease). In some patients with right ventricular failure, congestion of the hepatic veins

TABLE 10–3   Causes of right ventricular failure.

Left-sided failure
Precapillary obstruction
Congenital (shunts, obstruction)
Idiopathic pulmonary hypertension
Primary right ventricular failure
Right ventricular infarction
Cor pulmonale
Hypoxia-induced vasoconstriction
Pulmonary embolism
Chronic obstructive lung disease

with formation of ascites can impinge on normal diaphragmatic function and contribute to the sensation of dyspnea. In addition, reduced right-sided cardiac output alone can cause acidosis, hypoxia, and air hunger. If the cause of right-sided failure is a left-sided defect such as mitral stenosis, the onset of right heart failure can sometimes lessen the symptoms of pulmonary edema because of the decreased load placed on the left ventricle.

B. Elevated Jugular Venous Pressure—The position of venous pulsations of the internal jugular vein can be observed during examination of the neck (Figure 10–20A). The vertical distance above the heart at which venous pulsations are observed is an estimate of the right atrial or central venous pressure. Because the position of the right atrium cannot be precisely determined, the height of the jugular venous pulsation is measured relative to the angle of Louis on the sternum. Right atrial pressure can then be approximated by adding 5 cm to the height of the venous column (because the right atrium is approximately 5 cm inferior to the angle). Jugular venous pulsations are usually observed less than 7 cm above the right atrium. Elevated atrial pressures are present any time this distance is greater than 10 cm. Elevated atrial pressures indicate that the preload of the ventricle is adequate but ventricular function is decreased and fluid is accumulating in the venous system. Other causes of elevated jugular pressures besides heart failure include pericardial tamponade, constrictive pericarditis, and massive pulmonary embolism.

In addition to relative position, individual waveforms of the jugular venous pulse can be assessed. Three positive waves (*a, c,* and *v*) and two negative waves (*x* and *y*) can be recognized (Figure 10–20B). The *a* wave is caused by transmitted right atrial pressure from atrial contraction. The *c* wave is usually not present on bedside examination; it is thought to arise

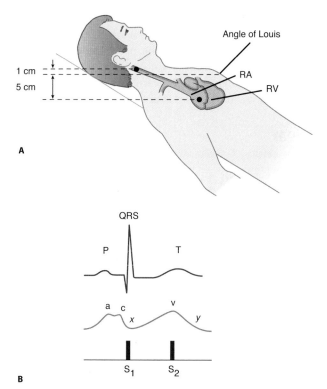

FIGURE 10–20 **A:** Examination of jugular venous pulse and estimation of venous pressure. (RA, right atrium; RV, right ventricle.) **B:** Jugular venous pressure waveforms in relation to the electrocardiogram (P wave, QRS, and T wave) and the first and second heart sounds (S_1 and S_2). The bottom of the x descent occurs coincident with the first heart sound (S_1). The v wave occurs just after the apical impulse is felt at the same time the second heart sound (S_2) is heard. See text for further explanation of jugular venous wave forms.

from bulging of the tricuspid valve during isovolumic contraction of the right ventricle. The x descent is thought to be due to atrial relaxation and downward displacement of the tricuspid annulus during systole. The v wave arises from continued filling of the right atrium during the latter part of systole. Once the tricuspid valve opens, blood flows into the right ventricle and the y descent begins. Evaluation of the individual waveforms will become particularly important when pericardial disease is discussed.

C. Anasarca, Ascites, Pedal Edema, Hepatojugular Reflux, Abdominal Pain—Elevated right-sided pressure leads to accumulation of fluid in the systemic venous circulation. Venous congestion can be manifested by generalized edema (anasarca), ascites (collection of fluid in the peritoneal space), and dependent edema (swelling of the feet and legs). Pressing on the liver for approximately 5 seconds can lead to displacement of blood into the vena cava; when the right ventricle cannot accommodate this additional volume, an increase in jugular venous pressure ("hepatojugular reflux") can be observed. Expansion of the liver from fluid accumulation can cause distention of the liver capsule with accompanying right upper quadrant abdominal pain.

CHECKPOINT

6. What are the clinical presentations of left ventricular CHF? Of right ventricular failure?
7. What are the four general categories that account for almost all causes of CHF?
8. Explain the differences between the pathophysiology of CHF resulting from systolic versus diastolic dysfunction.
9. What are the major clinical manifestations and complications of left- versus right-sided heart failure?

VALVULAR HEART DISEASE

Dysfunctional cardiac valves can be classified as either narrow (stenosis) or leaky (regurgitation). Although the tricuspid and pulmonary valves can become dysfunctional in patients with endocarditis, congenital lesions, or carcinoid syndrome, primary right-sided valvular abnormalities are relatively rare and are not discussed further here. In this section, the pathophysiologic mechanisms of stenotic and regurgitant aortic and mitral valves are addressed.

A general classification of heart murmurs is presented in Figure 10–21. Any disease process that creates turbulent flow in the heart or great vessels can cause a murmur. For instance, ventricular septal defect is associated with a systolic murmur because of the abnormal interventricular connection and the pressure difference between the left and right ventricles; patent ductus arteriosus is associated with a continuous murmur because of a persistent connection between the pulmonary artery and the aorta. However, valvular lesions are the principal cause of heart murmurs. Thus, an understanding of heart murmurs gives insight into the underlying pathophysiologic processes of specific valvular lesions.

Heart murmurs can be either systolic or diastolic. During systole, while the left ventricle is contracting, the aortic valve is open and the mitral valve is closed. Turbulent flow can occur either because of an incompetent mitral valve, leading to regurgitation of blood back into the atrium, or from a narrowed aortic valve. In diastole, the situation is reversed, with filling of the left ventricle through an open mitral valve while the aortic valve is closed. Turbulent flow occurs when there is narrowing of the mitral valve or incompetence of the aortic valve. Stenosis of valves usually develops slowly over time; lesions that cause valvular regurgitation can be either chronic or acute.

1. Aortic Stenosis

Clinical Presentation

For all causes of aortic stenosis, there is usually a long latent period of slowly increasing obstruction before symptoms appear. In descending order of frequency, the three characteristic symptoms of aortic stenosis are chest pain (angina pectoris), syncope, and congestive heart failure (see prior discussion).

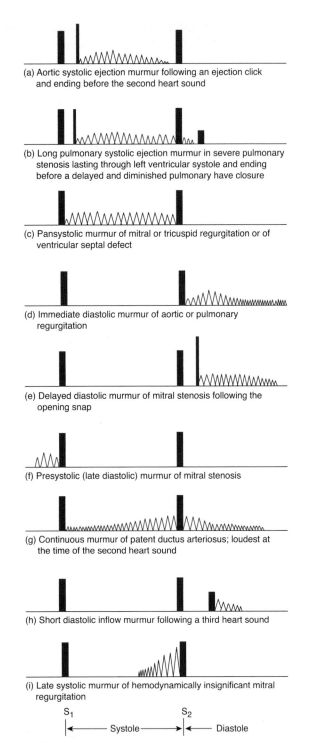

(a) Aortic systolic ejection murmur following an ejection click and ending before the second heart sound

(b) Long pulmonary systolic ejection murmur in severe pulmonary stenosis lasting through left ventricular systole and ending before a delayed and diminished pulmonary have closure

(c) Pansystolic murmur of mitral or tricuspid regurgitation or of ventricular septal defect

(d) Immediate diastolic murmur of aortic or pulmonary regurgitation

(e) Delayed diastolic murmur of mitral stenosis following the opening snap

(f) Presystolic (late diastolic) murmur of mitral stenosis

(g) Continuous murmur of patent ductus arteriosus; loudest at the time of the second heart sound

(h) Short diastolic inflow murmur following a third heart sound

(i) Late systolic murmur of hemodynamically insignificant mitral regurgitation

S_1 S_2

|← Systole →|← Diastole

FIGURE 10–21 The timing of the principal cardiac murmurs.

Once symptoms occur, the prognosis is poor if the obstruction is untreated, with average life expectancies of 2, 3, and 5 years for angina pectoris, syncope, and heart failure, respectively.

On physical examination, palpation of the carotid upstroke reveals a pulsation (pulsus) that is both decreased (parvus) and late (tardus) relative to the apical impulse. Palpation of the chest reveals an apical impulse that is laterally displaced

and sustained. On auscultation, a midsystolic murmur is heard, loudest at the base of the heart, and often with radiation to the sternal notch and the neck. Depending on the cause of the aortic stenosis, a crisp, relatively high-pitched aortic ejection sound can be heard just after the first heart sound. Finally, a fourth heart sound (S_4) is often present.

Etiology

Various causes of aortic stenosis are listed and described in Table 10–4.

Pathophysiology

The normal aortic valve area is approximately 3.5–4.0 cm². Critical aortic stenosis is usually present when the area is less than 0.8 cm². At this point, the systolic gradient between the left ventricle and the aorta can exceed 150 mm Hg, and most patients are symptomatic (Figure 10–22a). The fixed outflow obstruction places a large afterload on the ventricle. The compensatory mechanisms of the heart can be understood by examining Laplace's law for a sphere, where wall stress (T) is proportionate to the product of the transmural pressure (P) and cavitary radius (r) and inversely proportionate to wall thickness (W):

$$T \propto P \times \frac{r}{W}$$

In response to the pressure overload (increased P), left ventricular wall thickness markedly increases—while the cavitary radius remains relatively unchanged—by parallel replication of sarcomeres. These compensatory changes, termed "concentric hypertrophy," reduce the increase in wall tension observed in aortic stenosis (see Aortic Regurgitation). Analysis of pressure-volume loops reveals that, to

TABLE 10–4 Causes of aortic stenosis.

Type	Pathology	Clinical Presentation
Congenital	The valve can be unicuspid, bicuspid, or tricuspid with partially fused leaflets. Abnormal flow can lead to fibrosis and calcification of the leaflets.	Patient usually develops symptoms before age 30 years.
Rheumatic	Tissue inflammation results in adhesion and fusing of the commissures. Fibrosis and calcification of the leaflet tips can occur because of continued turbulent flow.	Patient usually develops symptoms between ages 30 and 70 years. Often the valve will also be regurgitant. Accompanying mitral valve disease is frequently present.
Degenerative	Leaflets become inflexible because of calcium deposition at the bases. The leaflet tips remain relatively normal.	The most likely cause of aortic stenosis in patients older than 70 years. Particularly prevalent in patients with diabetes or hypercholesterolemia.

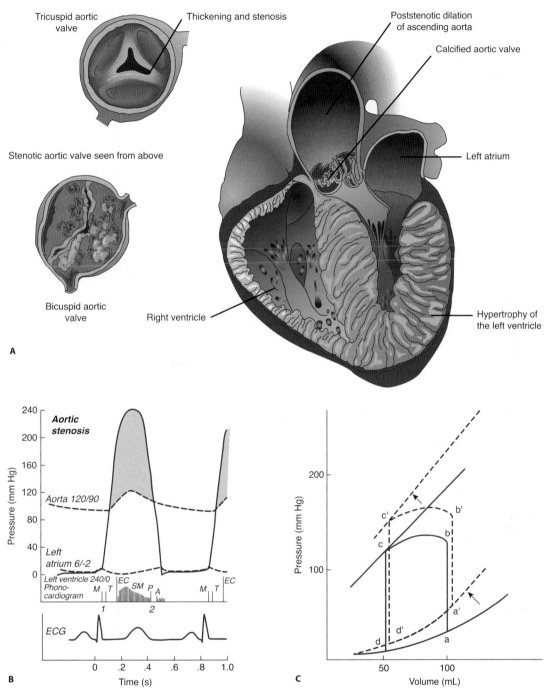

FIGURE 10–22 Aortic stenosis. **A:** Drawing of the left heart in left anterior oblique view showing anatomic features of aortic stenosis. Note structures enlarged: left ventricle (thickened); poststenotic dilation of the aorta. **B:** Drawing showing auscultatory and hemodynamic features of predominant aortic stenosis. Cardinal features include left ventricular hypertrophy; systolic ejection murmur. (EC, ejection click; SM, systolic murmur; P, pulmonary valve; A, aortic valve.)   (Redrawn, with permission, from Cheitlin MD, Sokolow M, McIlroy MB. *Clinical Cardiology,* 6th ed. Originally published by Appleton & Lange. Copyright © 1993 by the McGraw-Hill Companies, Inc.)   **C:** Pressure-volume loop in aortic stenosis. The left ventricle becomes thickened and less compliant, forcing the diastolic pressure-volume curve upward, which results in elevated left ventricular end-diastolic pressure (**a′**). Because the left ventricle must pump against a fixed gradient (increased afterload), **b** increases to **b′**. Finally, the hypertrophy of the ventricle results in increased inotropic force, which shifts the isovolumic pressure curve leftward.

maintain stroke volume and because of decreases in ventricular compliance, left ventricular end-diastolic pressure increases significantly (Figure 10–22c). The thick ventricle

leads to a prominent *a* wave on left atrial pressure tracings as the ventricle becomes more dependent on atrial contraction to fill the ventricle.

Clinical Manifestations

A. Symptoms

1. **Angina pectoris**—Angina can occur because of several mechanisms. First, approximately half of all patients with aortic stenosis have significant concomitant coronary artery disease. Even without significant coronary artery disease, the combination of increased oxygen demands because of ventricular hypertrophy and decreased supply as a result of excessive compression of the vessels can lead to relative ischemia of the myocytes. Finally, coronary artery obstruction from calcium emboli arising from a calcified stenotic aortic valve has been reported, although it is an uncommon cause of angina.

2. **Syncope**—Syncope in aortic stenosis is usually due to decreased cerebral perfusion from the fixed obstruction but may also occur because of transient atrial arrhythmias with loss of effective atrial contribution to ventricular filling. In addition, arrhythmias arising from ventricular tissues are more common in patients with aortic stenosis and can cause syncope.

3. **Congestive heart failure**—(See prior discussion of Heart Failure.) The progressive increase in left ventricular end-diastolic pressure can cause elevated pulmonary venous pressure and pulmonary edema.

B. Physical Examination—Because there is a fixed obstruction to flow, the carotid upstroke is decreased and late. Left ventricular hypertrophy causes the apical impulse to be displaced laterally and to become sustained. The increased dependence on atrial contraction is responsible for the prominent S_4. Flow through the restricted orifice gives rise to a midsystolic murmur. The murmur is usually heard best at the base of the heart but often radiates to the neck and apex. The murmur is usually crescendo-decrescendo, and in contrast to mitral regurgitation, the first and second heart sounds are usually easily heard. As aortic valve narrowing worsens, the murmur peaks later in systole. When calcified leaflets are present, the murmur tends to have a harsher quality. An aortic ejection sound, which is caused by the sudden checking of the leaflets as they open, is heard only when the leaflets remain fairly mobile, as in congenitally malformed valves.

Although obstruction of blood flow from the left ventricle is usually due to valvular disease, obstruction can also occur above or below the valve and can present in somewhat the same way as valvular aortic stenosis. A membranous shelf that partially obstructs flow just above the valve in the aorta can sometimes be present from birth. In this condition, the systolic murmur is usually heard best at the first intercostal space at the right sternal border. Subvalvular stenosis can occur in some patients who develop severe hypertrophy of the heart (Figure 10–23). This well-recognized clinical entity—hypertrophic cardiomyopathy—can also be manifested by a crescendo-decrescendo systolic murmur noted on physical examination. However, obstruction of the outflow tract in hypertrophic cardiomyopathy is dynamic, with greater obstruction when preload is decreased from decreased intraventricular volume. For this reason, having the patient stand or perform Valsalva's maneuver (expiratory effort against a closed glottis), both of which decrease venous return, causes the murmur to increase. Both of these maneuvers cause a decrease in the murmur due to valvular stenosis, because less absolute blood volume flows across the stenotic aortic valve.

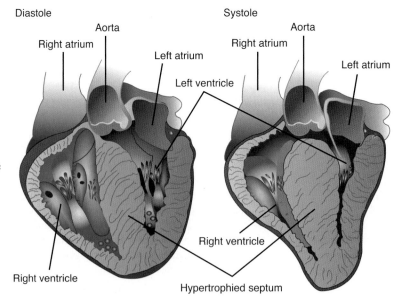

Cardinal features:
Left ventricular (especially septal) hypertrophy, diastolic dysfunction; systolic outflow obstruction, systolic anterior motion of mitral valve; excessive left ventricular emptying.

Variable factors:
Severity; level of peripheral resistance; low resistance and low blood volume lead to obstruction.

FIGURE 10–23 Hypertrophic cardiomyopathy (left lateral view). The cardinal features are displayed. (Redrawn, with permission, from Cheitlin MD, Sokolow M, McIlroy MB. *Clinical Cardiology*, 6th ed. Originally published by Appleton & Lange. Copyright © 1993 by the McGraw-Hill Companies, Inc.)

2. Aortic Regurgitation

Clinical Presentation

Aortic regurgitation can be either chronic or acute. In chronic aortic regurgitation, there is a long latent period during which the patient remains asymptomatic as the heart responds to the volume load. When the compensatory mechanisms fail, symptoms of left-sided failure become manifest. In acute aortic regurgitation, there are no compensatory mechanisms, so shortness of breath, pulmonary edema, and hypotension—often with cardiovascular collapse—occur suddenly.

Physical examination of patients with chronic aortic regurgitation reveals hyperdynamic (pounding) pulses. The apical impulse is hyperdynamic and displaced laterally. On auscultation, three murmurs may be heard: a high-pitched early diastolic murmur, a diastolic rumble called the Austin Flint murmur, and a systolic murmur. A third heart sound is often present. However, in acute aortic regurgitation, the peripheral signs are often absent, and in many cases the left ventricular impulse is normal. On auscultation, the diastolic murmur is much softer, and the Austin Flint murmur, if present, is short. The first heart sound will be soft and sometimes absent.

Etiology

Acute and chronic aortic regurgitation can be due to either valvular or aortic root abnormalities (Table 10–5).

Pathophysiology

Aortic regurgitation places a volume load on the left ventricle, because during diastole blood enters the ventricle both from the left atrium and from the aorta. If the regurgitation develops slowly, the heart responds to the increased diastolic pressure by fiber elongation and replication of sarcomeres in series, which leads to increased ventricular volumes. Because systolic pressure remains relatively unchanged, increased wall stress—by Laplace's law—can be compensated for by an additional increase in wall thickness. This response, "eccentric hypertrophy"—so named because the ventricular cavity enlarges laterally in the chest and becomes eccentric to its normal position—explains the different ventricular geometry observed in patients with aortic regurgitation versus those with aortic stenosis (concentric hypertrophy caused by the systolic pressure overload). Ultimately, chronic aortic regurgitation leads to huge ventricular volumes as demonstrated in the pressure-volume

TABLE 10–5 Causes of aortic regurgitation.

Site	Pathology	Causes	Time Course
Valvular	Cusp abnormalities	Endocarditis	Acute or chronic
		Rheumatic disease	Acute or chronic
		Ankylosing spondylitis	Usually chronic
		Congenital	Chronic
Aortic	Dilation	Aortic aneurysm	Acute or chronic
		Heritable disorders of connective tissue	Usually chronic
		Marfan's syndrome	
		Ehlers-Danlos syndrome	
		Osteogenesis imperfecta	
	Inflammation	Aortitis (Takayasu)	Usually chronic
		Syphilis	Usually chronic
		Arthritic diseases	Usually chronic
		Ankylosing spondylitis	
		Reiter's syndrome	
		Rheumatoid arthritis	
		Systemic lupus erythematosus	
		Cystic medial necrosis	Acute or chronic
	Tears with loss of commissural support	Trauma	Usually acute
		Dissection, often from hypertension	Usually acute

loops (Figure 10–24). The left ventricle operates as a low-compliance pump, handling large end-diastolic and stroke volumes, often with little increase in end-diastolic pressure. In addition, no truly isovolumic period of relaxation or contraction exists because of the persistent flow into the ventricle from the systemic circulation. Aortic pulse pressure is widened. Diastolic pressure decreases because of regurgitant flow back into the left ventricle and increased compliance of the large central vessels (in response to increased stroke volume); elevated stroke volume leads to increased systolic pressures (Figure 10–24C).

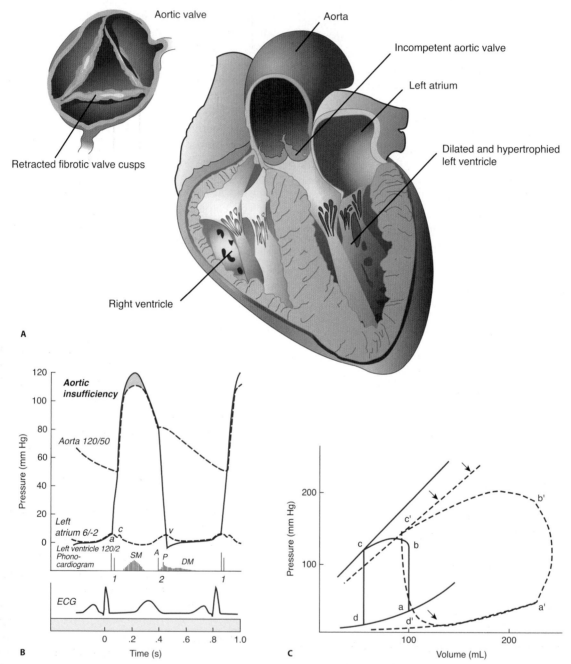

FIGURE 10–24 Aortic insufficiency (regurgitation). **A:** Drawing of the left heart in left anterior oblique view showing anatomic features of aortic insufficiency. Note structures enlarged: left ventricle, aorta. **B:** Drawing showing auscultatory and hemodynamic features of predominant aortic insufficiency. Cardinal features include large hypertrophied left ventricle; large aorta; increased stroke volume; wide pulse pressure; diastolic murmur. (SM, systolic murmur; A, aortic valve; P, pulmonary valve; DM, diastolic murmur.) (Redrawn, with permission, from Cheitlin MD, Sokolow M, McIlroy MB. *Clinical Cardiology*, 6th ed. Originally published by Appleton & Lange. Copyright © 1993 by the McGraw-Hill Companies, Inc.) **C:** Pressure-volume loop in chronic aortic insufficiency. Marked enlargement in left ventricular volume shifts the diastolic pressure-volume curve rightward. Hypertrophy of the ventricle shifts the isovolumic pressure-volume curve leftward (not shown), but ultimately the ventricle dilates and contractility decreases and the isovolemic pressure-volume curve shifts to the right. Stroke volume is enormous, although effective stroke volume may be minimally changed because much of the increase in stroke volume leaks back into the ventricle. Because the ventricle is constantly being filled from the mitral valve or the incompetent aortic valve, no isovolumic periods exist.

Clinical Manifestations

A. Shortness of Breath—Pulmonary edema can develop, particularly if the aortic regurgitation is acute and the ventricle does not have time to compensate for the sudden increase in volume. In chronic aortic regurgitation, compensatory mechanisms eventually fail and the heart begins to operate on the steeper portion of the diastolic pressure-volume relationship.

B. Physical Examination

1. **Hyperdynamic pulses**—In chronic aortic regurgitation, a widened pulse pressure is responsible for several characteristic peripheral signs. Palpation of the peripheral pulse reveals a sudden rise and then drop in pressure (water-hammer or Corrigan's pulse). Head bobbing (DeMusset's sign), rhythmic pulsation of the uvula (Müller's sign), and arterial pulsation seen in the nail bed (Quincke's pulse) have been described in patients with chronic aortic regurgitation.

2. **Murmurs**—Three heart murmurs can be heard in patients with aortic regurgitation: First, flow from the regurgitant volume back into the left ventricle can be heard as a high-pitched, blowing, early diastolic murmur usually perceived best along the left sternal border. Second, the rumbling murmur described by Austin Flint can be heard at the apex during any part of diastole. The Austin Flint murmur is thought to result from regurgitant flow from the aortic valve impinging on the anterior leaflet of the mitral valve, producing functional mitral stenosis. Finally, a crescendo-decrescendo systolic murmur, which is thought to arise from the increased stroke volume flowing across the aortic valve, can be heard at the left sternal border.

   In acute, severe aortic regurgitation, the early diastolic murmur may be softer because of rapid diastolic equalization of ventricular and aortic pressures. The first heart sound is soft because of early mitral valve closure from aortic regurgitation and elevated ventricular pressures.

3. **Third heart sound**—A third heart sound can be heard because of concomitant heart failure or because of the exaggerated early diastolic filling of the left ventricle.

4. **Apical impulse**—The apical impulse is displaced laterally because of the increased volume of the left ventricle.

3. Mitral Stenosis

Clinical Presentation

The symptoms of mitral stenosis include dyspnea, fatigue, and hemoptysis. Occasionally, the patient complains of palpitations or a rapid heartbeat. Finally, the patient with mitral stenosis may present with neurologic symptoms such as transient numbness or weakness of the extremities, sudden loss of vision, or difficulty with coordination.

The characteristic murmur of mitral stenosis is a late low-pitched diastolic rumble. In addition, an opening snap may be heard in the first portion of diastole (Figure 10–25). Auscultation of the lungs may reveal rales.

Etiology

Mitral stenosis is most commonly a sequela of rheumatic heart disease (Table 10–6). Infrequently, it may be caused by congenital lesions or calcium deposition. Atrial masses (myxomas) can cause intermittent obstruction of the mitral valve.

Pathophysiology

The mitral valve is normally bicuspid, with the anterior cusp approximately twice the area of the posterior cusp. The mitral valve area is usually 5–6 cm^2; clinically relevant mitral stenosis usually occurs when the valve area decreases to less than 1 cm^2. Because obstruction of flow protects the ventricle from pressure and volume loads, the left ventricular pressure-volume relationship shows relatively little abnormality other than decreased volumes. However, analysis of hemodynamic tracings shows the characteristic elevation in left atrial pressures (Figure 10–25B). For this reason, the main pathophysiologic abnormality in mitral stenosis is elevated pulmonary venous pressure and elevated right-sided pressures (pulmonary artery, right ventricle, and right atrium). Dilation and reduced systolic function of the right ventricle are commonly observed in patients with advanced mitral stenosis.

Clinical Manifestations

A. Symptoms

1. **Shortness of breath, hemoptysis, and orthopnea**—All of these symptoms occur because of elevated left atrial, pulmonary venous, and pulmonary capillary pressures (the actual mechanisms are described in the section on congestive heart failure).

2. **Palpitations**—Increased left atrial size predisposes patients with mitral stenosis to atrial arrhythmias. Chaotic atrial activity (ie, atrial fibrillation) is commonly observed. Because ventricular filling is particularly dependent on atrial contraction in patients with mitral stenosis, acute hemodynamic decompensation may occur when organized contraction of the atrium is lost.

3. **Neurologic symptoms**—Reduced outflow leads to dilation of the left atrium and stasis of blood flow. Thrombus in the left atrium is observed on echocardiography in approximately 20% of patients with mitral stenosis, and the prevalence increases with age, presence of atrial fibrillation, severity of stenosis, and any reduction in cardiac output. Embolic events that lead to neurologic symptoms occur in 8% of patients in sinus rhythm and in 32% of patients with chronic or paroxysmal atrial fibrillation. In addition, left atrial enlargement can sometimes impinge on the recurrent laryngeal nerve and lead to hoarseness (Ortner's syndrome).

B. Physical Examination—On auscultation of the heart, the diastolic rumble occurs because of turbulent flow across the narrowed mitral valve orifice. An opening snap, analogous to

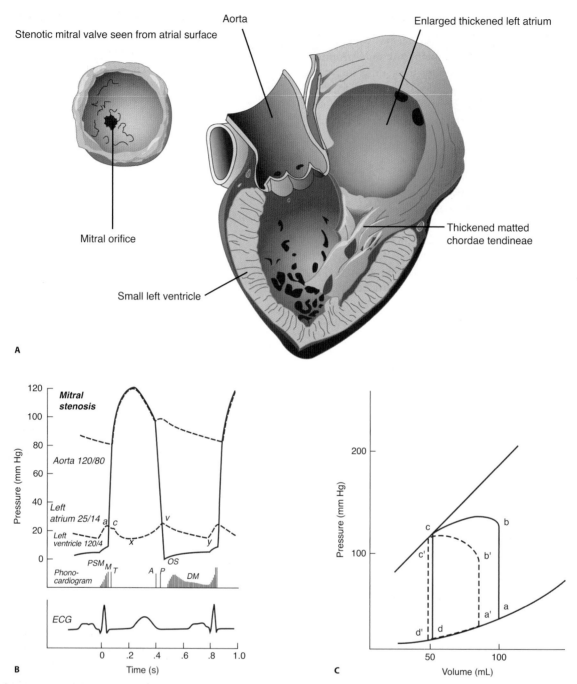

FIGURE 10–25 Mitral stenosis. **A:** Drawing of the left heart in left anterior oblique view showing anatomic features of mitral stenosis. Note enlarged left atrium, small left ventricle. **B:** Drawing showing auscultatory and hemodynamic features of mitral stenosis. Cardinal features include thickening and fusion of mitral valve cusps, elevated left atrial pressure, left atrial enlargement, opening snap, diastolic murmur. (PSM, presystolic murmur; OS, opening snap; M, mitral; T, tricuspid; A, aortic; P, pulmonary; DM, diastolic murmur.) (Redrawn, with permission, from Netter FH. *Heart* vol 5: CIBA Collection of Medical Illustrations, CIBA Pharmaceutical Co., 1969.) **C:** Pressure-volume loop in mitral stenosis. Filling of the left ventricle is restricted from **a** to **a'**, decreasing stroke volume to **b'c'**.

the ejection click described for aortic stenosis, may be heard in early diastole. The opening snap is heard only when the patient has relatively mobile leaflets.

Rales occur because elevated pulmonary capillary pressures lead to accumulation of intra-alveolar fluid.

4. Mitral Regurgitation

Clinical Presentation

The presentation of mitral regurgitation depends on how quickly valvular incompetence develops. Patients with chronic mitral regurgitation develop symptoms gradually over time. Common complaints include dyspnea, easy fatigability, and

TABLE 10–6 Causes of mitral stenosis.

Type	Comments
Rheumatic	Most common. Narrowing results from fusion and thickening of the commissures, cusps, and chordae tendineae. Symptoms usually develop 20 years after acute rheumatic fever.
Calcific	Usually causes mitral regurgitation but can cause mitral stenosis in some cases.
Congenital	Usually presents during infancy or childhood.
Collagen-vascular disease	Systemic lupus erythematosus and rheumatoid arthritis (rare).

TABLE 10–7 Causes of mitral regurgitation.

Type	Causes
Acute	
Ruptured chordae tendineae	Infective endocarditis
	Trauma
	Acute rheumatic fever
	"Spontaneous"
Ruptured or dysfunctional papillary muscles	Ischemia
	Myocardial infarction
	Trauma
	Myocardial abscess
Perforated leaflet	Infective endocarditis
	Trauma
Chronic	
Inflammatory	Rheumatic heart disease
	Collagen-vascular disease
Infection	Infective endocarditis
Degenerative	Myxomatous degeneration of the valve leaflets
	Calcification of the mitral annulus
Rupture or dysfunction of the chordae tendineae or papillary muscles	Infective endocarditis
	Trauma
	Acute rheumatic fever
	"Spontaneous"
	Ischemia
	Myocardial infarction
	Myocardial abscess
Congenital	
	Developmental anomalies

palpitations. Patients with acute mitral regurgitation present with symptoms of left heart failure: shortness of breath, orthopnea, and shock. Chest pain may be present in patients whose mitral regurgitation is due to coronary artery disease.

On physical examination, patients have a pansystolic regurgitant murmur that is heard best at the apex and often radiates to the axilla. This murmur often obscures the first and second heart sounds. When mitral valve incompetence is severe, a third heart sound is often present. In chronic mitral regurgitation, the apical impulse is often hyperdynamic and displaced laterally.

Etiology

In the past, rheumatic heart disease accounted for most cases of mitral regurgitation. Mitral valve prolapse is now probably the most common cause, followed by coronary artery disease. The tips of the anterior and posterior mitral valve leaflets are held in place during ventricular contraction by the anterolateral and posteromedial papillary muscles. The valves are connected to the papillary muscles via thin fibrous structures called chordae tendineae. In patients with mitral valve prolapse, extra tissue present on the valvular apparatus can undergo myxomatous degeneration by the fifth or sixth decade. Mitral regurgitation follows as a result of either poor coaptation of the valve leaflets or sudden rupture of the chordae tendineae. In coronary artery disease, obstruction of the circumflex coronary artery can lead to ischemia or rupture of the papillary muscles (Table 10–7).

Pathophysiology

When the mitral valve fails to close properly, regurgitation of blood into the left atrium from the ventricle occurs during systole. In chronic mitral regurgitation, the compensatory mechanism to this volume load is similar to the changes seen in aortic regurgitation. The left ventricle and atrium dilate, and to normalize wall stress in the ventricle there is also concomitant hypertrophy of the ventricular wall (see prior discussion of Laplace's law). Diastolic filling of the ventricle increases because it is now the sum of right ventricular output and the regurgitant volume from the previous beat. In acute mitral regurgitation, the sudden volume load on the atrium and ventricle is not compensated for by chamber enlargement and hypertrophy. The sudden

increase in atrial volume leads to prominent atrial v waves with transmission of this elevated pressure to the pulmonary capillaries and the development of pulmonary edema (Figure 10–26).

Clinical Manifestations

A. Symptoms

1. **Pulmonary edema**—Rapid elevation of pulmonary capillary pressure in acute mitral regurgitation leads to the sudden onset of pulmonary edema, manifested by shortness of breath, orthopnea, and paroxysmal nocturnal dyspnea. In chronic mitral regurgitation, the symptoms develop grad-

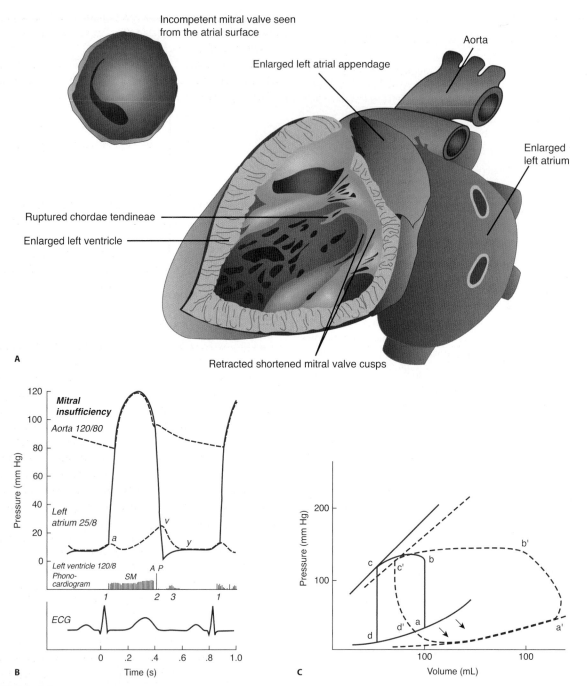

FIGURE 10–26 Mitral insufficiency (regurgitation). **A:** Drawing of the left heart in left lateral view showing anatomic features of mitral insufficiency. Note structures enlarged: left atrium, left ventricle. **B:** Drawing showing auscultatory and hemodynamic features of mitral insufficiency. Cardinal features include systolic backflow into left atrium, left atrial enlargement, left ventricular enlargement (hypertrophy in acute lesions), prominent *v* wave caused by filling from both the pulmonary veins and the regurgitant jet, holosystolic murmur. (3, third heart sound; SM, systolic murmur; A, aortic; P, pulmonary.) (Redrawn, with permission, from Cheitlin MD, Sokolow M, McIlroy MB. *Clinical Cardiology*, 6th ed. Originally published by Appleton & Lange. Copyright © 1993 by the McGraw-Hill Companies, Inc.) **C:** Pressure-volume loop in mitral insufficiency. Increased ventricular volumes shift the diastolic pressure-volume curve rightward. Stroke volume is increased because the ventricle can now eject blood into the low-pressure left atrium. With chronic volume loads, the isovolemic pressure-volume curve eventually shifts to the right.

ually, but at some point the compensatory mechanisms fail and pulmonary edema develops, particularly with exercise.

2. **Fatigue**—Fatigue can develop because of decreased forward blood flow to the peripheral tissues.

3. **Palpitations**—Left atrial enlargement may lead to the development of atrial fibrillation and accompanying palpitations. Patients with atrial fibrillation and mitral regurgitation have a 20% incidence of cardioembolic events.

B. Physical Examination

1. **Holosystolic murmur**—Regurgitant flow into the atrium produces a high-pitched murmur that is heard throughout systole. The murmur begins with the first heart sound, continues to the second heart sound, and is of constant intensity throughout systole. It finally ends when left ventricular pressure drops to equal left atrial pressure during isovolumic relaxation. Unlike with the murmur of aortic stenosis, there is little variation in the intensity of the murmur as the heart rate changes. In addition, the murmur does not change in intensity with respiration. It is usually heard best at the apex and often radiates to the axilla. If rupture of the anterior leaflet has occurred, the mitral regurgitation murmur will sometimes radiate to the back.

2. **Third heart sound**—A third heart sound is heard if heart failure is present. Because of increased and rapid filling of the ventricle during diastole, it may also be heard in the absence of overt failure in patients with severe mitral regurgitation.

3. **Displaced and hyperdynamic apical impulse**—The compensatory increase in left ventricular volume and wall thickness in patients with chronic mitral regurgitation is manifested by a laterally displaced apical impulse. Because the ventricle now has a low-pressure chamber (the left atrium) into which to eject blood, the apical impulse is often hyperdynamic. When mitral regurgitation develops suddenly, the apical impulse is not displaced or hyperdynamic, because the left ventricle has not had enough time for compensatory volume increases to occur.

CHECKPOINT

10. What are the clinical presentations of each of the four major categories of valvular heart disease?

11. What are the most common causes of each category of valvular heart disease?

12. What is the pathogenesis of each category of valvular heart disease?

13. What are the major clinical manifestations and complications of each category of valvular heart disease?

CORONARY ARTERY DISEASE

Clinical Presentation

Chest pain is the most common symptom associated with coronary artery disease. It is usually described as dull and can often radiate down the arm or to the jaw. It does not worsen with a deep breath and can be associated with shortness of breath, diaphoresis, nausea, and vomiting. This entire symptom complex has been termed **angina pectoris,** or "pain in the chest"; this phrase was first used by Heberden in 1744.

Clinically, angina is classified according to the precipitant and the duration of symptoms. If the pain occurs only with exertion and has been stable over a long period of time, it is termed **stable angina.** If the pain occurs at rest, it is termed **unstable angina.** Finally, regardless of the precipitant, if the chest pain persists without interruption for prolonged periods and irreversible myocyte damage has occurred, it is termed **myocardial infarction.**

On physical examination, the patient with coronary artery disease may have a fourth heart sound or signs of congestive heart failure and shock. However, more than any other cardiovascular problem, the initial diagnosis relies on patient history.

Etiology

Atherosclerotic obstruction of the large epicardial vessels is by far the most common cause of coronary artery disease. Spasm of the coronary arteries from various mediators such as serotonin and histamine has been well described and is more common in Japanese individuals. Rarely, congenital abnormalities can cause coronary artery diseases (Table 10–8).

Pathophysiology

Coronary blood flow brings oxygen to myocytes and removes waste products such as carbon dioxide, lactic acid, and hydrogen ions. The heart has a tremendously high metabolic requirement; although it accounts for only 0.3% of body weight, it is responsible for 7% of the body's resting oxygen consumption. Cellular ischemia occurs when there is either increased demand for oxygen relative to maximal arterial supply or an absolute reduction in oxygen supply. Although situations of increased demand such as thyrotoxicosis and aortic stenosis can cause myocardial ischemia, most clinical cases are due to decreased oxygen supply. Reduced oxygen supply can rarely arise from decreased oxygen content in blood—such as occurs in carbon monoxide poisoning or anemia—but more commonly stems from coronary artery abnormalities (Table 10–8), particularly atherosclerotic disease. Myocardial ischemia may arise from a combination of increased demand and decreased supply; cocaine abuse increases oxygen demand (by inhibiting

TABLE 10–8 Causes of coronary artery disease.

Type	Comments
Atherosclerosis	Most common cause. Risk factors include hypertension, hypercholesterolemia, diabetes mellitus, smoking, and a family history of atherosclerosis.
Spasm	Coronary artery vasospasm can occur in any population but is most prevalent in Japanese. Vasoconstriction appears to be mediated by histamine, serotonin, catecholamines, and endothelium-derived factors. Because spasm can occur at any time, the chest pain is often not exertion related.
Emboli	Rare cause of coronary artery disease. Can occur from vegetations in patients with endocarditis.
Congenital	Congenital coronary artery abnormalities are present in 1–2% of the population. However, only a small fraction of these abnormalities cause symptomatic ischemia.

reuptake of norepinephrine at adrenergic nerve endings in the heart) and can reduce oxygen supply by causing vasospasm.

Atherosclerosis of large coronary arteries remains the predominant cause of angina and myocardial infarction. Raised fatty streaks, which appear as yellow spots or streaks in the vessel walls, are seen in coronary arteries in almost all members of any population by 20 years of age (see Chapter 11). They are found mainly in areas exposed to increased shear stresses such as bending points and bifurcations and are thought to arise from isolated macrophage foam cell migration into areas of minimal chronic intimal injury. In many people this process progresses, with additional migration of foam cells, smooth muscle cell proliferation, and extracellular fat and collagen deposition (Figure 10–27). The extent and incidence of these advanced lesions vary among persons in different geographic regions and ethnic groups.

The underlying pathophysiologic processes differ for each clinical presentation of coronary artery disease. In patients with stable angina, fixed narrowing of one or several coronary arteries is usually present. Because the large coronary arteries usually function as conduits and do not offer resistance to flow, the arterial lumen must be decreased by 90% to produce cellular ischemia when the patient is at rest. However, with exercise, a 50% reduction in lumen size can lead to symptoms. In patients with unstable angina, fissuring of the atherosclerotic plaque can lead to platelet accumulation and transient episodes of thrombotic occlusion, usually lasting 10–20 minutes. In addition, platelet release of vasoconstrictive factors such as thromboxane A_2 or serotonin and endothelial dysfunction may cause vasoconstriction and contribute to decreased flow. In myocardial infarction, deep arterial injury from plaque rupture may cause formation of a relatively fixed and persistent thrombus. Recent research has emphasized that plaque composition mediated by inflammation has an important role in clinical presentation. Loss of the extracellular matrix and cellular necrosis due to the inflammatory response appear to be the key mediators for plaque rupture.

The heart receives its energy primarily from ATP generated by oxidative phosphorylation of free fatty acids, although glucose and other carbohydrates can be utilized. Within 60 seconds after coronary artery occlusion, myocardial oxygen tension in the affected cells falls essentially to zero. Cardiac stores of high-energy phosphates are rapidly depleted, and the cells shift rapidly to anaerobic metabolism with consequent lactic acid production. Dysfunction of myocardial relaxation and contraction occurs within seconds, even before depletion of high-energy phosphates occurs. The biochemical basis for this abnormality is not known. If perfusion is not restored within 40–60 minutes, an irreversible stage of injury characterized by diffuse mitochondrial swelling, damage to the cell membrane, and marked depletion of glycogen begins. The exact mechanism by which irreversible damage occurs is not clear, but severe ATP depletion, increased extracellular calcium concentrations, lactic acidosis, and free radicals have all been postulated as possible causes.

In experimental preparations, if ischemic myocardium is perfused within 5 minutes, systolic function returns promptly, whereas diastolic abnormalities may take up to 40 minutes to normalize. With prolonged episodes of ischemia—up to 1 hour—it may take up to 1 month to restore ventricular function. When the heart demonstrates this prolonged period of decreased function despite normal perfusion, the myocardium is said to be "stunned." The biochemical basis for stunning is poorly understood. If reperfusion occurs later or not at all, systolic function often will not return to the affected area.

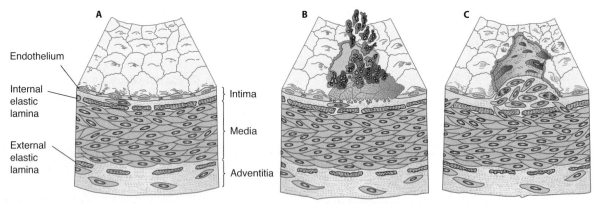

FIGURE 10–27 Mechanisms of production of atheroma. **A:** Structure of normal muscular artery. The adventitia, or outermost layer of the artery, consists principally of recognizable fibroblasts intermixed with smooth muscle cells loosely arranged between bundles of collagen and surrounded by proteoglycans. It is usually separated from the media by a discontinuous sheet of elastic tissue, the external elastic lamina. **B:** Platelet aggregates, or microthrombi, form as a result of adherence of the platelets to the exposed subendothelial connective tissue. Platelets that adhere to the connective tissue release granules whose constituents may gain entry into the arterial wall. Platelet factors thus interact with plasma constituents in the artery wall and may stimulate events shown in the next illustration. **C:** Smooth muscle cells migrate from the media into the intima through fenestrae in the internal elastic lamina and actively multiply within the intima. Endothelial cells regenerate in an attempt to re-cover the exposed intima, which thickens rapidly owing to smooth muscle proliferation and formation of new connective tissue. (Redrawn, with permission, from Ross R, Glomset JA. The pathogenesis of atherosclerosis. [Part 1.] N Engl J Med. 1976;295:369.)

Clinical Manifestations

A. Chest Pain

Chest pain has traditionally been ascribed to ischemia. However, more recent evidence suggests that, in patients with coronary artery disease, 70–80% of episodes of ischemia are actually asymptomatic. When present, the chest pain is thought to be mediated by sympathetic afferent fibers that richly innervate the atrium and ventricle. From the heart, the fibers traverse the upper thoracic sympathetic ganglia and the five upper thoracic dorsal roots of the spinal cord. In the spinal cord, the impulses probably converge with impulses from other structures. This convergence is probably the mechanism for the chest wall, back, and arm pain that sometimes accompanies angina pectoris. The importance of these fibers can be demonstrated in patients who have had a heart transplant. When these patients develop atherosclerosis, they remain completely asymptomatic, without development of angina.

Evidence suggests that the actual trigger for nerve stimulation is adenosine. Adenosine infusion into the coronary arteries can produce the characteristic symptoms of angina without evidence of ischemia. In addition, blocking the adenosine receptor (P_1) with aminophylline leads to reduced anginal symptoms despite similar degrees of ischemia.

Three factors probably account for the large proportion of asymptomatic episodes: dysfunction of afferent nerves, transient reduced perfusion, and differing pain thresholds among patients. Dysfunction of afferent nerves may cause silent ischemia. Patients with transplanted hearts do not sense cardiac pain despite significant atherosclerosis. Peripheral neuropathy in patients with diabetes may explain the increased episodes of silent ischemia described in this patient population. Transient reduced perfusion may also be an important mechanism for silent ischemia. Within a few seconds after cessation of perfusion, systolic and diastolic abnormalities can be observed. Angina is a relatively late event, occurring after at least 30 seconds of ischemia. Finally, differing pain thresholds between patients may explain the high prevalence of silent ischemia. The presence of angina is moderately correlated with a decreased pain tolerance. The mechanism for different pain thresholds is unknown but may be due to differences in plasma endorphins.

B. Fourth Heart Sound and Shortness of Breath

Both of these findings may occur because of diastolic and systolic dysfunction of the ischemic myocardium. (See prior discussion of congestive heart failure.)

C. Shock

The site of coronary artery occlusion determines the clinical presentation of myocardial ischemia or infarction. As a general rule, the more myocardium that is supplied by the occluded vessel, the more significant and severe are the symptoms. For example, obstruction of the left main coronary artery or the proximal left anterior descending coronary artery will usually present as severe cardiac failure, often with associated hypotension (shock). In addition, shock may be associated with coronary artery disease in several special situations. If necrosis of the septum occurs from left anterior descending artery occlusion, myocardial rupture with the formation of an interventricular septal defect can occur. Rupture of the anterior or lateral free walls from occlusion of the left anterior descending or circumflex coronary arteries, respectively, can lead to the formation of pericardial effusion and tamponade. Rupture of myocardial tissue usually occurs 4–7 days after the acute ischemic event, when the myocardial wall has thinned and is in the process of healing. Sudden hemodynamic decompensation during this period should arouse suspicion of these complications. Finally, circumflex artery occlusion may result in ischemia and dysfunction or overt rupture of the papillary muscles, which can produce severe mitral regurgitation and shock.

D. Bradycardia

Inferior wall myocardial infarctions usually arise from occlusion of the right coronary artery. Because the area of left ventricular tissue supplied by this artery is small, patients usually do not present with heart failure. However, the artery that provides blood supply to the AV node branches off the posterior descending artery, so that inferior wall myocardial infarctions are sometimes associated with slowed or absent conduction in the AV node. Besides ischemia, AV nodal conduction abnormalities can occur because of reflex activation of the vagus nerve, which richly innervates the AV node.

Dysfunction of the sinus node is rarely seen in coronary artery disease, because this area receives blood from both the right and the left coronary arteries.

E. Nausea and Vomiting

Nausea and vomiting may arise from activation of the vagus nerve in the setting of an inferior wall myocardial infarction.

F. Tachycardia

Levels of catecholamines are usually raised in patients with myocardial infarction. This helps to maintain stroke volume but leads to an increased heart rate.

CHECKPOINT

14. What is the clinical presentation of coronary artery disease along the continuum from stable angina to unstable angina to myocardial infarction?

15. What are the most common causes of coronary artery disease?

16. How do the pathophysiologies of stable angina, unstable angina, and myocardial infarction differ?

17. What are the major clinical manifestations and complications of coronary artery disease?

PERICARDIAL DISEASE

Pericardial disease may include inflammation of the pericardium (pericarditis) or abnormal amounts of fluid in the space between the visceral and parietal pericardium (pericardial effusion).

Pericarditis

Clinical Presentation

The patient presents with severe chest pain. Descriptions of the pain are variable, but the usual picture is of a sharp retrosternal onset with radiation to the back and worse with deep breathing or coughing. The pain is often position dependent: worse when lying flat and improved while sitting up and leaning forward.

On physical examination, the pericardial rub is pathognomonic of pericarditis. It is a high-pitched squeaking sound, often with two or more components.

Occasionally, continual inflammation of the pericardium leads to fibrosis and the development of constrictive pericarditis (Figure 10–28). Examination of the jugular venous pulsation is critical in the patient who may have constrictive pericarditis. The jugular venous pressure is elevated, and the individual waveforms are often quite prominent. In addition, there can be an inappropriate increase in the jugular venous pulsation level with inspiration (Kussmaul's sign). Hepatomegaly and ascites may be noted on physical examination. On auscultation of the heart, a high-pitched sound called a pericardial knock can be heard just after the second heart sound, often mimicking a third heart sound.

Etiology

Table 10–9 lists the causes of acute pericarditis. Viruses, particularly the coxsackieviruses, are the most common cause of acute pericarditis. Viruses are also probably responsible for "idiopathic" pericarditis.

Pathophysiology

In pericarditis, microscopic examination of pericardial specimens obtained at surgery (eg, stripping or window) or autopsy shows signs of acute inflammation, with increased numbers of polymorphonuclear leukocytes, increased vascularity, and deposition of fibrin. If the inflammation is of long duration, the pericardium can become fibrotic and scarred, with deposition of calcium.

The heavily fibrotic pericardium can inhibit the filling of the ventricles. At this point, signs of constrictive pericarditis appear (see following discussion).

Clinical Manifestations

A. Chest Pain—Chest pain is probably due to inflammation of the pericardium. Inflammation of adjacent pleura may account for the characteristic worsening of pain with deep breathing and coughing.

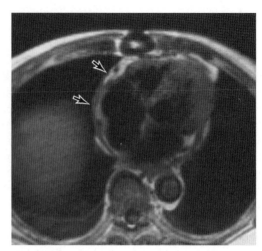

FIGURE 10–28 Magnetic resonance image of cross-section of thorax showing pericardial thickening (arrows) in a patient with constrictive pericarditis. (Courtesy of C Higgins. Reproduced, with permission, from Sokolow M, McIlroy MB. *Clinical Cardiology*, 6th ed. Originally published by Appleton & Lange. Copyright © 1993 by the McGraw-Hill Companies, Inc.)

TABLE 10–9 Causes of pericarditis.

Infections
Viral: coxsackievirus
Bacterial
Tuberculosis
Purulent: staphylococcal, pneumococcal
Protozoal: amebiasis
Mycotic: actinomycosis, coccidioidomycosis
Collagen-vascular disease
Systemic lupus erythematosus
Scleroderma
Rheumatoid arthritis
Neoplasm
Metabolic
Renal failure
Injury
Myocardial infarction
Postinfarction
Postthoracotomy
Trauma
Radiation
Idiopathic

B. Physical Examination

1. **Friction rub**—The pericardial friction rub is thought to arise from friction between the visceral and parietal pericardial surfaces. The rub is traditionally described as having three components, each associated with rapid movement of a cardiac chamber: The systolic component, which is probably related to ventricular contraction, is most common and most easily heard. During diastole, there are two components: one during early diastole, resulting from rapid filling of the ventricle, and another quieter component that occurs in late diastole, thought to be due to atrial contraction. The diastolic components often merge so that a two-component or "to-and-fro" rub is most commonly heard.

2. **Signs of constriction**—In the patient with constrictive pericarditis, early diastolic filling of the ventricle occurs normally, but the filling is suddenly stopped by the non-elastic thickened pericardium. This cessation of filling can be observed on the pressure-time curve of the ventricle and is probably responsible for the diastolic knock (Figure 10–29). In addition, the rapid emptying of the atrium leads to a prominent *y* descent that makes the *v* wave more noticeable on the atrial pressure tracing (Figure 10–30). Systemic venous pressure is elevated, because flow entering the heart is limited. Usually with inspiration, the decrease in intrathoracic pressure is transmitted to the heart, and filling of the right side of the heart increases with an accompanying fall in systemic venous pressure. In patients with constrictive pericarditis, this normal response is prevented and the patient develops Kussmaul's sign (Figure 10–31). Elevated systemic venous pressure can cause accumulation of fluid in the liver and intraperitoneal space, leading to hepatomegaly and ascites.

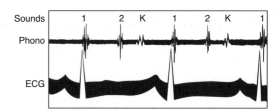

FIGURE 10–29 Phonocardiogram of typical sharp, early diastolic pericardial knock (K). (Courtesy Roche Laboratories Division of Hoffman-La Roche, Inc.)

PERICARDIAL EFFUSION & TAMPONADE

Clinical Presentation

Pericardial effusion may occur in response to any cause of pericarditis, so the patient may develop chest pain or pericardial rub as described previously. In addition, pericardial effusion may develop slowly and may be asymptomatic. However, sudden filling of the pericardial space with fluid can have catastrophic consequences by limiting ventricular filling (pericardial tamponade). Patients with pericardial tamponade often complain of shortness of breath, but the diagnosis is most commonly made by noting the characteristic physical examination findings associated with pericardial tamponade.

Pericardial tamponade is accompanied by characteristic physical signs that arise from the limited filling of the ventricle. The three classic signs of pericardial tamponade are called Beck's triad after the surgeon who described them in 1935: (1) hypotension, (2) elevated jugular venous pressure, and (3) muffled heart sounds. In addition, the patient may have a decrease in systemic pressure with inspiration (paradoxic pulse).

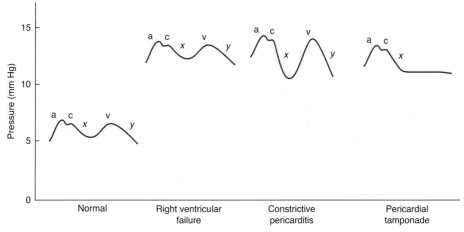

FIGURE 10–30 Jugular venous pressure waveforms in various kinds of heart disease. In right ventricular failure, mean jugular venous pressure is elevated, but the waveforms remain relatively unchanged. If right ventricular failure is accompanied by tricuspid regurgitation, the *v* wave may become more prominent (because the right atrium is receiving blood from both systemic venous return and the right ventricle). In constrictive pericarditis, the *y* descent becomes prominent because the right ventricle rapidly fills in early diastole. In contrast, in pericardial tamponade, the right ventricle only fills during early systole, so that only an *x* descent is observed. In both constrictive pericarditis and pericardial tamponade, mean jugular venous pressure is elevated.

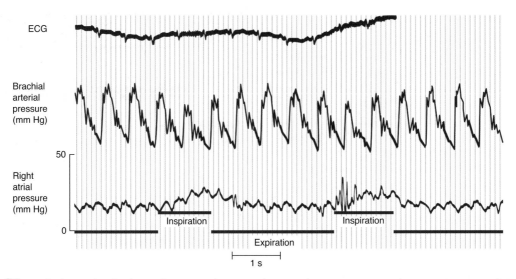

FIGURE 10–31 Brachial arterial and right atrial pressures showing pulsus paradoxus in a patient with constrictive pericarditis and an increase in right atrial pressure on inspiration (Kussmaul's sign). Both the systolic and diastolic atrial pressures rise with inspiration. (Redrawn, with permission, from Cheitlin MD, Sokolow M, McIlroy MB. *Clinical Cardiology*, 6th ed. Originally published by Appleton & Lange. Copyright © 1993 by the McGraw-Hill Companies, Inc.)

Etiology

Almost any cause of pericarditis can cause pericardial effusion.

Pathophysiology

The pericardium is normally filled with a small amount of fluid (30–50 mL) with an intrapericardial pressure that is usually about the same as the intrapleural pressure. With the sudden addition of fluid, the pericardial pressure can increase, at times to the level of the right atrial and right ventricular pressures. The transmural distending pressure of the ventricle decreases and the chamber collapses, preventing appropriate filling of the heart from systemic venous return. The four chambers of the heart occupy a relatively fixed volume in the pericardial sac, and evaluation of hemodynamics reveals equilibration of ventricular and pulmonary artery diastolic pressures with right atrial and left atrial pressures, all at approximately intrapericardial pressure.

Clinical Manifestations

Because the clinical manifestations of pericardial effusion without tamponade are similar to those of pericarditis, they are not described here. Instead, the pathophysiologic mechanisms for the symptoms and signs of pericardial tamponade are described.

A. Shortness of Breath—Dyspnea is the most common symptom of pericardial tamponade. The pathogenesis probably relates to a reduction in cardiac output and, in some patients, the presence of pulmonary edema.

B. Elevated Jugular Venous Pressure—Jugular venous pressure (Figure 10–30). In addition, cardiac tamponade alters the dynamics of atrial filling. Normally, atrial filling occurs first during ventricular ejection (*y* descent) and then later when the tricuspid valve opens (*x* descent). In cardiac tamponade, the atrium can fill during ventricular contraction so that the *x* descent can still be seen. However, when the tricuspid valve opens, further filling of the right atrium is prevented because chamber size is limited by the surrounding pericardial fluid. For this reason, the *y* descent is not seen in the patient with pericardial tamponade. Loss of the *y* descent in the setting of elevated jugular venous pressures should always arouse suspicion of pericardial tamponade.

C. Hypotension—Hypotension occurs because of reduced cardiac output.

D. Paradoxic Pulse—Arterial systolic blood pressure normally drops 10–12 mm Hg with inspiration. Marked inspiratory drop in systolic blood pressure (> 20 mm Hg) is an important physical finding in the diagnosis of cardiac tamponade but can also be seen in severe pulmonary disease and, less commonly, in constrictive pericarditis (Figure 10–31). Marked inspiratory decline in left ventricular stroke volume occurs because of decreased left ventricular end-diastolic volume. With inspiration, increased blood return augments filling of the right ventricle, which causes the interventricular septum to bow to the left and reduce left ventricular end-diastolic volume (reverse Bernheim effect). Also during inspiration, flow into the left atrium from the pulmonary veins is reduced, further reducing left ventricular preload.

E. Muffled Heart Sounds—Pericardial fluid can cause the heart sounds to become muffled or indistinct.

CHECKPOINT

18. What are the clinical presentations of each form of pericardial disease discussed previously?
19. What are the most common causes of pericarditis and pericardial effusion?
20. What are the major clinical manifestations and complications of pericarditis and pericardial effusion with tamponade?

CASE STUDIES

Eva M. Aagaard, MD, & Yeong Kwok, MD

(See Chapter 25, p. 691 for Answers)

CASE 48

A 59-year-old man is brought to the emergency department by ambulance after experiencing a syncopal episode. He states that he was running in the park when he suddenly lost consciousness. He denies any symptoms preceding the event, and he had no deficits or symptoms upon arousing. On review of systems, he does say that he has had substernal chest pressure associated with exercise for the last several weeks. Each episode was relieved with rest. He denies shortness of breath, dyspnea on exertion, orthopnea, and paroxysmal nocturnal dyspnea. His medical history is notable for multiple episodes of pharyngitis as a child. He is otherwise well. He has no significant family history. He was born in Mexico and moved to the United States at age 10 years. He does not smoke, drink alcohol, or use drugs. On examination, his blood pressure is 110/90 mm Hg, heart rate 95 beats/min, respiratory rate 15/min, and oxygen saturation 98%. Neck examination reveals both pulsus parvus and pulsus tardus. Cardiac examination reveals a laterally displaced and sustained apical impulse. He has a grade 3/6 midsystolic murmur, loudest at the base of the heart, radiating to the neck, and a grade 1/6 high-pitched, blowing, early diastolic murmur along the left sternal border. An S4 is audible. Lungs are clear to auscultation. Abdominal examination is benign. He has no lower extremity edema. Aortic stenosis is suspected.

Questions

A. What are the most common causes of aortic stenosis? Which is most likely in this patient? Why?
B. How does aortic stenosis cause syncope?
C. What is the pathophysiologic mechanism by which aortic stenosis causes angina pectoris?
D. How does aortic stenosis result in the physical findings described previously?
E. Based on the way this patient presented, what is his life expectancy if left untreated?

CASE 49

A 64-year-old man presents to the clinic with a 3-month history of worsening shortness of breath. He finds that he becomes short of breath after walking one block or one flight of stairs. He awakens at night, gasping for breath and has to prop himself up with pillows in order to sleep. On physical examination, his blood pressure is 190/60 and his pulses are hyperdynamic. His apical impulse is displaced to the left and downward. On physical examination, there are rales over both lower lung fields. On cardiac examination, there are three distinct murmurs: a high-pitched, early diastolic murmur loudest at the left lower sternal border, a diastolic rumble heard at the apex, and a crescendo-decrescendo systolic murmur heard at the left upper sternal border. Chest x-ray film shows cardiomegaly and pulmonary edema, and an echocardiogram shows severe aortic regurgitation with a dilated and hypertrophied left ventricle.

Questions

A. What accounts for the dilation and hypertrophy of the left ventricle in aortic regurgitation?
B. What is the pathophysiology of the wide pulse pressure (difference between the systolic and diastolic blood pressure) and the hyperdynamic pulses?
C. What explains the murmurs heard in this patient?
D. What are the underlying mechanisms responsible for the patient's shortness of breath with exertion and at night?

CASE 50

A 45-year-old man presents with a history of shortness of breath, irregular heart beat, and hemoptysis. He notes that over the past 2 weeks, he has become easily "winded" with minor activities. Also, he has coughed up some flecks of blood on a few occasions. He has noted a fast heartbeat and, on occasion, a pounding sensation in his chest. He gives a history of being ill for several weeks after a severe sore throat in childhood. On physical examination, his pulse rate is noted to be 120–130 beats/min and his rhythm, irregularly irregular. He has distended jugular venous pulses and rales at the bases of both lung fields. On cardiac examination, there is an irregular heart beat as well as a soft diastolic decrescendo murmur, loudest at the apex. An ECG shows atrial fibrillation as well as evidence of left atrial enlargement.

Questions

A. What is the likely diagnosis in this patient, and what are the elements in the history, physical examination, and ECG that support the diagnosis?
B. What is the main pathophysiologic mechanism in this condition, and how does it explain the irregular heart beat, shortness of breath, and hemoptysis?
C. What neurological complication can this patient develop?

CASE 51

A 59-year-old man presents to the emergency department with a 4-hour history of "crushing" chest pain. His cardiac examination is normal with no murmurs and normal heart sounds. An ECG reveals ST segment elevation in the lateral precordial leads and cardiac enzymes show evidence of myocardial injury. He undergoes emergent cardiac catheterization that shows a thrombus in the left circumflex artery. He undergoes successful angioplasty, and a stent is placed. He is monitored in the cardiac intensive care unit. He does well until the next day, when he develops sudden shortness of breath and decreasing oxygen saturations. Physical examination now reveals jugular venous distention, rales at both lung bases, and a blowing holosystolic murmur loudest at the apex, radiating into the axilla.

Questions

A. What likely accounts for this patient's sudden decompensation?
B. What is the main pathophysiologic derangement in this condition?
C. What changes in the heart take place if this condition develops slowly rather than suddenly?

CASE 52

A 55-year-old man presents to the clinic with complaints of chest pain. He states that for the last 5 months he has noted intermittent substernal chest pressure radiating to the left arm. The pain occurs primarily when exercising vigorously and is relieved with rest. He denies associated shortness of breath, nausea, vomiting, or diaphoresis. He has a medical history significant for hypertension and hyperlipidemia. He is taking atenolol for his high blood pressure and is eating a low-cholesterol diet. His family history is notable for a father who died of myocardial infarction at age 56 years. He has a 50-pack-year smoking history and is currently trying to quit. His physical examination is within normal limits with the exception of his blood pressure, which is 145/95 mm Hg, with a heart rate of 75 beats/min.

Questions

A. What is the likely diagnosis? How would you classify his diagnosis clinically?

B. What are the most common causes of this disease? Which is the most likely in this patient?

C. What are this patient's risk factors for coronary artery disease?

D. What is the hypothesized mechanism by which atherosclerotic plaques form?

E. What is the pathogenetic mechanism by which plaque formation results in the symptoms just mentioned?

CASE 53

A 35-year-old man presents to the emergency department with complaints of chest pain. The pain is described as 8 on a scale ranging from 1 to 10, retrosternal, and sharp in nature. It radiates to the back, is worse with taking a deep breath, and is improved by leaning forward. On review of systems, he has noted a "flu-like illness" over the last several days, including fever, rhinorrhea, and cough. He has no medical history and is taking no medications. He denies tobacco, alcohol, or drug use. On physical examination, he appears in moderate distress from pain, with a blood pressure of 125/85 mm Hg, heart rate 105 beats/min, respiratory rate 18/min, and oxygen saturation of 98% on room air. He is currently afebrile. His head and neck examination is notable for clear mucus in the nasal passages and a mildly erythematous oropharynx. The neck is supple, with shotty anterior cervical lymphadenopathy. The chest is clear to auscultation. Jugular veins are not distended. Cardiac examination is tachycardic with a three-component high-pitched squeaking sound. Abdominal and extremity examinations are normal.

Questions

A. What is the likely diagnosis?

B. What are the most common causes of this disease, and which is most likely in this patient?

C. What is the pathophysiologic mechanism for his chest pain?

D. What is the sound heard on cardiac examination? What is its cause?

E. What are two possible complications of this disease? What might you look for on physical examination to make certain that these complications are not present?

REFERENCES

General

Kusumoto FM. *Cardiovascular Pathophysiology.* Hayes Barton, 1999.

Arrhythmias

Antzelevitch C. Cellular basis and mechanism underlying normal and abnormal myocardial repolarization and arrhythmogenesis. Ann Med. 2004;36(Suppl 1):5–14. [PMID: 15176418]

Chou CC et al. New concepts in atrial fibrillation: mechanism and remodeling. Med Clin North Am. 2008 Jan;92(1):53–63. [PMID: 18060997]

Keating MT et al. Molecular and cellular mechanisms of cardiac arrhythmias. Cell. 2001 Feb 23;104(4):569–80. [PMID: 11239413]

McGuire MA. Paroxysmal supraventricular tachycardia: a century of progress. Heart Lung Circ. 2007 Jun;16(3): 222–8. [PMID: 17459770]

Ufberg JW et al. Bradydysrhythmias and atrioventricular conduction blocks. Emerg Med Clin North Am. 2006 Feb;24 (1):1–9. [PMID: 16308110]

Congestive Heart Failure

Aurigemma GP et al. Clinical Practice. Diastolic heart failure. N Engl J Med. 2004 Sep 9;351(11):1097–105. [PMID: 15356307]

Fukuta H et al. The cardiac cycle and a physiologic basis of left ventricular contraction, ejection, relaxation, and filling. Heart Fail Clin. 2008 Jan;4(1):1–11. [PMID: 18313620]

Haddad et al. Right ventricular function in cardiovascular disease, part II: Pathophysiology, clinical importance, and management of right ventricular failure. Circulation. 2008 Apr 1;117(13):1717–31. [PMID: 18378625]

Izzo JL et al. Mechanisms and management of hypertensive heart disease: From left ventricular hypertrophy to heart failure. Med Clin North Am. 2004 Sep;88(5):1257–71. [PMID: 15331316]

Kenchaiah S et al. Risk factors for heart failure. Med Clin North Am. 2004 Sep;88(5):1145–72. [PMID: 15331311]

Ouzounian M et al. Diastolic heart failure: Mechanisms and controversies. Nat Clin Pract Cardiovasc Med. 2008 Jul;5(7):375–86. [PMID: 18542106]

Young JB. Management of chronic heart failure: What do recent clinical trials teach us? Rev Cardiovasc Med. 2004;5(Suppl 1):S3–9. [PMID: 15184834]

Valvular Heart Disease

Aronow WS. Aortic stenosis. Compr Ther. 2007 Winter;33(4):174–83. [PMID: 18025609]

Boudoulas et al. Mitral valvular regurgitation: Etiology, pathophysiologic mechanisms, clinical manifestations. Herz. 2006 Feb;31(1):6–13. [PMID: 16502267]

Carabello BA. Aortic stenosis: from pressure overload to heart failure. Heart Fail Clin. 2006 Oct;2(4):435–42. [PMID: 17448430]

Carabello BA. The current therapy for mitral regurgitation. J Am Coll Cardiol. 2008 Jul 29;52(5):319–26. [PMID: 18652937]

Enriquez-Sarano M et al. Clinical practice. Aortic regurgitation. N Engl J Med. 2004 Oct 7;351(15):1539–46. [PMID: 15470217]

Ho SY. Anatomy of the mitral valve. Heart. 2002 Nov;88 (Suppl 4):iv5–10. [PMID: 12369589]

Rajamannan NM et al. Calcific aortic stenosis: an update. Nat Clin Pract Cardiovasc Med. 2007 May;4(5):254–62. [PMID: 17457349]

Coronary Artery Disease

Hansson GK. Inflammation, atherosclerosis, and coronary artery disease. N Engl J Med. 2005 Apr 21;352(16):1685–95. [PMID: 15843671]

Klein L et al. Coronary artery disease and prevention of heart failure. Med Clin North Am. 2004 Sep;88(5):1209–35. [PMID: 15331314]

Libby P. Atherosclerosis: Disease biology affecting the coronary vasculature. Am J Cardiol. 2006 Dec 18;98(12A):3Q–9Q. [PMID: 17169627]

Saigo M et al. Role of thrombotic and fibrinolytic factors in acute coronary syndromes. Prog Cardiovasc Dis. 2004 May–Jun;46(6):524–38. [PMID: 15224258]

Shah PK. Molecular mechanisms of plaque instability. Curr Opin Lipidol. 2007 Oct;18(5):492–9. [PMID: 17885418]

Pericardial Disease

Hoit BD. Pericardial disease and pericardial tamponade. Crit Care Med. 2007 Aug;35(8 Suppl):S355–64. [PMID: 17667460]

Shabetai R. Pericardial effusion: Haemodynamic spectrum. Heart. 2004 Mar;90(3):255–6. [PMID: 14966038]

...ascular Disorders: ...r Disease

...ID*

...normal structure and function of the ...he cardiovascular system and then ...ology of three common conditions

frequently seen by practicing physicians: atherosclerosis, hypertension, and shock.

...CULAR STRUCTURE & FUNCTION

...TOLOGY

...osed system of conduits that carry ...e tissues and back to the heart. All of ...e lungs, but the systemic circulation ...nt circuits in parallel (Figure 11–1). ...n in regional systemic blood flow ... systemic flow.

...e various types of blood vessels in ...in Figure 11–2. Note that as the ...creases, their number in the body ...ross-sectional area increases.

... lined by a single layer of endothe-...he endothelial cells constitute a ...cretes substances that affect the ...d provide for their growth, their ... the formation of new vessels that ...ues.

..., and the arterioles are made up of ...e tissue, the **adventitia;** a middle ... **media;** and an inner layer, the **intima,** containing the layer of endothelial cells and some sub-

endothelial connective tissue. The walls of the aorta and the large arteries contain abundant elastic tissue, much of it concentrated in the **internal elastic lamina,** a prominent band between the intima and the media, and another band, the **external elastic lamina,** between the media and the adventitia (Figure 11–3). The vessels are stretched by the force of cardiac ejection during systole, and the elastic tissue permits them to recoil during diastole. This maintains diastolic pressure and aids the forward motion of the blood. The walls of the arterioles contain less elastic tissue than the arteries but proportionately more smooth muscle (Figure 11–2). The muscle is extensively innervated by noradrenergic nerve fibers, which are constrictor in function. In some instances, there is a cholinergic innervation, which is vasodilator in function. The arteries and the arterioles offer considerable resistance to the flow of blood and are known as the **resistance vessels.**

Capillaries

The terminal portions of the arterioles, sometimes called metarterioles, drain into the **capillaries.** On the upstream side, the openings of the capillaries are surrounded by smooth muscle **precapillary sphincters.** There is debate about whether the metarterioles and sphincters are innervated. The capillaries themselves are made up of a single layer of endothelial cells. Outside these cells there are occasional pericytes, fibrous cells whose function is unknown (Figure 11–4). The capillaries anastomose extensively, and although each capillary is only 5–

---

*Adapted, with permission, from Ganong F. Cardiovascular Disease, Chapter 11 in McPhee SJ, Ganong WF. *Pathophysiology of Disease: An Introduction to Clinical Medicine,* 5th edition. New York, NY: McGraw-Hill; 2006.

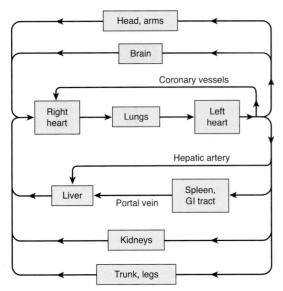

FIGURE 11–1   Diagram of the circulation in the adult.   (Redrawn, with permission, from Ganong WF. *Review of Medical Physiology*, 22nd ed. McGraw-Hill, 2005.)

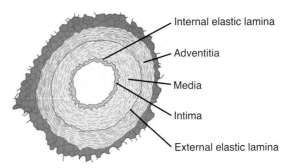

FIGURE 11–3   Cross section of a small artery.   (Redrawn, with permission, from Ganong WF. *Review of Medical Physiology*, 22nd ed. McGraw-Hill, 2005.)

9 μm in diameter, there are so many of them that the total cross-sectional area of all the capillaries is about 4500 cm².

Some substances cross capillary walls by vesicular transport, a process that involves endocytosis of plasma, movement of the vesicles formed in this way across the endothelial cell cytoplasm, and exocytosis on the tissue side. However, relatively little material is moved in this fashion, and most fluid and solute exchange occurs at the junctions between endothelial cells. In the liver, there are large gaps between endothelial cells (Chapter 14). In endocrine tissues, the small intestine, and the kidneys, tissues in which there is bulk flow of material across capillary walls, the cytoplasm of the endothelial cells is attenuated to form gaps called fenestrations. These gaps appear to be closed by a discontinuous membrane, which permits the passage of substances up to approximately 600 nm in diameter. In skeletal muscle, cardiac muscle, and many other tissues, there are no fenestrations, but the junctions between endothelial cells permit the passage of substances up to 10 nm in diameter. Finally, in brain capillaries, there are tight junctions between the endothelial cells. These

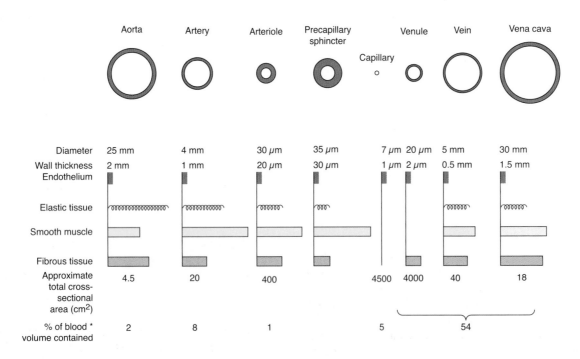

* In systemic vessels. There is an additional 12% in the heart and 18% in the pulmonary circulation.

FIGURE 11–2   Characteristics of systemic blood vessels. Cross sections of the vessels are not drawn to scale because of the huge range in size from aorta and vena cava to capillaries.   (Redrawn from Burton AC. Relation of structure to function of the tissues of the wall of blood vessels. Physiol Rev. 1954;34:619.)

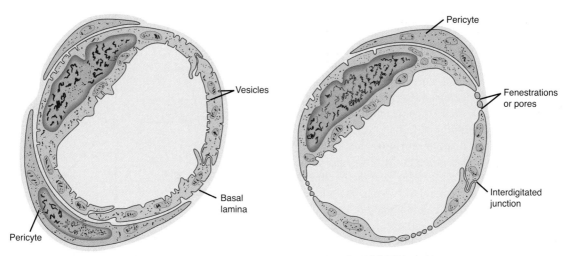

FIGURE 11–4 Cross sections of capillaries. Left: Continuous type of capillary found in skeletal muscle. Right: Fenestrated type of capillary. (Redrawn, with permission, from Orbison JL, Smith D eds: *Peripheral Blood Vessels,* Baltimore, Williams & Wilkins, 1962.)

tight junctions permit very little passive transport and are a key component of the blood-brain barrier. Water and CO_2 enter the brain with ease, but movement of most other substances in and out of brain tissue is mainly via transport proteins in the endothelial cells.

Venules & Veins

The venules are very similar to capillaries; they are about 20 µm in diameter, and their approximate total cross-sectional area is 4000 cm². They drain into veins that have modest amounts of smooth muscle and elastic tissue in their relatively thin walls and average 5 mm in diameter. The veins drain into the superior and inferior vena cavae, which in turn drain into the right atrium of the heart. The walls of the veins, unlike those of the arteries and arterioles, are easily distended and can expand to hold more blood without much increase in intravascular pressure. Therefore, they are known as **capacitance vessels.** They are innervated, and their smooth muscle can contract in response to noradrenergic stimulation, pushing blood into the heart and the arterial side of the circulation. The intima of the limb veins is folded at intervals to form the venous valves that prevent retrograde flow.

Lymphatics

The smallest lymphatic vessels are made up of endothelial tubes. Fluid appears to enter them through loose junctions between the endothelial cells. They drain into larger endothelial tubes that have valves and contractile walls containing smooth muscle, so that the fluid they contain moves centrally. The central lymphatics drain into the right and left subclavian veins. Thus, the lymphatic system drains excess fluid in the tissues back into the vascular system.

CHECKPOINT

1. How does the composition of the wall of an arteriole differ from that of an artery?
2. What are the modes of transport across the capillary wall? In what organ is transport greatest?
3. Why are veins termed capacitance vessels?

PHYSIOLOGY

Biophysical Considerations

In any system made up of a pump and a closed system of pipes such as the heart and the blood vessels, the flow of fluid between the two ends of the system depends on the pressure difference generated by the pump and the resistance to flow in the pipes:

$$Q = \frac{\Delta P}{R}$$

In the cardiovascular system, this translates into:

$$CO = \frac{MAP - Pra}{R}$$

where CO is cardiac output, MAP is mean arterial pressure, and Pra is the pressure in the right atrium. Since Pra is normally close to 0 mm Hg, this expression has the following corollary:

$$MAP = CO \times R$$

Thus, mean arterial pressure increases when there is an increase in cardiac output or when the diameter of the blood vessels (principally the arterioles) is decreased.

Flow in blood vessels is laminar (ie, an infinitely thin layer of blood next to the vessel wall does not move, the next layer moves slowly, and the next layer moves more rapidly, with the fastest flow in the center). Usually the flow is smooth, and no sound is generated. However, if flow is accelerated, it becomes turbulent when a **critical velocity** is reached. Constriction of a blood vessel or a heart valve causes faster flow in the constricted region because the kinetic energy of flow is increased and the potential energy is decreased (**Bernoulli's principle**). Therefore, critical velocity is more often reached. The turbulence causes noise. The examining physician hears this noise through the stethoscope as a **bruit** or **murmur.** The two terms are often used interchangeably, although the term "murmur" is more commonly applied to noise heard over the heart and the term "bruit" to noise heard over blood vessels. The sounds of Korotkoff heard over an artery below a blood pressure cuff (discussed later) are an example.

The main factors that determine flow in a blood vessel are the pressure difference between its two ends, the radius of the vessel, and the viscosity of the blood. The relation can be expressed mathematically by the **Poiseuille-Hagen formula:**

$$F = (P_A - P_B) \times \left(\frac{\pi}{8}\right) \times \left(\frac{1}{\eta}\right) \times \left(\frac{r^4}{L}\right)$$

where
  F = flow
  $P_A - P_B$ = pressure difference between the two ends of the tube
  η = viscosity
  r = radius of tube
  L = length of tube

Because flow is equal to pressure difference divided by resistance (R),

$$R = \frac{8\eta L}{\pi r^4}$$

Note that flow varies directly and pressure inversely with the fourth power of the radius of the vessel. This is why small changes in the diameter of the arterioles, the principal resistance vessels, cause large changes in pressure. For example, when the radius of a vessel is doubled, resistance is decreased to 6% of its previous value. Conversely, a small decrease in arterial diameter produces a relatively marked increase in blood pressure. Viscosity also has an effect, but, except at very high or very low values, the effect is small. Viscosity is high in polycythemia and low in anemia.

The relation between distending pressure and wall tension is shown in Figure 11–5. This relation is called the **law of Laplace.** It states that the wall tension (T) in a hollow viscus is equal to the product of the **transmural pressure** (P) and the radius * divided by the thickness of the wall (w):

$$T = \frac{Pr}{W}$$

In thin-walled structures, wall thickness is negligible, but in structures such as arteries it becomes a significant factor. The transmural pressure is the pressure inside the viscus minus the pressure outside the viscus, but in the body the latter is negligible. Therefore, in a distensible hollow viscus, transmural pressure at equilibrium is equal to wall tension

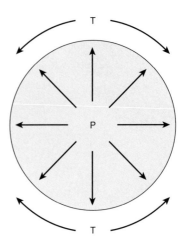

FIGURE 11–5 Law of Laplace. In a hollow object (eg, viscus, blood vessel), the distending pressure (P) equals the wall tension (T). (Redrawn, with permission, from Ganong WF. *Review of Medical Physiology,* 22nd ed. McGraw-Hill, 2005.)

divided by the two principal radii of curvature of the object $(r_1$ and $r_2)$:

$$P = T\left(\frac{1}{r_1} + \frac{1}{r_2}\right)$$

The operation of this law in the lungs is discussed in Chapter 9. In a cylinder such as a blood vessel, one radius is infinite, so

$$P = \frac{T}{r}$$

Thus, the smaller the radius of a vessel, the lower the wall tension that is necessary to balance the distending pressure. For example, the wall tension in the aorta is about 170,000 dynes/cm, whereas in capillaries it is about 16 dynes/cm. This is why the thin-walled, delicate capillaries do not collapse. The law of Laplace also applies to the heart. When the heart is dilated, it must develop more wall tension to function. Consequently, its work is increased.

With these principles and Figure 11–2 in mind, plus the fact that the major sites of vascular resistance are the arterioles, it is possible to understand the pressures in the various parts of the vascular system (Figure 11–6) and the velocity of flow in them. Systolic and diastolic pressures in the aorta and large arteries are stable, and there is a large pulse pressure. Normal pressure is about 120/80 mm Hg in healthy young adults. In the arterioles there is a sharp drop, so that pressure at the entrances to the capillaries is about 37 mm Hg and pulse pressure has disappeared. At the ends of the capillaries, it is about 17 mm Hg and falls steadily in the venous system to about 5 mm Hg at the entrance of the vena cavae into the right atrium. Velocity falls in the arterioles, is low in the capillaries because of the large total cross-sectional area, and increases again in the large veins.

The pressures mentioned previously are, of course, those recorded with patients in the supine position.

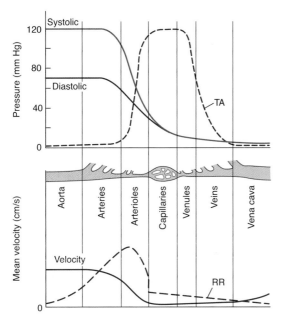

FIGURE 11–6 Diagram of the changes in pressure and velocity as blood flows through the systemic circulation. (TA, total cross-sectional area of the vessels, which increases from 4.5 cm^2 in the aorta to 4500 cm^2 in the capillaries [Figure 11–2]; RR, relative resistance, which is highest in the arterioles.) (Redrawn, with permission, from Ganong WF. *Review of Medical Physiology*, 22nd ed. McGraw-Hill, 2005.)

Because of the weight of the blood, there is a pressure increase in the standing position in both arteries and veins of 0.77 mm Hg for each centimeter below the heart it is measured and a corresponding decrease of 0.77 mm Hg for each centimeter above the heart. Thus, when the mean arterial pressure at the level of the heart is 100 mm Hg, the mean arterial pressure in a large artery in the foot of a standing averaged-sized adult is about 180 mm Hg; and in the head, it is about 62 mm Hg.

Measurement of Arterial Pressure

Arterial pressure can be measured directly by inserting a needle into an artery. Alternatively, it can be measured by the auscultatory method. The familiar inflatable cuff attached to a manometer is placed around the upper arm at the level of the heart and a stethoscope is placed over the brachial artery below the cuff. The cuff is inflated to well above the suspected systolic pressure and then deflated slowly. At the systolic pressure, a faint tapping sound is heard as blood first begins to pass beyond the cuff. With further lowering of the pressure, the sound becomes louder and then dull and muffled before finally disappearing. These are the **sounds of Korotkoff,** which are produced by turbulent flow in the brachial artery. The change from staccato to muffled sound occurs when blood first passes under the cuff continuously, even though the artery is still partially constricted. Continuous flow has a different auditory quality than interrupted flow. Finally, at the diastolic pressure, the sound disappears. Although diastolic pressure measured

directly with a catheter in the brachial artery correlates best with disappearance of sound in normal adults, in children and after exercise it correlates better with the change to a muffled sound.

Normal Arterial Pressure

Normal blood pressure in the brachial artery at heart level in healthy young adults is about 120/80 mm Hg. It is affected by many factors, including emotion and anxiety, and in some individuals blood pressure is higher when taken by a physician in the clinic than it is during normal activities at home ("**white-coat hypertension**"). Systolic and diastolic pressures normally fall by as much as 20 mm Hg during sleep. Therefore, normal subjects are called "dippers." In individuals with hypertension, the fall during sleep is reduced or absent (ie, hypertensives are "nondippers").

There is general agreement that blood pressure rises with advancing age, but there has been uncertainty about the magnitude of this rise because hypertension is a common disease whose incidence increases with advancing age. However, individuals who have systolic blood pressures < 120 mm Hg at age 50–60 years and never develop clinical hypertension still have systolic pressures that rise throughout life (Figure 11–7). This rise may be the closest approximation to the rise in normal individuals. Individuals with mild hypertension that is untreated show a significantly more rapid rise in systolic pressure. In both groups, diastolic pressure also rises but then starts to fall in middle age as the stiffness of arteries increases. Consequently, pulse pressure rises with advancing age.

It is interesting that systolic and diastolic blood pressures are lower in young women than in young men until the age of 55–65 years, after which they become comparable. Because there is a positive correlation between blood pressure and the incidence of heart attacks and strokes (discussed later), the lower blood pressure before menopause in women may be one reason why, on average, women live longer than men.

Capillary Circulation

In the capillaries, the velocity of blood flow is decreased because, although single-vessel diameter is small, there is a large total cross-sectional area. It is in the capillary bed that nutrients leave and wastes enter the circulation. The forces producing movement of solute and solvent across capillary walls are called **Starling forces** after the physiologist who first described them and analyzed their function. They are the hydrostatic pressure difference across the capillary wall (capillary pressure minus tissue pressure) and the osmotic pressure gradient across the capillary wall (capillary oncotic pressure minus tissue oncotic pressure). The hydrostatic pressure gradient is outward because tissue pressure is low, and the oncotic pressure gradient is inward because large molecules in the blood do not cross the capillary wall. Obviously, most of the net movement of substances out of a typi-

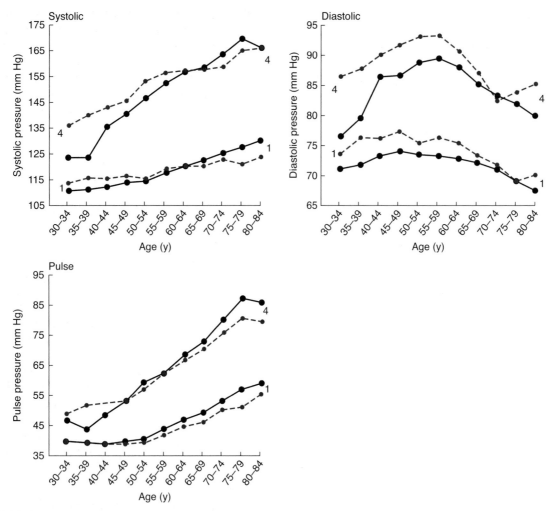

FIGURE 11–7 Effects of age and sex on systolic, diastolic, and pulse pressure in humans. Data are from a large group of individuals who were studied every 2 years throughout their adult lives. Group 1: individuals who had systolic blood pressures < 120 mm Hg at age 50–60. Group 4: Individuals who had systolic blood pressure ≥ 160 mm Hg at age 50–60 and had not received treatment for hypertension (ie, individuals with mild, untreated hypertension). Values for females are shown in the solid black lines and those for males are shown in the dashed red lines.   (Redrawn, with permission, from Franklin SS et al. Hemodynamic patterns of age-related changes in blood pressure: The Framingham Heart Study. Circulation. 1997;96:308.)

cal capillary occurs at its arteriolar end, where the net pressure gradient is outward primarily because hydrostatic pressure in the capillary (about 37 mm Hg, see Figure 11–8) is greater than the oncotic pressure. As the capillary resistance and the filtration progressively cause a decrease in the hydrostatic pressure along the length of the vessel, the inwardly directed oncotic pressure gradient becomes greater than the hydrostatic pressure gradient so that, at the venular end, fluid is reabsorbed. Thus, net flow is out of the capillary at the arteriolar end and into the capillary at the venular end. Any excess solute and solvent in the tissues is picked up by the lymph vessels and moved to the venous circulation by the main lymphatic ducts. Flow in the small lymphatics is passive, but in the larger lymphatic ducts there are valves and the walls contract.

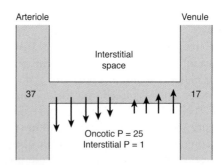

FIGURE 11–8 Schematic representation of pressure (P) gradients across the wall of a muscle capillary. The numbers at the arteriolar and venular ends of the capillary are the hydrostatic pressures in millimeters of mercury at these locations. The arrows indicate the approximate magnitude and direction of fluid movement. In this example, the pressure differential at the arteriolar end of the capillary is 11 mm Hg ([37 – 1] – 25) outward; at the opposite end, it is 9 mm Hg (25 – [17 – 1]) inward. (Redrawn, with permission, from Ganong WF. *Review of Medical Physiology*, 22nd ed. McGraw-Hill, 2005.)

REGULATION OF THE CARDIOVASCULAR SYSTEM

Given the vital nature of the cardiovascular system in maintaining blood flow to vital organs and adjusting flow so that it is increased in active tissues and decreased in inactive tissues, it is not surprising that multiple cardiovascular regulatory mechanisms have evolved. Cardiovascular adjustments are effected by altering the output of the pump (the heart), changing the diameter of the resistance vessels (chiefly the arterioles), and altering the amount of blood pooled in the capacitance vessels (the veins).

Regulation of cardiac output is discussed in Chapter 10. The caliber of the arterioles is regulated by vasodilator metabolites produced in metabolically active tissues, by the process of autoregulation, by a variety of vasoregulatory substances produced by endothelial cells, by circulating vasoactive hormones, and by a system of vasomotor nerves to the blood vessels and the heart. Discharge in the vasomotor nerves is regulated in feedback fashion by carotid sinus and aortic arch baroreceptors that monitor pressure in the arteries (high-pressure baroreceptor system) and baroreceptors in the cardiac atria and great veins (low-pressure baroreceptor system).

Vasodilator Metabolites

Various metabolic changes occurring in active tissues produce substances that dilate vessels supplying the tissues. This helps ensure the increased blood flow necessary to support the increased tissue activity. One important vasodilator is CO_2. Another is K^+, and adenosine dilates blood vessels in some tissues. In addition, the rise in temperature and the fall in pH that occur in some metabolically active tissues have a vasodilator effect.

Autoregulation

Many tissues have the ability to maintain a relatively constant blood flow during changes in perfusion pressure; this process is called **autoregulation.** The physiologic basis of autoregulation is unsettled. One factor is the myogenic response to stretch of the smooth muscle in arterioles; as pressure inside a vessel rises, its smooth muscle is stretched, and its response is to contract. Smooth muscle contracts in the absence of extrinsic innervation. Another factor may be accumulation of vasodilator metabolites; when flow to a tissue is reduced, the metabolites are not washed away, and they accumulate even in the absence of increased activity.

Substances Secreted by the Endothelium

The blood vessels are lined by a continuous layer of endothelial cells, and these cells play a vital role in the regulation of vascular function. They respond to flow changes (shear stress), stretch, a variety of circulating substances, and inflammatory mediators. In response to these stimuli, they secrete growth regulators and vasoactive substances. The growth factors regulate vascular development and are important in a number of diseases. The vasoactive substances produced by the endothelium generally act in a paracrine fashion to regulate local vascular tone. They include prostaglandins such as prostacyclin and also thromboxanes, nitric oxide, and endothelins.

A. Prostaglandins and Thromboxanes

Prostacyclin is produced by endothelial cells and thromboxane A_2 by platelets from their common precursor, arachidonic acid. Thromboxane A_2 produces platelet aggregation and vasoconstriction, whereas prostacyclin promotes vasodilation. The balance between the two is one of the mechanisms favoring local vasoconstriction and clot formation at sites of vascular injury while keeping the clot from extending, thereby maintaining normal flow in neighboring uninjured areas. The balance between platelet thromboxane A_2 and endothelial prostacyclin can be shifted by administration of low doses of aspirin. Thromboxane A_2 and prostacyclin are both produced from arachidonic acid by the cyclooxygenase pathway. Aspirin produces irreversible inhibition of cyclooxygenase. However, endothelial cells make more cyclooxygenase within a few hours, whereas circulating platelets do not, and new platelet cyclooxygenase appears only as new platelets enter the circulation over a period of days. Therefore, chronic administration of small doses of aspirin reduces intravascular clotting for prolonged periods and is of value in preventing myocardial infarctions, unstable angina, transient ischemic attacks, and stroke.

B. Nitric Oxide

The production of a potent vasodilator by endothelial cells was first suspected when it was noted that removal of the endothelium from rings of arterial tissue converted the normal dilator response to acetylcholine into a constrictor response. The responsible agent was first called **endothelium-derived relaxing factor,** but it is now known to be **nitric oxide (NO)**. NO is produced from arginine (Figure 11–9) in a reaction catalyzed by **nitric oxide synthase (NOS)**. Three forms of NOS have been cloned: NOS1, found in the nervous system; NOS2, found in macrophages and related immune cells; and NOS3, found in endothelial cells. NOS1 and NOS3 are activated by agents that increase intracellular Ca^{2+}, including the vasodilators acetylcholine and bradykinin, whereas NOS2 is activated by cytokines. The NO that is formed in endothelial cells diffuses to adjacent vascular smooth muscle cells, where it activates soluble guanylyl cyclase, producing cyclic guanosine monophosphate (cGMP; Figure 11–9). The cGMP mediates relaxation of vascular smooth muscle.

The vasodilators that act by way of NO in vivo include not only acetylcholine and bradykinin but vasoactive intestinal polypeptide (VIP), substance P, and some other polypeptides. In addition, various substances that produce vasoconstriction in vivo would have a much greater constrictor effect if they did not simultaneously release NO. Consequently, NO is a major local regulator of blood flow. Its widespread role in reg-

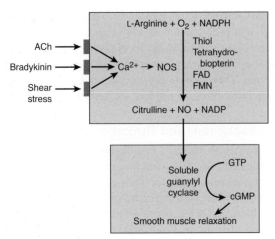

FIGURE 11–9 Synthesis of nitric oxide (NO) from arginine in endothelial cells and its action via stimulation of soluble guanylyl cyclase and generation of cyclic guanosine monophosphate (cGMP) to produce relaxation in vascular smooth muscle cells. The endothelial form of nitric oxide synthase (NOS) is activated by increased intracellular Ca^{2+}, and an increase in Ca^{2+} is produced by acetylcholine (ACh), bradykinin, or shear stress acting on the cell membrane. Thiol, tetrahydrobiopterin, flavin adenine dinucleotide (FAD), and flavin mononucleotide (FMN) are requisite cofactors. GTP, guanosine triphosphate. (Redrawn, with permission, from Ganong WF. *Review of Medical Physiology*, 22nd ed. McGraw-Hill, 2005.)

ulation of the vascular system is indicated by the fact that infusion of amino acid analogs of arginine that inhibit NOS cause blood pressure to rise. Thus, it appears that NOS is acting in a chronic fashion to keep the vascular system dilated.

NO is responsible in large part for reactive hyperemia, the vasodilation and increased blood flow that occur in tissues and organs after a transient obstruction of their blood supply is removed. It can be seen in the forearm after occlusion of the blood supply above the elbow, and it can be quantitated by measuring the increase in forearm volume by plethysmography. NO-dependent vasodilation can also be measured clinically by determining the dilator response to graded doses of acetylcholine injected intra-arterially.

Recent advances in the field of NO research have led to identification of asymmetric-dimethylarginine (ADMA), an endogenous inhibitor of NOS enzymes. Data are emerging linking ADMA to endothelial dysfunction, cardiovascular mortality and chronic kidney disease.

NO is present in many tissues in addition to the vascular system. Its function in some of these tissues is discussed in other chapters of this book.

C. Endothelins

Endothelial cells also produce endothelin-1 (ET-1), the most potent vasoconstrictor agent yet discovered. Three closely related endothelins have been identified in mammals: ET-1, endothelin-2 (ET-2), and endothelin-3 (ET-3). All are polypeptides related to the sarafotoxins, polypeptides found in snake venoms. They contain 21 amino acid residues and two disulfide

bonds (Figure 11–10). All are apparently released from larger prohormones (big endothelins) by endothelin-converting enzymes. ET-2 and ET-3 are found in the intestine and the kidneys, and ET-3 is found also in the brain. Their functions in these organs are unsettled. In the endothelial cells, some of the ET-1 that is produced enters the circulation, but most of it diffuses to smooth muscle in the vicinity. Thus, ET-1 is primarily a local vasoconstrictor acting in a paracrine manner.

Circulating Hormones That Affect Vascular Smooth Muscle

Hormones in the circulation that have general effects on the vascular system include vasoconstrictors and vasodilators. The principal vasoconstrictors are norepinephrine and epinephrine (see Chapter 12), vasopressin (Chapter 19), and angiotensin II (Chapter 21). The principal vasodilators are vasoactive intestinal peptide (VIP; see Chapter 13), kinins, and natriuretic peptides.

A. Kinins

The kinins are two related vasodilator polypeptides called **bradykinin** and **lysyl-bradykinin** (Figure 11–11). The de-

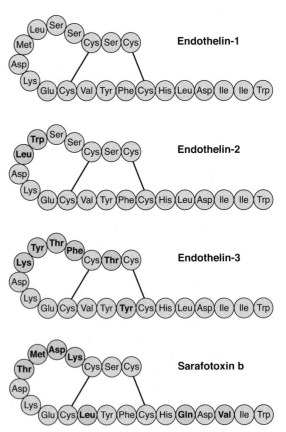

FIGURE 11–10 Structure of human endothelins and one of the snake venom sarafotoxins. The amino acid residues that differ from endothelin-1 are indicated in blue. (Redrawn, with permission, from Ganong WF. *Review of Medical Physiology*, 22nd ed. McGraw-Hill, 2005.)

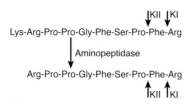

FIGURE 11–11   Kinins. Lysyl-bradykinin (top) can be converted to bradykinin (bottom) by aminopeptidase. The peptides are inactivated by kininase I (KI) or kininase II (KII) at the sites indicated by the short arrows. (Redrawn, with permission, from Ganong WF. *Review of Medical Physiology*, 22nd ed. McGraw-Hill, 2005.)

capeptide lysyl-bradykinin can be converted to the nonapeptide bradykinin by aminopeptidase. Both are metabolized to inactive fragments by the carboxypeptidase kininase I or the dipeptidylcarboxypeptidase kininase II. Kininase II and angiotensin-converting enzyme are the same enzyme, so inhibition of angiotensin-converting enzyme for the treatment of hypertension or heart failure increases plasma and tissue kinins.

Kinins are formed from two **kininogens:** high-molecular-weight (HMW) kininogen and low-molecular-weight (LMW) kininogen. These kinin precursor proteins are products of a single gene produced by alternative splicing. The proteases responsible for cleavage of kininogens are **kallikreins,** a family of enzymes encoded in humans by three genes situated on chromosome 19.

Lysyl-bradykinin and bradykinin are primarily tissue hormones produced, for example, by the kidneys and actively secreting glands, but small amounts are also found in the circulating blood. They act on two receptors, B$_1$ and B$_2$, both coupled to G proteins. Kinins increase blood flow to actively secreting glands by producing vasodilation, and when injected systemically they are relatively potent vasodilators.

B. Natriuretic Hormones

Atrial natriuretic peptide (ANP) is a polypeptide containing 28 amino acid residues that is secreted from the atria when atrial myocytes are stretched. **Brain natriuretic peptide (BNP)** was originally isolated from the brains of experimental animals, but in humans it is secreted by the ventricular myocytes and is commonly known as β-**type natriuretic peptide. CNP,** a third type of natriuretic peptide, is also found in humans. These peptides cause natriuresis, probably by increasing the glomerular filtration rate, which in turn causes excretion of salt and water, reducing blood volume and relieving the stretch on the atrial myocytes. They antagonize the pressor effects of angiotensin II and other pressor hormones. They act by increasing intracellular cGMP. All three have vasodilatory activity, but CNP differs in apparently having a greater effect on veins than arterioles. Their physiologic function is still unsettled. However, their circulating levels are increased in congestive heart failure, and measurement of circulating β-type natriuretic peptide is seeing increased use in the differential diagnosis and evaluation of heart failure. All three of these natriuretic peptides are found in various tissues other than the heart.

An additional natriuretic hormone that acts by inhibiting Na$^+$-K$^+$ adenosine triphosphatase (ATPase) is present in the circulation, but it raises rather than lowers blood pressure. There is substantial evidence that this hormone is actually ouabain and that it is secreted by the adrenal glands.

Neural Control Via the Sympathetic Vasomotor System

Factors affecting the caliber of the arterioles in the body and hence peripheral resistance and tissue blood flow are summarized in Table 11–1. This list includes the factors discussed previously plus a few additional polypeptides that have minor or special effects. It also includes the control of blood pressure by noradrenergic and in some instances cholinergic sympathetic vasomotor nerves to the arterioles. In addition to the extensive nerve supply to these resistance vessels, there is a moderate innervation of the capacitance vessels.

Discharge of the noradrenergic vasomotor nerves causes constriction of the arterioles innervated by the nerves, and if the discharge is general rather than local, there is an increase in blood pressure. In addition, discharge of sympathetic noradrenergic nerves innervating the heart increases blood pressure by increasing the force and rate of cardiac contraction (inotropic and chronotropic effects), increasing stroke volume and cardiac output. Noradrenergic stimulation also inhibits the effect of vagal stimulation, which normally slows the heart and decreases cardiac output.

The main control of vasomotor discharge is feedback regulation via the baroreceptors in the high-pressure and low-pressure portions of the circulatory system (Figure 11–12). The baroreceptors are stretch-sensitive nerve endings located in the carotid sinuses and aortic arch on the arterial side and in the walls of the great veins and the cardiac atria on the venous side. The nerve fibers relay impulses in cranial nerves IX and X to the medulla oblongata, where the fibers end in the nucleus tractus solitarius (Figure 11–13). From the nucleus, second-order neurons pass to the caudal portion of the ventrolateral medulla and environs. From there, third-order inhibitory neurons pass to the rostral ventrolateral medulla, the location of the cell bodies of the neurons that control blood pressure. The axons of these neurons descend into the spinal cord and innervate the cell bodies of the blood pressure-regulating preganglionic sympathetic neurons in the intermediolateral gray column of the spinal cord. The axons of the preganglionic neurons leave the spinal cord and synapse on the postganglionic neurons in the ganglionic chain and collateral ganglia as well as on the catecholamine-secreting cells in the adrenal medulla. The axons of the postganglionic noradrenergic neurons innervate the blood vessels and the heart. These pathways and the probable synaptic mediator at each synapse in the chain are shown in Figure 11–13. Note in particular that increased activity in the baroreceptor afferents produced by increases in blood pressure inhibits sympa-

TABLE 11–1 Summary of factors affecting the caliber of the arterioles.

Constriction
Local factors
Decreased local temperature
Autoregulation
Locally released platelet serotonin
Endothelial cell products
Endothelin-1
Hormones
Norepinephrine
Epinephrine (except in skeletal muscle and liver)
Arginine vasopressin
Angiotensin II
Circulating Na^+-K^+ ATPase inhibitor
Neuropeptide Y
Neural control
Increased discharge of noradrenergic vasomotor nerves
Dilation
Local factors
Increased CO_2, K^+, adenosine, lactate
Decreased O_2
Decreased local pH
Increased local temperature
Endothelial cell products
Nitric oxide
Hormones
Vasoactive intestinal peptide
CGRPα (calcitonin gene-related peptide, the α form)
Substance P
Histamine
Kinins
Natriuretic peptides (ANP, BNP, CNP)
Epinephrine in skeletal muscle and liver
Neural control
Activation of cholinergic dilator fibers to skeletal muscle
Decreased discharge of noradrenergic vasomotor nerves

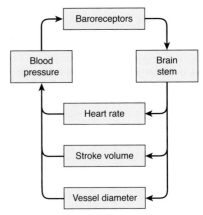

FIGURE 11–12 Feedback regulation of systemic blood pressure by baroreceptors. (Redrawn, with permission, from Ganong WF. *Review of Medical Physiology,* 22nd ed. McGraw-Hill, 2005.)

thetic vasomotor outflow, whereas decreased baroreceptor afferent discharge stimulates sympathetic vasomotor outflow. This is brought about by the inhibitory γ-aminobutyric acid–secreting neuron link between the caudal portion of the ventrolateral medulla and the rostral ventrolateral medulla. In addition, increased baroreceptor discharge stimulates afferents from the nucleus tractus solitarius to the dorsal motor nucleus of the vagus and the nucleus ambiguus. This increases vagal discharge to the heart, slowing the cardiac rate and decreasing cardiac output.

There are ancillary reciprocal circuits between the nucleus tractus solitarius and more dorsal portions of the brainstem and the hypothalamus that smooth and adjust the response of the baroreceptor pathway, but the primary neural regulation of blood pressure is mediated by the baroreceptor pathway in the medulla oblongata.

In addition to direct effects on vasomotor discharge, the baroreceptor pathway causes changes in endocrine function that augment the homeostatic value of baroreceptor responses. Adrenal medullary secretion is increased by discharge of the sympathetic nervous system, although the contributions of circulating catecholamines to the increase in blood pressure are relatively small. Increased sympathetic discharge also increases renin secretion from the kidneys, and the resultant increase in circulating angiotensin II not only acts directly on vascular smooth muscle to cause constriction but also increases aldosterone secretion. This in turn increases Na^+ and water retention, expanding extracellular fluid volume. Associated with increased vasomotor discharge, there is also an increase in vasopressin secretion. This is mediated by a pathway from the medulla to the hypothalamus. The vasopressin expands total body water and in this way helps restore extracellular fluid volume, although its contribution is relatively small.

Baroreceptor function can be tested in experimental animals and judiciously in humans by infusing the pressor drug phenylephrine at different doses and at each dose measuring the slowing of the heart rate by determining the interval

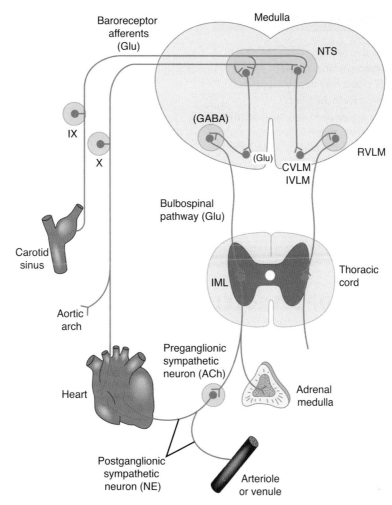

FIGURE 11–13   Basic pathways involved in the medullary control of blood pressure. The vagal efferent pathways to the heart are not shown. The probable neurotransmitters in the pathways are indicated in parentheses. (ACh, acetylcholine; GABA, γ-aminobutyric acid; Glu, glutamate; NE, norepinephrine; CVLM, IVLM, and RVLM, caudal, intermediate, and rostral ventrolateral medulla, respectively; IML, intermediolateral gray column; IX, glossopharyngeal nerve; NTS, nucleus tractus solitarius; X, vagus nerve.)   (Redrawn from Reis DJ et al. Role of adrenaline neurons of the ventrolateral medulla [the C group] in the tonic and phasic control of arterial pressure. Clin Exp Hypertens [A]. 1994;6:221.)

between the R waves (RR interval) of the ECG. An example of results of this type of testing is shown in Figure 11–14.

Sympathetic Vasodilator System

In addition to the sympathetic vasoconstrictor system, there appears to be a sympathetic vasodilator system consisting of anatomically sympathetic but functionally cholinergic neurons innervating blood vessels in skeletal muscle. This system is activated by a pathway that passes from the cerebral cortex through the hypothalamus and medulla without interruption to the intermediolateral gray column of the spinal cord. The function of the system and its importance in cardiovascular control remain a matter of debate, but it may be responsible for the sharp fall in blood pressure and fainting that can occur in association with intense emotion.

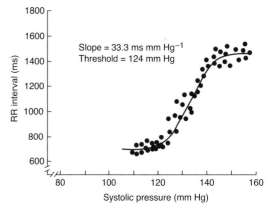

Slope = 33.3 ms mm Hg^{-1}
Threshold = 124 mm Hg

FIGURE 11–14   Baroreflex-mediated lowering of the heart rate during infusion of phenylephrine in a human subject. Note that the values for the RR interval of the ECG, which are plotted on the vertical axis, are inversely proportionate to the heart rate.   (Redrawn, with permission, from Kotrly K et al. Effects of fentanyl-diazepam-nitrous oxide anaesthesia on arterial baroreflex control of heart rate in man. Br J Anaesth. 1986;58:406.)

CHECKPOINT

4. Why do small changes in the diameter of the arterioles have relatively large effects on blood pressure?

5. Why does the velocity of blood flow decrease greatly in the capillaries and then increase in the veins?

6. What categories of factors are involved in regulating the diameter of arterioles?

7. By what mechanism does NO, produced by endothelial cells, act as a vasodilator?

8. What are the principal hormonal vasoconstrictors and vasodilators?

9. What is the role of baroreceptors in the feedback regulation of the high- and low-pressure portions of the circulatory system?

PATHOPHYSIOLOGY OF SELECTED VASCULAR DISORDERS

ATHEROSCLEROSIS

Prevalence & Significance

A condition that afflicts the large and medium-sized arteries of almost every human, at least in societies in which cholesterol-rich foodstuffs are abundant and cheap, is **atherosclerosis.** This condition begins in childhood and, in the absence of accelerating factors, develops slowly until it is widespread in old age. However, it is accelerated by a wide variety of genetic and environmental factors (see later discussion). It is characterized by localized fibrous thickenings of the arterial wall associated with lipid-infiltrated plaques that may eventually calcify. Old plaques are also prone to ulceration and rupture, triggering the formation of thrombi that obstruct flow. Therefore, atherosclerosis leads to vascular insufficiency in the limbs, abnormalities of the renal circulation, and dilations (aneurysms) and even rupture of the aorta and other large arteries. It also leads to common severe and life-threatening diseases of the heart and brain because of formation of intravascular clots at the site of the plaques.

In the United States and most other developed countries, it has been calculated that atherosclerosis is the underlying cause of about 50% of all deaths. Almost all patients with myocardial infarction—and most of those with stroke resulting from cerebral thrombosis—have atherosclerosis. The incidence of ischemic heart disease and strokes has been declining in the United States since 1963, but atherosclerosis is still very common. Thus, atherosclerosis underlies and is fundamentally responsible for a large portion of the clinical problems seen by physicians caring for adult patients.

Pathogenesis

The initial event in atherosclerosis is infiltration of low-density lipoproteins (LDLs) into the subendothelial region. The endothelium is subject to **shear stress,** the tendency to be pulled along or deformed by flowing blood. This is most marked at points where the arteries branch, and this is where the lipids accumulate to the greatest degree.

The LDLs are oxidized or altered in other ways. Thus, altered LDLs activate various components of innate immune system including macrophages, natural antibodies, and innate effector proteins such as C-reactive protein and complement. Altered LDLs are recognized by a family of **scavenger receptors** expressed on macrophages. These scavenger receptors mediate uptake of the oxidized LDL into macrophages and the formation of **foam cells** (Figure 11–15). The foam cells form **fatty streaks.** The streaks appear in the aorta in the first decade of life, in the coronary arteries in the second decade, and in the cerebral arteries in the third and fourth decades.

Oxidized LDLs have a number of deleterious effects, including stimulation of release of cytokines and inhibition of NO production. Vascular smooth muscle cells in the vicinity of foam cells are stimulated and move from the media to the intima, where they proliferate, lay down collagen and other matrix molecules, and contribute to the bulk of the lesion. Smooth muscle cells also take up oxidized LDL and become foam cells. Lipids accumulate both intracellularly and extracellularly.

As the atherosclerotic lesions age, T cells of the immune system as well as macrophages are attracted to them. The intercellular "soup" in the plaques contains a variety of cell-damaging substances, including ozone. Overall, the lesions have been shown to have many of the characteristics of a low-grade infection. Growth factors and cytokines involved in cell migration and proliferation are also produced by smooth muscle cells and endothelial cells, and there is evidence for

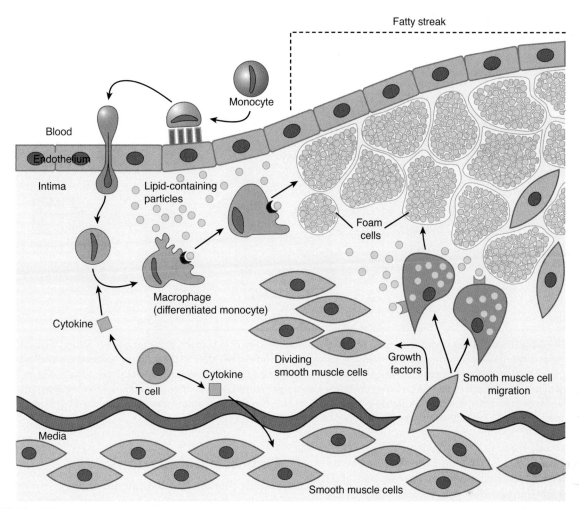

FIGURE 11–15 Formation of a fatty streak in an artery. After vascular injury, monocytes bind to the endothelium, then cross it to the subendothelial space, and become activated tissue microphages. The macrophages take up oxidized low-density lipoproteins (LDL), becoming foam cells. T cells release cytokines, which also activate macrophages. In addition, the cytokines cause smooth muscle cells to proliferate. Under the influence of growth factors, the smooth muscle cells then move to the subendothelial space where they produce collagen and take up LDL, adding to the population of foam cells. (Redrawn, with permission, from Hajjar DP, Nicholson AC. Atherosclerosis. Am Scientist. 1995;83:460.)

shear stress response elements in the flanking DNA of relevant genes in the endothelial cells. A number of investigators have searched for bacteria in plaques, and in a significant number *Chlamydophila pneumoniae*—an organism usually associated with respiratory infection—has been found. However, other organisms have also been found, and it is too early to say whether the chlamydiae are causative agents or merely coincidental tenants in the lesions.

As plaques mature, a fibrous cap forms over them. The plaques with defective or broken caps are most prone to rupture. The lesions alone may distort vessels to the point that they are occluded, but it is usually rupture or ulceration of plaques that triggers thrombosis, blocking blood flow.

A characteristic of atherosclerosis that is currently receiving considerable attention is its association with deficient release of NO and defective vasodilation. As noted, oxidized LDLs inhibit NO production. If acetylcholine is infused via catheter into normal coronary arteries, the vessels dilate; however, if it is infused when atherosclerosis is present, the vessels constrict. This indicates that endothelial secretion of NO is defective.

Relation to Dietary Cholesterol & Other Lipids

Transforming a monocyte into a lipid-ingesting macrophage involves the appearance on its surface of a unique type of oxidized LDL receptor, the **scavenger receptor,** and monocytes are stimulated to produce these receptors by the action of **macrophage colony-stimulating factor** secreted by endothelial cells and vascular smooth muscle cells. When oxidized LDL-receptor complexes are formed, they are internalized and the receptors recycle to the membrane while the lipid is stored.

Obviously, accumulation of lipid in foam cells is a key event in the progression of atherosclerotic lesions, and it is well established that lowering plasma cholesterol slows the progress of atherosclerosis. The main pathways for the metab-

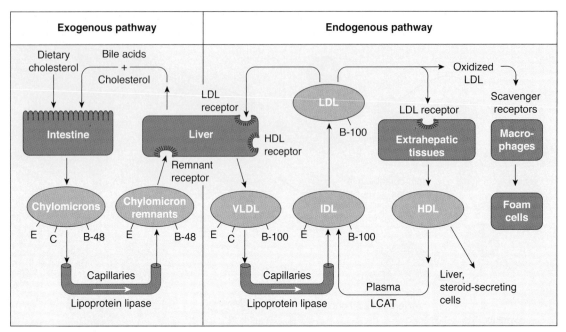

FIGURE 11–16 Simplified diagram of lipoprotein systems for transporting lipids in humans. In the exogenous system, chylomicrons rich in triglycerides of dietary origin are converted to chylomicron remnants rich in cholesteryl esters by the action of lipoprotein lipase. In the endogenous system, very low-density lipoproteins (VLDL) rich in triglycerides are secreted by the liver and converted to intermediate-density lipoproteins (IDL) and then to low-density lipoproteins (LDL) rich in cholesteryl esters. Some of the LDL enter the subendothelial space of arteries, are oxidized, and then taken up by macrophages, which become foam cells. LCAT, lecithin-cholesterol acyltransferase. The letters on the chylomicrons, chylomicron remnants, VLDL, IDL, and LDL identify the primary apoproteins found in them.

olism of ingested lipids are summarized in Figure 11–16. Because lipids are relatively insoluble, they are transported as special lipoprotein particles that increase their solubility. Dietary cholesterol and triglycerides are packaged in the protein-coated **chylomicrons** in intestinal epithelial cells. Under the influence of lipoprotein lipase, these particles release triglycerides to fat depots and muscles, and the resulting **chylomicron remnants** are taken up by the liver. The liver also synthesizes cholesterol and packages it with specific proteins to form **very-low-density lipoproteins (VLDLs)**. These lipoprotein particles enter the circulation and under the influence of lipoprotein lipase donate triglycerides to tissues. In this way, they become cholesterol-rich **intermediate-density lipoproteins (IDLs)** and **low-density lipoproteins (LDLs)**. The LDL supply cholesterol to the tissues. They provide all cells with the cholesterol for production of cell membranes and other uses. They also provide most of the cholesterol that is the precursor for all steroid hormones. As noted, oxidized LDLs are taken up by macrophages and smooth muscle cells in atherosclerotic lesions. On the other hand, **high-density lipoproteins (HDLs)** take cholesterol from peripheral cells and transport it to the liver where it is metabolized, keeping plasma and tissue cholesterol low. For this reason, it is referred to as "good cholesterol" as opposed to LDL cholesterol, which is "bad cholesterol." Efforts are being made to increase HDL by pharmaceutical means in the treatment of atherosclerosis.

Clinical Manifestations

Because atherosclerosis is an abnormality of arterial blood vessels, it can affect almost any organ in the body. Calcified atherosclerotic plaques are occasionally detected on x-ray film, and angiographic visualization of deformed arterial walls is possible. In general, however, atherosclerosis is asymptomatic until one of its complications develops.

In coronary arteries, atherosclerotic narrowing that reduces the lumen of a coronary artery more than 75% causes **angina pectoris,** the chest pain that results when pain-producing substances accumulate in the myocardium. Typically, the pain comes on during exertion and disappears with rest, as the substances are washed out by the blood. When atherosclerotic lesions cause clotting and occlusion of a coronary artery, the myocardium supplied by the artery dies (**myocardial infarction**). Myocardial infarction is also discussed in Chapter 10.

In the cerebral circulation, arterial blockage at the site of atherosclerotic plaques causes **thrombotic strokes.** Strokes are discussed in Chapter 7. In the abdominal aorta, extensive atherosclerosis can lead to aneurysmal dilation and rupture of the vessel. In the renal vessels, localized constriction of one or both renal arteries causes **renovascular hypertension** (see later discussion). In the circulation to the legs, vascular insufficiency causes **intermittent claudication** (fatigue and usually pain on walking that is relieved by rest). If the circulation of a limb is severely compromised, the skin can ulcerate, producing lesions that are slow to heal. Frank **gangrene** of the

TABLE 11–2 Conditions that accelerate the progression of atherosclerosis and the mechanisms responsible.

Condition	Mechanism
Male gender (and females after menopause)	Lack of LDL-lowering effect of estrogens; estrogens probably act by increasing the number of LDL receptors in the liver.
Family history of ischemic heart disease, stroke	Probably multiple genetic mechanisms.
Primary hyperlipidemia	Inherited disorders causing lipoprotein lipase deficiency (type I), defective LDL receptors (type IIa), abnormal apoprotein E (type III), deficiency of apoprotein C (type V), or unknown cause (types IIb and IV).
Secondary hyperlipidemia[1]	Increased circulating triglycerides produced by diuretics, β-adrenergic blocking drugs, excess alcohol intake.
Cigarette smoking	Probably carbon monoxide-induced hypoxic injury to endothelial cells.
Hypertension	Increased shear stress, with damage to endothelium.
Diabetes mellitus (types 1 and 2)	Decreased hepatic removal of LDL from the circulation; increased glycosylation of collagen, which increases LDL binding to blood vessel walls.
Obesity, particularly abdominal obesity	Unsettled, but obesity is associated with type 2 diabetes, hypertriglyceridemia, hypercholesterolemia, and hypertension, all of which are risk factors in their own right.
Nephrotic syndrome	Increased hepatic production of lipids and lipoprotein(a).
Hypothyroidism	Decreased formation of LDL receptors in the liver.
High lipoprotein(a)	Unsettled.
Elevated plasma homocysteine	Unsettled. Probably increased homocysteine provides more H_2O_2 and other reactive oxygen molecules that foster formation of oxidized LDL.

[1]Hypercholesterolemia and hypertriglyceridemia are both risk factors.

extremities may also occur. Less frequently, clot formation and obstruction may occur in vessels supplying the intestines or other parts of the body.

Risk Factors

As noted, the progression of atherosclerosis is accelerated by a wide variety of genetic and environmental factors (risk factors). These are summarized in Table 11–2. Obviously, treating the accelerating conditions that are treatable and avoiding those that are avoidable should reduce the incidence of myocardial infarctions, strokes, and other complications of atherosclerosis.

Estrogen increases cholesterol removal by the liver, and the progression of atherosclerosis is less rapid in premenopausal women that in men. In addition, epidemiologic evidence shows that estrogen replacement therapy protects the cardiovascular system in postmenopausal women. On the other hand, large doses of estrogens increase the incidence of blood clots, and even small doses produce a slight increase in clotting. In addition, in several studies, estrogen treatment of postmenopausal women failed to prevent second heart attacks. The reason for the discrepancies between the epidemiologic and experimental data is currently unsettled.

The effect of increased plasma levels of homocysteine and related molecules such as homocystine and homocysteine thiolactone, a condition sometimes called hyperhomocystin-

emia, deserves emphasis. These increases are associated with accelerated atherosclerosis, and the magnitude of the plasma elevation is positively correlated with the severity of the atherosclerosis. Markedly elevated levels resulting from documented mutations of relevant genes are rare, but mild elevations occur in 7% of the general population. The mechanism responsible for the accelerated vascular damage is unsettled, but homocysteine is a significant source of H_2O_2 and other reactive forms of oxygen, and this may accelerate the oxidation of LDL.

Homocysteine is an intermediate in the synthesis of methionine. It is metabolized by enzymes that are dependent on vitamin B_6, vitamin B_{12}, and folic acid. Supplementation of the diet with these vitamins reduces plasma homocysteine, usually to normal. Determining whether such supplements also reduce the incidence of the accelerated atherosclerosis will require prolonged, careful clinical trials, and the results of such studies to date are inconclusive.

Evidence is now overwhelming that lowering plasma cholesterol and triglyceride levels and increasing plasma HDL levels slows, and in some cases reverses, the atherosclerotic process. The desired decrease in lipids can sometimes be achieved with dietary restriction of cholesterol, saturated and trans fat alone, even though dietary restriction initiates a compensatory increase in cholesterol synthesis in the body. When dietary treatment is not adequate, reducing conversion of mevalonate to cholesterol with statins, drugs that inhibit hepatic 3-methylglutaryl coenzyme A (HMG-CoA) reductase, the enzyme which catalyzes this reaction, is beneficial. The currently available HMG-CoA reductase inhibitors include atorvastatin, lovastatin, pravastatin, simvastatin, fluvastatin, and rosuvastatin.

In cases in which there is severe hypercholesterolemia because of congenitally defective LDL receptors, gene therapy may be an option. However, despite promising preliminary results, gene therapy in humans appears to be unachievable until better means for gene transfer are developed. Other approaches to slowing or preventing development of atherosclerosis by molecular biologic techniques are under development.

Antioxidant treatment with agents such as α-tocopherol, vitamin E, and β-carotene has been used to inhibit oxidation of LDL, and this reduces the incidence of atherosclerotic changes in experimental animals. However, the results of antioxidant treatment in humans have generally been disappointing or negative.

Men who smoke a pack of cigarettes a day have a 70% increase in death rate from ischemic heart disease compared with nonsmokers, and there is also an increase in women. Smoking cessation lessens the risk of death and of myocardial infarction. The deleterious effects of smoking include endothelial damage caused by carbon monoxide-induced hypoxia. Other factors may also be involved. Thus, stopping smoking is a major way to slow the progress of atherosclerosis.

Because of the increased shear stress imposed on the endothelium by an elevated blood pressure, hypertension is another important modifiable risk factor for atherosclerosis. Lowering blood pressure has its greatest effect in reducing the incidence of stroke, but there are beneficial effects on ischemic heart disease as well. With modern methods of treatment, blood pressure in hypertensives can generally be reduced to normal or near-normal values, and the decrease in strokes, myocardial infarctions, and renal failure produced by such treatment is clear testimony to the value of reducing or eliminating this risk factor.

In diabetics, there are microvascular complications and macrovascular complications (see Table 18–9). The latter are primarily related to atherosclerosis. There is a twofold increase in the incidence of myocardial infarction compared with nondiabetics; severe circulatory deficiency in the legs with gangrene is relatively common; there are more thrombotic strokes; and renal failure is a serious problem (see Chapter 18). It is interesting in this regard that rigorous control of blood pressure in diabetics has been shown to be more efficacious in reducing cardiovascular complications than rigorous control of blood glucose.

The nephrotic syndrome and hypothyroidism also accelerate the progression of atherosclerosis and are treatable conditions.

CHECKPOINT

10. What is the most common cause of death in the United States among individuals older than 45 years?
11. What is the hypothesized mechanism of atherosclerotic plaque formation?
12. What are some ways in which atherosclerotic plaques can cause cardiovascular disease?
13. Name five treatable risk factors that accelerate the progression of atherosclerosis.

HYPERTENSION

Hypertension is not a single disease but a syndrome with multiple causes. In most instances, the cause remains unknown, and the cases are lumped together under the term **essential hypertension** (Table 11–3). However, mechanisms are continuously being discovered that explain hypertension in new subsets of the formerly monolithic category of essential hypertension, and the percentage of cases in the essential category continues to decline. Essential hypertension is often called **primary hypertension,** and hypertension in which the cause is known is called **secondary hypertension,** although this separation seems somewhat artificial. This chapter discusses the pathogenesis of hypertension and its complications in general terms and then discusses the specific causes of the currently defined subgroups and the unique features, if

TABLE 11–3   Estimated frequency of various forms of hypertension in the general hypertensive population.

	Percentage of Population
Essential hypertension	88
Renal hypertension	
Renovascular	2
Parenchymal	3
Endocrine hypertension	
Primary aldosteronism	5
Cushing's syndrome	0.1
Pheochromocytoma	0.1
Other adrenal forms	0.2
Estrogen treatment ("pill hypertension")	1
Miscellaneous (Liddle's syndrome, coarctation of the aorta, etc)	0.6

Modified from Williams GH. Hypertensive vascular disease. In: *Harrison's Principles of Internal Medicine,* 15th ed. Braunwald E et al (editors). McGraw-Hill, 2001.

any, that each adds to the general findings in patients with high blood pressure.

Pathogenesis

Current guidelines of the Joint National Committee on Prevention, Detection, Evaluation, and Treatment of High Blood Pressure define normal blood pressure as systolic pressure of < 120 mm Hg and diastolic pressure of < 80 mm Hg. Hypertension is defined as an arterial pressure greater than 140/90 mm Hg in adults on at least three consecutive visits to the doctor's office. People whose blood pressure is between normal and 140/90 mm Hg are considered to have pre-hypertension and people whose blood pressure falls in this category should appropriately modify their lifestyle to lower their blood pressure to below 120/80 mm Hg. As noted (Figure 11–7), systolic pressure normally rises throughout life, and diastolic pressure rises until age 50–60 years but then falls, so that pulse pressure continues to increase. In the past, emphasis has been on treating individuals with elevated diastolic pressure. However, it now appears that, particularly in elderly individuals, treating systolic hypertension is equally important or even more so in reducing the cardiovascular complications of hypertension.

The most common cause of hypertension is increased peripheral vascular resistance. However, because blood pressure equals total peripheral resistance times cardiac output, prolonged increases in cardiac output can also cause hypertension. These are seen, for example, in hyperthyroidism and beriberi. In addition, increased blood volume causes hypertension, especially in individuals with mineralocorticoid excess or renal failure (see later discussion); and increased blood viscosity, if it is marked, can increase arterial pressure.

Clinical Presentation

Hypertension by itself does not cause symptoms. Headaches, fatigue, and dizziness are sometimes ascribed to hypertension, but nonspecific symptoms such as these are no more common in hypertensives than they are in normotensive controls. Instead, the condition is discovered during routine screening or when patients seek medical advice for its complications. These complications are serious and potentially fatal. They include myocardial infarction, congestive heart failure, thrombotic and hemorrhagic strokes, hypertensive encephalopathy, and renal failure (Figure 11–17). This is why hypertension is called "the silent killer."

Physical findings are also absent in early hypertension, and observable changes are generally found only in advanced severe cases. These may include **hypertensive retinopathy** (ie, narrowed arterioles seen on funduscopic examination) and, in more severe cases, retinal hemorrhages and exudates along with swelling of the optic nerve head (papilledema). Prolonged pumping against an elevated peripheral resistance causes left ventricular hypertrophy, which can be detected by echocardiography, and cardiac enlargement, which can be detected on physical examination. It is important to listen with the stethoscope over the kidneys because in renal hypertension (see later discussion) narrowing of the renal arteries may cause bruits. These bruits are usually continuous throughout the cardiac cycle. It has been recommended that the blood pressure response to rising from the sitting to the standing position be determined. A blood pressure rise on standing sometimes occurs in essential hypertension presumably because of a hyperactive sympathetic response to the erect posture. This rise is usually absent in other forms of

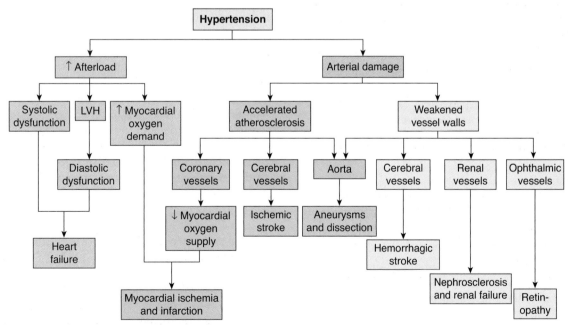

FIGURE 11–17 Pathogenesis of the complications produced by arterial hypertension. LVH, left ventricular hypertrophy. (Redrawn, with permission, from Deshmukh R et al. Chapter 13 in: *Pathophysiology of Heart Disease: A Collaborative Project of Medical Students and Faculty.* Lilly LS et al [editors]. 3rd edition. Williams & Wilkins, 2003.)

hypertension. Most individuals with essential hypertension (60%) have normal plasma renin activity, and 10% have high plasma renin activity. However, 30% have low plasma renin activity. Renin secretion may be reduced by an expanded blood volume in some of these patients, but in others the cause is unsettled, and low-renin essential hypertension has not yet been separated from the rest of essential hypertension as a distinct entity.

In many patients with hypertension, the condition is benign and progresses slowly; in others, it progresses rapidly. Actuarial data indicate that on average untreated hypertension reduces life expectancy by 10–20 years. Atherosclerosis is accelerated, and this in turn leads to ischemic heart disease with angina pectoris and myocardial infarctions (Chapter 10), thrombotic strokes and cerebral hemorrhages (Chapter 7), and renal failure (Chapter 16). Another complication of severe hypertension is **hypertensive encephalopathy,** in which there is confusion, disordered consciousness, and seizures. This condition, which requires vigorous treatment, is probably due to arteriolar spasm and cerebral edema.

In all forms of hypertension regardless of cause, the condition can suddenly accelerate and enter the malignant phase. In **malignant hypertension,** there is widespread fibrinoid necrosis of the media with intimal fibrosis in arterioles, narrowing them and leading to progressive severe retinopathy, congestive heart failure, and renal failure. If untreated, malignant hypertension is usually fatal in 1 year.

MANAGEMENT

A discussion of disease treatment is beyond the scope of this book. However, it should be noted that in all forms of hypertension modern treatment with adrenergic blocking drugs, inhibitors of the renin-angiotensin system, Ca^{2+} channel inhibitors, and diuretics reduce blood pressure, usually to normal levels. In addition, these treatments delay or prevent complications and lengthen life expectancy. However, they are not curative and must be continued indefinitely. Thus, essential hypertension is like diabetes mellitus: It can be controlled but not cured. If a cause of hypertension can be identified, its treatment may result in a cure. Consequently, it is important to identify such cases.

Etiology

A. Coarctation of the Aorta

Congenital narrowing of the aorta usually occurs just distal to the origin of the left subclavian artery. Peripheral resistance is increased above the constriction. Therefore, blood pressure is elevated in the arms, head, and chest but lowered in the legs. However, because the constriction is proximal to the renal arteries, renin secretion is increased in most cases of coarctation as a result of the reduction in arterial pressure in the renal arteries. This tends to increase blood pressure throughout the

TABLE 11–4 Salt sensitivity in humans.

	Percentage of Individuals	
	Normal	**Hypertensive**
White		
Salt-sensitive[1]	30	55
Salt-resistant	70	45
Black		
Salt-sensitive[1]	32	73
Salt-resistant	68	27

Courtesy of Weinberg MH. Data from Luft FC et al. Salt sensitivity and resistance of blood pressure. Hypertension. 1991;17(Suppl I): I102.

[1]Mean blood pressure decrease >10 mm Hg with furosemide and low-salt diet.

body. Elimination of the constriction by resecting the narrowed segment of the aorta usually cures the condition.

B. Salt Sensitivity

Through selective inbreeding, Dahl was able to develop two strains of rats: salt-sensitive rats that showed an increase in blood pressure when fed a high-salt diet and salt-resistant rats that did not. The genetic mechanisms responsible for these strain differences are currently under investigation. There may be a similar division of humans into salt-sensitive and salt-resistant groups, although obviously the lines between the groups are less distinct. As shown in Table 11–4, about 30% of whites with normal renal function and normal blood pressure are salt sensitive compared with 55% of whites with essential hypertension. For unknown reasons, a larger percentage of black hypertensives are salt sensitive. These figures have obvious significance in terms of recommendations about salt intake in hypertension.

It should be emphasized that the figures just cited refer to individuals with normal renal function and normal (or reduced) secretion of mineralocorticoid hormones. When renal function is reduced, mineralocorticoid secretion is increased, or the effects of mineralocorticoids are enhanced, there is abnormal retention of salt and water, and hypertension is produced on this basis (see later discussion).

Although the genetic mechanisms responsible for the differences in salt sensitivity are still unknown, recent studies have shed new light on our understanding of salt-mediated hypertension. Salt appears to activate two pathways which both lead to vascular smooth muscle contraction: 1) salt stimulates a subset of G proteins (G_{12-13}) that are responsible for the activation of myosin light chain kinase, which phosphorylates myosin to initiate contraction; and 2) salt stimulates the Rho/Rho kinase pathway, which inhibits myosin light chain phosphatase to prevent smooth muscle relaxation. Individual differences in these signaling pathways may indeed be behind the salt-related hypertension.

C. Renal Abnormalities

Goldblatt's observation that **renal artery constriction** increased blood pressure in experimental animals was rapidly followed by demonstration of the same event in humans. However, disappointment followed when it was found that **renal hypertension** resulting from constriction of one or both renal arteries accounted for only 2% of cases of clinical hypertension (Table 11–3). The narrowing can be due to atherosclerosis, fibroelastic overgrowth of the wall of the renal artery, or external pressure on the vessel. The initial constriction decreases renal arteriolar pressure, and this leads to increased renin secretion. The renin-angiotensin system is discussed in Chapters 16 and 21. However, in many cases, some other mechanism takes over chronically to maintain the hypertension. The nature of this other mechanism is unknown.

In rare instances, hypertension can be caused by tumors of the renin-secreting juxtaglomerular cells.

Ureteral obstruction can cause hypertension in animals and probably in humans by increasing renal interstitial pressure and thus decreasing the pressure gradient across the renin-secreting juxtaglomerular cells.

Acute and chronic glomerulonephritis and other forms of diffuse kidney disease can cause hypertension when loss of the ability to excrete salt is severe enough that Na^+ and water are retained and blood volume is expanded.

In **Liddle's syndrome,** there is abnormal sodium retention by the kidneys with expanded extracellular fluid volume, producing hypertension but no increase in circulating mineralocorticoids. The sodium retention is due to constitutive activation of the epithelial sodium channels (ENaC). The channels are inhibited by amiloride, and each has three subunits. Activating mutations in the genes for the β or the γ subunit have been documented in patients with Liddle's syndrome.

A mutation in the mineralocorticoid receptor that causes renal Na^+ retention and hypertension has also been described. This mutation makes the receptor constitutively active and causes progesterone and related steroids to act as agonists. The result is early-onset hypertension, which is markedly exacerbated during pregnancy.

D. Abnormalities of the Renin-Angiotensin System

Increased secretion of angiotensinogen from the liver can cause hypertension. Secretion of this angiotensin precursor (Chapter 21) is under endocrine control and is stimulated by estrogens. Consequently, it is increased in women taking contraceptive pills containing large amounts of estrogens. When circulating angiotensinogen is increased, more angiotensin II is formed and blood pressure rises. The normal compensation for this response is decreased secretion of renin because angiotensin II feeds back directly on the juxtaglomerular cells to reduce renin secretion. However, in some women, the compensation is incomplete and the estrogens cause a significant increase in blood pressure. The incidence of this **pill hypertension** in the general hypertensive population is about 1% (Table 11–3). Some of the women with the condition have underlying essential hypertension, which is triggered by the estrogens, but in others the hypertension is cured by stopping estrogen treatment. Mutations in the gene for angiotensinogen, which produce slight increases in circulating angiotensinogen, have been reported to be more common in patients with essential hypertension than in individuals with normal blood pressure.

E. Adrenal Gland Disorders

A remarkable number of adrenal abnormalities cause hypertension. These include mainly conditions in which mineralocorticoids are secreted in excess, but excess secretion of cortisol also causes hypertension, as does excess secretion of catecholamines by tumors of the adrenal medulla.

1. Mineralocorticoid excess—The classic form of mineralocorticoid excess hypertension (Conn's syndrome) is primary hyperaldosteronism caused by a tumor of the zona glomerulosa of the adrenal cortex (see Figure 21–17) that secretes large quantities of aldosterone. The elevated circulating aldosterone level leads to Na^+ retention with expansion of extracellular fluid volume and hypertension that is usually mild but can be severe. Because of the escape mechanism (see Chapter 21), edema does not occur, but there is chronic loss of K^+ and H^+. Consequently, the hallmark of primary hyperaldosteronism is hypertension with the added feature of hypokalemia. However, hypokalemia is not always present. Plasma renin activity is low, and there may be alkalosis.

Hypersecretion of deoxycorticosterone (DOC) can also cause mineralocorticoid-excess hypertension. DOC has less mineralocorticoid activity than aldosterone, but when present in increased amounts it can cause significant Na^+ retention. DOC secretion, unlike aldosterone secretion, is increased by chronic hypersecretion of adrenocorticotropic hormone (ACTH), so any condition that produces a chronic increase in ACTH secretion can also cause mineralocorticoid excess. This is the situation in **17α-hydroxylase deficiency;** the deficiency prevents the synthesis of cortisol, and ACTH secretion is consequently increased. However, the biosynthetic pathway leading to DOC is intact, and DOC secretion is increased. DOC is also the explanation of the hypertension found in the hypertensive form of **congenital adrenal hyperplasia.** This is due to 11β-hydroxylase deficiency, which prevents the conversion of DOC to corticosterone, causing circulating DOC to increase. In addition, the conversion of 11-deoxycortisol to cortisol is prevented, causing ACTH secretion to increase.

An interesting form of mineralocorticoid hypertension is **glucocorticoid-remediable aldosteronism (GRA).** In this autosomal dominant disorder, ACTH produces prolonged hypersecretion of aldosterone as well as glucocorticoids. The genes encoding aldosterone synthase and 11β-hydroxylase are 95% identical and located close together on chromosome 8. In GRA, there is unequal crossing over during development, and the regulatory 5′ portion of the 11-hydroxylase gene is fused to the coding region of the aldosterone synthase gene, so that

ACTH now causes induction of aldosterone synthase. The hypertension that results is variable in severity but is frequently more severe than the hypertension of primary hyperaldosteronism. Presumably this is because the tumors causing primary hyperaldosteronism develop later in life, whereas the congenital defect in GRA is present starting in early embryonic life. Strokes are common in GRA. GRA can be treated by administration of glucocorticoids in doses that suppress ACTH secretion. If the dose is chosen with care, inhibition of the secretion of ACTH can be achieved without producing the clinical features of Cushing's syndrome.

Another condition that mimics the effect of excess mineralocorticoid secretion is **apparent mineralocorticoid excess.** In vitro, mineralocorticoid receptors are as sensitive to glucocorticoids as they are to mineralocorticoids, but in vivo mineralocorticoid effects are produced only by mineralocorticoid hormones. This is because of the presence in the vicinity of the receptor of 11β-hydroxysteroid dehydrogenase type 2, an enzyme that converts the glucocorticoids cortisol and corticosterone to their relatively inactive 11-keto derivative (Figure 11–18). If this enzyme is congenitally absent or inhibited by substances such as licorice, which contains the enzyme

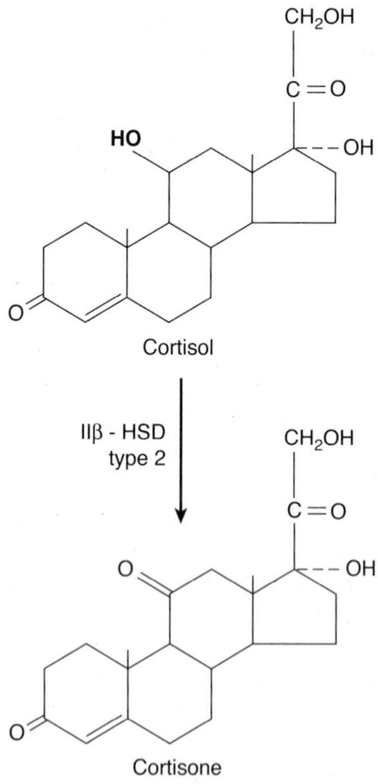

FIGURE 11–18 Conversion of cortisol to its 11-keto derivative, cortisone, by 11β-hydroxysteroid dehydrogenase (11β-HSD) type 2. This enzyme also catalyzes conversion of corticosterone to its 11-keto derivative, 11-dehydrocorticosterone. The keto derivatives do not bind to mineralocorticoid receptors. Similar reactions are catalyzed by 11β-HSD type 1 but are reversible, whereas those catalyzed by 11β-HSD type 2 are not.

inhibitor glycyrrhetinic acid, glucocorticoids have mineralocorticoid as well as glucocorticoid activity in vivo. Because glucocorticoids are normally present in much greater quantities than mineralocorticoids, their effect is relatively large.

2. Glucocorticoid excess—The incidence of hypertension is greater than normal in Cushing's syndrome, indicating that cortisol as well as mineralocorticoids can cause hypertension. The mechanism involved is unsettled, although there are a number of possibilities. First, glucocorticoids stimulate angiotensinogen secretion by the liver, and as noted, this increases circulating angiotensin II unless the feedback inhibition of renin secretion is able to compensate for the rise. Second, ACTH stimulates DOC secretion, and when present in increased amounts this steroid has appreciable mineralocorticoid activity. Third, there is evidence that glucocorticoids sensitize vascular smooth muscle to the contractile effect of catecholamines. Fourth, excess cortisol may overwhelm renal 11-hydroxysteroid dehydrogenase type 2, resulting in mineralocorticoid receptor activation by cortisol.

3. Excess secretion of catecholamines—Increases in adrenal medullary secretion of norepinephrine elevate systolic and diastolic pressure, and increases in epinephrine secretion may have the same effect. Tumors of the adrenal medulla (pheochromocytomas) cause hypertension. These tumors are discussed in more detail in Chapter 12. Norepinephrine-secreting tumors usually produce sustained hypertension, as do epinephrine-secreting tumors. However, about 15% of the tumors secrete episodically, producing intermittent bouts of palpitations, headache, glycosuria, and extreme systolic hypertension. The same symptoms are produced by acute injection of a large dose of epinephrine.

Pheochromocytomas can be diagnosed by measuring circulating catecholamines or their metabolites. Alternatively, one can administer clonidine, an α_2-adrenergic agonist that acts centrally to decrease sympathetic output. Therefore, it lowers blood pressure in patients with essential hypertension but has little or no effect on blood pressure in patients with pheochromocytomas. The mechanism by which clonidine acts centrally to decrease sympathetic discharge is unsettled and may involve imidazole receptors.

Surgical removal of a pheochromocytoma effects a cure in many cases. However, pheochromocytomas can be multiple, can recur, and may be malignant, with metastases.

F. Natriuretic Hormones

In view of the fact that Na$^+$ retention resulting from mineralocorticoid excess causes hypertension, it may seem surprising that a natriuretic hormone is also a suspected cause of hypertension. ANP and other natriuretic peptides of cardiac origin cause sodium loss in the urine and generally lower blood pressure. However, there is, in addition, a digitalis-like natriuretic substance in the circulation. Its source seems to be the adrenals, although it has also been claimed that it is secreted by the hypothalamus. This substance, which may be naturally occurring ouabain, inhibits Na^+-K^+ ATPase. This results in loss of Na^+ in the urine, but Ca^{2+} accumulates in cells because of the decrease in Na^+ gradient across the cell membrane. The increase in intracellular Ca^{2+} causes vascular smooth muscle to contract. Consequently, blood pressure is increased. However, the physiologic and pathophysiologic significance of this natriuretic hormone remains unsettled, and hypersecretion of it cannot as yet be considered a proved cause of clinical hypertension.

G. Neurologic Disorders

The nervous system plays a key role in maintaining blood pressure in normal individuals (see prior discussion). Clonidine and other drugs lower blood pressure by acting on the brain to decrease sympathetic discharge, and several of the most effective treatments for chronic hypertension act peripherally to reduce the effect of vasomotor sympathetic discharge to the blood vessels and heart. These and other observations suggest that clinical hypertension could be caused by CNS abnormalities. Interruption of the afferent input from the baroreceptors to the CNS in experimental animals causes increased blood pressure. However, emphasis has been placed on the variability of the blood pressure in such animals rather than on any consistent elevation of mean arterial pressure. There is some evidence that chronic pressure on the rostral ventrolateral medulla (Figure 11–13) caused by minor anatomic abnormalities can cause hypertension in humans. However, this evidence is controversial, and as yet it cannot be said that this is an established cause of hypertension.

H. Nitric Oxide

An intriguing observation in experimental animals is that administration of drugs that inhibit the production of NO increase blood pressure. Furthermore, there is a sustained elevation in blood pressure in knockout mice in which the genetic expression of the endothelial form of NOS has been disrupted. These observations suggest that there is a chronic blood pressure-lowering effect of NO and raise the possibility that inhibition of the production or effects of NO could be a cause of hypertension in humans.

I. Facilitation of Na^+-H^+ Exchange

In approximately 50% of patients with essential hypertension, the function of a ubiquitous pH-regulating Na^+-H^+ exchanger in cell membranes is enhanced. Evidence indicates that this is associated with a polymorphism in the gene for one of the β subunits of a G protein that facilitates the function of the G protein. However, the overall significance of this abnormality remains to be determined.

J. Relation to Insulin Resistance

There is a higher incidence of insulin resistance, hyperinsulinemia, hyperlipidemia, and obesity in patients with essential hypertension and in their normotensive relatives than in the general population or in patients with hypertension from known causes. This combination of abnormalities is sometimes called **syndrome X** and more recently the **metabolic syndrome.** There has been speculation that insulin resistance causes increased insulin secretion and that the resulting hyperinsulinemia stimulates the sympathetic nervous system, causing hypertension. However, correlation does not prove cause and effect, and patients with insulin-secreting pancreatic tumors (insulinomas) do not have an increased incidence of hypertension. Furthermore, in dogs and normal humans, prolonged infusions of insulin have a slight vasodilator rather than a vasoconstrictor effect, and in a careful study of obese patients with essential hypertension, prolonged infusion of insulin caused a small decrease rather than an increase in blood pressure. Thus, although the cause of the insulin resistance, hyperinsulinemia, obesity, and hyperlipidemia in hypertension remains unsettled, it seems unlikely that increased insulin resistance is a major cause of essential hypertension.

CHECKPOINT

14. Describe five physical findings in long-standing or severe hypertension.

15. Name 10 known causes of hypertension and a means by which each could be identified as the cause of hypertension in a patient.

16. What is the effect on blood pressure of disrupting the gene for the endothelial cell form of NOS in mice?

SHOCK

The term "shock" is used to denote various conditions, including the response to the passage of electric current through the body; the state that follows immediately after interruption of the spinal cord; and the stunned reaction to bad news. In the current context, it refers to an abnormality of the circulatory system in which there is inadequate tissue perfusion because of a relatively or absolutely inadequate cardiac output. The causes are divided into four groups: inadequate volume of blood to fill the vascular system (**hypovolemic shock**); increased size of the vascular system produced by vasodilation in the presence of a normal blood volume (**distributive, vasogenic, or low-resistance shock**); inadequate output of the heart as a result of myocardial abnormalities (**cardiogenic shock**); and inadequate cardiac output as a result of obstruction of blood flow in the lungs or heart (**obstructive shock**). Examples of the conditions or diseases that can cause each type are set forth in Table 11–5.

Hypovolemic Shock

Hypovolemic shock is characterized by hypotension; a rapid, thready pulse; cold, pale, clammy skin; intense thirst; rapid

TABLE 11–5 Types of shock, with examples of conditions or diseases that can cause each type.

Hypovolemic shock (decreased blood volume)
Hemorrhage
Trauma
Surgery
Burns
Fluid loss associated with vomiting or diarrhea
Distributive shock (marked vasodilation; also called vasogenic or low-resistance shock)
Fainting (neurogenic shock)
Anaphylaxis
Sepsis (also causes hypovolemia due to increased capillary permeability with loss of fluid into tissues)
Cardiogenic shock (inadequate output by a diseased heart)
Myocardial infarction
Congestive heart failure
Arrhythmias
Obstructive shock (obstruction of blood flow)
Tension pneumothorax
Pulmonary embolism
Cardiac tumor
Pericardial tamponade

respiration; and restlessness or, alternatively, torpor. Urine volume is markedly decreased. However, none of these findings are invariably present. Hypovolemic shock is commonly subdivided into categories on the basis of cause. The use of terms such as hemorrhagic shock, traumatic shock, surgical shock, and burn shock is of some benefit because although there are similarities between these various forms of shock, there are important features that are unique to each.

In hypovolemic and other forms of shock, inadequate perfusion of the tissues leads to increased anaerobic glycolysis, with production of large amounts of lactic acid. In severe cases, the blood lactate level rises from a normal value of about 1 mmol/L to 9 mmol/L or more. The resulting lactic acidosis depresses the myocardium, decreases peripheral vascular responsiveness to catecholamines, and may be severe enough to cause coma.

Multiple compensatory reactions come into play to defend extracellular fluid volume (Table 11–6). The large number of reactions that have evolved indicates the importance of maintaining blood volume for survival.

A decrease in pulse pressure or mean arterial pressure decreases the number of impulses ascending to the brain from the arterial baroreceptors, resulting in increased vasomotor discharge. The resulting vasoconstriction is generalized, sparing only the vessels of the brain and the heart. The coronary vessels are dilated because of the increased myocardial metabolism secondary to an increase in heart rate. Vasoconstriction in the skin accounts for the coolness and pallor, and vasoconstriction in the kidneys accounts for the shutdown in renal function.

The immediate cardiac response to hypovolemia is tachycardia. With more extensive loss of volume, tachycardia can be replaced by bradycardia, whereas with very severe hypovolemia, tachycardia reappears. Bradycardia may be due to unmasking of a vagally mediated depressor reflex, perhaps related to limiting blood loss.

Vasoconstriction in the kidney reduces glomerular filtration. This reduces water loss, but it reaches a point at which nitrogenous products of metabolism accumulate in the blood (**prerenal azotemia**). If hypotension is prolonged, there may be severe renal tubular damage, leading to acute renal failure.

The fall in blood pressure and the decreased O_2-carrying power of the blood caused by the loss of red cells results in stimulation of the carotid and aortic chemoreceptors. This not only stimulates respiration but increases vasoconstrictor discharge. In severe hypovolemia, the pressure is so low that there is no longer any discharge from the carotid and aortic baroreceptors. This occurs when the mean blood pressure is about 70 mm Hg. Under these circumstances, if the afferent discharge from the chemoreceptors via the carotid sinus and vagus nerves is stopped, there is a paradoxic further fall in blood pressure rather than a rise.

Hypovolemia causes a marked increase in the circulating levels of the pressor hormones angiotensin II, epinephrine, norepinephrine, and vasopressin. ACTH secretion is also

TABLE 11–6 Compensatory reactions activated by hypovolemia.

Vasoconstriction
Tachycardia
Venoconstriction
Tachypnea → Increased thoracic pumping
Restlessness → Increased skeletal muscle pumping (in some cases)
Increased movement of interstitial fluid into capillaries
Increased secretion of vasopressin
Increased secretion of glucocorticoids
Increased secretion of renin and aldosterone
Increased secretion of erythropoietin
Increased plasma protein synthesis

increased, and angiotensin II and ACTH both cause an acute increase in aldosterone secretion. The resulting retention of Na$^+$ and water helps reexpand blood volume.

Refractory Shock

Some patients with hypovolemia or septic shock die soon after the onset of the condition, and others recover as compensatory mechanisms gradually restore the circulation to normal. In an intermediate group of patients, shock persists for hours and gradually progresses. It eventually reaches a state in which there is no longer any response to vasopressor drugs and in which, even if the blood volume is returned to normal, cardiac output remains depressed. This condition is known as **refractory shock.** It used to be called **irreversible shock,** and patients still die despite vigorous treatment. However, more and more patients are saved as understanding of the pathophysiologic mechanisms increases and treatment is improved. Therefore, "refractory shock" seems to be a more appropriate term.

Various factors appear to make shock refractory. Precapillary sphincters are constricted for several hours but then relax while postcapillary venules remain constricted. Therefore, blood flows into the capillaries and remains there. Various positive feedback mechanisms contribute to the refractory state. For example, cerebral ischemia depresses vasomotor and cardiac discharge, causing blood pressure to fall and making the shock worse. This, in turn, causes a further reduction in cerebral blood flow. In addition, myocardial blood flow is reduced in severe shock. Myocardial failure makes the pumping action of the heart less effective and consequently makes the shock worse and further lowers myocardial blood flow.

A complication of shock that has a very high mortality rate is pulmonary damage with production of acute respiratory distress syndrome. The cause appears to be capillary endothelial cell damage and damage to alveolar epithelial cells with the release of cytokines (see Chapter 9).

Hypovolemic Shock

Hemorrhagic shock is probably the most carefully studied form of shock because it is easily produced in experimental animals. With moderate hemorrhage (5–15 mL/kg body weight), pulse pressure is reduced but mean arterial pressure may remain normal. With more severe hemorrhage, blood pressure always falls.

After hemorrhage, the plasma protein lost in shed blood is gradually replaced by hepatic synthesis, and the concentration of plasma proteins returns to normal in 3–4 days. The increase in circulating erythropoietin increases red blood cell formation, but it takes 4–8 weeks to restore red cell counts to normal.

Traumatic shock develops when there is severe damage to muscle and bone. This is the type of shock seen in battle casualties and automobile accident victims. Bleeding into the injured areas is the principal cause of such shock. The amount of blood that can be lost into a site of injury that appears relatively minor is remarkable; the thigh muscles can accommodate 1 L of extravasated blood, for example, with an increase in the diameter of the thigh of only 1 cm.

Breakdown of skeletal muscle is a serious additional problem when shock is accompanied by extensive crushing of muscle (**crush syndrome**). When pressure on tissues is relieved and they are once again perfused with blood, free radicals are generated, which cause further tissue destruction (**reperfusion-induced injury**). Increased Ca^{2+} in damaged cells can reach toxic levels. Large amounts of K$^+$ enter the circulation. Myoglobin and other products from reperfused tissue can accumulate in kidneys in which glomerular filtration is already reduced by hypotension, and the tubules can become clogged, causing anuria.

Surgical shock is due to combinations, in various proportions, of external hemorrhage, bleeding into injured tissues, and dehydration.

In **burn shock,** there is loss of plasma from burn surfaces and the hematocrit rises rather than falls, producing severe hemoconcentration. There are, in addition, complex metabolic changes. For these reasons, plus the problems of easy infection of burned areas and kidney damage, the mortality rate when third-degree burns cover more than 75% of the body is close to 100%.

Distributive Shock

In distributive shock, most of the symptoms and signs described previously are present. However, vasodilation causes the skin to be warm rather than cold and clammy. **Anaphylactic shock** is a good example of distributive shock. In this condition, an accelerated allergic reaction causes release of large amounts of histamine, producing marked vasodilation. Blood pressure falls because the size of the vascular system exceeds the amount of blood in it even though blood volume is normal.

A second type of distributive shock is **neurogenic shock,** in which a sudden loss of sympathetic autonomic activity (as seen in head and spinal cord injuries) results in vasodilation and pooling of blood in the veins. The resulting decrease in venous return reduces cardiac output and frequently produces fainting, or **syncope,** a sudden transient loss of consciousness. More benign and much more common form is **postural syncope,** which occurs on rising from a sitting or lying position. This is common in patients taking drugs that block sympathetic discharge or its effects on the blood vessels. Falling to the horizontal position restores blood flow to the brain, and consciousness is regained. Pressure on the carotid sinus produced, for example, by a tight collar can cause sufficient bradycardia and hypotension to cause fainting (carotid sinus syncope). Fainting caused by a variety of activities has been given appropriate names such as micturition syncope, cough syncope, deglutition syncope, and effort syncope.

Syncope resulting from neurogenic shock is usually benign. However, it must be distinguished from syncope resulting from other causes and, therefore, merits investigation. About 25% of syncopal episodes are of cardiac origin and are due either to transient obstruction of blood flow through the heart or to sudden decreases in cardiac output caused by various cardiac arrhythmias. In addition, fainting is the presenting symptom in 7% of patients with myocardial infarctions.

Another form of distributive shock is **septic shock.** This condition is discussed in detail in Chapter 4. It is now the most common cause of death in ICUs in the United States. It is a complex condition that includes elements of hypovolemic shock resulting from loss of plasma into the tissues ("third spacing") and cardiogenic shock resulting from toxins that depress the myocardium. It is associated with excess production of NO, and therapy with drugs that scavenge NO may be beneficial.

Streptococcal toxic shock syndrome is a particularly severe form of septic shock in which group A streptococci infect deep tissues; the M protein on the surface of those bacteria has an antiphagocytic effect. It also is released into the circulation, where it aggregates with fibrinogen.

Cardiogenic Shock

When the pumping function of the heart is impaired to the point that blood flow to tissues is no longer adequate to meet resting metabolic demands, **cardiogenic shock** results. This is most commonly due to extensive infarction of the left ventricle but can also be caused by other diseases that severely compromise ventricular function. The symptoms are those of hypovolemic shock plus congestion of the lungs and viscera resulting from failure of the heart to put out all the venous blood returned to it. Consequently, the condition is sometimes called "congested shock." The incidence of shock in pa-tients with myocardial infarction is about 10%, and the mortality rate is 60–90%.

Obstructive Shock

The picture of congested shock is also seen in **obstructive shock.** Causes include massive pulmonary emboli, tension pneumothorax with kinking of the great veins, and bleeding into the pericardium with external pressure on the heart (**cardiac tamponade**). In the latter two conditions, prompt surgery is required to prevent death. Pulsus paradoxus occurs in cardiac tamponade. Normally, blood pressure falls about 5 mm Hg during inspiration. In pulsus paradoxus, this response is exaggerated, and blood pressure falls 10 mm Hg or more as a result of increased pressure of the fluid in the pericardial sac on the external surface of the heart. However, pulsus paradoxus also occurs with labored respiration in severe asthma, emphysema, and upper airway obstruction.

CHECKPOINT

17. What are the four major pathophysiologic forms of shock?
18. Name three pathophysiologic consequences of lactic acidosis in shock.
19. Name three factors that tend to make shock refractory.
20. Describe five specific forms of hypovolemic shock.
21. Name three specific forms of distributive shock and distinguish them from hypovolemic shock.

CASE STUDIES

Eva M. Aagaard, MD, & Yeong Kwok, MD

(See Chapter 25, p. 694 for Answers)

CASE 54

A 56-year-old black man presents to the clinic for a routine physical examination. He has not seen a physician for 10 years. On arrival, he is noted to have a blood pressure of 160/90 mm Hg.

Questions

A. Does this man have hypertension? Why or why not?
B. What physical findings might be present if he has had long-standing hypertension?
C. What are some of the important complications of hypertension?
D. What are some causes of hypertension?

CASE 55

A young woman is brought to the emergency department by ambulance after a severe motor vehicle accident. She is unconscious. Her blood pressure is 64/40 mm Hg; heart rate is 150 beats/min. She is intubated and is being hand-ventilated. There is no evidence of head trauma. The pupils are 2 mm and reactive. She withdraws to pain. Cardiac examination reveals no murmurs, gallops, or rubs. The lungs are clear to auscultation. The abdomen is tense, with decreased bowel sounds. The extremities are cool and clammy, with thready pulses. Despite aggressive blood and fluid resuscitation, the patient dies.

Questions

A. What are the four major pathophysiologic causes of shock? Which was likely in this patient?

B. What pathogenetic mechanism accounts for this patient's unresponsiveness? For the cool, pale extremities?

C. What forms of hypovolemic shock may have been present in this patient? Why?

REFERENCES

General

Chen X et al. Tracking of blood pressure from childhood to adulthood: A systematic review and meta-regression analysis. Circulation. 2008 Jun 24;117(25):3171–80. [PMID: 18559702]

Dampney RA. Functional organization of central pathways regulating the cardiovascular system. Physiol Rev. 1994 Apr;74(2):323–64. [PMID: 8171117]

DiBona GF. Nervous kidney. Interaction between renal nerves and the renin-angiotensin system in the control of renal function. Hypertension. 2000 Dec;36(6):1083–8. [PMID: 11116129]

Ferrara N et al. Clinical applications of angiogenic growth factors and their inhibitors. Nat Med. 1999 Dec;5(12):1359–64. [PMID: 10581076]

Levin ER et al. Natriuretic peptides. N Engl J Med. 1998 Jul 30;339(5):321–8. [PMID: 9682046]

Mark DB et al. B-type natriuretic peptide—A biomarker for all seasons? N Engl J Med. 2004 Feb 12;350(7):718–20. [PMID: 14960748]

Palm F et al. Dimethylarginine dimethylaminohydrolase (DDAH): Expression, regulation, and function in the cardiovascular and renal systems. Am J Physiol Heart Circ Physiol. 2007 Dec;293(6):H3227–45. [PMID: 17933965]

Rubattu S et al. In the search for stroke genes: A long and winding road. Am J Hypertens. 2004 Feb;17(2):197–202. [PMID: 14751665]

Wright SJ. Human embryonic stem-cell research: Science and ethics. Am Sci. 1999;87(4):352.

Atherosclerosis

Anderson TJ et al. Systemic nature of endothelial dysfunction in atherosclerosis. Am J Cardiol. 1995 Feb 23;75(6):71B–74B. [PMID: 7863979]

Becker AE et al. The role of inflammation and infection in coronary artery disease. Annu Rev Med. 2001;52:289–97. [PMID: 11160780]

Brown BG et al. Nicotinic acid, alone and in combinations, for reduction of cardiovascular risk. Am J Cardiol. 2008 Apr 17;101(8A):58B–62B. [PMID: 18375243]

Chou MY et al. Oxidation-specific epitopes are important targets of innate immunity. J Intern Med. 2008 May;263(5):479–88. [PMID: 18410591]

De Caterina R et al. From asthma to atherosclerosis—5-lipoxygenase, leukotrienes, and inflammation. N Engl J Med. 2004 Jan 1;350(1):4–7. [PMID: 14702420]

Hausenloy DJ et al. Targeting residual cardiovascular risk: Raising high-density lipoprotein cholesterol levels. Heart. 2008 Jun;94(6):706–14. [PMID: 18480348]

Klett EL et al. Biomedicine. Will the real cholesterol transporter please stand up? Science. 2004 Feb 20;303(5661):1149–50. [PMID: 14976303]

Knopp RH et al. Comprehensive lipid management versus aggressive low-density lipoprotein lowering to reduce cardiovascular risk. Am J Cardiol. 2008 Apr 17;101(8A):48B–57B. [PMID: 18375242]

Lusis AJ. Atherosclerosis. Nature. 2000 Sep 14;407(6801):233–41. [PMID: 11001066]

Mazzone T et al. Cardiovascular disease risk in type 2 diabetes mellitus: Insights from mechanistic studies. Lancet. 2008 May 24;371(9626):1800–9. [PMID: 18502305]

Plutzky J. A cardiologist's perspective on cardiometabolic risk. Am J Cardiol. 2007 Dec 17;100(12A):3P–6P. [PMID: 18154744]

Steinhubl SR. Why have antioxidants failed in clinical trials? Am J Cardiol. 2008 May 22;101(10A):14D–19D. [PMID: 18474268]

Hypertension

Corvol P et al. Molecular genetics of human hypertension: Role of angiotensinogen. Endocr Rev. 1997 Oct;18(5):662–77. [PMID: 9331547]

Fyhrquist F et al. Renin-angiotensin system revisited. J Intern Med. 2008 Sep;264(3):224–36. [PMID: 18793332]

Gradman AH et al. Renin inhibition in hypertension. J Am Coll Cardiol. 2008 Feb 5;51(5):519–28. [PMID: 18237679]

Izzo JL, Black HR (editors). *Hypertension Primer*, 2nd ed. American Heart Association, 1999.

Lawes CM et al. International Society of Hypertension. Global burden of blood-pressure-related disease, 2001. Lancet. 2008 May 3;371(9623):1513–8. [PMID: 18456100]

Leeman L et al. Hypertensive disorders of pregnancy. Am Fam Physician. 2008 Jul 1;78(1):93–100. [PMID: 18649616]

Matchar DB et al. Systematic review: Comparative effectiveness of angiotensin-converting enzyme inhibitors and angiotensin II receptor blockers for treating essential hypertension. Ann Intern Med. 2008 Jan 1;148(1):16–29. [PMID: 17984484]

Reaven GM et al. Hypertension and associated metabolic abnormalities—The role of insulin resistance and the sympathoadrenal system. N Engl J Med. 1996 Feb 8;334(6):374–81. [PMID: 8538710]

Rubin PC (editor). *Hypertension in Pregnancy.* Elsevier, 2000.

The Seventh Report of the Joint National Committee on Prevention, Detection, Evaluation, and Treatment of Hypertension; the JNC 7 report. JAMA. 2003 May 21;289(19):2560–72. [PMID: 12748199]

Tullus K et al. Renovascular hypertension in children. Lancet. 2008 Apr 26;371(9622):1453–63. [PMID: 18440428]

Turnbull F et al. Effects of different regimens to lower blood pressure on major cardiovascular events in older and younger adults: Meta-analysis of randomised trials. BMJ. 2008 May 17;336(7653):1121–3. [PMID: 18480116]

Wilkinson IB et al. Mind the gap: Pulse pressure, cardiovascular risk, and isolated systolic hypertension. Am J Hypertens. 2000 Dec;13(12):1315–7. [PMID: 11130777]

Wirth A et al. G_{12}-G_{13}-LARG-mediated signaling in vascular smooth muscle is required for salt-induced hypertension. Nat Med. 2008 Jan;14(1):64–8. [PMID: 18084302]

Wolff T et al. Evidence for the reaffirmation of the U.S. Preventive Services Task Force recommendation on screening for high blood pressure. Ann Intern Med. 2007 Dec 4;147(11):787–91. [PMID: 18056663]

Shock

Brown EJ. The molecular basis of streptococcal toxic shock syndrome. N Engl J Med. 2004 May 13;350(20):2093–4. [PMID: 15141050]

Carlet J et al. Sepsis: Time to reconsider the concept. Crit Care Med. 2008 Mar;36(3):964–6. [PMID: 18431286]

Choi PT et al. Crystalloids vs. colloids in fluid resuscitation: A systematic review. Crit Care Med. 1999 Jan;27(1):200–10. [PMID: 9934917]

De Angelo J. Nitric oxide scavengers in the treatment of shock associated with the systemic inflammatory response syndrome. Expert Opin Pharmacother. 1999 Nov;1(1):19–29. [PMID: 11249560]

Dellinger RP et al. International Surviving Sepsis Campaign Guidelines Committee; American Association of Critical-Care Nurses; American College of Chest Physicians; American College of Emergency Physicians; Canadian Critical Care Society; European Society of Clinical Microbiology and Infectious Diseases; European Society of Intensive Care Medicine; European Respiratory Society; International Sepsis Forum; Japanese Association for Acute Medicine; Japanese Society of Intensive Care Medicine; Society of Critical Care Medicine; Society of Hospital Medicine; Surgical Infection Society; World Federation of Societies of Intensive and Critical Care Medicine. Surviving Sepsis Campaign: international guidelines for management of severe sepsis and septic shock: 2008. Crit Care Med. 2008 Jan;36(1):296–327. [PMID: 18158437]

Karlsson S et al. Finnsepsis Study Group. Vascular endothelial growth factor in severe sepsis and septic shock. Anesth Analg. 2008 Jun;106(6):1820–6. [PMID: 18499616]

Landry DW et al. The pathogenesis of vasodilatory shock. N Engl J Med. 2001 Aug 23;345(8):588–95. [PMID: 11529214]

Laupland KB et al. Polyclonal intravenous immunoglobulin for the treatment of severe sepsis and septic shock in critically ill adults: A systematic review and meta-analysis. Crit Care Med. 2007 Dec;35(12):2686–92. [PMID: 18074465]

Levi M et al. Disseminated intravascular coagulation. N Engl J Med. 1999 Aug 19;341(8):586–92. [PMID: 10451465]

O'Brien JM Jr et al. Sepsis. Am J Med. 2007 Dec;120(12):1012–22. [PMID: 18060918]

Pinsky MR. Hemodynamic evaluation and monitoring in the ICU. Chest. Chest. 2007 Dec;132(6):2020–9. [PMID: 18079239]

Topalian S, Ginsberg F, Parrillo JE. Cardiogenic shock. Crit Care Med. 2008 Jan;36(1 Suppl):S66–74. [PMID: 18158480]

Disorders of the Adrenal Medulla

Tobias Else, MD, Gary D. Hammer, MD, PhD, & Stephen J. McPhee, MD

The **adrenal medulla** secretes catecholamines (epinephrine, norepinephrine, and dopamine). The catecholamines help prepare the individual to deal with emergency situations. The major disorder of the adrenal medulla is **pheochromocytoma,** a neoplasm characterized by excessive catecholamine secretion.

NORMAL STRUCTURE & FUNCTION OF THE ADRENAL MEDULLA

ANATOMY

The adrenal medulla is the reddish-brown central portion of the adrenal gland (see Figure 21–2). Accessory medullary tissue is sometimes located in the retroperitoneum near the sympathetic ganglia or along the abdominal aorta (paraganglia) (Figure 12–1).

HISTOLOGY

The adrenal medulla is made up of polyhedral cells arranged in cords or clumps. Embryologically, the adrenal medullary cells derive from neural crest cells. Medullary cells are innervated by cholinergic preganglionic nerve fibers that reach the gland via the splanchnic nerves. The adrenal medulla can be regarded as a specialized sympathetic ganglion, where preganglionic sympathetic nerve fibers (using acetylcholine as a neurotransmitter) directly make contact with postganglionic cells, which secrete catecholamines directly into the circulation. This relationship is analogous to the other sympathetic paraganglions, which connect preganglionic cholinergic sympathetic nerve fibers with postganglionic fibers using catecholamines as neurotransmitters. Medullary parenchymal cells accumulate and store their hormone products in prominent, dense secretory granules, 150–350 nm in diameter. Histologically, these cells and granules have a high affinity for chromium salts (**chromaffin reaction**) and thus are called **chromaffin cells** and contain **chromaffin granules.** The granules contain the catecholamines epinephrine and norepineph-

rine. Morphologically, two types of medullary cells can be distinguished: epinephrine-secreting cells, which have larger, less dense granules, and norepinephrine-secreting cells, which have smaller, very dense granules. Separate dopamine-secreting cells have not been identified. Ninety percent of medullary cells are the epinephrine-secreting type and 10% are the norepinephrine-secreting type.

PHYSIOLOGY

The catecholamines help to regulate metabolism, contractility of cardiac and smooth muscle, and neurotransmission.

Formation, Secretion, & Metabolism of Catecholamines

The adrenal medulla secretes three catecholamines: epinephrine, norepinephrine, and dopamine. Secretion occurs after release of acetylcholine from the preganglionic neurons that innervate the medullary cells. The major biosynthetic pathways and hormonal intermediates for the catecholamines are shown in Figure 12–2. In humans, most (80%) of the catecholamine output of the adrenal medulla is epinephrine. Norepinephrine is principally found in nerve endings of the sympathetic nervous system and in the CNS, where it functions as a major neurotransmitter.

Approximately 70% of the epinephrine and norepinephrine and 95% of the dopamine found in plasma are conjugated to sulfate and inactive. In the supine state, the normal plasma

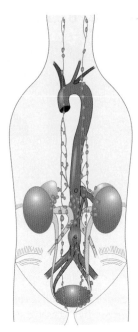

FIGURE 12–1   Anatomic distribution of extra-adrenal chromaffin tissue in the newborn.   (Redrawn, with permission, from Coupland R. *The Natural History of the Chromaffin Cell.* Longman, Green, 1965.)

level of free epinephrine is about 30 pg/mL (0.16 nmol/L); there is a 50–100% increase on standing. The normal plasma level of free norepinephrine is about 300 pg/mL (1.8 nmol/L), and the plasma free dopamine level is about 35 pg/mL (0.23 nmol/L).

Most catecholamine metabolism takes place within the same cells where they are synthesized, mainly because of leakage of catecholamines from vesicular stores into the cytoplasm. These vesicular stores exist in a dynamic equilibrium, with outward passive leakage counterbalanced by inward active transport that is controlled by vesicular monoamine transporters. In catecholaminergic neurons, the presence of monoamine oxidase in the cytoplasm leads to formation of reactive catecholaldehydes. Production of these toxic aldehydes is dependent on the dynamics of the vesicular-axoplasmic monoamine exchange and an enzyme-catalyzed conversion to nontoxic acids or alcohols. In sympathetic nerves, the aldehyde produced from norepinephrine is converted to 3,4-dihydroxyphenylglycol. Subsequent extraneuronal *O*-methylation leads to production of 3-methoxy-4-hydroxyphenylglycol, and its oxidation in the liver catalyzed by alcohol and aldehyde dehydrogenases leads to formation of vanillylmandelic acid (VMA). Compared with intraneuronal deamination, extraneuronal *O*-methylation of norepinephrine and epinephrine to metanephrines represents minor pathways of metabolism.

The single largest source of metanephrines is the adrenal medulla. In the circulation, the catecholamines have a short half-life of about 2 min. Normally, only very small quantities of free epinephrine (about 6 μg/d) and norepinephrine (about 30 μg/d) are excreted, but about 700 μg of VMA is excreted daily.

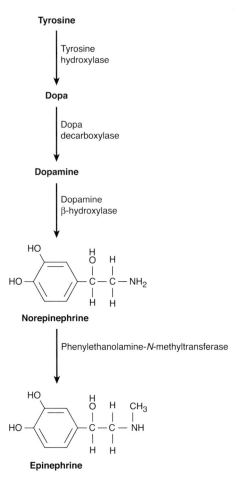

FIGURE 12–2   Biosynthesis of catecholamines.   (Redrawn, with permission, from Greenspan FS, Gardner DG [editors]. *Basic and Clinical Endocrinology,* 7th ed. McGraw-Hill, 2004.)

Regulation of Catecholamine Secretion

Physiologic stimuli affect medullary secretion through the nervous system. Medullary cells secrete catecholamines after release of acetylcholine from the preganglionic neurons that innervate them. Catecholamine secretion is low in the basal state and is reduced even further during sleep. In emergency situations, there is increased adrenal catecholamine secretion as part of a generalized sympathetic discharge that serves to prepare the individual for stress ("fight-or-flight" response). Physiological stress such as psychological, physical (eg, mechanical, thermal), and metabolic (eg, hypoglycemia, exercise) stress lead to catecholamine secretion.

Mechanism of Action of Catecholamines

The effects of epinephrine and norepinephrine are mediated by their actions on two classes of receptors: α- and β-adrenergic receptors (Table 12–1). Alpha receptors are subdivided into α_1 and α_2 receptors and β receptors into β_1, β_2, and β_3 receptors. Alpha$_1$ receptors mediate smooth muscle contraction in blood vessels and the genitourinary (GU) tract and increase glycogenolysis. Alpha$_2$ receptors mediate smooth muscle re-

TABLE 12–1 Physiologic effects of catecholamines on adrenergic receptors of selected tissues.

Organ or Tissue	Adrenergic Receptor	Effect
Heart (myocardium)	β_1	Increased force of contraction (inotropic)
	α_1, β_1	Increased rate of contraction (chronotropic)
	β_1	Increased excitability (predisposes to arrhythmia)
	β_1	Increased AV nodal conduction velocity
Blood vessels (vascular smooth muscle)	α_1, α_2	Vasoconstriction, hypertension
	β_2	Vasodilation
Kidney (juxtaglomerular cells)	β_1	Increased renin release
Gut (intestinal smooth muscle)	α_1	Increased sphincter tone (hyperpolarization); decreased motility (relaxation)
	β_2	Decreased motility (relaxation)
Pancreas (B cells)	α_2	Decreased insulin release
		Decreased glucagon release
	β_2	Increased insulin release
		Increased gluconeogenesis
Liver	α_1, β_2	Increased glucagon release
		Increased glycogenolysis
		Release of potassium
Adipose tissue	α	Decreased lipolysis
	β_1, β_3	Increased lipolysis
Skin (eg, apocrine glands on hands, axillas)	α_1	Increased sweating
Lung (bronchial smooth muscle)	β_2	Dilation of bronchi and bronchioles
Uterus (genitourinary smooth muscle)	α_1	Contraction
	β_2	Relaxation
Bladder (genitourinary smooth muscle)	α_1	Contraction
	β_2	Relaxation
Skeletal muscle	β_2	Vasodilation
		Increased glycogenolysis
		Increased release of lactic acid
Platelets	α_2	Aggregation
CNS	α	Increased alertness, anxiety, fear
Peripheral nerves	α_2	Decreased norepinephrine release
Most tissues	β_3	Increased calorigenesis
		Increased metabolic rate

Modified and reproduced, with permission, from Greenspan FS, Gardner DG (editors). *Basic and Clinical Endocrinology,* 7th ed. McGraw-Hill, 2004.

laxation in the GI tract and vasoconstriction of some blood vessels. Alpha$_2$ receptors also decrease insulin secretion. Beta$_1$ receptors mediate an increased rate and force of myocardial contraction and stimulate lipolysis and renin release. Beta$_2$ receptors mediate smooth muscle relaxation in the bronchi, blood vessels, GU tract, and GI tract and increase hepatic gluconeogenesis and glycogenolysis, muscle glycogenolysis, and release of insulin and glucagon.

Intracellular post-receptor signaling is different for each subclass of adrenergic receptor. Stimulation of α_1-adrenergic receptors results in an increase in intracellular Ca^{2+} concentrations. First, there is activation of phospholipase C by the guanine nucleotide binding stimulatory protein, G_s. Phospholipase C hydrolyzes the membrane-bound phospholipid, phosphatidylinositol-4,5-bisphosphate, to generate two second messengers: diacylglycerol and inositol-1,4,5-trisphosphate. Diacylglycerol in turn activates protein kinase C, which phosphorylates various cellular substrates. Inositol-1,4,5-trisphosphate stimulates release of intracellular Ca^{2+}, which then initiates various cellular responses.

Activation of α_2-adrenergic receptors results in a decrease in intracellular cyclic adenosine 3′,5′-monophosphate (cAMP). The mechanism involves receptor interaction with an inhibitory G protein, G_i, leading to inhibition of adenylyl cyclase. The fall in cAMP level leads to a decrease in activity of the cAMP-dependent protein kinase A. The G_i protein also stimulates K^+ channels and inhibits voltage-sensitive calcium channels.

On the other hand, β-adrenergic receptors stimulate adenylyl cyclase through the mediation of G_s. Activation of β-adrenergic receptors thus leads to an increase in cAMP, activation of the cAMP-dependent protein kinase A, and consequent phosphorylation of various cellular proteins. The G_s protein can also directly activate voltage-sensitive Ca^{2+} channels in the plasma membrane of cardiac and skeletal muscle.

The α_1- and β_1-adrenergic receptors are generally found in organs and tissues (eg, heart and gut) that are heavily innervated by—and situated so as to be readily activated by stimulation of—the sympathetic nerves. The α_1- and β_1-adrenergic receptors are preferentially stimulated by norepinephrine, especially that released by nerve endings. In contrast, the α_2- and β_2-adrenergic receptors are generally situated in postjunctional sites in organs and tissues (eg, uterine and bronchial skeletal muscle) remote from sites of norepinephrine release. The α_2- and β_2-adrenergic receptors are preferentially stimulated by circulating catecholamines, especially epinephrine.

Differences in tissue distribution, accessibility by nerve fibers, preferences for epinephrine versus norepinephrine, and differences in postreceptor signaling are thus responsible for the diverse effects of catecholamines in an organ- and cell-specific manner.

Effects of Catecholamines

The catecholamines have been termed fight-or-flight hormones because their effects on the heart, blood vessels, smooth muscle, and metabolism assist the organism in responding to stress. The principal physiologic effects of the catecholamines are shown in Table 12–1.

In the peripheral circulation, norepinephrine produces vasoconstriction in most organs (via α_1 receptors). Epinephrine produces vasodilation via β_2 receptors in skeletal muscle and liver and vasoconstriction elsewhere. The former usually outweighs the latter, and for that reason epinephrine usually lowers total peripheral resistance.

Norepinephrine causes both systolic and diastolic blood pressures to rise. The rise in blood pressure stimulates the carotid and aortic baroreceptors, resulting in reflex bradycardia and a fall in cardiac output. Epinephrine causes a widening of pulse pressure but does not stimulate the baroreceptors to the same degree, so the pulse rises and cardiac output increases.

Hence, pheochromocytomas or other tumors of the adrenal medulla, which usually secrete norepinephrine, lead to vasoconstriction and an increase in blood pressure.

The effects of catecholamines on metabolism include effects on glycogenolysis, lipolysis, and insulin secretion, mediated by both α- and β-adrenergic receptors. These metabolic effects result primarily from the action of epinephrine on four target tissues: liver, muscle, pancreas, and adipose tissue (see Table 12–1). The result is an increase in the levels of circulating glucose and free fatty acids. The increased supply of these two substances helps provide an adequate supply of metabolic fuel to the nervous system and muscle during physiologic stress.

The amount of circulating plasma epinephrine and norepinephrine needed to produce these various effects has been determined by infusing the catecholamines into resting subjects. For norepinephrine, the threshold for the cardiovascular and metabolic effects is a plasma level of about 1500 pg/mL, or about five times the basal level. In normal individuals, the plasma norepinephrine level rarely exceeds this threshold. However, for epinephrine, the threshold for tachycardia occurs at a plasma level of about 50 pg/mL, or about twice the basal level. The threshold for increasing systolic blood pressure and lipolysis is at about 75 pg/mL; for increasing glucose and lactate, about 150 pg/mL; and for increasing insulin secretion, about 40 pg/mL. In healthy individuals, plasma epinephrine levels often exceed these thresholds.

The physiologic effect of circulating dopamine is unknown. Centrally, dopamine acts to inhibit prolactin secretion. Peripherally, in small doses, injected dopamine produces renal vasodilation, probably by binding to a specific dopaminergic receptor. In moderate doses, it also produces vasodilation of the mesenteric and coronary circulation and vasoconstriction peripherally. It has a positive inotropic effect on the heart, mediated by action on the β_1-adrenergic receptors. Moderate to large doses of dopamine increase the systolic blood pressure without affecting diastolic pressure.

Overview of Adrenal Medullary Disorders

Pheochromocytoma is an uncommon tumor of adrenal medullary tissue that causes production of excessive amounts of catecholamines. Patients typically present with sustained or episodic hypertension or with a syndrome characterized by episodic palpitations, tachycardia, chest pain, headache, anxiety, blanching, excessive sweating, hyperglycemia, and glycosuria. Pheochromocytomas can usually be cured if diagnosed and treated properly. Autopsy series suggest that many pheochromocytomas are not clinically suspected.

PATHOPHYSIOLOGY OF SELECTED DISORDERS OF THE ADRENAL MEDULLA

Pheochromocytomas are the main pathological entity of the adrenal medulla. Other tumors of the adrenal medulla or its embryonic precursors include neuroblastomas and ganglioneuromas. Neuroblastomas are one of the most common tumors of early childhood. In response to therapy (or even spontaneously), neuroblastomas can differentiate into ganglioneuromas. Both of these tumors secrete catecholamines, but symptoms due to catecholamine excess are usually absent because they do not reach the levels observed with pheochromocytomas. Absence of the adrenal medulla (eg, after bilateral adrenalectomy) is usually well tolerated, though sometimes symptoms such as orthostatic hypotension may be observed. Closely related, but different from pheochromocytomas, are parasympathetic nervous system paragangliomas, which often arise in the affected patient's head and neck area.

PHEOCHROMOCYTOMA

Pheochromocytomas are neoplasms of the chromaffin cells of the adrenal medulla or extramedullary sites. These tumors secrete excessive amounts of epinephrine, norepinephrine, or both (rarely dopamine). Most pheochromocytomas secrete norepinephrine and cause sustained or, less commonly, episodic hypertension. Pheochromocytomas that secrete epinephrine cause hypertension less often; more frequently, they produce episodic hyperglycemia, glucosuria, and other metabolic effects.

Table 12–2 summarizes the clinical features of pheochromocytomas. Pheochromocytomas are uncommon, probably found in less than 0.1% of all patients with hypertension and in approximately two individuals per million population. Pheochromocytomas occur in both sexes and in all age groups but are most often diagnosed in the fourth or fifth decade of life. Compared with adults, children with pheo-

chromocytomas are more likely to have multifocal and extra-adrenal tumors, and a causal familial syndrome must always be excluded.

The diagnosis is important because sudden release of catecholamines from these tumors during surgery or obstetric delivery may prove fatal. Pheochromocytoma was classically referred to as "the 10% tumor" because 10% occur in extra-adrenal paraganglia, 10% are outside the abdomen, 10% are multiple, 10% are bilateral, about 10% are not associated with hypertension, 10% occur in children, and 10% are malignant. Recent research has revised some of these numbers. So, previ-

TABLE 12–2 Clinical features of pheochromocytoma.

Epidemiology	Adults; both sexes; all ages, especially 30–50 years
Biologic behavior	90% benign; 10% malignant
Secretion	High levels of catecholamines; most secrete norepinephrine
Clinical presentation	Sustained or less commonly episodic hypertension, sweating, palpitations, hyperglycemia, glycosuria
	Occasionally asymptomatic (found incidentally on CT scan or MRI)
Macroscopic features	Mass, often hemorrhagic; 10% bilateral, 9–23% extra-adrenal
Microscopic features	Nests of large cells, vascular stroma

TABLE 12–3 Major genetic syndromes associated with pheochromocytoma.

Syndrome	Clinical Features	Pheochromocytomas/Paragangliomas	Gene	Locus
MEN-2a	Medullary thyroid carcinoma	50% develop pheochromocytoma	*RET*	10q11.2
	Parathyroid hyperplasia	Bilateral, asynchronous pheochromocytoma		
	Pheochromocytoma			
MEN-2b	Medullary thyroid carcinoma			
	Pheochromocytoma			
	Ganglioneuromas			
	Marfanoid habitus			
NFI	Neurofibromas	0.1–5.0% develop pheochromocytoma (20–50% of hypertensive patients)	*NFI*	17q11.2
	Café-au-lait spots			
	Lisch nodules	90% benign		
	Plexiform neurofibromas			
	Sphenoid dysplasia	10% bilateral		
	Optic gliomas			
	Axillary and inguinal freckling	6% extra-adrenal		
	Pheochromocytoma			
VHL	Hemangioblastomas (brain, spine, retina)	20% develop pheochromocytoma	*VHL*	3p26-25
	Clear-cell renal cell cancer			
	Pheochromocytoma			
PGL1-4	Paraganglioma (parasympathetic or sympathetic)	30% of *SDHB* pheochromocytoma malignant	*PGL1-SDHD*	3p26-25
	Pheochromocytoma		*PGL3-SDHC*	
			PGL4-SDHB	

MEN, multiple endocrine neoplasia; NF1, neurofibromatosis type 1; VHL, von Hippel–Lindau syndrome; PGL, paraganglioma; SDH, succinate dehydrogenase.

Modified, with permission, from Bryant J et al. Pheochromocytoma: The expanding genetic differential diagnosis. J Natl Cancer Inst. 2003;95:1196.

ously, it was thought that about 10% occur as part of a familial syndrome, but now it appears that actually about 20–30% of cases are familial. Also, occurrence at extra-adrenal sites seems to be higher (9–23%) and multifocal pheochromocytomas can be found in roughly one third of childhood cases.

Etiology

Several genetic syndromes, all transmitted in an autosomal dominant fashion, are associated with an increased risk of pheochromocytoma and sympathetic or parasympathetic nervous system paragangliomas (occurring mainly in the head and neck area). Most familial cases are caused by one of four syndromes: neurofibromatosis type 1, von Hippel–Lindau syndrome, multiple endocrine neoplasia type 2 (MEN-2), and familial paraganglioma syndrome (Table 12–3). The genetic basis of these syndromes is now well defined. Patients with

neurofibromatosis type 1 (Recklinghausen's disease) have an increased incidence of pheochromocytoma caused by mutation of the *NF1* gene. Pheochromocytoma is a frequent occurrence in families with von Hippel–Lindau disease, which is caused by mutations of the *VHL* tumor suppressor gene.

In MEN-2a syndrome (Sipple's syndrome), pheochromocytomas occur in association with calcitonin-producing medullary carcinoma or C-cell hyperplasia of the thyroid and parathyroid hormone (PTH)–producing adenomas of the parathyroid. In MEN-2b, pheochromocytomas occur in association with medullary carcinoma of the thyroid and numerous oral mucosal neuromas. About 40% of patients with MEN-2a and MEN-2b have bilateral pheochromocytomas. The gene responsible for MEN-2a and MEN-2b has now been localized to chromosome 10q11.2. In 1993, more than two dozen different families with MEN-2a were found to have missense point mutations of the *RET* proto-oncogene, a tyrosine kinase receptor gene expressed at low levels in normal human thyroid tissue and at high levels in medullary thyroid carcinoma and pheochromocytoma tissue. Subsequently, it was documented that the position of the *RET* mutation is related to disease phenotype. Any mutation of the *RET* proto-oncogene at one specific position (codon 634) is associated with pheochromocytoma as part of MEN-2a and mutations at a different position (codon 918), with pheochromocytoma as part of MEN-2b. These germline mutations of the *RET* proto-oncogene were the first examples of a dominantly acting oncogenic point mutation causing a heritable neoplasm in humans. These missense mutations can be detected by DNA analysis, allowing identification of MEN carriers.

More recently, it has been determined that other familial cases of pheochromocytoma, also transmitted in autosomal dominant fashion, are caused by germline mutations in genes coding for subcomponents of the succinate-dehydrogenase complex (*SDHD, SDHB, SDHC*).

Germline mutations in *RET, VHL, SDHB, SDHC,* and *SDHD* taken together account for more than 20% of cases of isolated pheochromocytomas. Among all patients with pheochromocytoma, including those with known hereditary syndrome or a positive family history, the frequency of germline mutations in these four genes together approaches 30%. Given the high frequency of germline mutations, some experts now recommend genetic evaluation, genetic counseling, and perhaps genetic testing for all patients with pheochromocytomas, particularly those with a positive family history, multifocal disease, or a diagnosis before age 50 years. However, this age cutoff may not capture all hereditary cases; for example, the mean age at the diagnosis in *SDHD* pheochromocytomas is 43 years. Genetic testing may also be useful in screening families of carriers of mutations detected.

Almost all pheochromocytomas (about 90%) occur in the abdomen, and most of these (85%) are in the adrenal medulla. Extra-adrenal pheochromocytomas (including sympathetic and parasympathetic paragangliomas) are found in the perirenal area, the organ of Zuckerkandl, the urinary bladder, the heart, the neck, and the posterior mediastinum (Figure 12–1). Some of these tumors can lead to very specific symptoms (eg, urinary bladder pheochromocytoma can cause a hypertensive crisis with voiding). Extra-adrenal pheochromocytomas account for 10% of all pheochromocytomas in adults and 30–40% of pheochromocytomas in children. They are usually larger than adrenal pheochromocytomas.

Grossly, pheochromocytomas are generally well-circumscribed but vary in size, with weights ranging from less than 1 g to several kilograms (Figure 12–3). They are highly vascular tumors and frequently have cystic, necrotic, or hemorrhagic areas. Microscopically, the tumor consists of large pleomorphic cells arranged in sheets separated by a highly vascular stroma. In the cytoplasm, there are catecholamine-containing storage granules similar to those in normal adrenal medullary cells. Mitoses are rare, but tumor invasion of the adrenal capsule and blood vessels is common even in benign pheochromocytomas. About 10% of pheochromocytomas are

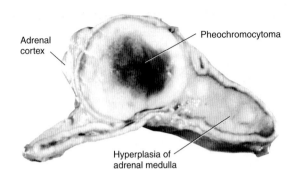

FIGURE 12–3 Cross section of adrenal, showing a pheochromocytoma associated with hyperplasia of the medulla in a patient with multiple endocrine neoplasia type IIa. He also had a medullary carcinoma of the thyroid and a large pheochromocytoma in the opposite adrenal. (Reproduced, with permission, from Chandrasoma P, Taylor CE. *Concise Pathology,* 3rd ed. Originally published by Appleton & Lange. Copyright © 1998 by the McGraw-Hill Companies, Inc.)

malignant. Malignancy is established only when a metastasis is found in a site where chromaffin cells are not usually demonstrated (eg, liver, lung, bone, or brain). Unfavorable prognostic factors suggesting a malignant course include large tumor size, local extension, younger age, DNA aneuploid tumors, and *SDHB* mutation.

Pathogenesis

Most pheochromocytomas release predominantly norepinephrine, but most also release epinephrine (Table 12–4). Rarely, a pheochromocytoma releases mostly or only epinephrine and very rarely mostly or only dopamine.

In about half of patients with pheochromocytoma, clinical manifestations vary in intensity and occur in an episodic or paroxysmal fashion. The paroxysms are related to sudden catecholamine discharge from the tumor. The sudden catecholamine excess causes hypertension, palpitations, tachycardia, chest pain, headache, anxiety, blanching, and excessive sweating. Such paroxysms usually occur several times a week but may occur only once every few months or up to 25 times daily. Paroxysms typically last for 15 minutes or less but may last for days. As time passes, the paroxysms usually become more frequent but generally do not change in character. A typical paroxysm may be produced by activities that compress the tumor (eg, bending, lifting, exercise, defecation, eating, or deep palpation of the abdomen) and by emotional distress or anxiety.

Other patients have persistently secreting tumors and more chronic symptoms, including sustained hypertension. However, such patients also usually experience paroxysms related to transient increases in catecholamine release. The long-term exposure to high levels of circulating catecholamines seems not to produce the classic hemodynamic responses observed after acute administration of catecholamines. This may be due in part to desensitization of the cardiovascular system to cate-

TABLE 12–4 Pathophysiologic and clinical manifestations of catecholamine excess.

Target Tissue	Physiologic Effect	Catecholamine Excess	
		Pathophysiologic Manifestations	Clinical Manifestations
Heart	Increased heart rate	Tachycardia	Palpitations
		Tachyarrhythmia	Angina pectoris
	Increased contractility	Increased myocardial O_2 consumption	Angina pectoris
		Myocarditis	Congestive heart failure
		Cardiomyopathy	
Blood vessels	Arteriolar constriction	Hypertension	Headache
			Congestive heart failure
			Angina pectoris
	Venoconstriction	Decreased plasma volume	Dizziness
			Orthostatic hypotension
			Circulatory collapse
Gut	Intestinal relaxation	Impaired intestinal motility	Ileus
			Obstipation
Pancreas (B cells)	Suppression of insulin release	Carbohydrate intolerance	Hyperglycemia
			Glucosuria
Liver	Increased glucose output	Carbohydrate intolerance	Hyperglycemia
			Glucosuria
Adipose	Lipolysis	Increased free fatty acids	Weight loss
Skin (apocrine glands)	Stimulation	Sweating	Diaphoresis
Bladder neck	Contraction	Elevated urethral pressures	Urinary retention
Most tissues	Increased basal metabolic rate	Increased heat production	Heat intolerance
			Sweating
			Weight loss

Modified, with permission, from Werbel SS, Ober KP. Pheochromocytoma: Update on diagnosis, localization, and management. Med Clin North Am. 1995;79:131.

cholamines and may explain why some patients with pheochromocytomas are entirely asymptomatic.

Clinical Manifestations

The clinical manifestations of pheochromocytoma are due to increased secretion of epinephrine and norepinephrine. Commonly reported manifestations are listed in Table 12–5.

The classical pentad of symptoms in patients with pheochromocytoma consists of: headache, palpitation, perspiration, pallor, and orthostasis. The most common presenting feature of pheochromocytoma is hypertension. In about half of cases, hypertension is sustained but the blood pressure shows marked fluctuations, with peak pressures during symptomatic paroxysms. During a hypertensive episode, the systolic blood pressure can rise to as high as 300 mm Hg. In about one third of cases, hypertension is truly intermittent. In some individuals with pheochromocytoma, hypertension is absent. The blood pressure elevation caused by the catecholamine excess results from two mechanisms: α receptor–mediated vasoconstriction of arterioles, leading to an increase in peripheral resistance; and $β_1$ receptor–mediated increases in cardiac output and in renin release, leading to increased circulating levels of angiotensin II. The increased total peripheral vascular resistance is probably primarily responsible for the maintenance of high arterial pressures.

TABLE 12–5 Clinical findings in pheochromocytoma.

Symptoms	Frequency (%)
Spells	67
Headache	59
Palpitations	50
Diaphoresis	50
Fainting episode	40
Bone pain	35
Weight loss	30
Anxiety	19
Nausea, vomiting	19
Dizziness	18
Flushing	14
Weakness, fatigue	14
Abdominal pain	14
Dyspnea	13
Paresthesias	13
Constipation	11
Chest pain	12
Flank pain	7
Visual symptoms	7
Diarrhea	6
Signs	
Hypertension	92
Sustained	48
Paroxysmal	44
Fever	28
Tachycardia	15
Orthostatic hypotension	12
Palpable mass	8
Shock	4
Laboratory findings	
Hyperglycemia	42
Hypercalcemia	4
Polycythemia	3

Modified, with permission, from Werbel SS, Ober KP. Pheochromocytoma: Update on diagnosis, localization, and management. Med Clin North Am. 1995;79:131.

Hypertensive crisis may be precipitated by a variety of drugs, including tricyclic antidepressants, antidopaminergic agents, metoclopramide, and naloxone. Beta-blockers should not be administered until alpha blockade has been established. Otherwise, blockade of β_2-adrenergic receptors, which promote vasodilation, will allow unopposed α-adrenergic receptor activation and produce marked vasoconstriction and hypertension.

Peripheral vasoconstriction, mediated by α receptors, causes both facial pallor and cool, moist hands and feet. Chronic vasoconstriction of the arterial and venous beds leads to a reduction in plasma volume and predisposes to postural hypotension. In others, orthostatic hypotension is associated with decreased cardiac stroke volume and an impaired response of total peripheral vascular resistance to changes in posture, perhaps indicative of diminished arteriolar and venous responsiveness. The reduced responsiveness of the vasculature to norepinephrine in patients with pheochromocytoma is probably related to downregulation of α-adrenergic receptors resulting from persistent elevations of norepinephrine levels.

Complications of pheochromocytoma are summarized in Table 12–6. If unrecognized and untreated, pheochromocytoma may be complicated by hypertensive retinopathy (retinal hemorrhages or papilledema); nephropathy; myocardial infarction, resulting from either myocarditis or coronary artery vasospasm; pulmonary edema, secondary either to left-sided congestive heart failure or noncardiogenic causes; and stroke from cerebral infarction, intracranial hemorrhage, or embolism. Cerebral infarction results from hypercoagulability, vasospasm, or both. Hemorrhage occurs secondary to severe arterial hypertension. Emboli can originate in mural thrombi in patients with dilated cardiomyopathy.

Ileus and obstipation are typical. However, diarrhea may occur as a result of rare adrenal production of vasoactive intestinal peptide (VIP) or dopamine.

In pregnancy, pheochromocytoma may lead to significant maternal morbidity and fetal demise.

The metabolic effects of excessive circulating catecholamines increase both blood glucose and free fatty acid levels. Increased glycolysis and glycogenolysis, combined with an α-adrenergic receptor–mediated inhibition of insulin release, cause the increase in blood sugar levels. In addition, epinephrine stimulates glucose production by gluconeogenesis and decreases insulin-mediated glucose uptake by peripheral tissues such as skeletal muscle. In pheochromocytoma, impaired glucose homeostasis may also result from β-adrenergic receptor desensitization, which produces relative insulin resistance. Glucose intolerance is common, and diabetes mellitus may occur.

Epinephrine raises blood lactate concentrations by stimulation of glycogenolysis and glycolysis. An increase in oxygen consumption from catecholamine stimulation of metabolism occurs in combination with a decrease in oxygen delivery to tissues from vasoconstriction, leading to lactate accumulation.

TABLE 12–6 Complications of pheochromocytoma.

Cardiovascular	**Renal**
Arrhythmias	Renal artery stenosis (resulting from kinking by adrenal mass)
Ventricular tachycardia	Renal infarction
Torsades de pointes	**Endocrine and metabolic**
Wolff-Parkinson-White syndrome	Hyperglycemia, glucose intolerance, diabetic ketoacidosis
Ventricular fibrillation	Hypoglycemia
ECG changes	Thyrotoxicosis (transient)
ST segment elevations or depressions	Reactivation of Graves' disease
Inverted or flattened T waves	Hypercalcemia
Prolonged QT intervals	Lactic acidosis
High or peaked P waves	Fever
Cardiomyopathy	**Skeletal**
Dilated	Osseous microthrombi (from hemoconcentration)
Hypertrophic	Brachydactyly
Left ventricular hypertrophy	**Skin**
Myocarditis	Leukocytoclastic vasculitis
Subendocardial, intramyocardial hemorrhages	**Crisis**
Acute myocardial infarction	Obtundation, shock, disseminated intravascular coagulation, seizures, rhabdomyolysis, acute renal failure, death
Pulmonary	
Pulmonary edema (noncardiogenic)	
Gastrointestinal	
Ileus	
Obstipation	
Megacolon	
Acute abdominal pain	

Occasionally, pheochromocytomas may also produce peptide hormones leading to specific paraneoplastic phenomena. For example, hypercalcemia may occur, related to excessive production of PTH-related peptide (PTHrP) in cases of malignant pheochromocytomas (as in some other malignancies) or to excessive production of PTH itself in cases of pheochromocytoma associated with MEN-2a–related hyperparathyroidism. Occasionally, ectopic production of adrenocorticotropic hormone (ACTH) by pheochromocytoma may lead to "ectopic" Cushing's syndrome. Rare cases have been described in which a pheochromocytoma produces vasoactive intestinal peptide (VIP) (causing severe diarrhea), growth hormone–releasing hormone (GHRH) (causing acromegaly), corticotropin-releasing hormone (CRH) (Cushing's syndrome), insulin (hypoglycemia), or other peptide hormones.

An increase in metabolic rate may cause weight loss (or, in children, lack of weight gain), and impaired heat loss from peripheral vasoconstriction may cause a mild elevation of basal body temperature, heat intolerance, flushing, or increased sweating.

During paroxysms, patients may experience marked anxiety, and when episodes are prolonged or severe, there may be visual disturbances, paresthesias, or seizures. A feeling of fatigue or exhaustion usually follows these episodes. Some patients present with psychosis or confusion.

There may be abdominal discomfort resulting from a large adrenal mass. Remarkably, some patients with pheochromocytomas are entirely asymptomatic.

Somewhat different clinical manifestations occur with predominantly epinephrine-releasing pheochromocytomas. Symptoms and signs include hypotension, prominent tachycardia, widened pulse pressure, cardiac arrhythmias, and noncardiogenic pulmonary edema. Acute hemorrhagic necrosis of the tumor may present initially as acute abdominal pain with marked hypertension, followed by hypotension, shock, and sudden death as a consequence of sudden cessation of catecholamine production ("fulminant pheochromocytoma crisis"). Death may also result from cardiovascular collapse secondary to prolonged vasoconstriction and loss of blood volume into the interstitium.

Patients with pure epinephrine-producing pheochromocytomas may be hypotensive because of epinephrine-induced peripheral vasodilation. Other patients with severe arterial vasoconstriction may appear to be in shock. In still others, the prolonged vasoconstriction of a hypertensive crisis may lead to shock.

Pheochromocytoma is diagnosed by demonstrating abnormally high concentrations of catecholamines or their breakdown products in the plasma or urine. Increases in plasma metanephrine concentrations are greater and more consistent than increases in plasma catecholamines or urinary metanephrines. This is perhaps because metanephrines persist in plasma longer than catecholamines and exhibit less variability in response to changes in posture. A reliable assay showing increased plasma or urine levels of metanephrines is usually sufficient to establish the diagnosis. If the patient has paroxysmal symptoms, sampling of blood or timed urine collections during an episode may be needed to establish the diagnosis. Studies have shown significant positive correlations between excretion of catecholamine metabolites and tumor volume.

Pheochromocytoma tumor cells produce large amounts of metanephrines from catecholamines leaking from stores and metabolized by catechol-*O*-methyltransferase (COMT) present in pheochromocytoma cells. Thus, these metabolites are particularly useful for detecting pheochromocytomas. Thus, the elevated plasma levels of free meta-nephrines in patients with pheochromocytoma are probably due mostly to metabolism before and not after release of the catecholamines into the circulation.

Plasma levels of chromogranin A (found in chromaffin granules) are significantly higher in patients with malignant pheochromocytomas than in those with benign tumors. Thus, markedly elevated chromogranin A levels may point to the diagnosis of a malignant pheochromocytoma. Serum chromogranin A levels can also be monitored during chemotherapy of malignant pheochromocytomas to gauge tumor response and to detect relapse.

Administration of the antihypertensive agent clonidine can be used to differentiate essential hypertension from hypertension caused by pheochromocytoma. This potent α_2 agonist stimulates α_2 receptors in the brain, reducing sympathetic outflow and blood pressure. A dose of 0.3 mg is given orally, and blood pressure and plasma catecholamine levels are determined periodically over the next 3 hours. Essential hypertension is partly dependent on centrally mediated catecholamine release. Administering clonidine normally suppresses sympathetic nervous system activity and substantially lowers plasma norepinephrine levels, reducing blood pressure. However, in patients with pheochromocytoma, the drug has little or no effect on plasma catecholamine levels because these tumors, which are not thought to be innervated, behave autonomously. Thus, the blood pressure remains unchanged.

Once a diagnosis of pheochromocytoma is made, the next step is to localize the neoplasm or neoplasms radiographically to permit surgical removal. Computed tomography (CT) or magnetic resonance imaging (MRI) can be used in tumor localization. CT and MRI have good sensitivity but poor specificity for detecting pheochromocytomas. Nuclear imaging studies such as iodine-131–metaiodobenzylguanidine scintigraphy or indium-111–DTPA-D-Phe-pentetreotide scanning have limited sensitivity but better specificity in diagnosis. For example, the specificity of ^{131}I-metaiodobenzylguanidine scintigraphy is very good for confirming that a tumor is a pheochromocytoma and for ruling out metastatic disease. In addition, 6-[fluorine-18]-fluorodopamine positron emission tomography can aid in both diagnosis and localization of the tumor in patients with positive biochemical test results. Some pheochromocytomas also express somatostatin receptors and can be imaged with an OctreoScan, which uses radiolabeled somatostatin receptor agonists.

Surgery in patients with pheochromocytoma, including resection of the tumor itself, involves the risk of significant complications. Operative and postoperative complications are directly associated with preoperative systolic blood pressure, tumor size, excretion of urinary catecholamines and their metabolites, duration of anesthesia, and number of surgeries. Understanding the pathophysiology of pheochromocytoma is critically important in preparing the patient for surgery. For example, as noted previously, it is important that hypertension not be treated with beta-blockers, which could cause paradoxic worsening of hypertension by allowing unopposed α stimulation. Instead, an α receptor blocker, such as phenoxybenzamine, can be used effectively.

CHECKPOINT

7. What genetic mutations are found in patients with pheochromocytoma?
8. What are the symptoms and signs of pheochromocytoma?
9. What are some complications of untreated pheochromocytoma?
10. What are the metabolic and neurologic effects of pheochromocytoma?
11. How is the diagnosis of pheochromocytoma made?

CASE STUDIES

Eva M. Aagaard, MD, & Yeong Kwok, MD

(See Chapter 25, p. 694 for Answers)

CASE 56

A 39-year-old woman comes to the office complaining of episodic anxiety, headache, and palpitations. She states that without dieting she has lost 15 pounds over the past 6 months. Physical examination is normal except for a blood pressure of 200/100 mm Hg and a resting pulse rate of 110 bpm. Chart review shows that prior blood pressures have always been normal, including one 6 months ago. A diagnosis of pheochromocytoma is entertained.

Questions

A. What other features of the history should be elicited? Why is family history important?

B. What laboratory tests should be ordered, and what results should be anticipated? If the laboratory tests are nondiagnostic and suspicion is high, what other test can be done?

C. What is the pathogenesis of the symptoms of anxiety, headache, palpitations, and weight loss in pheochromocytomas?

REFERENCES

General

Eisenhofer G et al. Catecholamine metabolism: A contemporary view with implications for physiology and medicine. Pharmacol Rev. 2004 Sep;56(3):331–49. [PMID: 15317907]

Goldfien A. Adrenal medulla. In: *Basic and Clinical Endocrinology*, 6th ed. Greenspan FS, Gardner DG (editors). McGraw-Hill, 2001.

Parmer RJ et al. Catecholaminergic pathways, chromaffin cells, and human disease. Ann N Y Acad Sci. 2002 Oct;971:497–505. [PMID: 12438170]

Vaughan ED Jr. Diseases of the adrenal gland. Med Clin North Am. 2004 Mar;88(2):443–66. [PMID: 15049587]

Pheochromocytoma

Failor RA et al. Hyperaldosteronism and pheochromocytoma: New tricks and tests. Prim Care. 2003 Dec;30(4):801–20. [PMID: 15024897]

Karagiannis A et al. Pheochromocytoma: an update on genetics and management. Endocr Relat Cancer. 2007 Dec;14(4):935–56. [PMID: 18045948]

Martin M et al. Pheochromocytoma: Risk groups, diagnosis and management in primary care. Hospital Physician. 2006;42:17–24.

Pacak K et al. Recent advances in genetics, diagnosis, localization, and treatment of pheochromocytoma. Ann Intern Med. 2001 Feb 20;134(4):315–29. [PMID: 11182843]

Tischler AS. Pheochromocytoma and extra-adrenal paraganglioma: Updates. Arch Pathol Lab Med. 2008 Aug;132(8):1272–84.

Gastrointestinal Disease

Jason C. Mills, MD, PhD,
Thaddeus S. Stappenbeck, MD, PhD,
& Nigel Bunnett, PhD

Gastrointestinal (GI) diseases most often present with one or more of four common classes of symptoms and signs: (1) abdominal or chest pain; (2) altered ingestion of food (eg, resulting from nausea, vomiting, **dysphagia** [difficulty swallowing], **odynophagia** [painful swallowing], or **anorexia** [lack of appetite]); (3) altered bowel movements (ie, diarrhea or constipation); and (4) GI tract bleeding, either occurring without warning or preceded by one or more of the foregoing (Table 13–1). However, not all cases of a particular GI disease present in the same way. For example, peptic ulcer disease, although typically accompanied by abdominal pain, may be painless.

GI disease may be limited to the GI tract (eg, reflux esophagitis, peptic ulcer, diverticular disease), be a manifestation of a systemic disorder (eg, inflammatory bowel disease), or present as a systemic disease resulting from a primary GI pathologic process (eg, vitamin deficiencies resulting from malabsorption). Because different parts of the GI tract are specialized for certain functions, the most prominent causes, consequences, and manifestations of disease differ from one anatomic site to another.

Acutely, GI disease can be complicated by dehydration, sepsis, or bleeding or by their consequences, such as shock. **Dehydration** can occur as a consequence of even subtle alterations in fluid input or outflow because the volume of fluid traversing the GI tract daily is enormous (see later discussion). **Sepsis** can result from disruption of the barrier function against pathogens in the environment, including bacteria resident in the colon. The tendency for **bleeding** is a reflection of the tremendous vascularity of the GI tract and the difficulty of applying pressure at the site of bleeding.

Chronically, GI disease can be complicated by malnutrition and deficiency states. These occur because many primary GI diseases result in **malabsorption** (failure to absorb one or more necessary nutrients in ingested food).

GI tract disease can present as partial or complete **obstruction** (blockage of movement of contents down the GI tract) caused by **adhesions** and **stenosis** resulting from proliferation of connective tissue in response to inflammation. The symptoms and signs of obstruction can range from mild nausea, abdominal pain, and anorexia to projectile vomiting and rebound tenderness. In severe cases, obstruction can result in perforation, infarction and bleeding, hypotension, shock, sepsis, and death. The severity of symptoms depends on the extent of obstruction, the degree to which the obstruction compromises blood flow to the affected region, and the stage in the natural history of the process at which the patient presents for medical attention.

CHECKPOINT

1. What are the cardinal symptoms and signs of GI disease?
2. What are some acute systemic complications of primary GI disease?
3. What additional systemic manifestations can occur as a result of chronic GI disease?

STRUCTURE, FUNCTION, & CONTROL OF THE GI TRACT

STRUCTURE OF THE GI TRACT

The GI tract is one of the most complex and important organ systems. It comprises the alimentary canal, a hollow structure extending from the mouth to the anus, and associated glandular organs (salivary glands, pancreas, gallbladder, and liver) that empty their contents into the canal (Figure 13–1). The GI tract, which is 7–9 m in the adult, includes the mouth, esophagus

TABLE 13–1 Common presentations of GI disease.

Cardinal GI Symptom or Sign	Esophagus	Stomach	Intestines	Gallbladder
Pain	Achalasia, reflux	Gastric ulcer Gastric cancer	Duodenal ulcer Irritable bowel syndrome Diverticular disease	Cholelithiasis
Altered ingestion				
Dysphagia	Achalasia, reflux			
Nausea, vomiting	Achalasia, reflux Esophageal cancer	Gastroparesis	Acute gastroenteritis Obstruction	Cholelithiasis
Altered bowel movements				
Constipation			Diverticular disease Diabetic autonomic neuropathy	
Diarrhea (including steatorrhea)		Gastric surgery, dumping syndrome	Gastroenteritis Irritable bowel syndrome Inflammatory bowel disease Diabetic autonomic neuropathy	Cholelithiasis
Bleeding				
Hematemesis	Varices resulting from portal hypertension	Gastric ulcer Mucosal laceration (eg, after violent retching)	Duodenal ulcer	
Bloody stools (including melena, frank blood, and occult blood)	Varices	Gastric ulcer	Inflammatory bowel disease Duodenal ulcer Diverticular disease Colon cancer Gastroenteritis Infarction	

(23–25 cm), stomach, small intestine (duodenum, jejunum, ileum; 6–7 m), large intestine (cecum and colon; 1.0–1.5 m), rectum, and anus. The GI tract is connected to the salivary glands, the pancreas, and the gallbladder, the sources of **exocrine** secretions that play an essential role in digestion.

The wall of the GI tract is composed of four main layers. From the lumen outward, these include the **mucosa, submucosa, muscularis externa,** and **serosa** (Figure 13–2). The precise structure of some of these layers, most notably the mucosa, varies from one region of the GI tract to the next. The **mucosa** has three components: specialized epithelial cells that line the lumen; the underlying **lamina propria,** a layer of connective tissue that contains small blood and lymphatic vessels, immune cells and nerve fibers; and the **muscularis mucosa,** a thin layer of muscle cells. The muscularis mucosa is an important boundary in determining whether cancer of the GI tract is still local-

ized to its site of origin or is likely to have metastasized (ie, spread to distant regions of the body). The **submucosa** is a layer of loose connective tissue directly beneath the mucosa containing larger blood and lymphatic vessels and a nerve plexus of the intrinsic or **enteric nervous system,** termed the **submucosal nerve (Meissner's) plexus.** This nerve plexus is particularly important for control of secretion in the GI tract. In some areas, the submucosa also contains glands and lymphoid tissue. The **muscularis externa** is composed of an inner circular and an outer longitudinal layer of smooth muscle and is responsible for motility of the GI tract. Between these muscle layers lies the **myenteric nerve (Auerbach's) plexus,** a division of the enteric nervous system that regulates motility. The **serosa** is an outer sheath of squamous epithelial cells and connective tissues, where larger nerves and blood vessels travel in a bed of connective and adipose tissue.

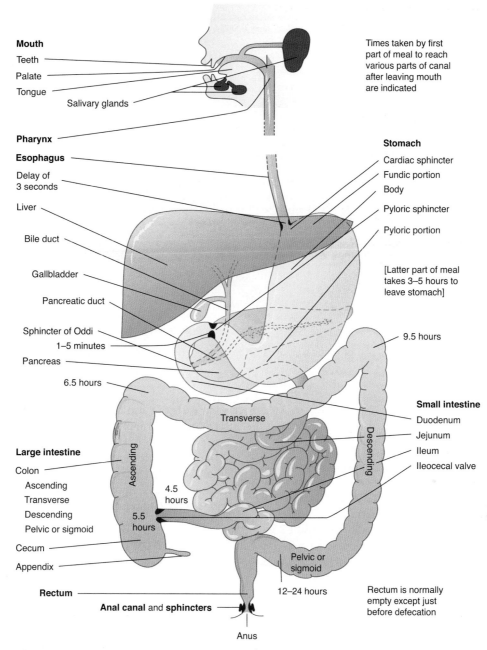

Mouth
Teeth
Palate
Tongue
Salivary glands

Pharynx

Esophagus
Delay of
3 seconds

Liver

Bile duct

Gallbladder

Pancreatic duct

Sphincter of Oddi
1–5 minutes

Pancreas

6.5 hours

Large intestine
Colon
    Ascending
    Transverse
    Descending
    Pelvic or sigmoid
Cecum
Appendix

Ascending

Transverse

Descending

4.5
hours

5.5
hours

Rectum

Anal canal and **sphincters**

Anus

Times taken by first
part of meal to reach
various parts of canal
after leaving mouth
are indicated

Stomach
Cardiac sphincter
Fundic portion
Body
Pyloric sphincter
Pyloric portion

[Latter part of meal
takes 3–5 hours to
leave stomach]

9.5 hours

Small intestine
Duodenum
Jejunum
Ileum
Ileocecal valve

Pelvic or
sigmoid

12–24 hours

Rectum is normally
empty except just
before defecation

FIGURE 13–1 Progress of food along the alimentary canal. Food undergoes mechanical as well as chemical changes to render it suitable for absorption and assimilation. (Redrawn, with permission, from Mackenna BR, Callander R. *Illustrated Physiology*, 6th ed. Churchill Livingstone, 1997.)

FUNCTIONS OF THE GI TRACT

The overall function of the GI tract is to take in nutrients and process them to a form that can be used by the body and to eliminate wastes. The major physiological processes that occur in the GI tract are **digestion, secretion, motility,** and **absorption.**

A. Digestion

Food is taken into the mouth as large particles containing macromolecules that are not immediately absorbable into the body. **Digestion** is the process that converts nutrients in food to products that can be **absorbed** by cells of the mucosa. Digestion includes **physical processes** (eg, chewing, GI contractions) that break up the food, mix it with digestive secretions, and propel it along the alimentary canal, and **chemical processes** (eg, digestive enzymes) that degrade food components (proteins, fats, polysaccharides) to products that can be absorbed (amino acids, fatty acids, monosaccharides). Digestive enzymes arise from exocrine glands (salivary gland, pancreas, gallbladder, and liver) and from cells and glands in the mucosa or are found on the apical surface of certain epithelial cells.

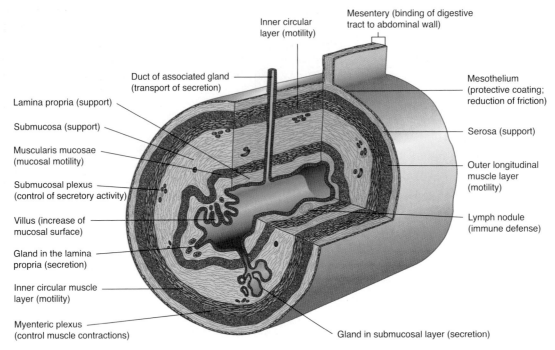

FIGURE 13–2 Schematic structure of a portion of the digestive tract with various possible components.   (Redrawn, with permission, from Bevelander G. *Outline of Histology*, 7th ed. Mosby, 1971.)

B. Secretion

During the process of digestion, large volumes of fluid are **secreted** into the lumen of the GI tract. Secretions arise from exocrine glands (salivary glands, pancreas, gallbladder) and from epithelial cells lining the gastrointestinal lumen (or glands that connect to the lumen). The daily fluid load in the GI tract is approximately 2 L of oral intake and 7 L of secretions (1.5 L saliva, 2.5 L gastric juice, 0.5 L bile, 1.5 L pancreatic juice, and 1 L intestinal secretions). From this total of 9 L, approximately 100 mL ends up in stool daily; the balance is recycled (Figure 13–3).

C. Motility

Secretions and luminal contents are moved from mouth to anus and mixed by a process termed **motility,** because of the coordinated contractions of smooth muscle. Smooth muscle cells have a resting membrane potential (small excess of negative charge) in their interior as a result of the activity of pumps in the plasma membrane. When a cell is depolarized, this potential difference is transiently abolished, generating a signal that (1) triggers events within that cell, leading to sliding of actin and myosin filaments, and (2) is propagated to neighboring cells, resulting in the coordinated response of muscle contraction. Depolarization of a cell can occur spontaneously or in response to a neural or hormonal stimulus depending on the specific characteristics of different cells. GI smooth muscle displays differences in contractile properties in different regions of the tract. "Slow-wave" oscillating depolarizations occur in some areas and rapid "spike" depolarizations in other areas. Each type occurs with a characteristic intrinsic frequen-

cy, but each can also be triggered by specific stimuli such as stretch, neuronal input, or hormones. Short bursts of spikes cause phasic motor activity; longer bursts cause tonic muscle contraction. Tonic contraction occurs at **sphincters** ("gates" that allow further movement down the GI tract only during relaxation). Phasic electrical activity occurs at the intervening regions of the GI tract (between sphincters).

D. Absorption

The products of digestion (amino acids, small peptides, monosaccharides, fatty acids) are taken into the body by the process of **absorption.** Absorbed molecules can pass across (**transcellular**

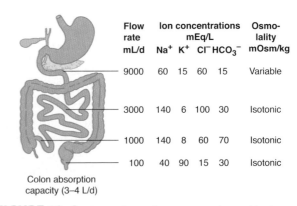

	Flow rate mL/d	Ion concentrations mEq/L				Osmolality mOsm/kg
		Na⁺	K⁺	Cl⁻	HCO₃⁻	
	9000	60	15	60	15	Variable
	3000	140	6	100	30	Isotonic
	1000	140	8	60	70	Isotonic
	100	40	90	15	30	Isotonic

Colon absorption capacity (3–4 L/d)

FIGURE 13–3   Approximate flow rates per day and ionic constituents of fluid passing through different levels of the intestine.   (Redrawn, with permission, from Fine KD, Krejs GJ, Fordtran JS. Diarrhea. In: *Gastrointestinal Disease*, 5th ed. Sleisenger MH, Fordtran JS [editors]. Saunders, 1993.)

route) or between (**paracellular route**) the epithelial cells lining the intestine to enter the blood or lymphatic systems. In general, this transport can occur by either a **passive,** energy-independent mechanism that occurs down an **electrochemical gradient** (of charge or concentration), or by an **active,** energy-requiring process that occurs against an electrochemical gradient. **Passive transport** can occur by simple **diffusion** (random molecular motion) of uncharged molecules that readily pass the lipid layer plasma membrane. In this manner, short-chain fatty acids are absorbed in the small intestine. Charged molecules that cannot cross the plasma membrane diffuse through specialized **channels** (transmembrane proteins) within the apical and basolateral membrane of epithelial cells. For instance, water is absorbed by diffusion through water channels or aquaporins in the small intestine. Some molecules that are absorbed by diffusion bind to transporter proteins in the plasma membrane that facilitate their transfer into the cell (**facilitated diffusion**). For example, fructose is absorbed into epithelial cells of the small intestine by facilitated diffusion through the apical membrane GLUT-5 transporter.

Active transport requires metabolic energy. There are two classes of active transport. In **primary active transport,** the transport molecule itself hydrolyzes adenosine triphosphate (ATP). An example of primary active transport is the Na-K ATPase found in the basolateral membrane of intestinal epithelial cells, which expels three Na^+ ions from cells in exchange for two K^+ ions that are pumped into the cell. This unequal transport of ions generates a transmembrane potential (negative inside; ie, transport is **electrogenic**). In **secondary active transport,** the

transporter itself does not hydrolyze ATP, but transport depends on an electrochemical gradient that has been established by primary active transport. The Na-K ATPase maintains a low intracellular Na^+ concentration and an inside negative potential in epithelial cells, thereby providing the electrochemical gradient for secondary active transport of many absorbed molecules. For example, glucose is absorbed against a concentration gradient across the apical membrane of epithelial cells in the small intestine by secondary active transport with Na^+ ions by the SGLT1 transporter. Two Na^+ ions are transported down their electrochemical gradient (generated by the Na-K ATPase), dragging with them one glucose molecule. For large molecules such as proteins, transport occurs by pinching off from, and fusion of membrane vesicles with, the plasma membrane. These processes are termed **endocytosis** (uptake into epithelial cells) and **exocytosis** (export out of epithelial cells).

In addition to the major roles of the GI tract that are related to digestion and absorption, the digestive tract has other functions that are essential for maintenance of health and homeostasis.

E. Defense

The mucosa of the GI tract is the largest surface of the body that is exposed to the environment, and the gut, like the skin, must protect the body from the external environment. Defense involves protection against ingested toxins, bacteria, and viruses, as well as the bacteria and toxins that normally exist in the large intestine (Table 13–2). The magnitude of the problem

TABLE 13–2 Mechanisms of defense of the GI tract (and features of structure and function involved).

Forms of Defense	Structural Adaptations	Functional Adaptations	Mechanism of Defense
Defense from acid			
Mucus production	Large numbers of mucus-secreting stomach surface cells	Mucin gene expression	Prevents direct contact of acid with epithelium
Bicarbonate production (alkaline tide)	Duodenal Brunner's glands		Neutralizes any acid that breaches epithelium
Prostaglandin production	Specialized prostaglandin-producing cells in lamina propria	Cyclo-oxygenase 1 and 2 (COX1/2) gene expression	Attenuates acid production
Tight junctions	Tight junction formation		Prevents breach of epithelium
Bicarbonate from pancreas	Pancreatic duct opening into duodenum	Response of secretin to gastric acid	Neutralizes acid leaving stomach
Defense from infection			
Secretory immune system	Mucosa-associated lymphoid tissue and transcytotic epithelial cells	Machinery for transcytosis of immunoglobulin	Extends to GI tract lumen the protective umbrella of blood-borne immunity
Rapid epithelial cell turnover	Cell proliferation in glands/crypts; cell release into lumen		Limits the consequences of enterocyte infection
Normal colonic microbiota		Induce expression of specific antimicrobial proteins (angiogenin4, Reg3γ)	
Stomach acid	Gastric glands containing parietal cells	Multiple humoral controls on acid secretion (histamine, acetylcholine, and gastrin)	Kills pathogenic organisms on ingestion

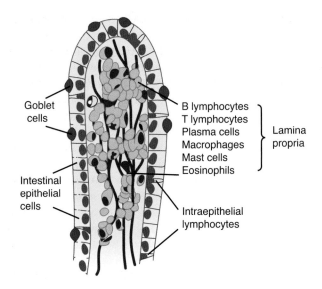

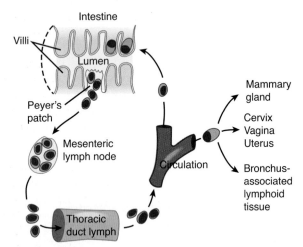

FIGURE 13–4 Systemic and local features of gut immunology. (Redrawn, with permission, from Kagnoff M. Immunology and disease of the gastrointestinal tract. In: *Gastrointestinal Disease*, 6th ed. Sleisenger MH, Fordtran JS [editors]. Saunders, 1998.)

is illustrated by the observation that there are more bacterial cells in the human colon than cells in the entire body. Defense involves two mechanisms.

1. **Immunologic defense**—The mucosal immune system or gut-associated lymphoid tissue (GALT) comprises Peyer's patches (aggregates of lymphoid cells in the small intestine) and diffuse populations of mucosal immune cells (Figure 13–4). The GALT protects against bacteria, viruses, and toxins and allows tolerance to potentially immunogenic dietary substances and bacteria.

2. **Nonimmunologic defense**—These mechanisms include secretion of gastric and intestinal fluid, electrolytes and mucus, and the tight junctions between epithelial cells. The secretions neutralize and flush away potentially damaging bacteria and macromolecules, and the tight junctions prevent their ingress into tissues.

Certain peptides secreted into the intestinal lumen contribute to defense and healing. **Defensins** are antimicrobial peptides that are secreted by epithelial cells in the intestine. They form holes in bacterial cell walls and prevent them from colonizing the small intestine. **Trefoil peptides** are secreted into the lumen of the GI tract with mucus. Among their many effects, they appear to promote healing of mucosal lesions.

F. Regulation of Fluid and Electrolyte Balance

The small intestine receives 8–9 L of fluid with electrolytes per day and secretes a further 1 L and electrolytes per day. Most of the fluid is absorbed. Thus, secretion and absorption must be regulated to maintain balance. Increased secretion or diminished absorption causes diarrhea, which can be fatal because of fluid and electrolytes loss.

G. Excretion

Undigested food products, bacteria, and certain heavy metals (eg, copper and iron excreted in bile) are excreted in feces.

CHECKPOINT

4. What are the major functions of the GI tract?
5. Describe the four major layers of a cross-section through the GI tract.
6. What volumes of fluid are transferred into and out of the GI tract each day?
7. Describe the general mechanism of electrolyte transport across epithelial cells.
8. Describe the defense mechanism of the GI tract.

MECHANISMS OF REGULATION OF THE GI TRACT

The processes of motility, secretion, digestion, and absorption are under close physiologic regulation by nerves, hormones, and paracrine substance (Figure 13–5).

A. Neural Control

There are two components of GI innervation.

1. **Intrinsic innervation by the enteric nervous system**—The enteric nervous system is the third division of the autonomic nervous system (Figure 13–6). An enteric neuron has its cell body within the wall of the GI tract and is thus intrinsic to the gut. The enteric nervous system comprises a series of ganglionated nerve plexuses that extend from the esophagus to the rectum, which are organized into two principal components: 1) the myenteric, or Auerbach's, plexus, which

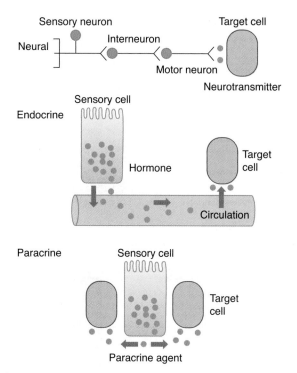

FIGURE 13–5 Neural, endocrine, and paracrine mechanisms of control in the GI tract.

is sandwiched between the layers of the muscularis externa; and 2) the submucosal or Meissner's plexus, which lies in the submucosa. The enteric nervous system is very extensive, containing as many neurons as are present in the spinal cord. It contains sensory or afferent neurons (sometimes called intrinsic primary afferent neurons [**IP-ANs**]) that sense the environment (eg, intestinal pH, osmolality, wall stretch), interneurons (the connectors), and

secretomotor or efferent neurons that control many cell types to stimulate or inhibit motility, secretion, absorption, and immune function of the GI tract. In this manner, the enteric nervous system can regulate the GI tract in a reflex manner without input from the CNS. For this reason, it is often called the "little brain." Enteric neurons use many neurotransmitters, most notably **neuropeptides.**

The degree to which the CNS regulates the enteric nervous system varies with region. The characteristic functions of structures derived from the embryonic foregut (eg, esophageal peristalsis, relaxation of the lower esophageal sphincter, gastric accommodation and peristalsis, pyloric sphincter function) are more dependent on CNS control. However, functions of structures derived from the embryonic midgut and hindgut (eg, intestinal peristalsis and mucosal secretion) can continue without input from the CNS.

The clinical importance of the enteric nervous system is seen in clinical syndromes in which its function is lost, which can occur at several levels. In esophageal achalasia, for example, as a result of enteric nervous system defects, the body of the esophagus is quiet and the lower sphincter is tonically contracted, making ingestion of food difficult or impossible. Similarly, loss of enteric nervous system function in syndromes of pseudo-obstruction of the small bowel or Hirschsprung's disease in the colon have severe clinical consequences, including abdominal pain, distension, and a risk of catastrophic intestinal perforation.

2. **Extrinsic innervation by parasympathetic and sympathetic nerves**—Extrinsic neurons that innervate the GI tract have cell bodies outside of the gut wall and allow a bidirectional communication between the brain and the gut (**the brain-gut axis**) (Figure 13–7). This communication can regulate the function of the enteric nervous system or directly control the activity of other cell types.

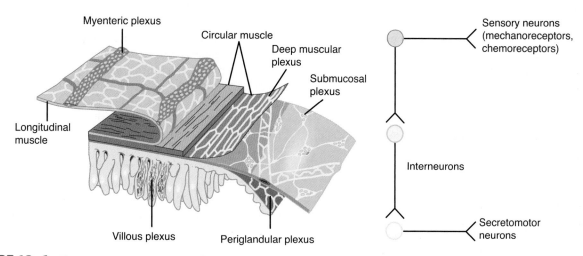

FIGURE 13–6 The enteric nervous system. **Left:** Enteric nervous system of the small intestine shows that enteric neurons are organized in two nerve plexuses, the submucosal plexus and myenteric plexus, with other plexuses including the deep muscular, periglandular, and villous plexus. (Redrawn with permission from Costa M, Furness JB, Llewellyn-Smith IJ. Histochemistry of the enteric nervous system. In: *Physiology of the Gastrointestinal Tract*, 2nd ed, Johnson LR [editor]. Raven Press, 1987.) **Right:** The enteric nervous system includes sensory neurons, interneurons, and motor neurons. Complete reflex arcs exist within the enteric nervous system.

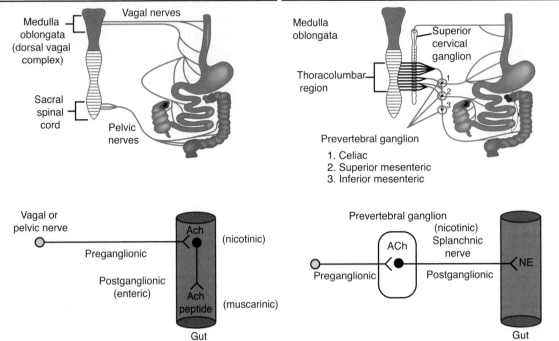

FIGURE 13–7 The extrinsic innervation of the GI tract by the parasympathetic and sympathetic nerves. Preganglionic parasympathetic nerves from the medulla and the sacral spinal cord project fibers in the vagal and pelvic nerves, respectively, to the wall of the GI tract and innervate enteric neurons that serve as postganglionic parasympathetic nerves. Preganglionic sympathetic nerves project fibers from the thoracolumbar regions of the spinal cord to the prevertebral ganglia, where they innervate postganglionic sympathetic nerves that project to the GI tract. Both the parasympathetic and sympathetic preganglionic nerves release acetylcholine (ACh), which activates nicotinic receptors on postganglionic nerves. Postganglionic parasympathetic nerves release acetylcholine and peptides, whereas postganglionic sympathetic nerves release norepinephrine (NE).

In **parasympathetic innervation**, the vagus nerve (cranial nerve X) innervates the esophagus, stomach, gallbladder, pancreas, and the first part of intestine, cecum, and proximal colon. The pelvic nerve from the sacral spinal cord innervates the distal colon and the rectum. Preganglionic cell bodies in the medulla (vagus) or sacral spinal cord (pelvic nerve) project fibers to some enteric neurons in the gut wall, which are thus in a sense postganglionic parasympathetic nerves. The preganglionic nerves use acetylcholine as a neurotransmitter, which activates **nicotinic receptors** on enteric neurons. The postganglionic enteric nerves use acetylcholine (acting on **muscarinic receptors**) and neuropeptides as neurotransmitters. Parasympathetic stimulation can stimulate and inhibit GI functions.

In **sympathetic innervation**, preganglionic sympathetic nerves arise from cell bodies in the thoracic spinal cord and project fibers to prevertebral ganglia (celiac, cranial, and caudal mesenteric ganglion). They release acetylcholine as a neurotransmitter that interacts with **nicotinic** receptors on the postganglionic nerves. Postganglionic fibers innervate some enteric neurons or directly innervate effector cells in the GI tract, such as vascular smooth muscle cells. Norepinephrine is

the major postganglionic neurotransmitter. Sympathetic innervation is often inhibitory to GI functions.

Regarding **extrinsic sensory nerves,** parasympathetic and sympathetic nerves tracts also carry sensory fibers from the gut to cell bodies that are located in nodose ganglia and the dorsal root ganglia, respectively. Cell bodies in the nodose and dorsal root ganglia then project fibers to the brain stem (from nodose ganglia) or spinal cord (from dorsal route ganglia). Sensory nerve fibers in the wall of the GI tract detect mucosal pH and osmolality and can respond to amino acids or glucose, temperature, tension, and touch. In this manner, the extrinsic sensory nerves sense changes in the environment of the intestine and trigger central reflexes that initiate secretomotor changes to maintain normal homeostasis. Extrinsic sensory nerves also contribute to GI inflammation and pain. Sensory nerve endings in the wall of the gut detect noxious chemical and mechanical stimuli, including acid, inflammatory agents, and distension. These stimuli trigger the release of the neuropeptides, substance P, and calcitonin gene-related peptide, from the endings of sensory nerves within the gut wall, where they induce extravasation of plasma proteins and infiltration of granulocytes and arteriolar vasodilatation to cause neurogenic inflammation. The same stimuli induce release of neuropeptides from the central projections of these neurons, where they participate in pain transmission. Additional research is required to define the mechanisms of neurogenic inflammation and GI pain.

B. Hormonal Control

Hormones are blood-borne messengers released from endocrine cells or glands into the circulation, which carries them to distant target cells (Figure 13–5). This mechanism of endocrine regulation was discovered in the GI tract in 1902, when Bayliss and Starling discovered the hormone **secretin** in the small intestine and showed that it stimulates secretion from the exocrine pancreas. Since then, a large number of hormones have been identified in all regions of the GI tract. In this respect, the GI tract is the largest endocrine organ.

GI hormones have several characteristics in common. They are secreted from endocrine cells that are scattered throughout the mucosa of the stomach and intestine rather than being concentrated in specialized glands. This diffuse distribution made purification a truly Herculean task: Many hundreds of kilograms of intestine were required to isolate a few milligrams of pure hormone. GI hormones are invariably peptides, and many of these peptides are present not only in endocrine cells but also in nerves of the enteric system and CNS (Table 13–3). Thus, they have dual functions as hormones and neurotransmitters. After feeding, there are elevated levels of many GI hormones in the circulation. When administered to reproduce postprandial plasma concentrations, these hormones have multiple biological effects, ranging from the stimulation of gastric acid secretion to the suppression of appetite. The physiologic role of some GI hormones has been clearly established by demonstration that antagonists of hormone receptors block certain physiologic processes. However, in many cases, such antagonists are not available, and the physiologic relevance of hormones that cannot be antagonized remains to be determined.

C. Paracrine Control

Many substances that are used for intercellular signaling are rapidly removed from the extracellular fluid by uptake into nearby cells or by enzymatic degradation. Such substances have a short half-life in the extracellular fluid and are consequently only capable of regulating neighboring cells. Paracrine substances are released from nonneuronal sensory cells and neurons and regulate the function of neighboring cells rather than influencing distant organs by passage through the circulation (Figure 13–5 and Table 13–3). Examples include **histamine** and **somatostatin**, which are released from cells in the stomach to control acid secretion, and **serotonin (5-hydroxytryptamine** [5-HT]), which is released in the small intestine to control activity of the vagus nerve.

CHECKPOINT

9. What are the three general mechanisms of control observed in the GI tract?
10. What are the two components of the enteric nervous system?
11. What are the three general types of enteric neuron?
12. Describe the parasympathetic and sympathetic innervation of the GI tract.
13. What is the relationship between the enteric and central nervous systems?

GI Smooth Muscle

A. Structure of GI Smooth Muscle

The two principal muscle layers that control motility of the GI tract are the inner circular layer and the outer longitudinal layer of the muscularis externa. They vary in thickness in different regions of the GI tract. For example, the muscles are thickened in the gastric antrum, where strong contractions break up food before it can enter the small intestine, and muscle layers are thickened to form sphincters. Most of the GI muscle is **smooth muscle,** except the pharynx, parts of the esophagus, and the external anal sphincter, which are made up of **striated** (skeletal) muscle. GI smooth muscle is similar to smooth muscle in other organs: Fusiform cells are packed together in bundles by connective tissue sheaths. **Gap junctions** between cells allow signals to readily pass from cell to cell so that the contraction of bundles occurs synchronously. **Interstitial cells of Cajal** form an extensive network of stellate cells in the muscle layers of the stomach and intestine that are intimately associated with smooth muscle cells and enteric neurons (Figure 13–8). They may have two functions. First, they transmit information from enteric neurons to the smooth muscle cells. Second, they are the **pacemaker cells,** which have the capacity to generate the basic electrical rhythm or slow waves that are a consistent feature of GI smooth muscle. Animals lacking interstitial cells of Cajal show markedly abnormal GI motility, including defective gastric emptying and intestinal stasis or ileus. Defects in interstitial cells of Cajal may be associated with motility disturbances in patients, and this is an area of active investigation.

B. Electrophysiology of GI Smooth Muscle

GI smooth muscle cells have a resting membrane potential of –40 to –80 mV as a result of the relative conductances of K^+, Na^+, and Cl^- ions. An electrogenic Na^+-K^+ ATPase contributes significantly to the resting membrane potential. Less is known about the electrophysiological properties of interstitial cells of Cajal, in part because of difficulties in isolating these cells for study. The resting membrane potential of smooth muscle cells varies characteristically with time and is called a slow wave or basic electrical rhythm. Slow waves occur at 3–5/min in the stomach and at 12–20/min in the intestine. Interstitial cells of Cajal set the frequency of the slow waves, and slow waves are

TABLE 13–3 **Secretory products of the GI tract.**

Products	Physiologic Actions	Site of Release	Stimulus for Release	Disease Association
True hormones				
Gastrin	Stimulates acid secretion and growth of gastric oxyntic gland mucosa	Gastric antrum (and duodenum)	Peptides, amino acids, distension, vagal stimulation	Zollinger-Ellison syndrome, peptic ulcer disease
CCK	Stimulates gallbladder contraction, pancreatic enzyme and bicarbonate secretion, and growth of exocrine pancreas	Duodenum and jejunum	Peptides, amino acids, long-chain fatty acids, (acid)	
Secretin	Stimulates pancreatic bicarbonate secretion, biliary bicarbonate secretion, growth of exocrine pancreas, pepsin secretion; inhibits gastric acid secretion, trophic effects of gastrin	Duodenum	Acid (fat)	
GIP	Stimulates insulin release; (inhibits gastric acid secretion)	Duodenum and jejunum	Glucose, amino acids, fatty acids	
Candidate hormones				
Motilin	Stimulates gastric and duodenal motility	Duodenum and jejunum	Unknown	Irritable bowel syndrome; diabetic gastroparesis
Pancreatic polypeptide	Inhibits pancreatic bicarbonate and enzyme secretion	Pancreatic islets of Langerhans	Protein (fat and glucose)	
Enteroglucagon	Elevates blood glucose?	Ileum	Glucose and fat	
Paracrines				
Somatostatin	Inhibits release of most other peptide hormones	GI tract mucosa, pancreatic islets of Langerhans	Acid stimulates, vagus inhibits release	Gallstones
Prostaglandins	Promote blood flow, increase mucus and bicarbonate secretion from gastric mucosa	Multiple	Various	NSAID-induced gastritis and ulcer disease
Histamine	Stimulates gastric acid secretion	Oxyntic gland mucosa	Gastrin and unknown others	
Neurocrines				
VIP	Relaxes sphincters and gut circular muscle; stimulates intestinal and pancreatic secretion	Mucosa and smooth muscle of GI tract	Enteric nervous system	Secretory diarrhea
Bombesin	Stimulates gastrin release	Gastric mucosa	Enteric nervous system	
Enkephalins	Stimulate smooth muscle contraction; inhibit intestinal secretion	Mucosa and smooth muscle of GI tract	Enteric nervous system	
Other products				
Intrinsic factor	Binds vitamin B_{12} to facilitate its absorption	Parietal cells of the stomach	Constitutive secretion	Autoimmune destruction resulting in pernicious anemia
Mucin	Lubrication and protection	Goblet cells along entire intestinal mucosa and surface cells in stomach	GI tract irritation	Viscid mucus in cystic fibrosis. Attenuation in some cases of peptic ulcer
Acid	Prevents infection; initiates digestion	Parietal cells of the stomach	Gastrin, histamine, acetylcholine, NSAIDs (indirectly)	Acid-peptic disease

Parentheses indicate minor components and effects.

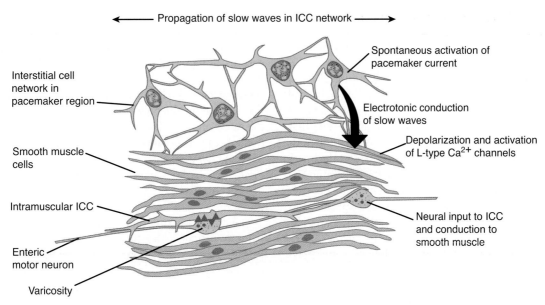

← Propagation of slow waves in ICC network →

Interstitial cell network in pacemaker region

Smooth muscle cells

Intramuscular ICC

Enteric motor neuron

Varicosity

Spontaneous activation of pacemaker current

Electrotonic conduction of slow waves

Depolarization and activation of L-type Ca^{2+} channels

Neural input to ICC and conduction to smooth muscle

FIGURE 13–8 Diagrammatic view of interstitial cells of Cajal (ICC) in the intestine, showing their interaction with enteric nerves and smooth muscle cells.

transmitted between cells through gap junctions. Nerves and hormones modulate the amplitude of slow waves. Depending on the amplitude of the slow waves and the excitability of the smooth muscle, slow waves can give rise to action potentials. If the slow-wave depolarization reaches a threshold, a train of action potentials will fire. Action potentials depolarize the membrane of the smooth muscle cells and induce an influx of Ca^{2+} ions into the cytoplasm through voltage-sensitive Ca^{2+} channels in the plasma membrane and from intracellular stores, causing contraction. What causes an action potential to occur? The presence of neurotransmitters or hormones that are released close to the smooth muscle cells alters the resting membrane potentials of the cells, which makes the oscillations in membrane potential (the slow waves) more or less likely to reach threshold and initiate an action potential. However, not all slow waves induce action potentials and resultant contractions. The explanation is that inhibitory motor neurons of the GI tract are highly active and thus prevent generation of action potentials and contractions. Action potentials and contractions can only occur when these inhibitory motor neurons are switched off by input from interneurons. Thus, the tonic inhibition serves to contrail the inherent excitability of the pacemaker cells.

C. Mechanical Properties of GI Smooth Muscle

Several characteristic patterns of contraction can be observed in GI smooth muscle. **Tonic contractions** are best represented by sphincters that act as one-way valves to prevent retrograde movement of material from distal to more proximal regions and thus to facilitate flow in an aboral direction. The proximal parts of the stomach and the gallbladder also exhibit tonic contractions. **Peristaltic contractions** are moving waves of contraction that propel digesta along the GI tract. Peristalsis involves neurally mediated contraction of smooth muscle on

the oral side of a bolus of digesta and a neurally mediated relaxation of muscle on the anal side of the digesta. Peristalsis occurs in the pharynx, esophagus, gastric antrum, and small and large intestine. **Segmental contractions** produce narrow contracted segments between relaxed segments. These movements allow mixing of the luminal contents with GI tract secretions and increase exposure to mucosal surfaces where absorption occurs. Segmentation occurs in the stomach and intestine. **Pathologic patterns of motility** include **spasms,** which are very strong and often painful contractions that occur continuously in a dysregulated manner, and **ileus,** where there is a markedly decreased or absent contractile activity. Ileus often results from irritation of the peritoneum involved in surgery, peritonitis, and pancreatitis. Further research is required to understand the mechanisms of these abnormal contractions, which may lead to improved therapies.

CHECKPOINT

14. What are the positive and negative regulators of smooth muscle cell action potentials?
15. What are the functions of interstitial cells of Cajal?
16. What are the general types of contractions observed in the GI tract after feeding?

OROPHARYNX & ESOPHAGUS

Anatomy & Histology

The oropharynx provides entry to the GI tract during swallowing and to the respiratory tract during breathing. It includes the vocal cords, which separate the two tracts and provide the structural basis for speech. Much of the oropharynx is lined with a respiratory-type ciliated pseudocolumnar epithelium.

The esophagus is a hollow tube (25–30 cm long, 2–3 cm wide). The wall of the esophagus consists of an epithelial cell layer, an inner layer of circular muscle, a myenteric nerve plexus, and an outer layer of longitudinal muscle. The first third of esophagus is composed of striated muscle, the middle third is mixed striated and smooth muscle, and the lower third is purely smooth muscle. The esophagus is delimited by an **upper esophageal sphincter** (a distinct thickening of striated circular muscle) and a **lower esophageal sphincter** (a tonically contracted 3–4 cm ring of smooth muscle). The two sphincters generate small luminal zones of high pressure, whereas the rest of the esophageal lumen is at a pressure equal to the surrounding body cavities. Between swallows, the two sphincters are closed, preventing entry of air and gastric acid into the esophagus. Regulation of the lower esophageal sphincter is especially important because it controls the passage of digesta into the stomach and prevents the reflux of gastric contents into the esophagus, where they can damage the mucosa. Between swallows, the lower esophageal sphincter is contracted, in large part by vagal cholinergic mechanisms. During swallowing, vagal inhibitory fibers allow the lower esophageal sphincter to relax, possibly because of release of inhibitory neurotransmitters from enteric nerves, including nitric oxide and vasoactive intestinal peptide (VIP).

Swallowing Reflex

Swallowing begins as a voluntary process that rapidly becomes an involuntary reflex mechanism. During the voluntary oral phase, the tongue pushes a bolus of food to the back of the mouth and into the oropharynx. From there on, the process is involuntary. In the **pharyngeal phase,** the food bolus stimulates touch receptors in the pharynx. Sensory signals pass by the glossopharyngeal, vagal, and trigeminal nerves to the swallowing center in the medulla and pons. Motor impulses pass through cranial nerves to control an involuntary process that directs food into the esophagus and away from the airway. Breathing is interrupted and the soft palate is elevated, closing the pharyngeal opening of the nasopharynx and preventing food from entering the internal openings of the nostrils. The tongue is pressed against the hard palate, closing the oral opening of the pharynx. The glottis is pulled under the epiglottis, which blocks the laryngeal opening. Cartilages around the larynx are pulled together, further restricting food from entering the respiratory tract. When all openings to the pharynx are closed, a wave of muscular contraction pushes the bolus of food toward the opening of the esophagus. As the food reaches the esophagus, the upper esophageal sphincter relaxes to accept the material and then closes after the bolus has moved through. The **esophageal phase** of swallowing begins when the bolus passes through the upper esophageal sphinc-

ter. Vagal stretch receptors in the wall of the esophagus detect distension by the bolus and induce a **vagovagal** reflex, during which vagal motor nerves induce a wave of contraction that spreads along the esophagus at 3–5 cm/s. This is termed **primary peristalsis** (Figure 13–9). As the wave of primary peristalsis reaches the lower esophageal sphincter, the sphincter relaxes to allow the bolus to enter the stomach. Distension of the esophagus by the bolus can initiate another wave of contraction called **secondary peristalsis.** Often repetitive waves of secondary peristalsis are required to clear the esophagus of food. Various hormones and neurotransmitters, foods, and drugs can affect the tone of the lower esophageal sphincter pressure.

The importance of oropharyngeal motility and its control is seen in patients who have had strokes or are demented. Inability to swallow properly often makes them unable to manage their own oral secretions, resulting in aspiration of oral contents into the lungs with development of pneumonia. This is a common cause of death in individuals with these kinds of CNS disorders. Disordered lower esophageal sphincter tone is a major cause of esophageal reflux, presenting as heartburn.

CHECKPOINT

17. What is the histologic difference between the proximal one third and the distal two thirds of the esophagus?
18. What are the functions of the upper and lower esophageal sphincters, and how are they regulated?
19. Describe the three phases of the swallowing reflex.

STOMACH

Anatomy & Histology

The stomach is a complex glandular organ that is guarded by two sphincters: the lower esophageal sphincter and the **pyloric sphincter** (Figure 13–10). The mucosa is composed of simple glands, consisting of a pit, neck, and a base, that markedly increase the surface area and are lined with specialized epithelial cells. The stomach can be divided into several regions on the basis of structure and function. The **cardia** is a small region just distal to the lower esophageal sphincter that does not secrete acid. The **corpus,** or **body,** is the major part of the stomach. Gastric glands in the corpus contain **parietal cells,** which secrete **hydrochloric acid** and **intrinsic factor,** and **chief cells,** which secrete **pepsinogen.** The corpus is a reservoir that is a major site of gastric digestion. The **pyloric antrum** is the distal region of the stomach that secretes the hormone **gastrin** from G cells. It is highly muscular, grinds food, and regulates gastric emptying. All regions of the stomach secrete mucus and bicarbonate.

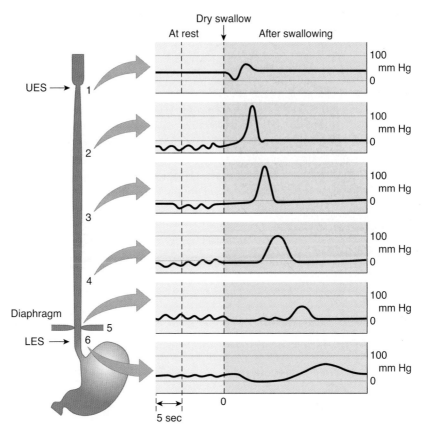

FIGURE 13–9 Primary peristalsis of the esophagus. The tracings show pressures in the indicated regions of the esophagus at rest and at various times after swallowing. UES, upper esophageal sphincter; LES, lower esophageal sphincter. (Redrawn from data in Conklin JL, Christensen J. Motor functions of the pharynx and esophagus. In: *Physiology of the Gastrointestinal Tract*, 3rd ed., Johnson LR [editor]. New York, LIppincott-Raven, 1994.)

Gastric Acid Secretion

A number of products are secreted from the stomach. Of these, hydrochloric acid is perhaps the most important from a pathophysiologic standpoint. Secretion of acid by the parietal cells of the gastric glands occurs in a basal diurnal pattern but can be stimulated by such diverse factors as the thought of food, distension of the stomach, and protein ingestion.

A. Molecular Mechanisms of HCl Secretion

The mechanisms by which parietal cells secrete HCl into the stomach have been intensively studied because of the importance of acid secretion to digestion and in disease states. Parietal cells are pyramidal in shape. Their membranes express a **H^+-K^+ ATPase**, a primary active transporter that is responsible for the secretion of HCl. Parietal cells undergo a remarkable change in appearance when stimulated to secrete HCl (Figure 13–11). In the unstimulated state, a tubulovesicular network that contains the H^+-K^+ ATPase characterizes the cells. On activation, the tubulovesicular membranes fuse with the plasma membrane to form a canalicular membrane with microvilli. The result is an increase in the area of the apical membrane by 50–100 fold and insertion of more H^+-K^+ ATPase pumps into the plasma membrane. This rearrangement promotes HCl secretion.

The H^+-K^+ ATPase is a heterodimer of an α-subunit (the catalytically active unit) and a β-subunit (involved in determining the intracellular location). The H^+-K^+ ATPase pumps H^+ ions from the cell across the apical membrane in exchange for K^+ ions (Figure 13–11). This is an example of primary active transport that is driven by ATP, which pumps H^+ ions against an enormous concentration gradient (1 million:1). Tight junctions between cells prevent the reentry of H^+ ions into the mucosa. The K^+ ions that have entered the cells then recycle to the lumen or enter interstitial fluid by K^+ channels. To maintain electroneutrality, Cl^- ions are secreted passively across the apical membrane into the lumen through Cl^- channels, forming HCl. The secreted H^+ ions are provided by H_2O and CO_2, which form H_2CO_3. Carbonic anhydrase generates H^+ ions for secretion and HCO_3^- ions, which enter the interstitial fluid by exchange for Cl^- ions. Cl^- ions enter against their electrochemical gradient, driven by efflux of HCO_3^- down an electrochemical gradient. The secretion of HCO_3^- into the blood forms the **"alkaline tide,"** which can lead to alkalosis when H^+ ion secretion is excessive. Water movement maintains the osmotic balance in all regions.

An understanding of the mechanisms of HCl secretion by parietal cells permitted the development of **proton pump inhibitors** (**PPIs**), a class of drugs that inhibit the H^+-K^+ ATPase. Drugs such as omeprazole, a benzimidazole, are

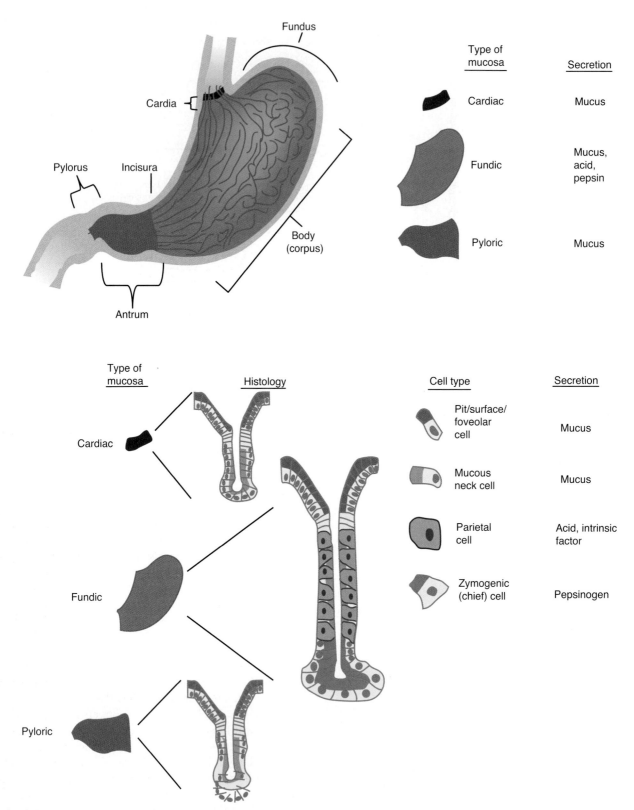

FIGURE 13–10   Anatomy and histology of the stomach.   (Redrawn, with permission, from Boron WF, Boulpaep EL [editors]. *Medical Physiology.* Saunders, 2003.)

inactive at neutral pH levels but, when acidified (in the stomach), bind to sulfhydryl groups of cysteine residues on the external surface of the H^+-K^+ ATPase, irreversibly inhibiting activity and blocking hypersecretion of gastric acid. Other experimental drugs, termed **acid pump antagonists,** competitively interfere with K^+ ion binding to block acid secretion. These drugs are widely used to inhibit the hypersecretion of gastric acid, which causes ulcer disease.

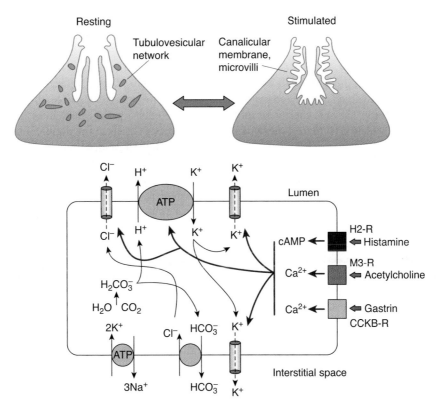

FIGURE 13–11 Acid secretion by parietal cells. **Top:** Upon stimulation, tubulovesicular network in the parietal cell fuses to form an extensive canalicular membrane with microvilli, which increases the surface area. **Bottom:** The mechanisms of HCl secretion by parietal cells, stimulated by histamine, acetylcholine, and gastrin, are demonstrated. For abbreviations, see legend for Figure 13–12.

B. Stimulants and Inhibitors of HCl Secretion

The three main stimulants of H^+ ion secretion are acetylcholine, gastrin, and histamine, all of which stimulate HCl secretion and induce characteristic shape changes of the stimulated parietal cell. **Acetylcholine** is released from vagal postganglionic or enteric neurons during feeding. It binds to muscarinic M3-type muscarinic receptors on parietal cells to stimulate H^+ ion secretion. **Gastrin** is a peptide hormone of 17 or 34 amino acids that is secreted from G cells in the gastric antrum during feeding. Gastrin binds to cholecystokinin (CCK) type B receptors on parietal cells, which also stimulates H^+ ion secretion.

Both acetylcholine and gastrin receptors activate the same signal transduction pathways: activation of phospholipase Cβ, leading to generation of inositol trisphosphate that mobilizes Ca^{2+} from intracellular stores, and diacylglycerol, which activates protein kinase C. Because both acetylcholine and gastrin act through similar intracellular pathways, the combined effects of gastrin and acetylcholine are additive.

Histamine is a paracrine substance secreted by enterochromaffin-like (ECL) and mast cells in the corpus mucosa during feeding. Histamine binds to H_2 receptors on parietal cells to activate adenylyl cyclase and increase cAMP. The cAMP activates protein kinase A to stimulate H^+ ion secretion. The combination of histamine and acetylcholine or gastrin can increase the rate of acid production by up to 10-fold over basal levels, a much greater effect than simple addition of

the effects of the agonists would predict. This effect is known as **potentiation.** Potentiation requires that two different signal molecules bind to receptors that act through different intracellular mechanisms. Increased intracellular Ca^{2+} and cAMP activate K^+ channels on the apical membrane of parietal cells, thereby promoting K^+ ion efflux from the cell. This hyperpolarizes the cell (more negative inside) to promote Cl^- ion secretion across the apical membrane. Ca^{2+} and cAMP also increase insertion of Cl^- channels and H^+-K^+ ATPase into the apical membrane. The combined effects are to stimulate HCl secretion.

Gastrin also regulates growth of the gastric epithelium. Excess gastrin produced by certain tumors causes hyperproliferation of gastric glands and parietal cells and excess secretion of gastric acid. The excess acid in the small intestine can lead to ulceration of the mucosa, steatorrhea as a result of inactivation of pancreatic lipases, and diarrhea. This condition is termed **Zollinger-Ellison syndrome.** Excessive administration of proton pump inhibitors can result in prolonged high luminal pH, which stimulates hypersecretion of gastric acid and increased mucosal growth. Termination of drug treatment then results in an acid production rebound because of the increased content of parietal cells and G cells.

In addition to the direct mechanisms by which acetylcholine, gastrin, and histamine stimulate HCl secretion from parietal cells, acetylcholine and gastrin also indirectly stimulate secretion by acting on enterochromaffin-like cells to promote the release of histamine, which in turn stimulates parietal cells. The importance of histamine to H^+ ion secretion is illustrated by studies with **histamine H_2 receptor antagonists,** such as cimetidine. These drugs not only inhibit histamine-stimulated H^+ ion secretion but also block the effects of acetylcholine and gastrin, thus confirming the indirect pathway. They are effective as they prevent the potentiation and are widely used to treat the hypersecretion of gastric acid.

Somatostatin, a peptide of 14 or 28 amino acids, is an important inhibitor of gastric acid secretion. Somatostatin directly inhibits proton secretion by activating receptors on parietal cells, which couple to produce inhibition of cAMP. Somatostatin also inhibits gastrin and histamine secretion, which indirectly inhibits proton secretion. Somatostatin is secreted by **D cells** in the gastric antrum and corpus. D cells in the gastric antrum have direct content with the stomach lumen (open endocrine cells), allowing them to sense the luminal contents. Protons in the antrum stimulate somatostatin secretion, which acts as a paracrine agent to inhibit gastrin secretion from neighboring G cells and to thereby indirectly reduce gastric acid secretion. This is an example of **negative-feedback regulation**. D cells in the corpus do not have contact with the lumen (closed cells) and thus cannot sense luminal protons. Instead, multiple neurohumoral factors (eg, noradrenalin, CCK, VIP) increase release of corpus somatostatin, which in turn inhibits acid production indirectly by decreasing histamine release from ECL cells and directly by inhibiting parietal cells. Vagal ACh and the T_H1 cytokine interferon-γ inhibit somatostatin release and promote acid secretion.

C. Integrated Regulation of Gastric Acid Secretion

Secretion of gastric acid between meals is low. Three phases of acid secretion occur during feeding (Figure 13–12). **The cephalic phase** (~30% of response) of secretion is initiated by the sight, smell, taste, and swallowing of food. These stimuli activate the dorsal motor nucleus of the vagal nerve in the medulla and result in vagal discharge and parasympathetic motor nerves. Stimulation has several consequences. In the corpus, postganglionic nerves release acetylcholine, which directly activates parietal cells by M3 receptors. Acetylcholine also induces histamine release from enterochromaffin cells, which indirectly stimulates H^+ ion secretion by parietal cells. In the antrum, vagal stimulation induces release of the peptide, **gastrin-releasing peptide,** from postganglionic fibers, which stimulates gastrin release and thus indirectly stimulates secretion of H^+ ion secretion. Acetylcholine also inhibits somatostatin release from D cells in the corpus and pylorus to stimulate secretion of H^+ ions.

The **gastric phase** (~70% of response) of secretion is induced by stimuli within the stomach. Vagal sensory nerves detect gastric distension with food and trigger a vagovagal reflex during which vagal motor nerves release acetylcholine in the stomach to promote acid secretion. Partially digested proteins and amino acids stimulate gastrin release from G cells in the pylo-

rus. G cells are open-type endocrine cells that have a brush border, allowing them to directly sense the contents of the stomach. Gastrin then stimulates acid secretion. Acidification of the pylorus stimulates somatostatin release, which inhibits acid secretion by a negative-feedback loop as described.

During the **intestinal phase**, the products of protein digestion, on entering the small intestine, can stimulate gastrin release from G cells in the duodenum. Many substances, most notably fat and acid, stimulate the secretion of hormones from the small intestine that inhibit gastric acid secretion. Examples include secretin and cholecystokinin.

Helicobacter pylori infection is responsible for almost all gastric and duodenal ulcers that are not caused by medications (eg, aspirin-like drugs). *H pylori* lives in the mucous layer of the stomach where the enzyme urease is active, converting urea to CO_2 and ammonia. Ammonia buffers luminal acid and protects the organism. *H pylori* also secretes proteins that modulate immune responses and directly alter mucosal cell signaling pathways. More than half of the world population is infected with *H pylori*. In most cases, the infection is mild and not detectable. In some people, however, the infection leads to symptomatic inflammation, ulceration, and increased risk of gastric cancer.

Other Gastric Secretions

Chief cells in the glands of the gastric corpus secrete **pepsinogen,** an inactive precursor (zymogen) of the active protease, pepsin. Acetylcholine is the main stimulant of pepsinogen secretion, although other factors (eg, gastrin) also stimulate secretion. Once released into the lumen of the stomach, gastric acid and preexisting pepsin convert pepsinogen to pepsin. Pepsin has a pH optimum of 3.0 and is thus active in the stomach. It is an endopeptidase that begins the degradation of dietary proteins to peptides. However, pepsin accounts for only 10% of the total protein digestion.

Mucins are high-molecular-weight glycoproteins secreted by mucous cells of gastric glands in the corpus and antrum. The peptide backbone of mucins is densely populated with carbohydrate side chains enriched with sulfate groups. Mucins combine with phospholipids, bicarbonate, and water to form the mucus gel layer that adheres to the surface of epithelial cells of the stomach. This layer forms physical protection for epithelial cells from damage by contractile grinding of food as well as noxious substances such as acid, pepsin, and bile acids. Acetylcholine and mucosal irritation stimulate secretion of mucin.

Epithelial cells of the corpus and antrum secrete HCO_3^- ions. Although the secretion of HCO_3^- is minor compared with H^+ ion secretion, HCO_3^- plays a major role in epithelial defense. HCO_3^- ions are trapped in the mucous gel to form an "unstirred layer" in proximity to the epithelium, where the pH is 7.0 compared with 1.0 to 3.0 in the lumen. Acetylcholine and intraluminal acid stimulate HCO_3^- secretion.

Intrinsic factor is a glycoprotein secreted by parietal cells that is required for vitamin B_{12} absorption. Vitamin B_{12}

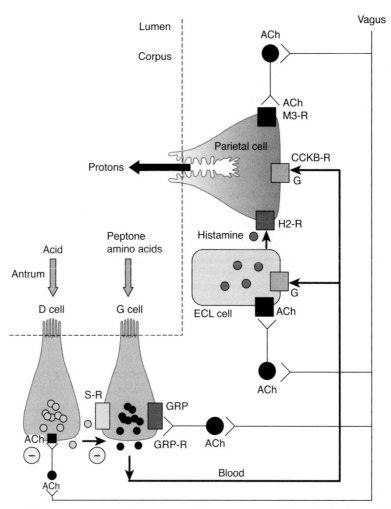

FIGURE 13–12 Regulation of gastric acid secretion by nerves and hormones. During the cephalic phase of digestion, vagal cholinergic nerves directly stimulate parietal cells and induce release of histamine from ECL cells, which also stimulate parietal cells. Vagal fibers also release gastrin-releasing peptide (GRP) in the antrum to induce gastrin secretion, which is carried in the bloodstream to induce release of histamine and stimulate parietal cells. During the gastric phase of digestion, food in the stomach triggers vagovagal reflexes and also stimulates gastrin secretion. Acidification of the gastric antrum stimulates the release of somatostatin, which inhibits gastrin release and thus acid secretion; vagal ACh inhibits somatostatin release. (ACh, acetylcholine; G, gastrin; S, somatostatin; M3-R, muscarinic 3 receptor; H2-R, histamine 2 receptor; CCKB-R, cholecystokinin B receptor; ECL, enterochromaffin-like; GRP-R, GRP receptor; GRP, gastrin-releasing peptide.)

(cobalamin) is not made in mammalian cells, and the only source is the diet: meat, fish, dairy products, but not vegetables or fruit. In the stomach, acid and pepsin release B_{12} from dietary carrier proteins. The acid environment permits binding of B_{12} to **haptocorrin** (R factor), a glycoprotein produced by salivary glands and gastric glands. The B_{12}-haptocorrin complex enters the duodenum, where pancreatic proteases digest the haptocorrin. Free intrinsic factor also enters the duodenum. Intrinsic factor combines with B_{12} in the less acidic environment of the small intestine, forming a degradation-resistant complex for transport to the ileum. Specific receptors on epithelial cells lining the ileum bind the vitamin B_{12}–intrinsic factor complex, which is taken into cells by endocytosis. The absorbed complex dissociates within the epithelial cells, and then vitamin B_{12} binds to transcobalamin II, a protein required for exocytosis and transport to the liver.

Destruction of parietal cells by autoimmune mechanisms results in vitamin B_{12} deficiency and **pernicious anemia,** resulting from impaired synthesis of purines and thymine for which vitamin B_{12} is required. The only reliable therapy is regular intramuscular injections of vitamin B_{12}.

GASTRIC MOTILITY

A. Patterns of Gastric Motility

In terms of motility, the proximal and distal regions of the stomach are distinct. The gastric corpus is a reservoir for gastric digestion. During each swallow, stretch of the esophagus induces a vagovagal reflex that causes the gastric corpus to relax in preparation to receive the food, a phenomenon known as **receptive relaxation**. When food enters the stomach, it relaxes further to accommodate a meal of 1.5 L without any increase in pressure, a phenomenon called **accommodation,** which involves vagovagal and local enteric reflexes. Thus, the stomach is a reservoir for ingested food. The antrum of the stomach is highly muscular, and here contractions serve to break food to smaller pieces and thereby facilitate digestion. The pyloric sphincter controls the rate at which the antral contractions propel partially digested food, or **chyme,** into the duodenum. During fasting, the antrum is relatively quiescent, with occasional forceful contractions that occur every 75–90 min. These intense contractions, of 5- to 10-min duration, are part of a general wave of contractions that sweep the entire length of the GI tract during fasting: the **migrating myoelectric complex.** Feeding disrupts the migrating myoelectric complex, and now the antrum contracts frequently at a rate of about three contractions per minute. These slow waves of peristaltic contraction originate from spontaneously active interstitial cells of Cajal in the pacemaker zone in the middle of the body of the stomach, and they sweep toward the antrum. When the membrane potential of muscle cells depolarizes to reach threshold, action potentials fire. Contractions occur during the plateau phase of the action potential. Gastrin and acetylcholine stimulate contraction by increasing the magnitude and duration of the action potentials.

B. Gastric Emptying

Immediately after a meal, the stomach may contain up to 1 L of material, which empties slowly into the small intestine. Regulation of gastric emptying occurs by alterations in motility of the proximal and distal stomach, pylorus, and duodenum. Gastric emptying is brought about by an increase in tone (intraluminal pressure) in the proximal stomach, increase in strength of antral contractions, opening of the pylorus, and inhibition of duodenal segmental contractions.

The rate of gastric emptying depends on the chemical and physical composition of chyme that enters the duodenum through the stimulation of both neural and hormonal pathways. Solids and liquids empty at different rates: Liquids empty rapidly, and solids empty only after a lag phase. Acid, fat, and hyperosmolar solutions entering the duodenum slow gastric emptying through stimulation of neuronal and hormonal mechanisms. Sensory neurons in the duodenum, both vagal and spinal, respond to nutrients, H^+ ions, and hyperosmolar content of chyme. Vagal motor nerves decrease antral contractions, contract the pylorus, and decrease proximal gastric motility. This results in **intestinal feedback inhibition (slowing) of gastric emptying.** The main vagal mediator that stimulates contraction is acetylcholine. VIP and nitric oxide are neuronal mediators that inhibit contraction. Many hormones that are released by endocrine cells in the small intestine have been implicated in the feedback inhibition of gastric emptying. **Secretin,** the release of which is stimulated by acid, inhibits antral contractions and stimulates contraction of the pyloric sphincter to slow emptying. **Cholecystokinin,** the release of which is stimulated by fat, acts on receptors on vagal sensory nerves to produce a vagovagal reflex that decreases gastric emptying.

The importance of nervous system control over gastric motility is reflected in the high incidence of the **dumping syndrome** (nausea, bloating, flushing, and explosive diarrhea) that occurs as a consequence of stomach dysmotility in some patients who have undergone surgical procedures such as partial gastrectomy or nonselective vagotomy.

CHECKPOINT

20. Describe the cell types found in the mucosa of the gastric corpus and antrum, and indicate the products of each cell type.
21. What are the roles of the proximal and distal stomach?
22. Describe the ionic basis of secretion of HCl from the gastric parietal cells.
23. Name a neurotransmitter, hormone, and paracrine agent that stimulates acid secretion from parietal cells.
24. Name a peptide that inhibits acid secretion from the parietal cells.
25. Describe the mechanisms of the cephalic, gastric, and intestinal phases of gastric acid secretion.
26. Name two types of drugs with distinct mechanisms of action that can be used to treat hypersecretion of gastric acid.
27. What is the role of the parietal cell in absorption of vitamin B_{12}?
28. Describe two processes by which the gastric mucosa is protected from acid in the lumen.
29. What are the patterns of motility in the corpus and the antrum?
30. How does the composition of the digesta in the lumen of the small intestine affect the rate of gastric emptying?

GALLBLADDER

Anatomy & Histology

The gallbladder is a muscular sac with a resting volume of about 50 mL that lies on the inferior surface of the liver. It is connected to the hepatic biliary system by the cystic duct, which leads to the common bile duct whose opening into the proximal duodenum is controlled by the sphincter of Oddi. The common bile duct and the pancreatic duct usually join just proximal to this sphincter.

Physiology

A. Bile Secretion

Bile, which is produced by the liver, flows down the hepatic duct and into the gallbladder through the cystic duct. It is stored there until stimulation of gallbladder contraction expels the contents of the gallbladder back through the cystic duct into the common bile duct and through the sphincter of Oddi into the duodenum. Stimuli for gallbladder contraction and sphincter of Oddi relaxation necessary for proper bile flow include both hormones and neural inputs. Fat in the intestine stimulates secretion of the hormone CCK from I cells. CCK causes contraction of the gallbladder and relaxation of the sphincter of Oddi. Depending on how long it remains in the gallbladder, bile becomes concentrated. Bile composition is further modified by mucin production under the control of prostaglandins and by saturation of bile cholesterol controlled in part by estrogens. The most prominent disorders of the gallbladder involve gallstone formation (see later discussion).

SMALL INTESTINE

Anatomy & Histology

Three regions can be distinguished along the approximately 6–7 m length of the small intestine. The pyloric sphincter marks the beginning of the **duodenum,** which is largely retroperitoneal and fixed in its location and is 20–25 cm in length. Because of this sphincter, stomach contents normally enter the duodenum in small spurts containing tiny suspended particles. In the duodenum, gastric contents are mixed with the secretions of the common bile duct and pancreatic duct. Beyond the duodenum, the small intestine is mobile and suspended in the peritoneal cavity by a mesentery. The proximal two fifths is the **jejunum.** The distal three fifths is the **ileum,** which ends at the ileocecal valve at the start of the large intestine.

The most striking gross structural features of the small intestine are the numerous **villi** (projections of the mucosa approximately 1 mm in height) (Figure 13–13). Each villus contains a single terminal branch of the arterial, venous, and lymphatic trees. Villi increase the absorptive capacity 5-fold and allow efficient transfer to the circulatory system of substances absorbed from the gut lumen by **enterocytes** (surface epithelial cells). By electron microscopy, each enterocyte contains 3000–5000 **microvilli,** plasma membrane evaginations on the apical side of the cell that further increase the absorptive surface area by 200-fold. Many digestive enzymes expressed by intestinal epithelial cells are located at the tips of these microvilli. As a group, these densely packed microvilli make up a "brush border" facing the intestinal lumen.

Invaginations of the intestinal epithelium that surround villi are called crypts of Lieberkühn. These structures are the location of epithelial intestinal stem cells and their proliferative daughters that together constantly produce new differentiated epithelial cells that form the epithelial lining of the intestine. Each crypt contains tetrapotential stem cells at or near the crypt base that produces the four mature epithelial cell types: absorptive enterocytes, mucus-secreting goblet cells; hormone-secreting enteroendocrine cells, and antimicrobial peptides and growth factor–secreting Paneth cells. Enterocytes, goblet, and enteroendocrine cells migrate out of crypts and onto adjacent villi. These cells then die by apoptosis at the tips of villi and are extruded into the lumen of the intestine; the average life span is about 4–6 days. On the other hand, Paneth cells are much longer lived (~60 days) and they migrate to the crypt base where they are in close contact with epithelial stem cells.

Digestion & Absorption in the Small Intestine

The small intestine is the main site of digestion and the principal site for nutrient absorption. Thus, it is appropriate to review all steps of digestion in the GI tract and then to consider the mechanisms by which these nutrients are absorbed.

A. Carbohydrates

Carbohydrates, which are mainly present in the diet as polysaccharides and disaccharides, must be digested to monosaccharides for absorption. Intestinal microbes contain a large repertoire of glycoside hydrolases that aid in the breakdown of complex plant polysaccharides. Alpha-amylases in salivary and pancreatic secretions cleave interior α-1,4 glucose linkages in large polymers of starch to form fragments (disaccharides, trisaccharides, and oligosaccharides). Oligosaccharidases and disaccharidases in the brush border of enterocytes digest small fragments to the monosaccharides, glucose, galactose, and fructose. Glucose and galactose, along with two Na^+ ions, are absorbed across the apical membrane of enterocytes by the same transporter, SGLT1. Passive uptake of water also occurs, maintaining osmolality on both sides of the cell membrane. The extrusion of Na^+ out of the basolateral membrane by the Na^+-K^+ ATPase provides an electrochemical Na^+ gradient that drives the absorption of glucose and galactose against their concentration gradients. Fructose is absorbed into the cell by facilitated diffusion through the apical membrane by a different transporter, GLUT-5. All three hexoses leave the cell by facilitated diffusion through a common transporter, GLUT-2, located in the basolateral membrane.

Lactose intolerance is the most common problem of carbohydrate digestion. It results mainly from the reduction of lactase activity in adults. Lactase is expressed normally at high levels in the jejunum of neonatal and infant humans. In many parts of the world, lactase levels are gradually reduced after weaning. However, lactase levels do not decrease significantly in populations where milk products are an important part of the adult diet. Lactase activity is rate limiting for lactose digestion in most adults throughout other regions of the world. If lactase is deficient, nondigested lactose is not absorbed. The nonabsorbed lactose retains water in the lumen to maintain the osmolality of chyme equivalent to that of plasma. This retention of fluid causes abdominal pain (cramps), nausea, and diarrhea. Bacterial fermentation of lactose in the distal small intestine and colon further exacerbates these symptoms.

Mutations of the gene encoding SGLT1 impair glucose and galactose absorption in some patients. Affected individuals

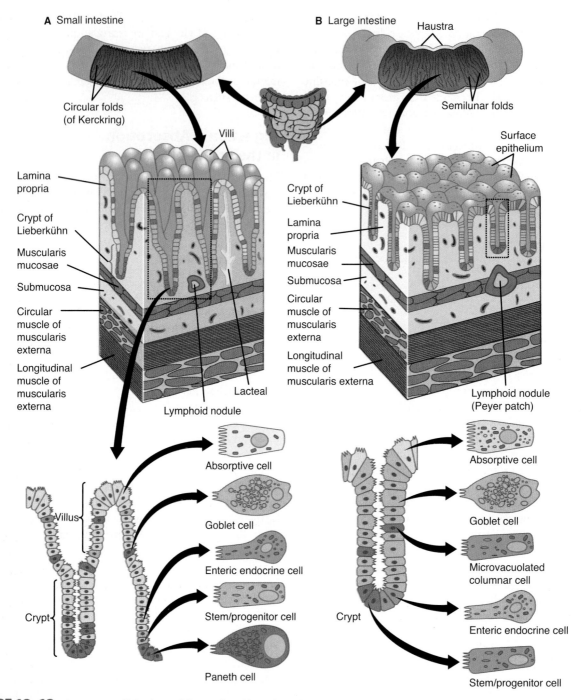

FIGURE 13–13   Anatomy and histology of the small and large intestine.   (Redrawn, with permission, from Boron WF, Boulpaep EL [editors]. *Medical Physiology*. Saunders, 2003.)

develop diarrhea when they consume sugars that are normally absorbed by SGLT1, because of defects in absorption of Na^+, monosaccharides, and water. In contrast, fructose, which is absorbed by GLUT-5, does not cause diarrhea.

B. Proteins

Proteins entering the intestine derive from the diet and also from cells shed from the mucosa. Protein digestion begins in the stomach by the action of pepsin, but most protein digestion

occurs in the lumen of duodenum and jejunum by the action of pancreatic proteases (**trypsin, chymotrypsin, carboxypeptidases**), yielding small oligopeptides and free amino acids. Peptidases on the surfaces of intestinal epithelial cells are required for the digestion of larger oligopeptides to yield smaller peptides and additional amino acids. Dipeptides and tripeptides are absorbed into enterocytes by secondary active cotransport with H^+ ions by the oligopeptide cotransporter, PepT1. The H^+ ions in the lumen are provided by a Na^+-K^+ transporter in the apical membrane. Amino acid uptake from the lumen occurs through several different transporters. Each transporter is specific for various side chain groups: acidic, basic, neutral, and imino. Uptake of most amino acids into enterocytes is coupled to cotransport with Na^+ ions that is driven by the Na^+-K^+ ATPase in the basolateral membrane. Absorbed dipeptides and tripeptides are hydrolyzed to amino acids within the enterocytes by independent cytosolic peptidases. Amino acids exit the cell through the basolateral membrane by cation-independent amino acid transporters. Infants can absorb proteins by endocytosis, providing a mechanism for transfer of immunoglobulins, and thus passive immunity, from mother to child.

C. Lipids

Triglycerides constitute about 90% of dietary lipid; cholesterol, phospholipids, sphingolipids, fatty acids, and fat-soluble vitamins make up the balance. Dietary lipids are first emulsified by mechanical digestion (chewing, antral contractions, segmentation), which produces fine droplets that are suspended in aqueous fluid. Digestion of lipids begins in the stomach by the combined action of swallowed **lingual lipase** from salivary glands, and **gastric lipase** secreted by gastric gland chief cells in the fundus. These lipases convert triglycerides to fatty acids and diglycerides. Most lipid digestion occurs in the duodenum and jejunum. Lipids in the lumen form micelles as a result of the emulsifying properties of bile salts, phospholipids, and mixing contractions of the stomach and intestine. The most important enzyme in lipid digestion is **pancreatic lipase.** Lipase is secreted as an active enzyme, but full activity requires an alkaline pH and binding to a cofactor called **colipase.** Procolipase is also secreted in pancreatic juice and is converted to colipase by trypsin in the intestinal lumen. Lipase is only active at the oil-water interface of the triglyceride droplets. Colipase promotes binding of lipase to the surface of micelles and thereby facilitates digestion. Lipase cleaves the fatty acid ester linkages at the 1 and 3 positions of the glycerol backbone of triglycerides to yield free fatty acids and a 2-monoglyceride.

The major barrier to lipid absorption is an **unstirred layer** on the surface of the enterocytes that is not readily mixed with the bulk fluid in the intestinal lumen because of the highly convoluted surface of the epithelium. The short- and medium-chain fatty acids that are water soluble and the long-chain fatty acids, monoglycerides, lysophospholipids, and cholesterol in the micelles diffuse through the unstirred layer to the surface of the enterocytes. Proton secretion creates an acidic microenvironment at the surface of enterocytes and promotes the protonation of fatty acids. Protonated fatty acids, monoglycerides, lysophospholipids, and cholesterol leave the micelles. Being uncharged (protonated) and thus lipid soluble, they readily diffuse into the cell. Fatty acids of <10 carbon atoms in length can pass through cells and enter the blood directly. Uptake of long-chain fatty acids (and some phospholipids) appears to be mediated by a specialized fatty acid transporter protein (microvillous membrane **fatty acid–binding protein**). Within the enterocyte, long-chain fatty acids bind to fatty acid–binding

proteins that transport the newly absorbed long-chain fatty acids to the smooth endoplasmic reticulum for reassembly into triglycerides with absorbed 2-monoglycerides. The triglycerides, cholesterol esters, and phospholipids are combined with specific proteins in the Golgi apparatus of enterocytes and assembled into **chylomicrons,** which are exported from the basolateral membrane of the cell. They enter the lymphatic system through the large intraendothelial channels and subsequently are delivered to the bloodstream. During a relatively brief circulation, they are partially lipolyzed by cell-surface lipases and acquire more protein components. The liver is the main destination for chylomicron remnants. Note that chylomicrons serve as the primary transporters of fat-soluble vitamins in the circulation.

D. Fluid and Electrolytes

The small intestine is the major site of water absorption. Water moves into and out of the lumen of the intestine to keep its contents iso-osmotic with plasma. Water transport in either direction is thus passive, being secondary and proportional to the movement of ions (especially Na^+ and Cl^- ions) and nutrients. In the small intestine, water absorption is greatest in mature epithelial cells at villous tips. Water secretion is greatest in immature cells at villous crypts. Most passage of water (and ions) occurs by transcellular transport through aquaporins, a family of water channels. There is also some paracellular transport of water and ions. Epithelial cells lining the GI tract are interconnected by tight junctions. Junctions are somewhat leaky, allowing some water and small ions to move between the lumen and the mucosa via paracellular transport. The resistance of tight junctions is an important determinant of the relative degree that transcellular transport occurs, and this resistance varies throughout the intestines. Tight junctions are most leaky in the duodenum and jejunum, becoming progressively less leaky (tighter) in the ileum and colon. Larger ions and organic solutes are more restricted in their movement across tight junctions.

The jejunum is the main site of absorption of Na^+ ions. Na^+ absorption is mainly transcellular, either by **cotransport** with nutrients (sugars, amino acids) or by **Na^+-K^+ exchange.** There is also **parallel Na^+ and Cl^- absorption** by a paracellular route. HCO_3^- ions are secreted in the proximal duodenum, but in the jejunum HCO_3^- and Cl^- ions are absorbed in large amounts. In the ileum, HCO_3^- is secreted and Cl^- is absorbed. K^+ ion absorption from the lumen of the small intestine occurs mainly by passive paracellular transport. The Na^+-coupled glucose transporter (SGLT1) in the apical membrane of the small intestine takes up two Na^+ ions with each glucose molecule. This property is central to the development of effective therapeutic oral rehydration solutions that contain glucose, Na^+, Cl^-, and HCO_3^- to enhance water and electrolyte uptake during severe diarrhea (eg, cholera).

The absorption of electrolytes and water is regulated by hormones and neurotransmitters. For example, angiotensin II and aldosterone, which are generated and released during dehydration, promote absorption of NaCl in the intestine.

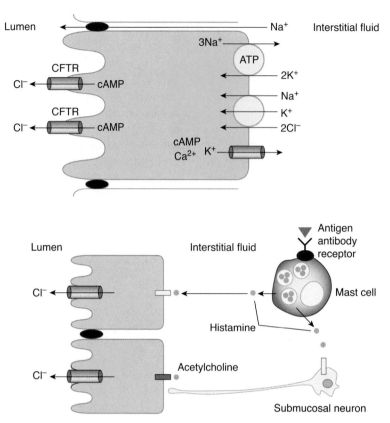

FIGURE 13–14 Mechanisms of fluid and electrolyte secretion by epithelial cells of the intestinal crypts. **Top:** Ionic basis of secretion of Cl⁻ and Na⁺ ions. **Bottom:** Regulation of fluid and electrolyte secretion by submucosal neurons and mast cells of the lamina propria. Activated mast cells release histamine, which either directly acts on epithelial cells or acts on submucosal neurons to stimulate release of acetylcholine, which then acts on epithelial cells.

Secretion in the Small Intestine

The cells of the crypts of Lieberkühn are important sites of electrolyte and water secretion. The Na⁺-K⁺ ATPase in the basolateral membrane of epithelial cells provides the electrochemical gradients for secondary active transport and diffusion of other ions. An Na-K-2Cl⁻ transporter in the basolateral membrane mediates the uptake of Na⁺, Cl⁻, and K⁺ ions into the cell (Figure 13–14). This is an example of secondary active transport: with the entry of Na⁺ ions, an electrochemical gradient drives the uptake of K⁺ and Cl⁻ ions against electrochemical gradients. Excess K⁺ ions leave the cell by basolateral K⁺ channels that can be regulated by Ca²⁺ and cAMP. Cl⁻ ions diffuse across the apical membrane of the enterocytes and into the intestinal lumen through a Cl⁻ channel that is regulated by cAMP. This electrogenic secretion of Cl⁻ ions provides a small negative charge to the lumen relative to the interstitial fluid, which drives the secretion of Na⁺ ions by a paracellular route. Water follows by transcellular and paracellular routes to maintain iso-osmolality with plasma. The net result is thus the secretion of NaCl and water.

Fluid and electrolyte secretion flushes bacterial products and toxins away from the surface of the epithelium and thus plays a role in mucosal defense. Numerous substances, termed **secretagogues,** stimulate fluid and electrolyte secretion in both health and diseases (Figure 13–14). **Neurotransmitter secretagogues** from the submucosal plexus include VIP and acetylcholine.

Paracrine secretagogues include bradykinin, serotonin, histamine, and prostaglandins. Some products from immune cells indirectly stimulate secretion by acting on submucosal neurons to induce release of acetylcholine or VIP, which then act on enterocytes to stimulate secretion. **Luminal secretagogues** include bacterial toxins. A toxin from **cholera** modifies G proteins and thereby permanently activates adenylyl cyclase and increases intracellular levels of cAMP. Strong activation of the apical Cl⁻ channels of crypt cells results in massive secretion of Cl⁻ ions and, in consequence, of water and Na⁺ ions. Patients with cholera may excrete 20 L of diarrhea per day, leading to rapid dehydration and death. An inexpensive and effective treatment is oral rehydration with glucose-containing solutions. The glucose drives the sodium-glucose cotransporter to transport both molecules into enterocytes, and with them chloride and water, thereby offsetting the fluid efflux mediated by the bacterial toxin. Because these cotransporters are lacking in the colon, its maximum absorptive capacity (5 L/d) is considerably less than that of the small intestine (12 L/d).

One type of Cl⁻ ion channel in the apical membrane is encoded by the gene for cystic fibrosis and is termed the **cystic fibrosis conductance regulator,** or **CFTR.** The CFTR is expressed in many epithelial cells throughout the body. Mutations in the channel result in improper folding and premature degradation of the channel protein. The secretion of Cl⁻ ions and, in consequence, of

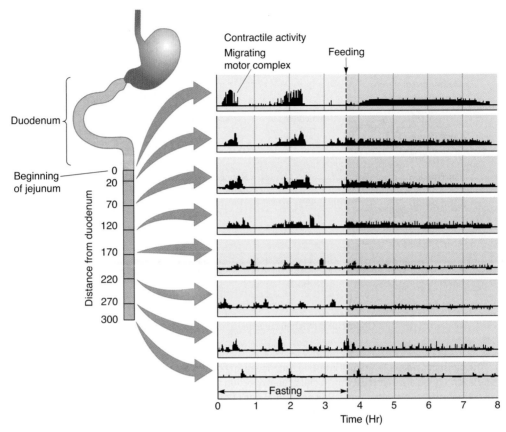

FIGURE 13-15 Mechanical activity of the small intestine during fasting and after feeding. The recordings are of intraluminal pressures measured at indicated regions of the intestine from a conscious dog. The migrating myoelectric complexes in the fasting state are disrupted by feeding, which induces segmentation and peristaltic contractions. (Redrawn, with permission, from Boron WF, Boulpaep EL [editors]. *Medical Physiology*. Saunders, 2003.)

Na$^+$ ions and water is diminished. In the airway, this results in production of thick secretions that impair ventilation.

Motility of the Small Intestine

A. Electrical Activity of Small Intestinal Muscle

In the human duodenum, slow waves occur at a frequency of 11–13/min. The slow-wave frequency declines to the ileum. The slow waves may or may not be associated with action potentials. In the intestine, slow waves alone do not cause contractions. However, when action potentials fire, they give rise to strong but highly localized contractions, the magnitude of which depends on the frequency of the action potentials. The slow waves are entirely intrinsic: They are generated within the intestine and probably depend on the unstable membrane potentials of the interstitial cells of Cajal. The frequency with which action potentials fire depends on the excitability of the muscle cells, which is influenced by circulating hormones, extrinsic nerves, and the enteric nervous system.

B. Mechanical Activity of Small Intestinal Muscle

During periods of fasting, the intestine is quiescent. However, every 90–120 min, there are bursts of action potentials in the muscle that induce waves of contraction lasting about 5 min.

These **migrating myoelectric complexes** take 90 min to traverse the small intestine. By the time the migrating myoelectric complex reaches the ileum, another begins in the stomach. These waves of contraction clear the small intestine of its contents, acting as a "housekeeper" to keep the lumen relatively clean, thereby minimizing bacterial overgrowth (Figure 13–15). The migrating myoelectric complex is associated with cycling levels of **motilin**, a 22-amino acid peptide hormone secreted by endocrine cells in the duodenum. Motilin may act on the enteric nervous system to regulate the migrating myoelectric complex. Its release appears to be under neural control, although luminal contents can also stimulate motilin release. The effect of motilin is to stimulate contraction of gastric and intestinal smooth muscle during the interdigestive period between meals.

During feeding, the migrating myoelectric complexes cease, probably because of the action of the vagus and gut hormones such as gastrin and cholecystokinin (Figure 13–15). The migrating myoelectric complexes are replaced by **phasic contractions** that are brief (a few seconds at each site) and restricted to short lengths of intestine (a few centimeters). Phasic contractions serve both to mix and propel food through the small intestine. **Rhythmic segmented contractions** provide the major local mixing activity in the small intestine. In this process, a short segment contracts while adjacent segments are relaxed. Then, the contracted segment relaxes while previously

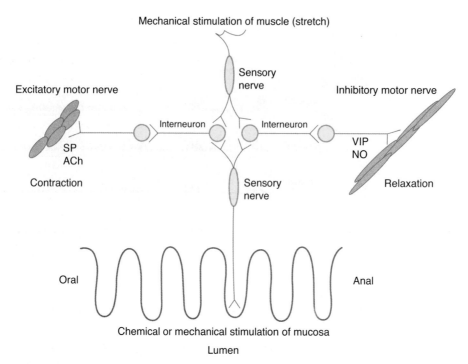

FIGURE 13–16 The peristaltic reflex of the small intestine. Enteric sensory nerves detect chemical or mechanical stimulation of the mucosa or stretch of the muscle layer. Signals are transmitted in an oral or anal direction by interneurons. Excitatory motor nerves release acetylcholine (ACh) and substance P (SP), which cause muscle contraction on the oral side of the stimulus. Inhibitory motor nerves release vasoactive intestinal peptide (VIP) and nitric oxide (NO), which cause muscle relaxation on the anal side of the stimulus.

relaxed adjacent segments contract. As these contractions alternate, chyme is forced in both directions, mixed with cell secretions, and brought into contact with cells lining the lumen. Short waves of **peristalsis** propel chyme distally, mixing chyme in successive segments and propelling it through the intestine.

C. Peristaltic Reflex

Localized chemical or mechanical stimulation of the small intestine results in a contraction on the oral side of the stimulus and relaxation on the anal side. These responses are controlled by the enteric nervous system. Sensory neurons that respond to chemicals (eg, acids) or mechanical stimuli (stroking the mucosa or stretch of the muscle with a bolus of digesta) activate excitatory ascending interneurons, which then innervate excitatory motor neurons (Figure 13–16). These neurons release excitatory neurotransmitters, acetylcholine, and the neuropeptide substance P, which activates receptors on circular muscle cells to trigger contraction. The sensory neurons also excite descending interneurons that innervate inhibitory motor neurons. They, in turn, release inhibitory neurotransmitters, VIP, and nitric oxide, which relax circular muscle.

Opiate drugs such as morphine, which are highly effective for relief of chronic pain (eg, cancer pain), have the detrimental side effect of inhibiting motility of the small intestine. Opioids act on enteric nerves to inhibit secretion of excitatory neurotransmitters to thereby inhibit peristalsis. The inhibition of motility slows down intestinal transit, allowing for a

more complete absorption, so the volume entering the colon is diminished and constipation results.

CHECKPOINT

31. Describe the hormonal reflex by which fat in the intestine stimulates the secretion of bile.

32. Describe the mechanism by which glucose is absorbed across the apical and basolateral membranes of an enterocyte.

33. What is the mechanism of absorption of tripeptides across an intestinal epithelial cell?

34. What is the role of bile in lipid absorption in the intestine?

35. List three general mechanisms of absorption of Na^+ ions in the small intestine.

36. Describe the mechanism of fluid and electrolyte secretion in the crypts of Lieberkühn.

37. Name two neurotransmitters that are secretagogues.

38. How do certain bacterial toxins stimulate fluid and electrolyte secretion in the crypts of Lieberkühn?

39. Describe the pattern of intestinal motility during fasting and after feeding.

40. Name one hormone that maintains the fasting pattern of motility and one that induces the fed pattern of motility in the small intestine.

41. Name the neurotransmitters that mediate the ascending and descending limbs of the peristaltic reflex.

COLON

Anatomy & Histology

The adult colon is 1.0–1.5 m in length. Its various segments (cecum, ascending, transverse, descending, sigmoid colon, and rectum) are involved in absorption of water and electrolytes, secretion of mucus, and formation, propulsion, and storage of unabsorbed material (feces). The colon is also the home of the majority of the intestinal microbes.

The surface of the colon consists of a columnar epithelium with no villi and few folds except in the distal rectum (Figure 13–13). The epithelial cells include absorptive cells and contain microvilli on their surface as well as mucus-secreting goblet cells. Colonic crypts contain goblet cells, endocrine cells, absorptive cells, and epithelial stem cells.

Digestion & Absorption of the Colon

Digestion in the colon occurs as a consequence of the action of the colonic microbiota. Short-chain fatty acids released by microbial action on dietary fiber are an important source of energy for the colon. More importantly, these short-chain fatty acids promote survival of healthy colonic epithelium while inducing apoptosis (programmed cell death) in epithelial cells that are progressing toward malignant transformation.

Absorption of fluid and electrolytes has been well studied and is a major function of the colon. Up to 5 L of water can be absorbed per day across the colonic epithelium. Furthermore, the colonic epithelium can also take up sodium against a considerable concentration gradient. Aldosterone, a hormone involved in fluid and electrolyte homeostasis, increases colonic sodium conductance in response to volume depletion, thus playing an important role in maintaining fluid and electrolyte balance.

Secretion of the Colon

The major secretory product of the colon is mucin, a complex glycoprotein conjugate that serves to lubricate and prevent the opposing sides of the intestinal tube from sticking together (thus collapsing the tube). In addition, mucin performs a protective function as antimicrobial peptides and immunoglobulins bind to mucin molecules, thus forming a barrier to intestinal microbes and pathogens.

Motility of the Colon

Unlike the stomach and small intestine, the colon is rarely inactive, although its activity is less easily characterized than that of the stomach, which has the pattern known as receptive relaxation, or than that of the small intestine, which displays the pattern known as the migrating motor complex and segmental to-and-fro action. Some patterns are discernible, however, such as the gastrocolic reflex (colonic mass peristalsis after a meal). Disorders of colonic motility are common complications of autonomic neuropathy in patients with diabetes mellitus and can cause severe GI complaints. Continence of stool requires contraction of the puborectalis muscle and the anal sphincter. Defecation involves relaxation of the puborectalis by the sacral parasympathetic nerves, resulting in straightening of the anorectal angle. Rectal distension results in reflex sympathetic-mediated internal and external sphincter relaxation.

CHECKPOINT

42. How does colonic motility differ from that in the small intestine?
43. What is the major secretory product of the colon?
44. What volume of water is the colon capable of absorbing per day?

OVERVIEW OF GI DISORDERS

DISORDERS OF MOTILITY

Disorders of motility affect all major regions of the GI tract. Because GI tract motility is a complex result of smooth muscle contraction under neural and hormonal control, abnormal motility of the GI tract can occur through damage to GI smooth muscle or to the neural and hormonal mechanisms by which it is controlled, or both. An example of muscle damage leading to abnormal motility is seen in esophageal stricture as a result of caustic ingestions or acid reflux. Abnormal neural control of motility is seen in esophageal achalasia. Esophageal motility disorders are typically characterized by dysphagia and odynophagia. An example of a neural defect that affects motility is Hirschsprung's disease. These patients are typically younger than 2 years and either present after birth with the inability to pass meconium or later develop severe constipation. The structural defect is a lack of myenteric neurons in the distal colon due to a congenital defect whereby the migration of neural crest precursor cells does not occur properly.

Motility disorders of the stomach include gastroparesis, a complication of diabetes mellitus, and dysmotility as a consequence of stomach surgery, from either resection of part of the stomach or **vagotomy.** Vagotomy entails surgical transection of the vagus nerve trunks, which prevents vagus-stimulated acid secretion and regulation of gastric motility. Before the availability of histamine H_2 receptor antagonists and proton pump inhibitors, selective vagotomy of the stomach was used as a treatment for the hypersecretion of gastric acid. Vagotomy is still sometimes performed as treatment for Zollinger-Ellison syndrome (ie, acid hypersecretion and severe peptic ulcer disease caused by a gastrin-secreting tumor).

The symptoms and signs of motility disorders in the stomach depend on their cause. Because vagotomy cuts fibers influencing the enteric nervous system as well as the intended fibers that influence acid secretion, a classic complication of vagotomy is disordered gastric motility. This may present clinically as either partial outlet obstruction or as too-rapid emptying of gastric contents into the duodenum, with resulting fluid shifts and vasomotor symptoms ("**dumping syndrome**"). Sometimes, however, patients may develop symptoms of stomach distension, nausea, early satiety, and vomiting suggestive of partial gastric outlet obstruction. To ameliorate the latter symptoms, **pyloroplasty** (severing the fibers of the pyloric sphincter) is done to render the sphincter less competent, so that food can pass more easily into the duodenum. Intrinsic neuropathy (eg, in diabetes mellitus) results in delayed gastric emptying, nausea, vomiting, and constipation rather than the classic dumping syndrome. The pathophysiologic basis for these differences is not known.

In the small intestine and colon, disordered motility occurs in **irritable bowel syndrome.** Irritable bowel syndrome is characterized by recurrent episodes of abdominal pain, bloating, and diarrhea alternating with constipation in the absence of detectable organic disease or structural abnormalities. The cause of this condition is still unclear.

DISORDERS OF SECRETION

Clinically recognized disorders of secretion involve the production of acid, intrinsic factor, or mucus by the stomach, digestive enzymes and bicarbonate by the pancreas, bile by the liver, and water and electrolytes by the small intestine in response to secretagogues.

Either elevated gastric acid secretion or diminished mucosal defense can predispose to development of **peptic ulcers.** These are discrete regions of erosion through the mucosa that are surrounded by apparently normal tissue. Acid-induced damage may occur in the form of an ulcer either in the stomach (**gastric ulcer**) or in the first part of the small intestine (**duodenal ulcer**). Acid-induced injury may also occur in the form of more diffuse and less clearly demarcated inflammation anywhere along the GI tract from the lower esophagus

through the duodenum. It appears that elevated acid secretion is relatively more important in the development of duodenal ulcer, whereas diminished mucosal defense (eg, from diminished mucus secretion in some cases) is a more crucial factor in development of gastric ulcer. Disorders of secretion involving the liver and pancreas are discussed in Chapters 14 and 15, respectively. Diarrhea, the major secretory disorder of the small intestine, is discussed later.

DISORDERS OF DIGESTION & ABSORPTION

Physiologically significant digestion and absorption can occur throughout the GI tract. Indeed, the effectiveness of sublingual nitroglycerin therapy for patients with angina is a testimonial to the efficacy of sublingual absorption. Nevertheless, the clinically prominent disorders of digestion and absorption focus on the small intestine and colon and the accessory organs (pancreas and liver) whose secretions (digestive enzymes, bicarbonate, and bile) are necessary for digestion and absorption in the small intestine.

GI MANIFESTATIONS OF SYSTEMIC DISEASE

A wide range of systemic conditions and diseases may produce symptoms and signs in the GI tract. These include endocrine disorders that alter control of GI tract functions or that predispose to pancreatitis or peptic ulcer disease; complications of diabetes mellitus, including autonomic neuropathy and ketoacidosis; pregnancy; deficiency disorders, including deficiency of zinc, niacin, and iron; and neoplastic, rheumatologic, and other syndromes (Table 13–4).

CHECKPOINT

45. What are some common symptoms of esophageal dysmotility?

46. Why does vagotomy often create motor disorders in the stomach?

PATHOPHYSIOLOGY OF DISORDERS OF THE ESOPHAGUS

The major disorders of the esophagus are related to motor functions: Disordered peristalsis and increased lower esophageal sphincter tone are seen in esophageal achalasia, whereas inappropriate lower esophageal sphincter relaxation results in reflux esophagitis.

ESOPHAGEAL ACHALASIA

Clinical Presentation

Esophageal achalasia is a motor disorder in which the lower esophageal sphincter fails to relax properly. As a result, a **functional obstruction** (ie, obstruction from abnormal function in

TABLE 13–4 GI manifestations of systemic diseases and their pathophysiologic mechanisms.

Disease or Condition	Commonly Associated GI Manifestations	Mechanism
Thyroid disease		
Autoimmune thyroiditis	Achlorhydria and pernicious anemia	Autoimmune destruction of parietal cells
Hypothyroidism	Esophageal reflux	Lower esophageal sphincter dysfunction
	Bezoars	Gastric dysmotility
	Constipation	Intestinal dysmotility
	Malabsorption	Villous atrophy and pancreatic insufficiency
Hyperthyroidism	Diarrhea and weight loss	Intestinal hypermotility with rapid transit and malabsorption
Adrenal disease		
Adrenal insufficiency	Abdominal pain	Unknown
	Diarrhea	Malabsorption resulting from loss of trophic effect of corticosteroids on enterocyte brush border
Parathyroid disease		
Primary hyperparathyroidism	Nausea and vomiting	Hypercalcemia-induced alteration in signal transduction resulting in gastric atony and dysmotility
	Pancreatitis	Hypercalcemia-induced premature activation of pancreatic enzymes
	Acid-peptic disease	Hypercalcemia-induced increased acid secretion
Diabetes mellitus		
	Esophageal, gastric, small and large intestinal, and rectal dysfunction	Autonomic neuropathy
	Nausea, vomiting, abdominal pain	Ketoacidosis with gastric atony
Pregnancy		
	Esophageal reflux; nausea and vomiting; hematemesis; constipation and hemorrhoids	Pressure effects of gravid uterus on lower esophageal sphincter, gastric emptying, intestinal transit time, and venous return
Deficiency states		
Zinc, niacin	Malabsorption syndrome	Altered enterocyte brush border
Cancer		
	Pain, fever, bleeding, ascites, obstruction, perforation	Metastases (most commonly breast cancer, melanoma, bronchogenic carcinoma of lung)
	Paraneoplastic syndromes and hypercalcemia	Tumor-produced peptides
Hematologic conditions		
Bleeding disorders	Intramural hematoma	Hemorrhage
Hypercoagulable states	Bowel infarction	Intestinal ischemia
Dysproteinemias	Hemorrhage, obstruction, amyloidosis	Infiltration
Rheumatologic disorders		
Scleroderma	Dysphagia, esophageal reflux, obstruction, bleeding, perforation, pseudo-obstruction, pancreatitis, malabsorption	Inflammation, vasculitis, vascular obliteration, villous atrophy
Systemic lupus erythematosus	Nausea, vomiting, mucosal ulceration	Inflammation, vasculitis, vascular obstruction, villous atrophy
Rheumatoid arthritis	Gastric ulcers, gastritis	Aspirin or NSAID use

(continued)

TABLE 13–4 GI manifestations of systemic diseases and their pathophysiologic mechanisms. (Continued)

Disease or Condition	Commonly Associated GI Manifestations	Mechanism
Metabolic and infiltrative disorders		
(dyslipidemias; sarcoidosis, amyloidosis)	Malabsorption	Infiltration, muscle atrophy, dysmotility
	Infarction	Infiltration, mucosal ischemia, infarction
Renal disorders		
(including chronic renal failure and transplantation)	Abdominal pain, GI bleeding, intestinal perforation	Gastritis, duodenitis, pancreatitis
Neurologic disorders		
(including spinal cord injury, myotonic dystrophy, CNS disease)	Impaired gut motility with nausea, vomiting, chronic constipation	Disordered central and enteric nervous system communication
	Gastroduodenal (Cushing) ulcers	Hemodynamic changes and/or increased vagal activity
Pulmonary disorders		
Asthma	Esophageal reflux	Nocturnal aspiration
Cystic fibrosis	Diarrhea, malabsorption, and weight loss	Pancreatic exocrine insufficiency

Reproduced, with permission, from Hunter TB, Bjeilard JC. Gastrointestinal complications of leukemia and its treatment. AJR Am J Roentgenol. 1984;143:513; Riley SA, Tumberg LA. Maldigestion and malabsorption. In: *Gastrointestinal Disease,* 4th ed. Sleisenger MH, Fordtran JS (editors). Saunders, 1989; and Sack TL, Sleisenger MH. Effects of systemic and extraintestinal disease on the gut. In: *Gastrointestinal Disease,* 4th ed. Sleisenger MH, Fordtran JS (editors). Saunders, 1989.

the absence of a visible mass or lesion) is created that is manifested as dysphagia (inability to swallow), regurgitation, and chest pain. It is a progressive disease in which severe radiographic distortion of the esophagus develops.

Etiology

The underlying cause of esophageal achalasia, which occurs with an incidence of 0.5–1.0 per 100,000 population per year, is unknown. Degeneration of the myenteric plexus and loss of inhibitory neurons that release VIP and nitric oxide, which dilate the lower esophageal sphincter, may contribute. Esophageal involvement in Chagas' disease, resulting from damage of the neural plexuses of the esophagus by the parasite *Trypanosoma cruzi,* bears a striking resemblance to esophageal achalasia. A number of other disorders, including malignancies, may present with manometric pressure characteristics or radiographic features similar to those observed in idiopathic esophageal achalasia.

Pathology & Pathogenesis

Although achalasia is manifested as a motor disorder of esophageal smooth muscle, it is actually due to defective innervation of smooth muscle in the esophageal body and lower esophageal sphincter. Lower esophageal sphincter tone is normally characterized by tonic contraction with intermittent relaxation resulting from a neural reflex arc (see earlier discussion). In achalasia, it is even more tightly contracted and does not relax properly in response to swallowing because of partial loss of neurons in the wall of the esophagus. Thus, achalasia can be thought of as a disorder caused by defective in-

hibitory pathways of the esophageal enteric nervous system. Interestingly, injection of botulinum toxin into the lower esophageal sphincter diminishes the excitatory pathways and thereby ameliorates symptoms. In addition to dysfunction of the lower esophageal sphincter, loss of normal peristalsis in the esophageal body is often seen in achalasia, consistent with the hypothesis of myenteric plexus degeneration. Variations of achalasia also exist in which normal peristalsis is replaced by simultaneous contractions of large or small amplitude.

Clinical Manifestations

Over months and years, lower esophageal sphincter dysfunction results in tremendous enlargement of the esophagus. Normally intended as a direct conduit to the stomach, the esophagus in advanced cases of achalasia can hold as much as 1 L of putrid, infected material, imposing a high risk of aspiration pneumonia. Without treatment, patients display progressive severe weight loss with worsening chest pain, mucosal ulceration, infection, and occasional esophageal rupture, culminating in death.

REFLUX ESOPHAGITIS

Clinical Presentation

The predominant presenting symptom of reflux is burning chest pain (heartburn) resulting from recurrent mucosal injury, often worse at night, when lying supine, or after consumption of foods or drugs that diminish lower esophageal sphincter tone.

TABLE 13–5 Factors influencing lower esophageal sphincter pressure.

	Increase	Decrease
Hormones	Gastrin	Secretin
	Motilin	Cholecystokinin
	Substance P	Glucagon
		Somatostatin
		Gastric inhibitory peptide (GIP)
		Vasoactive intestinal peptide (VIP)
		Progesterone
Neural agents	Alpha-adrenergic agonists	Beta-adrenergic agonists
		Alpha-adrenergic antagonists
	Beta-adrenergic antagonists	Anticholinergic agents
	Cholinergic agonists	
Foods	Protein meals	Fat
		Chocolate
		Ethanol
		Peppermint
Other	Histamine	Theophylline
	Antacids	Caffeine
	Metoclopramide	Gastric acidification
	Domperidone	Smoking
	Prostaglandin F_2	Pregnancy
	Migrating motor complex	Prostaglandins E_2, I_2
		Serotonin
	Raised intraabdominal pressure	Meperidine, morphine
		Dopamine
		Calcium channel blocking agents
		Diazepam
		Barbiturates

Reproduced with permission, from Diamant NE. Physiology of the esophagus. In: *Gastrointestinal Disease*, 5th ed. Sleisenger MH, Fordtran JS (editors). Saunders, 1993.

Etiology

Common causes of reflux esophagitis are those conditions that result in persistent or repetitive acid exposure to the esophageal mucosa. These include disorders that increase the rate of spontaneous transient lower esophageal sphincter relaxations (Table 13–5) or impair reflexes that normally follow

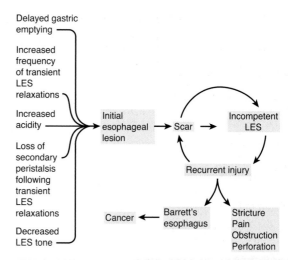

FIGURE 13–17 Pathophysiology of esophageal reflux disease. (LES, lower esophageal sphincter.)

transient lower esophageal sphincter relaxations with a secondary wave of esophageal peristalsis. Conditions that increase gastric volume or pressure (eg, partial or complete gastric outlet obstruction and conditions that increase acid production) also contribute. Occasionally, reflux esophagitis can be caused by alkaline injury (eg, pancreatic juice refluxing through both an incompetent pyloric sphincter and a relaxed lower esophageal sphincter). Hiatal hernia, a disorder in which a portion of the proximal stomach slides into the chest cavity with upward displacement of the lower esophageal sphincter, can contribute to the development of reflux.

Pathology & Pathogenesis

Normally, the tonically contracted lower esophageal sphincter provides an effective barrier to reflux of acid from the stomach back into the esophagus. This is reinforced by secondary esophageal peristaltic waves in response to transient lower esophageal sphincter relaxation. Effectiveness of that barrier can be altered by loss of lower esophageal sphincter tone (ie, the opposite of achalasia), increased frequency of transient relaxations, loss of secondary peristalsis after a transient relaxation, increased stomach volume or pressure, or increased production of acid, all of which can make more likely reflux of acidic stomach contents sufficient to cause pain or erosion. Recurrent reflux can damage the mucosa, resulting in inflammation, hence the term "reflux esophagitis." Recurrent reflux itself predisposes to further reflux because the scarring that occurs with healing of the inflamed epithelium renders the lower esophageal sphincter progressively less competent as a barrier.

Although typically a consequence of acid reflux, esophagitis can also result from reflux of pepsin or bile. In most cases of esophageal reflux disease, a common pathophysiologic thread can be identified (Figure 13–17). Recurrent mucosal damage results in infiltration of granulocytes and eosinophils, hyperplasia of basal cells, and eventually the development of friable, bleeding ulcers and exudates over the mucosal surface. These pathologic changes set the stage for scar formation and sphincter incompetence, predisposing to recurrent cycles of inflammation.

Increased frequency of transient lower esophageal sphincter relaxations may be partly in response to increased gastric distension. Normally, transient lower esophageal sphincter relaxations are accompanied by increased esophageal peristalsis. Individuals with defects in excitatory pathways that promote peristalsis may, therefore, be at increased risk for the development of esophageal reflux. Changes in the types of prostaglandins produced by the esophagus have been noted in reflux esophagitis, perhaps contributing to impairment of healing and predisposing to recurrences. In contrast to other forms of acid-mediated injury, *H pylori* infection does not appear to contribute to the development of reflux or esophagitis.

Clinical Manifestations

Heartburn is the usual symptom of reflux esophagitis, typically worsening on lying prone. With recurrent reflux, a range of complications may develop. The most common complication is the development of stricture in the distal esophagus. Progressive obstruction, initially to solid food and later to liquid, presents as dysphagia. Other complications of recurrent reflux include hemorrhage or perforation; hoarseness, coughing, or wheezing; and pneumonia as a result of aspiration of gastric contents into the lungs, particularly during sleep. Epidemiologic studies suggest that cigarette smoking and alcohol abuse associated with recurrent reflux result in a change in the esophageal epithelium from squamous to columnar histology, termed **Barrett's esophagus.** In 2–5% of cases, Barrett's esophagus leads to the development of adenocarcinoma.

CHECKPOINT

47. What are the roles of the lower esophageal sphincter structure in achalasia and in reflux esophagitis?
48. What are possible causes of achalasia?
49. What is the relationship of esophageal reflux to Barrett's esophagus and cancer?

PATHOPHYSIOLOGY OF DISORDERS OF THE STOMACH

Common disorders involving the stomach reflect the importance of its role as a secretory organ, in particular of acid and intrinsic factor. Disorders of acid secretion result in acid-peptic disease, whereas loss of intrinsic factor secretion results in inability to absorb vitamin B_{12}, manifesting as **pernicious anemia.** The major motility disorder of the stomach is gastroparesis.

ACID-PEPTIC DISEASE

Clinical Presentation

Patients with acid-peptic disease typically present with chronic, mild, gnawing or burning abdominal or chest pain resulting from superficial or deep erosion of the GI mucosa. Sudden complications include GI tract bleeding, resulting in hematemesis or melena, and perforation and infection, resulting in severe abdominal pain and signs of acute abdomen (absence of bowel sounds, guarding, rebound tenderness). The latter presentation reflects the fact that in some cases acid-peptic disease can be painless in the early stages and can be detected only when it leads to an intra-abdominal catastrophe.

Classically, duodenal ulcer presents as gnawing or burning epigastric pain occurring 1–3 hours after meals, often waking the patient at night, with antacids or food producing relief. However, many patients later documented to have duodenal ulcer do not fit this symptom profile. Elderly patients in particular often present with a complication of duodenal ulcer but no history of pain.

Etiology

Various causes of absolute or relative increased acid production (Figure 13–12) or decreased mucosal defenses (Table 13–2) predispose to acid-peptic disease. A specific infectious agent, the bacterium **Helicobacter pylori,** has been implicated in predisposition to a number of forms of acid-peptic disease, including duodenal ulcer, gastric ulcer, and gastritis (Figure 13–18).

Pathology & Pathogenesis

Corrosive agents (acid and pepsin) secreted by the stomach play a key role in gastric ulcer, duodenal ulcer, and acute erosive gastritis. Each of these diseases has a distinctive but overlapping pathogenesis with the common themes of either excessive acid secretion or diminished mucosal defense. Exactly why one but not another form of acid-peptic disease should develop in a given individual remains unclear. *H pylori* infection can cause acid-peptic disease by multiple mechanisms, including direct alteration of signal transduction in mucosal and immune cells, which in turn can increase acid secretion and diminish mucosal defenses. The complex interactions of the *H pylori* infection and its location and virulence, along with its clinical consequences (eg, inflammation, increased or decreased acid secretion), are illustrated in Figure 13–19.

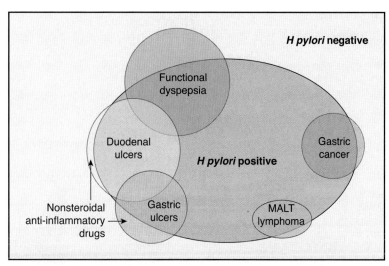

FIGURE 13–18 Relation of *H pylori* infection to upper GI tract conditions. The figure shows that most patients with gastroduodenal ulcers or gastric lymphoma or adenocarcinoma have also been infected with *H pylori*. Note, however, that the circles are not to scale, because gastric cancer occurs in < 1% of those infected with *H pylori*. Note, too, that relationships among the different conditions are more complex than depicted, because patients with cancer also often have had ulcers. (Redrawn, with permission, from Calam J, Baron JH. Pathophysiology of duodenal and gastric ulcer and gastric cancer. BMJ. 2001;323:980.)

H pylori is an extremely common pathogen, found in over half of the world's population; rates of infection are even higher in the poorest countries, where sanitation facilities and standards of personal hygiene are low. The most likely route of spread from person to person is fecal-oral. As many as 90% of infected individuals show signs of inflammation (gastritis or duodenitis) on endoscopy, although many of these individuals are clinically asymptomatic. Despite this high rate of association of inflammation with *H pylori* infection, the important role of other factors is indicated by the fact that only about 15% of infected individuals ever develop a clinically significant ulcer. These other factors (both genetic and environmental, such as cigarette smoking) must account for the individual variations and are pathophysiologically important. Nevertheless, the role of *H pylori* is of particular clinical importance because, of patients who do develop acid-peptic disease, especially among those with duodenal ulcers, the vast majority have *H pylori* infection. Furthermore, treatment that does not eradicate *H pylori* is associated with rapid recurrence of acid-peptic disease in most patients. There are numerous strains of *H pylori* that vary in their production of toxins such as CagA and VacA that directly alter cellular signaling pathways. Variations in bacterial strains as well as natural variation in the balance of inflammatory mediators (eg, T_H1 vs. T_H2 vs. T_H17 cytokines) triggered by infection may explain why *H pylori* infection is asymptomatic in most patients, causes peptic ulcers in some, and increases risk for development of lymphoma and adenocarcinoma in a few.

1. Gastric Ulcer

Gastric ulcer is distinguished from erosive gastritis by the depth of the lesion, with gastric ulcers penetrating through the mucosa. The actual ulcer crater is often surrounded by an area of intact but inflamed mucosa, suggesting that gastritis is a predisposing lesion to development of gastric ulcer. Most gastric ulcers occur on the lesser curvature of the stomach. It is likely that gastric ulcer represents the outcome of a number of different abnormalities summarized next.

Some gastric ulcers are believed to be related to impaired mucosal defenses, because the acid and pepsin secretory capacity of some affected patients is normal or even below normal.

Motility defects have been proposed to contribute to development of gastric ulcer in at least three ways. First, they contribute because of a tendency of duodenal contents to reflux back through an incompetent pyloric sphincter. Bile acids in the duodenal reflux material act as an irritant and may be an important contributor to a diminished mucosal barrier against acid and pepsin. Second, they may contribute as a result of delayed emptying of gastric contents, including reflux material, into the duodenum. Third, they may contribute as a result of delayed gastric emptying and hence food retention, causing increased gastrin secretion and gastric acid production. It is not known whether these motility defects are a cause or a consequence of gastric ulcer formation.

Mucosal ischemia may play a role in the development of a gastric ulcer. Prostaglandins are known to increase mucosal blood flow as well as bicarbonate and mucus secretion and to stimulate mucosal cell repair and renewal. Thus, their deficiency, resulting from nonsteroidal anti-inflammatory drug (NSAID) ingestion or other insults, may predispose to gastritis and gastric ulcer, as might diminished bicarbonate or mucus secretion resulting from other causes. Subsets of gastric ulcer patients with each of these defects have been identified. Thus, the risk factors (NSAID ingestion, smoking, psychologic stress, *H pylori* infection) that have been associated

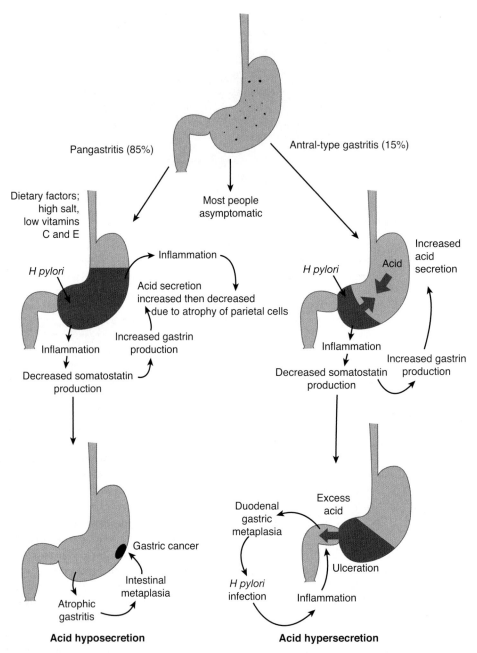

Pangastritis (85%)

Antral-type gastritis (15%)

Most people
asymptomatic

Dietary factors;
high salt,
low vitamins
C and E

H pylori

Inflammation

Acid secretion
increased then decreased
due to atrophy of parietal cells

Inflammation

Increased gastrin
production

Decreased somatostatin
production

H pylori

Acid

Increased
acid
secretion

Inflammation

Increased gastrin
production

Decreased somatostatin
production

Gastric cancer

Intestinal
metaplasia

Atrophic
gastritis

Excess
acid

Duodenal
gastric
metaplasia

Ulceration

H pylori
infection

Inflammation

Acid hyposecretion

Acid hypersecretion

FIGURE 13–19 Patterns of chronic *H pylori* infection with respect to acid production and pathology. **Left:** Acid hyposecretion. *H pylori* infection of the stomach body causes suppression of parietal cells, low acid secretion, atrophic gastritis, intestinal metaplasia, and predisposition to gastric cancer. **Right:** Acid hypersecretion. *H pylori* infection primarily of the stomach antrum causes decreased somatostatin and increased gastrin secretion, increasing acid secretion and predisposition to duodenal ulceration. (Redrawn from Calam J, Baron JH. Pathophysiology of duodenal and gastric ulcer and gastric cancer. BMJ. 2001;323:980.)

with gastric ulcer probably act by diminishing one or more mucosal defense mechanisms.

Gastritis (inflammation of the gastric mucosa) as a result of aspirin and other NSAIDs, bile salts, alcohol, or other insults may predispose to ulcer formation by (1) attenuating the barrier created by the epithelial cells or the mucus and bicarbonate they secrete or (2) reducing the quantity of prostaglandins the epithelial cells produce that might otherwise diminish acid secretion.

2. Acute Erosive Gastritis

Acute erosive gastritis includes inflammation resulting from superficial mucosal injury, mucosal erosion, or shallow ulcers caused by a wide variety of insults, most notably alcohol, drugs, and stress. Ethanol ingestion predisposes to gastritis but not to gastric ulcer. Unlike gastric or duodenal ulcers, in erosive gastritis the submucosa and muscularis mucosa are not penetrated. Acid hypersecretion, gastric anoxia, altered natural defenses (especially diminished mucus secretion), epithelial renewal, tissue mediators (eg, prostaglandins), reduced intramucosal pH, and intramucosal energy deficits have been suggested as factors in the development of superficial gastric mucosal injury.

3. Chronic Atrophic Gastritis

This heterogeneous group of syndromes is characterized by inflammatory cell infiltration with gastric mucosal atrophy and loss of glands. In chronic disease, unlike acute erosive gastritis, endoscopic abnormalities may not be grossly apparent. The capacity to secrete gastric acid is progressively reduced, and the serum levels of gastrin are elevated. Autoantibodies to parietal cells, intrinsic factor, and gastrin are common findings. Chronic atrophic gastritis is associated with *H pylori* infection, development of pernicious anemia, gastric adenocarcinoma, and GI endocrine hyperplasia with carcinoids (neuroendocrine tumors of the GI tract).

4. Duodenal Ulcer

Even more commonly than gastric ulcers, duodenal ulcers are sequelae of *H pylori* infection, caused by altered mucosal inflammatory responses and excessive acid secretion. Various other risk factors, including diet, smoking, and excessive alcohol consumption, may influence the development of duodenal ulcers, although specific associations (eg, between coffee or spicy foods and the development of ulcers) have not been demonstrated. Genetic factors also play a role; studies support the existence of a heritable component in duodenal ulcers distinct from that involved in gastric ulcer. Likewise, psychologic stress has been implicated in duodenal ulcer disease, perhaps by an autonomic-mediated influence on acid secretion (Figure 13–12). Interestingly, duodenal ulcers are associated with decreased risk for development of gastric adenocarcinoma, suggesting that duodenal ulceration indicates a distinct type of chronic *H pylori* infection (Figure 13–19).

Clinical Manifestations

Those forms of acid-peptic disease characterized by exclusively superficial mucosal lesions (eg, acute erosive gastritis) can result in either acute or chronic GI tract bleeding, accompanied by a significant drop in hematocrit and related complications (eg, precipitating angina in a patient with coronary artery disease). Patients with acute massive bleeding present with hematemesis (vomiting of blood), rectal bleeding, or melena (tarry stools from the effect of acid on blood) depending on the site of origin, the rate of transit of blood through the GI tract, and the extent of hemorrhage. Acute massive hemorrhage (> 10% of blood volume over minutes to hours) is manifested by hypotension, tachycardia, and orthostatic blood pressure and heart rate changes on standing, often with dizziness.

In addition to hemorrhage, complications of duodenal ulcer and gastric ulcer include life-threatening perforation and obstruction.

CHECKPOINT

50. How does pernicious anemia result from a secretory disorder of the stomach?
51. What is the typical acid secretion status of patients with pernicious anemia?
52. In which acid-peptic disorder are diminished mucosal defenses more important than acid hypersecretion?
53. How might motility defects contribute to gastric ulcer?
54. What factors may predispose a patient to duodenal ulcer disease?
55. How do NSAIDs contribute to acid-peptic disease?
56. What evidence indicates the importance of *H pylori* infection in acid-peptic disease?
57. What evidence suggests that other factors besides *H pylori* infection contribute to acid-peptic disease?

GASTROPARESIS

Clinical Presentation

A common complication of stomach disorders is delayed gastric emptying (Table 13–6). Known as gastroparesis, it is manifested by nausea, bloating, vomiting, and either constipation or diarrhea. The condition can also occur silently, producing metabolic derangements (eg, of blood glucose in patients with diabetes mellitus) in the absence of somatic symptoms.

Etiology

Gastroparesis is a common complication of poorly controlled diabetes mellitus, with consequent autonomic neuropathy.

Pathology & Pathogenesis

Disorders of gastric motility result from alterations in a number of normal gastric functions. These include (1) serving as a reservoir for ingested solids and liquids (eg, alteration caused by resection of the stomach); (2) mixing and homogenizing ingested food; and (3) functioning as a barrier that allows only small spurts of well-mixed chyme beyond the pyloric sphincter. The resulting disorders span the range from partial or complete gastric outlet obstruction to excessively rapid emptying and typically result from interference with the normal mechanisms by which these functions are controlled. These include the intrinsic contractility of gastric smooth muscle, the enteric nervous system, the autonomic nervous system's control over enteric nervous system function, and gut hormones.

Because the pyloric sphincter, like all sphincters, displays tonic contraction with intermittent transient relaxation, loss of vagal control results in excessive tonic contraction and symptoms of various degrees of gastric outlet obstruction. Disorders that affect the enteric nervous system such as the

TABLE 13–6 Conditions producing symptomatic gastric motor dysfunction.

Acute Conditions	Chronic Conditions	
Abdominal pain, trauma, inflammation	Mechanical	Pseudo-obstruction
Postoperative state	Gastric ulcer	Idiopathic, hollow visceral myopathy
Acute infections, gastroenteritis	Duodenal ulcer	Secondary (eg, amyloidosis, Chagas' disease, muscular dystrophies, cancer-associated syndrome)
Acute metabolic disorders:	Idiopathic hypertrophic pyloric stenosis	
Acidosis, hypokalemia, hypercalcemia or hypocalcemia, hepatic coma, myxedema	Superior mesenteric artery syndrome	Postgastric surgery
	Acid-peptic disease	Postvagotomy or postgastric resections
Immobilization	Gastroesophageal reflux	Medications
Hyperglycemia (glucose > 200 mg/dL)	Gastric ulcer disease, nonulcer dyspepsia	Anticholinergics, narcotic analgesics, levodopa, tricyclic antidepressants
Pharmaceutical agents and hormones	Gastritis	Hormones (pharmacologic studies)
Opioids, including endorphins and narcotics (eg, morphine)	Atrophic gastritis with or without pernicious anemia	Gastrin, cholecystokinin, somatostatin
Anticholinergics	Viral gastroenteritis (acute or chronic gastritis)	Anorexia nervosa: bulimia
Tricyclic antidepressants	Metabolic and endocrine	Idiopathic
Beta-adrenergic agonists	Diabetic ketoacidosis (acute)	Gastric dysrhythmias: tachygastria
Levodopa	Diabetic gastroparesis (chronic)	Gastroduodenal dyssynchrony
Aluminum hydroxide antacids	Addison's disease	Central nervous system: tabes dorsalis, depression
Gastrin	Hypothyroidism	
Cholecystokinin	Pregnancy?	
Somatostatin	Uremia?	
	Collagen-vascular diseases	
	Scleroderma	
	Dermatomyositis	
	Polymyositis	
	Systemic lupus erythematosus?	

Reproduced with permission, from McCallum RW. Motor function of the stomach in health and disease. In: *Gastrointestinal Disease,* 4th ed. Sleisenger MH, Fordtran JS (editors). Saunders, 1989.

neuropathy of diabetes mellitus and surgical cutting of the stomach wall or vagal trunk typically cause delayed emptying. However, it is important to remember that, in some cases, delayed emptying can result in symptoms expected from excessively rapid emptying. For example, an excessively contracted pylorus that can open completely but does so infrequently can result in entry into the duodenum of too large a bolus of chyme from the excessively distended stomach. Such a bolus may not be efficiently handled by the small intestine, resulting in poor absorption and diarrheal symptoms characteristic of the dumping syndrome.

Hormones play an ill-defined but important role in regulation of GI motility in health and disease. For example, the antibiotic erythromycin is recognized by the receptor for the GI hormone motilin, affecting GI motility. Some patients with gastroparesis are observed to have substantial improvement with erythromycin analogs, especially when complaints related to partial gastric outlet obstruction, such as bloating, nausea, and constipation, are prominent.

Because different patients have different relative contributions of the intrinsic nervous system, enteric nervous system, autonomic nervous system, higher centers of the CNS, and hormones over control of their GI tract motility, not all treatments for gastroparesis are effective for a majority of patients even with the same initial complaints.

Clinical Manifestations

Complications of gastroparesis include the development of bezoars from retained gastric contents, bacterial overgrowth, erratic blood glucose control, and, when nausea and vomiting are profound, weight loss. Elevated blood glucose can be either a cause or a consequence of delayed gastric emptying. Bacterial overgrowth itself can result in both malabsorption and diarrhea. For unknown reasons, the symptoms of gastroparesis are variable from patient to patient as well as over time in a given patient and often correlated poorly with delayed gastric emptying. In some cases, serotonin antagonists that decrease visceral perception may be more helpful than prokinetic agents in alleviating symptoms.

CHECKPOINT

58. What are the symptoms of delayed versus rapid gastric emptying?
59. What are the complications of gastroparesis?
60. Why might erythromycin improve diabetic gastroparesis?

DISORDERS OF THE GALLBLADDER

Gallbladder disease is most commonly due to gallstones (cholelithiasis).

1. Cholelithiasis

Clinical Presentation

Gallstones are most often asymptomatic, discovered incidentally at autopsy or during surgery for an unrelated condition. Of patients who do have symptoms referable to cholelithiasis, presentations range from mild nausea or abdominal discomfort after eating fatty or fried foods to severe right upper quadrant or midepigastric abdominal pain and jaundice. A history of chronic mild symptoms with dietary association typically predates an acute episode of abdominal pain. The typical patient with gallstones is female, has a history of high dietary fat intake, has had prior pregnancies (reflecting the role of estrogens in gallstone pathogenesis), and is in her 40s (reflecting the time necessary for progression to symptomatic disease).

Etiology

Gallstones come in several varieties. Most are composed largely of cholesterol with or without calcium deposits. Occasionally, especially in patients with a chronic hemolytic disease, bilirubin stones may form. Depending on the cause and the pathophysiologic mechanism involved, patients can have one or more of the following: a few large individual stones; many smaller stones; or "sludge," a thickened viscous gel resulting from concentration of bile that is believed to be highly prone to formation of stones.

Pathology and Pathogenesis

Cholelithiasis is of multifactorial origin. However, the formation of cholesterol gallstones usually requires the formation of bile whose cholesterol concentration is greater than its percentage solubility. The normal processes that prevent gallstone formation probably include the fact that bile does not normally stay in the gallbladder long enough to become lithogenic (prone to stone formation). Thus, loss of gallbladder muscular wall motility (resulting from either intrinsic disease of the muscle wall, altered levels of hormones such as CCK, or altered neural control) and excessive sphincteric contraction, impairing emptying, are important predisposing factors. One consequence of decreased gallbladder emptying is excessive concentration of bile, leading to heightened lithogenicity. This can occur from decreased absorption of water or altered bile composition resulting from increased cholesterol content or saturation. Other factors can cause an increased tendency to form stones at any given degree of concentration and saturation, including the presence of nucleating versus antinucleating factors in bile and the size and composition of the bile acid pool. Figure 13–20 summarizes the factors that predispose to gallstone formation, including estrogens, prostaglandins, increased mucus and glycoprotein production by the gallbladder epithelium, and chronic bacterial colonization or infection. Estrogens may play multiple roles, first affecting bile composition (increasing cholesterol and its saturation in bile) but also diminishing gallbladder motility (hence predisposing to stasis, sludge formation, and lithogenicity). Prostaglandins, which are protective in the stomach by increasing mucus production, actually may contribute to lithogenicity by the same mechanism. Thus, NSAIDs that block prostaglandin production are often beneficial for the prevention of gallstones in patients so predisposed, probably by decreasing mucus production.

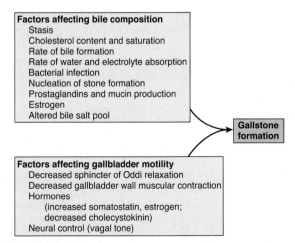

FIGURE 13–20 Pathophysiology of cholelithiasis.

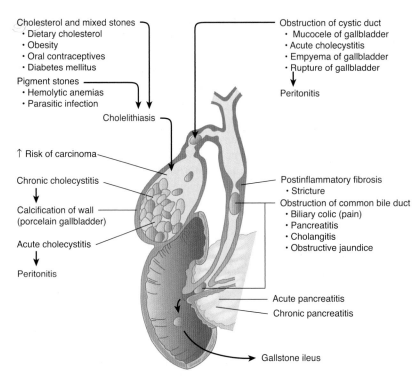

FIGURE 13–21   Clinical and pathologic effects of cholelithiasis.   (Redrawn, with permission, from Chandrasoma P, Taylor CE. *Concise Pathology*, 3rd ed. Originally published by Appleton & Lange. Copyright © 1998 by the McGraw-Hill Companies, Inc.)

Clinical Manifestations

The major clinical presentation of gallstones is inflammation of the gallbladder, or **cholecystitis.** Cholecystitis can be either acute, chronic, or acute against a background of chronic disease. An episode of acute cholecystitis can progress to acute pancreatitis if a stone travels down the common bile duct but fails to clear the sphincter of Oddi, thereby blocking the pancreatic duct. Likewise, an inflamed gallbladder can become infected or can undergo infarction and necrosis, setting the stage for systemic sepsis if the patient does not receive systemic broad-spectrum antibiotics and undergo emergency cholecystectomy (Figure 13–21).

PATHOPHYSIOLOGY OF DISORDERS OF THE SMALL INTESTINE & COLON

Diseases of the small and large intestine include diarrhea, inflammatory bowel disease, and diverticular disease. **Diarrhea** is a symptom that has many causes and diverse pathogenetic mechanisms, including altered motility, secretion, digestion, and absorption. Although intestinal disorders are particularly prominent causes, disease of the stomach, pancreas, and biliary tract can also cause diarrhea. **Inflammatory bowel diseases** are poorly understood chronic autoimmune processes in the small intestine, colon, or both, with malabsorption as a prominent feature and important systemic manifestations. **Diverticular disease** occurs most prominently in the colon, in part as a direct or indirect consequence of altered motor function. **Irritable bowel syndrome** is not a disease per se but a functional disorder manifested by abdominal pain with diarrhea or constipation in the absence of organic disease or gross structural changes of the intestine.

DIARRHEA

Clinical Presentation

Symptoms of diarrhea are an increased stool frequency, increased stool volume, and a decrease in stool consistency. Any process that increases the frequency of defecation or volume of stool makes it looser, because time-dependent absorption of water is responsible for the normal soft but formed consistency of stool. Infectious diarrheas are discussed in Chapter 4. This chapter focuses on general aspects of diarrhea and diarrheas from other causes.

Patients' subjective assessments of bowel movements are colored by their baseline bowel habits. An individual with chronic constipation, with bowel movements once every 3 days or so, may regard three soft stools in a day as diarrhea. In contrast, an individual on a high-fiber diet may normally have bowel movements twice or even three times a day.

Diarrhea can be acute (less than 2 weeks' duration) or chronic (over 4 weeks). Acute diarrhea is usually due to an infectious cause. The most common noninfectious causes are side effects of medications.

The simplest idea is that diarrhea is due to too much secretion or not enough absorption. **Osmotic (malabsorptive) diarrhea** is due to malabsorbed nutrients or poorly absorbed electrolytes that retain water in the lumen. Malabsorption occurs when the ability to digest or absorb a particular nutrient is defective and can be due to disordered mixing (altered motility), pancreatic insufficiency (altered digestion), or damage to enterocytes or their surface transporters (altered absorption). This type of diarrhea stops when the patient fasts. **Secretory diarrhea** results when secretagogues maintain elevated rates of fluid transport out of epithelial cells into the GI tract lumen. This type of diarrhea does not stop when the patient fasts. These physiologic distinctions are useful in both diagnosis and therapy of diarrheal disorders. In transport capacity, the small intestine far exceeds the colon (owing to the enormous surface area of the brush border). Thus, infectious, toxic, or other causes of heightened secretion in the small intestine can overwhelm absorptive mechanisms in the colon, resulting in diarrhea.

Etiology

Flow in the GI tract is a steady state involving massive fluid secretion into and absorption from the GI lumen. Each process is controlled by both extrinsic and intrinsic factors. Subtle aberrations in input or output at any of several levels can result in diarrhea with or without nutrient malabsorption. Thus, an excessive osmotic load, increased secretion, or diminished fluid resorption may result in diarrhea (Table 13–7).

An excessive osmotic load in the GI tract may come about in three different ways: by direct oral ingestion of excessive osmoles, by ingestion of a substrate that may be converted into excessive osmoles (eg, when bacterial action on the nondigestible carbohydrate lactulose generates a diarrhea-causing osmotic load in the colon), and as a manifestation of a genetic disease such as an enzyme deficiency in the setting of a particular diet (eg, milk consumption by a lactase-deficient individual).

Secretion is increased by either blood-borne or intraluminal secretagogues. These include endogenous endocrine products (eg, overproduction of VIP by a tumor), exotoxins resulting from direct ingestion (eg, acute food poisoning) or infection (eg, cholera), or GI luminal substances (eg, bile acids) that stimulate secretion.

Absorption of fluid, electrolytes, and nutrients can be diminished by many factors, including the toxic effects of alcohol and mucosal damage from infectious agents and from cytokines and prokinetic agents. Cytokines are released by immune and other cells (eg, in response to infection). Prokinetic agents speed up GI motility, thereby diminishing the time available for absorption of any given nutrient, fluid, or electrolyte load. Finally, inflammatory and other disorders resulting in loss of mucus, blood, or protein from the GI tract

TABLE 13–7 Mechanisms of diarrhea and major specific causes.

Mechanisms of Diarrhea	Specific Causes
Osmotic/malabsorption	Disaccharidase deficiencies (eg, lactase deficiency)
	Glucose-galactose or fructose malabsorption
	Mannitol, sorbitol ingestion
	Lactulose therapy
	Some salts (eg, magnesium sulfate)
	Some antacids (eg, Maalox)
	Generalized malabsorption
	Pancreatic enzyme inactivation (eg, by excess acid)
	Defective fat solubilization (disrupted enterohepatic circulation or defective bile formation)
	Ingestion of nutrient-binding substances
	Bacterial overgrowth
	Loss of enterocytes (eg, radiation, infection, ischemia)
	Lymphatic obstruction (eg, lymphoma, tuberculosis)
	Pancreatic enzyme deficiency
Secretory	Enterotoxins
	Tumor products (eg, VIP, serotonin)
	Laxatives
	Bile acids
	Fatty acids
	Congenital defects
Motility disorder	Diabetes mellitus
	Postsurgical
Inflammatory exudation	Inflammatory bowel disease
	Infection (eg, shigellosis)

Data from Fine KD, Krejs GJ, Fordtran JS. Diarrhea. In: *Gastrointestinal Disease*, 4th ed. Sleisenger MH, Fordtran JS (editors). Saunders, 1989.

may be manifested as diarrhea. Symptoms and signs suggesting specific causes of diarrhea are listed in Table 13–8.

Pathology & Pathogenesis

Recognition of pathophysiologic subtypes of secretory (Tables 13–9 and 13–10) and osmotic diarrheas provides a means of approaching diagnosis and therapy of diarrheal disorders. For example, nonbloody diarrhea that continues in the absence of oral intake must be due to a secretory mechanism, whereas diar-

TABLE 13–8 **Clues to diagnosis of diarrhea from other symptoms and signs.**

Symptoms or Signs Associated with Diarrhea	Diagnoses To Be Considered
Arthritis	Ulcerative colitis, Crohn's disease, Whipple's disease, enteritis resulting from *Yersinia enterocolitica*, gonococcal proctitis
Liver disease	Ulcerative colitis, Crohn's disease, colon cancer with metastases to liver
Fever	Ulcerative colitis, Crohn's disease, amebiasis, lymphoma, tuberculosis, Whipple's disease, other enteric infections (especially viral or toxin-producing bacterial)
Marked weight loss	Malabsorption, inflammatory bowel disease, colon cancer, thyrotoxicosis
Eosinophilia	Eosinophilic gastroenteritis, parasitic disease (particularly *Strongyloides*)
Lymphadenopathy	Lymphoma, Whipple's disease, AIDS
Neuropathy	Diabetic diarrhea, amyloidosis
Postural hypotension	GI bleeding, diabetic diarrhea, Addison's disease, idiopathic orthostatic hypotension
Flushing	Malignant carcinoid syndrome, pancreatic cholera syndrome
Erythema	Systemic mastocytosis, glucagonoma syndrome
Proteinuria	Amyloidosis
Collagen-vascular disease	Mesenteric vasculitis
Peptic ulcers	Zollinger-Ellison syndrome
Chronic lung disease	Cystic fibrosis
Systemic arteriosclerosis	Ischemic injury to gut
Frequent infections	Immunoglobulin deficiency
Hyperpigmentation	Whipple's disease, celiac disease, Addison's disease
Good response to corticosteroids	Ulcerative colitis, Crohn's disease, Whipple's disease, Addison's disease, eosinophilic gastroenteritis, celiac disease
Good response to antibiotics	Blind loop syndrome, tropical sprue, Whipple's disease

Reproduced and modified, with permission, from Fine KD, Krejs GJ, Fordtran JS. Diarrhea. In: *Gastrointestinal Disease*, 4th ed. Sleisenger MH, Fordtran JS (editors). Saunders, 1989.

rhea that diminishes as oral intake is curtailed (eg, in a patient receiving intravenous hydration) suggests an osmotic/malabsorptive cause. Likewise, the presence of white blood cells in the stool suggests an infectious or inflammatory origin of diarrhea, although their absence does not rule out such causes.

Of the many causes of diarrhea (Table 13–11), infectious agents are among the most important because they cause acute, sometimes life-threatening diseases whose pathogenesis is relatively well understood and because they are usually treatable. The symptoms of diarrhea caused by infectious agents are due to either toxins that alter small bowel secretion and absorption or direct mucosal invasion. The noninvasive toxin-producing bacteria are generally small bowel pathogens, whereas the invasive organisms are localized typically to the colon. Diarrheas caused by infectious agents are discussed in Chapter 4.

Evidence suggests that infectious causes of diarrhea can interface more intimately with normal mechanisms of secretory control than had been previously realized. Thus, in addition to its direct effect on the G protein controlling Cl^- ion secretion in the crypts of the small intestinal epithelium, cholera activates the enteric nervous system to cause fluid and electrolyte secretion in the colon.

Clinical Manifestations

Dehydration, malnutrition, weight loss, and specific vitamin deficiency syndromes (eg, glossitis, cheilosis, and stomatitis) are common signs in diarrhea depending on its cause, severity, and chronicity (Tables 13–8 and 13–10). In certain circumstances (eg, in young children), viral gastroenteritis is associated with a high mortality rate from dehydration when supportive measures (ie, oral or intravenous rehydration) are not promptly provided. Some individuals with diarrhea from parasitic infections remain relatively asymptomatic, whereas others may develop more severe symptoms and complications, including intestinal perforation.

CHECKPOINT

61. By what mechanisms do infectious agents cause diarrhea?
62. Name three ways in which an excessive osmotic load can occur in the GI tract.

INFLAMMATORY BOWEL DISEASE

Clinical Presentation

Noninfectious inflammatory bowel disease is distinguished from infectious entities by exclusion: recurrent episodes of mucopurulent (ie, containing mucus and white cells) bloody diarrhea characterized by lack of positive cultures for infectious organisms and failure to respond to antibiotics alone. Because inflammatory bowel disease is characterized by exacerbations and remissions, favorable responses to therapy are difficult to distinguish from spontaneous remissions occurring as part of the natural history of the disease.

TABLE 13–9 Histologic features of small intestinal diseases causing malabsorption.

Disease	Pathologic Features	Pattern of Distribution
Celiac (nontropical) sprue	Villus flattening, crypt hyperplasia, increased lymphocytes and plasma cells in lamina propria	Diffuse in proximal jejunum
Tropical sprue	Shortened villi, increased lymphocytes and plasma cells in lamina propria	Diffuse in proximal jejunum
Crohn's disease	Noncaseating granulomas with or without giant cells	Patchy lesions throughout GI tract but particularly affecting terminal ileum
Collagenous sprue	Subepithelial collagen deposits	Diffuse
Primary lymphoma	Malignant lymphocytes or histiocytes in lamina propria, variable villus flattening	Patchy
Whipple's disease	Lamina propria laden with PAS-staining foamy macrophages, bacilli in macrophages	Diffuse
Amyloidosis	Amyloid deposition in blood vessels, muscle layers	Diffuse in muscularis mucosae, mucosal sparing
Abetalipoproteinemia	Lipid-laden, vacuolated epithelial cells, normal villi	Diffuse
Radiation enteritis	Flattened villi, mucosal inflammation, fibrosis, ulceration	Patchy
Lymphangiectasia	Dilated lymphatics in lamina propria	Patchy
Eosinophilic gastroenteritis	Eosinophilic infiltrate in the intestinal wall	Patchy
Hypogammaglobulinemia	Villus flattening, *Giardia* trophozoites often present, few plasma cells	Patchy
Giardiasis	Trophozoites may be present, variable villus flattening	Patchy
Opportunistic infections	Organisms may be seen (*Isospora belli*, cryptosporidia, Microsporida), PAS-staining macrophages (*Mycobacterium avium* complex)	Patchy

TABLE 13–10 Symptoms and signs of malabsorption.

Clinical Features	Pathophysiology	Laboratory Findings
Diarrhea	Increased secretion and decreased absorption of water and electrolytes; unabsorbed fatty acids and bile salts	Increased fat excretion, decreased serum carotene, "osmotic gap" in stool electrolytes
Weight loss with hyperphagia	Decreased absorption of fat, protein, and carbohydrate	Increased fat excretion
Bulky, foul-smelling stools	Decreased fat absorption	Increased fat excretion
Muscle wasting, edema	Decreased protein absorption	Decreased serum albumin
Flatulence, borborygmi, abdominal distension	Fermentation of carbohydrates by intestinal bacteria	Increased fat excretion Decreased D-xylose absorption
Abdominal pain	Small intestinal stricture, infiltration of the pancreas, intestinal ischemia	Increased fat excretion
Paresthesias, tetany	Decreased vitamin D and calcium absorption	Hypocalcemia, hypomagnesemia
Bone pain	Decreased calcium absorption	Hypocalcemia, increased alkaline phosphatase
Muscle cramps, weakness	Excess potassium loss	Hypokalemia, abnormal ECG
Easy bruisability, petechiae, hematuria	Decreased vitamin K absorption	Prolonged prothrombin time, increased fat excretion
Hyperkeratosis, night blindness	Decreased vitamin A absorption	Decreased serum carotene, increased fat excretion
Pallor	Decreased vitamin B_{12}, folate, or iron absorption	Macrocytic anemia, microcytic anemia
Glossitis, stomatitis, cheilosis	Decreased vitamin B_{12}, folate, or iron absorption	Decreased serum vitamin B_{12}, RBC folate, or serum iron
Acrodermatitis	Zinc deficiency	Decreased serum zinc

Reproduced, with permission, from Wright TL, Heyworth MF. Maldigestion and malabsorption. In: *Gastrointestinal Disease,* 4th ed. Sleisenger MH, Fordtran JS (editors). Saunders, 1989.

TABLE 13–11   Most likely causes of diarrhea in seven different clinical categories.

1. Acute diarrhea (< 2–3 weeks' duration)	**5. Chronic and recurrent diarrhea**
Viral, bacterial, parasitic, and fungal infections	Irritable bowel syndrome
Food poisoning	Inflammatory bowel disease
Drugs[1] and food additives	Parasitic and fungal infections
Fecal impaction	Malabsorption syndromes
Pelvic inflammation	Drugs,[1] food additives, sorbitol
Heavy metal poisoning (acute or chronic)	Colon cancer
2. Traveler's diarrhea	Diverticulitis
Bacterial infections	Fecal impaction
Mediated by enterotoxins produced by *E coli*	Heavy metal poisoning (acute or chronic)
Mediated mainly by invasion of mucosa and inflammation (eg, invasive *E coli, Shigella*)	Raw milk-related diarrhea
Mediated by combinations of invasion and enterotoxins (eg, *Salmonella*)	**6. Chronic diarrhea of unknown origin (previous workup failed to reveal diagnosis)**
Viral and parasitic infections	Surreptitious laxative abuse
3. Diarrhea in homosexual men without AIDS	Defective anal sphincter competence masquerading as diarrhea
Amebiasis	Microscopic colitis syndrome
Giardiasis	Previously unrecognized malabsorption
Shigellosis	Pseudopancreatic cholera syndrome
Campylobacter	Idiopathic fluid malabsorption
Rectal syphilis	Hypermotility-induced diarrhea
Rectal spirochetosis other than syphilis	Neuroendocrine tumor
Rectal gonorrhea	**7. Incontinence**
Chlamydia trachomatis infection (lymphogranuloma venereum and non-LGV serotypes D–K)	Causes of sphincter dysfunction:
Herpes simplex	Anal surgery for fissures, fistulas, or hemorrhoids
4. Diarrhea in patients with AIDS	Episiotomy or tear during childbirth
Cryptosporidium	Anal Crohn's disease
Amebiasis	Diabetic neuropathy
Giardiasis	Causes of diarrhea: same as under 5 and 6 above.
Isospora belli	
Herpes simplex, cytomegalovirus	
Mycobacterium avium-intracellulare complex	
Salmonella typhimurium	
Cryptococcus	
Candida	
AIDS enteropathy	

Reproduced and modified, with permission, from Fine KD, Krejs GJ, Fordtran JS. Diarrhea. In: *Gastrointestinal Disease,* 5th ed. Sleisenger MH, Fordtran JS (editors). Saunders, 1993.

[1]Digitalis, propranolol, quinidine, diuretics, colchicine, antibiotics, lactulose, antacids, laxatives, chemotherapeutic agents, bile acids, Meclomen, and many others. (See drug compendiums for adverse effects of drugs the patient has been taking.)

Etiology

The cause of noninfectious inflammatory bowel disease is unknown despite progress in understanding its pathogenesis.

There are two forms of chronic inflammatory bowel disease: **Crohn's disease,** which is transmural and granulomatous in character, occurring anywhere along the GI tract, and **ulcerative colitis,** which is superficial and limited to the colonic mucosa. The causes of inflammatory bowel disease are unknown despite progress in understanding its pathogenesis.

Pathology & Pathogenesis

A combination of genetic risk and environmental factors are recognized key elements in the pathogenesis of inflammatory bowel disease. An explosion of newly recognized susceptibility genes for both Crohn's disease and ulcerative colitis have been discovered through genome-wide associations. These studies evaluated thousands of single nucleotide polymorphisms (SNPs) in thousands of patients with inflammatory bowel disease and compared them to people without the disease. These studies have found that several categories of susceptibility genes that include modulators of immune function and interaction with microorganisms.

Many environmental factors have been speculated to contribute to the development of Crohn's disease, including microorganisms (bacteria and viruses), dietary factors, genetic factors, defective immune responses, and psychosocial factors. The normal gut is able to modulate frank inflammatory responses to its constant bombardment with dietary and microbial antigens in the lumen. This modulation may be defective in Crohn's disease, resulting in uncontrolled inflammation. There has been considerable interest in the role of cytokines, such as interleukins and tumor necrosis factor, in Crohn's disease. Cytokine profiles of T_H1 and T_H17 categories have been implicated in Crohn's disease. Mice lacking the T_H1-inhibiting cytokine interleukin-10 have a T_H1 cytokine profile and develop a Crohn's disease-like inflammation of the intestine. Monoclonal antibodies to tumor necrosis factor (TNF) reduce inflammation in these animals and patients. Similar factors may contribute to the pathogenesis of ulcerative colitis, including infections, allergies to dietary components, immune responses to bacteria and self-antigens, and psychosocial factors. In mice, targeted disruption of the genes for the T-cell receptor and the cytokine IL-2 results in GI tract disease resembling ulcerative colitis.

The two forms of inflammatory bowel disease have characteristic differences and in many cases considerable overlap in manner of presentation (Table 13–12). The features common to all forms of inflammatory bowel disease are mucosal ulceration and inflammation of the GI tract, indistinguishable, in fact, from that which can occur acutely during invasive infectious diarrhea. Other factors besides the presence of key gene products, including infectious agents, altered host immune responses, immune-mediated intestinal damage, psychologic

factors, and dietary and environmental factors, may contribute to a final common pathway of disordered immune response.

Clinical Manifestations

A. Crohn's Disease

Crohn's disease most typically occurs in the distal ileum. However, the distribution of the disease can also involve the colon or less commonly any other region of the GI tract (including the oral cavity, esophagus, stomach, and proximal small intestine). A characteristic feature is that areas of ulceration and inflammation occur in a discontinuous fashion and involve the entire thickness of the bowel wall. Recurrence of disease can occur in previously uninvolved regions of the intestine and can even involve adjacent mesentery and lymph nodes. The combination of deep mucosal ulceration and submucosal thickening gives the involved mucosa a characteristic "cobblestone" appearance.

Perforation, fistula formation, abscess formation, and small intestinal obstruction are frequent complications of Crohn's disease, although an indolent course occurs in most patients. The full-thickness involvement of the bowel wall may predispose to these complications. Frank bleeding from the mucosal ulcerations can be either insidious or massive, as can **protein-losing enteropathy.** Another important complication is a possible increased incidence of intestinal cancer.

Patients with Crohn's disease often manifest symptoms outside of the GI tract. Most commonly, inflammatory disorders of the joints (arthritis), skin (erythema nodosum), eye (uveitis, iritis), mucous membranes (aphthous ulcers of the buccal mucosa) bile ducts (sclerosing cholangitis), and liver (autoimmune chronic active hepatitis) are also observed in these patients. Renal disorders, especially nephrolithiasis, are observed in one third of patients with Crohn's disease, probably related to increased oxalate absorption associated with steatorrhea. Amyloidosis is a serious complication of Crohn's disease, as is thromboembolic disease. Both of these complications are probably reflections of the systemic character of the inflammatory process. Patients are often malnourished and show evidence of nutrient deficiency states.

B. Ulcerative Colitis

In contrast to Crohn's disease, inflammation in ulcerative colitis is restricted to the mucosa of the colon and rectum. It typically begins at the anorectal junction and extends proximally. At one time it was believed that ulcerative colitis and Crohn's disease were distinct entities. This view was based on the observation of characteristic necrotic lesions of the colonic crypts of Lieberkühn, termed "crypt abscesses" in patients with ulcerative colitis. However, it is now recognized that in 10% of patients, regions characteristic of both Crohn's disease and ulcerative colitis are present. The diseases are similar in presentation (eg, bloody diarrhea and malabsorption) and in at least some of the complications (eg, protein-losing enteropathy and malnutrition), reflecting widespread involvement

TABLE 13–12 Similarities and differences between ulcerative colitis and Crohn's disease.

	Ulcerative Colitis	Crohn's Disease
Clinical features		
Rectal bleeding	> 90%	< 50%
Diarrhea	10–30%	> 70%
Abdominal mass	< 1%	30%
Perianal abscesses, sinuses, and fistulas	2%	30%
Bowel perforation (free)	2–3%	< 1%
Toxic megacolon	5–10%	< 5%
Cancer of colon	Definite increase (5%)	Possible increase
Pyoderma gangrenosum	< 5%	1%
Erythema nodosum	5%	15%
Renal stones	< 5% (uric acid stones)	10% (oxalate stones)
Stomatitis	10%	10%
Aphthous ulceration	4%	4%
Uveitis	45%	5–10%
Spondylitis	< 5%	15–20%
Peripheral arthritis	10%	20%
Thromboembolism with increased platelets and increased coagulant activity	Occurs	Occurs
Radiologic, endoscopic, and pathologic findings		
Rectal involvement	Almost 100%	< 50%
Ulcers	Superficial, multiple	Solitary ulcers in the rectum
	Irregular	Linear, serpiginous, and aphthoid ulcers
		Collar-button ulcers
Crypt abscesses, pseudopolyps, diminished goblet cells	> 70%	< 40%
Lymphoid aggregates and noncaseating granulomas	< 10%	60–70%
Extent of disease	Mucosal and continuous	Transmural and discontinuous with "skip lesions"
Ileal involvement	Nonspecific with mild inflammation and dilation (backwash ileitis)	Ulcers, fissures, and stenosis
Fatty liver	39–40%	30–40%
Pericholangitis	30%	20%
Sclerosing cholangitis	30%	20–30%
Cirrhosis	Rare	<1%
Gallstones	Rare	10–15%
Treatment		
General	Supportive and symptomatic	Supportive and symptomatic
Definitive (drugs)	Sulfasalazine, mesalamine, or olsalazine and corticosteroids	Sulfasalazine, corticosteroids, mercaptopurine

Modified and reproduced, with permission, from Gopalswamy N. Inflammatory bowel disease. In: *Clinical Medicine: Selected Problems with Pathophysiologic Correlations.* Barnes HV et al (editors). Year Book, 1988.

of the mucosa in both entities. However, because ulcerative colitis generally is limited to the mucosa, obstruction, perforation, and fistula formation are not typical complications. Most patients have mild disease, and, as with Crohn's disease, some patients will have only one or two episodes during their lifetimes. For unknown reasons, the risk of carcinoma appears even higher in ulcerative colitis than in Crohn's disease. Toxic megacolon is the one complication of ulcerative colitis that carries a high risk of perforation. Its cause is unknown.

Both ulcerative colitis and Crohn's disease can go into remission after treatment with first-line anti-inflammatory agents such as sulfasalazine and glucocorticoids. Crohn's disease also responds to therapy that utilizes monoclonal antibodies against the inflammatory cytokine, TNF. These antibodies bind to and inhibit this cytokine. Recently, therapy with anti-TNF monoclonal antibodies has been used in patients with ulcerative colitis as well. Because of potential complication of serious, even life-threatening infection, these drugs are utilized only for severe cases. The natural history of both diseases is of periods of remission interrupted by active disease; medical therapy during exacerbations is directed toward supportive measures and attempts at inducing remission. Because these diseases can recur after resection of involved regions of the GI tract, operative management is generally limited to relief of life-threatening intestinal obstruction or bleeding. Because of the variable response rate and the high risk of side effects, therapy with immunosuppressive agents such as mercaptopurine and azathioprine are limited to cases that have failed to respond to sulfasalazine and glucocorticoids.

CHECKPOINT

63. How is inflammatory bowel disease distinguished from infectious diarrhea?
64. What are the differences between ulcerative colitis and Crohn's disease?
65. What are the complications of inflammatory bowel disease?

DIVERTICULAR DISEASE

Clinical Presentation

Nearly 80% of patients with diverticula are asymptomatic except for chronic constipation. Of those who develop other symptoms, the most common presentation is an intermittent and unpredictable griping lower abdominal pain (diverticulitis). Additional features of the presentation depend on which of the two major complications of diverticula that the patient develops.

A patient who develops diverticulitis (see later discussion) may present with fever and with symptoms and signs of peri-

toneal irritation (guarding, rebound tenderness, absence of bowel sounds). A patient who develops diverticular bleeding may present with either frankly bloody stools or stools that are positive for occult blood.

Etiology

Diverticulosis results from an acquired deformity of the colon in which the mucosa and submucosa herniate through the underlying muscularis (Figure 13–22). This is a disease of modern affluent life. A rarity at the turn of the century, today it afflicts 30% of adults in the U.S. population. Its incidence increases with age, starting from about 40 years. Epidemiologic studies suggest that the consumption of highly refined foods and less fiber, with resulting increased prevalence of chronic constipation, may be responsible for the increased prevalence of diverticular disease.

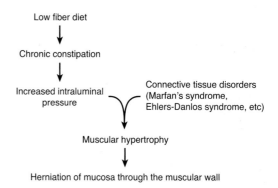

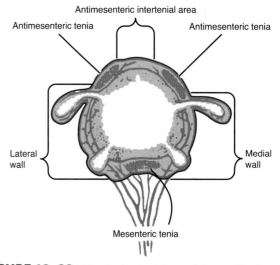

FIGURE 13–22 **Top:** Pathophysiology of diverticular disease. **Bottom:** Cross-sectional drawing of the colon, showing principal points of diverticula formation between mesenteric and antimesenteric teniae. (Redrawn, with permission, from Goligher JC. *Surgery of the Anus, Rectum and Colon*, 5th ed. Baillière Tyndall, 1984.)

Pathology & Pathogenesis

A. Diverticulosis

Most acquired diverticula occur in the colon; the descending colon and sigmoid (left side) are involved in > 90% of cases. Both structural and functional factors are believed to contribute to the development of diverticulosis. Acquired abnormalities in colonic wall connective tissue are believed to be the structural basis of diminished resistance to mucosal and submucosal herniation (Figure 13–22). The functional abnormality is believed to be related to chronic constipation and the development of a transmural pressure gradient from colonic lumen to peritoneal space as a result of vigorous muscle contraction of the colonic wall. This functional abnormality is most likely related to the change in dietary habits; decreased dietary fiber makes forward propulsion of feces at normal transmural pressures more difficult. This increased muscle contraction, which contributes to the development of diverticular disease, is also believed to cause the abdominal pain that is the cardinal symptom of uncomplicated diverticular disease. The pain may last hours to days, with sudden relief on passing flatus or feces. Constipation or diarrhea and flatulence are common findings during such episodes, leading to the suggestion that there is a relationship between irritable bowel syndrome and the development of diverticulosis. Treatment of the pain of diverticular disease with opioids is contraindicated because they directly raise intraluminal pressure and hence may increase the risk of perforation.

B. Diverticular Bleeding

Diverticula are a source of bleeding in 3–5% of patients with diverticulosis. Branches of the colonic intramural arteries (vasa recta) are closely associated with the diverticular sac, presumably leading to occasional rupture and bleeding. This is the most common cause of massive lower GI bleeding in the elderly. Diverticular bleeding is typically painless and not believed to be associated with a focus of inflammation.

C. Diverticulitis

This most common complication of diverticulosis develops when a focal area of inflammation occurs in the wall of a diverticulum in response to irritation by fecal material. The patient develops symptoms of abdominal pain and fever with a risk of progression to abscess with or without perforation. The perforations usually are self-contained, but the potential for subsequent fistula formation and intestinal obstruction is high.

Clinical Manifestations

About one fifth of all individuals with diverticular disease develop one of the two major complications—diverticular bleeding or diverticulitis—which must be distinguished from carcinoma, inflammatory bowel disease, and ischemic injury resulting from diffuse atherosclerosis.

IRRITABLE BOWEL SYNDROME

Irritable bowel syndrome is the most common cause of referral to gastroenterologists. It is characterized by altered bowel habits with abdominal pain in the absence of any detectable organic pathological process or specific motility or structural abnormalities.

A change in bowel habits, commonly alternating between diarrhea and constipation, is the principal characteristic of irritable bowel syndrome. Abdominal pain, which may be caused by intestinal spasms, is also common to all patients with irritable bowel syndrome. Bloating or perceived abdominal distension is another common feature. Intraluminal gas can result from swallowing air, diminished absorption of gas, and bacterial fermentation, although the cause in irritable bowel syndrome is unknown. Stress appears to have a considerable influence on these symptoms. Symptoms of irritable bowel syndrome frequently occur during or after a stressful event, and stressful events in early life may predispose to the development of irritable bowel syndrome.

Much of our understanding of the pathophysiology of irritable bowel syndrome derives from study of motility. In normal persons, high-amplitude peristaltic contractions occur 6–8 times per day. In constipated patients with irritable bowel syndrome, the frequency of high-amplitude peristaltic contractions of the intestine is diminished compared with normal subjects, suggesting that the constipation may be due to diminished motility. Visceral hyperalgesia may also occur in patients with irritable bowel syndrome. In patients with irritable bowel syndrome, distension of the colon with a balloon, to a degree that is not painful in normal individuals, can induce pain, indicative of visceral hyperalgesia.

Irritable bowel syndrome is a complex disorder, and its cause is poorly understood. Several theories have been proposed to explain the disorder, including alterations in sensitivity of the extrinsic and intrinsic nervous systems of the intestine, which may contribute to exaggerated sensations of pain and to abnormal control of intestinal motility and secretion. An alteration in the balance of secretion and absorption is also a potential cause. Although there is no gross inflammation of the intestine, there are reports of an increased influx of inflammatory cells (mast cells) into the colon of affected individuals as well as destruction of enteric neurons. The intestinal microbes that normally inhabit the small intestine and colon may be altered as well. One proposed theory is that irritable bowel syndrome develops as a result of an earlier and resolved bout of interstitial inflammation. In experimental animals, induction of intestinal inflammation induces visceral hyperalgesia and altered intestinal motility and secretion that persists many months after the inflammation is resolved. A similar mechanism may occur in a subset of patients who develop irritable bowel syndrome after an infection causes intestinal inflammation.

CASE STUDIES

Eva M. Aagaard, MD, & Yeong Kwok, MD

(See Chapter 25, p. 695 for Answers)

CASE 57

A 60-year-old man presents to the clinic with a 3-month history of gradually worsening dysphagia (difficulty swallowing). At first, he noticed the problem when eating solid food such as steak, but now it happens even with drinking water. He has a sensation that whatever he swallows becomes stuck in his chest and does not go into the stomach. He has also developed worsening heartburn, especially upon lying down, and has had to prop himself up at night to lessen the heartburn. He has lost 10 kg as a result of his swallowing difficulties. His physical examination is unremarkable. A barium swallow x-ray reveals a decrease in peristalsis of the body of the esophagus along with dilatation of the lower esophagus and tight closure of the lower esophageal sphincter. There is a beaked appearance of the distal esophagus involving the lower esophageal sphincter. There is very little passage of barium into the stomach.

Questions

A. What is the likely diagnosis in this patient, and what is the underlying pathophysiology of this condition?
B. Botulinum toxin can be used to treat this disorder. How does it help ameliorate the symptoms?
C. What are the possible complications of this disorder, and how do they arise?

CASE 58

A 32-year-old woman presents to her primary care provider complaining of a persistent burning sensation in her chest and upper abdomen. The symptoms are worse at night while she is lying down and after meals. She has tried drinking hot cocoa to help her sleep. She is a smoker and frequently relies on benzodiazepines for insomnia. She notes a sour taste in her mouth every morning. Physical examination is normal.

Questions

A. What is the pathogenetic mechanism of her GI disorder?
B. How may her lifestyle impact her symptoms?
C. What are some complications of chronic esophageal reflux disease?

CASE 59

A 74-year-old man with severe osteoarthritis presents to the emergency department reporting two episodes of melena (black stools) without hematochezia (bright red blood in the stools) or hematemesis (bloody vomitus). He takes 600 mg of ibuprofen three times a day to control his arthritis pain. He denies alcohol use. On examination his blood pressure is 150/70 Hg and his resting pulse is 96/min. His epigastrium is minimally tender to palpation. Rectal examination reveals black tarry stool in the vault, grossly positive for occult blood. Endoscopy demonstrates a 3 cm gastric ulcer. *Helicobacter pylori* is identified on biopsies of the ulcer site.

Questions

A. What are some of the proposed mechanisms for acid-peptic disease and specifically gastric ulcer disease?
B. How may this patient's analgesic use predispose him to acid-peptic disease?
C. What role does *H pylori* infection play in the pathogenesis of ulcer disease? How should this be taken into account when treating this patient?

CASE 60

A 67-year-old man with type 2 diabetes is seen by his primary care provider for frequent nausea, bloating, and intermittent diarrhea over the preceding 2 weeks. The vomiting typically occurs approximately 1–2 hours after eating. He states that over the past year he has become increasingly depressed after the death of his wife and has been less adherent to his oral hypoglycemic regimen and evening insulin. He also reports 6 months of worsening neuropathic pain in his feet. His fasting fingerstick blood glucose level is 253 mg/dL.

Questions

A. How may diabetes contribute to the development of gastroparesis? Is his poor control a cause or consequence of gastroparesis?
B. How can delayed gastric emptying cause diarrhea?

CASE 61

A 40-year-old woman presents to the emergency department with a history of worsening right upper quadrant pain. The pain started after she had pizza for dinner 2 days ago and is described as a sharp, stabbing sensation under her right ribs. She has also felt ill, developed slight nausea, and had a low-grade fever. There has been no vomiting or diarrhea. Physical examination reveals an obese woman with a low-grade fever and tenderness to palpation of the right upper quadrant of her abdomen. An abdominal ultrasound reveals a 2 cm gallstone lodged in the cystic duct with swelling of the gallbladder and thickening of the gallbladder wall.

Questions

A. What are the mechanisms involved in gallstone formation?
B. What factors in the pathogenesis of gallstones may be responsible for the fact that it is more common in premenopausal women?
C. What local complications can ensue from gallstone disease?

CASE 62

On a cruise ship sailing in the Caribbean, a number of passengers develop acute onset of nonbloody diarrhea approximately 24 hours after their land excursion to a small Mexican village where they sampled local cuisine. They deny fever, nausea, or vomiting but report 8 to 10 loose watery stools a day despite significant anorexia. Fecal leukocytes do not appear in the stool samples of the affected passengers. Enterotoxigenic *E coli* infection is identified during an outbreak investigation. Symptoms are self-limited in most of the affected passengers, improving after 48 hours.

Questions

A. Which mechanism of diarrhea may be attributed to this infection?
B. What clinical cues help you in distinguishing the type of diarrhea?
C. How should the passengers be treated?

CASE 63

A 42-year-old man with long-standing Crohn's disease presents to the emergency department with a 1-day history of increasing abdominal distension, pain, and obstipation. He is nauseated and has vomited bilious material. He has no history of abdominal surgery and has had two exacerbations of his disease this year. He is febrile with a temperature of 38.5 °C. Examination reveals multiple oral aphthous ulcers, hyperactive bowel sounds, and a grossly distended, diffusely tender abdomen without an appreciable mass. Abdominal radiographs reveal multiple air-fluid levels in the small bowel with minimal colonic gas consistent with a small bowel obstruction.

Questions

A. Describe the significance of the oral aphthous ulcers in the distribution of Crohn's disease.
B. What factors are thought to be involved in the pathogenesis of Crohn's disease? What is the evidence to support the role of cytokines in the pathogenesis of Crohn's disease?
C. What are the GI complications of Crohn's disease?
D. Describe some of the extraintestinal manifestations of Crohn's disease.

CASE 64

A 76-year-old woman with chronic constipation reports a 4-day history of "achy" left lower quadrant abdominal pain, graded 7/10, accompanied by low-grade fever and nausea. A colonoscopy performed 2 years ago revealed sigmoid diverticular disease. On examination she has a temperature of 38.6 °C. Her abdomen has a tender 3 × 2 cm mass in the left lower quadrant. Bowel sounds are normal. Her stool is positive for occult blood. An abdominal series shows a bowel gas pattern consistent with ileus and no evidence of free peritoneal air. A CT scan with contrast of the abdomen and pelvis shows pericolonic fat stranding with no evidence of an abscess. She is started on antibiotics and intravenous fluids with significant improvement in her symptoms.

Questions

A. Describe the pathogenesis of diverticular disease.
B. Why should opioids be avoided in the treatment of her abdominal pain?
C. What are the complications of diverticular disease?

CASE 65

A 32-year-old woman comes to the clinic complaining of a 3-month history of abdominal bloating, crampy abdominal pain, and a change in her bowel habits. Previously she had regular bowel movements, but 4 months ago, she developed gastroenteritis with nausea and vomiting after a cruise. The constant diarrhea and vomiting went away after a week, but since then she has had periods of constipation, lasting up to 3 days, alternating with periods of diarrhea. During the diarrheal episodes, she can have three to four loose bowel movements per day, though without blood or mucus in the stool. She describes diffuse abdominal cramping and bloating that are somewhat relieved by bowel movements. Her symptoms worsen during periods of stress. There has been no weight loss or fever. There is no association with particular foods (eg, wheat or dairy products). Her physical examination is unremarkable except for mild abdominal tenderness with no rebound or guarding. Serologic tests for celiac sprue are negative. Stool cultures and examinations are negative for bacterial or parasitic infections. A colonoscopy is unremarkable.

Questions

A. What is the likely diagnosis?

B. What are the theories about the pathophysiology of this condition?

REFERENCES

General

Camilleri M. Integrated upper gastrointestinal response to food intake. Gastroenterology. 2006 Aug;131(2):640–58. [PMID: 16890616]

Dimaline R et al. Attack and defence in the gastric epithelium—a delicate balance. Exp Physiol. 2007 Jul;92(4):591–601. [PMID: 17412751]

Farrugia G. Interstitial cells of Cajal in health and disease. Neurogastroenterol Motil. 2008 May;20(Suppl 1):54–63. [PMID: 18402642]

Grundy D. Signalling the state of the digestive tract. Auton Neurosci. 2006 Apr 30;125(1–2):76–80. [PMID: 16473562]

Merchant JL. Inflammation, atrophy, gastric cancer: Connecting the molecular dots. Gastroenterology. 2005 Sep;129(3):1079–82. [PMID: 16143144]

Merchant JL. Tales from the crypts: Regulatory peptides and cytokines in gastrointestinal homeostasis and disease. J Clin Invest. 2007 Jan;117(1):6–12. [PMID: 17200701]

Orlando LA et al. Chronic hypergastrinemia: Causes and consequences. Dig Dis Sci. 2007 Oct;52(10):2482–9. [PMID: 17415644]

Sanger GJ et al. Hormones of the gut-brain axis as targets for the treatment of upper gastrointestinal disorders. Nat Rev Drug Discov. 2008 Mar;7(3):241–54. [PMID: 18309313]

Wood JD. Enteric nervous system: Reflexes, pattern generators and motility. Curr Opin Gastroenterol. 2008 Mar;24(2):149–58. [PMID: 18301264]

Xu J et al. Evolution of symbiotic bacteria in the distal human intestine. PLoS Biol. 2007 Jun 19;5(7):e156. [PMID: 17579514]

GI Disease

Di Nardo G et al. Review article: molecular, pathological and therapeutic features of human enteric neuropathies. Aliment Pharmacol Ther. 2008 Jul;28(1):25–42. [PMID: 18410560]

Egan BJ et al. *Helicobacter pylori* gastritis, the unifying concept for gastric diseases. Helicobacter. 2007 Nov;12(Suppl 2):39–44. [PMID: 17991175]

Furness JB. The enteric nervous system: Normal functions and enteric neuropathies. Neurogastroenterol Motil. 2008 May;20(Suppl 1):32–8. [PMID: 18402640]

Kandulski A et al. *Helicobacter pylori* infection: A clinical overview. Dig Liver Dis. 2008 Aug;40(8):619–26. [PMID: 18396114]

Peter S et al. *Helicobacter pylori* and gastric cancer: The causal relationship. Digestion. 2007;75(1):25–35. [PMID: 17429205]

Sanghi S et al. Cyclooxygenase-2 inhibitors: A painful lesson. Cardiovasc Hematol Disord Drug Targets. 2006 Jun;6(2):85–100. [PMID: 16787194]

Achalasia & Esophageal Reflux

Dogan I et al. Esophageal motor disorders: Recent advances. Curr Opin Gastroenterol. 2006 Jul;22(4):417–22. [PMID: 16760760]

Fass R. Erosive esophagitis and nonerosive reflux disease (NERD): Comparison of epidemiologic, physiologic, and therapeutic characteristics. J Clin Gastroenterol. 2007 Feb;41(2):131–7. [PMID: 17245209]

Pohl D et al. Achalasia: An overview of diagnosis and treatment. J Gastrointestin Liver Dis. 2007 Sep;16(3):297–303. [PMID: 17925926]

Richter JE. How to manage refractory GERD. Nat Clin Pract Gastroenterol Hepatol. 2007 Dec;4(12):658–64. [PMID: 18043675]

Acid-Peptic Disease

Louw JA. Peptic ulcer disease. Curr Opin Gastroenterol. 2006 Nov;22(6):607–11. [PMID: 17053437]

Palmer K. Acute upper gastrointestinal haemorrhage. Br Med Bull. 2007;83:307–24. [PMID: 17942452]

Paran TS et al. Enteric nervous system and developmental abnormalities in childhood. Pediatr Surg Int. 2006 Dec;22(12):945–59. [PMID: 17001489]

Rokkas T et al. *Helicobacter pylori* and non-malignant diseases. Helicobacter. 2007 Oct;12(Suppl 1):20–2. [PMID: 17727456]

Schubert ML et al. Control of gastric acid secretion in health and disease. Gastroenterology. 2008 Jun;134(7):1842–60. [PMID: 18474247]

Gastroparesis & Ileus

Batke M et al. Adynamic ileus and acute colonic pseudo-obstruction. Med Clin North Am. 2008 May;92(3):649–70. [PMID: 18387380]

Jones MP et al. Small intestinal motility. Curr Opin Gastroenterol. 2008 Mar;24(2):164–72. [PMID: 18301266]

Ordög T. Interstitial cells of Cajal in diabetic gastroenteropathy. Neurogastroenterol Motil. 2008 Jan;20(1):8–18. [PMID: 18173559]

Patrick A et al. Review article: gastroparesis. Aliment Pharmacol Ther. 2008 May;27(9):724–40. [PMID: 18248660]

Sanjeevi A. Gastric motility. Curr Opin Gastroenterol. 2007 Nov;23(6):625–30. [PMID: 17906438]

Gallstone Disease

Sanders G et al. Gallstones. BMJ. 2007 Aug 11;335(7614):295-9. [PMID: 17690370]

Wittenburg H et al. Genetic predisposition to gallbladder stones. Semin Liver Dis. 2007 Feb;27(1):109–21. [PMID: 17295180]

Diarrhea

Barrett KE. New ways of thinking about (and teaching about) intestinal epithelial function. Adv Physiol Educ. 2008 Mar;32(1):25–34. [PMID: 18334565]

Holt PR. Intestinal malabsorption in the elderly. Dig Dis. 2007;25(2):144–50. [PMID: 17468550]

Turner JR. Molecular basis of epithelial barrier regulation: From basic mechanisms to clinical application. Am J Pathol. 2006 Dec;169(6):1901–9. [PMID: 17148655]

Inflammatory Bowel Disease

Arseneau KO et al. Innate and adaptive immune responses related to IBD pathogenesis. Curr Gastroenterol Rep. 2007 Dec;9(6):508–12. [PMID: 18377804]

Cho JH. The genetics and immunopathogenesis of inflammatory bowel disease. Nat Rev Immunol. 2008 Jun;8(6):458-66. [PMID: 18500230]

Rosenstiel P et al. NOD-like receptors: Ancient sentinels of the innate immune system. Cell Mol Life Sci. 2008 May;65(9):1361–77. [PMID: 18204816]

Sartor RB. Microbial influences in inflammatory bowel diseases. Gastroenterology. 2008 Feb;134(2):577–94. [PMID: 18242222]

Shih DQ et al. Immunopathogenesis of inflammatory bowel disease. World J Gastroenterol. 2008 Jan 21;14(3):390–400. [PMID: 18200661]

Stenson WF. Toll-like receptors and intestinal epithelial repair. Curr Opin Gastroenterol. 2008 Mar;24(2):103–7. [PMID: 18301257]

Vanderpool C et al. Mechanisms of probiotic action: Implications for therapeutic applications in inflammatory bowel diseases. Inflamm Bowel Dis. 2008 Nov;14(11):1585–96. [PMID: 18623173]

Xavier RJ, Podolsky DK. Unraveling the pathogenesis of inflammatory bowel disease. Nature. 2007 Jul 26;448(7152):427–34. [PMID: 17653185]

Diverticular Disease

Jacobs DO. Clinical practice. Diverticulitis. N Engl J Med. 2007 Nov 15;357(20):2057–66. [PMID: 18003962]

Parra-Blanco A. Colonic diverticular disease: Pathophysiology and clinical picture. Digestion. 2006;73(Suppl 1):47–57. [PMID: 16498252]

Irritable Bowel Syndrome

Mayer EA. Clinical practice. Irritable bowel syndrome. N Engl J Med. 2008 Apr 17;358(16):1692–9. [PMID: 18420501]

Videlock EJ et al. Irritable bowel syndrome: Current approach to symptoms, evaluation, and treatment. Gastroenterol Clin North Am. 2007 Sep;36(3):665–85. [PMID: 17950443]

Liver Disease

Mandana Khalili, MD, Charles E. Liao, MD,
& Tung Nguyen, MD

Although many different pathogenic agents and processes can affect the liver (Table 14–1), they are generally manifested in individual patients in a limited number of ways that can be assessed by evaluation of some key parameters. Liver disease can be acute or chronic, focal or diffuse, mild or severe, and reversible or irreversible. Most cases of **acute liver disease** (eg, caused by viral hepatitis) are so mild that they never come to medical attention. Transient symptoms of fatigue, loss of appetite, and nausea are often ascribed to other causes (eg, flu), and minor biochemical abnormalities referable to the liver that would be identified in blood studies are not discovered. The patient recovers without any lasting medical consequences. In other cases of acute liver injury, symptoms and signs are severe enough to call for medical attention. The entire range of liver functions may be affected or only a few, as is the case with liver injury resulting from certain drugs that cause isolated impairment of the liver's role in bile formation (**cholestasis**). Occasionally, viral and other causes of acute liver injury occur in an overwhelming manner, resulting in massive liver cell death. This syndrome of **fulminant hepatic failure** carries a high mortality rate; however, if the patient survives, liver function returns to normal and there is no residual evidence of liver disease.

Liver injury may continue beyond the initial acute episode or may be recurrent (chronic hepatitis). In some cases of chronic hepatitis, liver function remains stable or the disease process ultimately resolves altogether. In other cases, there is progressive and irreversible deterioration of liver function.

Cirrhosis is ultimately the consequence of progressive liver injury. Cirrhosis can occur in a subset of cases of chronic hepatitis that do not resolve spontaneously or after repeated episodes of acute liver injury, as in the case of chronic alcoholism. In cirrhosis, the liver becomes hard, shrunken, and nodular and displays impaired function and diminished reserve because of a decreased amount of functioning liver tissue. More importantly, the physics of blood flow is altered such that the pressure in the portal vein is elevated. As a result, the blood is *diverted around* the liver rather than *filtered through* the liver. This phenomenon, termed **portal-to-systemic** (or **portosystemic**) **shunting,** has profound effects on the function of various organ systems and sets the stage for certain devastating complications of liver disease that are described later.

Although liver disease resulting from many different causes may present in common ways, the reverse is also true (ie, liver disease from specific causes may have distinctly different presentations in different patients). For example, consider two patients with acute viral hepatitis: One may present with yellow eyes and skin—a manifestation of impaired liver function—complaining of nothing more than itching, fatigue, and loss of appetite, whereas the other may be brought to the emergency room moribund, with massive GI bleeding and encephalopathy. Such variations in the severity of liver disease are probably due to genetic, immunologic, and environmental (including perhaps nutritional) factors that are currently poorly understood.

The consequences of liver disease can be either reversible or irreversible. Those arising directly from acute damage to the functional cells of the liver, most notably **hepatocytes,** without destruction of the liver's capacity for regeneration, are generally reversible. Like many organs of the body, the liver normally has both a huge reserve capacity for the various biochemical reactions it carries out and the ability to regenerate fully differentiated cells and thereby recover completely from acute injury. Thus, only in the most fulminant cases or in end-stage disease are there insufficient residual hepatocytes to maintain minimal essential liver functions. More commonly, patients display transient signs of liver cell necrosis and disordered function followed by full recovery. The symptoms and signs of this sort of acute liver injury can best be understood as an impairment of normal biochemical functions of the liver.

Other consequences of liver disease are irreversible, typically seen in the patient with cirrhosis. These are best

TABLE 14–1 Categories of liver disease by presentation.

Cholestasis	Chronic hepatitis
Reactions to certain classes of drugs (including anabolic steroids, oral contraceptives, phenothiazines, erythromycins, oral hypoglycemic and antithyroid drugs)	Viral hepatitis (types B, C, and D)
	Primary autoimmune disorders (idiopathic autoimmune chronic hepatitis, primary biliary cirrhosis, and sclerosing cholangitis)
Direct causes (intrahepatic biliary atresia, cholangiocarcinoma, viral hepatitis, alcoholic hepatitis, primary biliary cirrhosis, pericholangitis)	Therapeutic drug–induced (methyldopa, nitrofurantoin, oxyphenisatin-containing laxatives)
Secondary causes (postoperative, endotoxins, total parenteral nutrition, sickle cell crisis, hypophysectomy, some porphyrias)	Genetic diseases (Wilson's disease, α_1-antiprotease deficiency)
Acute hepatitis	Infiltrative disorders (sarcoidosis, amyloidosis, hemochromatosis)
Viral and bacterial, including hepatitis viruses A, B, C, D, and E, herpes simplex virus, cytomegalovirus, Epstein-Barr virus, yellow fever virus, brucella, leptospira	**Cirrhosis**
	Infectious (viral hepatitis types B, C, and D and toxoplasmosis)
Reactions to certain classes of drugs (anesthetics such as halothane, anticonvulsants such as phenytoin, antihypertensives such as methyldopa, chemotherapeutic agents such as isoniazid, and thiazide diuretics such as hydrochlorothiazide)	Genetic diseases (Wilson's disease, hemochromatosis, α_1-antiprotease deficiency, glycogen storage diseases, Fanconi's syndrome, cystic fibrosis)
	Drugs and poisons (eg, methotrexate, alcohol)
Poisons (such as ethanol); reactions to drugs	Miscellaneous (sarcoidosis, graft-versus-host disease, inflammatory bowel disease, cystic fibrosis, jejunoileal bypass, diabetes mellitus)
Fulminant hepatic failure	**Focal or extrinsic diseases with variable manifestations in the liver**
Infections (with hepatitis viruses A, B, and D, yellow fever virus, cytomegalovirus; herpes simplex virus, and *Coxiella burnetii*)	Vascular (hepatic vein thrombosis, occlusion by parasites such as echinococcus or schistosoma)
Poisons and toxins, chemicals, herbal remedies, and drugs (*Amanita phalloides* toxin, phosphorus, ethanol; solvents, including carbon tetrachloride and dimethylformamide; anesthetics, including halothane; analgesics, including acetaminophen; antimicrobials, including tetracycline and isoniazid; and other drugs, including methyldopa, monoamine oxidase inhibitors, valproate, methylenedioxymethamphetamine [ecstasy])	Biliary (duct obstruction due to stones or tumor or bacterial infection)
	Infectious (systemic sepsis; bacterial, fungal, or parasitic abscesses)
	Granulomatous diseases (sarcoidosis, tuberculosis)
Ischemia and hypoxia (vascular occlusion, circulatory failure, heat stroke, gram-negative sepsis with shock, congestive heart failure, pericardial tamponade, Budd-Chiari syndrome)	Infiltrative diseases (hemochromatosis, amyloidosis, Gaucher's disease and other lysosomal storage diseases, lymphoma)
Miscellaneous metabolic anomalies (acute fatty liver of pregnancy, Reye's syndrome, Wilson's disease, galactosemia, tyrosinemia)	

Data from Isslebacher KJ, Podolsky DK. Biological and clinical approach to liver disease. In: *Harrison's Principles of Internal Medicine,* 12th ed. Wilson JD et al (editors). McGraw-Hill, 1991.

understood as a result of portosystemic shunting of blood flow. They include a heightened sensitivity to noxious substances absorbed from the GI tract (encephalopathy), an increased risk of massive GI bleeding (development of varices and coagulopathy), and malabsorption of fat in the stool (as a result of decreased bile flow). In contrast to the consequences of acute hepatitis, those of cirrhosis are generally irreversible. Nevertheless, some of these consequences are treatable. Commonly, patients with cirrhosis present with superimposed acute liver injury (eg, caused by an alcoholic binge or other drug exposure). Because they have a decreased hepatocyte mass and much less functional reserve, they are more sensitive to acute liver injury than patients with a normal liver.

CHECKPOINT

1. What parameters must you consider in assessing a patient with liver disease?
2. What factors may determine the difference in severity of liver disease between two patients with acute hepatitis resulting from the same cause?
3. In what ways is the patient with underlying cirrhosis who presents with acute hepatitis likely to be different from the patient with a previously normal liver and acute hepatitis?

STRUCTURE & FUNCTION OF THE LIVER

ANATOMY, HISTOLOGY, & CELL BIOLOGY

The liver is located in the right upper quadrant of the abdomen in the peritoneal space just below the right side of the diaphragm and under the rib cage (Figure 14–1). It is anatomically separated into two predominant lobes, a right and a left lobe. The right lobe has two lesser segments, the posterior caudate lobe and the inferior quadrate lobe. The liver can also be differentiated functionally via the portal blood flow into four sectors, which are further subdivided into eight segments. The liver weighs approximately 1400 g in the adult and is covered by a fibrous capsule. It receives nearly 25% of the cardiac output, approximately 1500 mL of blood flow per minute, via two sources: venous flow from the **portal vein,** which is crucial to performance of the liver's roles in bodily functions, and arterial flow from the **hepatic artery,** which is important for liver oxygenation and which supplies the biliary system via the cystic artery. These vessels converge within the liver, and the combined blood flow exits via the so-called **central veins** (also called terminal veins or hepatic venules) that drain into the hepatic vein and ultimately the inferior vena cava.

The portal vein carries venous blood from the small intestine, rich in freshly absorbed nutrients—as well as drugs and poisons—directly to the liver. Also flowing into the portal vein before its entry into the liver is the pancreatic venous drainage, rich in pancreatic hormones (insulin, glucagon, somatostatin, and pancreatic polypeptide). The portal vein forms a specialized capillary bed that allows individual hepatocytes to be bathed directly in portal blood. In part because of this system of blood supply, the liver is a prime site for metastatic spread of cancer, especially from the GI tract, breast, and lung.

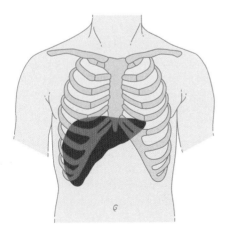

FIGURE 14–1 Location of the liver. (Redrawn, with permission, from Wolf DC. Evaluation of the size, shape and consistency of the liver. In: *Clinical Methods,* 3rd ed. Walker HK, Hall WD, Hurst JW [editors]. Butterworth, 1990.)

Concepts of Liver Organization

The substance (**parenchyma**) of the liver is organized into plates of hepatocytes lying in a cage of supporting cells termed **reticuloendothelial cells** (Figure 14–2A). The plates of hepatocytes are generally only one cell thick, and individual plates are separated from each other by vascular spaces called **sinusoids.** It is in these sinusoids that blood from the hepatic artery is mixed with blood from the portal vein on the way to the central vein. The reticuloendothelial cell meshwork in which the hepatocytes reside includes diverse cell types, most importantly the **endothelial cells** that make up the walls of the sinusoids; specialized macrophages, termed **Kupffer cells,** which are anchored in the sinusoidal space; and stellate cells or **lipocytes,** fat-storing cells involved in vitamin A metabolism, which lie between the hepatocytes and the endothelial cells. Approximately 30% of all cells in the liver are reticuloendothelial cells, and about 33% of these are Kupffer cells. Yet, because reticuloendothelial cells are smaller than hepatocytes, the reticuloendothelial system accounts for only 2–10% of the total protein in the liver. The reticuloendothelial cells are much more than just a cage for hepatocytes. They perform specific functions, including phagocytosis and secretion of cytokines, and communicate with each other as well as with hepatocytes. Their dysfunction contributes to both hepatocyte necrosis in acute liver disease and to hepatic fibrosis in chronic liver disease.

A. Lobules

Under the microscope at low-power magnification, liver architecture has been traditionally described in terms of the **lobule** (Figure 14–2B). Neat arrays of hepatocyte plates are organized around individual central veins to form hexagons with **portal triads** or **tracts** (sheathlike structures containing a portal venule, hepatic arteriole, and bile canaliculus) at their corners. The hepatocytes adjacent to the portal triad are termed the **limiting plate.** Disruption of the limiting plate is a significant diagnostic marker of some forms of immune-mediated liver disease. This may be seen in liver biopsies from patients with liver disease of unknown cause.

B. Functional Zonation

Physiologically, it is more useful to think of liver architecture in terms of the portal-to-central direction of blood flow: Blood entering the sinusoids from a terminal portal venule or hepatic arteriole flows past hepatocytes closest to those vessels first (termed zone 1 hepatocytes) and then percolates past zone 2 hepatocytes (so called because they are not the first hepatocytes reached by blood entering the hepatic parenchyma). The last hepatocytes reached by the blood before it enters the central vein are termed zone 3 hepatocytes. Thus, the microscopic organization of the liver can be viewed in terms of functional zones. A liver **acinus** is defined as the unit of liver tissue centered around the portal venule and hepatic arteriole whose

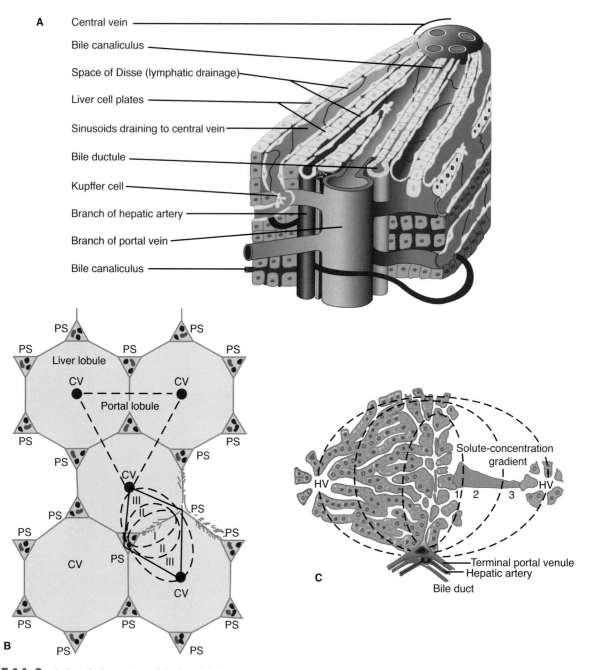

FIGURE 14–2   A: Detailed structure of the liver lobule.   (Redrawn, with permission, from Chandrasoma P, Taylor CE. *Concise Pathology,* 3rd ed. Originally published by Appleton & Lange. Copyright © 1998 by the McGraw-Hill Companies, Inc.)   **B:** Relationship of lobule to acinus. (CV, central vein; PS, portal space [or triad].)   (Redrawn, with permission, from Junqueira LC, Carneiro J, Kelley RO. *Basic Histology,* 9th ed. Originally published by Appleton & Lange. Copyright © 1998 by the McGraw-Hill Companies, Inc.)   **C:** Hepatic acinus. (HV, hepatic venule.)   (Redrawn, with permission, from Leeson CR. *Histology,* 2nd ed. Saunders, 1970.)

hepatocytes can be imagined to form concentric rings of cells in the order in which they come into contact with portal blood, first to last (Figure 14–2C). Hepatocytes at either extreme of the acinus (zones 1 and 3) appear to differ in both enzymatic activity and physiologic functions. Zone 1 hepatocytes, exposed to the highest oxygen concentrations, are particularly active in gluconeogenesis and oxidative energy metabolism. They are also the major site of urea synthesis (because freely diffusible substances such as ammonia ab-

sorbed from protein breakdown in the gut are largely extracted in zone 1). Conversely, zone 3 hepatocytes are more active in glycolysis and lipogenesis (processes requiring less oxygen). Zone 2 hepatocytes display attributes of both zone 1 and zone 3 cells.

C. Receptor-Mediated Uptake

Functional zonation applies only to processes driven by the presence of diffusible substances. The liver, however, is also

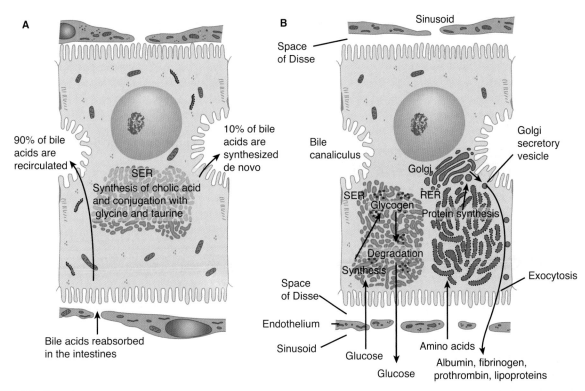

FIGURE 14–3 **A:** Mechanism of secretion of bile acids. About 90% of these compounds derive from bile acids absorbed in the intestinal epithelium and recirculated to the liver. The remainder are synthesized in the liver by conjugating cholic acid with the amino acids glycine and taurine. This process occurs in the smooth endoplasmic reticulum (SER). **B:** Protein synthesis and carbohydrate storage in the liver. Protein synthesis occurs in the rough endoplasmic reticulum, which explains why liver cell lesions or starvation leads to a decrease in the amounts of albumin, fibrinogen, and prothrombin in a patient's blood. In several diseases, glycogen degradation is depressed, with abnormal intracellular accumulation of this compound. (SER, smooth endoplasmic reticulum; RER, rough endoplasmic reticulum.) (Redrawn, with permission, from Junqueira LC, Carneiro J. *Basic Histology*, 10th ed. McGraw-Hill, 2003.)

involved in many pathways participating in receptor-mediated uptake and active transport of substances that are unable to diffuse freely into cells. These substances enter whichever hepatocytes have the appropriate transporters regardless of their zone. Similarly, substances that are tightly bound to carrier proteins for which the liver does *not* have receptors are cleared equally poorly by hepatocytes in all three zones.

Hepatocytes: Polarized Cells with Segregation of Functions

All surfaces of a hepatocyte are not the same. Hepatocytes have three sides. One side, the **apical surface,** forms the wall of the bile canaliculus. The second side, the **basolateral surface,** is in contact with the bloodstream via the sinusoids. The last side, the **lateral domain,** is bordered by the two other surfaces. Very different activities go forward at these regions of the hepatocyte plasma membrane; **tight junctions** between hepatocytes serve to maintain segregation of apical and basolateral plasma membrane domains. Processes related to bile transport and excretion act at the apical plasma membrane (Figure 14–3A). Uptake from and secretion into the bloodstream are activities that occur across the basolateral membrane (Figure 14–3B).

Effects of Hepatocyte Dysfunction

In view of this organization, it is perhaps not surprising that hepatocyte dysfunction can sometimes involve disruption of bile flow (cholestasis) with relative preservation of other functions. There is, however, no clear line between the consequences of disturbed apical and basolateral functions: Cholestasis, although initially a disorder of apical bile flow, is ultimately manifested at the basolateral surface. This is because it is at the basolateral surface that bilirubin and other substances to be excreted across the apical plasma membrane into the bile must first be taken up from the bloodstream. Similarly, disruption of energy metabolism or protein synthesis, although initially impinging on the secretory and metabolic processes of the hepatocyte, will ultimately affect the bile transport machinery in the apical plasma membrane as well.

Capacity for Regeneration

Although the normal liver contains very few cells in mitosis, when hepatocytes are lost, poorly understood mechanisms stimulate proliferation of the remaining hepatocytes. This is why in most cases of fulminant hepatic failure with massive hepatocellular death, if the patient survives the acute period of hepatic dysfunction (usually with medical therapy in the hospital), recovery will be complete. Similarly, surgical resection of liver tissue is followed by proliferation of the remaining hepatocytes (**hyperplasia**). Numerous growth factors (eg, HGF, TGF-α) and cytokines (eg, TNF, IL-1, IL-6) are involved in positioning the liver on a continuum between cell proliferation and cell death.

CHECKPOINT

4. From which vascular beds do the hepatic central veins derive their blood flow?

5. Why is the liver a major site for metastasis of malignant neoplasms from other parts of the body?

6. What cell types make up the liver, and what are their distinguishing characteristics?

7. What is the difference between the lobule concept and the acinus concept of liver subarchitecture?

8. What are some physiologic consequences of functional zonation in the liver?

9. What activities are found in zone 1 hepatocytes? In zone 3 hepatocytes?

10. What structures normally maintain the separation of apical and basolateral plasma membrane domains of the hepatocyte?

11. What happens to the remaining hepatocytes when part of the liver is surgically resected?

LIVER BLOOD FLOW & ITS CELLULAR BASIS

The portal blood flow, being venous in nature, is normally under low hydrostatic pressure (about 10 mm Hg). Accordingly, there must be little resistance to its flow within the liver, allowing the blood to percolate through the sinusoids and achieve maximal contact—for exchange of substances—with hepatocytes. Two unique features—fenestrations in the endothelial cells and lack of a typical basement membrane between endothelial cells and hepatocytes—aid in making the liver a low-pressure circuit for the flow of portal blood. These features are altered in cirrhosis, resulting in increased portal pressure and profound changes in liver blood flow, with devastating clinical consequences.

Fenestrations are spaces between the endothelial cells that make up the walls of the portal capillary system, which allow plasma and its proteins, but not red blood cells, free and direct access to the surface of the hepatocytes. This feature is crucial to the liver's function of uptake from and secretion into the bloodstream. This feature also contributes to the efficiency of the liver as a filter of portal blood. Most of the capillary beds in the body lack such fenestrations.

PHYSIOLOGY

The diverse functions of the liver are listed as four broad categories in Table 14–2. Although there is considerable overlap between them, systematic consideration of each category is a useful way of approaching the patient with liver disease.

TABLE 14–2 Functions of the normal liver.

Energy metabolism and substrate interconversion
Glucose production through gluconeogenesis and glycogenolysis
Glucose consumption by pathways of glycogen synthesis, fatty acid synthesis, glycolysis, and the tricarboxylic acid cycle
Cholesterol synthesis from acetate, triglyceride synthesis from fatty acids, and secretion of both in VLDL particles
Cholesterol and triglyceride uptake by endocytosis of HDL and LDL particles with excretion of cholesterol in bile, beta-oxidation of fatty acids, and conversion of excess acetyl-CoA to ketones
Deamination of amino acids and conversion of ammonia to urea via the urea cycle
Transamination and de novo synthesis of nonessential amino acids
Protein synthetic functions
Synthesis of various plasma proteins, including albumin, clotting factors, binding proteins, apolipoproteins, angiotensinogen, and insulin-like growth factor I
Solubilization, transport, and storage functions
Drug and poison detoxification through phase I and phase II biotransformation reactions and excretion in bile
Solubilization of fats and fat-soluble vitamins in bile for uptake by enterocytes
Synthesis and secretion of VLDL and pre-HDL lipoprotein particles and clearance of HDL, LDL, and chylomicron remnants
Synthesis and secretion of various binding proteins, including transferrin, steroid hormone–binding globulin, thyroid hormone–binding globulin, ceruloplasmin, and metallothionein
Uptake and storage of vitamins A, D, and B_{12} and folate
Protective and clearance functions
Detoxification of ammonia through the urea cycle
Detoxification of drugs through microsomal oxidases and conjugation systems
Synthesis and export of glutathione
Clearance of damaged cells and proteins, hormones, drugs, and activated clotting factors from the portal circulation
Clearance of bacteria and antigens from the portal circulation

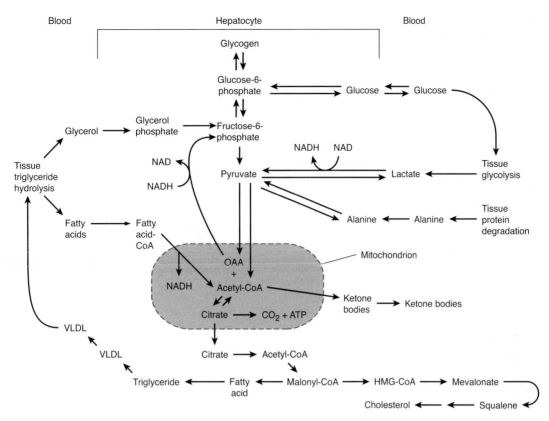

FIGURE 14–4 Pathways of hepatic carbohydrate and lipid metabolism. ATP, adenosine triphosphate; CoA, co-enzyme A; HMG, hepatic 3-methylglutaryl; OAA, oxaloacetic acid; VLDL, very low-density lipoproteins. (Redrawn from Schwartz CC. Hepatic metabolism. In: *Textbook of Medicine.* Kelley WN [editor]. Lippincott, 1989.)

Energy Generation & Substrate Interconversion

Much of the body's carbohydrate, lipid, and protein is synthesized, metabolized, and interconverted in the liver; products are removed from or released into the bloodstream in response to the energy and substrate needs of the body.

A. Carbohydrate Metabolism

After a meal, the liver achieves net glucose consumption (eg, for glycogen synthesis and generation of metabolic intermediates via glycolysis and the tricarboxylic acid cycle). This occurs as a result of a confluence of several effects. First, the levels of substrates such as glucose increase. Second, the levels of hormones that affect the amount and activity of metabolic enzymes change. Thus, when blood glucose increases, the ratio of insulin to glucagon in the bloodstream increases. The net effect is increased glucose utilization by the liver. In times of fasting (low blood glucose) or stress (when higher blood glucose is needed), hormone and substrate levels in the bloodstream drive metabolic pathways of the liver responsible for net glucose production (eg, the pathways of glycogenolysis and gluconeogenesis). As a result, blood glucose levels are raised to, or maintained in, the normal range in spite of wide and sudden changes in the rate of glucose input (eg, ingestion

and absorption) and output (eg, utilization by tissues) from the bloodstream (Figure 14–4).

B. Protein Metabolism

Related to its important role in protein metabolism, the liver is a major site for processes of oxidative deamination and transamination (Figure 14–5). These reactions allow amino groups to be shuffled among molecules in order to generate substrates for both carbohydrate metabolism and amino acid synthesis. Likewise, the urea cycle allows nitrogen to be excreted in the form of urea, which is much less toxic than free amino groups in the form of ammonium ions. Impairment of this function in liver disease is discussed in greater detail later.

C. Lipid Metabolism

The liver is the center of lipid metabolism. It manufactures nearly 80% of the cholesterol synthesized in the body from acetyl-CoA via a pathway that connects metabolism of carbohydrates with that of lipids (Figure 14–4). Moreover, the liver can synthesize, store, and export triglycerides (Figure 14–4). The liver is also the site of keto acid production via the pathway of fatty acid oxidation that connects lipid catabolism with activity of the tricarboxylic acid cycle.

In the process of controlling the body's level of cholesterol and triglycerides, the liver assembles, secretes, and takes up

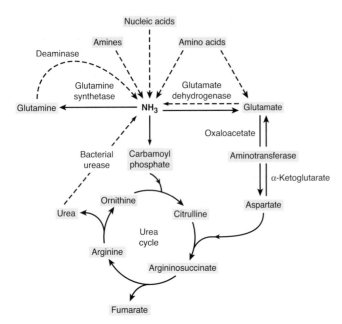

FIGURE 14–5 Urea cycle. Dashed lines signify pathways whose extent of involvement varies from patient to patient depending on genetic, dietary, and other factors. (Redrawn, with permission, from Powers-Lee SG, Meister A. Urea synthesis and ammonia metabolism. In: *The Liver: Biology and Pathology,* 3rd ed. Arias IM et al [editors]. Raven Press, 1994.)

various lipoprotein particles (Figure 14–6). Dietary fat is first absorbed into the small intestine then packaged into chylomicrons. Following removal of triglycerides, the chylomicron remnant is taken up by the liver via **low-density lipoprotein (LDL)** receptor–mediated endocytosis. To distribute lipids systemically, **very-low-density lipoproteins (VLDLs)** are secreted by the liver and transport triglycerides and cholesterol to adipose tissue for storage or to other tissues for immediate use. As triglycerides are removed, the structure of VLDL particles is modified by loss of lipid and protein components rendering intermediate-density lipoprotein (IDL) and further downstream LDL. LDL particles are then returned to the liver via the **LDL receptor**. On the other hand, **high-density lipoproteins (HDLs)**, a lipoprotein synthesized and secreted from the liver, scavenge excess cholesterol and triglycerides from other tissues and from the bloodstream, returning them to the liver where they are excreted. Thus, secretion of HDL and removal of LDL are both mechanisms by which cholesterol in excess of that needed by various tissues is removed from the circulation (Figures 14–6B and 14–6C).

Synthesis & Secretion of Plasma Proteins

The liver manufactures and secretes many of the proteins found in plasma, including albumin, several of the clotting factors, a number of binding proteins, and even certain hormones and hormone precursors. By virtue of the actions of these proteins, the liver has important roles in maintaining plasma oncotic pressure (serum albumin), coagulation (clotting factor synthesis and modification), blood pressure (an-

giotensinogen), growth (insulin-like growth factor-1), and metabolism (steroid and thyroid hormone-binding proteins). Table 14–3 lists some of the proteins synthesized by the liver and their physiologic functions.

Solubilizing, Transport, & Storage Functions

The liver plays an important role in solubilizing, transporting, and storing a variety of very different substances that would

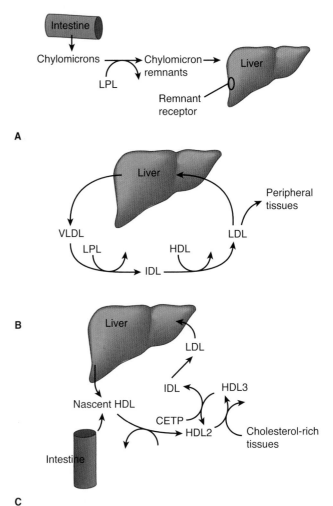

FIGURE 14–6 Lipoprotein metabolism in the liver. **A:** Exogenous fat transport pathway. **B:** Endogenous fat transport pathway. **C:** Pathway of reverse cholesterol transport. In each of these three pathways, lipoprotein particles are used to solubilize cholesteryl esters (and triglyceride), either for the purpose of import from the GI tract **(A)**, distribution to various tissues **(B)**, or transport to the liver for excretion in bile **(C)**. During their circulation, specific lipoprotein particles are transformed by addition and removal of apoproteins and by the action of enzymes in plasma or in tissues (eg, LPL, lipoprotein lipase; CETP, cholesteryl ester transfer protein). Intermediate-density lipoproteins (IDL) are intermediates in the conversion of VLDL to LDL. (HDL, high-density lipoproteins; LDL, low-density lipoproteins.) (Redrawn from Breslow JL. Genetic basis of lipoprotein disorders. J Clin Invest. 1989;84:373.)

TABLE 14–3 **Proteins synthesized by the liver: Physiologic functions and properties.**

Name	Principal Function	Binding Characteristics	Serum or Plasma Concentration
Albumin	Binding and carrier protein; osmotic regulator	Hormones, amino acids, vitamins, fatty acids	4500–5000 mg/dL
Orosomucoid	Uncertain; may have a role in inflammation		Trace; rises in inflammation
α_1-Antiprotease	Trypsin and general protease inhibitor	Proteases in serum and tissue secretions	1.3–1.4 mg/dL
α-Fetoprotein	Osmotic regulation; binding and carrier protein[1]	Hormones, amino acids	Found normally in fetal blood
α_2-Macroglobulin	Inhibitor of serum endoproteases	Proteases	150–240 mg/dL
Antithrombin	Protease inhibitor of intrinsic coagulation system	1:1 binding to proteases	17–30 mg/dL
Ceruloplasmin	Transport of copper	Six atoms copper/mol	15–60 mg/dL
C-reactive protein	Uncertain; has role in tissue inflammation	Complement C1q	< 1 mg/dL; rises in inflammation
Fibrinogen	Precursor to fibrin in hemostasis		200–450 mg/dL
Haptoglobin	Binding, transport of cell-free hemoglobin	Hemoglobin 1:1 binding	40–180 mg/dL
Hemopexin	Binds to porphyrins, particularly heme for heme recycling	1:1 with heme	50–100 mg/dL
Transferrin	Transport of iron	Two atoms iron/mol	3.0–6.5 mg/dL
Apolipoprotein B	Assembly of lipoprotein particles	Lipid carrier	
Angiotensinogen	Precursor to pressor peptide, angiotensin II		
Proteins, coagulation factors II, VII, IX, X	Blood clotting		20 mg/dL
Protein C	Inhibition of blood clotting		
Insulin-like growth factor I	Mediator of anabolic effects of growth hormone	IGF-I receptor	
Steroid hormone–binding globulin	Carrier protein for steroid hormones in bloodstream	Steroid hormones	3.3 mg/dL
Thyroxine-binding globulin	Carrier protein for thyroid hormones in bloodstream	Thyroid hormones	1.5 mg/dL
Transthyretin (thyroid-binding prealbumin)	Carrier protein for thyroid hormones in bloodstream	Thyroid hormones	25 mg/dL

Adapted from Donohue TM et al. Synthesis and secretion of plasma proteins by the liver. In: *Hepatology: A Textbook of Liver Disease.* Zakim D, Boyer TD (editors). Saunders, 1990.
[1]The function of alpha-fetoprotein is uncertain, but because of its structural homology to albumin it is often assigned these functions.

otherwise be difficult for the tissues to obtain or to move in and out of cells. Specific cells in the liver perform these functions by manufacturing specialized proteins that serve as receptors, binding proteins, or enzymes.

A. Enterohepatic Circulation of Bile Acids

Bile is a detergent-like substance synthesized by the liver that permits a variety of otherwise insoluble substances to be dissolved in an aqueous environment for transport into or out of the body. Bile acids are a major component of bile and are recycled via the so-called **enterohepatic circulation** between the liver and the intestines. After synthesis and active transport from hepatocyte cytoplasm into the bile canaliculus (across the apical plasma membrane of the hepatocyte), bile is collected in the biliary tract (and sometimes stored in the gallbladder) and excreted via the common bile duct into the duodenum. While still in the cytoplasm of the hepatocyte, many bile acids are conjugated to sugars, which increases their water solubility. Once in the duodenum, bile acids serve to solubilize lipids, facilitating digestion and absorption of fats. In the terminal ileum, both conjugated and deconjugated bile acids are taken up and transported from enterocytes to portal blood flow. Portal blood returns them to the liver, where specialized bile acid transporters (predominantly sodium taurocholate cotransporter, or Ntcp) return them to the hepatocyte cytosol via the basolateral plasma membrane facing the space of Disse. There they are subject to reconjugation and secretion across the apical membrane along with other components (eg, pigment, cholesterol) to form new bile. Thereafter, they engage in another cycle of enterohepatic transport.

B. Drug Metabolism and Excretion

Most of the enzymes that catalyze metabolic processes necessary for the detoxification and excretion of drugs and other substances are located in the smooth endoplasmic reticulum of hepatocytes. These pathways are used not only for metabolism of exogenous drugs but also for many endogenous substances that would otherwise be difficult for cells to excrete (eg, bilirubin and cholesterol). In most cases, this metabolism involves the conversion of **hydrophobic** (lipophilic) substances (which are difficult to excrete from cells because they tend to partition into cellular membranes) into more **hydrophilic** (polar) substances. This process involves catalysis of covalent modifications to make the substance more charged, so that it will partition more readily into an aqueous medium or at least be solubilized sufficiently in bile. As a result of these processes, collectively termed biotransformations, some substances that would otherwise be retained in cellular membranes can be excreted directly in the urine or transported into the bile for excretion in feces.

C. Phases of Biotransformation

Biotransformation generally occurs in two phases. **Phase I reactions** involve oxidation reductions in which an oxygen-containing functional group is added to the substance to be excreted. While oxidation itself does not necessarily have a major effect on water solubility, it usually introduces into the drug a reactive "handle" that makes possible other reactions that do render the modified substance water soluble. These **phase II reactions** usually involve covalent attachment of the drug to a water-soluble carrier molecule such as the sugar glucuronic acid or the peptide glutathione. Unfortunately, by making substances more chemically reactive, phase I oxidation reactions often convert mildly toxic drugs into more toxic reactive intermediates. If conjugation by phase II enzymes is impaired for some other reason, the reactive intermediate can sometimes react with and damage other cellular structures. This feature of drug detoxification has important clinical implications.

D. Role of Apolipoprotein in Solubilization and Transport of Lipids

The detoxification and bile transport pathways allow hepatocytes to convert a wide range of hydrophobic low-molecular-weight substances (eg, drugs and bilirubin) into a more hydrophilic and hence water-soluble form in which they can be excreted (eg, in bile or by the kidney). However, these are not the only solubilization challenges facing the body. The body also needs a mechanism that makes lipids available to various tissues (eg, to synthesize membranes) and one that removes any excess lipid the tissues do not use. For these processes to occur, lipid must be solubilized in a dispersed form that can be carried through the bloodstream. For this purpose, hepatocytes synthesize a class of specialized **apolipoproteins.** Apolipoproteins assemble into a variety of lipoprotein particles that transport lipids to and from various tissues by receptor-mediated endocytosis (see prior discussion of lipid metabolism).

E. Role in Production of Binding Proteins

Various cells in the liver synthesize proteins that bind certain substances very tightly (eg, some vitamins, minerals, and hormones). In some cases, this allows their transport in the bloodstream, where they would otherwise not be soluble (eg, steroids bound to steroid-binding globulin, which is synthesized and secreted by hepatocytes). In other cases, binding proteins made by the liver (eg, thyroid hormone–binding globulin) allow transport of specific substances (eg, thyroxine) in a form not fully accessible to tissues. In this way, the effective concentration of the substance is limited to its free concentration at equilibrium, and the tightly bound fraction forms a reservoir of the substance that is made available slowly as the free fraction is metabolized, thereby prolonging its half-life.

In some cases, binding proteins allow the liver to accumulate specific substances in relatively high concentrations and store them in a nontoxic form. Consider iron, for example, an essential nutrient. Free iron can be quite toxic to cells both directly as an oxidant and indirectly as an essential nutrient needed by infectious agents. Control of body iron occurs at the level of the enterocyte in the duodenum (see Chapter 13). Thus, the primary defect in the iron overload disorder hemochromatosis probably involves the enterocyte. Nevertheless, the liver has the responsibility of making a variety of proteins crucial for the binding and metabolism of iron. Through the actions of these proteins, the body gets the iron it needs without allowing excess free iron to cause damage or support pathogens.

Transferrin is an iron-binding protein synthesized and secreted into the bloodstream by the liver. On binding of free iron at normal pH, transferrin undergoes a conformational change that gives it high affinity for a specific membrane receptor of the hepatocyte (**transferrin receptor**). On receptor binding, the transferrin–transferrin receptor complex is internalized into the endocytic pathway, a progressively more acidic environment. There, at low pH, iron no longer remains bound to transferrin. However, conformational changes that occur at low pH allow transferrin to maintain high-affinity binding to its receptor even in the absence of bound iron. Thus, when the receptor recycles back to the surface, it brings the "empty" transferrin with it. On presentation to the pH 7.4 environment of the bloodstream, transferrin lacking bound iron is released from the receptor, and the cycle can start over again. In this way, transferrin and its receptor keep the bloodstream free of unbound iron. Meanwhile, the free iron released from transferrin in the acidic environment of the endosome is transported into the cytoplasm of the hepatocyte, where it binds to **ferritin,** a cytoplasmic iron storage protein. This provides a reservoir that can be mobilized in response to the body's needs but makes iron inaccessible to pathogens and keeps it from causing direct toxic effects. Similar dynamics of plasma-binding proteins, receptors, or cytosolic storage proteins occur for many other substances, including fat-soluble vitamins and steroid hormones.

Whereas most solubilization functions are performed in hepatocytes, some of the binding and storage functions involve accessory cells. Thus, vitamin A storage occurs in fat droplets seen in the **lipocytes** of the reticuloendothelial system. Lipocytes have been implicated in the pathogenesis of chronic liver injury and cirrhosis. Injury to other cells releases cytokines, which activate the lipocytes. The lipocytes respond by proliferating and by synthesizing collagen and other basement membrane components, leading to an increase in the extracellular matrix and contributing to hepatic fibrosis.

Protective & Clearance Functions

Many of the functions of the liver already discussed (eg, drug detoxification and excretion of excess cholesterol by conversion to and solubilization in bile) can also be considered protective. Nevertheless, it is useful to conceptualize the protective function as a separate category because of its clinical importance in ameliorating the consequences of liver disease.

A. Phagocytic and Endocytic Functions of Kupffer Cells

The liver helps remove bacteria and antigens that breach the defenses of the gut to enter the portal blood and also participates in clearing the circulation of endogenously generated cellular debris. It appears that specialized receptors on the Kupffer cell surface bind to glycoproteins (via carbohydrate receptors), to material coated with immunoglobulin (via the Fc receptor), or to complement (via the C3 receptor), thus allowing damaged plasma proteins, activated clotting factors, immune complexes, senescent blood cells, and so on to be recognized and removed.

B. Endocytic Functions of Hepatocytes

Hepatocytes have a number of specific receptors for damaged plasma proteins distinct from the receptors present on Kupffer cells (eg, the asialoglycoprotein receptor that specifically binds glycoproteins whose terminal sialic acid sugar residues have been removed). The precise physiologic significance of this metabolic action remains unclear.

C. Ammonia Metabolism

Ammonia generated from deamination of amino acids is metabolized within hepatocytes into the much less toxic substance urea. Loss of this function results in altered mental status, a common manifestation of severe or end-stage liver disease.

D. Hepatocyte Synthesis of Glutathione

Glutathione is the major intracellular (cytoplasmic) reducing reagent and thus is crucial for preventing oxidative damage to cellular proteins. This molecule is a nonribosomally synthesized tripeptide (γ-glutamyl-cystinyl-glycine) that is also a substrate for many phase II drug detoxification conjugation reactions. The liver may also export glutathione for use by other tissues.

Some additional indirect liver functions (eg, its role in maintaining normal sodium and water balance) are inferred from the derangements observed in patients with liver disease, as discussed in the following section.

Liver Function Tests

A number of tests are commonly used to assess liver injury. Often called liver function tests, serum aspartate aminotransferase (AST) and alanine aminotransferase (ALT) are measurements of levels of enzymes normally situated within hepatocytes. Their presence in the serum is thus actually a sign of liver cell necrosis rather than a true indication of liver function.

To assess liver function more directly, a number of other tests can be used. The levels of albumin, clotting factors, and bilirubin can be measured in blood samples. Each of these tests has advantages and disadvantages, and no one of them serves as an ideal sole indicator of liver function. For example, albumin has a relatively long half-life (18–20 days); its synthesis can be stimulated in excess of need, and it can be lost via the kidneys in renal disease. Furthermore, about two thirds of body albumin is located in the extravascular, extracellular space, so changes in fluid distribution can alter serum albumin concentration. Likewise, the simplest measure of clotting factor levels, the prothrombin time (PT), is a relatively insensitive measure because it does not become abnormal until more than 80% of hepatic synthetic capacity is lost. Furthermore, vitamin K deficiency, occurring in patients with nutritional deprivation, chronic cholestasis, or fat malabsorption, can prolong the PT. Serum bilirubin is a good measure of cholestasis, and determination of conjugated (direct) versus unconjugated (indirect) bilirubin provides a good assessment of whether cholestasis is intrinsic to the liver or due solely to obstruction (eg, by a stone in the common bile duct). Furthermore, cholestasis, even when caused by liver disease, often does not reflect the degree to which other hepatic functions are lost, and unconjugated hyperbilirubinemia can occur for other reasons (eg, hemolysis).

For these reasons, an accurate assessment of liver function requires several blood tests (eg, AST, ALT, albumin, PT, bilirubin) as well as clinical assessment of the patient.

The two most common schemes for grading liver function is the modified Child-Turcotte-Pugh (CTP) score (Table 14–4) and the Model for End-Stage Liver Disease (MELD score = 3.78[Ln serum bilirubin (mg/dL)] + 11.2[Ln INR] + 9.57[Ln serum creatinine (mg/dL)] + 6.43). The CTP score predicts 1- and 2-year survival and the MELD score.

TABLE 14–4 Grading liver function using the modified Child-Turcotte-Pugh score.

Parameter	Points		
	1	**2**	**3**
Albumin	> 3.5 g/dL	2.8–3.5 g/dL	< 2.8 g/dL
Bilirubin	< 2.0 mg/dL	2.0–3.0 mg/dL	> 3.0 mg/dL
Prothrombin time prolongation	< 4.0 s	4.0–6.0 s	> 6.0 s
Ascites	Absent	Controlled	Refractory
Encephalopathy	None	Controlled	Refractory

Modified Child-Pugh classification of the severity of liver disease according to the degree of ascites, the plasma concentrations of bilirubin and albumin, the prothrombin time, and the degree of encephalopathy. A total score of 5 to 6 is considered grade A (well-compensated disease); a score of 7–9 is grade B (significant functional compromise); and a score of 10–15 is grade C (decompensated disease). These grades correlate with one- and two-year patient survival: grade A is 100–85%; grade B, 80–60%; and grade C, 45–35%.

CHECKPOINT

12. What are the roles of the liver in carbohydrate, protein, and lipid metabolism?
13. What are two physiologic mechanisms by which the body transports cholesterol?
14. Explain phase I and phase II reactions in drug detoxification.
15. Name and explain four clearance or protective functions of the liver.
16. What specializations allow the liver normally to be a low-pressure conduit for blood flow?

OVERVIEW OF LIVER DISEASE

TYPES OF LIVER DYSFUNCTION

Most of the clinical consequences of liver disease can be understood either as a failure of one of the liver's four broad functions (summarized in Table 14–2) or as a consequence of portal hypertension, the altered hepatic blood flow of cirrhosis.

Hepatocyte Dysfunction

One mechanism of liver disease, particularly in acute liver injury, is dysfunction of the individual hepatocytes that make up the liver parenchyma. The pathway and extent of hepatocellular dysfunction determine the specific manifestations of liver disease. The outcomes to be anticipated when normal hepatic functions fail are described later.

Portal Hypertension

Some consequences of liver disease, particularly of cirrhosis, are best understood in terms of what we know about hepatic blood flow. Of greatest clinical importance are the existence under normal circumstances of a low-pressure portal venous capillary bed throughout the liver parenchyma and the functional zonation of portal blood flow.

When pathologic processes (eg, fibrosis) result in elevation of the normally low intrahepatic venous pressure, blood backs up and a substantial fraction of it finds alternative routes back to the systemic circulation, bypassing the liver. Thus, blood from the GI tract is, in effect, filtered less efficiently by the liver before entering the systemic circulation. The consequences of this portal-to-systemic shunting are loss of the protective and clearance functions of the liver, functional abnormalities in renal salt and water homeostasis, and a greatly increased risk of GI hemorrhage from the development of engorged blood vessels carrying venous blood bypassing the liver (eg, **esophageal, gastric, umbilical varices, etc**).

Even in the absence of any intrinsic parenchymal liver disease, portal-to-systemic shunting of blood can produce or contribute to **encephalopathy** (altered mental status resulting from failure to clear poisons absorbed from the GI tract), GI bleeding (resulting from esophageal varices), and malabsorption of fats and fat-soluble vitamins (caused by loss of enterohepatic recirculation of bile), with associated coagulopathy. In Table 14–5, the syndromes observed in liver disease are categorized as being a consequence of hepatocyte dysfunction, portal-to-systemic shunting, or both.

Pathophysiology of Functional Zonation

The fact that hepatocytes in the different zones of the acinus "see" blood in a particular sequence has great pathophysiologic significance. Because zone 1 hepatocytes see blood that has just left the portal venule or hepatic arteriole, they have access to the highest concentrations of various substances, both good (eg, oxygen and nutrients) and bad (eg, drugs and toxins absorbed from the GI tract). Zone 2 hepatocytes receive blood containing less of these substances, and zone 3 hepatocytes are bathed in blood largely depleted of them. However, zone 3 hepatocytes see the highest concentrations of products (eg, drug metabolites) released into the bloodstream by hepatocytes of zones 1 and 2. Thus, direct poisons have their most severe impact on zone 1 hepatocytes, whereas poisons that are generated as a result of hepatic metabolism cause more damage to those of zone 3. Similarly, because sinusoidal blood around zone 3 has the lowest oxygen concentration, hepatocytes of this zone are at greatest risk of injury under conditions of hypoxia.

MANIFESTATIONS OF LIVER DYSFUNCTION

Whether a result of hepatocyte dysfunction or portal-to-systemic shunting, prominent features of liver disease are manifestations of failure of normal functions. An understanding of these mechanisms offers insight into the probable causes of illness in a patient with acute or chronic liver disease.

Diminished Energy Generation & Substrate Interconversion

A first category of altered liver function involves the intermediary metabolism of carbohydrates, fats, and proteins.

A. Carbohydrate Metabolism

Severe liver disease can result in either hypoglycemia or hyperglycemia. Hypoglycemia results largely from a decrease in functional hepatocyte mass, whereas hyperglycemia is a result of portal-to-systemic shunting, which decreases the efficiency of postprandial extraction of glucose from portal blood by hepatocytes, thus elevating systemic blood glucose concentration.

B. Lipid Metabolism

Disturbance of lipid metabolism in the liver can result in syndromes of fat accumulation within the liver early in the course

TABLE 14–5 Pathophysiology of syndromes of aberrant function in liver disease.

Syndromes of Aberrant Function in Liver Disease	Hepatocellular Dysfunction	Portal-to-Systemic Shunting
Energy metabolism and substrate conversion		
Alcoholic hypoglycemia	✓	
Alcoholic ketoacidosis	✓	
Hyperglycemia		✓
Familial hypercholesterolemia	✓	
Hepatic encephalopathy	✓	✓
Fatty liver	✓	
Solubilization, transport, and storage function		
Reactions to drugs	✓	
Drug sensitivity	✓	✓
Steatorrhea	✓	✓
Fat-soluble vitamin deficiency	✓	✓
Coagulopathy	✓	✓
Protein synthetic function		
Edema due to hypoalbuminemia	✓	
Protective and clearance functions		
Hypergammaglobulinemia		✓
Hypogonadism and hyper-estrogenism	✓	✓
Renal dysfunction		
Sodium retention		✓
Impaired water excretion		✓
Impaired renal concentrating ability		✓
Deranged potassium metabolism		✓
Prerenal azotemia		✓
Acute renal failure		✓
Glomerulopathies		✓
Impaired renal acidification		✓
Hepatorenal syndrome		✓

of liver injury. Perhaps this is because the complex steps in assembly of lipoprotein particles for export of cholesterol and triglycerides from the liver are more sensitive to disruption than the pathways of lipid synthesis. Such disruption results in a buildup of fat that cannot be exported in the form of VLDL.

In certain chronic liver diseases such as primary biliary cirrhosis, bile flow decreases as a result of destruction of bile ducts. The decrease in bile flow results in decreased lipid clearance via bile, with consequent hyperlipidemia. These patients often develop subcutaneous accumulations of cholesterol termed **xanthomas.**

C. Protein Metabolism

Any disturbance of protein metabolism in the liver can result in a syndrome of altered mental status and confusion known as **hepatic encephalopathy.** As with carbohydrate metabolism, altered protein metabolism can result from either hepatocyte failure or portal-to-systemic shunting, with the net effect of elevation of blood concentrations of centrally acting toxins, including ammonia generated by amino acid metabolism.

Loss of Solubilization & Storage Functions

A. Disordered Bile Secretion

The clinical significance of bile synthesis can be seen in the prominence of cholestasis—failure to secrete bile—in many forms of liver disease. Cholestasis can occur as a result of extrahepatic obstruction (eg, from a gallstone in the common bile duct) or selective dysfunction of the bile synthetic and secretory machinery within the hepatocytes themselves (eg, from a reaction to certain drugs). The mechanisms responsible for cholestatic drug reactions are not well understood. Regardless of the mechanism, however, the clinical consequences of severe cholestasis may be profound: A failure to secrete bile results in a failure to solubilize substances such as dietary lipids and fat-soluble vitamins, resulting in **malabsorption** and deficiency states, respectively. Retained bile salts are also cytotoxic, but in the setting of cholestasis hepatocytes adapt to decrease uptake of bile salts by downregulating Na$^+$-bile acid cotransporter while maintaining bile salt excretion. As a result, hepatic necrosis is minimized in predominantly cholestatic syndromes, with the typical laboratory findings of minimally elevated levels of AST and ALT in the presence of marked jaundice and high levels of bilirubin. However, prolonged exposure to bile salts in chronic cholestatic diseases such as primary biliary cirrhosis leads to portal tract cytotoxic injury and inflammation, leading eventually to fibrosis and cirrhosis.

The solubilization function of bile works both to excrete and to absorb substances. Thus, in cholestasis, endogenous substances that are normally excreted via the biliary tract can accumulate to high levels. One such substance is bilirubin, a product of heme degradation (Figure 14–7). The buildup of bilirubin results in **jaundice** (**icterus**), which is a yellow discoloration of the scleras and skin. In the adult, the most significant feature of jaundice is that it serves as a readily monitored index of cholestasis, which may occur alone or with other abnormalities in hepatocyte function (ie, as part of the presentation of acute hepatitis). In the neonate, however, elevated bilirubin concentrations can be toxic to the developing nervous system, producing a syndrome termed **kernicterus.**

Similarly, cholesterol is normally excreted either by conversion into bile acids or by forming complexes, termed micelles, with preexisting (recycled) bile acids. In cholestasis, the resultant buildup of bile acids can lead to their deposition in the skin. This is believed to cause intense itching, or **pruritus.** Data suggest that, in at least some patients, cholestasis results in altered levels of endogenous opioids. Instead of skin deposition of bile acids altered endogenous opioid-mediated neurotransmission may be responsible for pruritus. Disorders of bile production are a basis for the formation of cholesterol gallstones. Nevertheless, as mentioned, other hepatocyte functions are often relatively well preserved in the face of significant cholestasis. The syndromes that produce jaundice are summarized in Table 14–6.

Hemolysis causes an unconjugated hyperbilirubinemia because the hepatic capacity to take up and conjugate bilirubin is exceeded. Gilbert's syndrome reflects a genetic defect in bilirubin conjugation. Thus, the findings in blood and urine are different from what is observed in hemolytic jaundice even though the pathway of bilirubin metabolism is backed up at a similar initial point. Extrahepatic biliary tract obstruction presents the other extreme, in which the actual pathway of bile formation is entirely intact, at least initially. In obstruction, the bilirubin level in the urine is high because the backed-up metabolite is conjugated and hence much more water soluble than unconjugated bilirubin, which accumulates in hemolysis. Most forms of jaundice that result from liver dysfunction caused by hepatocellular damage reflect variable degrees of overlap between unconjugated and conjugated hyperbilirubinemia.

B. Impaired Drug Detoxification

Two features of the mechanisms of drug detoxification are of particular clinical importance. One is the phenomenon of **enzyme induction.** It is observed that the presence in the bloodstream of any of the large class of drugs inactivated by phase I enzymes increases the amount and activity of these enzymes in the liver. This property of enzyme induction makes physiologic sense (as a response to the body's need for increased biotransformation) but can have undesired effects as well: A patient who chronically consumes large amounts of a substance that is metabolized by phase I enzymes (eg, ethanol) will induce high levels of these enzymes and thus speed up the metabolism of other substances metabolized by the same detoxifying enzymes (eg, antiseizure or anticoagulant medications, resulting in subtherapeutic blood levels of the drugs).

A second clinically important phenomenon in drug metabolism is that phase I reactions often convert relatively benign compounds into more reactive and hence more toxic ones. Normally, this heightened reactivity of phase I reaction products serves to facilitate phase II reactions, making detoxification more efficient. However, under certain conditions when phase II reactions are impaired (eg, during glutathione deficiency from inadequate nutrition), continued phase I enzyme activity can cause increased liver injury. This is because the

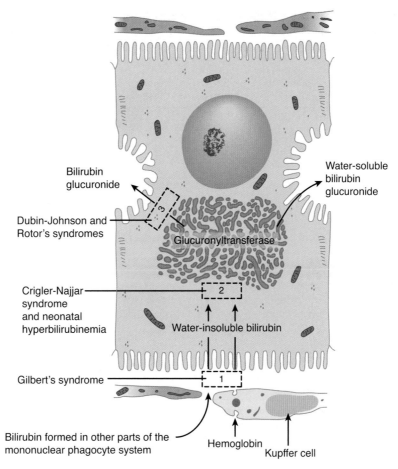

Bilirubin
glucuronide

Water-soluble
bilirubin
glucuronide

Dubin-Johnson and
Rotor's syndromes

Glucuronyltransferase

Crigler-Najjar
syndrome
and neonatal
hyperbilirubinemia

Water-insoluble bilirubin

Gilbert's syndrome

Bilirubin formed in other parts of the
mononuclear phagocyte system

Hemoglobin

Kupffer cell

FIGURE 14–7 The secretion of bilirubin. This water-insoluble compound is derived from the metabolism of hemoglobin in macrophages of the mononuclear phagocyte system. Glucuronyl transferase activity in the hepatocytes causes bilirubin to be conjugated with glucuronide in the smooth endoplasmic reticulum, forming a water-soluble compound. Accumulation of bilirubin and bilirubin glucuronide in the tissues produces jaundice. Several defective processes in the hepatocytes can cause diseases that produce jaundice: a defect in the capacity of the cell to trap and absorb bilirubin (rectangle 1), the inability of the cell to conjugate bilirubin because of a deficiency in glucuronyl transferase (rectangle 2), or problems in the transfer and excretion of bilirubin glucuronide into the biliary canaliculi (rectangle 3). One of the most frequent causes of jaundice, however—unrelated to hepatocyte activity—is the obstruction of bile flow as a result of gallstones or tumors of the pancreas. This causes jaundice primarily as a result of accumulation of bilirubin glucuronide in the tissues. (Redrawn, with permission, from Junqueira LC, Carneiro J. *Basic Histology*, 10th ed. McGraw-Hill, 2003.)

products of many phase I reactions, in the absence of glutathione, react with and damage cellular components. Such damage rapidly kills the hepatocyte.

Thus, the combined effects of certain common conditions can make the individual abnormally sensitive to the toxic effects of drugs. For example, the combination of induced phase I activity (eg, caused by alcoholism) with low phase II activity (eg, caused by low glutathione levels from nutritional deprivation) can result in heightened generation of reactive intermediates with an inadequate capacity to conjugate and detoxify them. A classic example of this phenomenon is acetaminophen toxicity. As little as 2.5 g of acetaminophen can produce significant liver damage in such susceptible individuals, whereas normal individuals have the capacity to detoxify 10 g/d or more. Table 14–7 lists common drugs and chemicals that cause morphologically distinctive changes in the liver.

C. Lipoprotein Dynamics and Dyslipidemias

The liver's role in lipid metabolism is illustrated by the genetic defect causing familial hypercholesterolemia. Lack of a functional LDL receptor in such cases renders the liver unable to clear LDL cholesterol from the bloodstream, resulting in markedly elevated serum cholesterol and accelerated atherosclerosis and coronary artery disease. Heterozygotes with one normal LDL receptor allele can be treated with drugs (eg, HMG-CoA reductase inhibitors) that inhibit endogenous cholesterol synthesis and thus upregulate LDL receptor levels. However, there is no effective drug therapy for homozygotes because they have no normal LDL receptors. Hepatic transplantation is effective therapy for homozygous familial hypercholesterolemia because it provides a genetically different liver with normal LDL receptors.

In acquired liver diseases, the serum cholesterol is elevated in biliary tract obstruction as a result of blockage of cholesterol

TABLE 14–6 Laboratory findings in the differential diagnosis of jaundice.

Type of Jaundice	Blood						Stool Color	Urine	
	Hct	Unconjugated Bilirubin (Indirect)	Conjugated Bilirubin (Direct)	Alkaline Phosphatase	Aminotransferases	Cholesterol		Bilirubin	Urobilinogen
Hemolytic	↓	↑↑	N	N	N	N	N	NP	↑
Hepatocellular									
Gilbert's syndrome	N	↑	N	N	N	N	N	NP	N or ↓
Abnormal conjugation	N	↑	N	N	N	N	N	NP	N or ↓
Hepatocellular damage	N	↑	↑	N or ↑	↑↑	N	N	↑	↑
Obstructive									
Defective excretion	N	N	N	N	N	N	N	↑	N
Intrahepatic cholestasis	N	N	↑	N	N	N or ↑	Pale	↑	↓
Extrahepatic biliary obstruction	N	N	↑↑	↑↑	N or ↑	↑	Pale	↑	↓

Key: N = normal; NP = not present in significant amounts due to insolubility in water; ↑ = increased compared with normal; ↓ = decreased compared with normal.

Modified and reproduced, with permission, from Chandrasoma P, Taylor CR. *Concise Pathology,* 3rd ed. Originally published by Appleton & Lange. Copyright © 1998 by the McGraw-Hill Companies, Inc.

excretion in bile, and it is diminished in severe alcoholic cirrhosis, in which fat malabsorption prevents cholesterol intake.

D. Altered Hepatic Binding and Storage Functions

Liver disease influences the liver's ability to store various substances. As a result, patients with liver disease are at high risk for certain deficiency states such as folic acid and vitamin B_{12} deficiency. Because these vitamins are needed for DNA synthesis, their deficiency results in **macrocytic anemia** (low red blood cell count with large red cells reflecting abnormal nuclear maturation), a common finding in patients with liver disease.

Diminished Synthesis & Secretion of Plasma Proteins

The clinical significance of liver protein synthesis and secretion derives from the wide range of functions carried out by these proteins. For example, because albumin is the major contributor to plasma oncotic pressure, hypoalbuminemia as a consequence of liver disease or nutritional deficiency presents with marked edema formation. Other important proteins synthesized and secreted by the liver include clotting factors and hormone-binding proteins.

Loss of Protective & Clearance Functions

A crucial protective function of the liver is its role as a filter of blood from the GI tract, by which various substances are removed from portal blood before it reenters the systemic circulation.

A. Clearance of Bacteria and Endotoxin

Clearance of bacteria by Kupffer cells of the liver is the final line of defense in keeping gut-derived bacteria out of the systemic circulation. Loss of this capacity in liver disease as a result of portal-to-systemic shunting may help to explain why, in patients with severe liver disease, infections can rapidly become systemic and result in sepsis.

B. Altered Ammonia Metabolism

Impairment of the liver's ability to detoxify ammonia to urea leads to hepatic encephalopathy, manifested as an altered mental status. This may be an early manifestation of acute fulminant hepatitis with massive hepatocellular dysfunction even before the development of maximal hepatocellular necrosis. It can be a final step in progressive chronic liver disease with diminished hepatocyte functional capacity. Most often it is a consequence of an increased ammonia load in a patient with marginal liver function or significant portal-to-systemic shunting. Thus, encephalopathy may occur as a first sign of renewed GI bleeding (as a result of increased

TABLE 14–7 Principal alterations of hepatic morphology produced by some commonly used drugs and chemicals.

Principal Morphologic Change	Class of Agent	Example[1]	Principal Morphologic Change	Class of Agent	Example[1]
Cholestasis	Anabolic steroid	Methyltestosterone[2]	Hepatitis (continued)	Antibiotic	Isoniazid[3]
	Antithyroid	Methimazole			Rifampin
	Antibiotic	Erythromycin estolate			Nitrofurantoin
		Nitrofurantoin		Diuretic	Chlorothiazide
	Oral contraceptive	Norethynodrel with mestranol		Laxative	Oxyphenisatin[3]
	Oral hypoglycemic	Chlorpropamide		Antidepressant	Amitriptyline
	Tranquilizer	Chlorpromazine[2]			Imipramine
	Oncotherapeutic	Anabolic steroids			Nefazodone
		Busulfan			Venlafaxine
		Tamoxifen		Anti-inflammatory	Ibuprofen
	Immunosuppressive	Cyclosporine			Indomethacin
	Anticonvulsant	Carbamazepine		Antifungal	Ketoconazole
	Calcium channel blocker	Diltiazem			Fluconazole
		Nifedipine		Antiviral	Ritonavir
		Verapamil			Efavirenz
	Angiotensin-converting enzyme inhibitor	Captopril			Nevirapine
		Enalapril			Zidovudine
	Antidepressant	Trazodone			Dideoxyinosine
Fatty liver	Antibiotic	Tetracycline		Calcium channel blocker	Nifedipine
	Anticonvulsant	Sodium valproate			Verapamil
	Antiarrhythmic	Amiodarone			Diltiazem
	Oncotherapeutic	Asparaginase		Leukotriene receptor antagonist	Zafirlukast
		Methotrexate			
Hepatitis	Anesthetic	Halothane[3]		Antipsychotic	Clozapine
	Anticonvulsant	Phenytoin	Mixed hepatitis and cholestasis	Immunosuppressive	Azathioprine
		Carbamazepine		Lipid lowering	Nicotinic acid
		Lamotrigine			Lovastatin, atorvastatin, other
		Felbamate			HMG-CoA reductase inhibitors
	Antihypertensive	Methyldopa[3]			
		Captopril			
		Enalapril			

(continued)

TABLE 14–7 Principal alterations of hepatic morphology produced by some commonly used drugs and chemicals. (Continued)

Principal Morphologic Change	Class of Agent	Example[1]	Principal Morphologic Change	Class of Agent	Example[1]
Toxic (necrosis)	Hydrocarbon	Carbon tetrachloride	Granulomas	Anti-inflammatory	Phenylbutazone
	Metal	Yellow phosphorus		Antibiotic	Sulfonamides
	Mushroom	*Amanita phalloides*		Xanthine oxidase inhibitor	Allopurinol
	Analgesic	Acetaminophen		Antiarrhythmic	Quinidine
	Solvent	Dimethylformamide		Anticonvulsant	Carbamazepine

Data from Isselbacher K et al (editors). *Harrison's Principles of Internal Medicine*, 13th ed. McGraw-Hill, 1994.

[1]Several agents cause more than one type of liver lesion and appear under more than one category.

[2]Rarely associated with a primary biliary cirrhosis-like lesion.

[3]Occasionally associated with chronic active hepatitis or bridging hepatic necrosis or cirrhosis.

production of ammonia and other products caused by breakdown of blood protein by GI tract microbes) or may simply be due to increased protein intake (eg, a cheeseburger eaten by a patient with cirrhosis). Finally, the development of sepsis in these patients results in increased endogenous protein catabolism and, therefore, elevated ammonia production in the face of a decreased capacity for ammonia detoxification because of the liver disease. Thus, the development of encephalopathy in a patient with chronic liver disease calls for investigation of possible acute GI bleeding as well as potentially catastrophic infection. Pending the outcome of diagnostic studies (eg, serial hematocrit measurements and cultures of blood, urine, and ascitic fluid), therapy is designed to improve mental status by diminishing the absorption of ammonia and other noxious substances from the GI tract. When the patient is given the nonabsorbable carbohydrate **lactulose,** whose metabolism by microbes creates an acidic environment, ammonia is trapped as the charged NH_4^+ species in the gut lumen and excreted by the resultant osmotic diarrhea. Thus, this toxin is prevented from ever entering the portal circulation, and the patient's mental status gradually improves. Lactulose also selects for a gut bacterial flora that produces less ammonia.

Furthermore, the resulting elevated blood ammonia and other nitrogen-containing compounds can upregulate peripheral receptors for endogenous benzodiazepine-like products. These effects may contribute to altered systemic hemodynamics in liver disease.

C. Altered Hormone Clearance in Liver Disease

Normally, the liver removes from the bloodstream the fraction of steroid hormones not bound to steroid hormone-binding globulin. On uptake by hepatocytes, these steroids are oxidized, conjugated, and excreted into bile, where a fraction undergoes enterohepatic circulation. In liver disease

accompanied by significant portal-to-systemic shunting, steroid hormone clearance is diminished, extraction of the enterohepatic circulated fraction is impaired, and enzymatic conversion of androgens to estrogens (peripheral aromatization) is increased. The net effect is an elevation of blood estrogens, which in turn alters hepatocyte protein synthesis and secretion and microsomal P450 activity. Synthesis of some hepatic proteins increases, whereas synthesis of others is diminished. P450 activity increases as the liver attempts to partially compensate for the higher blood estrogen levels by increased metabolism. Thus, male patients with liver disease display both gonadal and pituitary suppression as well as feminization.

Sodium & Water Balance

Patients with liver disease often display renal abnormalities and complications, most commonly sodium retention and difficulty excreting water. An intrinsic renal lesion is apparently not involved, because the kidneys of patients with liver disease typically function normally when transplanted into patients whose liver is normal. Instead, renal abnormalities associated with liver disease are functional, occurring because liver disease induces altered intravascular pressures and perhaps because of elevated nitric oxide levels or loss of as yet poorly understood factors secreted from the liver or the endothelium. By whatever homeostatic mechanisms, intravascular volume is perceived as being inadequate when it is actually only maldistributed. Renal mechanisms of salt and water retention are then stimulated to correct what has been sensed as volume depletion. Some of the factors influencing renal sodium retention in liver disease are summarized in Table 14–8. Patients with severe liver disease are at risk for renal failure related to these hemodynamic alterations.

TABLE 14–8 Factors influencing renal sodium retention in liver disease.

Hormonal
Elevated renal endothelin production
Hyperaldosteronism due to diminished clearance by the liver
Diminished angiotensinogen synthesis by the liver
Diminished renin and angiotensin II clearance by the liver
Altered kallikrein-kinin system
Loss of hepatic humoral natriuretic factors
Atrial natriuretic factor
Elevated blood estrogens
Prolactin
Vasoactive intestinal peptide
Elevated peripheral nitric oxide production
Neural
Increased sympathetic nervous system activity
Hemodynamic
Alterations in intrarenal blood flow
Portal-to-systemic shunting
Hypoalbuminemia

Modified and reproduced, with permission, from Epstein M. Functional renal abnormalities in cirrhosis: Pathophysiology and management. In: *Hepatology: A Textbook of Liver Disease*, 2nd ed. Zakim D, Boyer JD (editors). Saunders, 1990.

CHECKPOINT

17. Under what circumstances is hypoglycemia seen in liver disease?
18. Name three clinical consequences of cholestasis.
19. The development of hepatic encephalopathy in a patient with chronic liver disease should lead you to investigate what possible precipitating factors?
20. By what mechanisms can coagulation defects be a consequence of liver disease?
21. What is an explanation for hypogonadism in male patients with liver disease?

PATHOPHYSIOLOGY OF SELECTED LIVER DISEASES

ACUTE HEPATITIS

Acute hepatitis is an inflammatory process causing liver cell death either by necrosis or by triggering apoptosis (programmed cell death). A wide range of clinical entities can cause global hepatocyte injury of sudden onset. Worldwide, acute hepatitis is most commonly caused by infection with one of several types of viruses. Although these viral agents can be distinguished by serologic laboratory tests based on their antigenic properties, all produce clinically similar illnesses. Other less common infectious agents can result in liver injury (Table 14–1). Acute hepatitis is also sometimes caused by exposure to drugs (eg, isoniazid) or poisons (eg, ethanol).

Clinical Presentation

The severity of illness in acute hepatitis ranges from asymptomatic and clinically inapparent to fulminant and fatal. The presentation of acute hepatitis can be quite variable. Some patients are relatively asymptomatic, with abnormalities noted only by laboratory studies. Others may have a range of symptoms and signs, including anorexia, fatigue, weight loss, nausea, vomiting, right upper quadrant abdominal pain, jaundice, fever, splenomegaly, and ascites. The extent of hepatic dysfunction can also vary tremendously, correlating roughly with the severity of liver injury. The relative extent of cholestasis versus hepatocyte necrosis is also highly variable. The potential interrelationship of acute hepatitis, chronic hepatitis, and cirrhosis is illustrated in Figure 14–8.

Etiology

A. Viral Hepatitis

Acute hepatitis is commonly caused by one of five major viruses (Table 14–9): hepatitis A virus (HAV), hepatitis B virus (HBV), hepatitis C virus (HCV), hepatitis D virus (HDV), and hepatitis E virus (HEV).

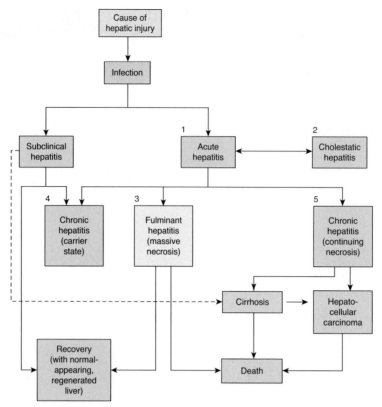

FIGURE 14–8 Clinical syndromes associated with hepatitis: acute hepatitis (1), which is sometimes associated with intrahepatic cholestasis (2). Fulminant hepatitis (3) is associated with massive necrosis and has a high mortality rate. Chronic viral hepatitis may lead to a carrier state without (4) or with (5) continuing hepatocyte necrosis. Chronic hepatitis associated with continuing necrosis often progresses to cirrhosis, whereas that associated simply with a carrier state does not.   (Redrawn, with permission, from Chandrasoma P, Taylor CE. *Concise Pathology*, 3rd ed. Originally published by Appleton & Lange. Copyright © 1998 by the McGraw-Hill Companies, Inc.)

Table 14–9 summarizes important characteristics of these viral agents. Other viral agents that can cause acute hepatitis, though less commonly, include the Epstein-Barr virus (cause of infectious mononucleosis), cytomegalovirus, varicella virus, measles virus, herpes simplex virus, rubella virus, and yellow fever virus. A newly discovered DNA virus, SEN virus, may be associated with transfusion-associated acute hepatitis not attributable to other viruses.

HAV, a small RNA virus, causes liver disease both by direct killing of hepatocytes and by the host's immune response to infected hepatocytes. It is spread by the fecal-oral route from infected individuals. Although most cases are mild, hepatitis A occasionally causes fulminant liver failure and massive hepatocellular necrosis, resulting in death. Regardless of the severity, patients who recover do so completely, show no evidence of residual liver disease, and have antibodies that protect them from reinfection.

HBV is a DNA virus that is transmitted by sexual contact or by contact with infected blood or other bodily fluids. This virus does not kill the cells it infects. Rather, the infected hepatocytes die almost exclusively as a consequence of attack by the immune system after recognition of viral antigens on the hepatocyte surface. Although most cases of hepatitis B infection are asymptomatic or produce only mild disease before clearance of the virus,

an excessive immune response may produce fulminant hepatic failure. In even fewer patients—typically those with mild acute disease—the immune response is inadequate to clear the virus completely, and chronic hepatitis develops. It is estimated that approximately 1.25 million Americans are infected with HBV, and an estimated 70,000 new infections occur each year. Additionally, complications of HBV-induced liver disease results in up to 5000 deaths each year in the United States.

HCV is a RNA virus, also transmitted by blood and body fluids, causes a form of hepatitis similar to HBV infection but with a far greater proportion of cases (60–85%) progressing to chronic hepatitis. Approximately 4 million Americans are infected with HCV, and about 30,000 new infections occur each year. End-stage liver disease from HCV accounts for 8000–10,000 deaths each year. End-stage liver disease due to HCV is the most common indication for liver transplantation in the United States.

HDV, also known as delta agent, is a defective RNA virus that requires helper functions of HBV to cause infection. Thus, individuals who are chronically infected with HBV are at high risk for HDV infection, whereas those who have been vaccinated against HBV are at no risk. HDV infection occurs either as coinfection with HBV or superinfection in the setting of chronic HBV. HDV infection causes a much more

TABLE 14–9   Characteristics of various types of viral hepatitis.

	Hepatitis A	Hepatitis B	Hepatitis C	Hepatitis D	Hepatitis E
Clinical presentation					
Onset	Abrupt	Insidious	Insidious	Insidious	Abrupt
Incubation period					
Range (days)	15–50	28–160	14–160	30–180	15–60
Mean (days)	30	8	50		40
Symptoms					
Arthralgia, rash	Uncommon	Common	Uncommon	Uncommon	Common
Fever	Common	Uncommon	Uncommon	Common	Common
Nausea, vomiting	Common	Common	Common	Common	Common
Jaundice	Uncommon in children	More common in hepatitis A	Uncommon	Common	Common
Laboratory data					
Duration of enzyme elevation	Short	Prolonged	Like hepatitis B	Like hepatitis B	
Virus type	RNA	DNA	RNA	RNA	RNA
	Picornavirus	Hepadnavirus	Flavivirus	Defective virus	Unclassified
Serologic tests					
Antigen	Yes	Yes	No	No	Yes
Antibody	Yes	Yes	Yes	Yes	Yes
Location of virus					
Blood	Transient	Prolonged	Prolonged	Prolonged	?Transient
Stool	Yes	No	No	No	Yes
Elsewhere	?	Yes	?	?	?
Outcome					
Severity of acute disease	Mild	Moderate	Mild	Moderate to severe	Severe
Mortality rate	Low (< 0.1%)	Low (< 0.5%)	None (in acute disease)	High (5%)	Moderate (+ 3%)
Chronic hepatitis	No	Yes	Yes	Yes	No
Chronic carrier	No	Yes	Yes	Yes	No
Associated with malignancy	No	Yes	Yes	Yes	No
Transmission					
Oral	+	±	?No	?No	+
Percutaneous	Rare	+	+	+	–
Sexual	+	+	–	+	?
Perinatal	–	+	±	–	?
Vaccine	Yes	Yes	No	No (vaccinate against HBV)	No

Data from Seeff LB. Diagnosis, therapy, and prognosis of viral hepatitis. In: *Hepatology: A Textbook of Liver Disease,* 2nd ed. Zakim D, Boyer JD (editors). Saunders, 1990.

TABLE 14–10   **Idiosyncratic drug reactions and the cells that are affected.**

Type of Reaction	Effect on Cells	Examples of Drugs
Hepatocellular	Direct effect or production by enzyme-drug adduct leads to cell dysfunction, membrane dysfunction, cytotoxic T-cell response	Isoniazid, trazodone, diclofenac, nefazodone, venlafaxine, lovastatin
Cholestasis	Injury to canalicular membrane and transporters	Chlorpromazine, estrogen, erythromycin and its derivatives
Immunoallergic	Enzyme-drug adducts on cell surface induce IgE response	Halothane, phenytoin, sulfamethoxazole
Granulomatous	Macrophages, lymphocytes infiltrate hepatic lobule	Diltiazem, sulfa drugs, quinidine
Microvesicular fat	Altered mitochondrial respiration, oxidation leads to lactic acidosis and triglyceride accumulation	Didanosine, tetracycline, acetylsalicylic acid, valproic acid
Steatohepatitis	Multifactorial	Amiodarone, tamoxifen
Autoimmune	Cytotoxic lymphocyte response directed at hepatocyte membrane components	Nitrofurantoin, methyldopa, lovastatin, minocycline
Fibrosis	Activation of stellate cells	Methotrexate, excess vitamin A
Vascular collapse	Causes ischemic or hypoxic injury	Nicotinic acid, cocaine, methylene-dioxymethamphetamine
Oncogenesis	Encourages tumor formation	Oral contraceptives, androgens
Mixed	Cytoplasmic and canalicular injury, direct damage to bile ducts	Amoxicillin-clavulanate, carbamazepine, herbs, cyclosporine, methimazole, troglitazone

Modified and reproduced, with permission, from Lee WM. Drug-induced hepatotoxicity. N Engl J Med. 2003;349:474.

severe form of hepatitis both in terms of the proportion of fulminant cases and in the percentage of cases that progress to chronic hepatitis. In North America, HDV coinfection primarily occurs in high-risk groups such as injection drug users and hemophiliacs, and in up to 9% of those high-risk patients who are HBV-coinfected individuals. In the United States, the prevalence of HDV coinfection in the general HBV-infected population is not well known.

HEV is an unclassified RNA virus, and like HAV, it is spread via the fecal-oral route. The clinical disease resembles hepatitis A, but HEV infection may result in fulminant hepatitis in pregnant women.

B. Toxic Hepatitis

Most cases of drug-induced liver disease present as acute hepatitis, although some present as cholestasis or other patterns (Table 14–7). The incidence of drug-induced hepatitis has been rising; acetaminophen is now the most common cause of fulminant hepatitis in the United States and the United Kingdom. Hepatic toxins can be further subdivided into those for which hepatic toxicity is predictable and dose dependent for most individuals (eg, acetaminophen) and those that cause unpredictable (idiosyncratic) reactions without relationship to dose. Tables 14–10 and 14–11 summarize speculations on the mechanisms of idiosyncratic and dose-related drug-induced hepatic disease. Idiosyncratic reactions to drugs may be due to genetic predisposition in susceptible individuals to certain pathways of drug metabolism that generate toxic interme-

diates. Prominent examples of drugs causing acute liver failure that have been withdrawn from the U.S. market include bromfenac, a nonsteroidal anti-inflammatory drug (NSAID), and

TABLE 14–11   Postulated mechanisms of drug-induced liver disease.

Effect	Example
Alteration of the physical properties of membranes	Estrogens
Inhibition of membrane enzymes (eg, Na⁺-K⁺ ATPase)	Chlorpromazine metabolites
Interference with hepatic uptake processes	Rifampin
Impairment of cytoskeletal function	Chlorpromazine metabolites
Formation of insoluble complexes in bile	Chlorpromazine
Conversion to reactive intermediates	Acetaminophen
Electrophils producing covalent modifications of tissue macromolecules	
Free radicals producing lipid peroxidation	Carbon tetrachloride
Redox cycling with production of oxygen radicals	Nitrofurantoin

Reproduced, with permission, from Bass NM, Ockner RK. Drug-induced liver disease. In: *Hepatology: A Textbook of Liver Disease,* 2nd ed. Zakim D, Boyer JD (editors). Saunders, 1990.

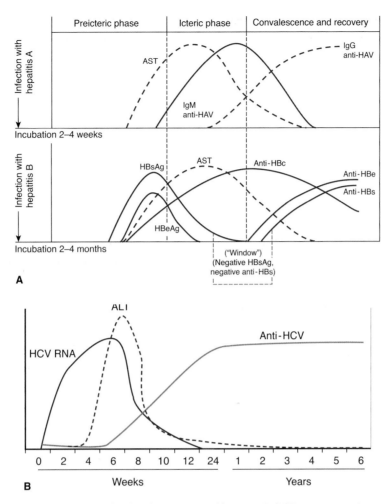

FIGURE 14–9 **(A)** Serum antibody and antigen levels in hepatitis A and hepatitis B. (AST, aspartate amino-transferase, a marker for hepato-cellular injury and necrosis; IgM anti-HAV, early antibody response to hepatitis A infection; IgG anti-HAV, late antibody response to hepatitis A infection; HBsAg, hepatitis B surface antigen, a marker of active viral gene expression; HBeAg, hepatitis B early antigen, a marker of infectivity.) Antibodies to the surface or early antigens (anti-HBs or anti-HBe) indicate immunity. (Redrawn, with permission, from Chandrasoma P, Taylor CE. *Concise Pathology*, 3rd ed. Originally published by Appleton & Lange. Copyright © 1998 by the McGraw-Hill Companies, Inc.) **(B)** Course of acute, resolving HCV infection. ALT, Alanine aminotransferase, HCV RNA, hepatitis C viral load, anti-HCV, HCV antibody. (Redrawn, with permission, from Hoofnagle JH. Course and outcome of hepatitis C. Hepatology. 2002 Nov;36(5 Suppl 1):S21–9.)

troglitazone sulfate, a thiazolidinedione used as an insulin-sensitizing agent in diabetes mellitus. Other thiazolidinedi-ones such as rosiglitazone and pioglitazone do not seem to have the same complication, although routine testing of trans-aminases has been recommended for those taking the drugs. HMG-CoA reductase inhibitors such as atorvastatin, lovastatin, and others are associated with elevated levels of transami-nases in less than 3% of patients and with few cases of acute liver failure.

The time course of acute hepatitis is highly variable. In hep-atitis A jaundice is typically seen 4–8 weeks after exposure, whereas in hepatitis B jaundice occurs usually from 8–20 weeks after exposure (Figure 14–9). Drug- and toxin-induced hepatitis typically occurs at any time during or shortly after exposure and resolves with discontinuance of the offending agent. This is usually the case for both idiosyncratic and dose-dependent reactions.

Acute hepatitis typically resolves in 3–6 months. Hepatic injury continuing for more than 6 months is arbitrarily defined as chronic hepatitis and suggests, in the absence of continued exposure to a noxious agent, that immune or other mechanisms are at work.

Pathogenesis

A. Viral Hepatitis

The viral agents responsible for acute hepatitis first infect the hepatocyte. During the incubation period, intense viral repli-cation in the liver cell leads to the appearance of viral compo-nents (first antigens, later antibodies) in urine, stool, and body fluids. Liver cell death and an associated inflammatory re-sponse then ensue, followed by changes in laboratory tests of liver function and the appearance of various symptoms and signs of liver disease.

1. **Liver damage**—The host's immunologic response plays an important though incompletely understood role in the pathogenesis of liver damage. In hepatitis B, for example, the virus is probably not directly cytopathic. Indeed, there are asymptomatic HBV carriers who have normal liver function and histologic features. Instead, the host's cellular immune response has an important role in causing liver cell injury. Patients with defects in cell-mediated immunity are more likely to remain chronically infected with HBV than to clear the infection. Histologic specimens from patients with HBV-related liver injury demonstrate lymphocytes next to necrotic liver cells. It is thought that cytolytic T lymphocytes become sensitized to recognize hepatitis B viral antigens (eg, small quantities of hepatitis B surface antigen [HBsAg]) and host antigens on the surfaces of HBV-infected liver cells.

2. **Extrahepatic manifestations**—Immune factors may also be important in the pathogenesis of the extrahepatic manifestations of acute viral hepatitis. For example, in hepatitis B, a serum sickness-like prodrome characterized by fever, urticarial rash and angioedema, and arthralgias and arthritis appears to be related to immune complex–mediated tissue damage. During the early prodrome, circulating immune complexes are composed of HBsAg in high titer in association with small quantities of anti-HBs. These circulating immune complexes are deposited in blood vessel walls, leading to activation of the complement cascade. In patients with arthritis, serum complement levels are depressed, and complement can be detected in circulating immune complexes containing HBsAg, anti-HBs, immunoglobulin (Ig) G, IgM, IgA, and fibrin. Cryoglobulinemia is a common finding in chronic hepatitis C infection.

Immune factors are thought to be important in the pathogenesis of some clinical manifestations in patients who become chronic HBsAg carriers after acute hepatitis. For example, in patients developing glomerulonephritis with nephrotic syndrome, histopathologic investigation demonstrates deposition of HBsAg, immunoglobulin, and complement in the glomerular basement membrane. In patients developing polyarteritis nodosa, similar deposits have been demonstrated in affected small and medium-sized arteries.

Other, more rare, extrahepatic manifestations include papular acrodermatitis, and Guillain-Barré syndrome for HBV, and idiopathic thrombocytopenic purpura, lichen planus, Sjögren's syndrome, and porphyria cutanea tarda for HCV.

B. Alcoholic Hepatitis

Ethanol has both direct and indirect toxic effects on the liver as well as effects on many other organ systems of the body. Its direct effects may result from increasing the fluidity of biologic membranes and thereby disrupting cellular functions. Its indirect effects on the liver are in part a consequence of its metabolism. Ethanol is sequentially oxidized to acetaldehyde and then to acetate, with the generation of NADH and adenosine triphosphate (ATP). As a result of the high ratio of reduced to oxidized NAD that is generated, the pathways of fatty acid oxidation and gluconeogenesis are inhibited, whereas fatty acid synthesis is promoted. Ethanol can also quantitatively and qualitatively alter the pattern of gene expression in various tissues but especially in the liver, resulting in impaired homeostasis and greater sensitivity to other toxins. These and other biochemical mechanisms may contribute to the common observation of fat accumulation in the liver of alcoholics and the tendency of hypoglycemia to develop in alcoholics whose liver glycogen has been depleted by fasting. Ethanol metabolism also affects the liver by generating acetaldehyde, which reacts with primary amino groups to inactivate enzymes, resulting in direct toxicity to the hepatocyte in which it is generated. Furthermore, proteins so modified may activate the immune system against antigens that were previously tolerated as "self."

There is considerable variation among individuals in the amount of ethanol required to cause acute liver injury. Whether nutritional, genetic, or other factors are responsible for these differences has not been determined. The mechanisms thought to be responsible for ethanol-induced liver injury are listed in Table 14–12.

Pathology

In uncomplicated acute hepatitis, the typical histologic findings consist of (1) focal liver cell degeneration and necrosis, with cell dropout, ballooning, and acidophilic degeneration (shrunken cells with eosinophilic cytoplasm and pyknotic nuclei); (2) inflammation of portal areas, with infiltration by mononuclear cells (small lymphocytes, plasma cells, eosinophils); (3) prominence of Kupffer cells and bile ducts; and (4) cholestasis (arrested bile flow) with bile plugs. Characteristically, although the regular pattern of the cords of hepatocytes is disrupted, the reticulin framework is preserved. This reticular framework provides scaffolding for liver cells when they regenerate.

Recovery from acute hepatitis from any cause is characterized histologically by regeneration of hepatocytes, with numerous mitotic figures and multinucleated cells, and by a largely complete restoration of normal lobular architecture.

Less commonly in acute hepatitis (1–5% of patients), there will be a more severe histologic lesion called **bridging hepatic necrosis** (also called subacute, submassive, or confluent necrosis). Bridging is said to occur between lobules because necrosis involves contiguous groups of hepatocytes, resulting in large areas of hepatic cell loss and collapse of the reticulin framework. Necrotic zones ("bridges") consisting of condensed reticulin, inflammatory debris, and degenerating liver cells link adjacent portal or central areas or may involve entire lobules.

Rarely, in massive hepatic necrosis or fulminant hepatitis (< 1% of patients), the liver becomes small, shrunken, and soft (acute yellow atrophy). Histologic examination reveals massive hepatocyte necrosis in most of the lobules, leading to extensive collapse and condensation of the reticulin framework and portal structures (bile ducts and vessels).

TABLE 14–12 Mechanisms of hepatocyte injury by ethanol.

Disorganizes the lipid portion of cell membranes, leading to adaptive changes in their composition
Increased fluidity and permeability of membranes
Impaired assembly of glycoproteins into membranes
Impaired secretion of glycoproteins
Impaired binding and internalization of large ligands
Formation of abnormal mitochondria
Impairment of transport of small ligands
Impairment of membrane-bound enzymes
Adaptive changes in lipid composition, leading to increased lipid peroxidation
Abnormal display of antigens on the plasma membrane
Alters the capacity of liver cells to cope with environmental toxins
Induces xenobiotic metabolizing enzymes
Directly inhibits xenobiotic metabolizing enzymes
Induces deficiency in mechanisms protecting against injury due to reactive metabolites
Enhances the toxicity of O_2
Oxidation of ethanol produces acetaldehyde, a toxic and reactive intermediate
Inhibits export of proteins from the liver
Modifies hepatic protein synthesis in fasted animals
Alters the metabolism of cofactors essential for enzymatic activity—pyridoxine, folate, choline, zinc, vitamin E
Alters the oxidation-reduction potential of the liver cell
Induces malnutrition

Reproduced, with permission, from Zakim D, Boyer TD, Montgomery C. Alcoholic liver disease. In: *Hepatology: A Textbook of Liver Disease,* 2nd ed. Zakim D, Boyer JD (editors). Saunders, 1990.

The pathology of alcoholic hepatitis is different from that of viral hepatitis in some ways. The specific pathologic features of alcoholic hepatitis include accumulation of Mallory's hyalin and infiltration of polymorphonuclear leukocytes.

Clinical Manifestations

A. Viral Hepatitis

Acute viral hepatitis usually is manifested in three phases: the prodrome, the icteric phase, and the convalescent phase.

1. **Prodrome**—The prodrome, typically lasting 3 or 4 days, is characterized by three sets of symptoms and signs: (1) non-specific constitutional symptoms and signs: malaise, fatigue, and mild fever; (2) GI symptoms and signs: anorexia, nausea, vomiting, altered senses of olfaction and taste (loss of taste for coffee or cigarettes), and right upper quadrant abdominal discomfort (reflecting the enlarged liver); and (3) extrahepatic symptoms and signs: headache, photophobia, cough, coryza, myalgias, urticarial skin rash, arthralgias or arthritis (10–15% of patients with HBV), and, rarely, hematuria and proteinuria.

2. **Icteric phase**—The icteric phase typically lasts for 1–4 weeks. The constitutional symptoms usually improve, although mild weight loss may occur. Pruritus occurs if cholestasis is severe. Right upper quadrant abdominal pain as a result of the enlarged and tender liver, which was present in the prodromal phase, continues. Splenomegaly is noted in 10–20% of patients.

Jaundice may be observed as a yellowing of the scleras, skin, or mucous membranes. Jaundice is generally not appreciated on physical examination before the serum bilirubin rises above 2.5 mg/dL (41.75 μmol/L). **Direct hyperbilirubinemia** is elevation of the level of conjugated bilirubin in the bloodstream. Its occurrence indicates unimpaired ability of hepatocytes to conjugate bilirubin but a defect in the excretion of bilirubin into the bile as a result of intrahepatic cholestasis or posthepatic obstructive biliary tract disease, with overflow of conjugated bilirubin out of hepatocytes and into the bloodstream.

Changes in stool color (lightening) and urine color (darkening) often precede clinically evident jaundice. This reflects loss of bilirubin metabolites from the stool as a consequence of disrupted bile flow. Water-soluble (conjugated) bilirubin metabolites are excreted in the urine, whereas water-insoluble metabolites accumulate in tissues, giving rise to jaundice. Note that in most cases of acute viral hepatitis the degree of liver impairment is sufficiently mild that jaundice does not develop.

Ecchymoses suggest coagulopathy, which may be due to loss of vitamin K absorptive capacity from the intestine (caused by cholestasis) or decreased coagulation factor synthesis. Rarely, loss of clearance of activated clotting factors triggers disseminated intravascular coagulation. Coagulopathy in which the prothrombin time can be corrected by vitamin K injections but not by oral vitamin K suggests cholestatic disease, because vitamin K uptake from the gut is dependent on bile flow. If the prothrombin time cannot be corrected with either oral or parenteral vitamin K, inability to synthesize clotting factor polypeptides (eg, as a result of massive hepatocellular dysfunction) should be suspected. Correction of prothrombin time with oral vitamin K alone suggests a nutritional deficiency rather than liver disease as the basis for the coagulopathy.

Tests for serum levels of various enzymes normally localized primarily within hepatocytes provide an indication of the extent of liver cell necrosis. For unclear reasons, perhaps related to liver cell polarity, certain forms of liver disease typically result in disproportionate elevations in some parameters. Thus, in alcoholic hepatitis but not in viral hepatitis, AST is often disproportionately elevated relative to ALT (AST:ALT

TABLE 14–13 **Commonly encountered serologic patterns in hepatitis B infection.**

HBsAg	Anti-HBs	Anti-HBc	HBeAg	Anti-HBe	Interpretation
+	–	IgM	+	–	Acute HBV infection, high infectivity
+	–	IgG	+	–	Chronic HBV infection, high infectivity
+	–	IgG	–	+	Late acute or chronic HBV infection, low infectivity
+	+	+	+/–	+/–	1. HBsAg of one subtype and heterotypic anti-HBs (common) 2. Process of seroconversion from HBsAg to anti-HBs (rare)
–	–	IgM	+/–	+/–	1. Acute HBV infection 2. Anti-HBc window
–	–	IgG	–	+/–	1. Low-level HBsAg carrier 2. Remote past infection
–	+	IgG	–	+/–	Recovery from HBV infection
–	+	–	–	–	1. Immunization with HBsAg (after vaccination) 2. Remote past infection (?) 3. False-positive

Reproduced, with permission, from Dienstag DL, Wards JR, Isselbacher KJ. Acute hepatitis. In: *Harrison's Principles of Internal Medicine*, 12th ed. Wilson JD et al (editors). McGraw-Hill, 1991.

ratio > 2.0). One hypothesis is that this is due to pyridoxine deficiency in alcoholics. Likewise, in cholestasis, alkaline phosphatase is commonly disproportionately elevated relative to AST or ALT.

Measurement of antigen and antibody titers is a convenient way to assess whether an episode of acute hepatitis is due to viral infection. Moreover, because IgM antibodies are produced early after exposure to antigens (ie, soon after onset of illness), the presence of IgM antibodies to either HAV or to core antigen of HBV (HBcAg) is strong evidence that an episode of acute hepatitis is due to the corresponding viral infection. Several months after onset of illness, IgM antibody titers wane and are replaced by antibodies of the IgG class, indicating immunity to recurrence of infection by the same virus. Presence of hepatitis B "e" antigen (HBeAg) correlates well with a high degree of infectivity (Table 14–13). However, more sensitive DNA tests have shown low levels of viral DNA in the blood of many who are HBeAg negative and who are thus still infectious. Subtle or profound mental status changes are seen in fulminant hepatic necrosis. Encephalopathy is believed to be related in part to failure of detoxification of ammonia, which normally occurs through the urea cycle. Other products such as γ-aminobutyric acid (GABA) may not be metabolized. Although ammonia is a neurotoxin, it remains unclear whether it is the major agent of CNS dysfunction or whether elevated blood levels of GABA (or other compounds) may act synergistically to alter mental status because of its role as a major inhibitory neurotransmitter.

In addition to encephalopathic changes caused by accumulation of toxins, acute hepatic failure is associated with encephalopathy from cerebral edema caused by increased intracranial pressure, perhaps related to alterations in the blood-brain barrier.

Renal dysfunction may complicate fulminant hepatic failure. Affected patients may develop prerenal azotemia when the glomerular filtration rate falls secondary to intravascular volume depletion. A state of intravascular volume depletion can be induced by the combination of decreased oral intake, vomiting, and formation of ascites. If uncorrected, this process can lead to acute tubular necrosis and acute renal failure. Other causes of renal dysfunction in fulminant hepatic failure include toxins (eg, acetaminophen or *Amanita* poisoning) or hepatorenal syndrome. Serum creatinine is a more accurate measure than blood urea nitrogen of renal impairment in fulminant hepatic failure resulting from decreased hepatic urea production. Other complications of fulminant hepatic failure include cardiovascular dysfunction as a result of systemic vasodilation and hypotension, pulmonary edema, coagulopathy, sepsis, and hypoglycemia.

3. **Convalescent phase**—The convalescent phase is characterized by complete disappearance of constitutional symptoms but persistent abnormalities in liver function tests. Symptoms and signs gradually improve.

CHECKPOINT

22. Describe the range of clinical presentations of acute hepatitis.
23. Which viruses can cause hepatitis?
24. What are some extrahepatic manifestations of viral hepatitis?
25. What is the basis for the extrahepatic manifestations of viral hepatitis?

TABLE 14–14 Simplified scoring system for chronic hepatitis.

1. Grade
A. Portal inflammation and interface hepatitis
0 Absent or minimal
1 Portal inflammation only
2 Mild or localized interface hepatitis
3 Moderate or more extensive interface hepatitis
4 Severe and widespread interface hepatitis
B. Lobular activity
0 None
1 Inflammatory cells but no hepatocellular damage
2 Focal necrosis or apoptosis
3 Severe hepatocellular damage
4 Damage includes bridging confluent necrosis
2. Stage
0 No fibrosis
1 Fibrosis confined to portal tracts
2 Periportal or portal–portal septa but intact vascular relationships
3 Fibrosis with distorted structure but no obvious cirrhosis
4 Probable or definite cirrhosis

Reprinted, with permission, from Jevon GP. Grade and stage for chronic hepatitis. Pediatr Dev Pathol. 2001;4:371.

CHRONIC HEPATITIS

Chronic hepatitis is a category of disorders characterized by the combination of liver cell necrosis and inflammation of varying severity persisting for more than 6 months. It may be due to viral infection; drugs and toxins; genetic, metabolic, or autoimmune factors; or unknown causes. The severity ranges from an asymptomatic stable illness characterized only by laboratory test abnormalities to a severe, gradually progressive illness culminating in cirrhosis, liver failure, and death. Based on clinical, laboratory, and biopsy findings, chronic hepatitis is best assessed with regard to (1) distribution and severity of inflammation, (2) degree of fibrosis, and (3) etiology, which has important prognostic implications. A simplified scoring system for assessment of liver biopsies for chronic hepatitis is presented in Table 14–14.

Clinical Presentation

Patients may present with fatigue, malaise, low-grade fever, anorexia, weight loss, mild intermittent jaundice, and mild hepatosplenomegaly. Others are initially asymptomatic and present late in the course of the disease with complications of cirrhosis, including variceal bleeding, coagulopathy, encephalopathy, jaundice, and ascites. In contrast to chronic persistent hepatitis, some patients with chronic active hepatitis, particularly those without serologic evidence of antecedent HBV infection, present with extrahepatic symptoms such as skin rash, diarrhea, arthritis, and various autoimmune disorders (Table 14–15).

Etiology

Either type of chronic hepatitis can be caused by infection with several hepatitis viruses (eg, hepatitis B with or without hepatitis D superinfection and hepatitis C); a variety of drugs and poisons (eg, ethanol, isoniazid, acetaminophen), often in amounts insufficient to cause symptomatic acute hepatitis; genetic and metabolic disorders (eg, α_1-antiprotease [α_1-antitrypsin] deficiency, Wilson's disease); or immune-mediated injury of unknown origin. Table 14–1 summarizes known causes of chronic hepatitis. Less than 5% of otherwise healthy adults with acute hepatitis B remain chronically infected with HBV; the risk is higher in those who are immunocompromised

TABLE 14–15 Autoimmune disorders and extrahepatic manifestations associated with chronic active hepatitis.

Thyroiditis
Thyrotoxicosis (rare)
Hypothyroidism
Autoimmune hemolytic anemia
Polyarthritis
Capillaritis
Glomerulonephritis
Pulmonary disorders
Fibrosing alveolitis
Primary pulmonary hypertension
Amenorrhea and other menstrual abnormalities
Ulcerative colitis
Monoclonal gammopathy
Hyperviscosity syndrome
Lichen planus
Polymyositis
Uveitis

Reproduced, with permission, from Maddrey WC. Chronic hepatitis. In: *Hepatology: A Textbook of Liver Disease,* 2nd ed. Zakim D, Boyer JD (editors). Saunders, 1990.

or of young age (eg, chronic infection develops in approximately 90% of neonates). Among those chronically infected, about two-thirds develop mild chronic hepatitis and one-third develop severe chronic hepatitis (see later discussion). Superinfection with HDV of a patient with chronic HBV infection is associated with a much higher rate of chronic hepatitis than is seen with isolated hepatitis B infection. Hepatitis D superinfection of patients with hepatitis B is also associated with a high incidence of fulminant hepatic failure. Finally, 60–85% of individuals with acute post-transfusional or community-acquired hepatitis C develop chronic hepatitis.

Pathogenesis

Many cases of chronic hepatitis are thought to represent an immune-mediated attack on the liver occurring as a result of persistence of certain hepatitis viruses or after prolonged exposure to certain drugs or noxious substances (Table 14–16). In some, no mechanism has been recognized. Evidence that the disorder is immune mediated is that liver biopsies reveal inflammation (infiltration of lymphocytes) in characteristic regions of the liver architecture (eg, portal versus lobular). Furthermore, a variety of autoimmune disorders occur with high frequency in patients with chronic hepatitis (Table 14–15).

A. Postviral Chronic Hepatitis

Viral hepatitis is the most common cause of chronic liver disease in the United States. In approximately 5% of cases of HBV infection and 60–85% of hepatitis C infections, the immune response is inadequate to clear the liver of virus, resulting in persistent infection. The individual becomes a chronic carrier, intermittently producing the virus and hence remaining infectious to others. Biochemically, these patients are often found

to have viral DNA integrated into their genomes in a manner that results in abnormal expression of certain viral proteins with or without production of intact virus. Viral antigens expressed on the hepatocyte cell surface are associated with class I HLA determinants, thus eliciting lymphocyte cytotoxicity and resulting in hepatitis. The severity of chronic hepatitis is largely dependent on the activity of viral replication and the response by the host's immune system.

Chronic hepatitis B infection predisposes the patient to the development of hepatocellular carcinoma even in the absence of cirrhosis. It remains unclear whether hepatitis B infection is the initiator or simply a promoter in the process of tumorigenesis. In hepatitis C infection, hepatocellular carcinoma develops only in the setting of cirrhosis.

B. Alcoholic Chronic Hepatitis

Chronic liver disease in response to some poisons or toxins may represent triggering of an underlying genetic predisposition to immune attack on the liver. In alcoholic hepatitis, however, repeated episodes of acute injury ultimately cause necrosis, fibrosis, and regeneration, leading eventually to cirrhosis (Figure 14–10). As in other forms of liver disease, there is considerable variation in the extent of symptoms before development of cirrhosis.

C. Nonalcoholic Fatty Liver Disease

In light of increasing obesity in the United States, there has been a significant increase in the prevalence of nonalcoholic fatty liver disease (NAFLD), a form of chronic liver disease that is associated with the metabolic syndrome. NAFLD occurs in disorders that cause predominantly macrovesicular fat accumulation in the liver. Conditions such as obesity, diabetes mellitus, hypertriglyceridemia, and insulin resistance are considered risk factors for development of NAFLD. An estimated 3–6% of the U.S. population with an aggressive form of NAFLD known as nonalcoholic steatohepatitis are, in particular, at higher risk of progressive liver disease, cirrhosis, and hepatocellular carcinoma.

D. Idiopathic Chronic Hepatitis

Some patients develop chronic hepatitis in the absence of evidence of preceding viral hepatitis or exposure to noxious agents (Figure 14–11). These patients typically have serologic evidence of disordered immunoregulation, manifested as hyperglobulinemia and circulating autoantibodies. Nearly 75% of these patients are women, and many have other autoimmune disorders. A genetic predisposition is strongly suggested. Most patients with autoimmune hepatitis show histologic improvement in liver biopsies after treatment with systemic corticosteroids. The clinical response, however, can be variable. Primary biliary cirrhosis and autoimmune cholangitis represent cholestatic forms of an autoimmune-mediated liver disease.

TABLE 14–16 Drugs implicated in the etiology of chronic hepatitis.

Drug	Use
Acetaminophen	Analgesic
Amiodarone	Antiarrhythmic
Aspirin	Analgesic
Ethanol	Abuse
Isoniazid	Antituberculous therapy
Methyldopa	Antihypertensive
Nitrofurantoin	Antibiotic
Propylthiouracil	Antithyroid therapy
Sulfonamides	Antibiotic

Modified and reproduced, with permission, from Bass NM, Ockner RK. Drug-induced liver disease. In: *Hepatology: A Textbook of Liver Disease*, 2nd ed. Zakim D, Boyer JD (editors). Saunders, 1990.

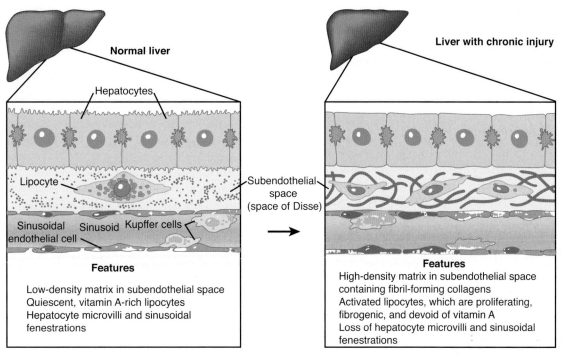

Normal liver

Hepatocytes

Lipocyte

Subendothelial space (space of Disse)

Sinusoidal endothelial cell   Sinusoid   Kupffer cells

Features

Low-density matrix in subendothelial space
Quiescent, vitamin A-rich lipocytes
Hepatocyte microvilli and sinusoidal fenestrations

Liver with chronic injury

Features

High-density matrix in subendothelial space containing fibril-forming collagens
Activated lipocytes, which are proliferating, fibrogenic, and devoid of vitamin A
Loss of hepatocyte microvilli and sinusoidal fenestrations

FIGURE 14–10 Changes in the hepatic subendothelial space during fibrosing liver injury. Cellular and matrix alterations in the space of Disse are critical events in the pathogenesis of hepatic fibrosis. The activation of lipocytes, characterized by proliferation and increased fibrogenesis, is associated with the replacement of the normal low-density matrix with a high-density matrix. These alterations are likely to underlie, at least in part, the loss of both endothelial fenestrations (pores) and hepatocytic microvilli typical of chronic liver injury. (Redrawn, with permission, from Bissell DM. The cellular basis of hepatic fibrosis. N Engl J Med. 1993;328:1828.)

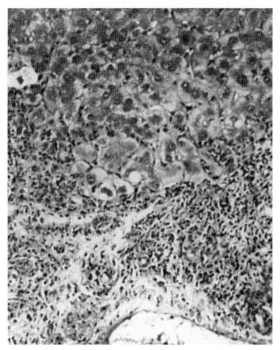

FIGURE 14–11 Chronic hepatitis, showing marked lymphocytic infiltration and fibrosis of the portal areas. The lymphocytes extend into the peripheral part of the lobule through the limiting plate. There is ongoing necrosis of hepatocytes in the peripheral part of the lobule (piecemeal necrosis). (Reproduced, with permission, from Chandrasoma P, Taylor CE. *Concise Pathology*, 3rd ed. Originally published by Appleton & Lange. Copyright © 1998 by the McGraw-Hill Companies, Inc.)

Pathology

All forms of chronic hepatitis share the common histopathologic features of (1) inflammatory infiltration of hepatic portal areas with mononuclear cells, especially lymphocytes and plasma cells, and (2) necrosis of hepatocytes within the parenchyma or immediately adjacent to portal areas (periportal hepatitis, or "piecemeal necrosis").

In mild chronic hepatitis, the overall architecture of the liver is preserved. Histologically, the liver reveals a characteristic lymphocyte and plasma cell infiltrate confined to the portal triad without disruption of the limiting plate and no evidence of active hepatocyte necrosis. There is little or no fibrosis, and what there is generally is restricted to the portal area; there is no sign of cirrhosis. A "cobblestone" appearance of liver cells is seen, indicating regeneration of hepatocytes.

In more severe cases of chronic hepatitis, the portal areas are expanded and densely infiltrated by lymphocytes, histiocytes, and plasma cells. There is necrosis of hepatocytes at the periphery of the lobule, with erosion of the limiting plate surrounding the portal triads (piecemeal necrosis; Figure 14–11). More severe cases also show evidence of necrosis and fibrosis between portal triads. There is disruption of normal liver architecture by bands of scar tissue and inflammatory cells that link portal areas to one another and to central areas (bridging necrosis). These connective tissue bridges are evidence of remodeling of hepatic architecture, a crucial step in the development of cirrhosis. Fibrosis may extend from the portal areas into the lobules, isolating hepatocytes into clusters and enveloping bile ducts. Regeneration of hepatocytes is seen with mitotic figures, multinucleated cells, rosette formation, and regenerative pseudolobules. Progression to cirrhosis is signaled by extensive fibrosis, loss of zonal architecture, and regenerating nodules.

Clinical Manifestations

Some patients with mild chronic hepatitis are entirely asymptomatic and identified only in the course of routine blood testing; others have an insidious onset of nonspecific symptoms such as anorexia, malaise, and fatigue or hepatic symptoms such as right upper quadrant abdominal discomfort or pain. Fatigue in chronic hepatitis may be related to a change in the hypothalamic-adrenal neuroendocrine axis brought about by altered endogenous opioidergic neurotransmission. Jaundice, if present, is usually mild. There may be mild tender hepatomegaly and occasional splenomegaly. Palmar erythema and spider telangiectases are seen in severe cases. Other extrahepatic manifestations are unusual. By definition, signs of cirrhosis and portal hypertension (eg, ascites, collateral circulation, and encephalopathy) are absent. Laboratory studies show mild to moderate increases in serum aminotransferase, bilirubin, and globulin levels. Serum albumin and the prothrombin time are normal until late in the progression of liver disease.

The clinical manifestations of chronic hepatitis probably reflect the role of a systemic genetically controlled immune disorder in the pathogenesis of severe disease. Acne, hirsutism, and amenorrhea may occur as a reflection of the hormonal effects of chronic liver disease. Laboratory studies in patients with severe chronic hepatitis are invariably abnormal to various degrees. However, these abnormalities do not correlate with clinical severity. Thus, the serum bilirubin, alkaline phosphatase, and globulin levels may be normal and aminotransferase levels only mildly elevated at the same time that a liver biopsy reveals severe chronic hepatitis. However, an elevated prothrombin time usually reflects severe disease.

The natural history and treatment of chronic hepatitis varies depending on its cause. The complications of severe chronic hepatitis are those of progression to cirrhosis: variceal bleeding, encephalopathy, coagulopathy, hypersplenism, and ascites. These are largely due to portosystemic shunting rather than diminished hepatocyte reserve (see later discussion).

CHECKPOINT

26. What are the categories of chronic hepatitis based on histologic findings on liver biopsy?
27. What are the causes of chronic hepatitis?
28. What are the consequences of chronic hepatitis?

CIRRHOSIS

Clinical Presentation

Cirrhosis is an irreversible distortion of normal liver architecture characterized by hepatic injury, fibrosis, and nodular regeneration. The clinical presentations of cirrhosis are a consequence of both progressive hepatocellular dysfunction and portal hypertension (Figure 14–12). As with other presentations of liver disease, not all patients with cirrhosis develop life-threatening complications. Indeed, in nearly 40% of cases of cirrhosis, it is diagnosed at autopsy in patients who did not manifest obvious signs of end-stage liver disease.

Etiology

The causes of cirrhosis are listed in Table 14–1. The initial injury can be due to a wide range of processes. A crucial feature is that the liver injury is not acute and self-limited but rather chronic and progressive. In the United States, alcohol abuse is the most common cause of cirrhosis. In other countries, infectious agents (particularly HBV and HCV) are the most common causes. Other causes include chronic biliary obstruction, drugs, metabolic disorders, chronic congestive heart failure, and primary (autoimmune) biliary cirrhosis.

Pathogenesis

Increased or altered synthesis of collagen and other connective tissue or basement membrane components of the extracellular matrix is implicated in the development of hepatic fibrosis and thus in the pathogenesis of cirrhosis. The role of the extracellular matrix in cellular function is an important area of research, and studies suggest that it is involved in modulating the activities of the cells with which it is in contact. Thus, fibrosis may affect not only the physics of blood flow through the liver but also the functions of the cells themselves.

Hepatic fibrosis appears to occur in three situations: (1) as an immune response, (2) as part of the process of wound healing, and (3) in response to agents that induce primary fibrogenesis. HBV and *Schistosoma* species are good examples of agents producing fibrosis on an immunologic basis. Agents such as carbon tetrachloride that attack and kill hepatocytes directly can produce fibrosis as part of wound healing. In both immune responses and wound healing, the fibrosis is triggered indirectly by the effects of cytokines released from invading inflammatory cells. Finally, certain agents such as ethanol and iron may cause primary fibrogenesis by directly increasing collagen gene transcription and thus increasing also the amount of connective tissue secreted by cells.

The actual culprit in all of these mechanisms of increased fibrogenesis may be the fat-storing cells (stellate cells) of the hepatic reticuloendothelial system. In response to cytokines, they differentiate from quiescent stellate cells in which vitamin A is stored into myofibroblasts, which lose their vitamin A storage capacity and become actively engaged in extracellular

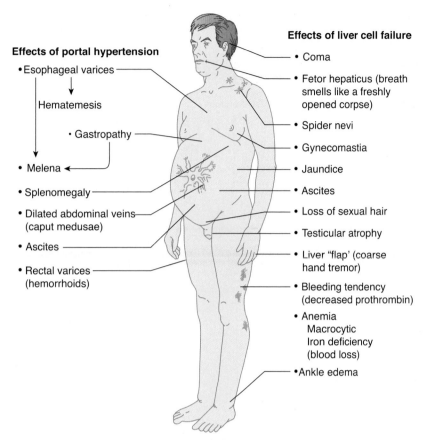

Effects of portal hypertension

- Esophageal varices

  → Hematemesis

- Gastropathy

- Melena

- Splenomegaly

- Dilated abdominal veins
  (caput medusae)

- Ascites

- Rectal varices
  (hemorrhoids)

Effects of liver cell failure

- Coma

- Fetor hepaticus (breath
  smells like a freshly
  opened corpse)

- Spider nevi

- Gynecomastia

- Jaundice

- Ascites

- Loss of sexual hair

- Testicular atrophy

- Liver "flap' (coarse
  hand tremor)

- Bleeding tendency
  (decreased prothrombin)

- Anemia
  Macrocytic
  Iron deficiency
  (blood loss)

- Ankle edema

FIGURE 14–12 Clinical effects of cirrhosis of the liver. (Redrawn, with permission, from Chandrasoma P, Taylor CE. *Concise Pathology*, 3rd ed. Originally published by Appleton & Lange. Copyright © 1998 by the McGraw-Hill Companies, Inc.)

matrix production. In addition to the stellate cells, fibrogenic cells are also derived from portal fibroblasts, circulating fibrocytes, bone marrow, and epithelial-mesenchymal cell transition. It appears that hepatic fibrosis occurs in two stages (Figure 14–13). The first stage is characterized by a change in extracellular matrix composition from non-cross-linked, non-fibril-forming collagen to collagen that is more dense and subject to cross-link formation. At this stage, liver injury is still reversible. The second stage involves formation of subendothelial collagen cross-links, proliferation of myoepithelial cells, and distortion of hepatic architecture with the appearance of regenerating nodules. Cirrhosis remains a dynamic state in which certain interventions, even at these advanced stages, may yield benefits such as regression of scar tissue and improvements in clinical outcomes.

Regardless of the possible effects on hepatocyte function, the increased fibrosis markedly alters the nature of blood flow in the liver, resulting in important complications discussed later.

The manner in which alcohol causes chronic liver disease and cirrhosis is not well understood. However, chronic alcohol abuse is associated with impaired protein synthesis and secretion, mitochondrial injury, lipid peroxidation, formation of acetaldehyde and its interaction with cellular proteins and membrane lipids, cellular hypoxia, and both cell-mediated and antibody-mediated cytotoxicity. The relative importance of each of these

factors in producing cell injury is unknown. Genetic, nutritional, and environmental factors (including simultaneous exposure to other hepatotoxins) also influence the development of liver disease in chronic alcoholics. Finally, acute liver injury (eg, from exposure to alcohol or other toxins) from which a person with a normal liver would fully recover may be sufficient to produce irreversible decompensation (eg, hepatorenal syndrome) in a patient with underlying hepatic cirrhosis.

Pathology

Grossly, the liver may be large or small, but it always has a firm consistency. Liver biopsy is the only method of definitively diagnosing cirrhosis.

Histologically, all forms of cirrhosis are characterized by three findings: (1) marked distortion of hepatic architecture, (2) scarring as a result of increased deposition of fibrous tissue and collagen, and (3) regenerative nodules surrounded by scar tissue. When the nodules are small (< 3 mm) and uniform in size, the process is termed **micronodular cirrhosis.** In **macronodular cirrhosis,** the nodules are > 3 mm and variable in size. Cirrhosis from alcohol abuse is usually micronodular but can be macronodular or both micronodular and macronodular. Scarring may be most severe in central regions, or dense bands of connective tissue may join portal and central areas.

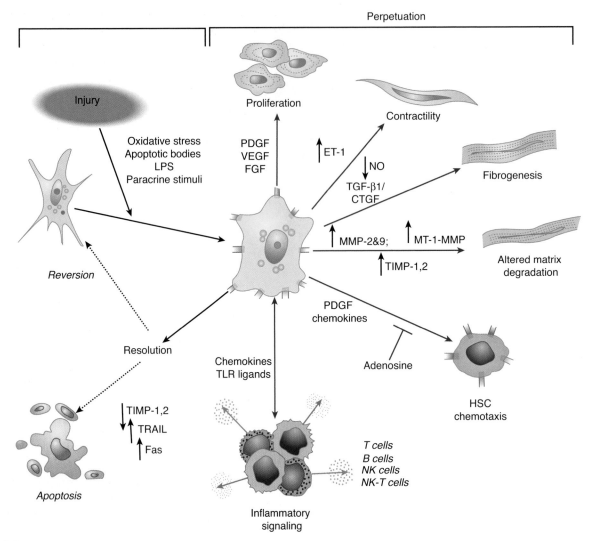

FIGURE 14–13   Pathways of hepatic stellate cell activation. Features of stellate cell activation can be distinguished between those that stimulate initiation and those that contribute to perpetuation. Initiation is provoked by soluble stimuli that include oxidant stress signals (reactive oxygen intermediates), apoptotic bodies, lipopolysaccharide (LPS), and paracrine stimuli from neighboring cell types including hepatic macrophages (Kupffer cells), sinusoidal endothelium, and hepatocytes. Perpetuation follows, characterized by a number of specific phenotypic changes including proliferation, contractility, fibrogenesis, altered matrix degradation, chemotaxis, and inflammatory signaling. FGF, fibroblast growth factor; ET-1, endothelin-1; NK, natural killer; NO, nitric oxide; MT, membrane type.   (Redrawn from Friedman SL. Mechanisms of hepatic fibrogenesis. Gastroenterology. 2008 May;134(6):1655-69.)

More specific histopathologic findings may help to establish the cause of cirrhosis. For example, invasion and destruction of bile ducts by granulomas suggests primary (autoimmune) biliary cirrhosis; extensive iron deposition in hepatocytes and bile ducts suggests hemochromatosis; and alcoholic hyalin and infiltration with polymorphonuclear cells suggest alcoholic cirrhosis.

Clinical Manifestations

The clinical manifestations of progressive hepatocellular dysfunction in cirrhosis are similar to those of acute or chronic hepatitis and include constitutional symptoms and signs: fatigue, loss of vigor, and weight loss; GI symptoms and signs:

nausea, vomiting, jaundice, and tender hepatomegaly; and extrahepatic symptoms and signs: palmar erythema, spider angiomas, muscle wasting, parotid and lacrimal gland enlargement, gynecomastia and testicular atrophy in men, menstrual irregularities in women, and coagulopathy.

Clinical manifestations of portal hypertension include ascites, portosystemic shunting, encephalopathy, splenomegaly, and esophageal and gastric varices with intermittent hemorrhage (Table 14–17).

A. Portal Hypertension

Portal hypertension is defined by a portal venous pressure gradient greater than 5 mm Hg. Portal hypertension is due to a rise in intrahepatic vascular resistance. The cirrhotic liver loses

TABLE 14–17 **Manifestations of cirrhosis.**

Due to portal hypertension with portal-to-systemic shunting
Ascites and increased risk of spontaneous bacterial peritonitis
Increased risk of sepsis
Increased risk of disseminated intravascular coagulation
Splenomegaly with thrombocytopenia
Encephalopathy
Varices
Drug sensitivity
Bile acid deficiency with malabsorption of fat and fat-soluble vitamins
Hyperestrogenemia
Hyperglycemia
Due to loss of hepatocytes
Hypoglycemia
Coagulopathy due to deficient clotting factor synthesis
Peripheral edema due to hypoalbuminemia
Hepatic coma
Other complications
Hepatorenal syndrome
Hepatocellular carcinoma
Hepatopulmonary syndrome

the physiologic characteristic of a low-pressure circuit for blood flow seen in the normal liver. The increased blood pressure within the sinusoids is transmitted back to the portal vein. Because the portal vein lacks valves, this elevated pressure is transmitted back to other vascular beds, resulting in splenomegaly, portal-to-systemic shunting, and many of the complications of cirrhosis discussed later.

B. Ascites

Ascites is the presence of excess fluid in the peritoneal cavity. Patients with ascites develop physical examination findings of increasing abdominal girth, a fluid wave, a ballotable liver, and shifting dullness. Ascites can develop in patients with conditions other than liver disease, including protein-calorie malnutrition (from hypoalbuminemia) and cancer (from lymphatic obstruction). In patients with liver disease, ascites is due to portal hypertension.

It is useful to recognize that liver disease with ascites formation occurs in a wide clinical spectrum. At one end is fully compensated portal hypertension with no ascites present because the volume of ascites generated is less than the approximately 800–1200 mL/d capacity of the peritoneal lymphatic drainage. At the other extreme is the typically fatal hepatorenal syndrome, in which patients with liver disease, usually with massive ascites, succumb to rapidly progressing acute renal failure. The hepatorenal syndrome seems to be precipitated by intense and inappropriate renal vasoconstriction and is characterized by extreme sodium retention typical of prerenal azotemia but in the absence of true volume depletion (see Chapter 16). Nonetheless, the presence of clinically apparent ascites in a patient with liver disease is associated with poor long-term survival.

Over the years, various mechanisms have been proposed to explain ascites formation. No single hypothesis of pathogenesis easily explains all findings at all points in time during the natural history of portal hypertension. Portal hypertension and inappropriate renal retention of sodium are important elements of all theories. The end result of ascites occurs when excess peritoneal fluid exceeds the capacity of lymphatic drainage, leading to increased hydrostatic pressure. The fluid can then be seen to visibly weep from the lymphatics and pool in the abdominal cavity as ascites.

The underfill/vasodilatation hypothesis proposes that the primary event in ascites formation is vascular, with reduced effective circulating volume leading to the activation of the renin-angiotensin system and subsequent renal sodium retention. The classic underfill hypothesis postulates that elevated hepatic sinusoidal pressure leads to sequestration of blood in the splanchnic venous bed. This results in underfilling of the central vein with diversion of intravascular volume to the hepatic lymphatics, which, like the central vein, drain the space of Disse. The peripheral arterial vasodilatation or splanchnic vasodilatation hypothesis adds the idea that, with portal-to-systemic shunting, vasodilatory products (eg, nitric oxide) that are normally cleared by the liver are instead delivered to the systemic circulation, where they cause peripheral arteriolar vasodilation, particularly in the splanchnic arterial bed. The resultant reduced arterial vascular resistance (Figure 14–14) is associated with decreased central filling pressures, decreased renal arterial perfusion, reflex renal arterial vasoconstriction, and increased renal tubular sodium resorption. Retention of sodium expands the intravascular volume, which exacerbates portal venous hypertension. The imbalance between hydrostatic versus oncotic pressure in the portal vein results in ascites formation. Although the splanchnic vasodilatation hypothesis accounts for many of the findings in ascites formation, the use of transhepatic intrajugular portal-to-systemic shunting (TIPS) as a means of decompressing the portal vein in patients with ascites provides a counterargument. As a result of the procedure, peripheral arteriolar vasodilation appears to increase (perhaps as a result of shunting of vasodilators such as nitric oxide that are normally cleared by the liver), yet ascites is generally dramatically improved.

Those who support the overflow hypothesis have proposed that the primary event in the development of ascites is inappropriate renal sodium retention. In this view, ascites is the consequence of overflow of fluid from the intravascular

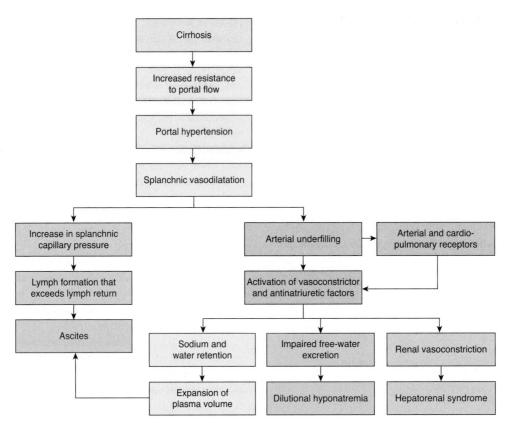

FIGURE 14–14   Proposed mechanism for ascites formation in cirrhosis through the splanchnic vasodilation hypothesis. This hypothesis incorporates elements of the underfill and vasodilation theories.   (Redrawn, with permission, from Gines P et al. Management of cirrhosis and ascites. N Engl J Med. 2004;350:1646.)

volume-expanded portal system into the peritoneal cavity. But what triggers the inappropriate renal sodium retention? One possibility is that there may exist a hepatorenal reflex by which elevated sinusoidal pressure triggers increased sympathetic tone or endothelin-1 secretion. Either of these pathways could cause an inappropriate degree of renal vasoconstriction, a decrease in glomerular filtration rate, and, by tubuloglomerular feedback (see Chapter 16), sodium retention. Note that endothelin-1 is both a renal vasoconstrictor and a stimulant of epinephrine secretion, which in turn stimulates more endothelin-1 secretion. Alternatively, it is possible that an as yet unidentified product from the diseased liver interferes with atrial natriuretic peptide (ANP) action at the kidney or is in some other way responsible for an inappropriate increase in renal sodium retention. Supporters of the overflow hypothesis point to the fact that many cirrhotic patients have sodium handling defects in the absence of ascites and do not have a measurable increase in renin-angiotensin activity. However, studies have shown that the renal sodium retention in these patients can be reversed by the use of an angiotensin II receptor antagonist.

Most likely, multiple mechanisms contribute to the development of ascites and to its perpetuation, worsening, or improvement in diverse clinical situations. Regardless of the initial events, once fully established, many if not all of the mechanisms described in Figure 14–14 are likely to contribute to ascites formation.

C. Hepatorenal Syndrome

Up to 10% of patients with liver disease can develop a poorly understood form of renal disease, called hepatorenal syndrome, which has a dismal prognosis. This disorder is distinct from both prerenal azotemia and acute tubular necrosis. It is characterized by a progressively rising serum creatinine that shows a lack of improvement after 48 hours of diuretic withdrawal and volume expansion with intravenous albumin, and diminished urine volume in the absence of shock, parenchymal renal disease, and use of nephrotoxic agents. Type 1 hepatorenal syndrome is rapidly progressive, with a doubling of the serum creatinine concentration to a level greater than 2.5 mg/dL in less than 2 weeks, whereas type 2 is slowly progressive. Hepatorenal syndrome typically occurs in patients with massive tense ascites and is often precipitated by overly aggressive attempts at diuresis in the hospital or an episode of spontaneous bacterial peritonitis. Hepatorenal syndrome is characterized by severe vasoconstriction of the renal circulation. The urine produced is notable for an extremely low sodium content (< 10 mmol/L) and an absence of casts, resembling the findings in prerenal azotemia. Yet when central venous pressures are measured, the patient does not show intravascular volume depletion and the disorder does not respond to hydration with normal saline. The renal abnormalities of the hepatorenal syndrome appear to be functional because no pathologic changes are identifiable in the kidney. In addition, when a kidney is transplanted from a patient dying of hepatorenal syndrome, it functions well in a recipient without liver disease. It remains to be determined whether this form of renal failure represents loss of an as yet unrecognized hormone produced by the liver that affects the kidneys or is the consequence of some combination of local hemodynamic effects resulting in diminished renal perfusion. Small nonrandomized studies showing some efficacy of vasoconstrictor drugs (vasopressin analogues or α-adrenergic agents) combined with albumin in treating hepatorenal syndrome suggest that hemodynamic changes may be the major cause.

The role of nitric oxide as an intracellular second messenger with vasodilatory effects on vascular beds and the role of endothelins, peptides synthesized by vascular endothelium that have vasoconstrictive properties, have been identified. A speculated role for nitric oxide–mediated peripheral arterial vasodilation combined with sympathetic nervous system and endothelin-mediated renal vasoconstriction has been proposed to explain the salt and water retention of cirrhosis. Those same mechanisms, in the extreme case, may give rise to the hepatorenal syndrome.

D. Hypoalbuminemia and Peripheral Edema

Progressive worsening of hepatocellular function in cirrhosis can result in a fall in the concentration of albumin and other serum proteins synthesized by the liver. As the concentration of these plasma proteins decreases, the plasma oncotic pressure is lowered, thereby tilting the balance of hemodynamic forces toward the development of both peripheral edema and ascites.

These hemodynamic changes further contribute to an avid sodium-retaining state despite total body water and sodium overload seen by urinalysis in the cirrhotic patient. Serum sodium may be low as a result of superimposed water retention caused by antidiuretic hormone release triggered by volume stimuli. A low serum potassium and metabolic alkalosis may be observed as a consequence of elevated aldosterone levels responding to renin release (and angiotensin II release) by the kidneys, which sense afferent intravascular depletion.

E. Spontaneous Bacterial Peritonitis

Spontaneous bacterial peritonitis is the development of infected ascites in the absence of a clear event (such as bowel perforation) that would account for the entry of pathogenic organisms into the peritoneal space. Symptoms and signs include fever, hypotension, abdominal pain or tenderness, decreased or absent bowel sounds, and abrupt onset of hepatic encephalopathy in a patient with ascites.

Patients with large-volume ascites or very low ascitic fluid protein levels are at increased risk for this complication. Ascitic fluid is an excellent culture medium for a variety of pathogens, including Enterobacteriaceae (chiefly *Escherichia coli*), group D streptococci (enterococci), *Streptococcus pneumoniae,* and viridans streptococci. The greater risk in patients with low ascitic fluid protein levels may be due to a low level of opsonic activity in the fluid.

The exact pathogenesis of spontaneous bacterial peritonitis is unknown. Peritonitis may occur because of bacterial seeding of the ascitic fluid via the blood or lymph or by bacteria traversing the gut wall. Enteric organisms may enter the portal venous blood via the portosystemic collaterals, bypassing the reticuloendothelial system of the liver.

F. Gastroesophageal Varices and Bleeding

As blood flow through the liver is progressively impeded, hepatic portal venous pressure rises. In response to the elevated portal venous pressure, there is a decrease in blood vessel wall thickness and enlargement of blood vessels that anastomose with the portal vein, such as those on the surface of the bowel and lower esophagus. These enlarged vessels are termed **varices.** Gastroesophageal varices occur in approximately 50% of patients with cirrhosis. Physical examination may reveal enlargement of hemorrhoidal and periumbilical vessels. Gastroesophageal varices are of more significance clinically, however, because of their tendency to rupture. The resulting massive bleeding is often life threatening because varices in these sites are not easy to tamponade. GI bleeding from varices and other sources (eg, duodenal ulcer, gastritis) in patients with cirrhosis is often exacerbated by concomitant coagulopathy (see later discussion).

G. Hepatic Encephalopathy

Hepatic encephalopathy is manifested by waxing and waning alterations in mental status that occur as a consequence of advanced decompensated liver disease or portal-to-systemic shunting (see Table 14–18 for a list of common precipitants). Abnormalities range from subtle alterations in mental status to profound obtundation. Changes in the sleep pattern starting with hypersomnia and progressing to reversal of the sleep-wake cycle are often an early sign. Cognitive changes include a full spectrum of mental abnormalities, ranging from mild confusion, apathy, agitation, euphoria, and restlessness, to marked confusion and even coma. Motor changes range from fine tremor, slowed coordination, and asterixis to decerebrate posturing and flaccidity. **Asterixis** is a phenomenon of intermittent myoelectrical silence manifested by many muscle groups and enhanced by fatigue. It is best demonstrated by asking the patient to flex the wrists with fingers extended ("stop traffic") and then observing a flapping motion of the fingers. It is thought to be due to decreased sensory input to the brainstem reticular formation, leading to transient lapses in posture. Cerebral edema, which is an important accompanying feature in patients with encephalopathy in acute liver disease, is not seen in cirrhotic patients with encephalopathy.

Common precipitants of encephalopathy are onset of GI bleeding, increased dietary protein intake, and an increased catabolic rate resulting from infection (including spontaneous

TABLE 14–18 Common precipitants of hepatic encephalopathy.

Increased nitrogen load
Gastrointestinal bleeding
Excess dietary protein
Azotemia
Constipation
Electrolyte imbalance
Hypokalemia
Alkalosis
Hypoxia
Hypovolemia
Drugs
Opioids, tranquilizers, sedatives
Diuretics
Miscellaneous
Infection
Surgery
Superimposed acute liver disease
Progressive liver disease

Reproduced, with permission, from Podolsky DK, Isselbacher KJ. Cirrhosis of the liver. In: *Harrison's Principles of Internal Medicine,* 12th ed. Wilson JD et al (editors). McGraw-Hill, 1991.

bacterial peritonitis). Similarly, because of compromised first-pass clearance of ingested drugs, affected patients are exquisitely sensitive to sedatives and other drugs normally metabolized in the liver. Other causes include electrolyte imbalance as a result of diuretics, vomiting, alcohol ingestion or withdrawal, or procedures such as TIPS.

The pathogenesis of hepatic encephalopathy is poorly understood. One proposed mechanism postulates that the encephalopathy is caused by toxins in the gut such as ammonia, derived from metabolic degradation of urea or protein; glutamine, derived from degradation of ammonia; or mercaptans, derived from degradation of sulfur-containing compounds. Because of anatomic or functional portal-systemic shunts, these toxins bypass the liver's detoxification processes and produce alterations in mental status. Increased levels of ammonia, glutamine, and mercaptans can be found in the blood and cerebrospinal fluid. However, blood ammonia and spinal fluid glutamine levels correlate poorly with the presence and severity of encephalopathy.

Alternatively, there may be impairment of the normal blood-brain barrier, rendering the CNS susceptible to various noxious agents. Increased levels of other substances, including metabolic products such as short-chain fatty acids and endogenous benzodiazepine-like metabolites, have also been found in the blood. Importantly, some patients show improvement in encephalopathy when treated with flumazenil, a benzodiazepine receptor antagonist.

A third proposed mechanism postulates a role for GABA, the principal inhibitory neurotransmitter of the brain. GABA is produced in the gut, and increased levels are found in the blood of patients with liver failure.

A fourth proposal postulates that there is an increased entry of aromatic amino acids into the CNS, resulting in increased synthesis of "false" neurotransmitters such as octopamine and decreased synthesis of normal neurotransmitters such as norepinephrine.

H. Coagulopathy

Factors contributing to coagulopathy in cirrhosis include loss of hepatic synthesis of clotting factors, some of which have a half-life of just a few hours. Under these circumstances, a minor or self-limited source of bleeding can become massive.

Hepatocytes are also functionally involved in the maintenance of a normal coagulation cascade through the absorption of vitamin K (a fat-soluble vitamin whose absorption is dependent on bile flow), which is necessary for the activation of some clotting factors (II, VII, IX, X). An ominous sign of the severity of liver disease is the development of a coagulopathy that does not respond to parenteral vitamin K, suggesting deficient clotting factor synthesis rather than impaired absorption of vitamin K because of fat malabsorption. Finally, loss of the liver's capacity to remove activated clotting factors and fibrin degradation products may play a role in the increased susceptibility to **disseminated intravascular coagulation,** a syndrome of coagulation factor consumption that results in uncontrolled simultaneous clotting and bleeding.

I. Splenomegaly and Hypersplenism

Enlargement of the spleen is a consequence of elevated portal venous pressure and consequent engorgement of the organ. Thrombocytopenia and hemolytic anemia occur because of sequestering of formed elements of the blood in the spleen, from which they are normally cleared as they age and are damaged.

J. Hepatocellular Carcinoma

Hepatocellular carcinoma (HCC) occurs in up to 5% of cirrhotic patients per year. There has been a rise in the incidence of HCC in the United States over the past few decades, which is likely secondary to an increased prevalence of NAFLD, HCV infections, and chronic hepatitis B infections due to immigration from countries with a high prevalence of HBV. Several etiologic factors have been identified in the development of this tumor.

1. Malignant transformation is heightened in any form of chronic liver disease, particularly cirrhosis.

2. The risk of developing HCC is increased 100-fold in chronic HBV carriers, even in the absence of cirrhosis. In the setting of chronic HBV infection, 30–50% of cases of HCC occur in the absence of cirrhosis.
3. The risk of developing HCC in the setting of HCV cirrhosis is approximately 1–4% per year.
4. Mycotoxins—metabolites of saprophytic fungi—are known hepatic carcinogens and have been proposed to act synergistically with cirrhosis and HBV infection in increasing the risk of liver cell cancer.
5. Hormonal factors have been implicated by experimental studies. The tumor is known to have a male predominance.

K. Pulmonary Complications

Up to one-third of patients with decompensated cirrhosis have problems associated with oxygenation. The hepatopulmonary syndrome is associated with advanced liver failure, hypoxemia, and intrapulmonary shunting as a result of vasodilatation. The cause of the vasodilatation is unknown, but substances such as nitric oxide, endothelin, and arachidonic acid are thought to be involved. As a result of ventilation-perfusion mismatch, patients often present with platypnea, dyspnea that worsens in the upright position. Liver transplantation leads to resolution of the hepatopulmonary syndrome. However, pulmonary hypertension affects some patients with advanced liver failure and is a contraindication to liver transplantation. Additionally, patients with cirrhosis may present with hepatic hydrothorax. Hepatic hydrothorax is defined as the presence of a pleural effusion due to small defects in the diaphragm of patients with cirrhosis without evidence of underlying cardiopulmonary disease.

L. Miscellaneous Manifestations

Other findings on physical examination of patients with cirrhosis include **spider angiomas** (prominent blood vessels with a central arteriole and small vessels radiating from it seen in the skin, particularly on the face and upper trunk), **Dupuytren's contractures** (fibrosis of the palmar fascia), testicular atrophy, **gynecomastia** (enlargement of breast tissue in men), palmar erythema, lacrimal and parotid gland enlargement, and diminished axillary and pubic hair (Figure 14–12). These findings are largely a consequence of estrogen excess resulting from decreased clearance of endogenous estrogens by the diseased liver combined with decreased hepatic synthesis of steroid hormone-binding globulin. Both of these mechanisms result in tissues receiving higher than normal concentrations of estrogens. In addition, a longer half-life of androgens may allow a greater degree of peripheral aromatization (conversion to estrogens by, eg, adipose tissue, hair follicles), further increasing estrogen-like effects in patients with cirrhosis. Xanthomas of the eyelids and extensor surfaces of tendons of the wrists and ankles can occur with chronic cholestasis such as occurs in primary biliary cirrhosis. Finally, profound muscle wasting and cachexia in cirrhosis probably reflect diminution of the liver's synthesis of carbohydrate, lipid, and amino acids.

CHECKPOINT

29. What are the defining features of cirrhosis?
30. What are the three categories of hepatic fibrosis? Name one agent causing each.
31. What are the two postulated stages in the development of cirrhosis?
32. What are some ways alcohol may injure the liver?
33. What are the major clinical manifestations of cirrhosis?
34. For each major clinical manifestation of cirrhosis, suggest a reasonable hypothesis to account for its pathogenesis.

CASE STUDIES

Jonathan Fuchs, MD, MPH, & Yeong Kwok, MD

(See Chapter 25, p. 697 for Answers)

CASE 66

A 28-year-old man, recently emigrating from the Philippines, was noted to have a positive tuberculin skin test result in the clinic. His chest radiograph showed no active tuberculosis, and he denied any symptoms of this infection, including weight loss, cough, or night sweats. To prevent future disease, daily dosing with isoniazid was recommended for the next 9 months. Two weeks after initiating therapy, the patient reported progressive fatigue, intermittent bouts of nausea, and abdominal pain. He also noticed darkening of his urine and light-colored stools. His sister noted a gradual yellowing of his eyes and skin. Blood tests showed a marked increase in serum bilirubin and aminotransferases. The isoniazid was discontinued, and his symptoms subsided with normalizing of his liver enzymes.

Questions

A. Describe the subtypes of toxic hepatitis.
B. What typical histologic findings are noted during uncomplicated acute hepatitis?
C. What is the pathogenesis of clinical jaundice seen in this patient?

CASE 67

A 44-year-old man is concerned about abnormal liver tests drawn for his preemployment physical 6 months ago. His serum aminotransferase levels were two times normal at that time and remain unchanged after repeat testing. On further questioning, he denies regular alcohol use but states that he used to inject heroin. Currently, he reports some fatigue but says he feels well otherwise. His primary care physician orders serologic testing, which reveals HBsAg-positive, anti-HBs-negative, and anti-HBc-positive IgG. Anti-HDV and anti-HCV test results are both negative.

Questions

A. Based on these antigen and antibody test results, what is the patient's diagnosis?
B. What percentage of patients with acute hepatitis B remain chronically infected with HBV? Of those patients, how many develop chronic active disease? What are the significant complications of chronic active infection?
C. What is the significance of hepatitis D superinfection?
D. What evidence exists supporting immune-mediated damage in chronic active hepatitis?

CASE 68

A 63-year-old man with a long history of alcohol use presents to his new primary care physician with a 6-month history of increasing abdominal girth. He has also noted easy bruisability and worsening fatigue. He denies any history of GI bleeding. He continues to drink three or four cocktails a night but says he is trying to cut down. Physical examination reveals a cachectic man who appears older than his stated age. Blood pressure is 108/70 mm Hg. His scleras are anicteric. His neck veins are flat, and chest examination demonstrates gynecomastia and multiple spider angiomas. Abdominal examination is significant for a protuberant abdomen with a detectable fluid wave, shifting dullness, and an enlarged spleen. The liver edge is difficult to appreciate. He has trace pitting pedal edema. Laboratory evaluation shows anemia, mild thrombocytopenia, and an elevated prothrombin time. Abdominal ultrasonogram confirms a shrunken, heterogeneous liver consistent with cirrhosis, significant ascites, and splenomegaly.

Questions

A. Describe possible mechanisms for alcohol-induced cirrhosis.

B. What is the proposed mechanism of portal hypertension, and how does it affect ascites formation?

C. Significant hematologic abnormalities exist. How might they be explained?

REFERENCES

General

Edmison J et al. Pathogenesis of non-alcoholic steatohepatitis: Human data. Clin Liver Dis. 2007 Feb;11(1):75–104. [PMID: 17544973]

Häussinger D et al. Pathogenetic mechanisms of hepatic encephalopathy. Gut. 2008 Aug;57(8):1156–65. [PMID: 18628377]

Kaplowitz, N. *Liver and Biliary Diseases,* 2nd ed. Williams & Wilkins, 1996.

Kolios G et al. Role of Kupffer cells in the pathogenesis of liver disease. World J Gastroenterol. 2006 Dec 14;12(46):7413–20. [PMID: 17167827]

Marra F et al. Molecular basis and mechanisms of progression of non-alcoholic steatohepatitis. Trends Mol Med. 2008 Feb;14(2):72–81. [PMID: 18218340]

Reuben A. Alcohol and the liver. Curr Opin Gastroenterol. 2008 May;24(3):328–38. [PMID: 18408461]

Sherlock S et al. *Diseases of the Liver and Biliary System,* 11th ed. Blackwell, 2002.

Stevens A et al. *Wheater's Functional Histology,* 5th ed. Churchill Livingstone, 2006.

Zakim D, Boyer TD (editors). *Hepatology: A Textbook of Liver Disease,* 4th ed. W.B. Saunders, 2003.

Acute Hepatitis

Baumert TF et al. Pathogenesis of hepatitis B virus infection. World J Gastroenterol. 2007 Jan 7;13(1):82–90. [PMID: 17206757]

Chang CY et al. Review article: Drug hepatotoxicity. Aliment Pharmacol Ther. 2007 May 15;25(10):1135–51. [PMID: 17451560]

Czaja AJ. Autoimmune liver disease. Curr Opin Gastroenterol. 2008 May;24(3):298–305. [PMID: 18408457]

Hay JE. Liver disease in pregnancy. Hepatology. 2008 Mar;47(3):1067–76. [PMID: 18265410]

Lee WM et al. Etiologies of acute liver failure. Curr Opin Crit Care. 2008 Apr;14(2):198–201. [PMID: 18388683]

Lee WM. Etiologies of acute liver failure. Semin Liver Dis. 2008 May;28(2):142–52. [PMID: 18452114]

Maheshwari A et al. Acute hepatitis C. Lancet. 2008 Jul 26;372(9635):321–32. [PMID: 18657711]

Norris W et al. Drug-induced liver injury in 2007. Curr Opin Gastroenterol. 2008 May;24(3):287–97. [PMID: 18408456]

Safioleas M et al. Hepatitis B today. Hepatogastroenterology. 2007 Mar;54(74):545–8. [PMID: 17523319]

Chronic Hepatitis

Antonelli A et al. HCV infection: Pathogenesis, clinical manifestations and therapy. Clin Exp Rheumatol. 2008;26(1 Suppl 48):S39–47. [PMID: 18570753]

Czaja AJ. Autoimmune liver disease. Curr Opin Gastroenterol. 2008 May;24(3):298–305. [PMID: 18408457]

Degertekin B et al. Update on viral hepatitis: 2007. Curr Opin Gastroenterol. 2008 May;24(3):306–11. [PMID: 18408458]

Gatta A et al. Hepatotropic viruses: New insights in pathogenesis and treatment. Clin Exp Rheumatol. 2008 Jan-Feb;26(1 Suppl 48):S33–8. [PMID: 18570752]

Krawitt EL. Clinical features and management of autoimmune hepatitis. World J Gastroenterol. 2008 Jun 7;14(21):3301–5. [PMID: 18528927]

Missiha SB et al. Disease progression in chronic hepatitis C: Modifiable and nonmodifiable factors. Gastroenterology. 2008 May;134(6):1699–714. [PMID: 18471548]

Hay JE. Liver disease in pregnancy. Hepatology. 2008 Mar;47(3):1067–76. [PMID: 18265410]

Köhnlein T et al. Alpha-1 antitrypsin deficiency: Pathogenesis, clinical presentation, diagnosis, and treatment. Am J Med. 2008 Jan;121(1):3–9. [PMID: 18187064]

Nguyen DH et al. Hepatitis B virus-cell interactions and pathogenesis. J Cell Physiol. 2008 Aug;216(2):289–94. [PMID: 18302164]

Wong CM et al. Molecular pathogenesis of hepatocellular carcinoma. Liver Int. 2008 Feb;28(2):160–74. [PMID: 18069974]

Cirrhosis

Adams PC et al. Haemochromatosis. Lancet. 2007 Dec 1;370(9602):1855–60. [PMID: 18061062]

Arroyo V et al. Pathogenesis and treatment of hepatorenal syndrome. Semin Liver Dis. 2008 Feb;28(1):81–95. [PMID: 18293279]

Fairbanks KD et al. Liver disease in alpha 1-antitrypsin deficiency: A review. Am J Gastroenterol. 2008 Aug;103(8):2136–41. [PMID: 18796107]

Friedman SL. Mechanisms of hepatic fibrogenesis. Gastroenterology. 2008 May;134(6):1655–69. [PMID: 18471545]

Jones DE. Pathogenesis of primary biliary cirrhosis. Clin Liver Dis. 2008 May;12(2):305–21. [PMID: 18456182]

Malhi H et al. Cellular and molecular mechanisms of liver injury. Gastroenterology. 2008 May;134(6):1641–54. [PMID: 18471544]

Preiss D et al. Non-alcoholic fatty liver disease: An overview of prevalence, diagnosis, pathogenesis and treatment considerations. Clin Sci (Lond). 2008 Sep;115(5):141–50. [PMID: 18662168]

Sanyal AJ et al. Portal hypertension and its complications. Gastroenterology. 2008 May;134(6):1715–28. [PMID: 18471549]

Schuppan D et al. Liver cirrhosis. Lancet. 2008 Mar 8;371(9615):838–51. [PMID: 18328931]

Disorders of the Exocrine Pancreas

15

Christopher J. Sonnenday, MD, MHS,
Diane M. Simeone, MD, & Stephen J. McPhee, MD

The pancreas is a gland with both exocrine and endocrine functions. The exocrine pancreas contains **acini,** which secrete pancreatic juice into the duodenum through the pancreatic ducts (Figure 15–1). Pancreatic juice contains a number of enzymes, some of which are initially made in an inactive form. Once activated, these enzymes help to digest food and prepare it for absorption in the intestine. Disorders interfering with normal pancreatic enzyme activity (pancreatic insufficiency) cause maldigestion of fat and steatorrhea (fatty stools). Dysfunction of the exocrine pancreas results from inflammation (acute pancreatitis, chronic pancreatitis), neoplasm (ductal adenocarcinoma, neuroendocrine tumors, and other pancreatic neoplasms), or duct obstruction by stones or abnormally viscid mucus (cystic fibrosis).

The endocrine pancreas is composed of the **islets of Langerhans.** The islets are distributed throughout the pancreas and contain several different hormone-producing cells. The islet cells manufacture hormones such as insulin that are important in nutrient absorption, storage, and metabolism. Dysfunction of the endocrine pancreas causes diabetes mellitus (see Chapter 18).

Both exocrine and endocrine pancreatic dysfunction occur together in some patients.

NORMAL STRUCTURE & FUNCTION OF THE EXOCRINE PANCREAS

ANATOMY

The pancreas is a solid organ that lies transversely in the retroperitoneum deep within the epigastrium. It is firmly fixed by fibrous attachments anterior to the suprarenal aorta and the first and second lumbar vertebrae. Thus, the pain of acute or chronic pancreatitis is situated deep in the epigastric region and frequently radiates to the back.

Normally, the pancreas is about 15 cm long, although it weighs less than 110 g. The organ is covered by a thin capsule of connective tissue that sends septa into it, separating it into lobules.

The pancreas can be divided into four parts: head, including the uncinate process; neck; body; and tail. The head is the thickest part of the gland (2–4 cm) and lies in the curved space between the first, second, and third portions of the duodenum. The uncinate process is the portion of the head that extends to the left behind the superior mesenteric vessels. The neck connects the head and body and sits immediately anterior to the superior mesenteric vessels. The body is situated transversely in the retroperitoneal space, bordered superiorly by the splenic artery and posteriorly by the splenic vein. The tail of the pancreas is less fixed in the retroperitoneum and extends toward, and often immediately adjacent to, the hilum of the spleen.

Embryologically, the pancreas develops as two separate endodermal buds from the developing foregut. These separate dorsal and ventral elements of the primordial pancreas initially develop opposite each other but, with rotation of the primitive gut, end up fusing together toward the left of the duodenum. The dorsal bud evolves to form the more cephalad and anterior portion of the pancreatic head, as well as the neck, body, and tail of the pancreas. The smaller ventral bud becomes the more caudal portion of the pancreatic head and the uncinate process. As cellular and mesenchymal elements develop, the dorsal and ventral buds evolve a conjoined ductal system, and the whole organ eventually takes its place in the retroperitoneum of the upper abdomen. Primitive neuroendocrine cells arise amid the developing ductal structures, and eventually form the interspersed islets of Langerhans.

The exocrine pancreas is drained by a major central duct called the **duct of Wirsung,** which runs the length of the

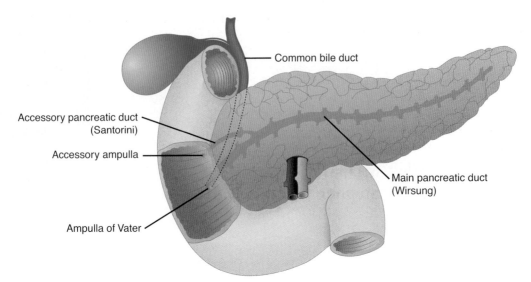

FIGURE 15–1   Anatomy of the pancreas. (Courtesy of W. Silen.)   (Redrawn, with permission, from Way LW [editor]. *Current Surgical Diagnosis & Treatment,* 10th ed. Originally published by Appleton & Lange. Copyright © 1998 by the McGraw-Hill Companies, Inc.)

gland. This duct is normally about 3–4 mm in diameter. In most individuals, the pancreatic duct enters the duodenum at the duodenal papilla alongside the common bile duct. The sphincter of Oddi surrounds both ducts. In about one third of individuals, the duct of Wirsung and the common bile duct join to form a common channel before terminating at the **ampulla of Vater** (Figure 15–1).

Many individuals also have a separate accessory pancreatic duct, called the **duct of Santorini,** that runs from the head and body of the gland to enter the duodenum about 2 cm proximal to the duodenal papilla (Figure 15–1). This structure is the embryologic remnant of the proximal ductal system of the dorsal pancreatic bud and often joins the main pancreatic duct in the body of the gland.

HISTOLOGY

The exocrine pancreas consists of clusters of acini, or **lobules,** which are drained by ductules. The islets of Langerhans of the endocrine pancreas are clusters of a few hundred cells, each located between the lobules.

Each pancreatic acinus is composed of several acinar cells surrounding a lumen (Figure 15–2). Centroacinar cells are centrally located in the acini, interpositioned between the acinar cells and ductal epithelium. The centroacinar cells are believed to have a primary role in the secretion of electrolytes and water into the pancreatic ductal system. The acinar cells synthesize and secrete enzymes. On histologic examination, acinar cells are typical exocrine glandular cells. They are pyramidal epithelial cells arranged in rows. Their apexes join to form the lumen of the acinus. **Zymogen granules** containing digestive enzymes or their precursors are found in the acinar cells. These granules are discharged by exocytosis from the apexes of the cells into the lumen. The number of zymogen granules in the cells varies; more are found during fasting and fewer after a meal.

Acini are centered on small branches of the pancreatic duct, which eventually converge to form the continuous lumen of the main pancreatic duct. The mature ducts are lined with a continuous layer of ductal epithelial cells, joined by tight junctions. The ductal epithelium contributes to the secretion of water and electrolytes into pancreatic secretions and forms the important epithelial barrier separating the pancreatic parenchyma from the enzyme-rich ductal secretions. Compromise of this epithelial barrier due to inflammation or trauma may be associated with significant peripancreatic inflammation and severe clinical sequelae.

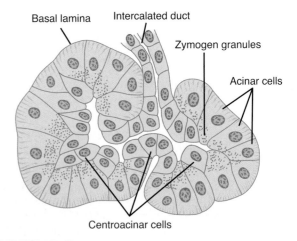

FIGURE 15–2   Schematic drawing of the pancreatic acini. Acinar cells are pyramidal in shape, with zymogen granules at their apexes. (Redrawn, with permission, from Junqueira LC, Carneiro J. *Basic Histology,* 10th ed. McGraw-Hill, 2003.)

PHYSIOLOGY

Composition of Pancreatic Juice

As much as 1500 mL of pancreatic juice is secreted each day. Pancreatic juice contains water, ions, and a variety of proteins. The principal ions in pancreatic juice are HCO_3^-, Cl^-, Na^+, and K^+. Of these, HCO_3^- is particularly important. At maximum flow rates, the concentration of HCO_3^- in pancreatic juice may reach 150 mEq/L (vs. 24 mEq/L in plasma), and the pH of the juice may reach 8.3. The alkaline nature of pancreatic juice plays a major role in neutralizing the gastric acid entering the duodenum with ingested food (chyme) from the stomach. The pH of the duodenal contents rises to 6.0–7.0, and by the time the chyme reaches the jejunum, its pH is nearly neutral.

Pancreatic enzymes aid in the intraluminal phase of digestion and absorption of fats, carbohydrates, and proteins. The rest of the proteins in pancreatic juice are plasma proteins, mucoproteins, and trypsin inhibitors (see later discussion).

Some of the pancreatic enzymes (lipase, amylase, deoxyribonuclease, and ribonuclease) are secreted by the acinar cells in their active forms. The remaining enzymes are secreted as inactive proenzymes or **zymogens** (trypsinogen, chymotrypsinogen, proelastase, procarboxypeptidase, and phospholipase A_2) that are activated in the lumen of the proximal intestine. Activation of zymogens within the acinar cell might otherwise lead to acute pancreatitis and pancreatic autodigestion.

When the pancreatic juice enters the duodenum, trypsinogen is converted to the active form trypsin by an enzyme found in the intestinal brush border called enteropeptidase (or enterokinase). Trypsin then converts the remaining proenzymes into active enzymes (eg, chymotrypsinogen into chymotrypsin). Trypsin can also activate its own precursor, trypsinogen, producing the potential for an autocatalytic chain reaction.

When trypsinogen is activated within the pancreas itself, two known protective mechanisms are available. First, there is inhibition of activated trypsin by pancreatic secretory trypsin inhibitor (PSTI), also known as serine protease inhibitor, Kazal type 1 (or SPINK1), which can inhibit approximately 20% of trypsin activity. If trypsin activity overwhelms the SPINK1/PSTI inhibitory capacity, then trypsin inactivation can occur through trypsin autolysis.

Regulation of Secretion of Pancreatic Juice

Between and after meals, pancreatic secretion is regulated by hormonal and neural actions and by neurohumoral interactions.

Secretion of pancreatic juice is controlled primarily by two different hormones—**secretin** and **cholecystokinin (CCK)**—that are produced by specialized enteroendocrine cells of the duodenal mucosa. These hormones act by distinct but synergistic intracellular pathways.

Secretion of secretin is triggered by gastric acid and by the products of protein digestion in the duodenum. Secretin acts chiefly on the pancreatic ductal epithelial, centroacinar, and to a lesser extent acinar cells to produce HCO_3^-, thus raising the pH of the pancreatic secretions. Secretion of H_2O is also increased in response to secretin, increasing the absolute volume of pancreatic juice. Mechanistic studies have demonstrated that secretin and the related hormone vasoactive intestinal peptide (VIP) act on ductal and acinar cells by activation of adenylate cyclase and subsequent cAMP-dependent protein kinase A.

Secretion of CCK is triggered by the products of protein and fat digestion (peptides, amino acids, and fatty acids) when they enter the duodenum. The release of CCK from specific intestinal cells is thought to be regulated by a cholecystokinin-releasing peptide in the proximal small intestine that is trypsin sensitive and active in the lumen. CCK acts chiefly on the acinar cells to cause release of enzymes from zymogen granules. Recent evidence has demonstrated that acinar cells in humans may not have CCK receptors, suggesting this hormone acts solely by neural stimulation. CCK release raises intracellular Ca^{2+} concentrations, which leads to release of pancreatic enzymes from the zymogen granules. Related enteric hormones acetylcholine and gastrin-releasing peptide (GRP) appear to act by similar calcium-dependent pathways. The integrated action of both secretin and CCK produces abundant secretion of enzyme-rich, alkaline pancreatic juice.

When both cAMP and calcium-dependent pathways are stimulated, the effect within the acinar cell is greater than the sum of their individual activities. Thus, CCK and secretin appear to act synergistically in response to a meal to stimulate the production of a large volume of alkaline pancreatic juice rich in digestive enzymes.

Digestive Functions of Pancreatic Juice

The secretion of pancreatic juice aids digestion in several ways. The large amount of bicarbonate in the juice helps to neutralize the acidic chyme from the stomach so that the pancreatic enzymes can function optimally in a neutral pH range.

Each of the enzymes also has an important digestive function. In digesting carbohydrates, pancreatic **amylase** splits straight-chain glucose polysaccharides (so-called amyloses in starch) into smaller α-limit dextrins, maltose and maltotriose. Brush border enzymes in the small intestine complete the hydrolysis of these smaller sugars into glucose, which is transported across the intestinal epithelium by Na^+-coupled transport. Pancreatic **lipase** contributes to fat metabolism by hydrolyzing triglycerides into fatty acids and a monoglyceride; this activity is most efficient in the presence of bile acids, which serve to emulsify the triglycerides. **Phospholipase A_2** splits a fatty acid off from lecithin to form lysolecithin. **Ribonuclease** and **deoxyribonuclease** attack the nucleic acids. The remaining enzymes help to digest proteins. **Trypsin,**

chymotrypsin, and **elastase** are endopeptidases (ie, they cleave peptide bonds in the middle of polypeptide chains). **Carboxypeptidase** is an exopeptidase (ie, it splits peptide bonds adjacent to the carboxyl terminals of peptide chains). Together, these proteases break down proteins into oligopeptides and free amino acids.

PATHOPHYSIOLOGY OF SELECTED EXOCRINE PANCREATIC DISORDERS

ACUTE PANCREATITIS

Clinical Presentations

Acute pancreatitis is a clinical syndrome resulting from acute inflammation and destructive autodigestion of the pancreas and peripancreatic tissues. Clinically, acute pancreatitis is a common and important cause of acute upper abdominal pain, nausea, vomiting, and fever. Data from the U.S. 2005 National Hospital Discharge Survey reveal that acute pancreatitis accounts for more than 237,000 hospital admissions, with more than 90% of cases occurring in adults. The incidence of acute pancreatitis appears to be increasing, and despite advances in critical care medicine, severe acute pancreatitis leads to death in a consistent 5% of incident cases.

Etiology

Acute pancreatitis has many causes (Table 15–1), but in all cases there is escape of activated proteolytic enzymes from the ducts, leading to local tissue injury, inflammation, necrosis, and in some cases infection.

The two most common conditions associated with acute pancreatitis are alcohol abuse and biliary tract disease.

Alcohol abuse is a common cause of acute pancreatitis in the United States, accounting for 65% of cases in some series. Acute pancreatitis usually occurs after an episode of heavy drinking. The exact mechanism by which alcohol damages the gland is not clear. Alcohol or its metabolite, acetaldehyde, may have a direct toxic effect on pancreatic acinar cells, leading to intracellular trypsin activation by the lysosomal enzymes, or may cause inflammation of the sphincter of Oddi, leading to retention of hydrolytic enzymes in the pancreatic duct and acini. Malnutrition may predispose to pancreatic injury in alcoholics. For example, deficiencies of trace elements such as zinc or selenium occur in alcoholic patients and are associated with acinar cell injury. Metalloenzymes such as superoxide dismutase, catalase, and glutathione peroxidase are important scavengers of free radicals.

In patients who do not drink alcohol, about 50% of cases of acute pancreatitis are associated with biliary tract disease. In such cases, the hypothesized mechanism is obstruction of the common bile duct and the main pancreatic duct when a gallstone or biliary sludge becomes lodged at the ampulla of Vater.

Reflux of bile or pancreatic secretions into the pancreatic duct lead to parenchymal injury. Others have proposed that bacterial toxins or free bile acids travel via lymphatics from the gallbladder to the pancreas, giving rise to inflammation. In either case, acute pancreatitis associated with biliary tract disease is more common in women because gallstones are more common in women.

A significant proportion of "gallstone" pancreatitis is not associated with discrete, measurable gallstones passing through the bile duct and obstructing the ampulla. Instead, biliary sludge, or **microlithiasis,** is believed to play an etiologic role in many cases of pancreatitis, which were previously classified as idiopathic. Endoscopic retrograde cholangiopancreatography (ERCP) performed in such cases often identifies the microlithiasis and viscous particulate bile in the distal common bile duct, which can cause transient biliary obstruction and activate the same mechanistic pathways that lead to pancreatitis as happens with larger gallstones. An alternative mechanism that has been proposed is recurrent passage of microlithiasis causing papillary stenosis or sphincter of Oddi dysfunction.

Thus, the absence of obvious gallstones on imaging studies does not definitively rule out a biliary cause of acute pancreatitis. Biliary microlithiasis may be suspected when an ultrasound shows low-level echoes that gravitate toward the dependent portion of the gallbladder without the acoustic shadowing typical of gallstones. Microlithiasis is documented when cholesterol monohydrate crystals and calcium bilirubinate granules are found on light microscopy of an endoscopically acquired, centrifuged specimen of bile. Risk factors for biliary microlithiasis include pregnancy, rapid weight loss, critical illness, prolonged fasting, total parenteral nutrition, administration of certain drugs (ceftriaxone and octreotide), and bone marrow or solid organ transplantation.

TABLE 15–1 Causes of acute pancreatitis.

Alcohol ingestion (acute or chronic alcoholism)	**Drugs**	
Biliary tract disease	Definite association	
Trauma	Immunosuppressives: azathioprine, mercaptopurine	
Blunt abdominal trauma	Diuretics: thiazides, furosemide	
Postoperative	Antimicrobials: sulfonamides, tetracyclines, pentamidine, didanosine, metronidazole, erythromycin	
Postendoscopic retrograde cannulation of pancreatic duct, injection of pancreatic duct	Steroids: estrogens, oral contraceptives, corticosteroids, ACTH	
Postelectric shock	Miscellaneous: valproic acid, metformin, intravenous lipid infusion	
Infections	Probable association	
Viral: mumps, rubella, coxsackievirus B, echovirus, viral hepatitis A, B, adenovirus, cytomegalovirus, varicella, Epstein-Barr virus, HIV	Immunosuppressives: asparaginase	
Bacterial: *Mycoplasma pneumoniae, Salmonella typhi,* group A streptococci (scarlet fever), staphylococci, actinomycosis, *Mycobacterium tuberculosis, Mycobacterium avium* complex, *Legionella, Campylobacter jejuni, Leptospira icterohaemorrhagiae*	Diuretics: ethacrynic acid, chlorthalidone	
	Miscellaneous: procainamide, cimetidine, ranitidine, sulfasalazine	
Parasitic: *Ascaris lumbricoides,* hydatid cyst, *Clonorchis sinensis*	Possible association	
Metabolic	Antimicrobials: isoniazid, rifampin, nitrofurantoin	
Hyperlipidemia, apolipoprotein CII deficiency syndrome, hypertriglyceridemia	Analgesics: acetaminophen, propoxyphene, salicylates, sulindac, other NSAIDs	
Hypercalcemia (eg, hyperparathyroidism)	Miscellaneous: methyldopa	
Uremia	**Vascular**	
Postrenal transplant	Vasculitis: systemic lupus erythematosus, polyarteritis nodosa, malignant hypertension, thrombotic thrombocytopenic purpura	
Pregnancy, eclampsia	Shock, hypoperfusion, myocardial or mesenteric infarction	
Hemochromatosis, hemosiderosis	Atheromatous embolism	
Malnutrition: kwashiorkor, sprue, postgastrectomy, Whipple's disease	**Mechanical**	
Diabetic ketoacidosis	Pancreas divisum with accessory duct obstruction	
Hereditary	Ampulla of Vater stenosis, tumor, obstruction (regional enteritis, duodenal diverticulum, duodenal surgery, worms, foreign bodies)	
Familial pancreatitis	Choledochocele	
Cystic fibrosis	Penetrating duodenal ulcer	
Poisons and toxins	Pancreatic carcinoma	
Venom: scorpion *(Tityus trinitatis)*	**Idiopathic**	
Inorganic: zinc, cobalt, mercuric chloride, saccharated iron oxide		
Organic: methanol, organophosphates		

Acute pancreatitis may result from a variety of infectious agents, including viruses (mumps virus, coxsackievirus, hepatitis A virus, HIV, or cytomegalovirus) and bacteria (*Salmonella typhi* or hemolytic streptococci). Patients with HIV infection can develop acute pancreatitis from the HIV infection itself, from related opportunistic infections, or from antiretroviral therapies. In HIV-infected patients, pancreatitis has

been associated with intravenous drug abuse, pentamidine therapy, *Pneumocystis jiroveci* and *Mycobacterium avium-intracellulare* infections, and gallstones.

Blunt or penetrating trauma and other injuries may cause acute pancreatitis. Pancreatitis sometimes occurs after surgical procedures near the pancreas (duodenal stump syndrome, pancreatic tail syndrome after splenectomy). Shock and hypothermia may cause decreased perfusion, resulting in cellular degeneration and release of pancreatic enzymes. Radiation therapy of retroperitoneal malignant neoplasms can sometimes cause acute pancreatitis, likely by injury to the microvasculature and acinar architecture.

Marked hypercalcemia, such as that associated with hyperparathyroidism, sarcoidosis, hypervitaminosis D, or multiple myeloma, causes acute pancreatitis in about 10% of cases. Two mechanisms have been hypothesized. The high plasma calcium concentration may cause calcium to precipitate in the pancreatic duct, leading to ductal obstruction. Alternatively, hypercalcemia may stimulate activation of trypsinogen in the pancreatic duct.

Pancreatitis is also associated with hyperlipidemia, particularly those types characterized by increased plasma levels of chylomicrons (types I, IV, and V). In these cases, it is postulated that free fatty acids liberated by the action of pancreatic lipase cause gland inflammation and injury. Alcohol abuse or oral contraceptive use increases the risk of acute pancreatitis in patients with hyperlipidemia.

A variety of drugs have been associated with pancreatitis, including corticosteroids, thiazide diuretics, immunosuppressants, and cancer chemotherapeutic agents.

Rarely, acute pancreatitis may be familial, occurring with an autosomal dominant inheritance pattern. **Hereditary pancreatitis** typically presents as recurring acute pancreatitis in childhood, progressing to chronic pancreatitis by young adulthood in >50% of cases. Hereditary recurrent acute pancreatitis has been associated with **mutations of the cationic trypsinogen gene** (*protease, serine, 1; PRSS1*) mapped to chromosome 7q35. Two point mutations, R122H and N29I, account for most cases and can be detected by genetic testing. Studies have suggested that the R122H mutation is associated with more severe acute pancreatitis, leading to more frequent attacks and hospital admissions. Other families have mutations in *SPINK1/PSTI*. It appears that mutations in cationic trypsinogen enhance trypsinogen autoactivation by altering calcium-mediated regulatory pathways, and mutations in *SPINK1/PSTI* diminish inhibition of active trypsinogen. Other mutations eliminate the trypsin autolysis site. Patients demonstrated to have hereditary pancreatitis should be enrolled in a pancreatic cancer surveillance program, and total pancreatectomy should be considered in select cases, as approximately 40% of affected patients develop pancreatic cancer by age 70 years.

Pancreas divisum is an anatomic variant in which the embryologic ventral and dorsal components of the pancreas fail to fuse, thus leaving two distinct ductal systems that do not communicate and that separately drain through two duodenal papillae. The smaller system drains through the major papilla, but the dominant dorsal system drains through the minor papilla, which can cause a relative obstruction to flow of pancreatic juice. Pancreas divisum occurs in up to 7% of autopsy series and may account for 2.7–7.5% of recurrent pancreatitis cases.

In about 15–25% of cases of acute pancreatitis, no etiologic factor can be identified. **Idiopathic acute recurrent pancreatitis** is seen in patients with more than one attack of acute pancreatitis when the underlying cause eludes detection despite a thorough search.

Pathology

The symptoms, signs, laboratory findings, and complications of acute pancreatitis can be explained on the basis of the pathologic damage to the ductules, acini, and islets of the pancreas. However, both the degree of damage and the clinical consequences are quite variable.

When the damage is limited in extent, the pathologic features consist of mild to marked swelling of the gland, especially the acini, and mild to marked infiltration with polymorphonuclear neutrophils. However, damage to tissue is usually only minimal to moderate, and there is no hemorrhage. In some cases, suppuration may be found along with edema, and this may result in tissue necrosis and abscess formation. In severe cases, massive necrosis and liquefaction of the pancreas occur, predisposing to pancreatic abscess formation. Vascular necrosis and disruption may occur, resulting in peripancreatic hemorrhage.

Severe cases of pancreatitis may be associated with the formation of ascites, which is likely a combination of serous fluid excreted by the inflamed peritoneal surface, liquefied peripancreatic fat, blood from peripancreatic tissues, and necrotic pancreatic debris. In rare cases associated with ductal disruption of the pancreas, the ascites may contain frank pancreatic secretions rich in amylase and other pancreatic enzymes. Documentation of amylase-rich peritoneal fluid establishes the diagnosis of so-called pancreatic ascites. In cases of severe acute pancreatitis, the peritoneal surfaces have a characteristic appearance upon surgical exploration or autopsy; fat necrosis, or saponification, may occur in and around the pancreas, omentum, and mesentery, appearing as chalky white foci that may later calcify.

Histologic studies of pancreas tissue obtained from patients with first attacks of acute alcoholic pancreatitis who underwent surgery for complications have found that the acute pancreatitis (pancreatic necrosis, steatonecrosis, infiltration by inflammatory cells) sometimes develops in a gland already affected by chronic pancreatitis (perilobular and intralobular fibrosis, loss of exocrine parenchyma and atrophy of residual lobules, dilated interlobular and intralobular ducts lined with cuboidal or flattened epithelium, and protein plugs within dilated ducts). It has been conjectured that, if acute alcoholic pancreatitis develops in a pancreas already affected by chronic pancreatitis, it is due to obstruction of the ducts by protein plugs, an early lesion of chronic pancreatitis.

Pathogenesis

The mechanism by which enzymes and bioactive substances become activated within the pancreas is a major unanswered question in acute pancreatitis.

One proposed theory of the pathogenesis of alcoholic pancreatitis emphasizes disordered agonist-receptor interaction on the membrane of pancreatic acinar cells. According to this theory, alcohol increases activation of intrapancreatic digestive enzymes either by sensitizing acinar cells to pathologic stimuli or by stimulating the release of the secretagogue, cholecystokinin (CCK), from duodenal cells. The hyperstimulation of pancreatic acinar cells and their muscarinic receptors mimics the mechanism of acute pancreatitis caused by scorpion stings, anti-acetylcholinesterase-containing insecticide poisoning, or administration of supramaximal doses of secretagogues such as acetylcholine and CCK. CCK receptor activation can initiate different patterns of zymogen activation in pancreatic acinar cells (see later discussion) and the extent of activation is enhanced by a distinct set of short-chain alcohols. Whether ethanol or other alcohols mediate these effects by interfering with acinar cell signaling pathways or by affecting acinar cell membrane fluidity is currently under investigation.

Another major theory postulates that intra-acinar cell activation of digestive zymogens is the earliest event in the development of acute pancreatitis and that those enzymes, once activated, cause acinar cell injury. Clinical and experimental studies demonstrate that zymogen activation is a very early feature of acute pancreatitis. The activation peptides of trypsinogen and carboxypeptidase A1, both markers of zymogen activation, can be detected in the serum with the first hours of acute pancreatitis. Both trypsin activity and trypsinogen activation peptide levels increase rapidly (within 15 minutes) after the induction of experimental pancreatitis.

Cathepsin B is capable of activating trypsinogen to trypsin, and it was once thought that cathepsin B activation of trypsinogen was the trigger for acute pancreatitis. However, it now appears that trypsin autoactivation is the key initiator. According to current theory, obstruction, bile reflux, and duodenal reflux disturb pancreatic acinar cell function, causing intracellular trypsin activation by the lysosomal enzymes. Other factors might also trigger this mechanism, including the toxic effects of alcohol and other drugs, the products of digestion of certain lipoproteins, ischemia and reperfusion injury, and increased intracellular calcium concentrations. Intracellular calcium ions are crucial messengers involved in normal acinar cell processes of stimulus-secretion coupling, enzyme processing, and zymogen secretion. It may be that the many different causes of pancreatitis are mediated by abnormal increases in intracellular calcium ions. Nonetheless, cathepsin B may play a role in amplification of the enzyme response.

The pathologic changes result from the action of activated trypsin and other pancreatic enzymes on the pancreas and surrounding tissues. Activated trypsin in turn activates the proenzymes of chymotrypsin, elastase, and phospholipase A_2, and those enzymes cause damage in several ways (Figure 15–3). For example, chymotrypsin activation leads to edema and vascular damage. Similarly, elastase, once activated from proelastase, digests the elastin in blood vessel walls and causes vascular injury and hemorrhage; damage to peripancreatic blood vessels can lead to hemorrhagic pancreatitis. Phospholipase A_2 splits a fatty acid off lecithin, forming lysolecithin, which is cytotoxic to erythrocytes and damages cell membranes. Formation of lysolecithin from the lecithin in bile may contribute to disruption of the pancreas and necrosis of surrounding fat. Phospholipase A_2 also liberates arachidonic acid, which is then converted to prostaglandins, leukotrienes, and other mediators of inflammation, contributing to coagulation necrosis.

Pancreatic lipase, released directly as a result of pancreatic acinar cell damage, acts enzymatically on surrounding adipose tissue, causing fat necrosis (Figure 15–3).

Furthermore, trypsin and chymotrypsin activate kinins, complement, coagulation factors, and plasmin, leading to edema, inflammation, thrombosis, and hemorrhage within the gland. For example, trypsin activation of the kallikrein-kinin

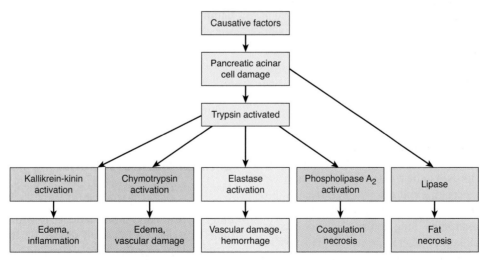

FIGURE 15–3 Hypothesized pathogenesis of acute pancreatitis. (Redrawn, with permission, from Marshall JB. Acute pancreatitis: A review with an emphasis on new developments. Arch Intern Med. 1993;153:1188.)

system leads to the release of bradykinin and kallidin, causing vasodilation, increased vascular permeability, edema, and inflammation (Figure 15–3).

The activated pancreatic enzymes also enter the bloodstream and may produce effects elsewhere in the body. Circulating phospholipases interfere with the normal function of pulmonary surfactant, contributing to the development of an adult respiratory distress syndrome in some patients with acute pancreatitis. Elevated serum lipase levels are sometimes associated with fat necrosis outside of the abdomen.

Finally, during acute pancreatitis, both the CC and CXC families of cytokines are implicated in the pathogenesis of the local and systemic inflammatory response. Cytokines and other inflammatory mediators such as tumor necrosis factor (TNF), interleukins (especially IL-1, IL-6, and IL-8), platelet-activating factor (PAF), and endotoxin are released rapidly and predictably from inflammatory cells. This release appears to be in response to the presence of active digestive enzymes, independent of the underlying cause. Production of cytokines during clinical pancreatitis begins shortly after pain onset and peaks 36–48 hours later. These agents are now thought to be principal mediators in the transformation of acute pancreatitis from a local inflammatory process to a systemic illness (Figure 15–4). The degree of TNF-induced inflammation correlates with the severity of pancreatitis. Cytokines rapidly enter the systemic circulation from the peritoneal cavity via the thoracic duct. In the systemic circulation, the cytokines affect many body systems and can produce the systemic inflammatory response syndrome (SIRS) and the multiorgan dysfunction syndrome typical of severe acute pancreatitis. Systemic complications of acute pancreatitis, such as respiratory failure, shock, and even multisystem organ failure, are accompanied by significant increases in monocyte secretion of TNF, IL-1, IL-6, and IL-8, and upregulation of the number of receptors for these cytokines on target cells. This finding suggests that TNF, IL-1, IL-6, and IL-8 play a central role in the pathophysiology of these manifestations.

Studies also suggest that substance P acting via neurokinin-1 (NK-1) receptors, PAF, and chemokines interacting with CCR1 receptors play important proinflammatory roles in determining the severity of acute pancreatitis. In particular, substance P and neurokinin-1 are involved in mediating acute lung injury. Substance P, a neuropeptide released from sensory afferent nerve endings, binds to the NK-1 receptor on the surface of effector cells and increases the permeability of vascular endothelium. The amount of substance P in the pancreas is increased during episodes of acute pancreatitis, and acinar cell expression of NK-1 receptors is markedly upregulated. Substance P appears to be a powerful proinflammatory mediator of both pancreatitis and associated lung injury. PAF also appears to play an important role in the development of pancreatitis and associated lung injury. Chemokines are chemoattractant cytokines that are involved in the activation and trafficking of various inflammatory cells. Chemokines acting via the chemokine receptor CCR1 appear to have a role in determining the severity of pancreatitis-associated lung

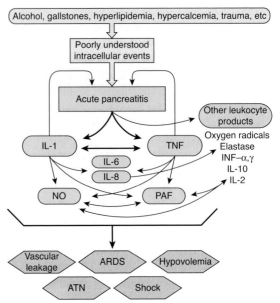

FIGURE 15–4 Inflammatory mediators of acute pancreatitis include interleukin-1B (IL-1) and tumor necrosis factor (TNF). As depicted, these two cytokines can induce other inflammatory mediators, such as IL-2, IL-6, IL-8, and IL-10; nitric oxide (NO); platelet activating factor (PAF); and interferon (INF)-α and INF-γ, while at the same time producing a direct noxious effect on the pancreas itself. Each of the mediators shown plays a role in development of the systemic manifestations of acute pancreatitis. ARDS, acute respiratory distress syndrome; ATN, acute tubular necrosis. (Redrawn, with permission, from Norman J. The role of cytokines in the pathogenesis of acute pancreatitis. Am J Surg. 1998;175:76.)

injury but no effect on the severity of the pancreatitis itself. On the other hand, complement factor 5a (C5a) appears to act as an anti-inflammatory agent during the development of pancreatitis.

Various factors play active roles as proinflammatory or anti-inflammatory agents in acute pancreatitis. Drugs or other interventions to counteract those agents that are proinflammatory (eg, TNF, IL-1, IL-6, IL-8, and PAF) or to stimulate those that are anti-inflammatory (eg, IL-10) may eventually prove useful in treating patients with clinical pancreatitis to prevent severe injury to the pancreas and to prevent associated systemic manifestations, such as lung injury. For example, lexipafant, a PAF antagonist, when administered within 48 hours of symptom onset, has demonstrated beneficial effects on outcome in clinical studies.

Clinical Manifestations

Acute pancreatitis may present in a highly variable manner, with the severity of inflammation and associated morbidity differing markedly among patients. Approximately 80% of patients experience a mild, self-limited illness to 2–3 days with no significant sequelae, but the remainder of patients may develop a life-threatening illness requiring intensive care and sometimes surgical intervention. Acute pancreatitis may recur,

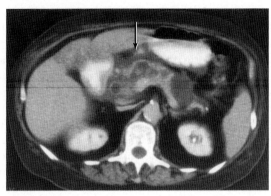

FIGURE 15–5 Acute pancreatitis on CT. Findings include enlargement and edema of the pancreas plus peripancreatic inflammatory change and fluid collections (arrow). (Used with permission from Henry I. Goldberg.)

depending primarily on its cause. With repeated attacks, the gland may eventually be permanently damaged, resulting in chronic pancreatitis or sometimes pancreatic insufficiency (see below). The distinction between acute pancreatitis and an acute exacerbation of chronic pancreatitis is determined by the clinical history and the characteristic finding on imaging of chronic pancreatitis. Acute and chronic pancreatitis have notably different management paradigms, so this distinction is important.

The diagnosis of pancreatitis is primarily clinical. Distinguishing pancreatitis from other, potentially lethal causes of abdominal pain and identifying those patients with severe pancreatitis who may develop serious complications from the remote systemic effects of the disease are major diagnostic concerns.

Computed tomography (CT) and magnetic resonance imaging (MRI) are useful in diagnosis (Figure 15–5). They are particularly useful in distinguishing between edematous and necrotizing forms and providing prognostic information by detecting extrapancreatic involvement.

A. Signs and Symptoms at Presentation

Abdominal pain is nearly universal and a hallmark presentation of acute pancreatitis. In rare cases, patients may present with occult pancreatic inflammation evident by hyperamylasemia—eg, following pancreatic trauma, medication administration, or other known precipitants. However, such presentations are unlikely to be associated with clinically significant pancreatitis.

The pain of acute pancreatitis is characteristic, often described as an intense, deep, searing pain that radiates to the back. Frank peritoneal inflammation may lead to diagnostic confusion with other, more immediate surgical emergencies such as a perforated peptic ulcer, appendicitis, or diverticulitis.

The pain of acute pancreatitis is thought to derive in part from stretching of the pancreatic capsule by distended ductules and parenchymal edema, inflammatory exudate, digested proteins and lipids, and hemorrhage. In addition, these materials may seep out of the parenchyma into the ret-

roperitoneum and lesser sac, where they irritate retroperitoneal and peritoneal sensory nerve endings and produce intense back and flank pain. The clinical findings of generalized peritonitis may follow.

Stretching of the pancreatic capsule may also produce **nausea and vomiting.** Increasing abdominal pain, peritoneal irritation, and electrolyte imbalance (especially hypokalemia) may cause a paralytic **ileus** with marked abdominal distention. If gastric motility is inhibited and the gastroesophageal sphincter is relaxed, there may be emesis. Both small and large bowel often dilate during an acute attack. Sometimes only a localized segment of bowel dilates. For example, there may be localized dilation of a segment of jejunum overlying the pancreas. In such cases, a plain x-ray film of the abdomen shows thickening of the valvulae conniventes and air-fluid levels ("sentinel loop"). In other cases, there may be segmental dilation of a portion of the overlying transverse colon. The x-ray film shows a sharply demarcated area of localized colonic dilation and edema ("colon cutoff sign").

Almost two thirds of patients with acute pancreatitis develop **fever.** The pathophysiologic mechanism responsible for fever involves the extensive tissue injury, inflammation, and necrosis and release of endogenous pyrogens, principally IL-1, from polymorphonuclear leukocytes into the circulation. In most cases of acute pancreatitis, fever does not indicate a bacterial infection. However, persistent fever beyond the fourth or fifth day of illness—or spiking temperatures to 40 °C or more—may signify development of infectious complications such as infected peripancreatic fluid collections, infected pancreatic necrosis, or ascending cholangitis.

The cardinal laboratory finding in acute pancreatitis is elevation of the **serum amylase,** often up to 10- to 20-fold. The serum amylase elevation occurs almost immediately (within hours), but it usually returns to normal within 48–72 hours even if symptoms continue. The sensitivity of the serum amylase in acute pancreatitis is estimated to be 70–95%, meaning that 5–30% of patients with acute pancreatitis have normal or minimally elevated serum amylase values. The specificity of the test is considerably lower. Patients with marked (more than 3-fold) elevations of serum amylase usually have acute pancreatitis. Patients with lesser elevations of serum amylase often have one of a variety of other conditions.

The serum amylase concentration reflects the steady state between the rates of amylase entry into and removal from the blood. Hyperamylasemia can result from either an increased rate of entry or a decreased rate of metabolic clearance of amylase in the circulation. The pancreas and salivary glands have much higher concentrations of amylase than any other organs and probably contribute almost all of the serum amylase activity in healthy persons. Amylase of pancreatic origin can be now be distinguished from that of salivary origin by a variety of techniques. Pancreatic hyperamylasemia results from injuries to the pancreas, ranging from minor (cannulation of the pancreatic duct) to severe (pancreatitis). In addition, injuries to the bowel wall (infarction or perforation) cause pancreatic hyperamylasemia as a result of enhanced absorption of amylase from the intestinal lumen. Salivary hyperamylasemia is observed in salivary gland diseases such as mumps parotitis but also (inexplicably) in a host of unrelated conditions such as chronic alcoholism, postoperative states (particularly after coronary artery bypass graft surgery), lactic acidosis, anorexia nervosa or bulimia nervosa, and certain malignancies. Hyperamylasemia can also result from decreased metabolic clearance of amylase caused by renal failure or macroamylasemia, a condition in which there are abnormally high-molecular-weight complexes of amylase bound to abnormal immunoglobulins in the serum.

Determination of **serum lipase** level is often helpful diagnostically. In acute pancreatitis, the serum lipase level is elevated, usually about 72 hours after onset of symptoms. The serum lipase measurement may be a better diagnostic test than serum amylase because it is just as easy to perform, may be more sensitive (85% vs. 79% sensitivity), is more specific for acute pancreatitis, and decreases to normal more slowly.

B. Early Complications of Acute Pancreatitis

Shock may occur in acute pancreatitis as a result of several interrelated factors. Hypovolemia results from massive exudation of plasma and hemorrhage into the retroperitoneal space and from accumulation of fluid in the gut as a result of ileus. Hypotension and shock may also result from release of kinins into the general circulation. For example, activation during acute inflammation of the proteolytic enzyme kallikrein results in peripheral vasodilation via liberation of the vasoactive peptides, bradykinin and kallidin. This vasodilation causes the pulse rate to rise and the blood pressure to fall. Cytokines like PAF, a very potent vasodilator and leukocyte activator, have been implicated in the development of shock and other manifestations of the SIRS. The contracted intravascular volume combined with the hypotension may lead to myocardial and cerebral ischemia, respiratory failure, metabolic acidosis, and decreased urinary output or renal failure as a result of acute tubular necrosis.

Tissue factor release and expression during proteolysis may cause activation of the plasma coagulation cascade and may lead to **disseminated intravascular coagulation** (DIC). In other cases, hypercoagulability of the blood is thought to be due to elevated concentrations of several coagulation factors, including factor VIII, fibrinogen, and perhaps factor V. Clinically affected patients may present with hemorrhagic discoloration (purpura) in the subcutaneous tissues around the umbilicus (Cullen's sign) or in the flanks (Grey Turner's sign). The splenic and portal veins are in close proximity to the pancreas and thus can become involved in the inflammatory process. Splenic vein thrombosis occurs in ~11% and portal vein thrombosis in ~2% of patients. Most thrombi are asymptomatic, but acute variceal bleeding may occur later in a small percentage of patients.

Pulmonary complications are a dreaded manifestation of severe acute pancreatitis and occur in 15–50% of patients. The severity of pulmonary complications can vary from mild hypoxia to respiratory failure (acute respiratory distress syndrome [ARDS]). It is estimated that 50% of early deaths in patients with severe acute pancreatitis are associated with respiratory failure due to profound acute lung injury. The pathophysiology of this acute lung injury appears to involve an increase in permeability of the alveolar-capillary membrane. The endothelial cell destruction in the alveolar capillaries may be mediated by circulating activated pancreatic enzymes including elastase and phospholipase A_2. Pulmonary surfactant, another important alveolar barrier, appears to be destroyed by phospholipase A_2. Additional pulmonary injury appears to be mediated by inflammatory leukocytes that are sequestered in the alveoli and interstitial tissues, with subsequent release of proinflammatory cytokines and chemokines that lead to further tissue destruction.

Quite often, acute pancreatitis is accompanied by a small (usually left-sided) **pleural effusion.** The effusion may be secondary to a direct effect of the inflamed, swollen pancreas on the pleura abutting the diaphragm or to tracking of exudative fluid from the pancreatic bed retroperitoneally into the pleural cavity through defects in the diaphragm. Characteristically, the pleural fluid is an exudate with high levels of protein, lactate dehydrogenase, and amylase. The effusion may contribute to segmental atelectasis of the lower lobes, leading to ventilation-perfusion mismatch and hypoxia.

Pancreatic necrosis may develop in approximately 10–20% of patients with acute pancreatitis and carries a 15–20% mortality rate. Dynamic contrast-enhanced CT, best performed within 24–48 hours of hospital admission, can help to determine the extent of necrosis and provide prognostic information about patient survival and need for surgical intervention. Sterile pancreatic necrosis, as documented by percutaneous aspiration, does not require operative intervention as long as it is associated with gradual clinical improvement.

Infected pancreatic necrosis occurs when there is bacterial infection of necrotic tissue in and around the inflamed pancreas. Infected necrosis occurs an average of 1–2 weeks or more after the onset of symptoms. This septic complication represents a serious, potentially life-threatening, complication of acute pancreatitis. Infected pancreatic necrosis carries a 20–50% mortality rate and is an indication for surgical debridement and drainage.

An **acute peripancreatic fluid collection** is a collection of enzyme-rich pancreatic secretions occurring 48 hours after symptom onset, located in or near the pancreas, and lacking a well-defined wall of granulation tissue or fibrous tissue. They occur in 30–50% of patients with acute pancreatitis and are often incorrectly called pseudocysts. Most resolve; only 10–15% evolve into pseudocysts with related complications.

C. Late Complications of Acute Pancreatitis

Pancreatic pseudocysts are nonepithelium-lined cavities that contain plasma, blood, pus, and pancreatic juice. They are the product of inflammatory fibrous or granulation tissue walling off a peripancreatic fluid collection. By definition, pseudocysts

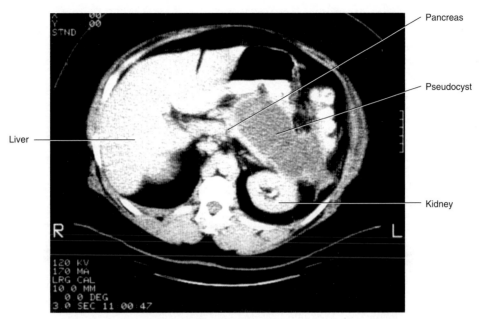

FIGURE 15–6 Pancreatic pseudocyst on CT. (Reproduced, with permission, from Way LW [editor]. *Current Surgical Diagnosis & Treatment,* 10th ed. Originally published by Appleton & Lange. Copyright © 1994 by the McGraw-Hill Companies, Inc.)

are distinguished from acute peripancreatic fluid collections by their persistence 4–6 weeks following an episode of acute pancreatitis. Pseudocysts generally occur after recovery from the acute attack and are the result of both parenchymal destruction and ductal obstruction or disruption. Some acini continue to secrete pancreatic juice, but because the juice cannot drain normally, it collects in an area of necrotic tissue, forming the ill-defined pseudocyst (Figure 15–6). As more juice is secreted, the cyst may grow progressively larger and may cause compression of nearby structures such as the portal vein (producing portal hypertension), common bile duct (producing jaundice or cholangitis), or gut (producing gastric outlet or bowel obstruction).

Most pancreatic pseudocysts will resolve spontaneously and no specific intervention is required when asymptomatic. Indications for surgical, endoscopic, or percutaneous intervention include persistent symptoms, large size (> 10 cm), and associated persistent ductal disruption. Treatment options for pseudocysts include external drainage either by surgical or percutaneous techniques or by internal drainage to the GI tract by surgical or endoscopic means.

Pancreatic abscess describes an infected peripancreatic fluid collection, typically one that has developed 4–6 weeks or more after an episode of acute pancreatitis. This term is often used interchangeably with infected pancreatic pseudocyst. However, unlike the local septic complications of pancreatitis that occur early, pancreatic abscess can often be treated successfully. Percutaneous drainage is the mainstay of therapy, with surgical drainage reserved for refractory cases.

Pancreatic ascites occurs when a direct connection develops between the pancreatic duct and the peritoneal cavity. Given its origin, it is not surprising that the ascitic fluid resembles pancreatic juice, characteristically an exudate with high protein and

extremely high amylase levels. Left untreated, massive pancreatic ascites may lead to pleural effusions, subcutaneous fat necrosis, or abdominal compartment syndrome.

Pancreatic fistulas, caused by disruption of the pancreatic duct, should be suspected in patients who develop pancreatic ascites or pleural effusions. Fistulas can be internal, connecting to pleural or pericardial spaces, colon, small intestine, or biliary tract, or external, draining through the skin.

Course & Prognosis

Most patients with acute pancreatitis recover completely with supportive medical management. The pancreas then regenerates and returns to normal except for some mild residual scarring. Diabetes mellitus almost never occurs after a single attack of pancreatitis. However, in some cases, one or more pancreatic pseudocysts form in the weeks to months after recovery.

The initial course of alcoholic pancreatitis is characterized by recurrent acute exacerbations and the later course by progressive pancreatic insufficiency. However, among individuals with recurrent acute alcoholic pancreatitis, two groups can be distinguished in terms of prognosis. About 75% of these cases progress to advanced chronic pancreatitis, typically with pancreatic calcification and pancreatic insufficiency. The remainder do not progress and do not develop pancreatic duct dilation. The factors responsible for progression have not yet been elucidated.

The severity of acute pancreatitis can be estimated by various methods: clinical assessment, biochemical tests, peritoneal lavage, CT, and prognostic criteria (Table 15–2).

Studies have shown that important predictors of mortality are (1) failure of more than one organ system in the early phase of acute pancreatitis or (2) pancreatic necrosis associated with

TABLE 15–2   Adverse prognostic signs in acute pancreatitis.

I. Ranson's criteria of severity of acute pancreatitis[1]

Criteria present at diagnosis or admission	Criteria developing during first 48 hours
Age > 55 years	Hematocrit fall > 10%
White blood cell count > 16,000/µL	Blood urea nitrogen rise > 5 mg/dL
Blood glucose > 200 mg/dL	Serum calcium < 8 mg/dL
Serum LDH > 350 IU/L	Arterial Po_2 < 60 mm Hg
AST > 250 IU/L	Base deficit > 4 mEq/L
	Estimated fluid sequestration > 6 L

Mortality rates correlate with number of criteria present

Number of criteria	Mortality rate
0–2	1%
3–4	16%
5–6	40%
7–8	100%

II. CT severity index[2]

A. Balthazar and Ranson's CT grade (based on non–contrast-enhanced appearance)	B. CT severity index (based on dynamic perfusion)		
	CT grade +	Necrosis	= Total score
0 = Normal pancreas	0	None	= 0
1 = Focal or diffuse enlargement	1	One third	= 2
2 = Gland abnormalities with mild peripancreatic enlargement	2	One half	= 4
3 = Fluid collection within a single location	3	> One half	= 6
4 = ≥ 2 fluid collections or gas in pancreas or surrounding inflammation	4	> One half	= 8

III. Other poor prognostic signs in acute pancreatitis[3]

A. Objective data	B. Organ failure
1. > 3 Ranson's criteria	C. Local complications
2. APACHE score > 8	1. Necrosis
3. Hemoconcentration, with hematocrit > 48%	2. Abscess
4. CT severity index > 6	3. Pseudocyst

[1]Modified from Way LW (editor). *Current Surgical Diagnosis & Treatment*, 10th ed. Originally published by Appleton & Lange. Copyright © 1994 by the McGraw-Hill Companies, Inc.

[2]Modified from Balthazar EJ et al. Acute pancreatitis: Value of CT in establishing prognosis. Radiology. 1990;174:331.

[3]Modified from Law NM et al. Emergency complications of acute and chronic pancreatitis. Gastroenterol Clin North Am. 2003;32:1169.

later development of multiple-organ failure. Organ failure, as defined by the 1992 Atlanta Symposium criteria, includes the following parameters: shock with systolic blood pressure < 90 mm Hg; respiratory failure with PaO_2 < 60 mm Hg; renal failure with serum creatinine > 2 mg/dL after fluid resuscitation; and GI bleeding with > 500 mL of blood loss within a 24-hour period. Multiple-organ failure is defined as a syndrome of progressive but potentially reversible organ failure, involving two or more systems remote from the original insult. The patient's prognosis is directly related to the number of failed organs. The pulmonary, renal, cardiovascular, CNS, and coagulation systems are most commonly involved.

About 20% of patients develop a severe or fatal attack. Severe acute pancreatitis is a systemic disease with two distinct phases. The first phase is SIRS, caused by the systemic effects of proinflammatory mediators discussed previously, which may lead to multiple-organ system dysfunctions within the first 72 hours. The second phase is uncontrolled decompensation, which includes progression to local pancreatic and intra-abdominal complications sometimes followed by irreversible multiple-organ system failure, culminating in death. Proper management of severe pancreatitis includes identification of patients at risk, aggressive treatment of identifiable causes (eg, emergency intervention by endoscopic retrograde cholangiopancreatography [ERCP] and sphincterotomy in gallstone pancreatitis), management of SIRS (eg, administration of lexipafant), and prevention and treatment of complications (eg, drainage and antibiotics for abscess).

The overall mortality rate for acute pancreatitis is 5–10%, but the rate increases to 35% or higher in complicated cases. Deaths often occur as a consequence of hemorrhagic shock, DIC, ARDS, or sepsis.

CHECKPOINT

5. What are the presenting symptoms and signs of acute pancreatitis?
6. What are the most common causes of acute pancreatitis?
7. Which drugs are commonly associated with pancreatitis?
8. What is the pathophysiologic mechanism by which hemorrhagic pancreatitis occurs?
9. What are the complications of severe pancreatitis?
10. What are the pathophysiologic mechanisms by which each of the complications of severe pancreatitis occurs?

CHRONIC PANCREATITIS

Clinical Presentations

Chronic pancreatitis is a relapsing disorder causing severe abdominal pain, exocrine and endocrine pancreatic insufficiency, severe duct abnormalities, and pancreatic calcifications. The prevalence of the disorder is about 30 cases per 100,000 individuals, and the yearly incidence ranges from 3.5 to 10 cases per 100,000. In chronic pancreatitis, there is chronic inflammation of the parenchyma, leading to progressive destruction of the acini, stenosis and dilation of the ductules, and fibrosis of the gland. Eventually, there is impairment of the gland's exocrine function (see Pancreatic Insufficiency later) and in severe cases loss of endocrine function as well (Chapter 18).

Etiology

It was at one time believed that chronic pancreatitis simply resulted from recurrent attacks of acute pancreatitis. However, there is some evidence that acute and chronic pancreatitis are

TABLE 15–3 Causes of chronic pancreatitis.

Alcohol abuse
Duct obstruction (eg, gallstones)
Pancreas divisum[1]
Tropical (malnutrition, toxin)
Hypercalcemia (eg, hyperparathyroidism)
Hyperlipidemia
Drugs
Trauma
Autoimmune
Hereditary
Cystic fibrosis (mucoviscidosis)
Idiopathic

[1]An anatomic variant that occurs with failure of normal fusion between the dorsal and ventral pancreatic ducts.

distinct pathogenetic entities. Patients developing acute pancreatitis are a mean 13 years older than those with onset of chronic calcified pancreatitis. Furthermore, the two diseases have been linked to different causes. Finally, in acute pancreatitis, the pancreas is normal before the attack and the pathologic changes are completely reversible if the patient survives, whereas in chronic pancreatitis the gland is abnormal before the attack and the pathologic changes are not reversible.

The major cause of chronic pancreatitis is chronic alcoholism, which accounts for about 70–80% of cases. The remainder are due to diverse causes listed in Table 15–3. In 1788, Cawley first reported the association of alcoholism with chronic pancreatitis. He described a "free living young man" with diabetes and emaciation. At autopsy, his pancreas was "full of stones." Patients with chronic pancreatitis resulting from alcohol abuse usually have a long history (6–12 years) of heavy alcohol consumption (150–175 g/d) before disease onset. In alcoholics, deficiencies of zinc and selenium may inhibit quenching of oxygen free radicals.

Long-term obstruction of the pancreatic duct can also cause chronic pancreatitis. The obstruction can be caused by a periampullary solid neoplasm, papillary stenosis, cystic lesions (cystic tumors or pseudocysts), scarring or stricture, or trauma. Pancreas divisum can cause chronic pancreatitis as a result of obstruction at the lesser papilla. Tropical chronic pancreatitis is a juvenile form of chronic calcific nonalcoholic pancreatitis. It is thought to be caused by protein or micronutrient deficiencies, which may cause impaired clearance of free radicals, or by ingestion of a toxic substance, such as cyanogens in cassava root. Chronic hypercalcemia may cause pancreatitis. For example, 10–15% of patients with hyperparathyroidism develop pancreatitis. Intraductal precipitation of calcium and stimulation of pancreatic enzyme secretion are thought to be important in pathogenesis. In some cases of chronic pancreatitis with features of Sjögren's syndrome, an autoimmune mechanism may be involved. Chronic hereditary pancreatitis, characterized by recurrent episodes of abdominal pain beginning in childhood, accounts for about 1% of cases. It is transmitted as an autosomal dominant genetic disorder with incomplete (~80%) penetrance. Hereditary chronic pancreatitis has also been associated with mutations in the cationic trypsinogen gene *PRSS1* or in the *SPINK1/PSTI* gene (discussed previously). Some cases are due to cystic fibrosis (mucoviscidosis; see later).

In some cases, no cause can be identified, and the disease is termed idiopathic chronic pancreatitis.

Pathology

As noted, in acute pancreatitis, peripancreatic and intrapancreatic fat necrosis is the key pathologic finding. In resolving acute pancreatitis, there is organization of fat necrosis with early perilobular fibrosis or peripancreatic pseudocysts. However, if acute pancreatitis is severe, and/or recurrent, it may perhaps evolve into chronic pancreatitis.

In the early stage of chronic pancreatitis, pseudocysts are present in half (52%) of patients, and there is a focally accentuated fibrosis of the perilobular and, to a lesser degree, intralobular type. Although intralobular and perilobular fibrosis of the pancreas is a hallmark of alcoholic pancreatitis, it is also common among patients with alcohol dependence and abuse who have no history of pancreatitis. Marked fibrosis, ductal distortions, and the presence of intraductal calculi are the main features of

TABLE 15–5 Proposed pathogenetic mechanisms for chronic pancreatitis.

"Big duct" mechanisms
Biliary-pancreatic reflux
Sphincter of Oddi obstruction or hypersecretion
Increased ductal permeability
"Small duct" mechanisms
Increased viscosity or hypersecretion of proteins
Increased lactoferrin
Decreased lithostathine (pancreatic stone protein)
Acinar cell mechanisms
Toxic metabolites
Unopposed free radical injury
Hyperstimulation of leukocytes
Lysosomal hyperactivity
Cholinergic hyperactivity
Abnormal protein trafficking
Stellate cell-induced fibrosis
Necrosis-fibrosis sequence

Data from Pitchumoni CS. Pathogenesis of alcohol-induced chronic pancreatitis: Facts, perceptions, and misperceptions. Surg Clin North Am. 2001;81:379.

TABLE 15–4 Pathogenetic classification of pancreatitis.

Pathogenetic Class	Subclassification	Pathologic Features
Acute pancreatitis	Mild pancreatitis	Fat necrosis
	Severe (necrotizing) pancreatitis	Coagulation necrosis
		Hemorrhagic necrosis
Chronic pancreatitis	Lithogenic pancreatitis	Protein plugs
	Obstructive pancreatitis	Calculi
	Inflammatory pancreatitis	Obstruction of main pancreatic duct
	Pancreatic fibrosis	
		Mononuclear cell infiltration
		Acinar cell necrosis
		Diffuse perilobular fibrosis

Modified, with permission, from Sidhu SS, Tandon RK. The pathogenesis of chronic pancreatitis. Postgrad Med J. 1995;71:67.

advanced chronic pancreatitis. Pseudocysts are less frequent (36%). CD4 and CD8 T lymphocytes are the predominant T-cell subsets in the inflammatory infiltrates in chronic pancreatitis.

Pathologically, chronic pancreatitis is characterized by scarring and shrinkage of the pancreas resulting from fibrosis and atrophy of acini and by stenosis and dilation of ductules. Grossly, the process usually involves the whole gland, but in about one third of cases it is localized, most often involving the head and body of the gland. The ductules and ducts are often filled with inspissated secretions or calculi. Between 36% and 87% of patients with chronic pancreatitis have ductal stones. The gland may be rock hard as a result of diffuse sclerosis and calcification, and biopsy may be required to differentiate chronic pancreatitis from pancreatic carcinoma (see Carcinoma of the Pancreas later). Microscopically, there are loss of acini, dilation of ductules, marked fibrosis, and a lymphocytic infiltrate. The islets of Langerhans are usually well preserved.

Pathogenesis

Table 15–4 presents a classification of pancreatitis based on pathogenesis, and Table 15–5 lists proposed pathogenetic mechanisms for chronic pancreatitis.

For chronic lithogenic pancreatitis, several different pathogenetic mechanisms have been postulated. One theory postulates **acinar protein (trypsinogen) hypersecretion** as an initial event (Figure 15–7A). Ultrastructural studies of exocrine pancreatic tissue from patients with chronic pancreatitis show signs of protein hypersecretion, including a larger diameter of cells, nuclei, and nucleoli; increased length of the endoplasmic reticulum; increased numbers of condensing vacuoles; and decreased numbers of zymogen granules. The hypersecretion of protein occurs without increased fluid or bicarbonate secretion by ductal cells. At the same time, there is an increase in the ratio of lysosomal hydrolases (cathepsin B) to digestive hydrolases (trypsinogen), resulting in activation of trypsinogen. Precipitation of intraductal protein into plugs is then thought to occur in the following fashion: **Lithostathines** (formerly called pancreatic stone proteins, or **PSPs**) are peptides secreted into pancreatic juice that normally inhibit the formation of protein plugs and the aggregation of calcium carbonate crystals to form stones. Acinar cell secretion of lithostathine is impaired by alcohol. Furthermore, when hydrolyzed by trypsin and cathepsin B, lithostathine H2/PSP-S1 is created. This insoluble peptide polymerizes into fibrils that form the matrix of protein plugs. At the same time, there is hypersecretion of calcium into the pancreatic juice. The calcium

hypersecretion is first triggered by neural (cholinergic, vagally mediated) or hormonal stimuli. Later, as the basal lamina of the pancreatic duct is eroded by contact with the protein plugs, there is transudation of serum protein and calcium into the pancreatic juice. The combination of protein plug formation in pancreatic juice that is thick, viscid, and protein rich and supersaturated with calcium carbonate leads to formation of **calculi** (stones) (Figure 15–7B). Lithostathine deficiency is unexplained but may be hereditary or acquired. Chronic alcoholism and malnutrition are acquired causes of lithostathine deficiency. Decreased levels of other nucleation-inhibitory factors, such as local trypsin inhibitor and citrate, in pancreatic juice further enhance formation of pancreatic plugs and stones. Lactoferrin, an iron-containing macromolecular protein, is elevated in the pancreatic secretions of alcoholic patients with pancreatitis. Lactoferrin can produce aggregation of large acidophilic proteins, such as albumin, and thus may be partly responsible for the formation of protein plugs. Similarly, GP2, a glycosylphosphatidylinositol-anchored protein, might have a role in protein plug formation. GP2 is released from the apical surface of acinar cells into the pancreatic ducts in relatively high concentrations. GP2 aggregates at pH < 7.0, and pancreatic juice from patients with chronic pancreatitis usually has a pH < 7.0. Eventually, the stones provoke formation of fibrotic ductal strictures and ductal ectasia, acinar cell atrophy, and parenchymal atrophy distal to obstructed ducts in the advanced stages of chronic pancreatitis.

Another theory postulates a **necrosis-fibrosis sequence,** in which focal necrosis during recurrent attacks of acute pancreatitis induces scarring and fibrosis, leading to chronic lithogenic pancreatitis (Figure 15–8A). In this scenario, vascular damage in acute pancreatitis causes cellular anoxia, necrosis, chronic inflammation, and subsequent fibrosis. In particular, periacinar and periductal fat necrosis induce periductal fibrosis, which partially obstructs the interlobular ducts. Stasis within the ductules then leads to protein plug and stone formation in the pancreatic juice (Figure 15–8B). Subsequently, total obstruction of ducts by calculi induces acinar cell necrosis, inflammation, and fibrosis (Figure 15–8C). Transforming growth factor-β (TGF-β) appears to be a mediator of collagen synthesis after pancreatic injury.

Oxidative stress may also be responsible for chronic pancreatitis. According to this theory, inappropriate activation of pancreatic cytochrome P450 enzymes (eg, by alcohol) results in lipid peroxidation by excess free radicals of oxygen. Resultant lipid deposition in the basal cytoplasm of acinar cells is thought to trigger the development of fibrosis. Oxidative stress and membrane lipid oxidation lead to an inflammatory process, perhaps mediated by chemokines attracting mononuclear cells.

In cases of chronic pancreatitis resulting from **obstruction of the pancreatic ducts,** the obstruction antedates the development of pancreatitis. The pathogenesis probably involves elevated pressures in the pancreatic duct, resulting in ischemia, necrosis, and inflammation of acinar cells. However, the ductal epithelium is preserved. Calcified protein plugs and stones are less often present. Many patients with idiopathic chronic pancreatitis also have ductal hypertension.

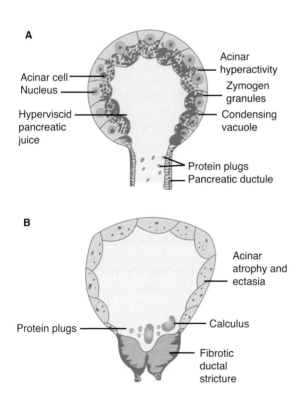

FIGURE 15–7 Proposed pathogenetic model of chronic pancreatitis emphasizing acinar protein hypersecretion. **A:** In early chronic pancreatitis, there are acinar cell hyperactivity and secretion of a hyperviscid pancreatic juice with an imbalance of pancreatic stone promoters and inhibitors, resulting in protein plug formation. **B:** In advanced chronic pancreatitis, there are acinar cell atrophy, ductal strictures and ectasia, and intraductal stones. (Redrawn, with permission, from Sidhu SS, Tandon RK. The pathogenesis of chronic pancreatitis. Postgrad Med J. 1995;71:67.)

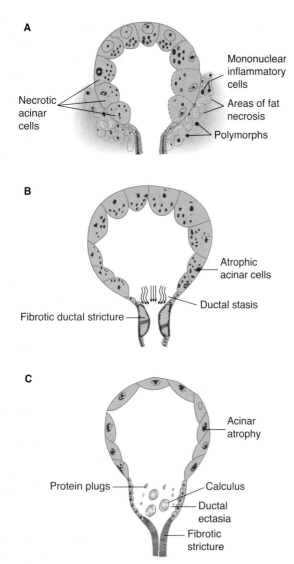

FIGURE 15–8 Proposed pathogenetic model of chronic pancreatitis emphasizing the sequence of acute pancreatitis followed by chronic pancreatitis. **A:** In acute pancreatitis, there are necrosis of acinar cells and fat and infiltration of inflammatory cells. **B:** Later, there are healing and fibrosis. **C:** Finally, changes of chronic pancreatitis appear, including acinar cell atrophy, formation of protein plugs and calculi, and ductal strictures and ectasia. (Redrawn, with permission, from Sidhu SS, Tandon RK. The pathogenesis of chronic pancreatitis. Postgrad Med J. 1995;71:67.)

Mutations of the cystic fibrosis transmembrane conductance regulator *(CFTR)* gene located on chromosome 7q32 are more common than expected among patients with chronic pancreatitis, particularly those with idiopathic chronic pancreatitis. This finding raises the possibility that *CFTR* mutations might increase the risk for pancreatitis after exposure to alcohol or certain drugs. In patients with chronic pancreatitis and cystic fibrosis, mutation of the *CFTR* gene causes inadequate function of *CFTR*, the chloride channel located on the luminal surface of the pancreatic duct cell that is highly involved in bicarbonate secretion. Major mutations in both alleles lead to loss of *CFTR* function and the inability to hydrate mucus, resulting in inspissated secretions and

obstruction of the ducts. Because pancreatic function may be maintained with *CFTR* function as little as 1% of normal, only severe *CFTR* mutations yielding little or no functional protein produce chronic pancreatitis and pancreatic insufficiency.

Finally, chronic inflammatory pancreatitis is sometimes produced by an **autoimmune** mechanism. Associated clinical features may include bilateral sialadenitis, intrahepatic cholestasis, and the nephrotic syndrome. Elevated levels of serum immune globulins are typical. In addition, the fact that different etiologic forms of chronic pancreatitis result in similar histologic features and comparable inflammatory cell reaction suggests that the disease, independent of underlying cause, reaches a common immunologic pathway beyond which it appears to progress as a single distinctive entity.

Pathophysiology

Maldigestion in chronic pancreatitis results from several factors. Long-standing inflammation and fibrosis of the pancreas can destroy exocrine tissue, leading to inadequate delivery of digestive enzymes to the duodenum in the prandial and postprandial periods. This maldigestion is worsened by inadequate delivery of bicarbonate to the duodenum, with consequent gastric acid inactivation of enzymes and bile acids. Gastric dysmotility and mechanical obstruction from fibrosis in the pancreatic head may also contribute. Chronic pancreatitis may thus result in the profound steatorrhea of pancreatic insufficiency. There is a direct correlation between severity of histologic findings and exocrine pancreatic dysfunction as estimated by the CCK-secretin test (see later).

Studies of patients with chronic pancreatitis have found no abnormalities in basal plasma levels of CCK and pancreatic polypeptide (PP), but impaired interdigestive cycling and postprandial release of CCK and PP have been noted. Chronic pancreatitis does not seem to have any effect on intestinal motility.

In chronic pancreatitis, fecal bile acid excretion has been found to be three times that of healthy individuals. Bile acid malabsorption is related to impairment of pancreatic bicarbonate secretion; it is generally not observed until bicarbonate output is markedly reduced (< 0.05 mEq/kg/h). Such bile acid malabsorption may cause the hypocholesterolemia seen in patients with chronic pancreatitis.

Impairment of exocrine function in chronic pancreatitis may also lead to increased CCK-mediated stimulation of the pancreas.

Hepatic insulin resistance has been demonstrated in patients with chronic pancreatitis, perhaps related to a decrease in high-affinity insulin receptors on the hepatocyte cell membrane. In rats, insulin binding improves after administration of pancreatic polypeptide.

Clinical Manifestations

The clinical manifestations of chronic pancreatitis are listed in Table 15–6. The major symptom of chronic pancreatitis is severe abdominal pain that can be either constant or intermittent.

TABLE 15–6 Clinical manifestations of chronic pancreatitis.

Abdominal pain
Nausea
Vomiting
Weight loss
Malabsorption
Hyperglycemia, diabetes mellitus
Jaundice

The abdominal pain often radiates to the midback or scapula and increases after eating. It is sometimes relieved by sitting upright or leaning forward. The pain is thought to derive from dilation of the duct system, causing ductal hypertension; inflammation of the parenchyma, causing pancreatic ischemia; or local enzymatic activity and destruction of the perineural sheath, exposing axons to cytokines released by inflammatory cells and ultimately causing perineural fibrosis. Evidence supporting ductal hypertension as a cause of pain in patients with chronic pancreatitis includes reports of significant pain relief (up to 75% of properly selected patients) with surgical decompression of a dilated main pancreatic duct. Patients may have recurrent attacks of severe abdominal pain, vomiting, and elevation of serum amylase (chronic relapsing pancreatitis). Continued alcohol intake may increase the frequency of painful episodes, at least when there is still relatively preserved pancreatic function; in severe pancreatic insufficiency, alcohol intake appears to have less influence on the development of abdominal pain. Pancreatic parenchymal pressure measurements have not been found to correlate with pain.

The classic triad of tropical chronic pancreatitis consists of abdominal pain, steatorrhea, and diabetes mellitus, often requiring insulin.

From 10% to 20% of patients have "painless pancreatitis," presenting with diabetes, jaundice, maldigestion, malabsorption, or steatorrhea. Anorexia and weight loss occur frequently, related to both poor nutrition and malabsorption from pancreatic insufficiency.

Physical findings include epigastric or upper abdominal tenderness. A fever or a palpable mass suggests a complication such as an abscess or a pseudocyst.

The diagnosis of chronic pancreatitis is based mainly on symptoms and signs. The serum amylase and lipase levels are elevated in only a minority of cases. In the remaining cases, the amylase and lipase levels are normal or low, probably because there is little residual functional pancreatic tissue. A finding of pancreatic calcifications on abdominal x-ray film is present in about 30% of cases and is pathognomonic of the condition. The calcifications are actually the intraductal pancreatic calculi composed of calcium carbonate and lithostathines. Endoscopic ultrasonography (EUS) typically reveals ductal dilation and may demonstrate pseudocysts in up to 10% of patients. CT scans may reveal calcifications and cystic areas not noted on plain abdominal x-ray films or ultrasonography.

About 5% of patients develop severe sclerosing pancreatitis involving the head of the pancreas, leading to obstruction of the common bile and pancreatic ducts. Obstruction of the common bile duct in the setting of chronic pancreatitis typically appears as a smooth, tapering stricture, rather than an abrupt cutoff, as is seen in bile duct obstruction due to pancreatic cancer. Obstruction may also be caused by a pseudocyst in the head of the pancreas. Common bile duct obstruction results in profound and persistent jaundice, resembling that produced by pancreatic carcinoma. The serum bilirubin and alkaline phosphatase are elevated.

ERCP is the best imaging procedure for assessing the severity and extent of ductal changes. ERCP findings include dilated ducts, frequently with adjacent areas of stricture, yielding a "chain of lakes" or "string of pearls" appearance, or ducts of normal caliber, with adjacent small ducts lacking side branches, yielding a "tree in winter" appearance. EUS and MRCP, alternative imaging techniques that provide visualization of the pancreatic ductal system, are increasingly being utilized to confirm a diagnosis of chronic pancreatitis.

Exocrine pancreatic function is estimated by the CCK-secretin test. In this test, measurements are made of pancreatic juice volume, amylase output, and bicarbonate concentration in the basal state, 30 minutes after intravenous injection of CCK, and 60 minutes after intravenous administration of secretin. Simpler, less invasive tests include the fecal elastase test, bentiromide test, pancreolauryl test, and cholesteryl-[^{14}C]octanoate breath test (see Pancreatic Insufficiency later).

Failure to secrete pancreatic juice results in malabsorption of fat (steatorrhea) and fat-soluble vitamins, leading to weight loss. Impairment of exocrine function is manifested by pancreatic insufficiency (see later). Studies screening patients with chronic pancreatitis have found that the majority develop exocrine dysfunction over time. One study documented that 63% developed exocrine dysfunction within 5 years and 94% after 10 years. Diabetes mellitus is a late complication of chronic pancreatitis and is not apparent until 80–90% of the gland is severely damaged.

The treatment of chronic pancreatitis is mainly symptomatic and directed toward relieving pain and treating exocrine and endocrine insufficiency (see below). Pain in these patients is often a serious clinical problem, leading to a significant compromise of quality of life and potential opioid tolerance and even addiction. If a precipitating factor such as an anatomic abnormality or metabolic condition is present, it may be treated with surgical or medical intervention. Methods of pain relief include abstinence from alcohol and use of conventional analgesics. If pain is not relieved, the use of opioids may be necessary. Invasive procedures, such as celiac plexus block, endoscopic procedures, and surgical drainage or resection may be indicated in select patients with debilitating symptoms.

The major complications of chronic pancreatitis are pseudocyst formation and mechanical obstruction of the common bile duct and duodenum. Less common complications include pancreatic fistulas with pancreatic ascites, pleural effusion, or sometimes pericardial effusion; splenic vein thrombosis and development of gastric varices; and formation of a pseudoaneurysm, with hemorrhage or pain resulting from expansion and pressure on adjacent structures. Fistulas result from disruption of the pancreatic duct. Splenic vein thrombosis occurs because the splenic vein, which courses along the posterior surface of the pancreas, may become involved in peripancreatic inflammation. Pseudoaneurysms may affect any of the arteries in proximity to the pancreas, most commonly the splenic, hepatic, gastroduodenal, and pancreaticoduodenal arteries.

In patients monitored for more than 10 years, the mortality rate is 22%; pancreatitis-induced complications account for 13% of the deaths. Older age at diagnosis, cigarette smoking, and alcohol intake are major predictors of mortality among individuals with chronic pancreatitis. Chronic pancreatitis of any cause has been associated with a 25-year cumulative risk of approximately 4% for the development of pancreatic cancer.

PANCREATIC INSUFFICIENCY

Clinical Presentations

Pancreatic exocrine insufficiency is the syndrome of maldigestion resulting from disorders interfering with effective pancreatic enzyme activity. Because pancreatic lipase is essential for fat digestion, its absence leads to steatorrhea (the occurrence of greasy, bulky, light-colored stools). On the other hand, although pancreatic amylase and trypsin are important for carbohydrate and protein digestion, other enzymes in gastric and intestinal juice can usually compensate for their loss. Thus, patients with pancreatic insufficiency seldom present with maldigestion of carbohydrate and protein (nitrogen loss).

Etiology

Pancreatic insufficiency usually results from chronic pancreatitis in adults or cystic fibrosis (mucoviscidosis) in children (Table 15–7). In some cases, it is a consequence of pancreatic resection or carcinoma of the pancreas. Pancreatic insufficiency occurs after bone marrow transplantation and appears to be related to prior acute or chronic graft-versus-host disease. Each of these conditions markedly reduces the amount of pancreatic enzymes secreted, often to less than 5% of normal.

Pancreatic exocrine insufficiency is also a common occurrence in patients recovering from severe acute pancreatitis, and its severity correlates with the extent of pancreatic necrosis. Its severity also correlates with the severity of concomitant endocrine insufficiency, manifested by the new onset of diabetes mellitus.

Less commonly, pancreatic insufficiency results from disease states that cause hypersecretion of gastric acid. For example, excessive gastrin secretion from a gastrinoma (an islet cell neoplasm composed of G cells) leads to continuous hyperse-

TABLE 15–7 Causes of pancreatic insufficiency.

Primary
A. Acquired decreased enzyme secretion
Chronic pancreatitis (alcohol abuse, trauma, hereditary, idiopathic)
Pancreatic, ampullary, and duodenal neoplasms
Pancreatic resection
Severe protein-calorie malnutrition, hypoalbuminemia
B. Congenital decreased enzyme secretion
Cystic fibrosis
Hemochromatosis
Shwachman's syndrome (pancreatic insufficiency with anemia, neutropenia, and bony abnormalities)
Enzyme deficiencies (trypsinogen, enterokinase, amylase, lipase, protease, and α_1-antiprotease deficiency)
Secondary
A. Intraluminal enzyme destruction: gastrinoma (Zollinger-Ellison syndrome)
B. Decreased pancreatic stimulation: small intestinal mucosal disease (nontropical sprue)
C. Mistiming of enzyme secretion: gastric surgery
1. Subtotal gastrectomy with Billroth I anastomosis
2. Subtotal gastrectomy with Billroth II anastomosis
3. Truncal vagotomy and pyloroplasty

cretion of gastric acid and a very low pH of gastric juice. In affected patients, the excess gastric acid overwhelms the normal pancreatic bicarbonate production and results in an abnormally acidic pH in the duodenum. This acid pH, in turn, causes decreased activity of otherwise adequate amounts of pancreatic enzymes.

Pathology & Pathogenesis

Normally, the activities of the various pancreatic enzymes decrease during their passage from the duodenum to the terminal ileum. However, the degradation rates of individual enzymes vary; lipase activity is lost rapidly and protease and amylase activity is lost slowly. Lipase activity is usually destroyed by proteolysis, mainly by the action of residual chymotrypsin. This mechanism persists in patients with pancreatic insufficiency, helping to explain why fat malabsorption develops earlier than protein or starch malabsorption.

Patients with destruction of the exocrine pancreas develop impaired digestion and absorption of fat. Clinically, fat malabsorption is manifested as steatorrhea. Although the steatorrhea is caused mostly by the deficiency of pancreatic lipase, the absence of pancreatic bicarbonate secretion also contributes to its occurrence. Without bicarbonate, acidic chyme from the stomach inhibits the activity of pancreatic lipase and causes precipitation of bile salts. Deficiency of bile salts in turn causes failure of micelle formation and interference with fat absorption.

Pathophysiology

Causes of maldigestion from exocrine pancreatic insufficiency include chronic pancreatitis, cystic fibrosis, pancreatic cancer, partial or total gastrectomy, and pancreatic resection. Each of these causes is associated with specific related changes in GI physiology, including changes in intraluminal pH, bile acid metabolism, gastric emptying, and intestinal motility.

For example, during the course of chronic pancreatitis, there is a close relationship among gastric acidity, exocrine pancreatic insufficiency, and impaired digestion. Postprandial gastric acidification has been found to be significantly greater among patients with severe pancreatic insufficiency than among those with mild or no insufficiency. Inhibition of gastric acid secretion by H_2 blockers such as cimetidine or proton pump inhibitors such as omeprazole improves the response to pancreatic enzyme replacement and decreases fecal fat excretion. However, it does not lead to complete elimination of steatorrhea.

On the other hand, loss of the stomach can cause considerable change in function of the exocrine pancreas. After total gastrectomy, patients frequently develop severe primary exocrine pancreatic insufficiency with maldigestion and weight loss. Postoperatively, pancreatic juice volume, bicarbonate output, and enzyme (amylase, trypsin, and chymotrypsin) secretion are reduced significantly compared with preoperative levels. These reductions probably result from changes in GI hormone secretion, altering regulation of pancreatic function. For example, after gastrectomy, most patients exhibit decreased baseline and postprandial gastrin and pancreatic polypeptide secretion and increased postprandial CCK secretion.

Clinical Manifestations

The symptoms and signs exhibited by patients with pancreatic insufficiency (Table 15–8) vary to some extent with the underlying disease.

A. Steatorrhea

Patients with steatorrhea usually describe their stools as voluminous or bulky, foul-smelling, greasy, frothy, pale yellow, and floating. However, significant steatorrhea may occur without any of these characteristics. It can be documented by placing the patient on a high-fat diet (50–150 g/d), collecting all stools for 3 days, and determining the average daily fecal fat excretion. A value of more than 7 g of fat per day is abnormal. Steatorrhea responds, often dramatically, to treatment with oral pancreatic enzymes, ingested with each meal and with snacks.

TABLE 15–8 Clinical manifestations of pancreatic insufficiency.

Symptoms and Signs	Percentage
Weight loss	90%
Steatorrhea (stool fat > 6 g/d)	48%
Edema, ascites	12%
Weakness	7%
Hypoproteinemia	14%
Malabsorption of vitamin B_{12}	40%

Modified from Evans WB, Wollaeger EE. Incidence and severity of nutritional deficiency states in chronic exocrine pancreatic insufficiency: Comparison with nontropical sprue. Am J Dig Dis. 1966;11:594.

B. Diarrhea

In patients with fat malabsorption, diarrhea may result from the cathartic action of hydroxylated fatty acids. These fatty acids inhibit the absorption of sodium and water by the colon. Less commonly, watery diarrhea, abdominal cramping, and bloating are due to carbohydrate malabsorption. Indeed, because salivary amylase production remains undisturbed and because pancreatic amylase production must be markedly reduced before intraluminal starch digestion is slowed, symptomatic carbohydrate malabsorption is uncommon in pancreatic insufficiency.

C. Hypocalcemia

Hypocalcemia, hypophosphatemia, tetany, osteomalacia, osteopenia (low bone mineral density), and osteoporosis can occur both from deficiency of the fat-soluble vitamin D and from the binding of dietary calcium to unabsorbed fatty acids, forming insoluble calcium-fat complexes (soaps) in the gut.

D. Nephrolithiasis

The formation of insoluble calcium soaps in the gut also prevents the normal binding of dietary oxalate to calcium. Dietary oxalate remains in solution and is absorbed from the colon, causing hyperoxaluria and predisposing to nephrolithiasis.

E. Vitamin B_{12} Deficiency

About 40% of patients with pancreatic insufficiency demonstrate malabsorption of vitamin B_{12} (cobalamin), although clinical manifestations of vitamin B_{12} deficiency are rare (anemia, subacute combined degeneration of the spinal cord, and dementia). The malabsorption of vitamin B_{12} appears to result from reduced degradation by pancreatic proteases of the normal complexes of vitamin B_{12} and its binding protein (R protein), resulting in less free vitamin B_{12} to bind to intrinsic factor in the small intestine.

F. Weight Loss

Long-standing malabsorption leads to protein catabolism and consequent weight loss, muscle wasting, fatigue, and edema. At times weight loss occurs in patients with chronic pancreatitis because eating exacerbates their abdominal pain or because narcotics used to control pain cause anorexia. In patients who develop diabetes mellitus, weight loss may be due to glycosuria.

Laboratory Tests & Evaluation

Because there is a direct correlation between duodenal (and therefore fecal) output of elastase 1 and duodenal output of lipase, amylase, trypsin, and bicarbonate, measurement of fecal elastase concentrations has been used as a screening test for exocrine pancreatic insufficiency. The diagnosis of pancreatic insufficiency is enhanced by several additional noninvasive tests of exocrine pancreatic function. These tests include the bentiromide test, pancreolauryl test, and cholesteryl-$[^{14}C]$octanoate breath test. In these tests, substrates for pancreatic digestive enzymes are administered orally and their products of digestion are measured. In the bentiromide test, N-benzoyl-L-tyrosine-p-aminobenzoic acid is administered as a substrate for chymotrypsin. Enzymatic cleavage yields p-aminobenzoic acid, which is absorbed from the gut and measured in the urine. In the pancreolauryl test, fluorescein dilaurate is administered and pancreatic esterases release fluorescein, which is then absorbed and measured in the urine. The cholesteryl-$[^{14}C]$octanoate breath test measures $^{14}CO_2$ output in the breath at 120 minutes after ingestion, allowing rapid detection of pancreatic exocrine insufficiency. Patients with chronic pancreatitis have markedly diminished excretion of p-aminobenzoic acid or fluorescein in the urine or output of $^{14}CO_2$ in the breath.

CHECKPOINT

11. How is chronic pancreatitis different from acute pancreatitis in terms of symptoms and signs?
12. What are the symptoms and signs of pancreatic insufficiency?

CARCINOMA OF THE PANCREAS

Epidemiology & Etiology

Pancreatic carcinoma has recently become the fourth leading cause of cancer-related death in the Unites States, with an annual incidence and mortality approaching 40,000 cases per year. Delay in diagnosis, relative resistance to chemotherapy and radiation, and intrinsic biological aggressiveness manifested by early metastatic disease all contribute to the abysmal prognosis associated with pancreatic adenocarcinoma. Pancreatic cancer usually occurs after age 50 years and increases in incidence with age, with most patients diagnosed between 60 and 80 years of age. It is somewhat more frequent in men than in women. Autopsy series document that pancreatic cancer has been identified in up to 2% of individuals undergoing a postmortem examination.

Many risk factors for pancreatic adenocarcinoma have been identified. Cigarette smoking has the strongest overall association and is thought to account for one-quarter of cases diagnosed. The association between cigarette smoking and pancreatic cancer is thought to be related to N-nitroso compounds present in cigarette smoke. Exposure to these agents leads to pancreatic ductal hyperplasia, a possible precursor to adenocarcinoma.

Other factors associated with an increased risk of pancreatic adenocarcinoma include a high dietary intake of saturated fat, exposure to nonchlorinated solvents, and the pesticide dichlorodiphenyl trichloroethane (DDT), although the overall contribution of these factors is likely small. Diabetes mellitus has also recently been identified as a risk factor for the disease. Chronic pancreatitis increases the risk of developing pancreatic adenocarcinoma by 10- to 20-fold. The role of other dietary factors (coffee, high fat intake, and alcohol use) is much debated. Diets containing fresh fruits and vegetables are thought to be protective. There is an increased incidence of pancreatic cancer among patients with hereditary pancreatitis, particularly among those who develop pancreatic calcifications. Rarely, pancreatic carcinoma is inherited in an autosomal dominant fashion in association with diabetes mellitus and exocrine pancreatic insufficiency. A genetic predisposition has also been identified in a number of familial cancer syndromes, including the syndromes listed in Table 15–9.

Pathology

Carcinomas occur more often in the head (70%) and body (20%) than in the tail (10%) of the pancreas. Although the cell of origin of pancreatic cancer is currently unknown, most pancreatic adenocarcinomas have a ductal phenotype. Recent reports suggest that the cell of origin may be an acinar or centroacinar cell that, when mutated, de-differentiates into this ductal phenotype. Pancreatic intraepithelial neoplasia (PanIN) and the mucin-producing cystic tumors, mucinous cystic neoplasms and intraductal papillary mucinous neoplasms, are thought to be precursor lesions of ductal adenocarcinoma of the pancreas. Results of molecular analyses (eg, for mutations in the proto-oncogene K-ras) suggest a monoclonal cellular origin in at least 95% of cases.

Grossly, pancreatic cancer presents as a profoundly desmoplastic, infiltrating tumor that obstructs the pancreatic duct and thus often causes fibrosis and atrophy of the distal gland. Carcinomas of the head of the pancreas tend to obstruct the common bile duct early in their course, leading to jaundice and, if the tumor is large, to widening of the duodenal C loop on contrast x-ray film or imaging studies. Tumors of the body and tail tend to present later in their course and thus tend to be very large when found.

TABLE 15–9 Genetic syndromes associated with pancreatic cancer.

Syndrome	Mode of Inheritance	Gene	Chromosomal Locus
Hereditary pancreatitis	AD	PRSS1 (cationic trypsinogen)	7q35
Hereditary nonpolyposis colorectal cancer	AD	MSH2	2p
		MLH1	2p
		PMS2	7p
		PMS1	2q
Familial breast/ovarian cancer	AD	BRCA2	13q
Familial atypical mole-melanoma	AD	P16	9p
Familial polyposis	AD	FAP	—
Ataxia-telangiectasia	AR	ATM	11q22-23
Peutz-Jeghers	AD	STK11	19p
Cystic fibrosis	AD	CFTR	7

Modified, with permission, from Sohn TA et al. The molecular genetics of pancreatic ductal carcinoma: A review. Surg Oncol. 2000;9:95.

Key: AD, autosomal dominant; AR, autosomal recessive.

Microscopically, 90% of pancreatic cancers are adenocarcinomas; the remainder are adenosquamous, anaplastic, and acinar cell carcinomas. Pancreatic cancer tends to spread into surrounding tissues, invading neighboring organs along the perineural fascia, causing severe pain, and via the lymphatics and bloodstream, causing metastases in regional lymph nodes, liver, and other more distant sites (Figure 15–9).

Pathogenesis

As with other malignancies, it appears that specific molecular genetic alterations occur during development of pancreatic cancer, including overexpression of receptor-ligand systems, activation of oncogenes, inactivation of tumor suppressor genes, and mutations of DNA mismatch repair genes. For example, activating point mutations in the proto-oncogene K-ras at codon 12 have been identified in > 90% of pancreatic cancers. Mutation in the *TP53* tumor suppressor gene has been detected in 50–75% of adenocarcinomas of the pancreas. Concurrent loss of *TP53* and K-ras function may contribute to the clinical aggressiveness of the cancer. In addition, in approximately 90% of cases, the *P16* tumor-suppressor gene, located on chromosome 9p, is inactivated. Mutations in DNA mismatch repair genes can also lead to pancreatic cancer. It appears that multiple mutations must occur for pancreatic cancer to develop. Familial pancreatic cancer syndromes arise from germline mutations. Examples include mutations in *STK11* in Peutz-Jeghers syndrome and in DNA mismatch repair genes. The mismatch repair gene *BRCA2* is inactivated in approximately 7–10% of pancreatic cancers. Familial syndromes and genetic alterations related to pancreatic cancer are summarized in Table 15–9.

In chronic pancreatitis, a common pathway for the development of pancreatic cancer may be through the chronic inflammatory process, including a pronounced stromal reaction. Mediators of chronic inflammation in the stroma likely support a transformation to malignancy, although the exact mechanisms remain unknown. Cytokines produced by the activated stroma appear to promote the aggressive behavior of pancreatic cancer cells.

Clinical Manifestations

The clinical presentation of pancreatic cancer may sometimes be indistinguishable from that of chronic pancreatitis, in part because inflammatory changes commonly occur in both chronic pancreatitis and pancreatic adenocarcinoma. The clinical manifestations (Table 15–10) of pancreatic cancer vary with location and histologic tumor type.

Patients with carcinoma of the head of the pancreas usually present with painless, progressive jaundice resulting from common bile duct obstruction (Figure 15–9). Sometimes the obstruction caused by carcinoma in the head of the pancreas is signaled by the presence of both jaundice and a dilated gallbladder palpable in the right upper quadrant (**Courvoisier's law**). Patients with carcinoma of the body or tail of the pancreas usually present with epigastric abdominal pain, profound weight loss, abdominal mass, and anemia. These patients usually present at later stages and often have distant metastases, particularly in the liver. Splenic vein thrombosis may occur as a complication of cancers in the body or tail of the gland.

About 70% of patients with pancreatic cancer have impaired glucose tolerance or frank diabetes mellitus. While

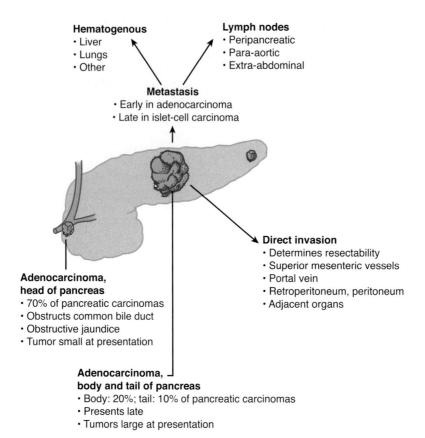

Hematogenous
• Liver
• Lungs
• Other

Lymph nodes
• Peripancreatic
• Para-aortic
• Extra-abdominal

Metastasis
• Early in adenocarcinoma
• Late in islet-cell carcinoma

**Adenocarcinoma,
head of pancreas**
• 70% of pancreatic carcinomas
• Obstructs common bile duct
• Obstructive jaundice
• Tumor small at presentation

Direct invasion
• Determines resectability
• Superior mesenteric vessels
• Portal vein
• Retroperitoneum, peritoneum
• Adjacent organs

**Adenocarcinoma,
body and tail of pancreas**
• Body: 20%; tail: 10% of pancreatic carcinomas
• Presents late
• Tumors large at presentation

FIGURE 15–9   Pancreatic cancer: location and pattern of spread.   (Redrawn, with permission, from Chandrasoma P, Taylor CR. *Concise Pathology,* 3rd ed. Originally published by Appleton & Lange. Copyright © 1998 by the McGraw-Hill Companies, Inc.)

this may be due to proximal ductal obstruction and atrophy of the distal gland, some patients appear to have resolution of impaired glucose tolerance or diabetes with surgical resection, suggesting that pancreatic cancers elaborate a yet unidentified diabetogenic substance.

Adenocarcinomas of the pancreas are sometimes associated with superficial thrombophlebitis or DIC, thought to be related to thromboplastins in the mucinous secretions of the adenocarcinoma. The uncommon acinar cell carcinomas sometimes secrete lipase into the circulation, causing fat necrosis in subcutaneous tissues (manifested as skin rashes) and bone marrow (manifested as lytic bone lesions) throughout the body.

A variety of tumor markers, such as carcinoembryonic antigen (CEA), CA 19-9, alpha-fetoprotein, pancreatic oncofetal antigen, and galactosyl transferase II, can be found in the serum of patients with pancreatic cancer. However, none of these tumor markers have sufficient specificity or predictive value to be useful in screening for the disease. CA 19-9 may be useful to predict recurrence in patients following surgical resection or to follow disease burden in patients who are being treated with systemic chemotherapy.

In evaluating patients who are suspected of having pancreatic cancer, the initial diagnostic test of choice is a contrast-enhanced, thin-cut helical CT scan. For patients with an equivocal or inconclusive CT scan, endoscopic ultrasound with or without fine needle aspiration is recommended to aid in diagnosis. Endoscopic retrograde cannulation of the pancreatic duct (ERCP) with stent placement is useful to relieve obstructive jaundice. In patients with pancreatic head lesions, brushing of the biliary or pancreatic duct during ERCP may confirm the diagnosis of pancreatic adenocarcinoma. With the new imaging technique of positron emission tomography (PET), an increased uptake of the radiolabeled tracer 2-[^{18}F]-fluoro-2-deoxy-D-glucose is seen in about 95% of patients with pancreatic cancer. Such uptake is not seen in patients with chronic pancreatitis. In addition to aiding in diagnosis, helical CT is useful for delineating the regional vascular anatomy and to look for major vascular invasion by tumor, a sign of unresectability, or to determine the presence of metastatic disease.

Clinical prognostic factors have been identified. These include tumor size, tumor site, clinical stage, lymph node metastasis, type of surgery, anemia requiring blood transfusion, performance status, and adjuvant radiation therapy. Prognosis is influenced also by histologic characteristics such as capsular invasion, blood vessel invasion, multicentricity of the tumor, epithelial atypia in the uninvolved areas of the pancreas, and a lymphocytic infiltrate at the tumor margin.

TABLE 15–10 Clinical manifestations of pancreatic carcinoma.

Manifestation	Percentage
Symptoms and signs	
Abdominal pain	73–74%
Anorexia	70%
Weight loss	60–74%
Jaundice[1]	65–72%
Diarrhea	27%
Weakness	21%
Palpable gallbladder	9%
Constipation	8%
Hematemesis or melena	7%
Vomiting	6%
Abdominal mass	1–38%
Migratory thrombophlebitis	< 1%
Abnormal laboratory tests[2]	
↑ Alkaline phosphatase	82%
↑ 5′-Nucleotidase	71%
↑ LDH	69%
↑ AST	64%
↑ Bilirubin	55%
↑ Amylase	17%
↑ α-Fetoprotein	6%
↑ Carcinoembryonic antigen (CEA)	57%
↓ Albumin	60%

Modified from Anderson A, Bergdahl L. Carcinoma of the pancreas. Am Surg. 1976;42:173; Hines LH, Burns RP. Ten years' experience treating pancreatic and peri-ampullary cancer. Am Surg. 1976;42:442.

[1]With carcinoma of the head of the pancreas.

[2]Modified from Fitzgerald PJ et al. The value of diagnostic aids in detecting pancreas cancer. Cancer. 1978;41:868.

Unfortunately, only about 15% of pancreatic carcinomas are diagnosed at an early stage when cure by surgical resection is possible. At present, the overall 5-year survival rate is less than 5%, and only 15–20% of patients undergoing curative tumor resections live longer than 5 years. The poor prognosis is mainly due to the advanced stage of disease by the time of presentation, its extraordinary local tumor progression, and its early systemic dissemination. Patients with metastatic disease have a short median survival (3–6 months), and those with locally advanced, nonmetastatic disease live on average only slightly longer (6–10 months).

CHECKPOINT

13. What are the risk factors for pancreatic cancer?
14. What are common symptoms and signs of pancreatic cancer?
15. How can you make the diagnosis of pancreatic cancer in a patient with suggestive symptoms and signs?

CASE STUDIES

Jonathan Fuchs, MD, MPH, & Yeong Kwok, MD

(See Chapter 25, p. 699 for Answers)

CASE 69

An admitting physician is called to the emergency department to evaluate a 58-year-old woman who presents with a 2-day history of fever, anorexia, nausea, and abdominal pain. Suspecting pancreatitis, the physician inquired about a history of similar symptoms. She was seen 2 months ago in the emergency department for an episode of unrelenting, achy right upper quadrant abdominal pain, at which time ultrasound imaging demonstrated multiple gallstones without evidence of cystic duct obstruction or gallbladder wall edema. At this time, serum amylase and lipase levels are both grossly elevated. On day 3 of her hospital course, the physician is called urgently to evaluate the patient for hypotension, increased shortness of breath, and ensuing respiratory failure. She requires endotracheal intubation and mechanical ventilation. A chest radiograph and severe hypoxia support the diagnosis of acute respiratory distress syndrome.

Questions

A. By what mechanism can biliary stones cause pancreatitis?
B. At the time of admission, what additional historic features and laboratory studies should be obtained to further clarify the etiology of her pancreatitis?
C. Describe how acute pancreatitis may be complicated by acute respiratory distress syndrome.

CASE 70

A 52-year-old man with a 20-year history of alcohol abuse presents to his primary care provider complaining of recurrent episodes of epigastric and left upper quadrant abdominal pain. Over the past month, the pain has become almost continuous, and he has requested morphine for better pain control. He also comments that recently his stool has been bulky and foul smelling. He has a history of alcohol-related acute pancreatitis. Examination reveals a 10-pound weight loss over the past 6 months. He has some mild muscle guarding over the epigastrium with tenderness to palpation. Bowel sounds are somewhat decreased. Serum amylase and lipase are mildly elevated. A plain film of the abdomen demonstrates pancreatic calcifications.

Questions

A. How often do heavy drinkers develop chronic pancreatitis?
B. What are the proposed mechanisms of alcohol-induced chronic pancreatitis?
C. Describe the pathogenesis of steatorrhea.
D. Why may a proton pump inhibitor be helpful for this patient?

CASE 71

During a family reunion, a 62-year-old widower describes to his son a 1-month history of lethargy. He attributed it to the stress of a recent move from a large three-bedroom house into an apartment. His granddaughter comments that his eyes appear "yellow" and that he has lost a significant amount of weight since their last visit with him. Corroborating the finding of painless jaundice, his internist orders a contrast-enhanced spiral CT, revealing a 3-cm mass in the head of the pancreas.

Questions

A. On physical examination, the patient has a palpable and mildly tender gallbladder. What is the significance of this finding?
B. What hematologic abnormalities may be associated with pancreatic cancer?
C. What are some important clinical prognostic factors?

REFERENCES

Acute Pancreatitis

Al Mofleh IA. Severe acute pancreatitis: Pathogenetic aspects and prognostic factors. World J Gastroenterol. 2008 Feb 7;14(5):675–84. [PMID: 18205255]

Alexakis N et al. When is pancreatitis considered to be of biliary origin and what are the implications for management? Pancreatology. 2007;7(2-3):131–41. [PMID: 17592225]

Badalov N et al. Drug-induced acute pancreatitis: An evidence-based review. Clin Gastroenterol Hepatol. 2007 Jun;5(6):648–61. [PMID: 17395548]

Browne GW et al. Pathophysiology of pulmonary complications of acute pancreatitis. World J Gastroenterol. 2006 Nov 28;12(44):7087–96. [PMID: 17131469]

Cappell MS. Acute pancreatitis: Etiology, clinical presentation, diagnosis, and therapy. Med Clin North Am. 2008 Jul;92(4):889–923. [PMID: 18570947]

Cosen-Binker LI et al. Recent insights into the cellular mechanisms of acute pancreatitis. Can J Gastroenterol. 2007 Jan;21(1):19–24. [PMID: 17225878]

De Campos T et al. From acute pancreatitis to end-organ injury: Mechanisms of acute lung injury. Surg Infect (Larchmt). 2007 Feb;8(1):107–20. [PMID: 17381402]

Delhaye M et al. Pancreatic ductal system obstruction and acute recurrent pancreatitis. World J Gastroenterol. 2008 Feb 21;14(7):1027–33. [PMID: 18286683]

Frossard JL et al. Acute pancreatitis. Lancet. 2008 Jan 12;371(9607):143–52. [PMID: 18191686]

Haney JC et al. Necrotizing pancreatitis: Diagnosis and management. Surg Clin North Am. 2007 Dec;87(6):1431–46. [PMID: 18053840]

Hughes SJ et al. Necrotizing pancreatitis. Gastroenterol Clin North Am. 2007 Jun;36(2):313–23. [PMID: 17533081]

Pandol SJ et al. Pathobiology of alcoholic pancreatitis. Pancreatology. 2007;7(2-3):105–14. [PMID: 17592222]

Vonlaufen A et al. The role of inflammatory and parenchymal cells in acute pancreatitis. J Pathol. 2007 Nov;213(3):239–48. [PMID: 17893879]

Witt H et al. Chronic pancreatitis: Challenges and advances in pathogenesis, genetics, diagnosis, and therapy. Gastroenterology. 2007 Apr;132(4):1557–73. [PMID: 17466744]

Zhang XP et al. The pathogenic mechanism of severe acute pancreatitis complicated with renal injury: A review of current knowledge. Dig Dis Sci. 2008 Feb;53(2):297–306. [PMID: 17597411]

Chronic Pancreatitis

Aghdassi A et al. Diagnosis and treatment of pancreatic pseudocysts in chronic pancreatitis. Pancreas. 2008 Mar;36(2):105–12. [PMID: 18376299]

Behrman SW et al. Pathophysiology of chronic pancreatitis. Surg Clin North Am. 2007 Dec;87(6):1309–24. [PMID: 18053833]

Klöppel G. Toward a new classification of chronic pancreatitis. J Gastroenterol. 2007 Jan;42 Suppl 17:55–7. [PMID: 17238028]

Okazaki K et al. Recent advances in autoimmune pancreatitis: Concept, diagnosis, and pathogenesis. J Gastroenterol. 2008;43(6):409–18. [PMID: 18600384]

Hart AR et al. Pancreatic cancer: A review of the evidence on causation. Clin Gastroenterol Hepatol. 2008 Mar;6(3):275–82. [PMID: 18328435]

Keller J et al. Idiopathic chronic pancreatitis. Best Pract Res Clin Gastroenterol. 2008;22(1):105–13. [PMID: 18206816]

Lankisch PG. Chronic pancreatitis. Curr Opin Gastroenterol. 2007 Sep;23(5):502–7. [PMID: 17762555]

Mariani A et al. Is acute recurrent pancreatitis a chronic disease? World J Gastroenterol. 2008 Feb 21;14(7):995–8. [PMID: 18286677]

Nair RJ et al. Chronic pancreatitis. Am Fam Physician. 2007 Dec 1;76(11):1679–88. [PMID: 18092710]

Teich N et al. Hereditary chronic pancreatitis. Best Pract Res Clin Gastroenterol. 2008;22(1):115–30. [PMID: 18206817]

Uomo G et al. Risk factors of chronic pancreatitis. Dig Dis. 2007;25(3):282–4. [PMID: 17827958]

Witt H et al. Chronic pancreatitis: Challenges and advances in pathogenesis, genetics, diagnosis, and therapy. Gastroenterology. 2007 Apr;132(4):1557–73. [PMID: 17466744]

Pancreatic Insufficiency

Andersen DK. Mechanisms and emerging treatments of the metabolic complications of chronic pancreatitis. Pancreas. 2007 Jul;35(1):1–15. [PMID: 17575539]

Domínguez-Muñoz JE. Pancreatic enzyme therapy for pancreatic exocrine insufficiency. Curr Gastroenterol Rep. 2007 Apr;9(2):116–22. [PMID: 17418056]

Stallings VA et al. Clinical Practice Guidelines on Growth and Nutrition Subcommittee; Ad Hoc Working Group. Evidence-based practice recommendations for nutrition-related management of children and adults with cystic fibrosis and pancreatic insufficiency: Results of a systematic review. J Am Diet Assoc. 2008 May;108(5):832–9. [PMID: 18442507]

Pancreatic Cancer

Albo D et al. Translation of recent advances and discoveries in molecular biology and immunology in the diagnosis and treatment of pancreatic cancer. Surg Oncol Clin N Am. 2008 Apr;17(2):357–76. [PMID: 18375357]

Goonetilleke KS et al. Current status of gene expression profiling of pancreatic cancer. Int J Surg. 2008 Feb;6(1):81–3. [PMID: 18359465]

Grocock CJ et al. Familial pancreatic cancer: A review and latest advances. Adv Med Sci. 2007;52:37–49. [PMID: 18217388]

Hart AR et al. Pancreatic cancer: A review of the evidence on causation. Clin Gastroenterol Hepatol. 2008 Mar;6(3):275–82. [PMID: 18328435]

Jensen RT et al. Inherited pancreatic endocrine tumor syndromes: Advances in molecular pathogenesis, diagnosis, management, and controversies. Cancer. 2008 Oct 1;113(7 Suppl):1807–43. [PMID: 18798544]

Koorstra JB et al. Pancreatic carcinogenesis. Pancreatology. 2008;8(2):110–25. [PMID: 18382097]

Korc M. Pancreatic cancer-associated stroma production. Am J Surg. 2007 Oct;194(4 Suppl):S84–6. [PMID: 17903452]

McKay CJ et al. Chronic inflammation and pancreatic cancer. Best Pract Res Clin Gastroenterol. 2008;22(1):65–73. [PMID: 18206813]

Mahadevan D et al. Tumor-stroma interactions in pancreatic ductal adenocarcinoma. Mol Cancer Ther. 2007 Apr;6(4):1186–97. [PMID: 17406031]

Maitra A et al. Pancreatic cancer. Annu Rev Pathol. 2008;3:157–88. [PMID: 18039136]

Saif MW et al. Genetic alterations in pancreatic cancer. World J Gastroenterol. 2007 Sep 7;13(33):4423–30. [PMID: 17724796]

Sarkar FH et al. Pancreatic cancer: Pathogenesis, prevention and treatment. Toxicol Appl Pharmacol. 2007 Nov 1;224(3):326–36. [PMID: 17174370]

Schneider G et al. Molecular biology of pancreatic cancer—New aspects and targets. Anticancer Res. 2008 May-Jun;28(3A):1541–50. [PMID: 18630509]

Singh M et al. Precursor lesions of pancreatic cancer: Molecular pathology and clinical implications. Pancreatology. 2007;7(1):9–19. [PMID: 17449961]

Strimpakos A et al. Pancreatic cancer: From molecular pathogenesis to targeted therapy. Cancer Metastasis Rev. 2008 Sep;27(3):495–522. [PMID: 18427734]

Renal Disease

Benjamin D. Parker, MD, & Joachim H. Ix, MD

16

Patients with renal disease who present early in the course of illness typically have abnormalities of urine volume or composition (eg, presence of red blood cells or abnormal amounts of protein). Later, they manifest systemic symptoms and signs of lost renal function (eg, edema, fluid overload, electrolyte abnormalities, and anemia). Depending on the nature of the renal disease, they may progress—rapidly or slowly—to display a wide range of chronic complications resulting from inadequate residual renal function.

Because there are no pain receptors within the substance of the kidney, pain is a prominent presenting complaint only in those renal diseases (eg, nephrolithiasis) in which there is involvement of the ureter or the renal capsule.

Because of the crucial role of the kidney in filtering blood, a wide range of systemic diseases and disease of other organ systems may be manifested most prominently in the kidney. Thus, renal disease is a prominent presentation of long-standing diabetes mellitus, hypertension, and autoimmune disorders such as systemic lupus erythematosus.

Without treatment, renal disease may result in sufficient loss of kidney function to be incompatible with life. However, not all renal disease has an inexorable downhill course and dismal outcome. The consequences of renal disease depend on the extent and nature of the injury and its natural history and time course. Some forms of renal disease are transient. Even when severe, they may be self-limited and reversible and, if managed properly, may have no permanent consequences. Other forms progress eventually to renal failure, either rapidly or slowly, with associated metabolic and hemodynamic consequences. When renal disease progresses, there can be loss of renal filtration capacity (eg, disordered regulation of body electrolyte and volume status) as well as loss of nonexcretory renal functions such as the production of erythropoietin, resulting in anemia.

CHECKPOINT

1. What are some important causes of renal disease?
2. What are some consequences of renal failure?

NORMAL STRUCTURE & FUNCTION OF THE KIDNEY

ANATOMY, HISTOLOGY, & CELL BIOLOGY

The kidneys are a pair of encapsulated organs located in the retroperitoneal area (Figure 16–1). A renal artery enters and a renal vein exits from each kidney at the hilum. Approximately 25% of cardiac output goes to the kidneys. Blood is filtered in the kidneys, removing wastes—in particular urea and nitrogen-containing compounds—and regulating extracellular electrolytes and intravascular volume. Because renal blood flow is from cortex to medulla and because the medulla has a relatively low blood flow for a high rate of metabolic activity, the normal oxygen tension in the medulla is lower than in other parts of the kidney. This makes the medulla particularly susceptible to ischemic injury.

The anatomic unit of kidney function is the **nephron,** a structure consisting of a tuft of capillaries termed the **glomerulus,** the site at which blood is filtered, and a **renal tubule** from which water and salts in the filtrate are reclaimed (Figure 16–2). Each human kidney has approximately 1 million nephrons.

A glomerulus consists of an **afferent** and an **efferent arteriole** and an intervening tuft of capillaries lined by endothelial

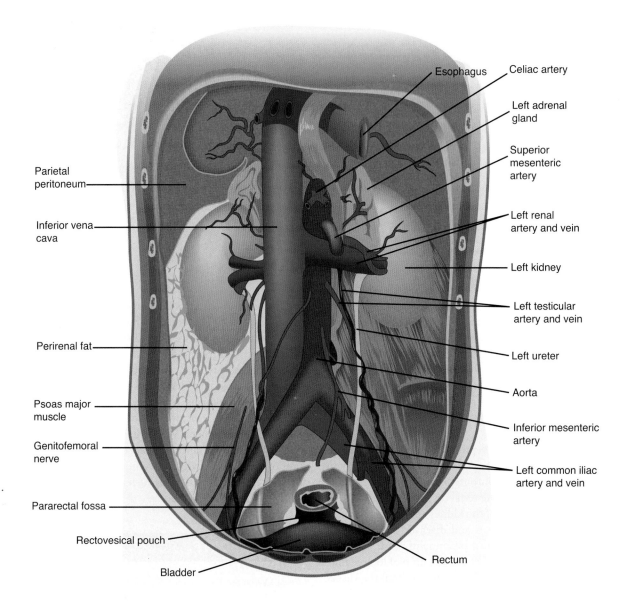

FIGURE 16–1   Vessels and organs of the retroperitoneum.   (Redrawn, with permission, from Lindner HH. *Clinical Anatomy.* Originally published by Appleton & Lange. Copyright © 1989 by the McGraw-Hill Companies, Inc.)

cells and covered by epithelial cells that form a continuous layer with those of **Bowman's capsule** and the renal tubule. The space between capillaries in the glomerulus is called the **mesangium.** Material comprising a basement membrane is located between the capillary endothelial cells and the epithelial cells (Figure 16–2).

Closer examination of glomerular histology and cell biology reveals features not found in most peripheral capillaries (Figure 16–2). First, the glomerular capillary endothelium is fenestrated. However, because the endothelial cells have a coat of negatively charged glycoproteins and glycosaminoglycans, they normally exclude plasma proteins such as albumin. On the other side of the glomerular basement membrane are the epithelial cells. Termed "podocytes" because of their numer-

ous extensions or foot processes, these cells are connected to one another by modified desmosomes.

The mesangium is an extension of the glomerular basement membrane but is less dense and contains two distinct cell types: intrinsic glomerular cells and tissue macrophages. Both cell types contribute to the development of immune-mediated glomerular disease by their production of, and response to, cytokines such as transforming growth factor-β (TGF-β).

The complex organization of the glomerulus is crucial not only for renal function but also for explaining the differences observed in glomerular disease. Thus, in some conditions immune complexes may accumulate under the epithelial cells, whereas in others they accumulate under the endothelial cells. Likewise, because immune cells are not able to cross the glo-

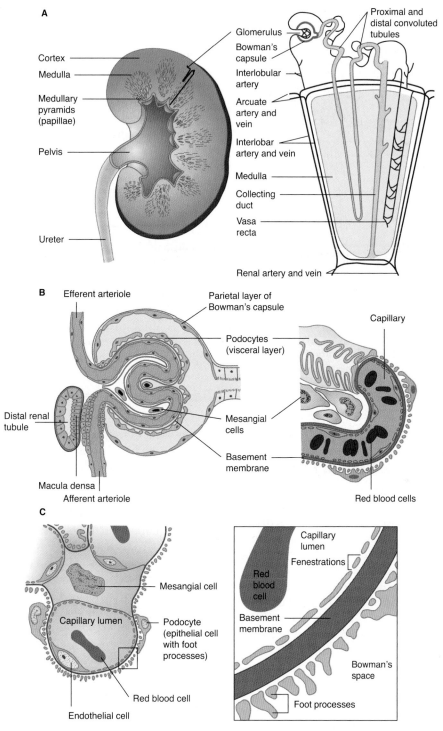

FIGURE 16–2 Structures of the kidney. **A:** Landmarks of the normal kidney. **B:** Glomerulus and glomerular capillary. **C:** Detailed structure of the glomerulus and the glomerular filtration membrane composed of endothelial cell, basement membrane, and podocyte. Note that for clarity the distal tubule is separated from the glomerulus in **A;** however, its true anatomic relationship, which is essential for physiologic function, is illustrated in **B.** (Redrawn, with permission, from Chandrasoma P, Taylor CE. *Concise Pathology,* 3rd ed. Originally published by Appleton & Lange. Copyright © 1998 by the McGraw-Hill Companies, Inc.)

merular basement membrane, immune complex deposition under the epithelial cells is generally not accompanied by a cellular inflammatory reaction (see later discussion).

The renal tubule itself has a number of different structural regions: the **proximal convoluted tubule,** from which approximately 80% of the electrolytes and water are reclaimed; the **loop of Henle;** and a **distal convoluted tubule** and **collecting duct** (Figure 16–3), where the urine is concentrated and additional electrolyte and water changes are made in response to hormonal control.

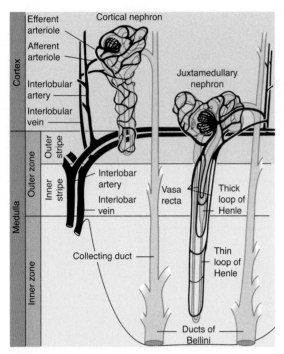

FIGURE 16–3   The vascular supply of the cortical and juxtamedullary nephrons.   (Redrawn, with permission, from Pitts RF. *Physiology of the Kidney and Body Fluids*, 3rd ed. Year Book, 1963.)

PHYSIOLOGY

Glomerular Filtration & Tubular Resorption

Approximately 120 mL/min of glomerular filtrate are generated in a normal person with two fully functional kidneys. The approximate mass cutoff of substances for filtration is 70 kDa. However, substances smaller than this are often retained, sometimes because of charge effects or because they are tightly bound to other proteins to give them a larger effective size.

After filtration at the glomerulus, most of the Na^+—and, under normal conditions, almost all of the K^+ and glucose—is actively resorbed from the tubular fluid in the proximal tubule. Water is resorbed osmotically. In addition to absorption, a number of substances are secreted into the tubular fluid through the action of transporters along the renal tubule. Examples of substances that are secreted include organic anions and cations such as creatinine, histamine, and many drugs and toxins.

Normally, about 30 mL/min of isotonic filtrate is delivered to the loops of Henle, where a countercurrent multiplier mechanism achieves concentration of the urine. The loop of Henle passes down into the medulla of the kidney, where secretion of Na^+ from the cells in the thick ascending limb establishes a hypertonic concentration gradient to reabsorb water from the tubular fluid across the cells of the descending limb.

Under normal circumstances, no more than 5–10 mL/min of glomerular filtrate is delivered to the collecting ducts. Water absorption in the collecting ducts occurs directly through water channels controlled by **vasopressin** (also known as **antidiuretic hormone [ADH]**). Under the control of aldosterone, Na^+ resorption from tubular fluid and K^+ and H^+ transport into tubular fluid occur in different types of cells in the renal collecting ducts. Phosphoric and sulfuric acid and other acids are not volatile and, therefore, cannot be excreted by the lungs. Instead, they must be excreted as salts by the kidney and are thus termed "fixed acids." Urinary excretion of fixed acids also occurs in the collecting duct. Even though it deals with less than one tenth of the total glomerular filtrate, the collecting duct is the site of regulation of urine volume and the site at which water, Na^+, acid-base, and K^+ balance are achieved. The crucial role of the collecting duct in regulation of kidney function depends on two features: First, the collecting duct is under hormonal control, in contrast to the proximal tubule, whose actions are generally a simple function of volume and composition of tubular fluid and constitutively active transporters. Second, the collecting duct is the last region of the renal tubule traversed before the remaining 1–2 mL/min of the original glomerular filtrate exits into the ureters as urine. Insight into the functional roles of the proximal and distal renal tubules can be seen in the clinical features of the various forms of renal tubular acidosis (Table 16–1).

Renal Regulation of Blood Pressure

The kidney plays an important role in blood pressure regulation by virtue of its effect on Na^+ and water balance, major determinants of blood pressure. First, the Na^+ concentration in the proximal tubular fluid is sensed at the macula densa (Figure 16–2), part of the **juxtaglomerular apparatus.** The juxtaglomerular apparatus also assesses the perfusion pressure of the blood, an important indicator of intravascular volume status under normal circumstances. Through the action of these two sensors, either low Na^+ or low perfusion pressure acts as a stimulus to renin release. **Renin,** a protease made in the juxtaglomerular cells, cleaves angiotensinogen in the blood to generate **angiotensin I,** which is then cleaved to **angiotensin II** by **angiotensin-converting enzyme** (**ACE**). Angiotensin II raises blood pressure by triggering vasoconstriction directly and by stimulating aldosterone secretion, resulting in Na^+ and water retention by the collecting duct. All of these effects expand the extracellular fluid (ECF) and hence renal perfusion pressure, completing a homeostatic negative feedback loop that alleviates the initial stimulus for renin release.

Intravascular volume depletion also triggers vasopressin release. Receptors in the carotid body and elsewhere sense a fall in blood pressure and activate autonomic neural pathways, including fibers that go to the hypothalamus, where vasopressin release is controlled. Vasopressin is released and travels via the bloodstream throughout the body. At the collecting duct renal tubular apical plasma membrane, vasopressin facilitates insertion of water channels, thereby increasing the number of water channels. This results in reabsorption of free water. Further discussions of water balance and the role of vasopressin are presented in Chapter 19.

TABLE 16–1 Characteristics of the different types of renal tubular acidosis.[1]

	Type 1 (Distal)	Type 2 (Proximal)	Type 4
Basic defect	Decreased distal acidification (eg, due to H^+-ATPase defect, reduced cortical Na^+ reabsorption, or increased membrane permeability)	Diminished proximal HCO_3^- reabsorption (eg, due to impaired Na^+-K^+ ATPase, Na^+-H^+ exchange, or carbonic anhydrase deficiency)	Aldosterone deficiency or resistance
Urine pH during acidemia	> 5.3	Variable: > 5.3 if above reabsorptive threshold; < 5.3 if below	Usually < 5.3
Plasma [HCO_3^-], untreated	May be below 10 mEq/L	Usually 14–20 mEq/L	Usually above 15 mEq/L
Fractional excretion of HCO_3^- at normal plasma [HCO_3^-]	< 3% in adults; may reach 5–10% in young children	> 15–20%	< 3%
Diagnosis	Response to $NaHCO_3$ or NH_4Cl	Response to $NaHCO_3$	Measure plasma aldosterone concentration
Plasma [K^+]	Usually reduced or normal; elevated with voltage defect	Normal or reduced	Elevated
Dose of HCO_3^- to normalize plasma [HCO_3^-], mEq/kg per day	1–2 in adults; 4–14 in children	10–15	1–3; may require no alkali if hyperkalemia corrected
Nonelectrolyte complications	Nephrocalcinosis and renal stones	Rickets or osteomalacia	None

Modified, with permission, from Rose BD. *Clinical Physiology of Acid-Base and Electrolyte Disorders,* 4th ed. McGraw-Hill, 1993.

[1]What was once called type 3 RTA is actually a variant of type 1.

From rat studies, it appears that nephron number is programmed in utero. Some have speculated that low nephron number at birth (normal range: 0.3–1.4 million per kidney) predisposes an individual to the development of essential hypertension in adulthood. Maternal malnutrition sufficiently severe to produce a small-for-gestational-age infant may also result in a nephron number at the lower end of the normal range, thus also predisposing to hypertension in adulthood.

Renal Regulation of Ca^{2+} Metabolism

The kidney plays a number of important roles in Ca^{2+} and phosphate homeostasis. First, the kidney is the site of 1α-hydroxylation or 24-hydroxylation of 25-hydroxycholecalciferol, the hepatic metabolite of vitamin D_3. This increases Ca^{2+} absorption from the gut. Second, the kidney is a site of action of **parathyroid hormone** (**PTH**), resulting in Ca^{2+} retention and phosphate wasting in the urine. Further discussion of the role of the kidney in Ca^{2+} and phosphate homeostasis is presented in Chapter 17.

Renal Regulation of Erythropoiesis

The kidney is the main site of production of the hormone **erythropoietin,** which stimulates bone marrow production and maturation of red blood cells. Thus, when untreated, patients with end-stage renal disease typically display a profound anemia, with hematocrit levels in the range of 20–25%, and they improve in response to erythropoietin (epoetin alpha) administration.

Regulation of Renal Function

There are a variety of physical, hormonal, and neural mechanisms by which the functions of the kidney are controlled. Vasopressin, together with the physics of the countercurrent multiplier in the loop of Henle and the hypertonic medullary interstitium, makes it possible to concentrate the urine under normal circumstances. This confers on the healthy kidney the ability to maintain fluid homeostasis under widely diverse conditions (by generating either a concentrated or dilute urine, depending on whether the body needs to conserve or excrete salt and water).

Tubuloglomerular feedback refers to the ability of the kidney to regulate the glomerular filtration rate (GFR) in response to the solute concentration in the distal renal tubule. When an excessive concentration of Na^+ in the tubular fluid is sensed by the **macula densa,** afferent arteriolar vasoconstriction is triggered. This diminishes the GFR so that the renal tubule has a smaller solute load per unit time, allowing Na^+ to be more efficiently reclaimed from tubular fluid. A variety of vasoactive substances, including adenosine, prostaglandins, nitric oxide, and peptides such as endothelin and bradykinin, contribute to the humoral control of tubuloglomerular feedback.

Another important challenge for the kidney is regulation of renal cortical versus medullary blood flow. Renal cortical blood flow needs to be sufficient to maintain a GFR high enough to clear renally excreted wastes efficiently without exceeding the capacity of the renal tubules for solute reabsorption. Likewise, medullary blood flow must be closely regulated. Excessive medullary blood flow can disrupt the osmolar gradient achieved by the countercurrent exchange mechanism. Insufficient medullary blood flow can result in anoxic injury to the renal tubule. From the perspective of individual nephrons, redistribution of blood flow from cortex to medulla involves preferentially supplying blood (and, therefore, oxygen) to those nephrons with long loops of Henle that dip down into the inner medulla.

Adaptations of the kidney to injury can also be thought of as a form of regulation. Thus, loss of nephrons results in compensatory **glomerular hyperfiltration** (increased GFR per nephron) and renal hypertrophy. Although hyperfiltration may be adaptive in the short term, allowing maintenance of the total renal GFR, it has been implicated as a common inciting event in further nephron destruction from a variety of causes.

There are other clinically important adaptations to injury. Poor renal perfusion from any cause results in responses that improve perfusion through afferent arteriolar vasodilation and efferent arteriolar vasoconstriction in response to hormonal and neural cues. These regulatory effects are reinforced by inputs sensing Na^+ balance. Alteration of Na^+ balance is another way to influence blood pressure and hence renal perfusion pressure. Sympathetic innervation by the renal nerves influences renin release. Renal prostaglandins play an important role in vasodilation, especially in patients with chronically poor renal perfusion.

CHECKPOINT

3. What are the parts of the nephron, and what role does each part play in renal function?
4. How is renal function regulated?
5. What are the nonexcretory functions of the kidney?
6. What are the relationships, if any, between each nonexcretory function named previously and the kidney's role in fluid, electrolyte, and blood pressure regulation?

OVERVIEW OF RENAL DISEASE

ALTERATIONS OF KIDNEY STRUCTURE & FUNCTION IN DISEASE

Renal disease can be categorized either by the site of the lesion (eg, glomerulopathy vs. tubulointerstitial disease) or by the nature of the factors that have led to kidney disease (eg, immunologic, metabolic, infiltrative, infectious, hemodynamic, or toxic).

Glomerular disease can be further categorized according to clinical presentation. Thus, some disorders present with profound proteinuria but no evidence of a cellular inflammatory reaction (nephrotic disorders), whereas others have variable degrees of proteinuria associated with red and white blood cells in the urine (nephritic disorders).

Nephrotic disorders typically show immune complex deposition at or under the epithelial cells, often with morphologic changes in the foot processes (Figure 16–4). This probably reflects damage to the selective nature of the glomerular filter (eg, by immune complex formation) or deposition of preformed complexes, in some cases with complement activation but without concomitant activation of a cellular immune response. Although the lack of a cellular immune response may limit the damage done, it also slows the resolution of the disorder, with proteinuria taking months or years to resolve even when the underlying disease has been brought under control.

Nephritic disorders show immune complex deposits either in a subendothelial location or in the glomerular basement membrane or mesangium (Figure 16–4). The cellular immune system has ready access to all of these locations, and the resulting inflammatory reaction can be a two-edged sword. Thus, when the underlying process can be controlled, phagocytosis of the subendothelial deposits speeds recovery. On the other hand, an uncontrolled or prolonged inflammatory response can result in a greater degree of destruction of glomerular architecture, in part because of the local production and action of cytokines.

Certain regions of the kidney are particularly susceptible to certain kinds of injury: (1) The renal medulla is a low oxygen tension environment, which makes it more susceptible to ischemic injury. (2) The glomerulus is the initial filter of blood entering the kidney and thus is a prominent site of injury related to immune complex deposition and complement fixation. (3) Hemodynamic factors regulating blood flow have profound effects on the kidney both because the GFR, a primary determinant of renal function, depends on blood flow and because the kidney is susceptible to hypoxic injury.

One useful organizing scheme that combines a consideration of both the site and the cause of renal disease in approaching patients with new renal failure is to first categorize the cause of the patient's renal failure as prerenal, intrarenal, or postrenal and then to subdivide each of these categories according to specific causes and anatomic locations (Table 16–2).

Prerenal causes of renal failure are those resulting from inadequate blood flow to the kidney. These include intravascular volume depletion, structural lesions of the renal arteries, drug effects on renal blood flow, and hypotension from any cause that results in renal hypoperfusion.

Intrarenal causes are those disorders that result in damage to the nephron directly rather than indirectly as a secondary consequence of inadequate perfusion or obstruction. As mentioned, intrarenal causes include specific disorders of the kidney as well as systemic diseases with prominent manifestations in the kidney. Some of these disorders are manifested as glomerular injury, whereas others involve primarily the tubules.

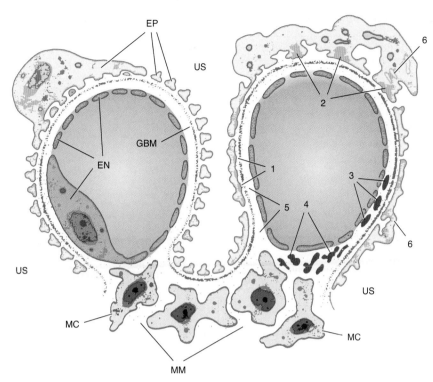

FIGURE 16–4 Anatomy of a normal glomerular capillary is shown on the left. Note the fenestrated endothelium (EN), glomerular basement membrane (GBM), and the epithelium with its foot processes (EP). The mesangium is composed of mesangial cells (MC) surrounded by extracellular matrix (MM) in direct contact with the endothelium. Ultrafiltration occurs across the glomerular wall and through channels in the mesangial matrix into the urinary space (US). Typical localization of immune deposits and other pathologic changes is depicted on the right. (1) Uniform subepithelial deposits as in membranous nephropathy. (2) Large, irregular subepithelial deposits or "humps" seen in acute postinfectious glomerulonephritis. (3) Subendothelial deposits as in diffuse proliferative lupus glomerulonephritis. (4) Mesangial deposits characteristic of immunoglobulin A nephropathy. (5) Antibody binding to the glomerular basement membrane (as in Goodpasture's syndrome) does not produce visible deposits, but a smooth linear pattern is seen on immunofluorescence. (6) Effacement of the epithelial foot processes is common in all forms of glomerular injury with proteinuria.   (Redrawn, with permission, from Luke RG et al. Nephrology and hypertension. In: *Medical Knowledge Self-Assessment Program IX.* American College of Physicians, 1992.)

Within each category, disorders can be approached according to their specific cause or their phenotype and manifestations.

Postrenal causes are those related to urinary tract obstruction, from either kidney stones, structural lesions (eg, tumors, prostatic hyperplasia, or strictures), or functional abnormalities (eg, spasm or drug effects).

MANIFESTATIONS OF ALTERED KIDNEY FUNCTION

The major manifestations of altered kidney function are the effects on excretion of urea and on maintenance of Na^+, K^+, water, and acid-base balance. Failure to excrete urea adequately, manifested as progressive elevation of blood urea nitrogen (BUN) and serum creatinine, results in uremia (see Chronic Renal Failure). Uremia can be characterized by a variety of clinical abnormalities (see Table 16–7), presumably caused by a buildup of one or more uncharacterized toxins. These toxins may be normally formed in the body and excreted in the urine, or a new substance may be formed as a consequence of altered

metabolism in kidney failure. In the absence of adequate renal clearance mechanisms, ingestion of excess amounts of Na^+, K^+, water, or acids results in electrolyte, volume, and acid-base abnormalities that can be life threatening. Furthermore, excess Na^+ ingestion in a patient with renal failure results in intravascular volume expansion, with complications of hypertension and congestive heart failure.

CHECKPOINT

7. What characteristics of various parts of the nephron make it particularly susceptible to certain types of injury?

8. What are the features that distinguish prerenal, intrarenal, and postrenal causes of renal failure?

9. What are the major categories of complications of inadequate renal function?

TABLE 16–2　**Major causes of kidney disease.**

Prerenal disease	Tubular disease
True volume depletion	Acute
Gastrointestinal, renal, or sweat losses or bleeding	Acute tubular necrosis
Heart failure	Multiple myeloma
Hepatic cirrhosis (including the hepatorenal syndrome)	Hypercalcemia
Nephrotic syndrome (particularly after diuretic therapy for edema)	Uric acid nephropathy
Hypotension	Chronic
Nonsteroidal anti-inflammatory drugs	Polycystic kidney disease
Bilateral renal artery stenosis (particularly after therapy with an angiotensin-converting enzyme inhibitor)	Medullary sponge kidney
Intrarenal disease	Interstitial disease
Vascular disease	Acute
Acute	Pyelonephritis
Vasculitis	Interstitial nephritis (usually drug-induced)
Malignant hypertension	Chronic
Scleroderma	Pyelonephritis (due primarily to vesicoureteral reflux)
Thromboembolic disease	Analgesic abuse
Chronic	**Postrenal disease**
Nephrosclerosis	Obstructive uropathy
Glomerular disease	Prostatic disease
Glomerulonephritis	Malignancy
Nephrotic syndrome	Calculi
	Congenital abnormalities

Data from Rose BD. Diagnostic approach to patient with renal disease. In: *Pathophysiology of Renal Disease,* 2nd ed. McGraw-Hill, 1987.

PATHOPHYSIOLOGY OF SELECTED RENAL DISEASES

ACUTE KIDNEY INJURY

Clinical Presentation

Acute kidney injury is produced by a heterogeneous group of disorders that have in common the rapid deterioration of renal function, resulting in accumulation in the blood of nitrogenous wastes that would normally be excreted in the urine. The patient presents with a rapidly rising BUN and serum creatinine. Depending on the cause and when the patient comes to medical attention, there may be other presenting features as well (Table 16–3). Thus, diminished urine volume (oliguria) is commonly but not always seen. Urine volume may be normal early or indeed at any time in milder forms of acute kidney injury. Patients presenting relatively late may display any of the clinical manifestations described later.

Etiology

The major causes of acute kidney injury are presented in Table 16–4.

A. Prerenal Causes

As demonstrated by the Starling equation, filtration across a glomerulus is determined by the hydrostatic and oncotic pressures in both the glomerular capillary and its surrounding tubular lumen as described by the relationship: filtration = $K_f [P_c -] P_t] - \sigma[\pi_c - \pi_t]$. K_f and σ are constants determined by

TABLE 16–3 Initial clinical and laboratory data base for defining major syndromes in nephrology.

Syndrome	Important Clues to Diagnosis	Common Findings Not of Diagnostic Value
Acute or rapidly progressive renal failure	Anuria	Hypertension
	Oliguria	Hematuria, proteinuria, pyuria, casts
	Documented recent decline in GFR	Edema
Acute nephritis	Hematuria, red cell casts	Proteinuria, pyuria
	Azotemia, oliguria	Circulatory congestion
	Edema, hypertension	
Chronic renal failure	Azotemia for > 3 months	Hematuria, proteinuria, casts
	Prolonged symptoms or signs of uremia	Oliguria, polyuria, nocturia
	Symptoms or signs of renal osteodystrophy	Edema, hypertension
	Kidneys reduced in size bilaterally	Electrolyte disorders
	Broad casts in urinary sediment	
Nephrotic syndrome	Proteinuria > 3.5 g/1.73 m^2 per 24 hours	Casts
	Hypoalbuminemia	Edema
	Hyperlipidemia	
	Lipiduria	
Asymptomatic urinary abnormalities	Hematuria	
	Proteinuria (below nephrotic range)	
	Sterile pyuria, casts	
Urinary tract infection	Bacteriuria > 10^5 colonies/mL	Hematuria
	Other infectious agent documented in urine	Mild azotemia
	Pyuria, leukocyte casts	Mild proteinuria
	Frequency, urgency	Fever
	Bladder tenderness, flank tenderness	
Renal tubular defects	Electrolyte disorders	Hematuria
	Polyuria, nocturia	Mild azotemia
	Symptoms or signs of renal osteodystrophy	Mild proteinuria
	Large kidneys	Fever
	Renal transport defects	
Hypertension	Systolic/diastolic hypertension	Proteinuria
		Casts
		Azotemia
Nephrolithiasis	History of stone passage or removal	Hematuria
	Stone seen by x-ray	Pyuria
	Renal colic	Frequency, urgency
Urinary tract obstruction	Azotemia, oliguria, anuria	Hematuria
	Polyuria, nocturia, urinary retention	Pyuria
	Slowing of urinary stream	Enuresis, dysuria
	Large prostate, large kidneys	
	Flank tenderness, full bladder after voiding	

TABLE 16–4 **Major causes of acute kidney injury.**

Disorder	Examples
Hypovolemia	Volume loss via the skin, gastrointestinal tract, or kidney. Hemorrhage. Sequestration of extracellular fluid (burns, pancreatitis, peritonitis).
Cardiovascular failure	Impaired cardiac output (infarction, tamponade). Vascular pooling (anaphylaxis, sepsis, drugs).
Extrarenal obstruction	Urethral occlusion: vesical, pelvic, prostatic, or retroperitoneal neoplasms. Surgical accident. Medication. Calculi. Pus, blood clots.
Intrarenal obstruction	Crystals (uric acid, oxalic acid, sulfonamides, methotrexate).
Bladder rupture	Trauma.
Vascular diseases	Vasculitis. Malignant hypertension. Thrombotic thrombocytopenia purpura. Scleroderma. Arterial or venous occlusion.
Glomerulonephritis	Immune complex disease. Anti-GBM disease.
Interstitial nephritis	Drugs. Hypercalcemia. Infections. Idiopathic.
Postischemic	All conditions listed above under hypovolemia and cardiovascular failure.
Pigment-induced	Hemolysis (transfusion reaction, malaria). Rhabdomyolysis (trauma, muscle disease, coma, heat stroke, severe exercise, potassium or phosphate depletion).
Poison-induced	Antibiotics. Contrast material. Anesthetic agents. Heavy metals. Organic solvents.
Pregnancy-related	Septic abortion. Uterine hemorrhage. Eclampsia.

Reproduced, with permission, from Andersen RJ, Schrier RW. Acute renal failure. In: *Harrison's Principles of Internal Medicine*, 12th ed. Wilson JD et al (editors). McGraw-Hill, 1991.

the permeability of a given glomerulus and the effective contribution of osmotic pressure, respectively; P_c = intracapillary hydrostatic pressure, π_c = intracapillary oncotic pressure, P_t = intratubular hydrostatic pressure, and π_t = intratubular oncotic pressure. Perturbations in any of the above factors may alter renal filtration. Of particular importance is the intracapillary hydrostatic pressure which is determined by relative blood flow into and out of the glomerular capillary. A normal kidney has the unique ability to autoregulate blood flow both in and out of the glomerular capillary through alterations in resistance of the afferent and efferent arterioles across a wide range of systemic blood pressure. Most capillary beds only possess the former. Lower relative flows into the glomerulus with decreased renal blood flow or afferent artery constriction may lower intracapillary hydrostatic pressure and diminish filtration. Likewise, higher relative flows out of glomerulus with efferent artery dilation may also lower intracapillary hydrostatic pressure. Some patients who are dependent on prostaglandin-mediated vasodilation to maintain renal perfusion can develop renal failure simply from ingestion of nonsteroidal anti-inflammatory drugs (NSAIDs). Similarly, patients

with renal hypoperfusion (eg, from renal artery stenosis, congestive heart failure, or intrarenal small vessel disease) who are dependent on angiotensin II–mediated vasoconstriction of the efferent renal arterioles to maintain renal perfusion pressure may develop acute kidney injury on ingesting ACE inhibitors.

B. Intrarenal Causes

The intrarenal causes can be further divided into specific **inflammatory diseases** (eg, vasculitis, glomerulonephritis, drug-induced injury) and **acute tubular necrosis** resulting from many causes (including ischemia, poisons, and hemolysis).

Notable among intrarenal causes are the toxic effects of aminoglycoside antibiotics and rhabdomyolysis, in which myoglobin, released into the bloodstream after crush injury to muscle, precipitates in the renal tubules. The former may be mitigated by close monitoring of renal function during antibiotic therapy, especially in elderly patients and those with some degree of underlying renal compromise. Rhabdomyolysis may be detected by obtaining a serum creatine kinase level in patients admitted to the hospital with trauma or altered mental status and may be mitigated by maintaining a vigorous alkaline diuresis to prevent myoglobin precipitation in the tubules.

Sepsis is one of the most common causes of acute kidney injury. As a complication of sepsis, acute kidney injury involves a combination of prerenal and intrarenal factors. The prerenal factor is renal hypoperfusion as a consequence of the hypotensive, low systemic vascular resistance septic state. The intrarenal component may be a consequence of the cytokine dysregulation that characterizes the sepsis syndrome (Chapter 4), including elevated blood levels of tumor necrosis factor, interleukin-1, and interleukin-6, which contribute to intrarenal inflammation, sclerosis, and obstruction. Patients with sepsis are often exposed also to nephrotoxic drugs such as aminoglycoside antibiotics.

C. Postrenal Causes

The postrenal causes are those that result in urinary tract obstruction, such as renal stones.

Pathology & Pathogenesis

Regardless of their origin, all forms of acute kidney injury, if untreated, result in acute tubular necrosis, with sloughing of cells that make up the renal tubule. Depending on the timing of intervention between onset of initial injury and eventual acute tubular necrosis, acute kidney injury may be irreversible or reversible, with either prevention of or recovery from acute tubular necrosis.

The precise molecular mechanisms responsible for the development of acute tubular necrosis remain unknown. Theories favoring either a tubular or vascular basis have been proposed (Figure 16–5). According to the tubular theory, occlusion of the tubular lumen with cellular debris forms a cast that increases intratubular pressure sufficiently to offset perfusion pressure and decrease or abolish net filtration pressure. Vascular theories propose that decreased renal perfusion pressure from the combination of afferent arteriolar vasoconstriction and efferent

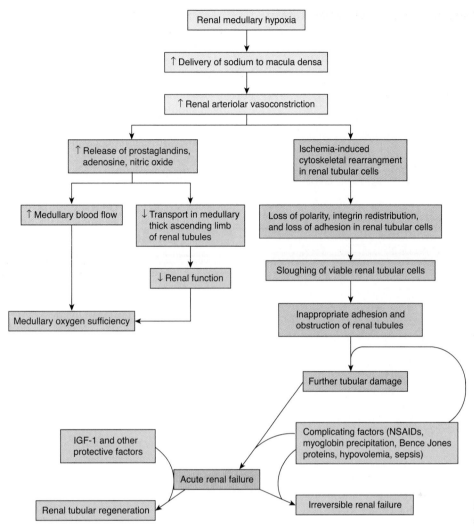

FIGURE 16–5 Pathophysiology of ischemia-induced acute kidney injury. Mild or uncomplicated medullary hypoxia results in tubuloglomerular reflex adjustments that restore medullary oxygen sufficiency at the price of diminished renal function. However, in the event of extreme renal medullary hypoxia or when associated with complicating factors such as those indicated in the figure, full-blown acute kidney injury develops. Whether acute kidney injury is reversible or irreversible depends on a balance of reparative and complicating factors.

arteriolar vasodilation reduces glomerular perfusion pressure and, therefore, glomerular filtration. It may be that both mechanisms act to produce acute kidney injury, varying in relative importance in different individuals depending on the cause and time of presentation. Studies suggest that one consequence of hypoxia is disordered adhesion of renal tubular epithelial cells, resulting both in their exfoliation and subsequent adhesion to other cells of the tubule, thereby contributing to tubular obstruction (Figure 16–5). Another consequence may be dysregulation of elements that secure tubular cells together resulting in leak of filtrate out of the tubular lumen and abnormal sorting of cellular transmembrane channels required for the normal function of the nephron. Renal damage, whether caused by tubular occlusion or vascular hypoperfusion, is potentiated by the hypoxic state of the renal medulla, which increases the risk of ischemia (Table 16–5). Research has implicated cytokines and endogenous peptides such as endothelins and the regulation of their production as possible explanations

for why, subjected to the same toxic insult, some patients develop acute kidney injury and others do not and why some with acute kidney injury recover and others do not. It appears that these products together with activation of complement and neutrophils increase vasoconstriction in the already ischemic renal medulla and in that way exacerbate the degree of hypoxic injury that occurs in acute kidney injury.

Clinical Manifestations

The initial symptoms are typically fatigue and malaise, probably early consequences of loss of the ability to excrete water, salt, and wastes via the kidneys. Later, more profound symptoms and signs of loss of renal water and salt excretory capacity develop: dyspnea, orthopnea, rales, a prominent third heart sound (S_3), and peripheral edema. Altered mental status reflects the toxic effect of uremia on the brain, with elevated blood levels of nitrogenous wastes and fixed acids.

TABLE 16–5 Agents and events that ameliorate or exacerbate hypoxia in the renal medulla.

Ameliorating effect
Decreased tubular transport
Decreased glomerular filtration rate
Prostaglandin E_2
Adenosine
Bradykinin
Nitric oxide
Exacerbating effect
Polyene antibiotics (eg, amphotericin B)
Renal hypertrophy
Nonsteroidal anti-inflammatory drugs
Angiotensin II
Calcium
Myoglobin
Radiographic contrast agents

Modified and reproduced, with permission, from Brezis M, Rosen S. Hypoxia of the renal medulla: Its implications for disease. N Engl J Med. 1995;332:647.

The clinical manifestations of acute kidney injury depend not only on the cause but also on the stage in the natural history of the disease at which the patient comes to medical attention. Patients with renal hypoperfusion (prerenal causes of acute kidney injury) first develop **prerenal azotemia** (elevated BUN without tubular necrosis), a direct physiologic consequence of a decreased GFR. With appropriate treatment, renal perfusion can typically be improved, prerenal azotemia can be readily reversed, and the development of acute tubular necrosis can be prevented. Without treatment, prerenal azotemia may progress to acute tubular necrosis. Recovery from acute tubular necrosis, if it occurs, will then follow a more protracted course, often requiring supportive dialysis before adequate renal function is regained.

A variety of clinical tests can help determine whether a patient with signs of acute kidney injury is in the early phase of prerenal azotemia or has progressed to full-blown acute tubular necrosis. However, the overlap in clinical presentation along the continuum between pre-renal azotemia and acute tubular necrosis is such that the results of any one of these tests must be interpreted in the context of other findings and the clinical history.

Perhaps the earliest manifestation of prerenal azotemia is an elevated ratio of BUN to serum creatinine. Normally 10–15:1, this ratio may rise to 20–30:1 in prerenal azotemia, with a normal or near-normal serum creatinine. If the patient proceeds to acute tubular necrosis, this ratio may return to normal but with a progressively elevated serum creatinine.

Likewise, a fluctuating but not inexorably rising serum creatinine suggests prerenal azotemia.

Urinalysis may also be useful. There are no typical abnormal findings in simple prerenal azotemia, whereas granular casts, tubular epithelial cells, and epithelial cell casts are found in acute tubular necrosis. Casts are formed when debris in the renal tubules (protein, red cells, or epithelial cells) takes on the cylindric, smooth-bordered shape of the tubule. Likewise, because hypovolemia is a stimulus to vasopressin release (see Chapter 19), the urine is maximally concentrated (up to 1500 mOsm/L) in prerenal azotemia. However, with progression to acute tubular necrosis, the ability to generate a concentrated urine is largely lost. Thus, a urine osmolality of less than 350 mOsm/L is a typical finding in acute tubular necrosis.

Finally, the fractional excretion of Na^+

$$FE_{Na^+}[\%] = \frac{Urine_{Na^+}/Plasma_{Na^+}}{Urine_{Cr}/Plasma_{Cr}} \times 100$$

is an important indicator in oliguric acute kidney injury to determine whether a patient has progressed from simple prerenal azotemia to frank acute tubular necrosis. In simple prerenal azotemia, more than 99% of filtered Na^+ is reabsorbed. This value allows accurate identification of Na^+ retention states (such as prerenal azotemia) even when there is water retention as a result of vasopressin release. With progression of prerenal azotemia to acute kidney injury with acute tubular necrosis, this ability of the kidney to retain sodium avidly is generally lost. However, there are some conditions in which the FE_{Na+} is less than 1% in patients with acute tubular necrosis (Table 16–6).

TABLE 16–6 Causes of acute kidney injury in which FE_{Na^+} may be below 1%.

Prerenal disease
Acute tubular necrosis
10% of nonoliguric cases
Superimposed upon chronic prerenal state
Hepatic cirrhosis
Heart failure
Severe burns
Myoglobinuria or hemoglobinuria
Radiocontrast media
Sepsis
Acute glomerulonephritis or vasculitis
Acute obstructive uropathy
Acute interstitial nephritis

Reproduced, with permission, from Rose BD. Acute renal failure—Prerenal disease vs acute tubular necrosis. In: *Pathophysiology of Renal Disease*, 2nd ed. McGraw-Hill, 1987.

CHRONIC RENAL FAILURE

Clinical Presentation

Patients with chronic renal failure and uremia show a constellation of symptoms, signs, and laboratory abnormalities in addition to those observed in acute kidney injury. This reflects the long-standing and progressive nature of their renal impairment and its effects on many types of tissues (Table 16–7). Thus, osteodystrophy, neuropathy, bilateral small kidneys shown by abdominal ultrasonography, and anemia are typical initial findings that suggest a chronic course for a patient newly diagnosed with renal failure on the basis of elevated BUN and serum creatinine.

Etiology

The most common cause of chronic renal failure is diabetes mellitus (Chapter 18), followed closely by hypertension and glomerulonephritis (Table 16–8). Polycystic kidney disease, obstruction, and infection are among the less common causes of chronic renal failure.

Pathology & Pathogenesis

A. Development of Chronic Renal Failure

The pathogenesis of acute renal disease is very different from that of chronic renal disease. Whereas acute injury to the kidney results in death and sloughing of tubular epithelial cells, often followed by their regeneration with reestablishment of normal architecture, chronic injury results in irreversible loss of nephrons. As a result, a greater functional burden is borne by fewer nephrons, manifested as an increase in glomerular filtration pressure and hyperfiltration. For reasons not well understood, this compensatory hyperfiltration, which can be thought of as a form of "hypertension" at the level of the individual nephron, predisposes to fibrosis and scarring (**glomerular sclerosis**). As a result, the rate of nephron destruction and loss increases, thus speeding the progression to **uremia,** the complex of symptoms and signs that occurs when residual renal function is inadequate.

Owing to the tremendous functional reserve of the kidneys, up to 50% of nephrons can be lost without any short-term evidence of functional impairment. This is why individuals with two healthy kidneys are able to donate one for transplantation. When GFR is further reduced, leaving only about 20% of initial renal capacity, some degree of azotemia (elevation of blood levels of products normally excreted by the kidneys) is

observed. Nevertheless, patients may be largely asymptomatic because a new steady state is achieved in which blood levels of these products are not high enough to cause overt toxicity. However, even at this apparently stable level of renal function, hyperfiltration-accelerated evolution to end-stage chronic renal failure is in progress. Furthermore, because patients with this level of GFR have little functional reserve, they can easily become uremic with any added stress (eg, infection, obstruction, dehydration, or nephrotoxic drugs) or with any catabolic state associated with increased turnover of nitrogen-containing products with reduction in GFR.

B. Pathogenesis of Uremia

The pathogenesis of chronic renal failure derives in part from a combination of the toxic effects of (1) retained products normally excreted by the kidneys (eg, nitrogen-containing products of protein metabolism), (2) normal products such as hormones now present in increased amounts, and (3) loss of normal products of the kidney (eg, loss of erythropoietin).

Excretory failure results also in fluid shifts, with increased intracellular Na^+ and water and decreased intracellular K^+. These alterations may contribute to subtle alterations in function of a host of enzymes, transport systems, and so on.

Clinical Manifestations

A. Na⁺ Balance and Volume Status

Patients with chronic renal failure typically have some degree of Na^+ and water excess, reflecting loss of the renal route of salt and water excretion. A moderate degree of Na^+ and water excess may occur without objective signs of extracellular fluid excess. However, continued excessive Na^+ ingestion contributes to congestive heart failure, hypertension, ascites, peripheral edema, and weight gain. On the other hand, excessive water ingestion contributes to hyponatremia. A common recommendation for the patient with chronic renal failure is to avoid excess salt intake and to restrict fluid intake so that it equals urine output plus 500 mL (insensible losses). Further adjustments in volume status can be made either through the use of diuretics (in a patient who still makes urine) or at dialysis.

Because these patients also have impaired renal salt and water conservation mechanisms, they are more sensitive than normal to sudden extrarenal Na^+ and water losses (eg, vomiting, diarrhea, and increased sweating with fever). Under these circumstances, they more easily develop ECF depletion, further deterioration of renal function (which may not be reversible), and even vascular collapse and shock. The symptoms and signs of dry mucous membranes, dizziness, syncope, tachycardia, and decreased jugular venous filling suggest progression of volume depletion.

B. K⁺ Balance

Hyperkalemia is a serious problem in chronic renal failure, especially for patients whose GFR has fallen below 5 mL/min. Above that level, as GFR falls, aldosterone-mediated K^+ trans-

TABLE 16–7 Clinical abnormalities in uremia.[1]

Fluid and electrolyte	Cardiovascular
Volume expansion and contraction (I)	Arterial hypertension (I or P)
Hypernatremia and hyponatremia (I)	Congestive heart failure or pulmonary edema
Hyperkalemia and hypokalemia (I)	Pericarditis (I)
Metabolic acidosis (I)	Cardiomyopathy (I or P)
Hypocalcemia (I)	Uremic lung (I)
Bone and mineral	Accelerated atherosclerosis (P or D)
Renal osteodystrophy (I or P)	Hypotension and arrhythmias (D)
Osteomalacia (D)	**Skin**
Metabolic	Skin pallor (I or P)
Carbohydrate intolerance (I)	Hyperpigmentation (I, P, or D)
Hypothermia (I)	Pruritus (P)
Hypertriglyceridemia (P)	Ecchymoses (I or P)
Protein-calorie malnutrition (I or P)	Uremic frost (I)
Impaired growth and development (P)	**Gastrointestinal**
Infertility and sexual dysfunction (P)	Anorexia (I)
Amenorrhea (P)	Nausea and vomiting (I)
Dialysis (amyloid, β_2-microglobulin) arthropathy (D)	Uremic fetor (I)
Neuromuscular	Gastroenteritis (I)
Fatigue (I)	Peptic ulcer (I or P)
Sleep disorders (P)	Gastrointestinal bleeding (I, P, or D)
Impaired mentation (I)	Hepatitis (D)
Lethargy (I)	Refractory ascites on hemodialysis (D)
Asterixis (I)	Peritonitis (D)
Muscular irritability (I)	**Hematologic**
Peripheral neuropathy (I or P)	Normocytic, normochromic anemia (P)
Restless legs syndrome (I or P)	Microcytic (aluminum-induced) anemia (D)
Paralysis (I or P)	Lymphocytopenia (P)
Myoclonus (I)	Bleeding diathesis (I or D)
Seizures (I or P)	Increased susceptibility to infection (I or P)
Coma (I)	Splenomegaly and hypersplenism (P)
Muscle cramps (D)	Leukopenia (D)
Dialysis disequilibrium syndrome (D)	Hypocomplementemia (D)
Dialysis dementia (D)	
Myopathy (P or D)	

Reproduced, with permission, from Lazarus JM, Brenner BM. Chronic renal failure. In: *Harrison's Principles of Internal Medicine,* 14th ed. Fauci AS et al (editors). McGraw-Hill, 1998.

[1]Virtually all the abnormalities contained in this table are completely reversed in time by successful renal transplantation. The response of these abnormalities to hemodialysis or peritoneal dialysis therapy is more variable. (I) denotes an abnormality that usually improves with an optimal program of dialysis and related therapy. (P) denotes an abnormality that tends to persist or even progress, despite an optimal program. (D) denotes an abnormality that develops only after initiation of dialysis therapy.

TABLE 16–8 Prevalence and incidence by etiology for United States Medicare–treated end-stage renal disease for 2005.

	Prevalence n = 485,012		Incidence n = 106,912	
	Count	Percent	Count	Percent
Diabetes	179,157	36.9	46,851	43.8
Hypertension	117,438	24.2	28,622	26.8
Glomerulonephritis	78,345	16.2	8,100	7.6
Cystic disease	22,458	4.6	2,495	2.3
Other urologic	13,581	2.8	2,158	2.0
Other cause	49,251	10.2	12,224	11.4
Unknown	18,827	3.9	4,590	4.3
Missing data	5,955	1.2	1,872	1.8

Data from the United States Renal Data System 2007 Annual Report, U.S. Department of Health and Human Services, Health Care Financing Administration (http://www.usrds.org).

port in the distal tubule increases in a compensatory fashion. Thus, a patient whose GFR is between 50 mL/min and 5 mL/min is dependent on tubular transport to maintain K^+ balance. Treatment with K^+-sparing diuretics, ACE inhibitors, or β-blockers—drugs that may impair aldosterone-mediated K^+ transport—can, therefore, precipitate dangerous hyperkalemia in a patient with chronic renal failure.

Patients with diabetes mellitus (the leading cause of chronic renal failure) may have a syndrome of **hyporeninemic hypoaldosteronism.** This syndrome is a condition in which lack of renin production by the kidney diminishes the levels of angiotensin II and, therefore, impairs aldosterone secretion. As a result, affected patients are unable to compensate for falling GFR by enhancing their aldosterone-mediated K^+ transport and, therefore, have relative difficulty handling K^+. This difficulty is usually manifested as hyperkalemia even before GFR has fallen below 5 mL/min.

Finally, not only are patients with chronic renal failure more susceptible to the effects of Na^+ or volume overload, but they are also at greater risk of hyperkalemia in the face of sudden loads of K^+ from either endogenous sources (eg, hemolysis, infection, trauma) or exogenous sources (eg, stored blood, K^+-rich foods, or K^+-containing medications).

C. Metabolic Acidosis

The diminished capacity to excrete acid and generate base in chronic renal failure results in metabolic acidosis. In most cases when the GFR is above 20 mL/min, only moderate acidosis develops before reestablishment of a new steady state of buffer production and consumption. The fall in blood pH in these individuals can usually be corrected with 20–30 mmol (2–3 g) of sodium bicarbonate by mouth daily. However, these patients are highly susceptible to acidosis in the event of a sudden acid load or the onset of disorders that increase the generated acid load.

D. Mineral and Bone

Several disorders of phosphate, Ca^{2+}, and bone metabolism are observed in chronic renal failure as a result of a complex series of events (Figure 16–6). The key factors in the pathogenesis of these disorders include (1) diminished absorption of Ca^{2+} from the gut, (2) overproduction of PTH, (3) disordered vitamin D metabolism, and (4) chronic metabolic acidosis. All of these factors contribute to enhanced bone resorption. Hypophosphatemia and hypermagnesemia can occur through overuse of phosphate binders and magnesium-containing antacids, although hyperphosphatemia is more common. Hyperphosphatemia contributes to the development of hypocalcemia and thus serves as an additional trigger for secondary hyperparathyroidism, elevating blood PTH levels. The elevated blood PTH further depletes bone Ca^{2+} and contributes to osteomalacia of chronic renal failure (see later discussion).

E. Cardiovascular and Pulmonary Abnormalities

Congestive heart failure and pulmonary edema can develop in the context of volume and salt overload. Hypertension is a common finding in chronic renal failure, also usually on the basis of fluid and Na^+ overload. However, hyperreninemia is also a recognized syndrome in which falling renal perfusion triggers the failing kidney to overproduce renin and thereby elevate systemic blood pressure.

Pericarditis resulting from irritation and inflammation of the pericardium by uremic toxins is a complication whose incidence in chronic renal failure is decreasing owing to earlier institution of renal dialysis.

Increased cardiovascular risk is a complication seen in patients with chronic renal failure and remains the leading cause of mortality in this population. It results in myocardial infarction, stroke, and peripheral vascular disease. Cardiovascular risk factors in these patients include hypertension, hyperlipidemia, glucose intolerance, chronic elevated cardiac

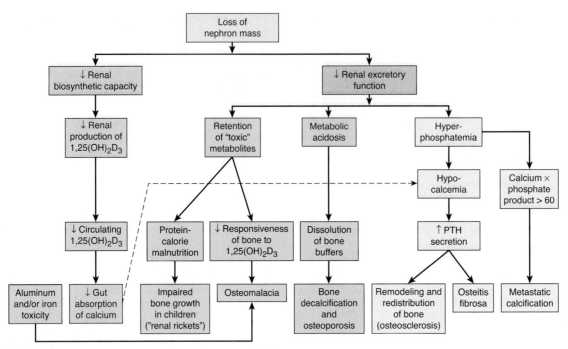

FIGURE 16–6 Pathogenesis of bone diseases in chronic renal failure. (Redrawn, with permission, from Brenner BM, Lazarus JM. Chronic renal failure. In: *Harrison's Principles of Internal Medicine,* 13th ed. Isselbacher KJ et al [editors]. McGraw-Hill, 1994.)

output, and valvular and myocardial calcification as a consequence of elevated $Ca^{2+} \times PO_4^3$ product as well as other, less well-characterized factors of the uremic milieu.

F. Hematologic Abnormalities

Patients with chronic renal failure have marked abnormalities in red blood cell count, white blood cell function, and clotting parameters. Normochromic, normocytic anemia, with symptoms of listlessness and easy fatigability and hematocrit levels typically in the range of 20–25%, is a consistent feature. The anemia is due chiefly to lack of production of erythropoietin and loss of its stimulatory effect on erythropoiesis. Thus, patients with chronic renal failure, regardless of dialysis status, show a dramatic improvement in hematocrit when treated with erythropoietin (epoetin alpha). Additional causes of anemia may include bone marrow suppressive effects of uremic poisons, bone marrow fibrosis due to elevated blood PTH, toxic effects of aluminum (from phosphate-binding antacids and dialysis solutions), and hemolysis and blood loss related to dialysis (while the patient is anticoagulated with heparin).

Patients with chronic renal failure display abnormal hemostasis manifested as increased bruising, increased blood loss at surgery, and an increased incidence of spontaneous GI and cerebrovascular hemorrhage (including both hemorrhagic strokes and subdural hematomas). Laboratory abnormalities include prolonged bleeding time, decreased platelet factor III, abnormal platelet aggregation and adhesiveness, and impaired prothrombin consumption, none of which are completely reversible even in well-dialyzed patients.

Uremia is associated with increased susceptibility to infections, believed to be due to leukocyte suppression by uremic toxins. The suppression seems to be greater for lymphoid cells than neutrophils and seems also to affect chemotaxis, the acute inflammatory response, and delayed hypersensitivity more than other leukocyte functions. Acidosis, hyperglycemia, malnutrition, and hyperosmolality also are believed to contribute to immunosuppression in chronic renal failure. The invasiveness of dialysis and the use of immunosuppressive drugs in renal transplant patients also contribute to an increased incidence of infections.

G. Neuromuscular Abnormalities

CNS symptoms and signs may range from mild sleep disorders and impairment of mental concentration, loss of memory, errors in judgment, and neuromuscular irritability (manifested as hiccups, cramps, fasciculations, and twitching) to asterixis, myoclonus, stupor, seizures, and coma in end-stage uremia. Asterixis is manifested as involuntary flapping motions seen when the arms are extended and wrists held back to "stop traffic." It is due to altered nerve conduction in metabolic encephalopathy from a wide variety of causes, including renal failure.

Peripheral neuropathy (sensory greater than motor, lower extremities greater than upper), typified by the restless legs syndrome (poorly localized sense of discomfort and involuntary movements of the lower extremities), is a common finding in chronic renal failure and an important indication for starting dialysis.

Patients receiving hemodialysis can develop aluminum toxicity, characterized by speech dyspraxia (inability to repeat words), myoclonus, dementia, and seizures. Likewise, aggressive acute dialysis can result in a disequilibrium syndrome characterized by nausea, vomiting, drowsiness, headache, and seizures in a patient with very high BUN levels. Presumably, this is an effect of rapid pH or osmolality change in ECF, resulting in cerebral edema.

H. GI Abnormalities

Nonspecific GI findings in uremic patients include anorexia, hiccups, nausea, vomiting, and diverticulosis. Although their precise pathogenesis is unclear, many of these findings improve with dialysis.

I. Endocrine and Metabolic Abnormalities

Women with uremia have low estrogen levels, which perhaps explains the high incidence of amenorrhea and the observation that they rarely are able to carry a pregnancy to term. Regular menses—but not a higher rate of successful pregnancies—typically return with frequent dialysis.

Similarly, low testosterone levels, impotence, oligospermia, and germinal cell dysplasia are common findings in men with chronic renal failure.

Finally, chronic renal failure eliminates the kidney as a site of insulin degradation, thereby increasing the half-life of insulin. This typically has a stabilizing effect on diabetic patients whose blood glucose was previously difficult to control.

J. Dermatologic Abnormalities

Skin changes arise from many of the effects of chronic renal failure already discussed. Patients with chronic renal failure may display pallor because of anemia, skin color changes related to accumulated pigmented metabolites or a gray discoloration resulting from transfusion-mediated hemochromatosis, ecchymoses and hematomas as a result of clotting abnormalities, and pruritus and excoriations as a result of Ca^{2+} deposits from secondary hyperparathyroidism. Finally, when urea concentrations are extremely high, evaporation of sweat leaves a residue of urea termed "uremic frost."

CHECKPOINT

13. What is uremia?
14. What are the most prominent symptoms and signs of uremia?
15. What is the mechanism by which altered sodium, potassium, and volume status develop in chronic renal failure?
16. What are the most common causes of chronic renal failure?

GLOMERULONEPHRITIS & NEPHROTIC SYNDROME

Clinical Presentation

A number of disorders result in structural alterations of the glomerulus and present with some combination of the following findings: hematuria, proteinuria, reduced GFR, and hypertension. Some of these disorders are specific to the kidney, whereas others are systemic diseases in which the kidney is primarily or prominently involved.

Disorders resulting in glomerular disease, whether manifestations of systemic injury or otherwise, fall into five categories:

1. **Acute glomerulonephritis,** in which there is an abrupt onset of hematuria and proteinuria with reduced GFR and renal salt and water retention, sometimes followed by recovery of renal function. Patients with acute glomerulonephritis are a subset of those with an intrarenal cause of acute kidney injury.

2. **Rapidly progressive glomerulonephritis,** in which recovery from the acute disorder does not occur. Worsening renal function results in irreversible and complete renal failure over weeks to months. Early in the course of rapidly progressive glomerulonephritis, these patients can be categorized as having a form of acute kidney injury. Later, with progression of their renal failure over time, they display all of the features described for chronic renal failure.

3. **Chronic glomerulonephritis,** in which renal impairment after acute glomerulonephritis progresses slowly over a period of years and eventually results in chronic renal failure.

4. **Nephrotic syndrome,** manifested as marked proteinuria, particularly albuminuria (defined as 24-hour urine protein excretion > 3.5 g), hypoalbuminemia, edema, hyperlipidemia, and fat bodies in the urine. Nephrotic syndrome may be either isolated (eg, minimal change disease) or part of some other glomerular syndrome (eg, with hematuria and casts).

5. **Asymptomatic urinary abnormalities,** including hematuria and proteinuria (usually in amounts below that seen in nephrotic syndrome) but no functional abnormalities associated with reduced GFR, edema, or hypertension. Many patients with these findings will develop chronic renal failure slowly over decades.

Etiology

Acute glomerulonephritis occurs most typically in the setting of infectious diseases, classically pharyngeal or cutaneous infections with certain "nephritogenic" strains of group A beta-hemolytic streptococci but also other pathogens (Table 16–9).

Rapidly progressive glomerulonephritis appears to be a heterogeneous group of disorders, all of which display pathologic features common to various categories of necrotizing vasculitis (Table 16–10; also see later discussion).

Chronic glomerulonephritis and nephrotic syndrome are largely of unclear origin. Progressive renal deterioration in patients with chronic glomerulonephritis proceeds slowly but inexorably, resulting in chronic renal failure as many as 20 years after initial discovery of an abnormal urinary sediment.

Some cases of nephrotic syndrome are variants of acute glomerulonephritis, rapidly progressive glomerulonephritis, or

TABLE 16–9 Causes of acute glomerulonephritis.

Infectious diseases
Poststreptococcal glomerulonephritis*
Nonstreptococcal postinfectious glomerulonephritis
Bacterial: infective endocarditis,* "shunt nephritis," sepsis,* pneumococcal pneumonia, typhoid fever, secondary syphilis, meningococcemia
Viral: hepatitis B, infectious mononucleosis, mumps, measles, varicella, echovirus, coxsackievirus
Parasitic: malaria, toxoplasmosis
Multisystem diseases: systemic lupus erythematosus,* vasculitis,* Henoch-Schönlein purpura,* Goodpasture's syndrome
Primary glomerular diseases: mesangiocapillary glomerulonephritis, Berger's disease (IgA nephropathy),* "pure" mesangial proliferative glomerulonephritis
Miscellaneous: Guillain-Barré syndrome, irradiation of Wilms' tumor, diphtheria-pertussis-tetanus vaccine, serum sickness

Reproduced, with permission, from Glassock RJ, Brenner BM. The major glomerulopathies. In: *Harrison's Principles of Internal Medicine,* 12th ed. Wilson JD et al (editors). McGraw-Hill, 1991.

*Most common causes.

chronic glomerulonephritis in which massive proteinuria is a presenting feature. Other cases of nephrotic syndrome fall into the category of **minimal change disease,** in which many of the pathologic consequences are due to proteinuria.

The most common cause of asymptomatic urinary abnormalities is **IgA nephropathy,** an immune complex disease characterized by diffuse mesangial IgA deposition. Other causes are listed in Table 16–11.

Pathology & Pathogenesis

The different forms of glomerulonephritis and nephrotic syndrome probably represent differences in the nature, extent, and specific cause of immune-mediated renal damage. A number of cytokines—in particular transforming growth factor-1 (TGF-1) and platelet-derived growth factor (PDGF)—are synthesized by mesangial cells, inciting an inflammatory reaction in some forms of glomerular disease. Classic associations between the natural history and defining fluorescence and electron microscopic observations have been made (Figure 16–4; Table 16–12). However, because it is not known exactly how the various forms of immune-mediated renal damage occur, each category is described separately with its associated findings.

A. Acute Glomerulonephritis

Postinfectious acute glomerulonephritis is due to immune attack on the infecting organism in which there is cross-reactivity between an antigen of the infecting organism (eg, of group A beta-hemolytic streptococci) and a host antigen. The result is deposition of immune complexes and complement (Figure

TABLE 16–10 Causes of rapidly progressive glomerulonephritis.

Infectious diseases
Poststreptococcal glomerulonephritis*
Infective endocarditis*
Occult visceral sepsis
Hepatitis B infection (with vasculitis or cryoimmunoglobulinemia)
Human immunodeficiency virus infection
Multisystem diseases
Systemic lupus erythematosus*
Henoch-Schönlein purpura*
Systemic necrotizing vasculitis (including Wegener's granulomatosis)*
Goodpasture's syndrome*
Essential mixed (IgG/IgM) cryoimmunoglobulinemia
Malignancy
Relapsing polychondritis
Rheumatoid arthritis (with vasculitis)
Drugs
Penicillamine*
Hydralazine
Allopurinol (with vasculitis)
Rifampin
Idiopathic or primary glomerular disease
Idiopathic crescentic glomerulonephritis*
Type I—with linear deposits of immunoglobulin (anti-GBM antibody–mediated)
Type II—with granular deposits of immunoglobulin (immune complex–mediated)
Type III—with few or no immune deposits of immunoglobulin ("pauci-immune")
Antineutrophil cytoplasmic antibody–induced? "forme fruste" of vasculitis
Superimposed on another primary glomerular disease
Mesangiocapillary (membranoproliferative glomerulonephritis)* (especially type II)
Membranous glomerulonephritis*
Berger's disease (IgA nephropathy)*

Reproduced, with permission, from Glassock RJ, Brenner BM. The major glomerulopathies. In: *Harrison's Principles of Internal Medicine,* 12th ed. Wilson JD et al (editors). McGraw-Hill, 1991.

*Most common causes.

TABLE 16–11 Glomerular causes of asymptomatic urinary abnormalities.

Hematuria with or without proteinuria
Primary glomerular diseases
Berger's disease (IgA nephropathy)*
Mesangiocapillary glomerulonephritis
Other primary glomerular hematurias accompanied by "pure" mesangial proliferation, focal and segmental proliferative glomerulonephritis, or other lesions
"Thin basement membrane" disease (? "forme fruste" of Alport's syndrome)
Associated with multisystem or heredofamilial diseases
Alport's syndrome and other "benign" familial hematurias
Fabry's disease
Sickle cell disease
Associated with infections
Resolving poststreptococcal glomerulonephritis*
Other postinfectious glomerulonephritides*
Isolated nonnephrotic proteinuria
Primary glomerular diseases
"Orthostatic" proteinuria*
Focal and segmental glomerulosclerosis*
Membranous glomerulonephritis*
Associated with multisystem or heredofamilial diseases
Diabetes mellitus*
Amyloidosis*
Nail-patella syndrome

Reproduced, with permission, from Glassock RJ, Brenner BM. The major glomerulopathies. In: *Harrison's Principles of Internal Medicine,* 12th ed. Wilson JD et al (editors). McGraw-Hill, 1991.

*Most common causes.

TABLE 16–12 Location of electron-dense deposits in glomerular disease.

Subepithelial
Amorphous (epimembranous) deposits
Membranous nephropathy
Systemic lupus erythematosus
Humps
Acute postinfectious glomerulonephritis (eg, post-streptococcal glomerulonephritis, bacterial endocarditis)
Intramembranous
Membranous nephropathy
Membranoproliferative glomerulonephritis type II
Subendothelial
Systemic lupus erythematosus
Membranoproliferative glomerulonephritis type I
Less commonly, bacterial endocarditis, IgA nephropathy, Henoch-Schönlein purpura, mixed cryoglobulinemia
Mesangial
Focal glomerulonephritis
IgA nephropathy
Henoch-Schönlein purpura
Systemic lupus erythematosus
Mild or resolving acute postinfectious glomerulonephritis
Subepithelial and subendothelial
Systemic lupus erythematosus
Membranoproliferative glomerulonephritis, type III
Postinfectious glomerulonephritis

Reproduced, with permission, from Rose BD. Pathogenesis, clinical manifestations and diagnosis of glomerular disease. In: *Pathophysiology of Renal Disease,* 2nd ed. McGraw-Hill, 1987.

16–4; Table 16–13) in glomerular capillaries and the mesangium. Symptoms and signs typically occur 7–10 days after onset of the acute pharyngeal or cutaneous infection and resolve over weeks after treatment of the infection.

B. Rapidly Progressive Glomerulonephritis

Immunofluorescence studies permit distribution into subgroups correlating with other features of the disease. Linear immunoglobulin deposits suggest antiglomerular basement membrane (GBM) antibody, which may coincident with pulmonary hemorrhage, characteristic of Goodpasture's syndrome. Granular immunoglobulin deposits are suggestive of immune complexes due to an underlying systemic disease, such as IgA nephropathy, postinfectious glomerulonephritis, lupus nephritis, or mixed cryoglobulinemia. Few or no immune deposits (pauci-immune) are often coincident with an autoantibody pattern (ANCA) typical of Wegener's granulomatosis or microscopic polyangiitis. ANCA-negative pauci-immune necrotizing glomerulonephritis is seen less frequently but is also a recognized clinical entity.

Immunofluorescence studies permit distribution into subgroups correlating with other features of the disease. From 5% to 20% of patients have linear anti-GBM antibody deposits in glomeruli and a tendency to hemoptysis reminiscent of

TABLE 16–13   Factors causing and mediators of glomerular injury.

Factors affecting immune complex deposition
Host immune response
Rate of complex clearance
In situ complex formation
Antigenic or complex charge
Renal hemodynamics
Mediators of glomerular damage
Complement
Neutrophils
Macrophages
Platelets
Vasoactive amines
Fibrin
Lymphokines

Modified and reproduced, with permission, from Rose BD. Pathogenesis, clinical manifestations and diagnosis of glomerular disease. In: *Pathophysiology of Renal Disease,* 2nd ed. McGraw-Hill, 1987.

Goodpasture's syndrome. Further, 30–40% have granular immunoglobulin deposits and an autoantibody pattern typical of Wegener's granulomatosis (antineutrophil cytoplasmic antibody). The latter patients are typically older, with more systemic constitutional symptoms.

C. Chronic Glomerulonephritis

Some patients with acute glomerulonephritis develop chronic renal failure slowly over a period of 5–20 years. Cellular proliferation, in either the mesangium or the capillary, is a pathologic structural hallmark in some of these cases, whereas others are notable for obliteration of glomeruli (**sclerosing chronic glomerulonephritis,** which includes both focal and diffuse subsets), and yet others display irregular subepithelial proteinaceous deposits with uniform involvement of individual glomeruli (**membranous glomerulonephritis**).

D. Nephrotic Syndrome

In patients with nephrotic syndrome, the glomerulus may appear intact or only subtly altered, without a cellular infiltrate as a manifestation of inflammation. Immunofluorescence with antibodies to immunoglobulin G (IgG) often demonstrates deposition of antigen-antibody complexes in the glomerular basement membrane. In the subset of patients with minimal change disease, in which proteinuria is the sole urinary sediment abnormality and in which (often) no changes can be seen by light microscopy, electron microscopy reveals obliteration of epithelial foot processes (Table 16–14).

TABLE 16–14   Clinical and histologic features of idiopathic nephrotic syndrome.

Glomerular Disease	Distinguishing Clinical and Laboratory Findings	Characteristic Morphologic Features
Minimal change disease	Commonest cause in children (75%); steroid- or cyclophosphamide-sensitive (80% of cases); nonprogressive; normal renal function; scant hematuria.	**LM:** normal **IF:** negative to trace IgM **EM:** podocyte effacement; no immune deposits
Focal and segmental glomerulosclerosis	Early-onset hypertension; microscopic hematuria; progressive renal failure (75% of cases).	**LM:** early, segmental sclerosis in some glomeruli with tubular atrophy; late, sclerosis of most glomeruli **IF:** focal and segmental IgM, C3 **EM:** foot process fusion, sclerosis, hyalin
Membranous nephropathy	Commonest cause in adults (40–50%); peak incidence fourth and sixth decades; male: female 2–3:1; microscopic hematuria (55%); early hypertension (30%); spontaneous remission (20%); progressive renal failure (30–40%).	**LM:** early, normal; late, GBM thickening **IF:** granular IgG and C3 **EM:** subepithelial deposits and GBM expansion
Membranoproliferative glomerulonephritis	Peak incidence second and third decades; mixed nephrotic-nephritic features; slowly progressive in most, rapid in some; hypocomplementemia.	**LM:** hypercellular glomeruli with duplicated GBM ("tramtracks") **IF:** type I, diffuse C3, variable IgG and IgM; type II, C3 capillary wall and mesangial nodules **EM:** type I, subendothelial immune deposits; type II, dense GBM

Data from Glassock RJ, Brenner BM. The major glomerulopathies. In: *Harrison's Principles of Internal Medicine,* 13th ed. Isselbacher KJ et al (editors). McGraw-Hill, 1994; and data from Hall PM. Nephrology and hypertension. In: *Medical Knowledge Self-Assessment Program 13.* American College of Physicians, 2003.

Key: EM = electron microscopy; GBM = glomerular basement membrane; IF = immunofluorescence; LM = light microscopy.

Clinical Manifestations

In glomerulonephritic diseases, damage to the glomerular capillary wall results in leakage of red blood cells and proteins, which are normally too large to cross the glomerular capillary, into the renal tubular lumen, giving rise to hematuria and proteinuria.

A fall in GFR results because either glomerular capillaries are infiltrated with inflammatory cells or contractile cells (eg, mesangial cells) respond to vasoactive substances by restricting blood flow to many glomerular capillaries.

Edema and hypertension are a direct consequence of fluid and salt retention secondary to the fall of GFR in the face of excess consumption of salt and water.

A transient fall in serum complement is observed as a result of immune complex and complement deposition in the glomerulus, as can be seen with lupus nephritis, membranoproliferative glomerulonephritis, and post-infectious glomerulonephritis.

An elevated titer of antibody to streptococcal antigens is observed in cases associated with group A β-hemolytic streptococcal infections. Another characteristic of the clinical course in poststreptococcal acute glomerulonephritis is a lag between clinical signs of infection and the development of clinical signs of nephritis.

Patients with the nephrotic syndrome have profoundly decreased plasma oncotic pressures because of the loss of serum proteins in the urine. This results in intravascular volume depletion and activation of the renin-angiotensin-aldosterone system and the sympathetic nervous system. The secretion of vasopressin is also increased. Such patients also have altered renal responses to atrial natriuretic peptide. Nevertheless, they may develop signs of intravascular volume depletion, including syncope, shock, and acute kidney injury despite often being edematous on clinical examination.

Hyperlipidemia associated with nephrotic syndrome appears to be a result of decreased plasma oncotic pressure, which stimulates hepatic very low-density lipoprotein synthesis and secretion.

Loss of other plasma proteins besides albumin in nephrotic syndrome may present as any of the following: (1) A defect in bacterial opsonization and thus increased susceptibility to infections (eg, as a result of loss of IgG); (2) hypercoagulability (eg, resulting from antithrombin deficiency, reduced levels of proteins C and S, hyperfibrinogenemia, and hyperlipidemia); (3) vitamin D deficiency state and secondary hyperparathyroidism (eg, resulting from loss of vitamin D–binding proteins); (4) altered thyroid function tests without any true thyroid abnormality (resulting from reduced levels of thyroxine-binding globulin).

CHECKPOINT

17. What are the categories of glomerulonephritis, and what are their common and distinctive features?

18. What are the pathophysiologic consequences of nephrotic syndrome?

RENAL STONES

Clinical Presentation

Patients with renal stones present with flank pain and hematuria with or without fever. Depending on the level of the stone and the patient's underlying anatomy (eg, if there is only a single functioning kidney or significant preexisting renal disease), the presentation may be complicated by obstruction (Table 16–15) with decreased or absent urine production.

Etiology

Although a variety of disorders may result in the development of renal stones (Table 16–16), at least 75% of renal stones con-

TABLE 16–15 Common mechanical causes of urinary tract obstruction.

Ureter	Bladder outlet
Ureteropelvic junction arrowing or obstruction	Bladder neck obstruction
Ureterovesical junction arrowing or obstruction	Ureterocele
	Benign prostatic hypertrophy
Ureterocele	Cancer of prostate
Retrocaval ureter	Cancer of bladder
Calculi	Calculi
Inflammation	Diabetic neuropathy
Trauma	Spinal cord disease
Sloughed papillae	Carcinomas of cervix, colon
Tumor	Trauma
Blood clots	**Urethra**
Uric acid crystals	Posterior urethral valves
Pregnant uterus	Anterior urethral valves
Retroperitoneal fibrosis	Stricture
Aortic aneurysm	Meatal stenosis
Uterine leiomyomas	Phimosis
Carcinoma of uterus, prostate, bladder, colon, rectum	Stricture
	Tumor
Retroperitoneal lymphoma	Calculi
Accidental surgical ligation	Trauma

Reproduced, with permission, from Seifter JL, Brenner BM. Urinary tract obstruction. In: *Harrison's Principles of Internal Medicine,* 14th ed. Fauci AS et al (editors). McGraw-Hill, 1998.

tain calcium. Most cases of calcium stones are due to idiopathic hypercalciuria, with hyperuricosuria and hyperparathyroidism as other major causes. Uric acid stones are typically caused by hyperuricosuria, especially in patients with a history of gout or excessive purine intake (eg, a diet high in organ meat products). Defective amino acid transport, as occurs in cystinuria, can result in stone formation. Finally, struvite stones, made up of magnesium, ammonium, and phosphate salts, are a result of chronic or recurrent urinary tract infection by urease-producing organisms (typically *Proteus*).

Pathology & Pathogenesis

Renal stones result from alterations in the solubility of various substances in urine, such that there is nucleation and precipitation of salts. A number of factors can tip the balance in favor of stone formation.

TABLE 16–16 Major causes of renal stones.

Stone Type and Causes	All Stones (%)	Occurrence of Specific Causes[1]	M:F Ratio	Etiology	Diagnosis	Treatment[3]
Calcium stones	75–85%		2:1 to 3:1			
Idiopathic hypercalciuria		50–55%	2:1	Hereditary (?)	Normocalcemia, unexplained hypercalciuria[2]	Thiazide diuretic agents
Hyperuricosuria		20%	4:1	Diet	Urine uric acid > 750 mg/24h (women), > 800 mg/24 h (men)	Allopurinol or diet
Primary hyperparathyroidism		5%	3:10	Neoplasia	Unexplained hypercalcemia	Surgery
Distal renal tubular acidosis		Rare	1:1	Hereditary	Hyperchloremic acidosis, minimum urine pH > 5.5	Alkali replacement
Intestinal hyperoxaluria		≈1–2%	1:1	Bowel surgery	Urine oxalate > 50 mg/24 h	Cholestyramine or oral calcium loading
Hereditary hyperoxaluria		Rare	1:1	Hereditary	Urine oxalate and glycolic or L-glyceric acid increased	Fluids and pyridoxine
Idiopathic stone disease		20%	2:1	Unknown	None of the above	Oral phosphate, fluids
Uric acid stones	5–8%					
Gout		≈ 50%	3:1 to 4:1	Hereditary	Clinical diagnosis	Alkali to raise urine pH
Idiopathic		≈ 50%	1:1	Hereditary (?)	Uric acid stones, no gout	Allopurinol if daily urine uric acid above 1000 mg
Dehydration		?	1:1	Intestinal, habit	History, intestinal fluid loss	Alkali, fluids, reversal of cause
Lesch-Nyhan syndrome		Rare	Men	Hereditary	Reduced hypoxanthine-guanine phosphoribosyl transferase level	Allopurinol
Malignant tumors		Rare	1:1	Neoplasia	Clinical diagnosis	Allopurinol
Cystine stones	1%		1:1	Hereditary	Stone type; elevated cystine excretion	Massive fluids, alkali, penicillamine if needed
Struvite stones	10–15%		2:10	Infection	Stone type	Antimicrobial agents and judicious surgery

Reproduced, with permission, from Asplin, JR, Coe FL, Favus MJ. Nephrolithiasis. In: *Harrison's Principles of Internal Medicine*, 14th ed. Fauci AS et al (editors). McGraw-Hill, 1998.

[1]Values are percentages of patients within each category of stone who display each specific cause.

[2]Urine calcium above 300 mg/24 h (men), 250 mg/24 h (women), or 4 mg/kg/24 h (either sex). Hyperthyroidism, Cushing's syndrome, sarcoidosis, malignant tumors, immobilization, vitamin D intoxication, rapidly progressive bone disease, and Paget's disease all cause hypercalciuria and must be excluded in diagnosis of idiopathic hypercalciuria.

[3]Besides fluids and dietary protein restriction, which are a mainstay of therapy in most forms of stone disease.

Dehydration favors stone formation, and a high fluid intake to maintain a daily urine volume of 2 L or more appears to be protective. The precise mechanism of this protection is unknown. Hypotheses include dilution of unknown substances that predispose to stone formation and decreased transit time of Ca^{2+} through the nephron, minimizing the likelihood of precipitation.

A high-protein diet predisposes to stone formation in susceptible individuals. A dietary protein load causes transient metabolic acidosis and an increased GFR. Although serum Ca^{2+} is not detectably elevated, there is probably a transient increase in calcium resorption from bone, an increase in glomerular calcium filtration, and inhibition of distal tubular calcium resorption. This effect appears to be greater in known stone-formers than in healthy controls.

A high-Na^+ diet predisposes to Ca^{2+} excretion and calcium oxalate stone formation, whereas a low dietary Na^+ intake has the opposite effect. Furthermore, urinary Na^+ excretion increases the saturation of monosodium urate, which can act as a nidus for Ca^{2+} crystallization.

Despite the fact that most stones are calcium oxalate stones, oxalate concentration in the diet is generally too low to support a recommendation to avoid oxalate to prevent stone formation. Similarly, calcium restriction, formerly a major dietary recommendation to calcium stone formers, is beneficial only to the subset of patients whose hypercalciuria is diet dependent. In others, decreased dietary calcium may actually increase oxalate absorption and predispose to stone formation.

A number of factors are protective against stone formation. In order of decreasing importance, fluids, citrate, magnesium, and dietary fiber appear to have a protective effect. Citrate may prevent stone formation by chelating calcium in solution and forming highly soluble complexes compared with calcium oxalate and calcium phosphate. Although pharmacologic supplementation of the diet with potassium citrate has been shown to increase urinary citrate and pH and decrease the incidence of recurrent stone formation, the benefits of a naturally high-citrate diet have not been investigated. However, some studies suggest that vegetarians have a lower inci-

dence of stone formation. Presumably, they avoid the stone-forming effect of high protein and Na^+ in the diet, combined with the protective effects of fiber and other factors.

Stone formation per se within the renal pelvis is painless until a fragment breaks off and travels down the ureter, precipitating ureteral colic. Hematuria and renal damage can occur in the absence of pain.

Clinical Manifestations

The pain associated with renal stones is due to distention of the ureter, renal pelvis, or renal capsule. The severity of pain is related to the degree of distention that occurs and thus is extremely severe in acute obstruction. Anuria and azotemia are suggestive of bilateral obstruction or unilateral obstruction of a single functioning kidney. The pain, hematuria, and even ureteral obstruction caused by a renal stone are typically self-limited. For smaller stones, passage usually requires only fluids, bed rest, and analgesia. The major complications are (1) hydronephrosis and permanent renal damage as a result of complete obstruction of a ureter, with resulting backup of urine and buildup of pressure; (2) infection or abscess formation behind a partially or completely obstructing stone, which can rapidly destroy the involved kidney; (3) renal damage subsequent to repeated kidney stones; and (4) hypertension resulting from increased renin production by the obstructed kidney.

CHECKPOINT

19. How do patients with renal stones present?
20. Why do renal stones form?
21. What are the common categories of renal stones (by composition)?

CASE STUDIES

Jonathan Fuchs, MD, MPH, & Yeong Kwok, MD

(See Chapter 25, p. 699 for Answers)

CASE 72

A healthy 26-year-old woman sustained a significant crush injury to her right upper extremity while on the job at a local construction site. She was brought to the emergency department and subsequently underwent pinning and reconstructive surgery and received perioperative broad-spectrum antibiotics. Her blood pressure remained normal throughout her hospital course. On the second hospital day, a medical consultant noted a marked increase in her creatinine, from 0.8 to 1.9 mg/dL. Her urine output dropped to 20 mL/h. Serum creatine kinase was ordered and reported as 3400 units/L.

Questions

A. What are the primary causes of this patient's acute kidney injury? How should her renal failure be categorized (as prerenal, intrarenal, or postrenal)?

B. Which two types are most likely in this patient? How might they be distinguished clinically?

C. How should she be treated?

CASE 73

A 58-year-old obese woman with hypertension, type 2 diabetes, and chronic renal insufficiency is admitted to hospital after a right femoral neck fracture sustained in a fall. Recently, she has been complaining of fatigue and was started on epoetin alfa subcutaneous injections. Her other medications include an angiotensin-converting enzyme inhibitor, a β-blocker, a diuretic, calcium supplementation, and insulin. On review of systems, she reports mild tingling in her lower extremities. On examination, her blood pressure is 148/60 mm Hg. She is oriented and able to answer questions appropriately. There is no evidence of jugular venous distention or pericardial friction rub. Her lungs are clear, and her right lower extremity is in Buck's traction in preparation for surgery. Asterixis is absent.

Questions

A. Describe the pathogenesis of bone disease in chronic renal failure. How could this explain her increased likelihood of sustaining a fracture after a fall?

B. Why was erythropoietin therapy initiated?

C. What is the significance of a pericardial friction rub in the setting of chronic renal failure?

CASE 74

A 40-year-old man with Hodgkin's lymphoma is admitted to the hospital because of anasarca. He has no known history of renal, liver, or cardiac disease. His serum creatinine level is slightly elevated at 1.4 mg/dL. Serum albumin level is 2.8 g/dL. Liver function test results are normal. Urinalysis demonstrates no red or white blood cell casts, but 3+ protein is noted and a 24-hour urine collection shows a protein excretion of 4 g/24 hours. He is diagnosed with nephrotic syndrome, and renal biopsy suggests minimal change disease. Steroids and diuretics are instituted, with gradual improvement of edema. The hospital course is complicated by deep venous thrombosis of the left calf and thigh that requires anticoagulation.

Questions

A. This patient suffers from generalized body edema (anasarca). By what mechanism does the edema form?

B. What are the characteristic morphologic features seen in minimal change disease? How does this differ from other forms of glomerulonephritis?

C. How does nephrotic syndrome predispose this patient to thromboembolic disease?

CASE 75

A 48-year-old white man presents to the emergency department with unremitting right flank pain. He denies dysuria or fever. He does report significant nausea without vomiting. He has never experienced anything like this before. On examination, he is afebrile, and his blood pressure is 160/80 mm Hg with a pulse rate of 110/min. He is writhing on the gurney, unable to find a comfortable position. His right flank is mildly tender to palpation, and abdominal examination is benign. Urinalysis is significant for 1+ blood, and microscopy reveals 10–20 red blood cells per high-power field. Nephrolithiasis is suspected, and the patient is intravenously hydrated and given pain medication with temporary relief.

Questions

A. What is the most likely cause of this patient's renal stone disease?

B. Describe your discharge instructions to the patient, reflecting on the pathogenesis of stone disease.

C. Why is this disorder painful?

REFERENCES

General

Bagshaw SM et al. Conventional markers of kidney function. Crit Care Med. 2008 Apr;36(4 Suppl):S152–8. [PMID: 18382187]

Barri YM. Hypertension and kidney disease: A deadly connection. Curr Hypertens Rep. 2008 Feb;10(1):39–45. [PMID: 18367025]

Beck LH Jr et al. Glomerular and tubulointerstitial diseases. Prim Care. 2008 Jun;35(2):265–96. [PMID: 18486716]

Berthoux FC et al. Natural history of primary IgA nephropathy. Semin Nephrol. 2008 Jan;28(1):4–9. [PMID: 18222341]

Petrie CJ et al. Broken pump or leaky filter? Renal dysfunction in heart failure: A contemporary review. Int J Cardiol. 2008 Aug 18;128(2):154–65. [PMID: 18191240]

Vanholder R et al. European Uremic Toxin Work Group. A bench to bedside view of uremic toxins. J Am Soc Nephrol. 2008 May;19(5):863–70. [PMID: 18287557]

Acute Kidney Injury

Endre ZH et al. Early detection of acute kidney injury: Emerging new biomarkers. Nephrology (Carlton). 2008 Apr;13(2):91–8. [PMID: 18275495]

Kellum JA. Acute kidney injury. Crit Care Med. 2008 Apr;36(4 Suppl):S141–5. [PMID: 18382185]

Liu KD et al. Renal repair and recovery. Crit Care Med. 2008 Apr;36(4 Suppl):S187–92. [PMID: 18382192]

McCullough PA. Acute kidney injury with iodinated contrast. Crit Care Med. 2008 Apr;36(4 Suppl):S204–11. [PMID: 18382195]

Naughton CA. Drug-induced nephrotoxicity. Am Fam Physician. 2008 Sep 15;78(6):743–50. [PMID: 18819242]

Palevsky PM. Indications and timing of renal replacement therapy in acute kidney injury. Crit Care Med. 2008 Apr;36(4 Suppl):S224–8. [PMID: 18382198]

Ronco C et al. Potential interventions in sepsis-related acute kidney injury. Clin J Am Soc Nephrol. 2008 Mar;3(2):531–44. [PMID: 18235149]

Rosen S et al. Acute tubular necrosis is a syndrome of physiologic and pathologic dissociation. J Am Soc Nephrol. 2008 May;19(5):871–5. [PMID: 18235086]

Schmitt R et al. Recovery of kidney function after acute kidney injury in the elderly: A systematic review and meta-analysis. Am J Kidney Dis. 2008 Aug;52(2):262–71. [PMID: 18511164]

Wan L et al. Pathophysiology of septic acute kidney injury: What do we really know? Crit Care Med. 2008 Apr;36(4 Suppl):S198–203. [PMID: 18382194]

Chronic Renal Failure

Cho MH et al. Pathophysiology of minimal change nephrotic syndrome and focal segmental glomerulosclerosis. Nephrology (Carlton). 2007 Dec;12 Suppl 3:S11–4. [PMID: 17995521

Dukkipati R, Adler S, Mehrotra R. Cardiovascular implications of chronic kidney disease in older adults. Drugs Aging. 2008;25(3):241–53. [PMID: 18331075]

Graves JW. Diagnosis and management of chronic kidney disease. Mayo Clin Proc. 2008 Sep;83(9):1064–9. [PMID: 18775206]

Moe SM et al. Mechanisms of vascular calcification in chronic kidney disease. J Am Soc Nephrol. 2008 Feb;19(2):213–6. [PMID: 18094365]

Raggi P et al. Contribution of bone and mineral abnormalities to cardiovascular disease in patients with chronic kidney disease. Clin J Am Soc Nephrol. 2008 May;3(3):836–43. [PMID: 18322050]

Singh P et al. The balance of angiotensin II and nitric oxide in kidney diseases. Curr Opin Nephrol Hypertens. 2008 Jan;17(1):51–6. [PMID: 18090670]

Stenvinkel P et al. Emerging biomarkers for evaluating cardiovascular risk in the chronic kidney disease patient: How do new pieces fit into the uremic puzzle? Clin J Am Soc Nephrol. 2008 Mar;3(2):505–21. [PMID: 18184879]

Glomerulonephritis

Beck LH Jr et al. Glomerular and tubulointerstitial diseases. Prim Care. 2008 Jun;35(2):265–96. [PMID: 18486716]

Catapano F et al. Antiproteinuric response to dual blockade of the renin-angiotensin system in primary glomerulonephritis: Meta-analysis and metaregression. Am J Kidney Dis. 2008 Sep;52(3):475–85. [PMID: 18468748]

Ferraccioli G et al. Renal interstitial cells, proteinuria and progression of lupus nephritis: New frontiers for old factors. Lupus. 2008;17(6):533–40. [PMID: 18539706]

Glassock RJ. IgA nephropathy: Challenges and opportunities. Cleve Clin J Med. 2008 Aug;75(8):569–76. [PMID: 18756838]

Jennette JC et al. New insight into the pathogenesis of vasculitis associated with antineutrophil cytoplasmic autoantibodies. Curr Opin Rheumatol. 2008 Jan;20(1):55–60. [PMID: 18281858]

Lavin PJ et al. Therapeutic targets in focal and segmental glomerulosclerosis. Curr Opin Nephrol Hypertens. 2008 Jul;17(4):386–92. [PMID: 18660675]

Novak J et al. IgA glycosylation and IgA immune complexes in the pathogenesis of IgA nephropathy. Semin Nephrol. 2008 Jan;28(1):78–87. [PMID: 18222349]

Kidney Stones

Asplin JR. Evaluation of the kidney stone patient. Semin Nephrol. 2008 Mar;28(2):99–110. [PMID: 18359391]

Mattoo A et al. Cystinuria. Semin Nephrol. 2008 Mar;28(2):181–91. [PMID: 18359399]

Sakhaee K. Nephrolithiasis as a systemic disorder. Curr Opin Nephrol Hypertens. 2008 May;17(3):304–9. [PMID: 18408483]

Sakhaee K et al. Metabolic syndrome and uric acid nephrolithiasis. Semin Nephrol. 2008 Mar;28(2):174–80. [PMID: 18359398]

Vezzoli G et al. Update on primary hypercalciuria from a genetic perspective. J Urol. 2008 May;179(5):1676–82. [PMID: 18343451]

Worcester EM et al. Nephrolithiasis. Prim Care. 2008 Jun;35(2):369–91, vii. [PMID: 18486720]

Worcester EM et al. New insights into the pathogenesis of idiopathic hypercalciuria. Semin Nephrol. 2008 Mar;28(2):120–32. [PMID: 18359393]

Disorders of the Parathyroids & Calcium & Phosphorus Metabolism

Dolores M. Shoback, MD,
& Deborah E. Sellmeyer, MD

This chapter presents a general overview of the key hormones involved in the regulation of calcium, phosphate, and bone mineral metabolism. These include **parathyroid hormone, vitamin D**—principally the 1,25-(OH)$_2$ vitamin D metabolite (1,25-dihydroxycholecalciferol)—**calcitonin**, and **fibroblast growth factor (FGF)-23.** The cycle of bone remodeling is described as a basis for understanding normal maintenance of skeletal integrity in adults and of mineral homeostasis. The symptoms and signs caused by excess or deficiency of the calciotropic hormones are presented along with the natural histories of **primary hyperparathyroidism, familial (benign) hypocalciuric hypercalcemia, hypercalcemia of malignancy,** different forms of **hypoparathyroidism,** and **medullary carcinoma of the thyroid.** Two of the most commonly encountered causes of low bone mass—**osteoporosis** and **osteomalacia**—are reviewed, along with discussions regarding their pathogenesis.

NORMAL REGULATION OF CALCIUM & PHOSPHORUS METABOLISM

PARATHYROID GLANDS

Anatomy

Normal parathyroid glands each weigh 30–40 mg and are gray-tan to yellow-gray. Each individual typically has four glands, so that the average total parathyroid tissue mass in the adult is 120–160 mg.

The superior pair of parathyroid glands arise from the fourth branchial pouches in the embryo. These glands are located near the point of intersection of the middle thyroid artery and the recurrent laryngeal nerve. The superior parathyroid glands may be attached to the thyroid capsule posteriorly or, rarely, embedded in the thyroid gland itself. Alternative locations include the tracheoesophageal groove and the retroesophageal space. The blood supply to the superior parathyroid glands is from the inferior thyroid artery or, less commonly, the superior thyroid artery.

The inferior parathyroid glands develop from the third branchial pouch, as does the thymus gland. These glands typically lie at or near the lower pole of the thyroid gland lateral to the trachea. The inferior glands receive their blood supply from the inferior thyroid arteries. The location of the inferior parathyroid glands is variable. When there are ectopic glands, they are typically found in association with thymic remnants.

A common site for ectopic glands is the anterior mediastinum. Less common ectopic locations are the carotid sheath, pericardium, and pharyngeal submucosa. About 10% of people have additional (supernumerary) parathyroid glands.

Histology

The parathyroid gland is composed of three different cell types: chief cells, clear cells, and oxyphil cells. **Chief cells** are small in diameter (4–8 μm) with central nuclei and are thought to be responsible for the synthesis and secretion of **parathyroid hormone (PTH).** In their active state, they have a prominent endoplasmic reticulum and dense Golgi regions where PTH is synthesized and packaged for secretion. **Clear cells** are probably chief cells with an increased glycogen content. **Oxyphil cells** appear in the parathyroid glands after puberty. They are larger than chief cells (6–10 μm), and their number increases with age. It is not clear whether these cells secrete PTH and whether they are derived from chief cells.

The normal adult parathyroid gland contains fat. The relative contribution of fat to the glandular mass increases with age and may reach 60–70% of gland volume in the elderly. If hyperplasia or adenomatous changes occur, the component of the gland that is fat decreases dramatically.

Physiology

Approximately 99% of total body calcium is found in the skeleton and teeth; the remainder is in the extracellular fluids. Calcium in these fluids exists in three forms: ionized, protein bound, and complexed. About 47% of total blood calcium is protein bound, predominantly to albumin but also to globulins. A similar fraction is ionized. The remainder is complexed to organic ions such as citrate, phosphate, and bicarbonate. Serum ionized calcium controls vital cellular functions such as hormone secretion and action, muscle contraction, neuromuscular transmission, and blood clotting. The binding of calcium to albumin is pH dependent, increasing with alkalosis and decreasing with

acidosis. Thus, if the ionized calcium is low, acidosis tends to protect against symptomatic hypocalcemia. Conversely, alkalosis predisposes to symptomatic hypocalcemia.

Circulating levels of PTH can change within seconds after an alteration in serum calcium. PTH secretory rates are related to the serum ionized calcium concentration by an inverse sigmoidal relationship (Figure 17–1). Low ionized calcium concentrations maximally stimulate secretion, whereas increases in calcium suppress the production and release of PTH. PTH secretion is exquisitely sensitive to very small changes in the calcium concentration, which have substantial effects on the rate of hormone synthesis and release.

The extracellular calcium-sensing receptor (CaSR), expressed by parathyroid cells, detects changes in the extracellular calcium concentration. This receptor is activated by increases in the calcium concentration and couples to intracellular pathways that produce inhibition of hormone secretion (Figure 17–2) and parathyroid cell proliferation. In addition to the parathyroid gland, CaSRs are expressed in the kidney, thyroid C cells, brain, and many other tissues. Chronic hypocalcemia is also a stimulus to the proliferation of parathyroid cells, which eventually results in glandular hyperplasia. PTH is produced in the parathyroid glands as a 115-amino-acid precursor molecule (preproPTH) that is successively cleaved within the cell to form the mature 84-amino-acid peptide PTH(1–84) (Figure 17–3). This form of the hormone is packaged into secretory granules and released into the circulation. PTH(1–84) is the biologically active form of PTH at target cells and has a very short half-life in vivo of approximately 10 minutes. PTH(1–84) is metabolized in the liver and other tissues to midregion and carboxyl terminal forms that are probably biologically inactive. These circulating fragments accumulate to very high levels in patients with renal failure, because the kidney is an important site for

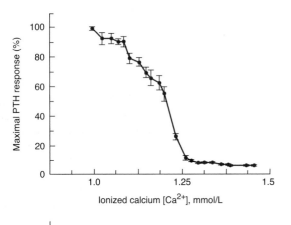

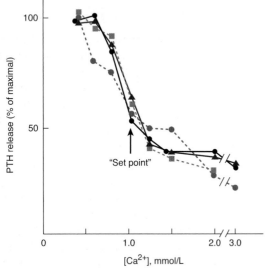

FIGURE 17–1 Inverse sigmoidal relationship between parathyroid hormone (PTH) release and the extracellular calcium concentration in human studies (upper panel) and in vitro in human parathyroid cells (bottom panel). Studies shown in the upper panel were performed by infusing calcium and the calcium chelator EDTA into normal subjects. Serum intact PTH was measured by a two-site immunoradiometric assay. In the lower panel, PTH was measured in the medium surrounding parathyroid cells in vitro by an assay for intact PTH. The midpoint between the maximal and minimal secretory rates is defined as the set point for secretion. (Redrawn, with permission, from Brown E. Extracellular Ca²⁺ sensing, regulation of parathyroid cell function, and role of Ca²⁺ and other ions as extracellular [first] messengers. Physiol Rev. 1991;71: 371.)

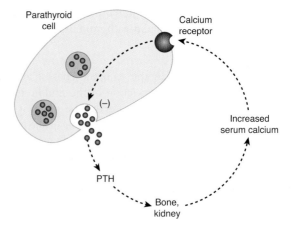

FIGURE 17–2 Sequence of events by which the calcium ion concentration is sensed by the parathyroid calcium-sensing receptor (CaSR). Activation of this receptor is eventually linked through intracellular signal transduction pathways to the inhibition of PTH secretion and parathyroid cell proliferation. (Redrawn with modification from Taylor R. A new receptor for calcium ions. J NIH Res. 1994;6:25.)

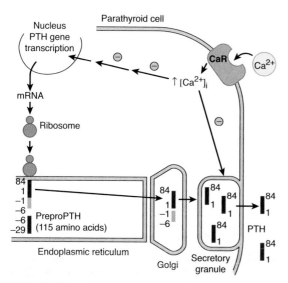

FIGURE 17–3 Biosynthetic events in the production of parathyroid hormone (PTH) within the parathyroid cell. PreproPTH gene is transcribed to its mRNA, which is translated on the ribosomes to preproPTH (amino acids –29 to +84). The presequence is removed within the endoplasmic reticulum, yielding proPTH (–6 to +84). An additional six-amino-acid fragment is removed in the Golgi. Mature PTH(1–84) released from the Golgi is packaged in secretory granules and released into the circulation in the presence of hypocalcemia. The calcium-sensing receptor (CaSR) or CaR is proposed to sense changes in extracellular calcium that affect both the release of PTH and the transcription of the preproPTH gene. High extracellular calcium concentrations also promote the intracellular degradation of PTH. (Redrawn, with permission, from Habener JF et al. Biosynthesis of parathyroid hormone. Recent Prog Horm Res. 1977;33:249.)

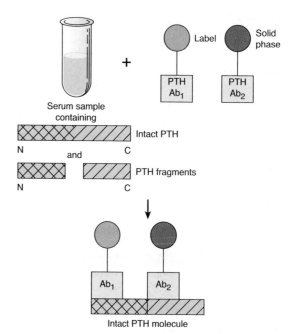

FIGURE 17–4 Schematic representation of the principle of the two-site assay for parathyroid hormone (PTH), in this case full-length, biointact PTH(1–84). The label may be a luminescent probe or ^{125}I in the immunochemiluminometric or immunoradiometric assay, respectively. Two different region-specific antibodies are used (Ab$_1$ and Ab$_2$). The epitope for Ab$_1$ is at the extreme N-terminus ensuring that only the hormone species containing both N- and C-terminal/midregion immunodeterminants are counted in the assay.

clearance of PTH from the body. Intact PTH assays in routine use measure PTH(1–84) using immunoradiometric or immunochemiluminometric methods that employ two antibodies: one directed against an amino terminal epitope, which is labeled, and the other directed against a carboxyl terminal epitope of PTH(1–84), which is immobilized (Figure 17–4). It is now clear that these "intact" PTH assays also detect amino-terminally truncated fragments of hormone such as PTH(7–84) that accumulate particularly in the serum of uremic patients. It is estimated that 30–50% of circulating "intact PTH" in uremic sera may represent these amino terminal fragments. This led to the development of "whole PTH" assays that only detect PTH(1–84). The amino terminal antibody in these assays specifically recognizes the first six amino acids of PTH(1–84). Such assays more accurately reflect secreted bioactive PTH produced in patients (Figure 17–4), although they have not as yet replaced the original intact assays.

Mechanism of Parathyroid Hormone Action

There are two types of PTH receptors. The type 1 receptor recognizes PTH and parathyroid hormone-related peptide

(PTHrP) and is also called the PTH-1 receptor. The type 2 receptor is specific for PTH. PTH and PTHrP (described later) bind to the type 1 receptor through residues in their amino terminal domains. This part of the molecule is also responsible for the activation of adenylyl cyclase and production of the second-messenger cAMP (Figure 17–5). The type 1 receptor also couples to the stimulation of phospholipase C activity, leading to the generation of inositol trisphosphate and diacylglycerol (Figure 17–5). Activation of this signal transduction pathway induces intracellular calcium mobilization and protein kinase C activation in PTH- and PTHrP-responsive cells. The type 2 PTH receptor is expressed in nonclassic PTH target tissues (ie, brain, pancreas, testis, and placenta). This receptor is not thought to be involved in mineral balance, and its natural ligand may be a hypothalamic peptide called tubuloinfundibular peptide.

Effects of Parathyroid Hormone

The serum ionized calcium and phosphate concentrations reflect the net transfer of these ions from bone, GI tract, and glomerular filtrate. PTH and 1,25-(OH)$_2$D play key roles in the regulation of calcium and phosphate balance (Figure 17–6). When the serum calcium concentration falls, PTH is rapidly released and acts quickly to promote calcium reabsorption in the distal tubule and the medullary thick ascending limb of

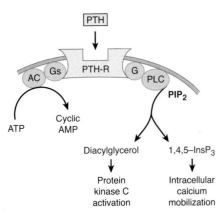

FIGURE 17–5 Signal transduction pathways activated by parathyroid hormone (PTH) binding to the PTH-1 receptor (PTH-R) in a target cell. PTH interacts with its receptor. This enhances guanosine triphosphate binding to the stimulatory G protein of adenylyl cyclase G_s, which activates the enzyme. Cyclic adenosine monophosphate (cAMP) is formed. PTH also increases G protein-dependent activation of phospholipase C (PLC), which catalyzes the breakdown of the membrane phospholipid phosphatidylinositol 4,5-bisphosphate (PIP$_2$). This produces the second messengers, inositol trisphosphate (1,4,5-InsP$_3$) and diacylglycerol. 1,4,5-InsP$_3$ mobilizes intracellular calcium, and diacylglycerol activates protein kinase C.

Henle's loop. PTH also stimulates the release of calcium from a rapidly exchangeable pool of bone calcium. These actions serve to restore serum calcium levels to normal.

The renal action of PTH is rapid, occurring within minutes after an increase in the hormone. The overall effect of PTH on the kidney, however, depends on several factors. When hypocalcemia is present and PTH is elevated, urinary calcium excretion is low. This reflects the full expression of the primary renal effect of PTH to enhance renal calcium reabsorption. When PTH levels are high in primary hyperparathyroidism, hypercalcemia results from increased mobilization of calcium from bone and enhanced intestinal calcium absorption. These events increase the delivery of calcium to the glomerular filtrate. Because more calcium is filtered, more is excreted in the urine, despite the high PTH levels. If the filtered load of calcium is normal or low in a patient with primary hyperparathyroidism—because of a low dietary calcium intake or demineralized bone—urinary calcium excretion may be normal or even low. Thus, there may be considerable variability in calcium excretion among patients with hyperparathyroidism.

If kidney function is normal, chronic elevation in serum PTH increases renal 1,25-(OH)$_2$D production. This steroid hormone stimulates both calcium and phosphate absorption across the small intestine (Figure 17–6). The effect requires at least 24 h to develop fully and begin to restore normal calcium levels. Achievement of eucalcemia then leads to a downward readjustment in the PTH secretory rate. Any increase in 1,25-(OH)$_2$D serves to inhibit further PTH synthesis.

The major effect of PTH on phosphate handling is to promote its excretion by inhibition of sodium-dependent phosphate transport in the proximal and distal tubules. Serum phosphate levels are thought to affect PTH secretion rates directly, with hyperphosphatemia serving as a stimulus to PTH secretion by an uncertain mechanism. Hypophosphatemia enhances the conversion of 25-(OH)D to 1,25-(OH)$_2$D in the kidney, which through its intestinal and renal effects promotes phosphate retention. Hyperphosphatemia also inhibits 1,25-(OH)$_2$D production (see below) and lowers serum calcium by complexing it.

PTH also increases urinary excretion of bicarbonate through its action on the proximal tubule. This can produce proximal renal tubular acidosis. These physiologic responses to PTH are the basis for the hypophosphatemia and hyperchloremic acidosis commonly observed in patients with hyperparathyroidism. Dehydration is also common in moderate to severe hypercalcemia of any origin. This is due to the effect of hypercalcemia on vasopressin action in the medullary thick ascending limb of the kidney. High calcium levels, presumably by interacting with renal CaSRs, blunt the ability of endogenous vasopressin to stimulate water reabsorption. Thus, hypercalcemia induces vasopressin-resistant nephrogenic diabetes insipidus.

In conjunction with 1,25-(OH)$_2$D, PTH increases bone resorption to restore normocalcemia (see below). PTH acts on bone in two steps. The first is to mobilize calcium and phosphate rapidly from a compartment in direct contact with extracellular fluids. The second step of calcium mobilization results from bone matrix dissolution and alterations in the bone remodeling process. The initial skeletal response to PTH occurs within 2–3 hours. Later effects require several hours to develop. In its initial action on bone, PTH enhances osteoclastic activity and thus bone resorption. Subsequently, PTH stimulates bone formation, because the processes of resorption and formation are coupled. In primary and secondary hyperparathyroidism, when PTH production rates are excessive, net bone loss may occur over time, perhaps because even though the processes of formation and resorption are coupled, they may not occur with 100% efficiency.

PARATHYROID HORMONE-RELATED PEPTIDE

PTHrP is a 141-amino-acid peptide that is homologous with PTH at its amino terminal region (Figure 17–7) and is recognized by the type 1 PTH receptor. Consequently, PTHrP has effects on bone and kidney similar to those of PTH; it increases bone resorption, increases phosphate excretion, and decreases renal calcium excretion. PTHrP is secreted by tumor cells and was originally identified as the cause of hypercalcemia of malignancy, a syndrome that can mimic primary hyperparathyroidism (see later).

Unlike PTH, which is exclusively produced by parathyroid cells, PTHrP is produced in many tissues. It functions mainly as a tissue growth and differentiation factor at the local level

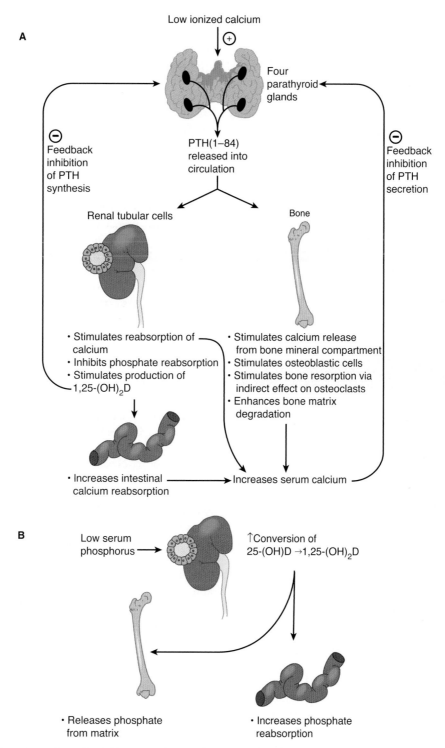

FIGURE 17–6   Main actions of parathyroid hormone (PTH) and 1,25-(OH)$_2$D in the maintenance of calcium and phosphate homeostasis. (Redrawn, with permission, from Chandrasoma P, Taylor CE. *Concise Pathology,* 3rd ed. Originally published by Appleton & Lange. Copyright © 1998 by the McGraw-Hill Companies, Inc.)

and a regulator of smooth muscle tone. In the normal development of cartilage and bone, PTHrP stimulates the proliferation of chondrocytes and inhibits the mineralization of cartilage. Embryos without PTHrP are nonviable, with multiple abnormalities of bone and cartilage. PTHrP also appears

to regulate the normal development of skin, hair follicles, teeth, and the breast. PTHrP plays an important role in determining the calcium content of the milk from lactating animals.

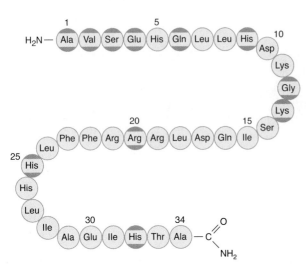

FIGURE 17–7   The amino acid sequence of the 34 amino acid residue at the N terminal parathyroid hormone (PTH)–related peptide. Amino acids that are identical to those in PTH are shown with dark yellow borders.   (Redrawn, with permission, from Felig P et al [editors]. *Endocrinology and Metabolism,* 3rd ed. McGraw-Hill, 1995.)

CHECKPOINT

1. Describe the cell types in the parathyroid gland.
2. How do serum albumin concentration and blood pH influence the distribution of calcium into ionized and protein-bound fractions?
3. What advances have occurred in two-site immunoassays for PTH that affect uremic patients?
4. What are the actions of PTH and 1,25-(OH)$_2$D on bone, kidney, and the GI tract?'
5. What is PTHrP? How is its action similar to and different from that of PTH?

BONE

Bone has two compartments. On the outside is **cortical** or **compact** bone, which makes up 80% of the skeletal mass. Beneath the cortex lies the other compartment: **trabecular** or **cancellous** bone, which makes up 20% of skeletal mass. Trabecular bone consists of interconnected plates, the trabeculae, which are covered by bone cells and are sites of active remodeling. The spaces in this irregular honeycomb are filled with bone marrow: either red marrow, in which hematopoiesis is active, or white marrow, which is mainly fat. Because of its high surface-to-volume ratio and abundant cellular activity, trabecular bone is remodeled more rapidly than cortical bone. Because of the low ratio of surface to volume, cortical bone is remodeled slowly.

To understand the remodeling process, it is important to know something about bone cells.

Osteocytes, the most abundant cells in bone, reside deep in the matrix, communicating and receiving nutrients via a sys-

tem of haversian canals. Osteocytes function as mechanoreceptors, detecting strain on the bone and signaling for changes in bone remodeling. **Osteoclasts,** multinucleated giant cells specialized for resorption of bone, are terminally differentiated cells that arise continuously from hematopoietic precursors in the monocyte lineage and do not divide. The formation of osteoclasts requires hematopoietic growth factors such as macrophage colony-stimulating factor (m-CSF) and also requires a signal from marrow stromal cells. A cell surface molecule on marrow stromal cells, which is required for osteoclast differentiation and activation is known as **RANK-L,** or the ligand for *receptor activator of nuclear factor kappa B.* RANK-L binds to its receptor **RANK** on osteoclast precursors and signals to the cell interior. A variety of cells, including those from the marrow, produce a soluble, secreted decoy receptor, **osteoprotegerin** (**OPG**), that binds RANK-L, thereby preventing its interaction with RANK and halting osteoclast differentiation and activation (Figure 17–8). As osteoclasts mature, they acquire the capacity to produce osteoclast-specific enzymes and finally fuse to produce the mature multinucleated cell. The maturation process is accelerated by bone-resorbing hormones such as PTH and vitamin D, presumably through their effects on the RANK-L/OPG system.

To resorb bone, the motile osteoclast alights on a bone surface and seals off an area by forming an adhesive ring in which cellular integrins bind tightly to bone matrix proteins (Figure 17–9). Having isolated an area of bone surface, the osteoclast develops above the surface an elaborately invaginated plasma membrane structure called the **ruffled border.** The ruffled border is a distinctive organelle, but it acts essentially as a huge lysosome, which dissolves bone mineral by secreting acid onto the isolated bone surface, and simultaneously breaks down the bone matrix by secretion of collagenase and catheptic proteases. The resulting collagen peptides have pyridinoline crosslinks that can be assayed in urine as a measure of bone resorption rates. Bone resorption can be controlled in two ways: by regulating the formation of osteoclasts and by regulating the activity of mature osteoclasts. The **osteoblast,** or bone-forming cell, arises from a mesenchymal precursor in the bone marrow stroma. When actively forming bone, the osteoblast is a tall, plump cell with an abundant Golgi apparatus. On active bone-forming surfaces, osteoblasts are found side by side, laying down bone matrix by secreting proteins and proteoglycans. The most important protein of bone matrix is type I collagen, which makes up 90% of bone matrix and is deposited in regular layers that serve as the main scaffold for deposition of minerals. There are many other constituents of bone matrix, including the protein **osteocalcin,** which is unique to bones and teeth and whose serum level used as a clinical measure of the rate of bone formation.

After laying down bone matrix, osteoblasts mineralize it by depositing hydroxyapatite crystals in an orderly array on the collagen layers to produce lamellar bone. The process of mineralization is poorly understood but requires an adequate supply of extracellular calcium and phosphate as well as the

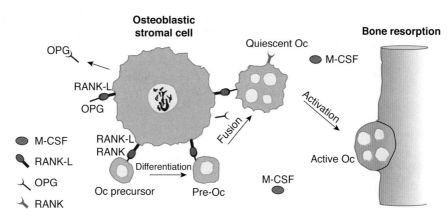

FIGURE 17–8 Cell-cell interactions and molecules essential for the differentiation and activation of osteoclasts. A cell surface molecule known as **RANK-L** on osteoblastic bone marrow stromal cells can interact with osteoclastic precursor cells in the bone marrow (derived from cells of the monocytic lineage) through their cell surface molecules designated **RANK.** This interaction, in the presence of sufficient mCSF, promotes the differentiation and fusion of these cells eventually to form mature osteoclasts and enables otherwise quiescent osteoclasts to resorb bone. These pathways are interfered with by the elaboration of a secreted decoy receptor molecule for RANK-L known as **OPG**, which blocks activation and differentiation of osteoclasts. (Oc, osteoclast.) (Redrawn, with permission, from Goltzman D. Osteolysis and cancer. J Clin Invest. 2001;107:1219.)

enzyme alkaline phosphatase, which is secreted in large amounts by active osteoblasts.

Bone remodeling occurs in an orderly cycle in which old bone is first resorbed and new bone then deposited. Cortical bone is remodeled from within by cutting cones (Figure 17–10), groups of osteoclasts that cut tunnels through the compact bone. They are followed by trailing osteoblasts, lining the tunnels and laying down a cylinder of new bone on their walls, so

that the tunnels are progressively narrowed until all that remains are the tiny haversian canals, by which the cells that are left behind as resident osteocytes are fed.

In trabecular bone, the remodeling process occurs on the surface (Figure 17–11). Osteoclasts first excavate a pit, and the pit is then filled in with new bone by osteoblasts. In a normal adult, this cycle takes ~200 days. At each remodeling site, bone resorption and new bone formation are ordinarily

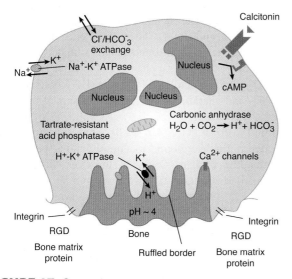

FIGURE 17–9 Schematic view of an active osteoclast. Calcitonin receptors, the ruffled border, and enzymes and channels involved in secretion of acid onto the bone surface are shown. Integrins are transmembrane-spanning receptors on osteoclasts, which bind to determinants (RGD) in bone matrix proteins such as fibronectins. The integrins are responsible for the tight attachment of osteoclasts to the bone surface. (Redrawn, with permission, from Felig P et al [editors]. *Endocrinology and Metabolism,* 3rd ed. McGraw-Hill, 1995.)

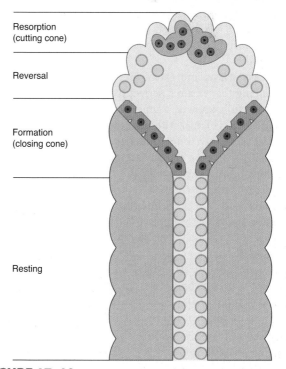

FIGURE 17–10 A cutting cone remodeling cortical bone. (Redrawn, with permission, from Felig P et al [editors]. *Endocrinology and Metabolism,* 3rd ed. McGraw-Hill, 1995.)

1. Osteoclast recruitment and activation

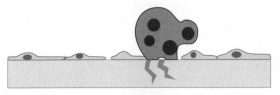

2. Resorption and osteoblast recruitment

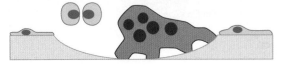

3. Osteoblastic bone formation

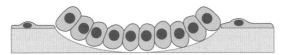

4. Completed remodeling cycle

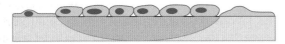

FIGURE 17–11 Sequential steps in remodeling of trabecular bone. (Redrawn, with permission, from Felig P et al [editors]. *Endocrinology and Metabolism*, 3rd ed. McGraw-Hill, 1995.)

tightly coupled, so that in a state of zero net bone balance, the amount of new bone formed is precisely equivalent to the amount of old bone resorbed. This degree of balance is brief, however. From age ~20–30, bone mass is consolidated after gains in growth and mineral deposition that were achieved during adolescence. After age 30, we begin to lose bone slowly.

How osteoclasts and osteoblasts communicate to achieve the coupling that ensures perfect (or near-perfect) bone balance is not fully known. It appears that the important signals are local, not systemic. Although they have not been identified with certainty, one candidate is RANK-L (described above). RANK-L is a cell-surface molecule on stromal cells that binds to osteoclast precursors and supports their development and differentiation. RANK-L also binds to RANK on mature osteoclasts, and this may mediate the coupling of bone formation and bone resorption. The process of bone remodeling does not absolutely require systemic hormones except to ensure an adequate supply of calcium and phosphate. However, systemic hormones use the bone as a source of minerals for regulation of extracellular calcium homeostasis. Osteoblasts have receptors for PTH and 1,25-$(OH)_2$ vitamin D, but osteoclasts do not. Isolated osteoclasts do not respond to PTH or vitamin D, except in the presence of osteoblasts. This coupling mechanism makes certain that when bone resorption is activated by PTH (eg, to provide calcium to correct hypocalcemia) bone formation will also increase, tending to replenish lost bone.

CHECKPOINT

6. Describe the two compartments of bone.
7. How is bone resorption by osteoclasts controlled?
8. What is the role of osteoblasts in bone formation? How are the actions of osteoblasts and osteoclasts coupled?

VITAMIN D

Vitamin D is actually a prohormone produced and metabolized to its active forms by the body. With exposure to normal amounts of sunlight, we synthesize enough vitamin D in our skin to meet our needs. The main natural source of vitamin D in the diet is in the livers of fish, which ingest ultraviolet-irradiated sterols (in phytoplankton and zooplankton) and store the vitamin D produced in their livers.

Physiology

7-Dehydrocholesterol, stored in the epidermis, is converted to vitamin D (cholecalciferol) by ultraviolet light (wavelengths 280–310 nm) (Figure 17–12). This step involves breakage of the B ring of the cholesterol structure to produce a secosteroid; hormones with an intact cholesterol nucleus (eg, estrogen) are called steroids.

Although cutaneous synthesis of vitamin D can be sufficient for our needs, persons in northern climates may become deficient in vitamin D at the end of the winter months, and the ill and infirm may not have adequate sunlight exposure. It is, therefore, recommended that the diet contain 200 IU of vitamin D per day for individuals up to age 50, 400 IU/day for those between the ages of 50 and 70, and 600 IU/day for those older than 70 years. In the United States, milk is supplemented with 400 IU of vitamin D per quart. Dietary supplements of vitamin D consist of vitamin D_2 (ergocalciferol) and vitamin D_3 (cholecalciferol). Vitamin D_2 and vitamin D_3 are activated in similar fashion to their active metabolites.

Vitamin D formed in the skin is a lipophilic substance that is transported to the liver bound to albumin and a specific vitamin D–binding protein (DBP). In the liver, vitamin D is hydroxylated to produce 25-hydroxyvitamin D (25-[OH]D) (Figure 17–12). This process, like cutaneous synthesis of vitamin D, is not closely regulated. 25-(OH)D is still rather lipophilic, and it is transported by DBP in the serum to target tissues. The blood contains most of the 25-(OH)D in the body. Therefore, a good clinical test for vitamin D deficiency is measurement of the serum level of 25-(OH)D.

The final metabolic processing step in the synthesis of the active hormone takes place principally in the kidney. The conversion of 25-(OH)D to 1,25-$(OH)_2$D by the 25-(OH)D 1-hydroxylase in the renal cortex is tightly regulated. The synthesis of 1,25-$(OH)_2$D is increased by PTH, thus linking the formation of 1,25-$(OH)_2$D closely to PTH in the integrated control of calcium homeostasis. The production of 1,25-$(OH)_2$D is also stimulated by hypophosphatemia, hypocalce-

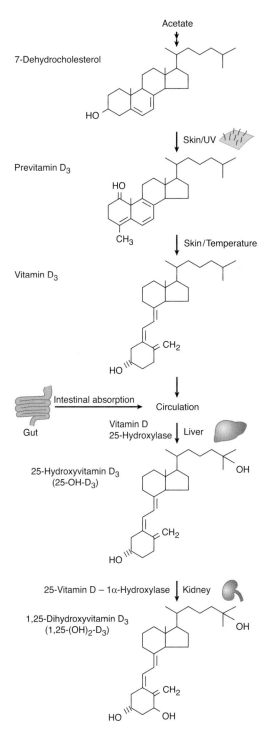

FIGURE 17–12 The formation and activation of vitamin D. (Redrawn, with permission, from Felig P et al [editors]. *Endocrinology and Metabolism*, 3rd ed. McGraw-Hill, 1995.)

mia, and FGF23 (described below). On the other hand, hypercalcemia, hyperphosphatemia, and decreased PTH will reduce 1,25-(OH)$_2$D production. As an additional control, 1,25-(OH)$_2$D induces the enzyme 24-hydroxylase, which catabolizes 25-(OH)D and 1,25-(OH)$_2$D, thus reducing their levels. The coordinated control by PTH, blood mineral levels,

and the vitamin D supply is very efficient. Levels of 1,25-(OH)$_2$D vary only slightly over an enormous range of vitamin D production rates but respond precisely to changes in the intake of calcium and phosphate within the normal range.

Vitamin D Action

The vitamin D receptor is a member of the steroid receptor superfamily of nuclear DNA-binding receptors. Upon ligand binding, the receptor attaches to enhancer sites in target genes and directly regulates their transcription. Thus, many of the effects of vitamin D involve new RNA and protein synthesis. Although many vitamin D metabolites are recognized by the receptor, 1,25-(OH)$_2$D has an affinity approximately 1000-fold greater than that of 25-(OH)D.

The primary target organs for 1,25-(OH)$_2$D are intestine and bone. The most essential action of 1,25-(OH)$_2$D is to stimulate the intestinal transport of calcium. Although calcium can be absorbed passively through a paracellular route, at low dietary calcium levels the active transport of calcium through the intestinal epithelial cells is required in a process that is regulated by 1,25-(OH)$_2$D. 1,25-(OH)$_2$D also induces the active transport of phosphate, but passive absorption dominates this process, and the net effect of 1,25-(OH)$_2$D is small.

In bone, 1,25-(OH)$_2$D regulates a number of osteoblastic functions. Vitamin D deficiency leads to rickets, a defect in mineralization. However, the defect in mineralization results mainly from decreased delivery of calcium and phosphate to sites of mineralization. 1,25-(OH)$_2$D also stimulates osteoclasts to resorb bone, releasing calcium to maintain the extracellular calcium concentration. This likely results from activation of the RANK-L/RANK signaling pathway by 1,25-(OH)$_2$D.

To demonstrate the interplay among calcium, phosphorus, PTH, and vitamin D, consider a person who switches from a high normal to a low intake of calcium and phosphate: from 1200 mg to 300 mg per day of calcium (the equivalent of leaving three glasses of milk out of the diet). The net absorption of calcium falls sharply, causing a transient decrease in the serum calcium level. This activates a homeostatic response led by an increase in PTH. The increased PTH level stimulates the release of calcium from bone and the retention of calcium by the kidney. In addition, the increase in PTH, the fall in calcium, and the concomitant fall in the serum phosphate level (because of both decreased intake and PTH-induced phosphaturia) activate renal 1,25-(OH)$_2$D synthesis. 1,25-(OH)$_2$D increases the fraction of calcium that is absorbed from the intestine, further increases calcium release from bone, and restores the serum calcium to normal.

FIBROBLAST GROWTH FACTOR 23 (FGF23)

FGF23 Biochemistry

FGF23 is a member of the large family of FGFs, local factors that are important in the control of cell proliferation and

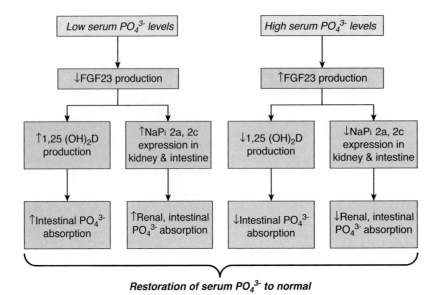

FIGURE 17–13   Phosphate homeostasis is maintained by the coordinated actions of FGF-23 and 1,25(OH)$_2$D. Low serum phosphate (PO$_4^{3-}$) levels suppress FGF-23 production, which increases 1,25(OH)$_2$D production and the expression of renal and intestinal phosphate transporters (NaPi 2a, 2c). As a result, intestinal and renal phosphate reabsorption rise to restore serum phosphate back to normal. When serum phosphate levels increase, FGF-23 levels rise, thereby suppressing these same biochemical pathways, and restoring serum phosphate balance.

differentiation. FGF23, in contrast to other FGF family members, plays a central role in the regulation of systemic phosphate homeostasis, vitamin D metabolism, and bone mineralization. Rapid advances in our understanding of FGF23 biology and its roles in normal physiology and bone disease are the result of astute analyses by many investigators of kindreds with rare genetic disorders and key transgenic and knockout mouse models, targeting essential molecules in FGF23 signaling cascades.

Physiology of FGF23

FGF23 is produced by many tissues in the body, but its primary source appears to be bone cells, particularly osteocytes. A critical regulator of FGF23 production is the serum phosphate level (Figure 17–13). When phosphate levels rise (eg, high-phosphate diet, renal failure), FGF23 levels increase. When serum phosphate levels fall (eg, phosphate depletion, low-phosphate diet), serum FGF23 levels decrease. In states of phosphate excess, FGF23 reduces the expression of the sodium phosphate co-transporters (NaPi 2a and 2c) in the kidney and intestine. This leads to the rapid excretion of phosphate by the kidney and reduced intestinal phosphate absorption, which in turn restore the serum phosphate level to normal. To further control the amount of phosphate being delivered to the circulation, FGF23 also inhibits the renal production of 1,25-(OH)$_2$D (see Figure 17–13). These direct actions of FGF23 are mediated by FGF receptors and their co-receptor transmembrane protein klotho.

Role of FGF23 in Disease

Several rare disorders have served to define the actions of FGF23 in phosphate and vitamin D metabolism in humans.

Disorders of FGF23 excess include **X-linked hypophosphatemic rickets, autosomal dominant hypophosphatemic rickets,** and **tumor-induced osteomalacia** (Table 17–12 and see the section on **osteomalacia**, below). Hypophosphatemia and osteomalacia resulting from phosphate wasting are hallmarks of these disorders. In contrast, loss of function of FGF23, due to rare genetic disorders, is associated with syndromes of ectopic calcification, abnormal mineralization, and hyperphosphatemia. The role of FGF23 in the hyperphosphatemia and osteodystrophy of chronic kidney disease is being actively investigated.

CHECKPOINT

9. How is vitamin D produced from 7-dehydrocholesterol?
10. Where is vitamin D stored?
11. Where does the final step in the activation of vitamin D take place, and how is it regulated?
12. What are the actions of vitamin D?

PARAFOLLICULAR CELLS (C CELLS)

Anatomy & Histology

C cells of the thyroid gland secrete the peptide hormone calcitonin. They constitute 0.1% or less of thyroid cell mass and are distributed in the central parts of the lateral lobes of the thyroid, especially between the upper and middle thirds of the lobes. C cells are neuroendocrine cells derived from the ultimobranchial body, a structure that fuses with the thyroid.

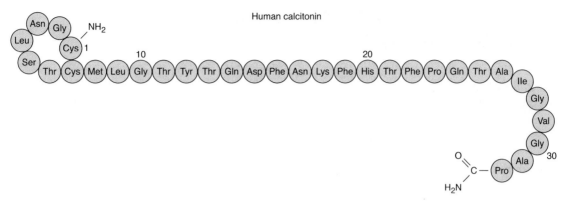

FIGURE 17–14 Amino acid sequence of human calcitonin, demonstrating its biochemical features, including an amino terminal disulfide bridge and carboxyl terminal prolineamide.

C cells are small spindle-shaped or polygonal cells distributed throughout the thyroid. They contain abundant granules, mitochondria, and Golgi. They may be present as single cells or arranged in nests, cords, and sheets within the thyroid parenchyma. They are often found within thyroid follicles, are larger than follicular cells, and stain positively for calcitonin.

Physiology

Calcitonin is a 32-amino-acid peptide hormone with a seven-member amino terminal disulfide ring and carboxyl terminal prolineamide (Figure 17–14). Differential processing of the calcitonin gene can lead to the production of either calcitonin in C cells or calcitonin gene-related peptide in neurons. Although calcitonin gene-related peptide has cardiovascular and neurologic effects in pharmacologic doses, the function of the peptide at normal physiologic levels is unknown. C-cell tumors may release both peptides.

Hypercalcemia stimulates the release of calcitonin through the activation of CaSRs in C cells. Substantial changes in serum calcium are normally required to modulate the release of calcitonin. It is not known whether small physiologic changes in serum calcium, which rapidly modulate PTH secretion, elicit significant changes in calcitonin levels. The GI hormones cholecystokinin and gastrin are also secretagogues for calcitonin.

Calcitonin secretion in vivo is assessed by measuring serum levels with a two-site radioimmunoassay. Calcitonin typically rises to very high levels in patients with medullary carcinoma of the thyroid.

Actions of Calcitonin

Calcitonin interacts with receptors in kidney and bone. This interaction stimulates adenylyl cyclase activity and the generation of cAMP (as shown in Figure 17–5 for PTH). In the kidney, receptors for calcitonin are localized in the cortical ascending limb of Henle's loop, whereas in bone calcitonin receptors are found on osteoclasts.

The main function of calcitonin is to lower serum calcium, and this hormone is rapidly released in response to hypercalcemia. Calcitonin inhibits osteoclastic bone resorption and rapidly blocks the release of calcium and phosphate from bone. The latter effect is apparent within minutes after the administration of calcitonin. These effects ultimately lead to a fall in serum calcium and phosphate.

Calcitonin acts directly on osteoclasts and blocks the resorption of bone induced by hormones like PTH and vitamin D. The potency of calcitonin depends on the underlying rate of bone resorption. Calcitonin also has a modest effect on the kidney to produce mild phosphaturia. With prolonged administration of calcitonin, "escape" from its effects occurs.

The overall importance of calcitonin in the maintenance of calcium homeostasis is unclear. Serum calcium concentrations are normal in patients after thyroidectomy, which removes all functioning C cells.

CHECKPOINT

13. What are the actions of calcitonin?
14. What is the effect of thyroidectomy on serum calcium?

PATHOPHYSIOLOGY OF SELECTED DISORDERS OF CALCIUM METABOLISM

PRIMARY & SECONDARY HYPERPARATHYROIDISM

Etiology

Primary hyperparathyroidism is due to excessive production and release of PTH by the parathyroid glands. The prevalence of hyperparathyroidism is approximately 1:1000 in the United States, and the incidence of the disease increases with age. The patient group most frequently affected is postmenopausal women.

Primary hyperparathyroidism may be caused by any of the following: adenoma, hyperplasia, or carcinoma (Table 17–1). **Chief cell adenomas** are the most common cause, accounting for almost 85% of all cases. The vast majority of parathyroid adenomas occur sporadically and are solitary.

Parathyroid hyperplasia refers to an enlargement or abnormality of all four glands. In atypical forms of hyperplasia, only one gland may be enlarged, but the other three glands typically show at least slight microscopic abnormalities such as increased cellularity and reduced fat content. The distinction between hyperplasia and multiple adenomas is challenging and usually requires the examination of all four glands. Key characteristics for judging whether a gland is normal or not are its size, weight, and histologic features.

Parathyroid hyperplasia may be part of the autosomal dominant **multiple endocrine neoplasia** (**MEN**) syndromes (Table 17–2). In patients with MEN-1, caused by mutations in the *MEN1* gene, which encodes the protein **menin**, there is high penetrance of hyperparathyroidism, affecting as many as 95% of patients. When their glands are examined microscopically, there are usually abnormalities in all four glands. Recurrent hyperparathyroidism, even after initially successful surgery, is common in these patients. Hyperparathyroidism also occurs in MEN-2, although at a much lower frequency in MEN-2a (about 20%) and rarely in MEN-2b. Familial hyperparathyroidism, without other features of MEN syndromes, characteristically involves all four glands. There is an increased risk of parathyroid cancer in these kindreds. Kindreds with isolated hyperparathyroidism and mutations in *menin* are considered to be allelic variants of MEN-1. Both the hyperparathyroidism-jaw tumor syndrome and familial

isolated hyperparathyroidism are causes for autosomal dominant hyperparathyroidism. The former often includes ossifying fibromas of the jaw and renal tumors and is caused by inactivating germline mutations in the *HRPT2* gene that encodes the protein **parafibromin**.

Parathyroid carcinoma is a rare malignancy, but the diagnosis should be considered in a patient with severe hypercalcemia and a palpable cervical mass. At surgery, cancers are firmer than adenomas and more likely to be attached to adjacent structures. It is sometimes difficult to distinguish parathyroid carcinomas from adenomas on histopathologic grounds. Vascular or capsular invasion by tumor cells is a good indicator of malignancy, but these features are not always present. In many cases, local recurrences or distant

TABLE 17–1   Causes of primary hyperparathyroidism.

Solitary adenomas	80–85%
Hyperplasia	10%
Multiple adenomas	≈2%
Carcinoma	≈2–5%

TABLE 17–2   Clinical features of multiple endocrine neoplasia syndromes.

MEN-1
Benign parathyroid tumors (very common)
Pancreatic tumors (benign or malignant)
Gastrinoma
Insulinoma
Glucagonoma, VIPoma (both rare)
Pituitary tumors
Growth hormone-secreting
Prolactin-secreting
ACTH-secreting
Other tumors: lipomas, carcinoids, adrenal and thyroid adenomas
MEN-2a
Medullary carcinoma of the thyroid
Pheochromocytoma (benign or malignant)
Hyperparathyroidism (uncommon)
MEN-2b
Medullary carcinoma of the thyroid
Pheochromocytoma
Mucosal neuromas, ganglioneuromas
Marfanoid habitus
Hyperparathyroidism (very rare)

Key: VIP, vasoactive intestinal polypeptide; ACTH, adrenocorticotropic hormone.

metastases to liver, lung, or bone are the clinical findings that support this diagnosis. Approximately 20% of patients with the hyperparathyroidism-jaw tumor syndrome and germline mutations in the *HRPT2* gene (described above) develop parathyroid cancer. Furthermore, mutations in *HRPT2* have also been found in familial isolated hyperparathyroidism and in sporadic parathyroid cancers. The normal cellular function of parafibromin is unknown.

Secondary hyperparathyroidism implies diffuse glandular hyperplasia resulting from a defect outside the parathyroids. Secondary hyperparathyroidism in patients with normal kidney function may be observed in patients with severe calcium and vitamin D deficiency states (see below). In patients with chronic renal failure, there are many causative factors that contribute to the often dramatic enlargement of the parathyroid glands. These include decreased $1,25\text{-}(OH)_2D$ production, reduced intestinal calcium absorption, skeletal resistance to PTH, and renal phosphate retention.

Pathogenesis

PTH secretion in primary hyperparathyroidism is excessive given the level of the serum calcium. At the cellular level, there is both increased cell mass and a secretory defect. The latter is characterized by reduced sensitivity of PTH secretion to suppression by the serum calcium concentration. This qualitative regulatory defect is more common than truly autonomous secretion. Thus, parathyroid glands from patients with primary hyperparathyroidism are typically enlarged and, in vitro, demonstrate a "shift to the right" in their calcium setpoint for secretion (Figure 17–15). How these two defects interact in the pathogenesis of the disease remains to be fully elucidated.

The genetic defects responsible for primary hyperparathyroidism have received considerable attention. Genes that regulate the cell cycle are thought to be important in the pathogenesis of a significant subset of parathyroid tumors. The *PRAD1* gene (parathyroid rearrangement adenoma), whose product is a D1 cyclin, has been implicated in parathyroid tumor development and also in the pathogenesis of several malignant tumors (B-cell lymphomas, breast and lung cancers, and squamous cell cancers of the head and neck). Cyclins are cell cycle regulatory proteins. The *PRAD1* gene is located on the long arm of chromosome 11, as is the gene encoding for PTH. Analysis of parathyroid tumor DNA suggests that a chromosome inversion event occurred, which led to juxtaposition of the 5-regulatory domain of the *PTH* gene upstream to the *PRAD1* gene (Figure 17–16). Because regulatory sequences in the *PTH* gene are responsible for its cell-specific transcription, this inversion was initially postulated to lead to a parathyroid cell-specific overproduction of the *PRAD1* gene product. Excessive cyclin would enhance the proliferative potential of the cells bearing this inversion and, given sufficient time, could induce PTH excess. A transgenic mouse model in which cyclin D1 is overexpressed in parathyroid tissue under the control of the *PTH* gene promoter provides proof for this pathogenetic mechanism of primary hyperparathyroidism.

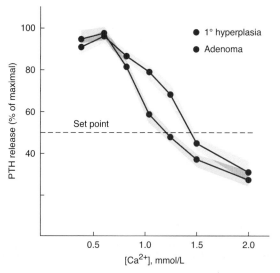

FIGURE 17–15 PTH secretion in vitro from human parathyroid cells from patients with parathyroid adenomas and hyperplasia. The set-point for secretion is the calcium concentration at which PTH release is suppressed by 50%. This is shifted to the right in the majority of parathyroid adenomas compared to normal tissues, in which the set-point is approximately 1.0 mmol/L ionized calcium. (Redrawn, with permission, from Brown EM et al. Dispersed cells prepared from human parathyroid glands: Distinct calcium sensitivity of adenomas vs primary hyperplasia. J Clin Endocrinol Metab. 1978;46:267.)

The gene responsible for MEN-1, which produces the protein product menin, was identified in 1997. It is thought to function as a tumor suppressor gene. In keeping with the "two-hit" hypothesis of oncogenesis, patients with MEN-1 inherit an abnormal or inactivated *MEN1* allele from one parent. This germline defect is present in all cells. During postnatal life, the other *MEN1* allele in a parathyroid cell, for example, undergoes spontaneous mutation or deletion. If this second mutation confers a growth advantage on the descendant cells, there is clonal outgrowth of cells bearing the second mutation, and eventually a tumor results. In approximately 25% of nonfamilial benign parathyroid adenomas, there is allelic loss of DNA from chromosome 11, where the *MEN-1* gene is located.

Menin localizes to the nucleus, where it binds to the transcription factor JunD in vitro and suppresses transcription. Menin's role in normal physiology and the mechanisms by which it promotes tumor formation in the pituitary, pancreas, and parathyroid glands are unknown. Mice with targeted deletion of both genes encoding the murine menin homologues (or *Men-1*) die in utero. Mice that are heterozygous for *Men-1* deletion survive but develop tumors in their pancreatic islets, adrenal cortices, and parathyroid, thyroid, and pituitary glands as they age, serving as a model for the MEN-1 syndrome.

Genetic testing is available to detect mutations in the *MEN1* gene so that appropriate case management and genetic counseling can be done.

The hyperparathyroidism in both MEN-2a and MEN-2b is caused by mutations in the RET protein. RET clearly plays an important role in the pathogenesis of the other endocrine tumors

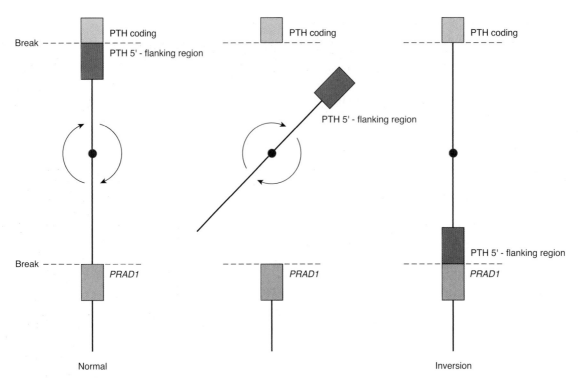

FIGURE 17–16 Proposed genetic rearrangement of chromosome 11 in a subset of sporadic parathyroid adenomas. An inversion of DNA sequence near the centromere of chromosome 11 places the 5′-regulatory region of the *PTH* gene (also on chromosome 11) adjacent to the *PRAD1* gene, whose product is involved in cell cycle control. This places the *PRAD1* gene under the control of *PTH* regulatory sequences, which would be predicted to be highly active in parathyroid cells. (Redrawn, with permission, from Arnold A. Molecular genetics of parathyroid gland neoplasia. J Clin Endocrinol Metab. 1993;77:1109.)

in these syndromes as well as in familial medullary carcinoma of the thyroid (see below). How RET mutations alter parathyroid cell growth or PTH secretion has not been elucidated.

Clinical Manifestations

Hyperparathyroidism may present in a variety of ways. Patients with this disease may be truly asymptomatic, and their diagnosis is made by screening laboratory tests. Other patients may have skeletal complications or nephrolithiasis. Because calcium affects the functioning of nearly every organ system, the symptoms and signs of hypercalcemia are protean (Table 17–3). Depending on the nature of the complaints, the patient with primary hyperparathyroidism may be suspected of having a psychiatric disorder, a malignancy, or, less commonly, a granulomatous disease such as tuberculosis or sarcoidosis.

Hyperparathyroidism is a chronic disorder in which long-standing PTH excess and hypercalcemia may produce increasing symptomatology, especially symptoms from renal stones or low bone mass. Recurrent stones containing calcium phosphate or calcium oxalate occur in 10–15% of patients with primary hyperparathyroidism. Nephrolithiasis may be complicated by urinary outflow tract obstruction, infection, and progressive renal insufficiency. Patients with significant PTH excess may experience increased bone turnover and progressive loss of bone mineral, especially in postmenopausal women. This is reflected in subperiosteal resorption, osteoporosis (particularly of cortical bone), and even pathologic fractures.

A sizable proportion of patients with primary hyperparathyroidism, however, are asymptomatic. These patients may experience no clinical deterioration if their hyperparathyroidism is monitored rather than treated surgically. Because it is difficult to identify these patients with certainty when the diagnosis of hyperparathyroidism is made, regular follow-up is mandatory. Recent studies indicate that bone mass may deteriorate significantly, especially at cortical sites (ie, hip, forearm) after conservative follow-up beyond 8–10 years. These observations have reopened the question of how presumed innocuous mild primary hyperparathyroidism may be deleterious to the skeleton.

Radiologic features of primary hyperparathyroidism are caused by the chronic effects of excess PTH on bone and the kidneys. These include subperiosteal resorption (evident most strikingly in the clavicles and distal phalanges), generalized low bone mass, and the characteristic but now rare brown tumors. Uncommonly, osteosclerosis may result from excessive PTH action on bone. Abdominal films may show nephrocalcinosis or nephrolithiasis.

The complete differential diagnosis of hypercalcemia should be considered in all patients with this abnormality (Table 17–4). Primary hyperparathyroidism accounts for most cases of hypercalcemia in the outpatient setting. The

TABLE 17–3 Symptoms and signs of primary hyperparathyroidism.

Systemic	Ocular	Skeletal and Rheumatologic
Weakness	Band keratopathy	Osteopenia
Easy fatigue	**Cardiac**	Pathologic fractures
Weight loss	Shortened QT interval	Brown tumors of bone
Anemia	Hypertension	Bone pain
Anorexia	**Renal**	Gout
Pruritus	Stones	Pseudogout
Ectopic calcifications	Polyuria, polydipsia	Chondrocalcinosis
Neuropsychiatric and Neuromuscular	Metabolic acidosis	Osteitis fibrosa cystica
Depression	Concentrating defects	**GI**
Poor concentration	Nephrocalcinosis	Peptic ulcer disease
Memory deficits		Pancreatitis
Peripheral sensory neuropathy		Constipation
Motor neuropathy		Nausea
Proximal and generalized muscle weakness		Vomiting

diagnosis of primary hyperparathyroidism is confirmed by at least two simultaneous measurements of calcium and intact PTH. An elevated or inappropriately normal PTH in the setting of hypercalcemia is the key feature in making the diagnosis of primary hyperparathyroidism (Table 17–5).

Patients with secondary hyperparathyroidism may have normal or subnormal calcium levels (see below). If renal function is normal, serum phosphate is also often reduced. Although serum PTH is elevated, the demineralized state of the bone and the chronic vitamin D deficiency combine to produce a low filtered load of calcium. Hence, urinary calcium excretion is often quite low. The 25-(OH)D level is also low or undetectable in vitamin D deficiency resulting from a variety of causes.

FAMILIAL (BENIGN) HYPOCALCIURIC HYPERCALCEMIA

Etiology

In patients with asymptomatic hypercalcemia, the diagnosis of **familial (benign) hypocalciuric hypercalcemia** should be considered. Individuals with this condition typically have an elevated serum calcium and magnesium, normal or mildly elevated PTH levels, and hypocalciuria (Table 17–5). This disorder is inherited in an autosomal dominant manner and is typically due to point mutations in one allele of the CaSR gene. In families with this form of benign hypercalcemia, there are rare occurrences of **neonatal severe primary hyperparathy-**

roidism. Infants with this form of hyperparathyroidism, usually the result of consanguinity, generally have inherited two copies of mutant CaSR genes.

Pathogenesis

The CaSR, a member of the G protein-coupled receptor superfamily, is highly expressed in the parathyroid gland and kidney. In the parathyroid, the molecule functions to detect changes in ambient serum calcium concentration and then adjust the rate of PTH secretion. In the kidney, the CaSR sets the level of urinary calcium excretion, based on its perception of the serum calcium concentration.

In familial hypocalciuric hypercalcemia and neonatal hyperparathyroidism, the ability to detect serum calcium is faulty in both the kidney and parathyroid. Familial hypocalciuric hypercalcemia is due to a partial reduction—and neonatal hyperparathyroidism to a marked reduction—in the ability to sense extracellular calcium. Parathyroid chief cells missense the serum calcium as "low," and PTH secretion occurs when it should be suppressed (Figure 17–2). This produces inappropriately normal or slightly high PTH levels. In the kidney, serum calcium concentrations are also detected (inappropriately) as low, and calcium is retained. This produces the hypocalciuria typical of this condition. Depending on the mutant gene dosage, the clinical symptoms tend to be mild in familial hypocalciuric hypercalcemia and severe and life-threatening in neonatal hyperparathyroidism.

TABLE 17–4 **Differential diagnosis of hypercalcemia.**

Primary hyperparathyroidism
Adenoma
Carcinoma
Hyperplasia
Familial (benign) hypocalciuric hypercalcemia
Inherited: CaSR mutations
Acquired: autoantibodies inhibiting the CaSR
Malignancy-associated hypercalcemia
Solid tumors (majority with excess PTHrP production)
Multiple myeloma
Adult T-cell leukemia and lymphoma
Other lymphomas
Thyrotoxicosis
Drugs
Thiazides
Lithium
Vitamin D or A intoxication
Granulomatous diseases
Sarcoidosis
Tuberculosis
Histoplasmosis (and other fungal diseases)
Milk-alkali syndrome
Adrenal insufficiency

Clinical Manifestations

Patients with familial hypocalciuric hypercalcemia typically have lifelong asymptomatic elevations in serum calcium. However, they are not thought to suffer the consequences of end-organ dysfunction characteristic of long-standing hyperparathyroidism and hypercalcemia. These individuals are generally spared the nephrolithiasis, low bone mass, and renal dysfunction that can occur in patients with primary hyperparathyroidism. Individuals with familial hypocalciuric hypercalcemia do not benefit from parathyroidectomy. Their hypercalcemia does not remit with surgery unless a total parathyroidectomy is performed. Surgery is not recommended because the condition is benign.

In contrast, infants with neonatal hyperparathyroidism have marked hypercalcemia, dramatic elevations in serum PTH, bone demineralization at birth, hypotonia, and pro-

found failure to thrive. These infants usually require total parathyroidectomy in the newborn period for survival.

In the asymptomatic hypercalcemic patient, a careful family history should be obtained in an effort to document hypercalcemia or the occurrence of failed parathyroidectomies in other family members. Simultaneous serum and urinary calcium and creatinine levels should be measured to rule out familial hypocalciuric hypercalcemia. In this condition, urinary calcium levels are typically low and almost always less than 100 mg/24 h (Table 17–5). The calcium-creatinine clearance ratio derived from spot or 24-hour urine collections is usually below 0.01. The ratio is calculated as urine calcium (mg/dL) × serum creatinine (mg/dL)/serum calcium (mg/dL) × urine creatinine (mg/dL). Genetic testing for CaSR gene mutations is commercially available in several reference laboratories and is the best approach to achieving a definitive diagnosis.

CHECKPOINT

15. What is the most common cause of primary hyperparathyroidism?
16. What is the occurrence of hyperparathyroidism in the multiple endocrine neoplasia syndromes?
17. In what conditions does secondary hyperparathyroidism occur? By what symptoms and signs is it distinguished from primary hyperparathyroidism?
18. What are the common symptoms and signs of primary hyperparathyroidism? How can primary hyperparathyroidism be distinguished from familial hypocalciuric hypercalcemia? What is the mechanism for this difference?

HYPERCALCEMIA OF MALIGNANCY

Etiology

Hypercalcemia occurs in approximately 10% of all malignancies. It is commonly seen in solid tumors, particularly squamous cell carcinomas (eg, lung, esophagus), renal carcinoma, and breast carcinoma. Hypercalcemia occurs in more than one third of patients with multiple myeloma but is unusual in lymphomas and leukemias.

Pathogenesis

Solid tumors usually produce hypercalcemia by secreting PTHrP, whose properties have been described previously. This is humoral hypercalcemia, which mimics primary hyperparathyroidism and results from a diffuse increase in bone resorption induced by high circulating levels of PTHrP. The syndrome is exacerbated by the ability of PTHrP to reduce renal excretion of calcium and the ability of hypercalcemia (acting via renal CaSRs) to blunt renal concentrating ability, which results in progressive dehydration.

TABLE 17–5 Laboratory findings in hypercalcemia from various causes.

	Serum Ca^{2+}	Serum PO$_4^{3-}$	Intact PTH	PTHrP	Serum 1,25 (OH)D	Urine Ca^{2+}
Primary hyperparathyroidism	↑	↓, N	↑	N, Und	N, ↑	N, ↑[1]
Malignancy-associated hypercalcemia	↑	↓, N	Und	↑[2]	N, ↓	↑
Familial (benign) hypocalciuric hypercalcemia	↑	N	N, ↑[3]	Und	N	↓
Vitamin D–dependent hypercalcemia	↑	N, ↑	↓	Und	N, ↑[4]	↑

[1]Can also be low depending on the dietary calcium and the filtered load of calcium.
[2]In the 70–80% of patients with cancer and a humoral basis for hypercalcemia.
[3]Mild increases in PTH have been reported in up to 25% of patients.
[4]1,25-(OH)$_2$D may not be frankly elevated in patients with vitamin D$_2$ or D$_3$ intoxication.
Key: N, normal; Und, undetectable; PTH, parathyroid hormone; PTHrP, PTH-related peptide.

Multiple myeloma produces hypercalcemia by a different mechanism; myeloma cells induce local bone resorption or osteolysis in the bone marrow, probably by releasing cytokines with bone-resorbing activity, such as interleukin-1 and tumor necrosis factor. Rarely, lymphomas produce humoral hypercalcemia by secreting 1,25-(OH)$_2$D.

Finally, even though many hypercalcemic patients have bone metastases, these may not contribute directly to the pathogenesis of hypercalcemia.

Clinical Manifestations

Unlike patients with primary hyperparathyroidism, who often are minimally symptomatic, patients with hypercalcemia of malignancy are typically very ill. Hypercalcemia typically occurs in advanced malignancy—the average survival of hypercalcemic patients is usually several weeks to months—and the tumor is almost invariably obvious on examination of the patient. In addition, hypercalcemia is often severe and symptomatic, with nausea, vomiting, dehydration, confusion, or coma. Biochemically, malignancy-associated hypercalcemia is characterized by a decreased serum phosphate and a suppressed level of intact PTH (Table 17–5). With most solid tumors, the serum level of PTHrP is increased. These findings, together with the differences in clinical presentation, usually make the differentiation of this syndrome from primary hyperparathyroidism relatively easy.

CHECKPOINT

19. What tumors commonly result in hypercalcemia?
20. What are the mechanisms by which a tumor may cause hypercalcemia?
21. What are the clinical symptoms and signs of hypercalcemia of malignancy?

HYPOPARATHYROIDISM & PSEUDOHYPOPARATHYROIDISM

Etiology

The total serum calcium includes the contributions from ionized, protein bound, and complexed forms of calcium. It should be recognized, however, that symptoms of hypocalcemia occur only if the ionized fraction of calcium is reduced. Furthermore, only patients with low ionized calcium levels should be evaluated for the possibility of a hypocalcemic disorder.

A common cause of low serum total calcium is hypoalbuminemia. A low serum albumin lowers only the protein-bound, and not the ionized, calcium. Thus, such patients need not be evaluated for mineral disorders. To determine whether a hypoalbuminemic patient has a low ionized calcium, this parameter can be measured directly. If this laboratory test is not readily available, a reasonable alternative is to correct the serum total calcium for the low serum albumin. This is done by adjusting the serum total calcium upward by 0.8 mg/dL for each 1 g/dL reduction in serum albumin. This simple correction usually brings the adjusted serum total calcium into the normal range.

The differential diagnosis of a low ionized calcium is lengthy (Table 17–6). Hypocalcemia can result from reduced PTH secretion caused by **hypoparathyroidism** or hypomagnesemia. It can also be due to decreased end-organ responsiveness to PTH despite adequate or even excessive levels of the hormone; this is termed **pseudohypoparathyroidism.**

All forms of hypoparathyroidism are uncommon (Table 17–7). Most cases are the result of inadvertent trauma to, removal of, or devascularization of the parathyroid glands during thyroid or parathyroid surgery. The incidence of postoperative hypoparathyroidism (range: 0.2–30%) depends on the extent of the antecedent surgery and the surgeon's skill in identifying normal parathyroid tissue and preserving its blood supply. Postoperative hypocalcemia may be transient or permanent. Some patients may also be left with diminished parathyroid reserve.

TABLE 17–6 Differential diagnosis of hypocalcemia.

Failure to secrete parathyroid hormone (PTH)
Hypoparathyroidism (see Table 17–7)
Resistance to PTH action
Pseudohypoparathyroidism (types 1a, 1b, 2)
Sepsis-associated hypocalcemia
Failure to secrete PTH and resistance to PTH action
Chronic magnesium depletion as a result of
Diarrhea, malabsorption
Alcoholism
Drugs: aminoglycoside antibiotics, loop diuretics, cisplatin, amphotericin B
Parenteral nutrition
Primary renal magnesium wasting
Failure to produce 1,25-(OH)$_2$D
Vitamin D deficiency as a result of nutritional causes
Liver disease
Cholestasis
Small intestinal disorders producing malabsorption
Renal failure
Vitamin D–dependent rickets type 1: defective 1α-hydroxylase activity (very rare)
Tumor-induced osteomalacia
Resistance to 1, 25-(OH)$_2$D action
Vitamin D–dependent rickets type 2: defect in vitamin D receptor (rate)
Vitamin D–dependent rickets type 3: overproduction of a hormone response element binding protein that interferes with binding of the vitamin D receptor-rentinoic acid receptor heterodimer to target DNA
Acute challenges to the homeostatic mechanisms
Pancreatitis (formation of calcium salts in retroperitoneal fat)
Drug-induced (eg, EDTA, citrate, plicamycin, bisphosphonates, phosphate, foscarnet)
Liver transplantation (citrate is not metabolized, thereby forming calcium citrate complexes and lowering ionized calcium)
Rhabdomyolysis
Hungry bone syndrome (increased deposition into demineralized bone)
Osteoblastic metastases (eg, breast or prostate cancer)
Tumor lysis syndrome (acute phosphate load released from tumor cells as a result of cytolytic therapy)

A variety of causes other than postsurgical complications may produce an absolute or relative state of PTH deficiency (Table 17–7). These include autoimmune glandular failure, magnesium depletion, autosomal dominant or recessive or X-linked hypoparathyroidism, hypoparathyroidism resulting from activating mutations of the CaSR or stimulating antibodies directed against the CaSR (see below), and hypoparathyroidism resulting from iron overload or Wilson's disease. Abnormal development of the glands resulting in varying degrees of severity of hypoparathyroidism is seen in the **DiGeorge syndrome.** This syndrome can present in infancy, childhood, or even adulthood and may be accompanied by defective cell-mediated immunity and other congenital anomalies (Table 17–7). Mutations in the gene for transcription factor GCMB (glial cell missing-B), which is essential in the development of the parathyroid glands, are linked to familial isolated hypoparathyroidism. Mutations in the transcription factor GATA3 cause abnormal otic vesicle, renal, and parathyroid gland development resulting in deafness, renal anomalies, and hypoparathyroidism.

There are two syndromes of **autoimmune polyendocrine failure syndrome** termed **APS.** Patients with APS-1 commonly have mucocutaneous candidiasis, Addison's disease (adrenal insufficiency), and hypoparathyroidism and less commonly ovarian failure and thyroid dysfunction. Various

TABLE 17–7 Causes of hypoparathyroidism.

Complication of thyroid, parathyroid or laryngeal surgery
Autoimmune destruction
Isolated
Autoimmune polyendocrine failure syndrome type 1 (APS-1)
Secondary to magnesium depletion or hypermagnesemia
Post-^{131}I therapy for Graves' disease or thyroid cancer
Secondary to accumulation of iron (thalassemia, hemochromatosis) or copper (Wilson's disease)
Genetic forms of hypoparathyroidism
DiGeorge or 22q deletion syndrome
Autosomal recessive or autosomal dominant mutations in pre-proPTH gene
X-linked hypoparathyroidism
Mutations in transcription factors involved in parathyroid development (eg, GCMB, GATA3)
Mitochondrial DNA mutations
Activating mutations of the CaSR
Acquired autoimmune syndrome caused by autoantibodies activating the CaSR
Tumor invasion (very rare)

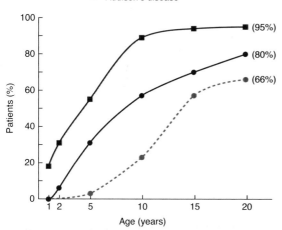

FIGURE 17–17 Cumulative incidence of three common manifestations of autoimmune polyglandular failure type 1 (APS-1) compared with age at onset in a cohort of 68 patients. The figures in parentheses reflect incidences at age 20. (Data plotted from Ahonen P et al. Clinical variation of autoimmune polyendocrinopathy-candidiasis-ectodermal dystrophy [APECED] in a series of 68 patients. N Engl J Med. 1990;322:1829.)

components of APS-1 present by the teens or early 20s (Figure 17–17).

Autoantibodies to adrenal and parathyroid tissue are seen in most of these patients. Eventually, other endocrine glands may become involved (eg, gonads, thyroid, and pancreas). APS-1 is an autosomal recessive disorder due to mutations in the autoimmune regulator (*AIRE*) gene. *AIRE* is expressed normally in a subpopulation of epithelial cells in the thymus that are thought to be involved in negative selection of autoreactive T cells during clonal selection. These T-cell clones are involved in self-recognition, and the failure to delete these T-cell clones is thought to underlie the autoimmune destruction of the endocrine cells affected in APS-1.

APS-2 or **Schmidt's syndrome** is characterized by hypothyroidism and adrenal insufficiency and does not involve the parathyroid glands (see Chapter 21).

Pathogenesis

The pathogenesis of hypoparathyroidism is straightforward. The mineral disturbance occurs because the amount of PTH released is inadequate to maintain normal serum calcium concentrations, mainly due to the loss of the renal calcium-conserving effects of PTH and the inability to generate 1,25-$(OH)_2D$. Hypocalcemia results, and hyperphosphatemia is also observed because the proximal tubular effect of PTH to promote phosphate excretion is lost. Because PTH is required to stimulate the renal production of 1,25-$(OH)_2D$, levels of 1,25-$(OH)_2D$ are low in patients with hypoparathyroidism. Hyperphosphatemia further suppresses 1,25-$(OH)_2D$ synthesis. Low 1,25-$(OH)_2D$ levels lead to reduced intestinal calcium

absorption. In the absence of adequate 1,25-$(OH)_2D$ and PTH, the mobilization of calcium from bone is abnormal. Because PTH is deficient, urinary calcium excretion is often high, despite the hypocalcemia.

Magnesium depletion is a common cause of hypocalcemia. The pathogenesis of hypocalcemia in this clinical setting relates to a functional and reversible state of hypoparathyroidism. There is also decreased renal and skeletal responsiveness to PTH. Magnesium depletion may occur from a variety of causes, including chronic alcoholism, diarrhea, and drugs such as loop diuretics, aminoglycoside antibiotics, amphotericin B, and cisplatin (Table 17–6). Magnesium is required to maintain normal PTH secretory responses. Once body magnesium stores are replete, PTH levels rise appropriately in response to the hypocalcemia, and the mineral imbalance is corrected.

In **pseudohypoparathyroidism**, PTH levels are usually elevated, but the ability of target tissues (particularly kidney) to respond to the hormone is subnormal. In pseudohypoparathyroidism type 1, the ability of PTH to generate an increase in the second-messenger cAMP is reduced. In patients with type 1a, this is due to a deficiency in the cellular content of the α subunit of the stimulatory G protein ($G_{s-\alpha}$), which couples the PTH receptor to the adenylyl cyclase enzyme. In patients with type 1b, $G_{s-\alpha}$ protein levels are normal, and in some cases there is altered regulation of the $G_{s-\alpha}$ gene transcription due to abnormal DNA methylation. In patients with pseudohypoparathyroidism type 2, urinary cAMP is normal but the phosphaturic response to infused PTH is reduced. The pathogenesis of this more rare form of PTH resistance remains obscure.

Patients with activating mutations of the CaSR typically present with autosomal dominant hypocalcemia and hypercalciuria. Both defects are due to overly sensitive CaSRs, which turn off PTH secretion and renal calcium reabsorption at subnormal serum calcium levels. These individuals rarely experience symptoms of their often mild hypocalcemia, but if given vitamin D, they are prone to develop marked hypercalciuria, nephrocalcinosis, and even renal failure.

Clinical Manifestations

The symptoms and signs of hypocalcemia are similar, regardless of the underlying cause (Table 17–8). Patients may be asymptomatic or may have latent or overt tetany. **Tetany** is defined as spontaneous tonic muscular contractions. Painful carpal spasms and laryngeal stridor are striking manifestations of tetany. Latent tetany may be demonstrated by testing for Chvostek's and Trousseau's signs. **Chvostek's sign** is elicited by tapping on the facial nerve anterior to the ear. Twitching of the ipsilateral facial muscles indicates a positive test. A positive **Trousseau's sign** is demonstrated by inflating the sphygmomanometer with the cuff around the arm above the systolic blood pressure for 3 min. In hypocalcemic individuals, this causes painful carpal muscle contractions and spasms (Figure 17–18). If hypocalcemia is severe and unrecognized, airway compromise, altered mental status, generalized seizures, and even death may occur.

TABLE 17–8 Symptoms and signs of hypocalcemia.

Systemic	Confusion
	Weakness
	Mental retardation
	Behavioral changes
Neuromuscular	Paresthesias
	Psychosis
	Seizures
	Carpopedal spasms
	Chvostek's and Trousseau's signs
	Depression
	Muscle cramping
	Parkinsonism
	Irritability
	Basal ganglia calcifications
Cardiac	Prolonged QT interval
	ST-T wave changes
	Congestive heart failure
Ocular	Cataracts
Dental	Enamel hypoplasia of teeth
	Defective root formation
	Failure of adult teeth to erupt
Respiratory	Laryngospasm
	Bronchospasm
	Stridor

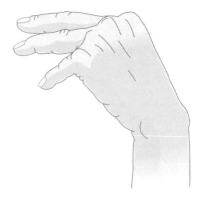

FIGURE 17–18   Position of fingers in carpal spasm resulting from hypocalcemic tetany.   (Redrawn, with permission, from Ganong WF. *Review of Medical Physiology*, 22nd ed. McGraw-Hill, 2005.)

Chronic hypocalcemia can produce intracranial calcifications that have a predilection for the basal ganglia. These may be detectable by CT scanning, MRI, or skull radiographs. Chronic hypocalcemia may also enhance calcification of the lens and the formation of cataracts.

In addition to the symptoms and signs of hypocalcemia, patients with pseudohypoparathyroidism type 1a may have a constellation of features collectively known as **Albright's hereditary osteodystrophy.** They include short stature, obesity, mental retardation, round facies, shortened fourth and fifth metacarpal and metatarsal bones, and subcutaneous ossifications. In considering the differential diagnosis of hypocalcemia, one must be guided by the clinical setting. A positive family history is very important in supporting a diagnosis of pseudohypoparathyroidism and other hereditary forms of hypoparathyroidism (Table 17–7). The patient with

hypocalcemia, hyperphosphatemia, and a normal serum creatinine most likely has hypoparathyroidism. A history of neck surgery should be sought. There may be a long latent period before symptomatic hypocalcemia presents in postsurgical hypoparathyroidism. The physical examination can be helpful if it identifies signs of hypocalcemia, stigmata of Albright's hereditary osteodystrophy, or other features of APS-1 (ie, vitiligo, mucocutaneous candidiasis, adrenal insufficiency). Patients with pseudohypoparathyroidism type 1a often have other endocrine abnormalities such as primary hypothyroidism or gonadal failure.

In the differential diagnosis of hypocalcemia, laboratory findings are extremely useful (Table 17–9). Serum phosphate is often (not invariably) elevated in hypoparathyroidism and pseudohypoparathyroidism. In magnesium depletion, serum phosphate is usually normal. In secondary hyperparathyroidism not due to renal failure, serum phosphate is typically low. Serum PTH levels are crucial in determining the cause of hypocalcemia. PTH is classically elevated in untreated pseudohypoparathyroidism but not in hypoparathyroidism or magnesium depletion. Intact PTH may be undetectable, low, or normal in patients with hypoparathyroidism depending on the parathyroid functional reserve. In patients with secondary hyperparathyroidism resulting from defects in the production or bioavailability of vitamin D, the clinical setting often suggests a problem with vitamin D (eg, regional enteritis, bowel resection, liver disease). The presence of a low 25-(OH)D level and an increased PTH confirms this diagnosis.

Measurement of serum magnesium is the first step in ruling out magnesium depletion as the cause of hypocalcemia and should be part of the initial evaluation. If urinary magnesium is inappropriately high relative to the serum magnesium, renal magnesium wasting is present. PTH levels in this setting are typically low or normal. Normal PTH levels, however, are inappropriate in the presence of hypocalcemia.

The diagnosis of pseudohypoparathyroidism can be confirmed by infusing synthetic human PTH(1–34) and measuring urinary cAMP and phosphate responses. This maneuver is designed to prove that there is end-organ resistance to PTH

TABLE 17–9 Laboratory findings in hypocalcemia.

	Serum Ca^{2+}	Serum PO_4^{3-}	Intact PTH	25-$(OH)D_3$	Urinary cAMP Response to PTH Infusion
Hypoparathyroidism	↓	↑, N	↓, N[1]	N	N
Pseudohypoparathyroidism	↓	↑, N	↑	N	↓[2]
Magnesium depletion	↓	N	↓, N[1]	N	N
Secondary hyperparathyroidism[3]	↓	N, ↓	↑	↓	N

[1]May be normal, but inappropriate to level of serum calcium.

[2]Urinary cAMP responses to PTH infusion are subnormal in pseudohypoparathyroidism type 1a and 1b.

[3]As a result of vitamin D deficiency, for example; urinary calcium excretion usually less than 50 mg/24 h.

Key: PTH, parathyroid hormone; cAMP, cyclic adenosine monophosphate.

and to determine whether the diagnosis is pseudohypoparathyroidism type 1 or type 2.

Hypoparathyroidism may vary in its severity and, therefore, in the need for therapy. In some patients with decreased parathyroid reserve, only situations of increased stress on the glands, such as pregnancy or lactation, induce hypocalcemia. In other patients, PTH deficiency is a chronic symptomatic disorder necessitating lifelong therapy with calcium supplements and vitamin D analogues. All patients so treated should have periodic monitoring of serum calcium, urinary calcium, and renal function. Patients with autoimmune hypoparathyroidism should also be examined regularly for the development of adrenal insufficiency, hypothyroidism, and diabetes mellitus as well as other complications of APS-1.

CHECKPOINT

22. What are the causes of hypoparathyroidism?
23. What is the mechanism of pseudohypoparathyroidism?
24. What are the symptoms and signs of hypocalcemia?
25. How can laboratory studies be used to distinguish various causes of hypocalcemia?

MEDULLARY CARCINOMA OF THE THYROID

Etiology

Medullary carcinoma of the thyroid gland, a C-cell neoplasm, accounts for only 5–10% of all thyroid malignancies. Approximately 80% are sporadic and 20% are familial, occurring in autosomal dominant MEN-2a and MEN-2b and in non-MEN syndromes. In sporadic cases, the tumor is usually unilateral. In hereditary forms, however, tumors are often bilateral and multifocal.

Pathogenesis

The growth pattern of medullary carcinoma is slow but progressive, and local invasion of adjacent structures is common. The tumor spreads hematogenously, with metastases typically to lymph nodes, bone, and lung. The clinical progression of this cancer is variable. Although there may be early metastases to cervical and mediastinal lymph nodes in as many as 70% of patients, the tumor still usually behaves in an indolent fashion. In a minority of cases, a more aggressive pattern of tumor growth has been noted. Early detection in high-risk individuals, such as those with a family history of medullary carcinoma or MEN-2a or MEN-2b, is crucial to prevent advanced disease and distant metastases. Overall survival is estimated to be 80% at 5 years and 60% at 10 years.

Patients with MEN-2 develop medullary carcinoma at frequencies approaching 100%. C-cell hyperplasia typically precedes the development of cancer. In MEN-2a and MEN-2b, the thyroid lesions are malignant. In contrast, pheochromocytomas associated with either MEN-2a or MEN-2b are infrequently malignant. Hyperparathyroidism in MEN-2a, which is uncommon, is usually due to diffuse hyperplasia and not to a malignancy. Chronic hypercalcitoninemia as a result of the tumor may also contribute to the pathogenesis of parathyroid hyperplasia. Parathyroid hyperplasia is rarely seen in patients with either MEN-2b or sporadic carcinoma. Germline mutations in the *RET* proto-oncogene on chromosome 10 are known to play a causal role in three forms of medullary carcinoma. These include cases of familial isolated medullary thyroid cancer, MEN-2a, and MEN-2b.

Clinical Manifestations

Sporadic medullary carcinoma occurs with about equal frequency in males and females and is typically found in patients older than 50 years. In MEN-2a or MEN-2b, the tumor occurs at a much younger age, often in childhood. In fact, medullary carcinoma in a patient younger than 40 years should suggest familial medullary carcinoma or MEN-2a or MEN-2b. Medullary carcinoma may present as a single nodule or as multiple thyroid nodules. Patients with sporadic medullary carcinoma often have palpable cervical lymphadenopathy.

Because C cells are neuroendocrine cells, these tumors have the capacity to release calcitonin and other hormones such as prostaglandins, serotonin, adrenocorticotropin, somatostatin, and calcitonin gene-related peptide. Serotonin, calcitonin, or the prostaglandins have been implicated in the pathogenesis of the secretory diarrhea observed in approximately 25% of patients with medullary carcinoma. If diarrhea is present, this usually indicates a large tumor burden or metastatic disease. Patients may also have flushing, which has been ascribed to the production by the tumor of substance P or calcitonin gene-related peptide, both of which are vasodilators.

In a patient suspected of having medullary carcinoma, a radionuclide thyroid scan may demonstrate one or more cold nodules. These nodules are solid on ultrasonography. Fine-needle aspiration biopsy shows the characteristic C-cell lesion with positive immuno-staining for calcitonin. Surprisingly, the diagnosis of medullary carcinoma is not suspected preoperatively in most cases and is made instead by frozen section at the time of surgery. The tumor has the propensity to contain large calcifications, which can be seen on x-ray films of the neck. Bone metastases may be lytic or sclerotic in their appearance, and pulmonary metastases may be surrounded by fibrotic reactions.

The most important laboratory test in determining the presence and extent of medullary carcinoma is the calcitonin level. Circulating calcitonin levels are typically elevated in most patients, and serum levels correlate with tumor burden. In C-cell hyperplasia, basal calcitonin may or may not be elevated. However, these patients usually demonstrate abnormal provocative testing. Intravenous calcium gluconate (2 mg/kg of elemental calcium) is injected over 1 minute, followed by pentagastrin (0.5 μg/kg) over 5 seconds. Provocative testing is based on the ability of calcium and the synthetic gastrin analogue pentagastrin to hyperstimulate calcitonin release in patients with increased C-cell mass resulting from either hyperplasia or carcinoma. An increase in serum calcitonin, more than twice the normal response, is considered abnormal. It must be borne in mind that false-positive provocative testing for calcitonin can occur.

Serial calcitonin levels are a useful parameter for monitoring therapeutic responses in patients with medullary carcinoma or for diagnosing a recurrence, along with clinical examination and imaging procedures. Calcitonin levels usually reflect the extent of disease. If the tumor becomes less differentiated, calcitonin levels may no longer reflect tumor burden. Another useful tumor marker for medullary carcinoma is carcinoembryonic antigen (CEA). This antigen is frequently elevated in patients with medullary carcinoma and is present at all stages of the disease. Rapid increases in CEA predict a worse clinical course.

Surgery is the mainstay of therapy for patients with medullary thyroid carcinoma. Total thyroidectomy is advocated because the tumors are often multicentric. Patients may also receive radioactive iodine ablation of any residual thyroid tis-

sue, because any C cells remaining may undergo malignant degeneration. Patients should be monitored indefinitely for recurrences because these tumors may be very indolent. All patients with medullary carcinoma of the thyroid, whether familial or sporadic, should be tested for *RET* oncogene mutations. This testing is commercially available and has supplanted calcitonin provocative testing in patients from families with isolated medullary carcinoma or MEN-2a or MEN-2b. More than 90% of patients with MEN-2 have been found to harbor *RET* mutations. Sporadic cases of medullary carcinoma of the thyroid should also be tested to detect the occurrence of a new mutation for which other family members can then be screened. Properly performed DNA testing is essentially unambiguous in predicting gene carrier status and can be used prospectively to recommend prophylactic thyroidectomy in young patients with MEN-2 before the development of C-cell hyperplasia or frank carcinoma.

Patients with MEN-2a or MEN-2b, even in the absence of symptoms, should undergo screening tests for the possibility of pheochromocytoma before thyroid surgery. These tests include the determination of urinary catecholamines and their metabolites and adrenal CT scanning. These tumors may be clinically silent at the time medullary carcinoma is diagnosed, and they should be removed before thyroidectomy (Chapter 12).

CHECKPOINT

26. How can you make the diagnosis of medullary carcinoma of the thyroid?
27. What is the treatment for medullary carcinoma?
28. Which patients are at high risk for medullary carcinoma?

OSTEOPOROSIS

Etiology

Osteoporosis is defined as low bone mass. The bone is normal in composition but reduced in amount. Bone mass accrues rapidly throughout childhood and very rapidly in adolescence; half of adult bone mineral density is achieved during the teenage years (Figure 17–19). Peak bone mass is accomplished at approximately age 25 years. Bone mass then remains relatively stable through the adult years, followed by a rapid loss of bone in women at the time of menopause. In the later stages of life, both men and women continue to lose bone, although at a slower rate than that seen at the time of menopause.

Achieving maximum peak bone mass depends on optimal nutrition, physical activity, general health, and hormonal exposure throughout childhood and adolescence. Inadequate nutrition and weightbearing exercise can negatively impact acquisition of insufficient peak bone mass. After bone growth is completed, the bone mass is determined by the level of peak

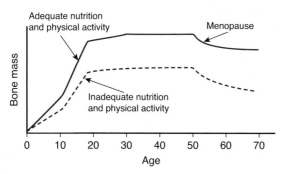

FIGURE 17–19 Bone mass in women as a function of age, demonstrating the potential effect of suboptimal nutrition and physical activity during the critical time of bone accrual in childhood and adolescence. (Redrawn, with permission, from Heaney RP et al. Peak bone mass. Osteo Int. 2000;11:985.)

bone mass that was attained and the subsequent rate of loss. Genetics are very important in determining bone mass. It has long been recognized that blacks have greater peak bone mass than whites or Asians and are relatively protected from osteoporosis. It now appears that, within the Caucasian population, more than half the variance in bone mass is genetically determined. However, a number of hormonal and environmental factors can reduce the genetically determined peak bone mass or hasten the loss of bone mineral and thus present important risk factors for osteoporosis (Figure 17–19, Table 17–10).

The most important etiologic factor in osteoporosis is sex steroid deficiency. The estrogen deficiency that occurs after menopause accelerates loss of bone mass; postmenopausal women consistently have lower bone mass than men and a higher incidence of osteoporotic fractures. With respect to bone remodeling in men, testosterone serves some of the same functions as estrogen in women, but recent work indicates that estradiol generated from the peripheral aromatization of testosterone is the critical sex steroid mediating the preservation of male bone mass. Hypogonadal men experience accelerated bone loss. Men on androgen deprivation therapy for prostate cancer are at increased risk for bone loss and fracture. Another important risk factor for bone loss is the use of corticosteroids or endogenous cortisol excess in Cushing's syndrome. Glucocorticoid-induced osteoporosis is one of the most devastating complications of chronic therapy with these agents. Certain other medications, including thyroid hormone, anticonvulsants, and chronic heparin therapy, immobilization, alcohol abuse, and smoking are also risk factors for osteoporosis. Diet is important as well. As discussed below, an adequate intake of calcium and vitamin D is necessary to build peak bone mass optimally and to minimize the rate of loss. Other dietary factors may also be important. Osteoporosis is most prevalent in Western societies, and it has been speculated that our high protein and sodium chloride intake or related factors may predispose to osteoporosis, perhaps by enhancing urinary calcium losses. Many additional disorders affecting the GI, hematologic, and connective tissue systems can contribute to the development of osteoporosis (Table 17–10).

TABLE 17–10 Causes of osteoporosis.

Primary osteoporosis
Aging (senile or involutional)
Juvenile
Idiopathic (young adults)
Connective tissue diseases
Osteogenesis imperfecta
Homocystinuria
Ehlers-Danlos syndrome
Marfan syndrome
Drug-induced
Corticosteroids
Alcohol
Thyroid hormone
Chronic heparin
Anticonvulsants
Hematologic
Multiple myeloma
Systemic mastocytosis
Immobilization
Endocrine
Hypogonadism
Hypercortisolism
Hyperthyroidism
Hyperparathyroidism
GI disorders
Subtotal gastrectomy
Malabsorption syndromes
Obstructive jaundice
Biliary cirrhosis

Pathogenesis

Because bone remodeling involves the coupled resorption of bone by osteoclasts and the deposition of new bone by osteoblasts, bone loss could result from increased bone resorption, decreased bone formation, or a combination. Postmenopausal osteoporosis is the consequence of accelerated bone resorption. The urinary excretion of calcium and breakdown products of type 1 collagen (eg, N- and C-telopeptides) increases, the serum PTH level is somewhat suppressed, and, if bone is biopsied, osteoclast numbers and resorption surfaces are increased. The bone formation rate is also enhanced, with an increase in serum alkaline phosphatase and the serum level of the bone matrix protein osteocalcin, both reflecting increased osteoblastic activity. This high-turnover state is the direct result of estrogen deficiency and can be reversed by estrogen replacement therapy.

The accelerated phase of estrogen-deficient bone loss begins immediately after menopause (natural or surgical). It is most evident in trabecular bone, the compartment that is remodeled most rapidly. As much as 5–10% of spinal trabecular bone mineral is lost yearly in postmenopausal women, and osteoporotic fractures in early post-menopausal women are often in the spine, a site of primarily trabecular bone. After 5–15 years, the rate of bone loss slows, so that after age 65 the rates are similar in both sexes.

The cellular basis for the activation of bone resorption in the estrogen-deficient state is not fully understood. Osteoclasts have estrogen receptors and could respond directly to estrogen deficiency, but there is strong evidence that cytokines such as interleukin-6 are released from cells in the bone microenvironment in estrogen deficiency. These cytokines increase the expression of RANK-L and decrease the expression of OPG on stromal cells and osteoblasts. These critical changes together promote an imbalance in bone remodeling that favors increased osteoclastogenesis and bone resorption.

The pathogenesis of age-related bone loss is less certain. It begins after age 30 years, is relatively slow, and occurs at first at a similar rate regardless of gender or race. It was once thought that elderly patients with osteoporosis ranged from low-turnover states, characterized by markedly decreased osteoblastic activity, to high-turnover states that resemble the accelerated phase of postmenopausal bone loss. It now appears that only a few such individuals are truly in a low-turnover state. For example, serum osteocalcin levels remain elevated throughout the latter decades of life, suggesting that osteoblast activity is not absolutely diminished. It is probable, however, that the balance of cellular activity is altered, with a reduced osteoblast response to continued bone resorption, so that resorption cavities are incompletely filled by new bone formation during the remodeling cycle.

One important factor in the pathogenesis of age-related bone loss is a relative deficiency of dietary calcium and 1,25-$(OH)_2D$. The capacity of the intestine to absorb calcium diminishes with age. Because renal losses of calcium are obligatory, a decreased efficiency of calcium absorption means that dietary calcium intake must be increased to prevent negative calcium balance. It is estimated that about 1200 mg/d of elemental calcium is required to maintain calcium balance in people over age 65 (Table 17–11). American women in this age group ingest 500–600 mg of calcium daily; the calcium intakes in men are somewhat higher. In addition, some older individuals may be deficient in vitamin D, further impairing their ability to absorb calcium. Particularly in northern climates, where sunlight exposure is reduced in the winter

TABLE 17–11 Recommended calcium and vitamin D intakes.

Age	Calcium (mg/day)	Vitamin D (IU/day)
0–6 months	210	200
7–12 months	270	200
1–3 years	500	200
4–8 years	800	200
9–18 years	1300	200
19–50 years	1000	200
51–70 years	1200–1500	400
70+ years	1200–1500	600

months, borderline low levels of 25-(OH)D and mild secondary hyperparathyroidism are evident by the end of winter.

The PTH level increases with age. This may be an example of secondary hyperparathyroidism that results from the following sequence of events: The well-known decrease in the mass of functioning renal tissue with age could lead to decreased renal synthesis of 1,25-$(OH)_2D$, which would directly release PTH secretion from its normal inhibition by 1,25-$(OH)_2D$. The reduced 1,25-$(OH)_2D$ level would also decrease calcium absorption, exacerbating an intrinsic inability of the aging intestine to absorb calcium normally. Secondary hyperparathyroidism would then result from the dual effects of 1,25-$(OH)_2D$ deficiency on the parathyroid gland and the intestine. In addition, the responsiveness of the parathyroid gland to inhibition by calcium is reduced with aging. The hyperparathyroidism of aging may thus result from the combined effects of age on the kidney, intestine, and parathyroid glands.

Provision of a dietary supplement with adequate vitamin D reduces the rate of age-related bone loss and protects against fracture. This suggests that reduced calcium absorption and secondary hyperparathyroidism play significant roles in the pathogenesis of osteoporosis in the elderly. However, the loss of bone continues after calcium supplementation, albeit at a lower rate, and it is thus likely that intrinsic changes in bone remodeling, perhaps having to do with a reduced osteoblastic response to ongoing osteoclastic bone resorption, also contribute to senile osteoporosis.

In secondary osteoporosis associated with glucocorticoid administration or alcoholism, there is a marked reduction in bone formation rates and serum osteocalcin levels. It is likely that glucocorticoids produce a devastating osteoporotic syndrome because of the rapid loss of bone that results from frankly depressed bone formation in the face of normal or even increased bone resorption.

The form of secondary osteoporosis associated with immobilization is another example of a resorptive state with marked uncoupling of bone resorption and bone formation and is

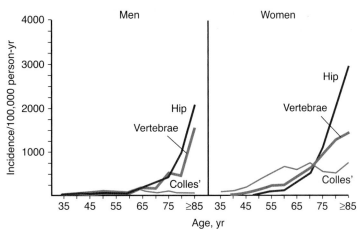

FIGURE 17–20 Age-specific incidence rates of wrist, hip, and vertebral fractures in men and women derived from Rochester, Minnesota data. (Redrawn, with permission, from Cooper C, Melton LJ. Epidemiology of osteoporosis. Trends Endo Metab. 1992;3:224.)

characterized by hypercalciuria and suppression of PTH. When individuals with a high preexisting state of bone remodeling (eg, adolescents and patients with hyperthyroidism or Paget's disease) are immobilized, bone resorption may be accelerated enough to produce hypercalcemia.

Clinical Manifestations

Osteoporosis is asymptomatic until it produces fractures and deformity. Typical osteoporotic fractures occur in the spine, the hip, and the wrist (Colles' fracture). In women, wrist fractures increase in incidence at menopause and then stay relatively stable at this increased rate with age. The incidence of hip and vertebral fractures increases rapidly with aging in both men and women (Figure 17–20). The vertebral bodies may be crushed, resulting in loss of height, or may be wedged anteriorly, resulting in height loss and kyphosis. The dorsal kyphosis of elderly women ("dowager's hump") results from anterior wedging of multiple thoracic vertebrae. Spinal fractures may be acute and painful or may occur gradually and be manifested only as kyphosis or loss of height.

The worst complication of osteoporosis is hip fracture. Hip fractures typically occur in the elderly, with a sharply rising incidence in both sexes after age 80 years. This is due to a variety of factors, including the tendency for a slower rate of bone loss in the cortical bone that makes up the hip compared with the predominantly trabecular bone of the spine. The personal and social costs of hip fracture are enormous. One third of American women who survive past age 80 years will suffer a hip fracture. The 6-month mortality rate is approximately 20%, much of it resulting from the complications of immobilizing frail persons in a hospital bed. The complications include pulmonary embolus and pneumonia. About half of elderly people with a hip fracture will never walk freely again. The long-term costs of chronic care for these persons are a major social concern.

The diagnosis of osteoporosis is sometimes made radiologically, but in general x-ray films are a poor diagnostic tool. A chest x-ray film will miss 30–50% of cases of spinal osteoporosis and, if overpenetrated, may lead to the diagnosis of osteoporosis in someone with a normal bone mass. The best way to diagnose osteoporosis is by measuring bone mineral density by dual-energy x-ray absorptiometry (DXA). The technique is precise, rapid, and relatively inexpensive. It delivers a considerably lower radiation dose than a chest x-ray. The relationship between bone mineral density and fracture risk is a continuous one (ie, the lower the bone mineral density, the higher the fracture risk). Osteoporosis has been defined by the World Health Organization (WHO) as a bone mineral density value 2.5 standard deviations or more below the young adult normal value (ie, a T score of −2.5 or less). This cutoff was selected based on the observation that 16% of postmenopausal Caucasian women at age 50 years will have femoral neck bone density values below −2.5, and this population has a 16% lifetime risk of hip fracture. However, it should be remembered that there is no threshold at this value and that bone mineral density measurements need to be interpreted in light of other risk factors for fracture such as age and propensity for falls. An absolute 10-year fracture risk calculation algorithm (termed FRAX) has recently been developed by the WHO. The algorithm incorporates hip bone mineral density values and several clinical risk factors to determine an individual's 10-year probability of a major osteoporotic or hip fracture. The URL www.shef.ac.uk/FRAX/index.htm provides access to the WHO absolute fracture risk calculator. This tool is useful for determining the need for treatment in lieu of just using the single DXA value.

It is additionally important to realize that not all of the risk for fracture is captured by measurements of bone mineral density because the strength of bone is also a function of bone quality. Bone quality, determined by the microarchitecture of a bone, its mechanical strength, its material properties, and its ability to withstand stress, may be substantially different in two individuals with the same bone mineral density. Techniques to assess bone quality noninvasively are being actively investigated.

Elderly persons with osteoporosis are unlikely to sustain a hip fracture unless they fall. Risk factors for falling include muscle weakness, impaired vision, impaired balance, sedative use, and environmental factors. Therefore, strategies to prevent falls are an important part of the approach to the osteoporotic patient.

Individuals at risk for osteoporosis benefit from calcium supplementation to a total intake of about 1200–1500 mg/d. This can be accomplished with dairy products or other calcium-rich foods, with calcium-fortified foods, or with a calcium supplement such as calcium carbonate. Vitamin D should be provided in age-appropriate doses (400–600 IU/d). The current recommended intakes for calcium and vitamin D are given in Table 17–11. Calcium supplementation in younger individuals may increase peak bone mass and decrease premenopausal bone loss, but its optimal role in this age group has not been determined. Estrogen replacement reduces bone loss, relieves hot flushes after menopause, and reduces fracture risk. It requires concomitant use of progestins in women who have not had a hysterectomy to prevent endometrial carcinoma and also increases the risk of breast cancer, stroke, myocardial infarction, and venous thromboembolism. The side-effect profile of estrogen has limited its use to short-term therapy at the time of menopause, typically in women suffering from hot flushes. Other antiresorptive agents available for treatment of osteoporosis include alendronate, risedronate, ibandronate, zoledronic acid, calcitonin, and raloxifene. The first four agents are bisphosphonates that directly inhibit osteoclastic bone resorption. Given therapeutically, calcitonin decreases bone resorption and may protect against bone loss and vertebral fractures. Raloxifene, a selective estrogen response modulator, inhibits bone resorption as estrogen does. Raloxifene does not induce endometrial changes, and it has estrogen antagonist actions in breast cells that may appear to decrease the incidence of breast carcinoma in postmenopausal women. The only agent currently available that can stimulate bone formation is parathyroid hormone (PTH1-34) (teriparatide). In contrast to the bone resorption that is caused by continuous elevations in PTH such as occur in hyperparathyroidism, a single daily injection of PTH stimulates bone formation and, to a lesser extent, bone resorption, resulting in net gains in bone density and decreased fracture risk.

CHECKPOINT

29. What is the relative importance of hereditary versus environmental or hormonal factors in contributing to osteoporosis?
30. What are the risk factors for osteoporosis?
31. What are the symptoms and signs of osteoporosis?
32. What are the risk factors for fracture in a patient with osteoporosis?
33. What treatments can prevent bone loss?

OSTEOMALACIA

Etiology

Osteomalacia is defined as a defect in the mineralization of bone. When it occurs in the young, it also affects the mineralization of cartilage in the growth plate, a disorder called **rickets**. Osteomalacia can result from a deficiency of vitamin D, a deficiency of phosphate, an inherited deficiency in alkaline phosphatase (hypophosphatasia), or agents that have adverse effects on bone (Table 17–12). Surprisingly, dietary calcium deficiency rarely produces osteomalacia, although a few cases have been reported.

Vitamin D deficiency is becoming more common in the United States because of decreased sunlight exposure, increased use of sunscreens, and limited dietary sources of vitamin D. Individuals of dark-skinned ethnicities are particularly vulnerable because they have less cutaneous synthesis

TABLE 17–12 **Causes of osteomalacia.**

Vitamin D deficiency
Nutritional
Malabsorption
Hereditary vitamin D–dependent rickets
Type I (renal 1α-hydroxylase deficiency)
Type II (absent or defective vitamin D receptor)
Phosphate deficiency
Renal phosphate wasting
X-linked hypophosphatemia
Autosomal dominant hypophosphatemic rickets
Autosomal recessive hypophosphatemic rickets
Fanconi syndrome
Renal tubular acidosis (type II)
Oncogenic osteomalacia (acquired, associated with mesenchymal tumors and prostate cancer)
Phosphate-binding antacids
Deficient alkaline phosphatase: hereditary hypophosphatasia
Drug toxicity
Fluoride
Aluminum (chronic renal failure)
Etidronate disodium
Phosphate-binding antacids
Chronic renal failure

of vitamin D in response to sunlight. Fortified milk is the main food source of vitamin D, but at 100 IU/cup of milk, it can be difficult to achieve the recommended 200–600 IU/d of vitamin D. Some cereals and other foods have been also been fortified with vitamin D. In addition to insufficient intake, vitamin D deficiency can be the result of malabsorption of this fat-soluble vitamin. Severe rickets also occurs as part of three rare heritable disorders of vitamin D action: renal 1α-hydroxylase deficiency, in which vitamin D is not converted to 1,25-$(OH)_2$D; mutant vitamin D receptors with reduced activity; and overproduction of a hormone response element binding protein that interferes with the activation (by the vitamin D receptor-retinoic acid receptor heterodimer) of vitamin D response elements on genes.

Phosphate deficiency with osteomalacia is usually caused by inherited or acquired renal phosphate wasting. Three hereditary forms of renal phosphate wasting include X-linked, autosomal dominant, or autosomal recessive hypophosphatemic rickets. Osteomalacia and hypophosphatemia can also result from tumors that are typically mesenchymal in origin and often located in the head and neck region. Many of these tumors overproduce FGF23 (see above) and induce renal phosphate wasting and low 1,25-$(OH)_2$D levels, eventually leading to osteomalacia. The *FGF23* gene is mutated in kindreds with autosomal dominant hypophosphatemic rickets. Families with X-linked hypophosphatemic rickets have mutations in the *PHEX* gene, which encodes an endopeptidase. This endopeptidase is thought to inactivate a postulated factor given the name "phosphatonin." Inactivation of the *PHEX* gene product is thought to enhance the in vivo activity of this phosphate-regulating factor. FGF23 levels are elevated in patients with XLH, but FGF23 does not appear to be a substrate for PHEX.

Pathogenesis

Vitamin D deficiency produces osteomalacia in stages. In the early stage, reduced calcium absorption produces secondary hyperparathyroidism, preventing hypocalcemia at the cost of increased renal phosphate excretion and hypophosphatemia. In later stages, hypocalcemia ensues, and hypophosphatemia progresses because of the combined effects of reduced absorption and the phosphaturic action of PTH. The poor delivery of minerals to bone (possibly coupled with the absence of direct effects of vitamin D on bone) impairs the mineralization of bone matrix. Since osteoblasts continue to synthesize bone matrix, unmineralized matrix or osteoid accumulates at bone-forming surfaces.

Clinical Manifestations

Patients with osteomalacia have bone pain, muscle weakness, and a waddling gait. Radiologically, they may have reduced bone mass, detectable by both x-ray and bone densitometry. The hallmark of the disorder, however, is the pseudofracture: local bone resorption that has the appearance of a nondisplaced fracture, classically in the pubic rami, clavicles, or scapulas. In children with rickets, the leg bones are bowed (osteomalacia means "softening of bones"), the costochondral junctions are enlarged ("rachitic rosary"), and the growth plates are widened and irregular, reflecting the increase in unmineralized cartilage. Biochemically, the hallmarks of vitamin D–deficient osteomalacia are hypophosphatemia, hyperparathyroidism, variable hypocalcemia, and marked reductions in urinary calcium to less than 50 mg/d. The 25-(OH)D level is reduced, indicative of decreased body stores of vitamin D. In vitamin D deficiency and other forms of osteomalacia, the alkaline phosphatase level is increased.

Although the disorder can be suspected strongly on clinical grounds and the biochemical changes summarized previously are confirmatory, a firm diagnosis of osteomalacia requires either the radiologic appearance of rickets or pseudofractures or a characteristic bone biopsy. If bone is biopsied for quantitative histomorphometry, thickened osteoid seams and a reduction in the mineralization rate are found. Treatment with vitamin D or aggressive phosphate replacement in patients with renal phosphate wasting will reverse osteomalacia or heal rickets.

CHECKPOINT

34. What are the causes of osteomalacia?
35. What are the two stages in which vitamin D deficiency produces osteomalacia?
36. What are the symptoms and signs of osteomalacia?

CASE STUDIES

Eva M. Aagaard, MD, & Yeong Kwok, MD

(See Chapter 25, p. 700 for Answers)

CASE 76

A 56-year-old woman presents to her primary care physician complaining of progressive fatigue, weakness, and diffuse bony pain. She says that her symptoms have been getting worse over the last 2 months. Her medical history is notable for well-controlled hypertension and recurrent renal stones. Physical examination is unremarkable. A serum calcium level is elevated.

Questions

A. What are some common causes of hypercalcemia? Which do you suspect in this patient, and why?

B. What is the pathogenesis of primary hyperparathyroidism? What genes have been implicated?

C. How would you make the diagnosis of primary hyperparathyroidism?

CASE 77

A 40-year-old woman comes to clinic to discuss some unexpected laboratory test abnormalities. She underwent these tests as part of a life insurance examination and was noted to have a mildly elevated serum calcium level. She has been healthy with no medical problems. She feels well and denies fatigue or pain. She does not take any medications or dietary supplements. There is no significant family history. Her physical examination is unremarkable. Repeated laboratory testing confirms a mildly elevated serum calcium level but also shows a normal serum phosphorus level, intact parathyroid hormone (PTH), and 1,25-OH$_2$D levels. A 24-hour urinary calcium test returns low, at 60 mg/24 h.

Questions

A. What is the likely diagnosis in this patient?

B. What is the underlying pathophysiology of this disorder, and how does this lead to the elevated serum calcium?

CASE 78

A 69-year-old man presents to his primary care physician complaining of fatigue, nausea, weakness, and diffuse bony pain. He states his symptoms have been getting progressively worse over the last 2 months. In addition, he has noted a 15-pound weight loss over approximately the same time span. His wife, who has accompanied him, also noted that he seems increasingly confused. His medical history is notable for well-controlled hypertension and chronic obstructive pulmonary disease. He has a 100 pack–year smoking history. On physical examination he is chronically ill appearing and thin. Vital signs are notable for a blood pressure of 120/85 mm Hg, a heart rate of 98 beats/min, and a respiratory rate of 16/min. Lungs have an increased expiratory phase, with mild expiratory wheeze. He has decreased breath sounds at the left base. The remainder of his examination is unremarkable. A serum calcium level is markedly elevated. Hypercalcemia of malignancy is suspected.

Questions

A. What tumors commonly cause hypercalcemia? Which is likely in this patient?

B. What would you expect his serum PTH level to be? What about his serum PTHrP? Why?

C. How does PTHrP secretion cause hypercalcemia?

CASE 79

A 32-year-old woman presents to the emergency department with complaints of involuntary hand spasms. She states that as she worked folding the laundry, she had a sudden severe spasm of her right hand such that her fingers flexed. The spasm was quite painful and lasted several minutes, resolving spontaneously. She is 6 months pregnant. Her medical history is otherwise notable for thyroid tumor status postthyroidectomy 3 years ago. She is taking synthetic thyroid hormone and a prenatal multivitamin. Family history is unremarkable. On physical examination, she has positive Chvostek's and Trousseau's signs. Examination is otherwise unremarkable. Serum calcium level is low. Hypoparathyroidism as a complication of the thyroid surgery is suspected.

Questions

A. What is the mechanism by which thyroid surgery can result in hypocalcemia? Why may she only now be symptomatic?

B. What is Chvostek's sign? Trousseau's sign? What does each represent?

C. What would you expect this patient's serum phosphate level to be? Serum PTH? Why?

CASE 80

A 23-year-old woman presents to her primary care physician complaining of diarrhea. The diarrhea is described as profuse and watery and has been getting progressively worse over the last 2 months. She has had no bloody or black bowel movements. The condition is not made worse by food and is not associated with fever, chills, sweats, nausea, or vomiting. On review of systems, she does note a 5-pound weight loss in the last 3 months. She also notes occasional flushing. She denies any significant family history. On physical examination, she is a thin white woman in no acute distress. She is afebrile, with a blood pressure of 100/60 mm Hg, heart rate of 100 beats/min, and respiratory rate of 14/min. Head examination is unremarkable. Neck examination reveals bilateral hard nodules of the thyroid, a 2-cm nodule on the right upper pole, and a 1.5-cm nodule on the left upper pole. She has a firm 1-cm lymph node in the right anterior cervical chain. Lungs are clear. Cardiac examination is mildly tachycardiac, with regular rhythm and no extra sounds. The abdomen has hyperactive bowel sounds and is soft, nontender, nondistended, and without masses. Skin examination discloses no rashes. Medullary carcinoma of the thyroid is suspected.

Questions

A. What is the cause of this patient's diarrhea? Flushing?

B. How would you make a diagnosis of medullary carcinoma of the thyroid?

C. What other tests would you like to order? Why?

CASE 81

A 72-year-old woman presents to the emergency room after falling in her home. She slipped on spilled water in her kitchen. She was unable to get up after her fall and was found on the floor in her kitchen by her son, stopping by after work. She complains of severe right hip pain. On examination, she has bruising over her right hip. Range of motion in her right hip is markedly decreased, with pain on both internal and external rotation. X-ray film reveals a hip fracture and probable low bone mass. The history raises concern about osteoporosis.

Questions

A. What are some important causes of osteoporosis?

B. What are the likely causes of osteoporosis in this patient and the underlying pathogenesis of each?

C. What are the risk factors for fractures in patients with osteoporosis?

D. What are common complications of hip fractures?

E. What treatments are available to prevent bone loss?

CASE 82

A 93-year-old woman is brought to the emergency department by ambulance for "failure to thrive." Today the woman's daughter was attempting to roll her to clean her, and the patient fell from the bed to the floor. They have been unable to pay for medications for several months. For many months, the patient has been eating only broth because of difficulty with chewing and swallowing. On examination, she is pale, with central obesity, wasting of her extremities, and flexion contractures of her right upper and lower extremities. On head-neck examination, she has temporal wasting, right facial droop, pale conjunctivas, and dry mucous membranes. Lungs are clear to auscultation. Cardiac examination is notable for an S4 gallop. She moans when her extremities are palpated. Laboratory reports show hypocalcemia, hypophosphatemia, and elevated alkaline phosphatase. X-ray films of her pelvis reveal low bone mass and "pseudofracture" of the pubic rami. Osteomalacia is suspected.

Questions

A. What are the causes of osteomalacia? Which do you suspect in this patient? Why?

B. What is the pathogenesis of osteomalacia in this patient?

C. What would you expect to see on a bone biopsy for quantitative histomorphometry?

REFERENCES

General Bone and Mineral Metabolism and Vitamin D

Bringhurst FR et al. Hormones and disorders of mineral metabolism. In: *Williams Textbook of Endocrinology*, 11th ed. Kronenberg HR et al (editors). Saunders, 2008.

Christakos S et al. Vitamin D: Molecular mechanism of action. Ann N Y Acad Sci. 2007 Nov;1116:340–8. [PMID: 18083936]

Duerr EM et al. Molecular genetics of neuroendocrine tumors. Best Pract Res Clin Endocrinol Metab. 2007 Mar;21(1):1–14. [PMID: 17382262]

Egbuna OI et al. Hypercalcaemic and hypocalcaemic conditions due to calcium-sensing receptor mutations. Best Pract Res Clin Rheumatol. 2008 Mar;22(1):129–48. [PMID: 18328986]

Holick MF. Vitamin D deficiency. N Engl J Med. 2007 Jul 19;357(3):266–81. [PMID: 17634462]

Jacobs TP et al. Rare causes of hypercalcemia. J Clin Endocrinol Metab. 2005 Nov;90(11):6316–22. [PMID: 16131579]

Lakhani VT et al. The multiple endocrine neoplasia syndromes. Annu Rev Med. 2007;58:253–65. [PMID: 17037976]

Strewler GJ. Humoral manifestations of malignancy. In: *Williams Textbook of Endocrinology*, 11th ed. Kronenberg HR et al (editors). Saunders, 2008.

Thakker RV. Genetics of endocrine and metabolic disorders: Parathyroid. Rev Endocr Metab Disord. 2004 Mar;5(1):37–51. [PMID: 14966388]

Hyperparathyroidism

Ambrogini E et al. Surgery or surveillance for mild asymptomatic primary hyperparathyroidism: A prospective randomized clinical trial. J Clin Endocrinol Metab. 2007 Aug;92(8):3114–21. [PMID: 17535997]

Andress DL. Bone and mineral guidelines for patients with chronic kidney disease: A call for revision. Clin J Am Soc Nephrol. 2008 Jan;3(1):179–83. [PMID: 18057310]

Bilezikian JP et al. Primary hyperparathyroidism: New concepts in clinical, densitometric and biochemical features. J Intern Med. 2005 Jan;257(1):6–17. [PMID: 15606372]

Bollerslev J et al. Medical observation, compared with parathyroidectomy, for asymptomatic primary hyperparathyroidism: A prospective, randomized trial. J Clin Endocrinol Metab. 2007 May;92(5):1687–92. [PMID: 17284629]

Hruska KA et al. Renal osteodystrophy, phosphate homeostais, and vascular calcification. Semin Dial. 2007 Jul-Aug;20(4):309–15. [PMID: 17635820]

Lee PK et al. Trends in the incidence and treatment of parathyroid cancer in the United States. Cancer. 2007 May 1;109(9):1736–41. [PMID: 17372919]

Lemos MC et al. Multiple endocrine neoplasia type 1 (MEN1): Analysis of 1336 mutations reported in the first decade following identification of the gene. Hum Mutat. 2008 Jan;29(1):22–32. [PMID: 17879353]

Machens A et al. Age-related penetrance of endocrine tumours in multiple endocrine neoplasia type 1 (MEN1): A multicentre study of 258 gene carriers. Clin Endocrinol (Oxf). 2007 Oct;67(4):613–22. [PMID: 17590169]

Martin KJ et al. Parathyroid hormone: New assays, new receptors. Semin Nephrol. 2004 Jan;24(1):3–9. [PMID: 14730504]

Moe SM et al. Chronic kidney disease-mineral-bone disorder: A new paradigm. Adv Chronic Kidney Dis. 2007 Jan;14(1):3–12. [PMID: 17200038]

Mosekilde L. Primary hyperparathyroidism and the skeleton. Clin Endocrinol (Oxf). 2008 Jul;69(1):1–19. [PMID: 18167138]

Palmer SC et al. Meta-analysis: Vitamin D compounds in chronic kidney disease. Ann Intern Med. 2007 Dec 18;147(12):840–53. [PMID: 18087055]

Rubin MR et al. The natural history of primary hyperparathyroidism with or without parathyroid surgery after 15 years. J Clin Endocrinol Metab. 2008 Sep;93(9):3462–70. [PMID: 18544625]

Silverberg SJ et al. The diagnosis and management of asymptomatic primary hyperparathyroidism. Nat Clin Pract Endocrinol Metab. 2006 Sep;2(9):494–503. [PMID: 16957763]

Familial (Benign) Hypocalciuric Hypercalcemia & Neonatal Severe Primary Hyperparathyroidism

Brown EM. Clinical lessons from the calcium-sensing receptor. Nat Clin Pract Endocrinol Metab. 2007 Feb;3(2):122–33. [PMID: 17237839]

Chattopadhyay N et al. Role of calcium-sensing receptor in mineral ion metabolism and inherited disorders of calcium-sensing. Mol Genet Metab. 2006 Nov;89(3):189–202. [PMID: 16919492]

Pallais JC et al. Acquired hypocalciuric hypercalcemia due to auto-antibodies against the calcium-sensing receptor. N Engl J Med. 2004 Jul 22;351(4):362–9. [PMID: 15269316]

Fibroblast Growth Factor-23

Antoniucci DM et al. Dietary phosphorus regulates serum fibroblast growth factor-23 concentrations in healthy men. J Clin Endocrinol Metab. 2006 Aug;91(8):3144–9. [PMID: 16735491]

Araya K et al. A novel mutation in fibroblast growth factor 23 gene as a cause of tumoral calcinosis. J Clin Endocrinol Metab. 2005 Oct;90(10):5523–7. [PMID: 16030159]

Burnett SM et al. Regulation of C-terminal and intact FGF-23 by dietary phosphate in men and women. J Bone Miner Res. 2006 Aug;21(8):1187–96. [PMID: 16869716]

Fukumoto S et al. FGF23 is a hormone-regulating phosphate metabolism—Unique biological characteristics of FGF23. Bone. 2007 May;40(5):1190–5. [PMID: 17276744]

Jonsson KB et al. Fibroblast growth factor 23 in oncogenic osteomalacia and X-linked hypophosphatemia. N Engl J Med. 2003 Apr 24;348(17):1656–63. [PMID: 12711740]

Urakawa I et al. Klotho converts canonical FGF receptor into a specific receptor for FGF23. Nature. 2006 Dec 7;444(7120):770–4. [PMID: 17086194]

Hypercalcemia of Malignancy

Clines GA et al. Hypercalcemia of malignancy and basic research on mechanisms responsible for osteolytic and osteoblastic metastasis to bone. Clin Adv Hematol Oncol. 2004 May;2(5):295–302. [PMID: 16163196]

Clines GA et al. Mechanisms and treatment for bone metastases. Clin Adv Hematol Oncol. 2004 May;2(5):295–302. [PMID: 16163196]

Mundy GR et al. PTH-related peptide (PTHrP) in hypercalcemia. J Am Soc Nephrol. 2008 Apr;19(4):672–5. [PMID: 18256357]

Ralston SH et al. Medical management of hypercalcemia. Calcif Tissue Int. 2004 Jan;74(1):1–11. [PMID: 14523593]

Stewart AF. Clinical practice. Hypercalcemia associated with cancer. N Engl J Med. 2005 Jan 27;352(4):373–9. [PMID: 15673803]

Hypoparathyroidism and Hypocalcemia

Alimohammadi M et al. Autoimmune polyendocrine syndrome type 1 and NALP5, a parathyroid autoantigen. N Engl J Med. 2008 Mar 6;358(10):1018–28. [PMID: 18322283]

Bastepe M. The GNAS locus and pseudohypoparathyroidism. Adv Exp Med Biol. 2008;626:27–40. [PMID: 18372789]

Cooper MS et al. Diagnosis and management of hypocalcaemia. BMJ. 2008 Jun 7;336(7656):1298–302. [PMID: 18535072]

Eisenbarth GS et al. Autoimmune polyendocrine syndromes. N Engl J Med. 2004 May 13;350(20):2068–79. [PMID: 15141045]

Goswami R et al. Prevalence of calcium sensing receptor autoantibodies in patients with sporadic idiopathic hypoparathyroidism. Eur J Endocrinol. 2004 Jan;150(1):9–18. [PMID: 14713274]

Kifor O et al. Activating antibodies to the calcium-sensing receptor in two patients with autoimmune hypoparathyroidism. J Clin Endocrinol Metab. 2004 Feb;89(2):548–56. [PMID: 14764760]

Kobrynski L et al. Velocardiofacial syndrome, DiGeorge syndrome: The chromosome 22q11.2 deletion syndromes. Lancet. 2007 Oct 20;370(9596):1443–52. [PMID: 17950858]

Mantovani G et al. Mutations in the Gs alpha gene causing hormone resistance. Best Pract Res Clin Endocrinol Metab. 2006 Dec;20(4):501–13. [PMID: 17161328]

Perheentupa J. Autoimmune polyendocrinopathy-candidiasis-ectodermal dystrophy. J Clin Endocrinol Metab. 2006 Aug;91(8):2843–50. [PMID: 16684821]

Shoback D. Clinical practice. Hypoparathyroidism. N Engl J Med. 2008 Jul 24;359(4):391–403. [PMID: 18650515]

Soderbergh A et al. Prevalence and clinical associations of 10 defined autoantibodies in autoimmune polyendocrine syndrome type I. J Clin Endocrinol Metab. 2004 Feb;89(2):557–62. [PMID: 14764761]

Medullary Carcinoma of the Thyroid

Fialkowski EA et al. Current approaches to medullary thyroid carcinoma, sporadic and familial. J Surg Oncol. 2006 Dec 15;94(8):737–47. [PMID: 17131404]

Hoff AO et al. Medullary thyroid carcinoma. Hematol Oncol Clin North Am. 2007 Jun;21(3):475–88. [PMID: 17548035]

Moore SW et al. Familial medullary carcinoma prevention, risk evaluation, and RET in children of families with MEN2. J Pediatr Surg. 2007 Feb;42(2):326–32. [PMID: 17270543]

Raue F et al. Multiple endocrine neoplasia type 2: 2007 update. Horm Res. 2007;68 (Suppl 5):101–4. [PMID: 18174721]

You YN et al. Medullary thyroid cancer. Surg Oncol Clin N Am. 2006 Jul;15(3):639–60. [PMID: 16882502]

Osteoporosis

Bischoff-Ferrari HA et al. Fracture prevention with vitamin D supplementation: A meta-analysis of randomized controlled trials. JAMA. 2005 May 11;293(18):2257–64. [PMID: 15886381]

Black DM et al; HORIZON Pivotal Fracture Trial. Once-yearly zoledronic acid for treatment of postmenopausal osteoporosis. N Engl J Med. 2007 May 3;356(18):1809–22. [PMID: 17476007]

Canalis E et al. Mechanisms of anabolic therapies for osteoporosis. N Engl J Med. 2007 Aug 30;357(9):905–16. [PMID: 17761594]

Dawson-Hughes B et al. Estimates of optimal vitamin D status. Osteoporos Int. 2005 Jul;16(7):713–6. [PMID: 15776217]

Dawson-Hughes B et al. National Osteoporosis Foundation Guide Committee. Implications of absolute fracture risk assessment for osteoporosis practice guidelines in the USA. Osteoporos Int. 2008 Apr;19(4):449–58. [PMID: 18292975]

Ebeling PR. Clinical practice. Osteoporosis in men. N Engl J Med. 2008 Apr 3;358(14):1474–82. [PMID: 18385499]

Geller JL et al. Vitamin D therapy. Curr Osteoporos Rep. 2008 Mar;6(1):5–11. [PMID: 18430394]

Holick MF et al. Prevalence of vitamin D inadequacy among postmenopausal North American women receiving osteoporosis therapy. J Clin Endocrinol Metab. 2005 Jun;90(6):3215–24. [PMID: 15797954]

Kanis JA et al. Assessment of fracture risk. Osteoporos Int. 2005 Jun;16(6):581–9. [PMID: 15616758]

Kanis JA et al. Ten year probabilities of osteoporotic fractures according to BMD and diagnostic thresholds. Osteoporos Int. 2001 Dec;12(12):989–95. [PMID: 11846333]

Kanis JA et al. The use of clinical risk factors enhances the performance of BMD in the prediction of hip and osteoporotic fractures in men and women. Osteoporos Int. 2007 Aug;18(8):1033–46. [PMID: 17323110]

Khosla S et al. Clinical practice. Osteopenia. N Engl J Med. 2007 May 31;356(22):2293–300. [PMID: 17538088]

Khosla S et al. Building bone to reverse osteoporosis and prevent fractures. J Clin Invest. 2008 Feb;118(2):421–8. [PMID: 18246192]

Lyles KW et al; HORIZON Recurrent Fracture Trial. Zoledronic acid and clinical fractures and mortality after hip fracture. N Engl J Med. 2007;357:1799–1809. [PMID: 18427590]

National Osteoporosis Foundation, 2008 Clinician's Guide to Prevention and Treatment of Osteoporosis. http://www.nof.org/professionals/Clinicians_Guide.htm.

Olszynski WP et al. Osteoporosis in men: Epidemiology, diagnosis, prevention, and treatment. Clin Ther. 2004 Jan;26(1):15–28. [PMID: 14996514]

Rosen CJ. Clinical practice. Postmenopausal osteoporosis. N Engl J Med. 2005 Aug 11;353(6):595–603. [PMID: 16093468]

Sambrook P et al. Osteoporosis. Lancet. 2006 Jun 17;367(9527):2010–8. [PMID: 16782492]

Seeman E et al. Bone quality—The material and structural basis of bone strength and fragility. N Engl J Med. 2006 May 25;354(21):2250–61. [PMID: 16723616]

U.S. Department of Health and Human Services. *Bone Health and Osteoporosis: A Report of the Surgeon General.* Rockville, MD: U.S. Department of Health and Human Services, Office of the Surgeon General, 2004. http://www.surgeongeneral.gov/library.

Osteomalacia and Rickets

Bergwitz C et al. SCL34A3 mutations in patients with hereditary hypophosphatemic rickets with hypercalciuria predict a key role for the sodium-phosphate cotransporter NaPi-IIc in maintaining phosphate homeostasis. Am J Hum Genet. 2006 Feb;78(2):179–92. [PMID: 16358214]

Brame LA et al. Renal phosphate wasting disorders: Clinical features and pathogenesis. Semin Nephrol. 2004 Jan;24(1):39–47. [PMID: 14730508]

Feng JQ et al. Loss of DMP1 causes rickets and osteomalacia and identifies a role for osteocytes in mineral metabolism. Nat Genet. 2006 Nov;38(11):1310–5. [PMID: 17033621]

Holick MF. Resurrection of vitamin D deficiency and rickets. J Clin Invest. 2006 Aug;116(8):2062–72. [PMID: 16886050]

Jan de Beur S. Tumor-induced osteomalacia. JAMA. 2005 Sep 14;294(10):1260–7. [PMID: 16160135]

Lewiecki EM et al. Tumor-induced osteomalacia: Lessons learned. Arthritis Rheum. 2008 Mar;58(3):773–7. [PMID: 18311810]

Lorenz-Depiereux B et al. Hereditary hypophosphatemic rickets with hypercalciuria is caused by mutations in the sodium-phosphate cotransporter SLC34A3. Am J Hum Genet. 2006 Feb;78(2):193–201. [PMID: 16358215]

Nasu T et al. Tumor-induced hypophosphatemic osteomalacia diagnosed by the combinatory procedures of magnetic resonance imaging and venous sampling for FGF23. Intern Med. 2008;47(10):957–61. [PMID: 18480582]

Pettifor JM. Rickets and vitamin D deficiency in children and adolescents. Endocrinol Metab Clin North Am. 2005 Sep;34(3):537–53. [PMID: 16085158]

Thacher TD et al. Nutritional rickets around the world: Causes and future directions. Ann Trop Paediatr. 2006 Mar;26(1):1–16. [PMID: 16494699]

Disorders of the Endocrine Pancreas

Janet L. Funk, MD

Insulin and **glucagon,** the two key hormones that orchestrate fuel storage and utilization, are produced by the islet cells in the pancreas. **Islet cells** are distributed in clusters throughout the exocrine pancreas. Together, they comprise the endocrine pancreas. **Diabetes mellitus,** a heterogeneous disorder that affects 8% of the population in the United States and more than 20% of individuals between the ages of 65 and 74 years, is the most common disease associated with disordered secretion of hormones of the endocrine pancreas. Pancreatic tumors that secrete excessive amounts of specific islet cell hormones are far less common, but their clinical presentations underscore the important regulatory roles of each hormone.

NORMAL STRUCTURE & FUNCTION OF THE PANCREATIC ISLETS

ANATOMY & HISTOLOGY

The endocrine pancreas is composed of nests of cells (**islets of Langerhans**) that are distributed throughout the exocrine pancreas. This anatomic feature allows for their enzymatic isolation from the exocrine pancreas for islet cell transplantation. Although numbering in the millions, the multicellular islets comprise only 1% of the total pancreas. The endocrine pancreas has great reserve capacity; more than 70% of the insulin-secreting β **cells** must be lost before dysfunction occurs. Each of the four major islet cell types produces a different secretory product (Table 18–1). Insulin-secreting β cells are the predominant cell type. The majority of the remaining islet cells, glucagon-secreting α cells and somatostatin-secreting δ **cells,** secrete hormones that counter the effects of insulin. A fourth major islet cell type, the pancreatic polypeptide-secreting **PP cell,** is primarily located in islets within the posterior lobe of the head of the pancreas, an embryologically distinct region receiving a different blood supply. Current limitations associated with islet cell transplantation have stimulated interest in the potential use of stem cell–derived islet cells and, with this, a renewed interest in elucidating transcription factors critical for the differentiation of specific endocrine (vs. exocrine) pancreatic cells from a single progenitor (Table 18–1).

The islets are much more highly vascularized than the exocrine pancreatic tissues. At least one major arteriole supplies each islet and is lined with islet cells whose secretory products exert intraislet, paracrine, or endocrine effects on hormone release (Figure 18–1). Blood from the islets then drains into the hepatic portal vein. Thus, the islet cell secretory products pass directly into the liver, a major site of action of glucagon and insulin, before proceeding into the systemic circulation.

The islets are also abundantly innervated. Both parasympathetic and sympathetic axons enter the islets and either directly contact cells or terminate in the interstitial space between the cells. Neural regulation of islet cell hormone release, both directly through the sympathetic fibers and indirectly through stimulation of catecholamine release by the adrenal medulla, plays a key role in glucose homeostasis during stress.

CHECKPOINT

1. What percentage of islets must be lost before endocrine pancreatic dysfunction becomes manifest?
2. Identify the major hormone-secreting cells in an islet of Langerhans.

TABLE 18–1   Islet cells of the endocrine pancreas.

Cell Type	Developmental Transcription Factors	Secretory Products	Islet Composition (%)
α	PAX6, MAFB	**Glucagon**, proglucagon, glucagon-like peptides (GLPs)	20%
β	PAX6, NKX2.2, NKX6.1, MAFB, PDX1	**Insulin,** C peptide, proinsulin, amylin, γ-aminobutyric acid (GABA)	70%
δ	PAX4, PDX1	**Somatostatin**	10%
PP		**Pancreatic polypeptide**	(< 1%)

PHYSIOLOGY

1. Insulin

Synthesis and Metabolism of Insulin

Insulin is a protein composed of two peptide chains (A and B chains) connected by two disulfide bonds (Figure 18–2). The precursor of insulin, **preproinsulin** (MW 11,500), is synthesized in the ribosomes and enters the endoplasmic reticulum of β cells, where it is promptly cleaved by microsomal enzymes to form proinsulin (MW 9000). **Proinsulin,** consisting of A and B chains joined by a 31-amino-acid **C peptide,** is transported to the Golgi apparatus, where it is packaged into secretory vesicles. While in the secretory vesicle, proinsulin is cleaved at two sites to form insulin (51 amino acids; MW 5808) and the C peptide fragment (Figure 18–2). Secretion of insulin is, therefore, accompanied by an equimolar secretion of C peptide and also by small amounts of proinsulin that escape cleavage.

Recombinant human insulin or its analogues, first introduced in 1982, have now replaced beef or pork insulin preparations whose sales in the United States were discontinued in 2006. Insulin has a circulatory half-life of 3–5 minutes and is catabolized in both the liver and the kidney. The liver catabolizes approximately 50% of insulin on its first pass through the liver after it is secreted from the pancreas into the portal vein. In contrast, both C peptide and proinsulin are catabolized only by the kidney and, therefore, have half-lives three to four times longer than that of insulin itself.

Regulation of Secretion

Glucose is the primary physiologic stimulant of insulin release (Figure 18–3). Glucose entry into β cells is facilitated by the **glucose transporter** GLUT-2, which is in excess and allows the bidirectional transport of glucose, thereby creating an equilibrium between extracellular and intracellular glucose concentrations. Once in the cell, the metabolism of glucose—rather than glucose itself—stimulates insulin secretion.

Glucokinase, an enzyme with low affinity for glucose whose activity is regulated by glucose, controls the first step in glucose metabolism: phosphorylation of glucose to form glucose 6-phosphate. This enzyme, by determining the rate of glycolysis, is thought to function as the β-cell **glucose sensor**. Glycolysis produces an increase in adenosine triphosphate (ATP), which blocks ATP-dependent K^+ channels (K_{ATP}) in the β-cell membrane. The resultant cell depolarization allows Ca^{2+} to enter, triggering exocytosis of insulin-containing granules. Sulfonylurea drugs used to treat diabetes also stimulate insulin secretion by binding to and blocking K_{ATP}.

Although glucose is the most potent stimulator of insulin release, other factors such as amino acids ingested with a meal or vagal stimulation can cause insulin release (Table 18–2). Glucose-stimulated insulin secretion can also be enhanced by several enteric hormones, such as **glucagon-like peptide-1 (GLP-1)**, which has led to interest in GLP-like drugs for dia-

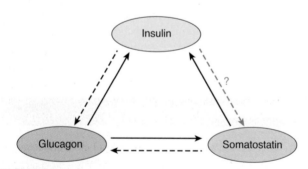

FIGURE 18–1 Schematic diagram indicating paracrine/endocrine regulation of islet cell hormones. Inhibition is indicated by a dashed line; stimulation by a solid line.

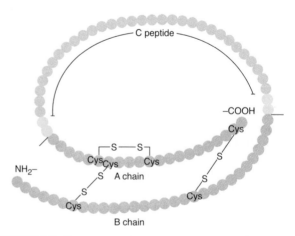

FIGURE 18–2 Amino acid sequence and covalent structure of human proinsulin. Converting enzymes separate C peptide from insulin (blue colored residues). (Redrawn from Kohler PO, Jordan RM [editors]. *Clinical Endocrinology.* Wiley, 1986.)

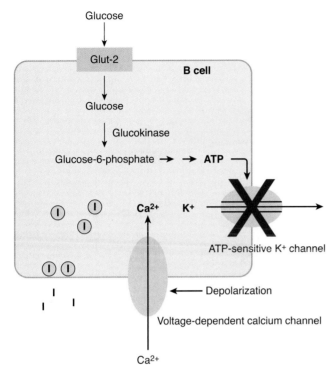

FIGURE 18–3 Schematic diagram of glucose-stimulated insulin release from β cell. Glucose enters the β cell via GLUT-2–mediated diffusion. Metabolism of glucose, the first step of which is controlled by glucokinase, results in ATP production. Cytosolic ATP blocks ATP-dependent K⁺ channels and thus K⁺ efflux, resulting in cell depolarization. This allows Ca^{2+} to enter via voltage-dependent calcium channels, stimulating the exocytosis of insulin-containing secretory granules.

TABLE 18–2 Regulation of islet cell hormone release.

	β-Cell Insulin Release	δ-Cell Somatostatin Release	α-Cell Glucagon Release
Nutrients			
Glucose	↑	↑	↓
Amino acids	↑	↑	↑
Fatty acids	—	—	↓
Ketones	—	—	↓
Hormones			
Enteric hormones	↑	↑	↑
Insulin	↓	↓?	↓
GABA	—	↓	↓
Somatostatin	↓	↓	↓
Glucagon	↑	↑	—
Cortisol	—	—	↑
Catecholamines	↓ (α-adrenergic)	—	↑ (β-adrenergic)
Neural			
Vagal	↑	—	↑
β-adrenergic	↑	—	↑
α-adrenergic	↓	—	↓

Key: ↑ = increased; ↓ = decreased; — = no effect or no known effect.

betes treatment. Insulin secretion is inhibited by catecholamines and by somatostatin.

Mechanism of Action

Insulin exerts its effects by binding to **insulin receptors** present on the surfaces of target cells (Figure 18–4). Insulin receptors are present in liver, muscle, and fat, the classic insulin-sensitive tissues responsible for fuel homeostasis. In addition, insulin can mediate other effects in nonclassic target tissues, such as the ovary, via interaction with insulin receptors or by cross-reactivity with **insulin-like growth factor-1** (IGF-1) receptors. Binding of insulin to its receptor causes activation of a tyrosine kinase region of the receptor and autophosphorylation of the receptor. Activation of the insulin receptor initiates a phosphorylation cascade within the cell, beginning with the phosphorylation of a network of docking proteins (**insulin receptor substrates [IRSs]**) that engage and amplify downstream signaling molecules, ultimately leading to the biologic effects of insulin (eg, translocation of GLUT-4 glucose transporter to the plasma membranes of muscle and fat cells and activation of glycogen synthase).

Effects

Insulin plays a major role in fuel homeostasis (Table 18–3). Insulin mediates changes in fuel metabolism through its effects on three main tissues: liver, muscle, and fat. In these tissues, insulin promotes fuel storage (anabolism) and prevents the breakdown and release of fuel that has already been stored (catabolism). The total lack of insulin is incompatible with life, and the same is true of excess insulin.

In the liver, insulin promotes fuel storage by stimulation of glycogen synthesis and storage. Insulin inhibits hepatic glucose output by inhibiting gluconeogenesis (glucose synthesis) and glycogenolysis (glycogen breakdown). By also stimulating glycolysis (metabolism of glucose to pyruvate), insulin promotes the formation of precursors for fatty acid synthesis. Moreover, insulin stimulates lipogenesis, leading to the increased synthesis of very low-density lipoproteins (VLDLs), particles that deliver triglycerides to fat tissue for storage. Insulin also inhibits fatty acid oxidation and the production of ketone bodies (ketogenesis), an alternative fuel produced only in the liver that can be used by the brain when glucose is not available.

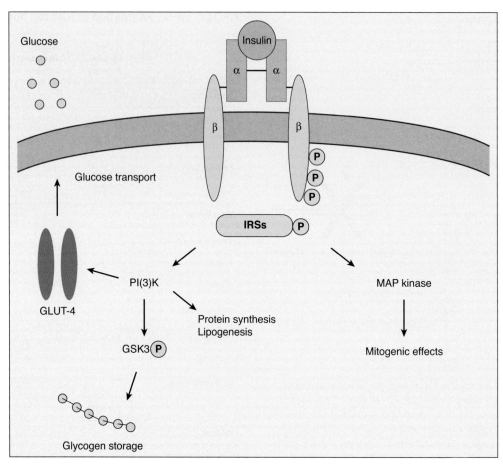

FIGURE 18–4   Model of insulin receptor signaling. The insulin receptor is composed of two α and two β subunits linked by disulfide bonds. Binding of insulin to the extracellular α subunits activates a tyrosine kinase present in the cytoplasmic domain of the β subunit. The activated kinase auto-phosphorylates specific tyrosine residues in the β subunit. Receptor kinase activation is also the critical first step in a cascade of intracellular events that begins with phosphorylation of multiple docking proteins (insulin receptor substrates [IRSs]). Once activated, these multifunctional proteins initiate complex intracellular signaling pathways. Binding of IRS to phosphatidylinositol 3-kinase (PI3-K) initiates one of the major pathways effecting carbohydrate, protein, and lipid metabolism, including translocation of the glucose transporter, GLUT-4, to the cell surface and the inactivation, by phosphorylation, of glycogen synthase kinase 3 (GSK3) and subsequent dephosphorylation and activation of glycogen synthase, thus stimulating glucose storage. In contrast, mitogenic effects of insulin are mediated by a MAP kinase pathway.

Although hepatic uptake of glucose is not regulated by insulin, insulin does stimulate glucose uptake both in muscle and in fat by causing the rapid translocation of an insulin-sensitive glucose transporter (GLUT-4) to the surface of these cells. Uptake of glucose by muscle accounts for the vast majority (85%) of insulin-stimulated glucose disposal. In muscle, insulin promotes the storage of glucose by stimulating glycogen synthesis and inhibiting glycogen catabolism. Insulin also stimulates protein synthesis in muscle.

Insulin stimulates fat storage by stimulating lipoprotein lipase, the enzyme that hydrolyzes the triglycerides carried in VLDLs and other triglyceride-rich lipoproteins to fatty acids, which can then be taken up by fat cells. Increased glucose uptake caused by upregulation of the GLUT-4 transporter also aids in fat storage because this increases the levels of glycerol phosphate, a substrate in the esterification of free fatty acids, which are then stored as triglycerides. In fat cells, insulin also inhibits lipolysis, preventing the release of fatty acids,

a potential substrate for hepatic ketone body synthesis. Insulin exerts this effect by decreasing the activity of hormone-sensitive lipase, the enzyme that hydrolyzes stored triglycerides to releasable fatty acids. Together, these changes result in increased fat storage.

CHECKPOINT

3. What is the half-life of insulin? How is it catabolized? What percentage is extracted on first pass through the liver?

4. How do the half-lives of C peptide and proinsulin compare with that of insulin?

5. List the main substances that stimulate insulin secretion.

6. What characteristics of the β-cell glucose transporter allow intracellular glucose levels to equal those of the extracellular space?

TABLE 18–3 Hormonal regulation of fuel homeostasis.

	Insulin	Somatostatin	Glucagon	Catecholamines	Cortisol	Growth Hormone
Liver						
Fuel storage						
Glycogenesis	↑		↓			
Lipid synthesis	↑		↓			
Fuel breakdown						
Glycogenolysis	↓		↑	↑		↑
Gluconeogenesis	↓		↑	↑	↑	↑
Fatty acid oxidation or ketogenesis	↓		↑			
Kidneys						
Fuel breakdown						
Gluconeogenesis	↓			↑		
Muscle						
Fuel storage						
Glucose uptake or glycogenesis	↑			↓	↓	↓
Fuel breakdown						
Protein catabolism	↓				↑	
Adipose tissue						
Fuel storage						
Lipoprotein lipolysis	↑					
Fatty acid esterification	↑					
Fuel breakdown						
Lipolysis of stored fat	↓			↑	↑	↑
Pancreas						
Secretion of:						
Insulin (β cell)	↓	↓	↑	↓		
Glucagon (α cell)	↓	↓		↑	↑	↑
Somatostatin (δ cell)	(↓?)	↓	↑			

Key: ↑ = increased, ↓ = decreased.

7. What is the probable "glucose sensor" in the β cell?
8. What are the major inhibitors of insulin secretion?
9. What are the current thoughts on the mechanisms of insulin action?
10. Which tissues are insulin dependent for glucose uptake?
11. What are three ways in which insulin stimulates fat storage?

2. Glucagon

Synthesis and Metabolism

Glucagon, a 29-amino-acid peptide, is produced in α cells of the pancreas by the proteolytic processing of proglucagon, a larger precursor protein. In addition to the pancreas, proglucagon is also expressed in the intestine and brain. While glucagon is the major bioactive metabolite produced in the

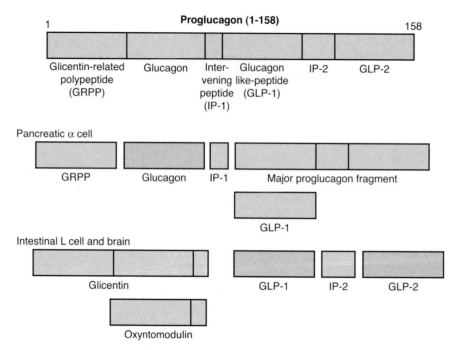

FIGURE 18–5 Organ-specific post-translational processing of proglucagon. Shading indicates major peptide produced.

pancreatic α cell, differential processing in the intestine results in the production of glucagon-like peptide (GLP)-1 and GLP-2 in response to a meal (Figure 18–5). This tissue-specific processing results in peptides with opposing effects on carbohydrate metabolism; pancreatic glucagon opposes the effects of insulin, whereas GLPs acts as **incretins,** gut-derived peptides that enhance glucose-stimulated insulin secretion. Long-acting analogues of GLP-1, which also stimulates β cell proliferation and increases β cell mass, are currently being studied for the treatment of Type 2 diabetes. The circulatory half-life of glucagon is 3–6 minutes. Like insulin, glucagon is metabolized in the liver and kidneys. However, the liver accounts for only 25% of glucagon clearance.

Regulation of Secretion

In contrast to the stimulation of insulin secretion by glucose, glucagon secretion is inhibited by glucose (Table 18–2). It is not known whether the α cell directly senses glucose, or whether its response is indirectly mediated by paracrine/endocrine effects of other pancreatic factors. Current opinion favors the later hypothesis whereby insulin plays the major role in modulating (ie, inhibiting) glucagon secretion. Other pancreatic factors inhibiting glucagon secretion include somatostatin and two additional β-cell secretory products, γ-**aminobutyric acid (GABA), and insulin-associated zinc.** Like insulin, glucagon secretion is stimulated by amino acids, an important regulatory feature in the metabolism of protein meals. In contrast, fatty acids and ketones inhibit glucagon secretion. Counter-regulatory hormones such as catecholamines (via a predominating β-adrenergic effect) and cortisol stimulate glucagon release.

Mechanism of Action

The liver is the major target organ for glucagon action. Glucagon binds to a glucagon receptor present on the cell surface of hepatocytes. Binding of glucagon promotes interaction of the receptor with a stimulatory G protein, which in turn activates adenylyl cyclase. Cyclic adenosine monophosphate, generated by adenylyl cyclase, activates protein kinase A, which then phosphorylates enzymes responsible for the biologic activity of glucagon in the liver. There is also some evidence that the glucagon receptor may act via an adenylyl cyclase-independent mechanism by stimulation of phospholipase C.

Effects

The actions of glucagon were first demonstrated in 1921 by Banting and Best when they observed a mild transient hyperglycemia preceding insulin-induced hypoglycemia when testing pancreatic extracts in vivo. Glucagon is a **counter-regulatory hormone,** acting in a catabolic fashion to oppose the effects of insulin. Indeed, glucagon injections are used clinically to treat severe hypoglycemia. Hepatic effects of glucagon (Table 18–3) include: (1) stimulation of both hepatic glucose synthesis (gluconeogenesis) and the release of glycogen stores (glycogenolysis) to increase hepatic glucose output; (2) stimulation of fatty acid oxidation and ketogenesis, thus providing an alternative fuel (**ketone bodies**) that can be used by the brain when glucose is not available; and (3) increased hepatic uptake of amino acids, which fuels gluconeogenesis.

3. Somatostatin

Synthesis, Metabolism, and Regulation of Secretion

Like preproglucagon, preprosomatostatin is synthesized in the pancreas, GI tract, and brain, where it is differentially processed in a tissue-specific fashion to produce several biologically active peptides. Somatostatin-14 (SS-14), the first somatostatin to be isolated, is a 14-amino-acid peptide that was initially discovered in the hypothalamus as the factor responsible for the inhibition of growth hormone release. Only later was it appreciated that δ cells of the pancreas also secrete SS-14. In brain and intestine, somatostatin-28 (SS-28), an amino-terminally extended peptide that includes the 14-amino-acid sequence of SS-14, is also produced from preprosomatostatin and has a range of action comparable to that of SS-14 but a potency that is somewhat greater. The half-life of somatostatin (< 3 minutes) is shorter than that of insulin or glucagon. Because somatostatin has been shown to inhibit the synthesis and secretion of most peptide hormones, synthetic somatostatin analogues, such as octreotide, that have a much longer half-life (hours) have been developed for clinical use in inhibiting ectopic peptide hormone production by a variety of tumors. The same secretagogues that stimulate insulin secretion also stimulate somatostatin (Table 18–2). These include glucose, amino acids, enteric hormones, and glucagon.

Mechanism of Action and Effects

Somatostatin exerts its effects via binding to a family of inhibitory G (G_i) protein–coupled receptors (SST1-5) that are distributed in a tissue-specific fashion. In all tissues where somatostatin is produced, it acts primarily in an inhibitory fashion. In the endocrine pancreas, somatostatin is thought to act via paracrine effects on the other islet cells, inhibiting the release of insulin, glucagon, and PP (Table 18–3). In addition, somatostatin acts in an autocrine fashion to inhibit its own release. In the GI tract, somatostatin retards the absorption of nutrients through multiple mechanisms, including the inhibition of gut motility, inhibition of several enteric peptides, and inhibition of pancreatic exocrine function. Consistent with the multiple inhibitory effects of this peptide, the synthetic somatostatin analogue octreotide has multiple clinical uses, including inhibition of hormone production by pituitary adenomas, inhibition of certain types of chronic diarrhea, inhibition of tumor growth, and inhibition of bleeding from esophageal varices.

4. Pancreatic Polypeptide

Pancreatic peptide (**PP**), a 36-amino-acid peptide is produced by the PP cells in the islets of the posterior lobe of the head of the pancreas, is released in response to a mixed meal, an effect that appears to be mediated by protein and vagal stimulation. While long known to affect gastrointestinal motility and secretions, recent evidence suggests that PP may also inhibit food intake and stimulate energy expenditure. These latter effects of PP (a member of the neuropeptide Y family of peptide hormones) are mediated via binding to a Y4 receptor and are thought to involve inhibition of hepatic vagal nerve afferent activity.

CHECKPOINT

12. What are some important stimulators and inhibitors of glucagon secretion?

13. What is the major target organ for glucagon? What are the mechanisms of glucagon action?

14. What metabolic pathways are sensitive to glucagon, and how are they affected?

15. What hormone antagonizes glucagon's effect on metabolic pathways?

16. Where else in the body besides the islets of Langerhans is glucagon made?

17. By what mechanisms can GLPs enhance glucose-stimulated insulin secretion?

18. What is the role of somatostatin in the islets of Langerhans?

5. Hormonal Control of Carbohydrate Metabolism

Carbohydrate metabolism is primarily controlled by the relative amounts of insulin and glucagon produced by the endocrine pancreas (Table 18–3; Figure 18–6). Conversely, disregulation of both of these hormones contributes to hyperglycemia in diabetes. Under normal conditions, when plasma glucose levels are high, the actions of insulin predominate,

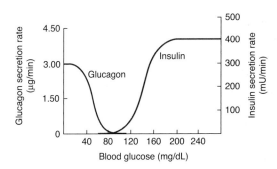

FIGURE 18–6 Mean rates of insulin and glucagon delivery from an artificial pancreas at various blood glucose levels. The device was programmed to establish and maintain normal blood glucose in insulin-requiring diabetic humans, and the values for hormone output approximate the output of the normal human pancreas. The shape of the insulin curve also resembles the insulin response of incubated β cells to graded concentrations of glucose. (Copyright © 1977 American Diabetes Association. Marliss EB et al. Normalization of glycemia in diabetics during meals with insulin and glucagon delivery by the artificial pancreas. Diabetes. 1977;26:663–72. Reprinted with permission from the American Diabetes Association.)

including insulin suppression of glucagon secretion. Fuel storage is promoted by insulin stimulation of glycogen storage in the liver; glucose uptake, glycogen synthesis, and protein synthesis by muscle; and fat storage by adipose tissue. Insulin inhibits the mobilization of substrates from peripheral tissues and opposes any effects of glucagon on the stimulation of hepatic glucose output.

In contrast, when glucose levels are low, plasma insulin levels are suppressed and the effects of glucagon predominate in the liver (ie, increased hepatic glucose output and ketone body formation). In the absence of insulin, muscle glucose uptake is markedly decreased, muscle protein is catabolized, and fat is mobilized from adipose tissue. Therefore, with insulinopenia, glucose loads cannot be cleared, and substrates for hepatic gluconeogenesis (amino acids, glycerol) and ketogenesis (fatty acids)—processes that are stimulated by glucagon—are increased.

Fasting State

After an overnight fast, the liver plays a primary role in maintaining blood glucose by producing glucose at the same rate at which it is used by resting tissues (Table 18–4). Glucose uptake and utilization occur predominantly in tissues that do not require insulin for glucose uptake, such as the brain. Hepatic glucose output is stimulated by glucagon and is primarily due to glycogenolysis, which can provide, on average, an 8-hour supply of glucose. The low levels of insulin that are present (basal secretion of 0.25–1.0 unit/h) are insufficient to block the release of fatty acids from fat, which provide fuel for muscles (fatty acid oxidation) and substrate for hepatic ketogenesis. However, these levels of insulin are sufficient to prevent excessive lipolysis, ketogenesis, and gluconeogenesis, thus preventing hyperglycemia and ketoacidosis.

With prolonged fasting (> 24–60 h), liver glycogen stores are depleted. Glucagon levels rise slightly, and insulin levels decline further. Gluconeogenesis now becomes the sole source of hepatic glucose production, using substrates such as amino acids that are mobilized from the periphery at a greater rate. With starvation, a switch occurs from gluconeogenesis to the production of ketones, an alternative fuel source that provides 90% of the energy used by the brain, a critical organ that accounts for 25% of basal metabolic energy needs. In this manner, survival is prolonged as muscle protein is conserved in favor of increased mobilization of fatty acids from adipose tissue, a process made possible by increased insulinopenia. The liver then converts fatty acids to ketone bodies, a process that is stimulated by glucagon.

Fed State

With ingestion of a carbohydrate load, insulin secretion is stimulated and glucagon is suppressed (Table 18–4). Hepatic glucose production and ketogenesis are suppressed by the high ratio of insulin to glucagon. Insulin stimulates hepatic glycogen storage. Insulin-mediated glucose uptake, which oc-

TABLE 18–4 Insulin-glucagon (I:G) molar ratios in blood in various conditions.

Condition	Hepatic Glucose Storage (S) or Production (P)[1]	I:G
Glucose availability	++++ (S)	70
Large carbohydrate meal	++ (S)	25
IV glucose	+ (S)	7
Small meal		
Glucose need	+ (P)	2.3
Overnight fast	++ (P)	1.8
Low-carbohydrate diet	++++ (P)	0.4
Starvation		

Courtesy RH Unger. Reproduced, with permission, from Ganong WF. *Review of Medical Physiology*, 22nd ed. McGraw-Hill, 2005.

[1]+ to ++++ indicate relative magnitude.

curs primarily in muscle, is also stimulated, as is muscle glycogen synthesis. Fat storage occurs in adipose tissue.

With ingestion of a protein meal, both insulin and glucagon are stimulated. In this way, insulin stimulates amino acid uptake and protein formation by muscle. However, stimulation of hepatic glucose output by glucagon counterbalances the tendency of insulin to cause hypoglycemia.

Conditions of Stress

During severe stress, when fuel delivery to the brain is in jeopardy, **counter-regulatory hormones,** in addition to glucagon, act synergistically. They maintain blood glucose levels by maximizing hepatic output of glucose and peripheral mobilization of substrates and by minimizing fuel storage (Table 18–3). **Glucagon** and **epinephrine** act within minutes to elevate blood glucose, whereas the counterregulatory effects of **cortisol** and **growth hormone** are not seen for several hours. Epinephrine, cortisol, and growth hormone stimulate glucagon release, whereas epinephrine inhibits insulin, thus maximally increasing the glucagon-insulin ratio. In addition, these three hormones act directly on the liver to increase hepatic glucose production and peripherally to stimulate lipolysis and inhibit insulin-sensitive glucose uptake. During severe stress, hyperglycemia may actually result from the combined effects of counterregulatory hormones.

Similar but less marked effects occur in response to exercise when glucagon, catecholamines, and, to a lesser extent, cortisol help meet the several-fold increase in glucose utilization rates due to exercising muscle by increasing hepatic glucose output and lipolysis of fat stores, effects that are made possible by a lowering of insulin levels. Low insulin levels also allow muscles to use glycogen stores for energy.

Role of Renal Gluconeogenesis in Glucose Homeostasis

Kidney and liver both express the enzymes required to augment the glucose pool by gluconeogenesis and the secretion of glucose stored as glycogen. While the kidney contributes little to the glucose pool during an overnight fasting, it contributes approximately 50% of endogenous glucose production during a prolonged (> 40 hour) fast. Gluconeogenesis predominates in the kidney as its glycogen stores are minimal, a process that is stimulated by epinephrine, inhibited by insulin, and unaffected by glucagon.

CHECKPOINT

19. In insulinopenic states, why are substrates for hepatic gluconeogenesis and ketogenesis increased?
20. What is the effect of a protein meal on insulin versus glucagon secretion?
21. What is the difference in time course of action of the various counterregulatory hormones?

PATHOPHYSIOLOGY OF SELECTED ENDOCRINE PANCREATIC DISORDERS

DIABETES MELLITUS

Clinical Presentation

Diabetes mellitus is a heterogeneous disorder defined by the presence of **hyperglycemia.** Diagnostic criteria for diabetes include (1) a fasting plasma glucose ≥ 126 mg/dL, (2) symptoms of diabetes plus a random plasma glucose ≥ 200 mg/dL, or (3) a plasma glucose level ≥ 200 mg/dL after an oral dose of 75 g of glucose (**oral glucose tolerance test, OGTT**).

Hyperglycemia in all cases is due to a functional deficiency of insulin action. Deficient insulin action can be due to a decrease in insulin secretion by the β cells of the pancreas, a decreased response to insulin by target tissues (**insulin resistance**), or an increase in the counterregulatory hormones that oppose the effects of insulin. The relative contributions of each of these three factors not only form the basis of classification of this disorder into subtypes but also help to explain the characteristic clinical presentations of each subtype (Table 18–5).

Diabetes prevalence in the United States, which has been increasing over the last decade, reached 10% in 2007 in those aged 20 years or older. More than 90% of cases of diabetes are regarded as primary processes for which individuals have a genetic predisposition and are classified as either **Type 1** or **Type 2** (Tables 18–5 and 18–6). Type 1 diabetes mellitus (Type 1 DM) is less common than Type 2, accounting for 5-10% of cases of primary diabetes. Type 1 DM is characterized by autoimmune destruction of pancreatic β cells with resultant severe insulin deficiency. In a minority of patients, the cause of Type 1 DM is unknown. The disease commonly affects individuals younger than 30 years; a bimodal peak in incidence occurs around age 5–7 years and at puberty. Although autoimmune destruction of the β cells does not occur acutely, clinical symptoms do. Patients present after only days or weeks of polyuria, polydipsia, and weight loss with markedly elevated serum glucose concentrations. **Ketone bodies** are also increased because of the marked lack of insulin, resulting in severe, life-threatening acidosis (**diabetic ketoacidosis**). Patients with Type 1 DM require treatment with insulin.

Type 2 diabetes mellitus (Type 2 DM) differs from Type 1 in several distinct ways (Table 18–6): It accounts for the overwhelming majority of diabetes (90–95%); has a stronger genetic component; occurs most commonly in adults; increases in prevalence with age (eg, 20% in individuals older than 65 years); occurs more commonly in Native Americans, Mexican Americans, and African Americans; and is associated with increased resistance to the effects of insulin at its sites of action as well as a decrease in insulin secretion by the pancreas. It is often (85% of cases) associated with obesity, an additional factor that increases insulin resistance. **Insulin resistance** is the hallmark of Type 2 DM. Because these patients often have varying amounts of residual insulin secretion that prevent severe hyperglycemia or ketosis, they often are asymptomatic and are diagnosed 5–7 years after the actual onset of disease by the discovery of an elevated fasting glucose on routine screening tests. Population screening surveys show that a remarkable 30% of cases of Type 2 DM in the United States are undiagnosed. Once identified, most individuals (70%) are managed with lifestyle modification (eg, diet, exercise, weight management) alone or in combination with medications that: (1) enhance endogenous glucose-independent or -dependent insulin secretion (sulphonylureas or incretins, respectively), (2) decrease insulin resistance in hepatic or peripheral tissues (eg, metformin or glitazones, respectively), or (3) interfere with intestinal absorption of carbohydrates (eg, intestinal α-glycosidase inhibitors). These patients, therefore, do not require insulin treatment for survival. However, some patients with Type 2 DM are treated with insulin to achieve optimal glucose control.

An epidemic of Type 2 DM is occurring worldwide, particularly in non-European populations; it has been estimated that 1 in 3 children born after 2000 will develop diabetes in their lifetime. In addition, Type 2 DM is also now being diagnosed with increased frequency in children. For example,

TABLE 18–5 **Etiologic classification of diabetes mellitus.**

I. Type 1 diabetes (β-cell destruction, usually leading to absolute insulin deficiency)	4. Cystic fibrosis	F. Infections
A. Immune mediated	5. Hemochromatosis	1. Congenital rubella
B. Idiopathic	6. Fibrocalculous pancreatopathy	2. Cytomegalovirus
II. Type 2 diabetes (may range from predominant insulin resistance with relative insulin deficiency to a predominant secretory defect with insulin resistance)	7. Others	3. Others
	D. Endocrinopathies	G. Uncommon forms of immune-mediated diabetes
III. Other specific types	1. Acromegaly	1. "Stiff-man" syndrome
A. Genetic defects of β-cell function	2. Cushing's syndrome	2. Anti-insulin receptor antibodies
1. Chromosome 12, HNF-1α (MODY 3)	3. Glucagonoma	3. Others
2. Chromosome 7, glucokinase (MODY 2)	4. Pheochromocytoma	H. Other genetic syndromes sometimes associated with diabetes
3. Chromosome 20, HNF-4α (MODY 1)	5. Hyperthyroidism	1. Down syndrome
4. Chromosome 13, insulin promoter factor-1 (IPF-1; MODY 4)	6. Somatostatinoma	2. Klinefelter's syndrome
5. Chromosome 17, HNF-1β (MODY 5)	7. Aldosteronoma	3. Turner's syndrome
6. Chromosome 2, *NeuroD1* (MODY 6)	8. Others	4. Wolfram's syndrome
7. Mitochondrial DNA	E. Drug- or chemical-induced	5. Friedreich's ataxia
8. Others	1. Vacor (N-3-pyridylmethyl-N′-p-nitrophenyl urea [PNU])	6. Huntington's chorea
B. Genetic defects in insulin action	2. Pentamidine	7. Laurence-Moon-Biedl syndrome
1. Type A insulin resistance	3. Nicotinic acid	8. Myotonic dystrophy
2. Leprechaunism	4. Glucocorticoids	9. Porphyria
3. Rabson-Mendenhall syndrome	5. Thyroid hormone	10. Prader-Willi syndrome
4. Lipoatrophic diabetes	6. Diazoxide	11. Others
5. Others	7. β-adrenergic agonists	IV. Gestational diabetes mellitus
C. Diseases of the exocrine pancreas	8. Thiazides	
1. Pancreatitis	9. Dilantin	
2. Trauma, pancreatectomy	10. α-Interferon	
3. Neoplasia	11. Others	

Modified and reproduced, with permission, from the American Diabetes Association. Diagnosis and classification of diabetes mellitus. Diabetes Care. 2008;31(Suppl 1):S55–60.

while Type 1 DM remains the most common cause of diabetes in children younger than 10 years (regardless of ethnicity) and in older, non-Hispanic white children, Type 2 DM accounts for more than 50% of the diagnoses in older children of Hispanic, African American, Native American, and Asian Pacific Islander ancestry. In all age groups and ethnicities, this increased incidence of Type 2 DM is associated with obesity.

Other causes of diabetes, accounting for less than 5% of cases, include processes that destroy the pancreas (eg, pancreatitis), specifically inhibit insulin secretion (eg, genetic B-cell defects [MODY]), induce insulin resistance (eg, certain HIV protease inhibitors), or increase counter-regulatory hormones

(eg, Cushing's syndrome) (Table 18–5, part III). Clinical presentations in these cases depend on the exact nature of the process and are not discussed here.

Gestational diabetes mellitus occurs in pregnant women with an incidence ranging from 3–8% in the general population to up to 16% in Native American women (Table 18–5, part IV), may recur with subsequent pregnancies, and tends to resolve at parturition. Up to 50% of these women can go on to develop diabetes (predominantly Type 2 DM). Gestational diabetes usually occurs in the second half of gestation, precipitated by the increasing levels of hormones such as chorionic somatomammotropin, progesterone, cortisol, and prolactin

TABLE 18–6 Some features distinguishing type 1 diabetes mellitus from type 2 diabetes mellitus.

	Type 1 DM	Type 2 DM
Epidemiology		
Age at diagnosis	Childhood	Adult
		(incidence increasing with obesity in children)
Prevalence (in USA)	0.2%, age < 20 years	11%, age > 20 years
Phenotype		
β-cell insulin secretion abnormal	Absolute deficiency	Impaired secretion
Insulin resistance	No	Yes
Obese	No	Yes
(BMI = body mass index = weight [kg]/height² [m²])		*(85% have BMI > 25; 50% have BMI > 30)*
Autoimmune disease	Yes *(90% have islet cell antibodies)*	No
Postulated environmental triggers	Viral infections, dietary exposures (cow's milk, cereal)	Obesity (diet, exercise)
Genotype		
Concordance in monozygotic twins	< 50%	> 70%
Incidence in offspring		
Single parent affected	2–5%	15%
Both parents affected	10%	50%
Genetic loci associated with risk	HLA class II genes	Heterogeneous sets of interacting genes

that have counterregulatory anti-insulin effects. Because of its potential adverse effects on fetal outcome, gestational diabetes is currently diagnosed or ruled out by routine screening with an oral glucose load at the first prenatal visit in high-risk populations—obese, age > 25 years, family history of diabetes, or member of an ethnic group with a high prevalence of diabetes—or at 24 weeks gestation in those with average risk.

Etiology

A. Type 1 Diabetes Mellitus (Type 1 DM)

Type 1 diabetes is an autoimmune disease caused by the selective destruction of pancreatic β cells by T lymphocytes targeting ill-defined β cell antigens. In early disease, lymphocytic infiltrates of macrophage-activating CD4+ cells and cytokine-secreting, cytotoxic CD8+ cells surround the necrotic β cells. Autoimmune destruction of the β cell occurs gradually over several years until sufficient β cell mass is lost to cause symptoms of insulin deficiency. At the time of diagnosis, ongoing inflammation is present in some islets, whereas other islets are atrophic and consist only of glucagon-secreting α cells and somatostatin-secreting δ cells. Autoantibodies against islet cells and insulin, while appearing early in the course of disease, are thought to serve as markers, rather than mediators, of β cell

destruction. As such, they have been used to aid in the differential diagnosis of Type 1 DM vs. Type 2 DM in children (particularly with the rising incidence of Type 2 DM in this population) and to assess the probability for development of Type 1 DM in first-degree relatives who are at increased risk for Type 1 DM (2–6% incidence).

Islet cell antibodies (ICA), which include those directed against **glutamic acid decarboxylase (GAD)** and **tyrosine phosphatase-2 protein (IA2)**, and antibodies against insulin (**insulin autoantibody [IAA]**) are each present in 50% of newly diagnosed diabetics and are highly predictive of disease onset in first-degree relatives (70% of first-degree relatives positive for both develop disease within 5 years). Because the appearance of autoantibodies is followed by progressive impairment of insulin release in response to glucose (Figure 18–7), both criteria have been used with great success to identify at-risk first-degree relatives with the ultimate, but as yet unmet, goal of intervening to prevent diabetes. However, because only 10% of individuals newly diagnosed with Type 1 DM have a positive family history, these screening methods cannot be used to identify the vast majority of individuals developing this low-incidence disease.

At least 50% of the genetic susceptibility for Type 1 DM has been linked to the genes of the major histocompatibility

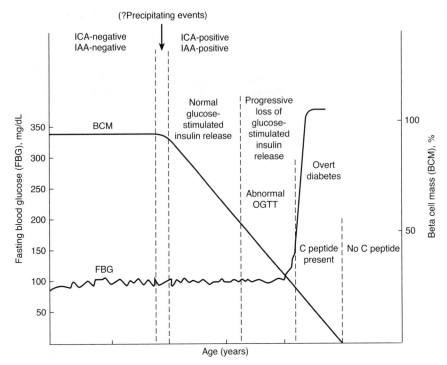

FIGURE 18–7   Stages in development of type 1 diabetes. BCM, basal cell mass; FBG, fasting blood glucose; IAA, insulin autoantibodies; ICA, islet cell antibodies; OGTT, oral glucose tolerance test.   (Redrawn, with permission, from Eisenbarth GS. Autoimmune beta cell insufficiency—Diabetes mellitus type I. Triangle. 1984;23;111. Copyright © 1984 Novartis.)

complex (MHC) that encode class II human leukocyte antigens (HLAs), molecules expressed on the surface of specific antigen-presenting cells such as macrophages. Class II molecules form a complex with processed foreign antigens or autoantigens, which then activates CD4 T lymphocytes via interaction with the T-cell receptor. Alleles at the class II HLA-DR or HLA-DQ loci have the strongest influence on the risk of Type 1 DM. However, identification of HLA haplotypes remains a research tool at this time.

While genetic susceptibility clearly plays a role in Type 1 DM, the 50% concordance rate in identical twins, as well as the continuing increase in the incidence of Type 1 DM since World War II, suggests that environmental factors may also play a critical role. Evidence suggests that viral infections, such as congenital exposure to rubella, may precipitate disease, particularly in genetically susceptible individuals. It is hypothesized that an immune response to foreign antigens may also incite β-cell destruction if these foreign antigens have some homology with islet cell antigens (**molecular mimicry**). For example, one identified islet cell antigen (GAD) shares homology with a coxsackievirus protein and another with bovine serum albumin, a protein present in cow's milk, consumption of which in early childhood may be associated with an increased incidence of Type 1 DM.

B. Type 2 Diabetes (Type 2 DM)

Given the current epidemic of Type 2 DM associated with rising rates of obesity, environmental factors are clearly critical for the development of this disorder. And yet, the genetic components underlying Type 2 DM are even stronger than those associated with Type 1 DM. In Type 2 DM, in contrast to the absolute lack of insulin in Type 1 DM, two metabolic defects are responsible for hyperglycemia: (1) target tissue resistance to the effects of insulin, and (2) inadequate pancreatic β cell insulin secretion in the setting of insulin resistance.

Whether the primary lesion in Type 2 DM is insulin resistance or defective β cell insulin secretion, continues to be debated. Several decades before the onset of clinical diabetes, insulin resistance and high insulin levels are present. This has led researchers to hypothesize that **insulin resistance** could be the primary lesion, resulting in a compensatory increase in insulin secretion that ultimately cannot be maintained by the pancreas. When the pancreas becomes "exhausted" and cannot keep up with insulin demands, clinical diabetes results.

Insulin resistance is a key factor in the link between obesity and Type 2 DM. Adipose tissue is the primary source of mediators of insulin resistance. The mechanisms by which fat tissue, particularly **central (abdominal) adiposity,** increases insulin resistance continues to be elucidated and appears to include: (1) toxic effects of excess free fatty acids (**lipotoxicity**), which decrease skeletal muscle insulin sensitivity by interfering with IRS signaling; and (2) dysregulated secretion of cytokines produced in the fat tissue (**adipokines**), such as the anti-diabetogenic hormone, **leptin,** which acts centrally to control satiety and enhance insulin sensitivity. Evidence also suggests a critical role for local inflammation in this process. For example, **tumor necrosis factor** (**TNF**) secretion from hypertropic adipocytes and macrophages attracted into the fat tissue by other inflammatory adipocyte secretory products (eg, **macrophage chemoattractant protein-1** [MCP-1]) is thought to block **peroxisome proliferator-activated receptor gamma** (**PPARγ**). PPARγ, whose activity is enhanced by the glitzaone class of diabetes drugs, is an adipose transcription factor that decreases insulin resistance by altering adipokine secretion and decreasing FFA release.

The importance of obesity in the etiology of Type 2 DM (85% of Type 2 DM patients are obese) is underscored by the fact that weight loss in obese Type 2 diabetics can ameliorate or even terminate the disorder. However, while all obese individuals are hyperinsulinemic and insulin resistant, most do not develop diabetes. Therefore, alternatively or additionally, a **primary pancreatic β-cell defect** is also postulated in the pathogenesis of Type 2 DM. Beta-cell mass normally increases with obesity. However, in those who develop impaired glucose tolerance and, later, frank diabetes, **β-cell apoptosis** causes a decline in β-cell mass. Local deposition of **amylin,** a β-cell product, is thought to contribute to this process. Impairment of the acute release of insulin (**first phase insulin release**) that precedes sustained insulin secretion in response to a meal occurs well before the onset of frank diabetes. Chronic exposure to hyperglyemia and elevated free fatty acids also contributes to the impairment of β-cell insulin secretion (**glucolipotoxicity**).

In the last 2 decades, a great deal of work has been directed toward identifying the genes that account for the strong genetic component of Type 2 DM. Initial efforts targeting specific candidate genes have been followed by genome wide approaches, all of which have yielded useful information, including the identification of a small subset of cases of Type 2 DM that are monogenic in origin. One monogenetic form of Type 2 DM is maturity-onset diabetes of the young (**MODY**). This autosomal dominant disorder accounts for 1–5% of cases of Type 2 DM and is characterized by the onset of mild diabetes in lean individuals before the age of 25 years. MODY is caused by mutations in one of six pancreatic genes, glucokinase, the β-cell glucose sensor, or five different transcription factors. In contrast, the vast majority of cases of Type 2 DM are thought to be polygenic in origin, due to the inheritance of an interacting set of susceptibility genes. The list of genes linked to increased risk of Type 2 DM is extensive and growing. Among the most cited mutated/polymorphic genes to date are transcription factor 7-like 2 gene (*TCF7L2*), which has the highest documented attributable risk (odds ratio of 1.4), calpain-10 (odds ratio, 1.2) and PPARγ2 (odds ratio, 1.2). **TCF7L2,** a nuclear receptor that mediates Wnt (wingless) signaling, may effect β-cell insulin secretion directly or indirectly via induction of intestinal GLP-1 production and alter insulin resistance via effects on adipocyte maturation. **Calpain** may regulate both insulin secretion by modulation of β-cell apoptosis, and insulin sensitivity by altering GLUT-4 expression and activity in skeletal muscle. **PPARγ2,** a member of the previously discussed transcription factor family that is critical to adipose cytokine regulation, is also expressed in

pancreatic β cells where it mediates high-fat diet–induced increases in β-cell mass.

CHECKPOINT

22. What are the key characteristics of Type 1 DM and Type 2 DM?
23. What is the role of heredity versus the environment in each of the two major types of diabetes mellitus?
24. What are two possible mechanisms of insulin resistance in Type 2 DM?
25. What is the role of obesity in Type 2 DM?

Pathology & Pathogenesis

No matter what the origin, all types of diabetes result from a relative deficiency of insulin action. In addition, in Type 2 DM, glucagon levels can be inappropriately high. This high **glucagon-insulin ratio** creates a state similar to that seen in fasting and results in a superfasting milieu that is inappropriate for maintenance of normal fuel homeostasis (Table 18–3; Figure 18–6).

The resulting metabolic derangements depend on the degree of loss of insulin action. Adipose tissue is most sensitive to insulin action. Therefore, low insulin activity is capable of suppressing lipolysis and enhancing fat storage. Higher levels of insulin are required to oppose glucagon effects on the liver and block hepatic glucose output. In normal individuals, basal levels of insulin activity are capable of mediating these responses. However, the ability of muscle and other insulin-sensitive tissues to respond to a glucose load with insulin-mediated glucose uptake requires the stimulated secretion of insulin from the pancreas.

Mild deficiencies in insulin action are, therefore, manifested first by an inability of insulin-sensitive tissues to clear glucose loads. Clinically, this results in **postprandial hyperglycemia.** Such individuals, most commonly Type 2 diabetics with residual insulin secretion but increased insulin resistance, will have abnormal oral glucose tolerance test results. However, fasting glucose levels remain normal because sufficient insulin action is present to counterbalance the glucagon-mediated hepatic glucose output that maintains them. When a further loss of insulin action occurs, glucagon's effects on the liver are not sufficiently counter-balanced. Individuals, therefore, have both postprandial hyperglycemia and **fasting hyperglycemia.**

Although Type 2 diabetics usually have some degree of residual endogenous insulin action, Type 1 diabetics have none. Therefore, untreated or inadequately treated Type 1 diabetics manifest the most severe signs of insulin deficiency. In addition to fasting and postprandial hyperglycemia, they also develop **ketosis** because a marked lack of insulin allows maximal lipolysis of fat stores to supply substrates for unopposed glucagon stimulation of ketogenesis in the liver.

Fatty acids liberated from increased lipolysis, in addition to being metabolized by the liver into ketone bodies, can also be reesterified and packaged into VLDLs. Furthermore, insulin deficiency causes a decrease in lipoprotein lipase, the enzyme responsible for hydrolysis of VLDL triglycerides in preparation for fatty acid storage in adipose tissue, thereby slowing VLDL clearance. Therefore, both Type 1 and Type 2 diabetics can have elevations in VLDL levels as a result of both an increase in VLDL production and a decrease in VLDL clearance.

Because insulin stimulates amino acid uptake and protein synthesis in muscle, the decrease in insulin action in diabetes results in decreased muscle protein synthesis. Marked insulinopenia, such as occurs in Type 1 DM, can cause negative nitrogen balance and marked protein wasting. Amino acids not taken up by muscle are instead diverted to the liver where they are used to fuel gluconeogenesis.

In Type 1 DM or Type 2 DM, the superimposition of stress-induced counterregulatory hormones on what is already an insulinopenic state exacerbates the metabolic manifestations of deficient insulin action. The stress of infection, for example, can, therefore, induce diabetic ketoacidosis in both Type 1 and some Type 2 diabetics.

In addition to the metabolic derangements discussed previously, diabetes causes other chronic complications that are responsible for the high morbidity and mortality rates associated with this disease. Diabetic complications are largely the result of vascular disease affecting both the microvasculature (retinopathy, nephropathy, and some types of neuropathy) and the macrovasculature (coronary artery disease, peripheral vascular disease).

Clinical Manifestations

A. Acute Complications

1. Hyperglycemia—When elevated glucose levels exceed the renal threshold for reabsorption of glucose, **glucosuria** results. This causes an osmotic diuresis manifested clinically by **polyuria,** including **nocturia.** Dehydration results, stimulating thirst that results in **polydipsia.** A significant loss of calories can result from glucosuria, because urinary glucose losses can exceed 75 g/d (75 g × 4 kcal/g = 300 kcal/d). **Polyphagia** also accompanies uncontrolled hyperglycemia. The three "polys" of diabetes—polyuria, polydipsia, and polyphagia—are common presenting symptoms in both type 1 and symptomatic Type 2 patients. Weight loss can also occur as a result of both dehydration and loss of calories in the urine. Severe weight loss is most likely to occur in patients with severe insulinopenia (Type 1 DM) and is due to both caloric loss and muscle wasting. Increased protein catabolism also contributes to the growth failure seen in children with Type 1 DM.

Elevated glucose levels raise plasma osmolality:

$$\text{Osmolality (mOsm/L)} = 2[\text{Na}^+(\text{mEq/L}) + \text{K}^+(\text{mEq/L})]$$
$$+ \frac{\text{Glucose (mg/dL)}}{18} + \frac{\text{BUN (mg/dL)}}{2.8}$$

Changes in the water content of the lens of the eye in response to changes in osmolality can cause blurred vision.

In women, glucosuria can lead to an increased incidence of candidal vulvovaginitis. In some cases, this may be their only presenting symptom. In uncircumcised men, candidal balanitis (a similar infection of the glans penis) can occur.

2. Diabetic ketoacidosis—A profound loss of insulin activity leads not only to increased serum glucose levels because of increased hepatic glucose output and decreased glucose uptake by insulin-sensitive tissues but also to ketogenesis. In the absence of insulin, lipolysis is stimulated, providing fatty acids that are preferentially converted to ketone bodies in the liver by unopposed glucagon action. Typically, profound hyperglycemia and ketosis (diabetic ketoacidosis) occur in Type 1 diabetics, individuals who lack endogenous insulin. However, diabetic ketoacidosis can also occur in Type 2 DM, particularly during infections, severe trauma, or other causes of stress that increase levels of counterregulatory hormones, thus producing a state of profound inhibition of insulin action.

Severe hyperglycemia with glucose levels reaching an average of 500 mg/dL can occur if compensation for the osmotic diuresis associated with hyperglycemia fails. Initially, when elevated glucose levels cause an increase in osmolality, a shift of water from the intracellular to the extracellular space and increased water intake stimulated by thirst help to maintain intravascular volume. If polyuria continues and these compensatory mechanisms cannot keep pace with fluid losses—particularly decreased intake as a result of the nausea and increased losses resulting from the vomiting that accompany ketoacidosis—the depletion of intravascular volume leads to decreased renal blood flow. The kidney's ability to excrete glucose is, therefore, reduced. Hypovolemia also stimulates counter-regulatory hormones. Therefore, glucose levels rise acutely owing to increased glucose production stimulated by these hormones and decreased clearance by the kidney, an important source of glucose clearance in the absence of insulin-mediated glucose uptake.

In diabetic ketoacidosis, coma occurs in a minority of patients (10%). Hyperosmolality (not acidosis) is the cause of coma. Profound cellular dehydration occurs in response to the marked increase in plasma osmolality. A severe loss of intracellular fluid in the brain leads to coma. Coma occurs when the effective plasma osmolality reaches 340 mOsm/L (normal: 280–295 mOsm/L). Because urea is freely diffusible across cell membranes, blood urea nitrogen is not used to calculate the effective plasma osmolality:

$$\text{Effective osmolality} = 2[\text{Na}^+(\text{mEq/L}) + \text{K}^+(\text{mEq/L})]$$
$$+ \frac{\text{Glucose (mEq/L)}}{18}$$

The increase in **ketogenesis** caused by a severe lack of insulin action results in increased serum levels of ketones and ketonuria. Insulinopenia is also thought to decrease the ability of tissues to use ketones, thus contributing to the maintenance

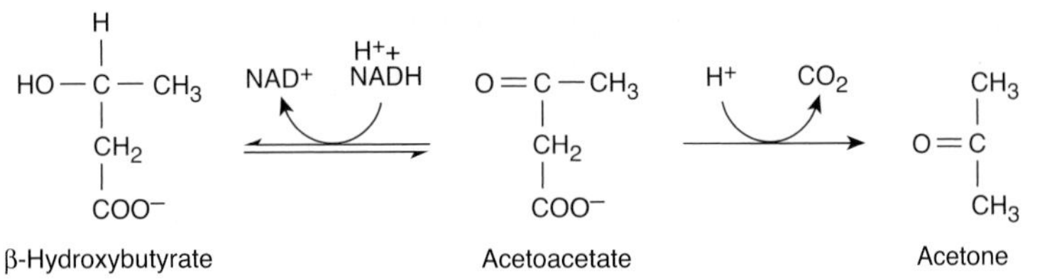

FIGURE 18–8 Interconversion of ketone bodies. (Redrawn, with permission, from Stryer L. *Biochemistry*, 3rd ed. Freeman, 1988.)

of ketosis. **Acetoacetate** and **β-hydroxybutyrate,** the chief ketone bodies produced by the liver, are organic acids and, therefore, cause metabolic acidosis, decreasing blood pH and serum bicarbonate (Figure 18–8). Respiration is stimulated, which partially compensates for the metabolic acidosis by reducing PCO_2. When the pH level is lower than 7.20, characteristic deep, rapid respirations occur (**Kussmaul breathing**). Although acetone is a minor product of ketogenesis (Figure 18–8), its fruity odor can be detected on the breath during diabetic ketoacidosis.

Na^+ is lost in addition to water during the osmotic diuresis accompanying diabetic ketoacidosis. Therefore, total body Na^+ is depleted. Serum levels of Na^+ are usually low owing to the osmotic activity of the elevated glucose, which draws water into the extracellular space and in that way decreases the Na^+ concentration (serum Na^+ falls approximately 1.6 mmol/L for every 100 mg/dL increase in glucose).

Total body stores of K^+ are also depleted by diuresis and vomiting. However, acidosis, insulinopenia, and elevated glucose levels cause a shift of K^+ out of cells, thus maintaining normal or even elevated serum K^+ levels until acidosis and hyperglycemia are corrected. With administration of insulin and correction of acidosis, serum K^+ falls as K^+ moves back into cells. Without treatment, K^+ can fall to dangerously low levels, leading to potentially lethal cardiac arrhythmias. Therefore, K^+ supplementation is routinely given in the treatment of diabetic ketoacidosis. Similarly, phosphate depletion accompanies diabetic ketoacidosis, although acidosis and insulinopenia can cause serum phosphorus levels to be normal before treatment. Phosphate replacement is provided only in cases of extreme depletion given the risks of phosphate administration. (Intravenous phosphate may complex with Ca^{2+}, resulting in hypocalcemia and Ca^{2+} phosphate deposition in soft tissues.)

Marked **hypertriglyceridemia** can also accompany diabetic ketoacidosis because of the increased production and decreased clearance of VLDL that occurs in insulin-deficient states. Increased production is due to the increased hepatic flux of fatty acids, which, in addition to fueling ketogenesis, can be repackaged and secreted as VLDL; decreased clearance is due to decreased lipoprotein lipase activity. Although serum Na^+ levels can be decreased owing to the osmotic effects of glucose, hypertriglyceridemia can interfere with some common procedures used to measure serum Na^+. This causes pseudohyponatremia (ie, falsely low serum Na^+ values, due to overestimation of actual serum volume).

Nausea and vomiting often accompany diabetic ketoacidosis, contributing to further dehydration. Abdominal pain, present in 30% of patients, may be due to gastric stasis and distention. Amylase is frequently elevated (90% of cases), in part because of elevations of salivary amylase, but it is usually not associated with symptoms of pancreatitis. Leukocytosis is frequently present and does not necessarily indicate the presence of infection. However, because infections can precipitate diabetic ketoacidosis in Type 1 DM and Type 2 DM, other manifestations of infection should be sought, such as fever, a finding that cannot be attributed to diabetic ketoacidosis.

Diabetic ketoacidosis is treated by replacement of water and electrolytes (Na^+ and K^+) and administration of insulin. With fluid and electrolyte replacement, renal perfusion is increased, restoring renal clearance of elevated blood glucose, and counter-regulatory hormone production is decreased, thus decreasing hepatic glucose production. Insulin administration also corrects hyperglycemia by restoring insulin-sensitive glucose uptake and inhibiting hepatic glucose output. Rehydration is a critical component of the treatment of hyperosmolality. If insulin is administered in the absence of fluid and electrolyte replacement, water will move from the extracellular space back into the cells with correction of hyperglycemia, leading to vascular collapse. Insulin administration is also required to inhibit further lipolysis, thus eliminating substrates for ketogenesis, and to inhibit hepatic ketogenesis, thereby correcting ketoacidosis.

During treatment of diabetic ketoacidosis, measured serum ketones may transiently rise instead of showing a steady decrease. This is an artifact because of the limitations of the nitroprusside test that is usually used at the bedside to measure ketones in both serum and urine. Nitroprusside only detects acetoacetate and not β-hydroxybutyrate. During untreated diabetic ketoacidosis, accelerated fatty acid oxidation generates large quantities of NADH in the liver, which favors the formation of β-hydroxybutyrate over acetoacetate (Figure 18–8). With insulin treatment, fatty acid oxidation decreases and the redox potential of the liver shifts back in favor of acetoacetate formation. Therefore, although the absolute amount of hepatic ketone body production is decreasing with treatment of diabetic ketoacidosis, the relative amount of acetoacetate production is increasing, leading to a transient increase in measured serum ketones by the nitroprusside test.

3. Hyperosmolar coma—Severe hyperosmolar states in the absence of ketosis can occur in Type 2 DM. These episodes are frequently precipitated by decreased fluid intake such as can occur during an intercurrent illness or in older debilitated patients who lack sufficient access to water and have abnormal renal function hindering the clearance of excessive glucose loads. The mechanisms underlying the development of hyperosmolality and **hyperosmolar coma** are the same as in diabetic ketoacidosis. However, because only minimal levels of insulin activity are required to suppress lipolysis, these individuals have sufficient insulin to prevent the ketogenesis that results from increased fatty acid flux. Because of the absence of ketoacidosis and its symptoms, patients often present later and, therefore, have more profound hyperglycemia and dehydration; glucose levels often range from 800–2400 mg/dL. Therefore, the effective osmolality exceeds 340 mOsm/L more frequently in these patients than in those presenting with diabetic ketoacidosis, resulting in a higher incidence of coma.

Although ketosis is absent, mild ketonuria can be present if the patient has not been eating. K^+ losses are less severe than in diabetic ketoacidosis. Treatment is similar to that of diabetic ketoacidosis. Mortality is 10 times higher than in diabetic ketoacidosis because the Type 2 diabetics who develop hyperosmolar nonketotic states are older and often have other serious precipitating or complicating illnesses. For example, myocardial infarction can precipitate hyperosmolar states or can result from the alterations in vascular blood flow and other stressors that accompany severe dehydration.

4. Hypoglycemia—Hypoglycemia is a complication of insulin treatment in both Type 1 DM and Type 2 DM, but it can also occur with oral hypoglycemic drugs that stimulate glucose-independent insulin secretion (eg, sulfonylureas). Hypoglycemia often occurs during exercise or with fasting, states that normally are characterized by slight elevations in counterregulatory hormones and depressed insulin levels. Low insulin levels in these conditions are permissive for the counterregulatory hormone-mediated mobilization of fuel substrates, increased hepatic glucose output, and inhibition of glucose disposal in insulin-sensitive tissues. These responses normally would increase blood glucose. However, hypoglycemia is precipitated in diabetic patients in these circumstances by inappropriate dosing with exogenous insulin or by induction of endogenous insulin.

The acute response to hypoglycemia is mediated by the counterregulatory effects of glucagon and catecholamines (Table 18–7). Initial symptoms of hypoglycemia occur secondary to **catecholamine release** (shaking, sweating, palpitations). As glucose drops further, **neuroglycopenic symptoms** also occur from the direct effects of hypoglycemia on CNS function (confusion, coma). A characteristic set of symptoms (night sweats, nightmares, morning headaches) also accompanies hypoglycemic episodes that occur during sleep (**nocturnal hypoglycemia**).

Type 1 diabetics are especially prone to hypoglycemia. In individuals with deficient endogenous insulin production, the glucagon response to hypoglycemia is virtually absent for reasons that are unclear. Moreover, recent episodes of hypoglycemia reduce the catecholamine response to subsequent

TABLE 18–7 Symptoms of hypoglycemia.

Autonomic	
Adrenergic	**Cholinergic**
Tremor/shakiness	Sweating
Anxiety	Hunger
Palpitations/tachycardia	
Neuroglycopenic	
Weak/fatigued/drowsy	Diplopia
Headache	Difficulty speaking
Behavioral changes	Seizures
Confusion	Coma
Associated with nocturnal hypoglycemia	
Night sweats	Morning headaches
Nightmares	Lassitude
Restlessness	Difficulty awakening

hypoglycemia and cause hypoglycemia unawareness by reducing the sympathoadrenal response and resulting neurogenic symptoms. This hypoglycemia-induced autonomic failure, which is distinct from diabetic autonomic neuropathy, is reversed by avoidance of hypoglycemia but exacerbated by exercise or sleep, both of which can further decrease the catecholamine response to a given level of hypoglycemia.

Acute treatment of hypoglycemia in diabetic individuals consists of rapid oral or intravenous administration of glucose at the onset of warning symptoms or the administration of glucagon intramuscularly. Rebound hyperglycemia can occur after hypoglycemia because of the actions of counterregulatory hormones (**Somogyi phenomenon**), an effect that can be aggravated by excessive glucose administration.

B. Chronic Complications

Over time, diabetes results in damage and dysfunction in multiple organ systems (Table 18–8). Vascular disease is a major cause of many of the sequelae of this disease. Both **microvascular disease** (retinopathy, nephropathy, neuropathy) that is specific to diabetes and **macrovascular disease** (coronary artery disease, peripheral vascular disease) that occurs with increased frequency in diabetes contribute to the high morbidity and mortality rates associated with this disease. **Neuropathy** also causes increased morbidity, particularly by virtue of its role in the pathogenesis of foot ulcers.

Although Type 1 DM and Type 2 DM both suffer from the complete spectrum of diabetic complications, the incidence varies with each type and with treatment. Macrovascular disease is the major cause of death in Type 2 DM. With the advent of intensive glucose control strategies and the use of

TABLE 18–8 Chronic complications of diabetes mellitus.

Microvascular disease
Nephropathy
Neuropathy
Sensorimotor distal symmetric neuropathy
Autonomic neuropathy
Focal and multifocal neuropathies
Vascular
Nonvascular (entrapment)
Macrovascular disease
Coronary artery disease
Cerebrovascular disease
Peripheral vascular disease
Associated complications
Foot ulcers
Infections

angiotensin-converting enzyme inhibitors, renal failure secondary to **nephropathy** is no longer the most common cause of death in individuals with Type 1 DM who now, with increased longevity, are increasingly suffering from macrovascular complications. Although blindness occurs in both types, proliferative changes in retinal vessels (**proliferative retinopathy**) are a major cause of blindness in Type 1 DM, whereas macular edema is the most important cause in Type 2 DM. **Autonomic neuropathy,** one of the manifestations of diabetic neuropathy, is more common in Type 1 DM.

1. Role of glycemic control in preventing complications— A paradigm shift in diabetes treatment occurred in 1993 with publication of the results of the Diabetes Control and Complications Trial (**DCCT**), the first major trial to examine the effects of attempted glucose normalization (**tight** or **intensive diabetic control**) on the incidence of complications. In this study of individuals with Type 1 DM, intensive (vs. conventional) treatment reduced microvascular complications (retinopathy, nephropathy, neuropathy) by 60%. A subsequent study in Type 2 DM (United Kingdom Prospective Diabetes Study [**UKPDS**]) demonstrated a 25% decrease in microvascular complications (retinopathy, nephropathy) with improved glycemic control. In contrast, the role of glycemic control in preventing macrovascular disease, the major cause of death in Type 2 DM, is less clear. With the publication in 2008 of three major clinical trials demonstrating either no improvement, or indeed an increase (**ACCORD** trial), in mortality and macrovascular complications with intensive treatment

in Type 2 DM, discussions regarding the most appropriate treatment goals (eg, degree of glucose normalization) and modalities (eg, therapeutics that minimize risk of hypoglycemia and/or weight gain) in Type 2 DM continue.

While the importance of glycemic control in influencing the occurrence of microvascular complications is undisputed, genetic factors also clearly play a role. For example, evidence from a variety of studies suggests that approximately 40% of type 1 diabetics may be particularly susceptible to the development of severe microvascular complications. The identity of responsible genetic factors is not known but is the subject of investigation. However, this observation suggests that not all individuals with Type 1 DM may achieve the same benefits from intensive control regimens, which are both inconvenient and associated with an increased risk of hypoglycemia.

2. Microvascular complications—Consistent with clinical evidence defining the critical role of hyperglycemia in microvasular disease, data indicate that high intracellular levels of glucose in cells that cannot down-regulate glucose entry (glomeruli, endothelium and nerve cells) result in microvascular damage via four distinct, diabetes-specific pathways that were sequentially discovered (Figure 18–9): (1) increased polyol pathway flux, (2) increased formation of advanced glycation end-product (AGE), (3) activation of protein kinase C (PKC), and (4) increased hexosamine pathway flux. More recent information suggests that increased flux through these four pathways is induced by a common factor, overproduction of mitochondrial-derived reactive oxygen species generated by increased flux of glucose through the TCA cycle (Figure 18–9). The end result of these changes in the microvasculature is an increase in protein accumulation in vessel walls, a loss of endothelial cells, and, ultimately, occlusion.

The **polyol pathway** has been extensively studied in diabetic nerve cells and is also present in endothelial cells (Figure 18–9). Many cells contain aldose reductase, an enzyme that converts toxic aldehydes to their respective alcohols (polyol pathway). While aldose reductase has a low affinity for glucose, under conditions of intercellular hyperglycemia, this pathway can account for up to one third of glucose flux, converting glucose to sorbitol. The excess **sorbitol** produced from this reaction was originally thought to result in osmotic damage to the microvasculature. More recent data instead suggest that the real culprit leading to vascular damage is the consumption of NADPH that accompanies glucose reduction. As NADPH is required to regenerate reduced glutathione (GSH), a thiol that detoxifies reactive oxygen species (ROS), consumption of NADPH in the polyol pathway is thought to result in decreased clearance of damaging free radicals within the cell. While polyol pathway-mediated damage appears to be a prominent feature in nerve cells, its role in the vasculature is less clear.

The formation of irreversibly glycated proteins called **advanced glycosylation end-products** (AGEs) also causes microvascular damage in diabetes (Figure 18–9). When present in high concentrations, glucose can react reversibly

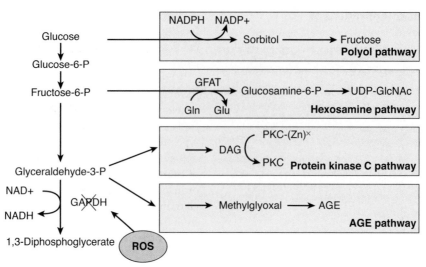

FIGURE 18–9 Mechanisms of microvascular damage initiated by intracellular hyperglycemia. Overproduction of reactive oxygen species (ROS) in response to high glucose is thought to inhibit glyceraldehyde-3-phosphate dehydrogenase (GAPDH), thus increasing the concentration of upstream glycolytic metabolites that are shunted into alternative pathways. Among these (1) conversion of glucose to sorbitol depletes NADPH, thus preventing the regeneration of ROS scavengers; (2) conversion of fructose-6-phosphate to uridine diphosphate-N-acetylglucosamine (UDP-GLcNAc) leads to protein modifications that alter gene expression; (3) glyceraldehyde-3 phosphate is metabolized to form diacylglycerol (DAG), which in turn activates protein kinase C (PKC), resulting in altered vascular hemodynamics; and (4) carbonyls formed by multiple mechanisms, including oxidation of glyceraldehyde-3 phosphate to form methylglyoxal, react irreversibly with proteins to form dysfunctional products (advanced glycation products, AGE) that cause intracellular and extracellular vascular changes.   (Redrawn from Kronenberg [editor]. *Williams Textbook of Endocrinology*, 11th edition. Copyright Elsevier [2008].)

and nonenzymatically with protein amino groups to form an unstable intermediate, a Schiff base, which then undergoes an internal rearrangement to form a more stable glycated protein, also known as an early glycosylation product (**Amadori product**) (Figure 18–10). Such a reaction accounts for the formation of **glycated HbA**, also known as HbA_{1c}. In diabetics, elevated glucose leads to increased glycation of HbA within red blood cells. Because red blood cells circulate for 120 days, measurement of HbA_{1c} in diabetic patients serves as an index of glycemic control over the preceding months. Early glycosylation products can undergo a further series of chemical reactions and rearrangements, often involving the formation of reactive **carbonyl** intermediates, leading to the irreversible formation of AGE. Dicarbonyl formation from direct autooxidation of glucose also contributes to AGE formation (Figure 18–10). AGE damage the microvasculature via 3 major pathways: (1) intracellular AGE formation from proteins involved in transcription alters endothelial gene expression; (2) irreversible cross linking of AGE adducts formed from matrix proteins results in vascular thickening and stiffness; and (3) binding of extracellular AGE adducts to AGE receptors (RAGE) on macrophages and endothelium stimulates NF-κB-regulated inflammatory cascades and resultant vascular dysfunction.

Intracellular endothelial hyperglycemia stimulates glycolysis and, with this, an increase in the de novo synthesis of diacylglycerol (DAG) from the glycolytic intermediate, glyceraldehyde-3-phosphate (Figure 18–9). DAG, in turn, activates several isoforms of **protein kinase C (PKC)** that are present in these cells. This inappropriate activation of PKC alters blood flow and changes endothelial permeability, in part via effects on nitric oxide pathways, and also contributes to thickening of the extracellular matrix.

Last, increased shunting of glucose through the **hexosamine pathway** via diversion of the glycolytic intermediate, fructose-6-phosphate, is also postulated to play a role in microvascular disease (Figure 18–9). The **hexosamine pathway** contributes to insulin resistance, producing substrates that, when covalently linked to transcription factors, stimulate the expression of proteins, such as transforming growth factor and plasminogen activator inhibitor, that enhance microvascular damage.

Evidence suggests that all four of these pathways may actually be linked by a common mechanistic element: hyperglycemia-induced **oxidative stress.** In particular, the increase in electron donors that results from shunting glucose through the tricarboxylic acid cycle increases mitochondrial membrane potential by pumping proteins across the mitochondrial inner membrane. This increased potential prolongs the half-life of superoxide generating enzymes, thus increasing the conversion of O_2 to O_2^-. These increased **reactive oxygen species (ROS)** lead to inhibition of the glycolytic enzyme, glyceraldehyde-3-phosphate dehydrogenase (GADPH), and a resultant increase in upstream metabolites that can now be preferentially diverted into the four mechanistic pathways (Figure 18–9).

a. Retinopathy—Diabetes is the leading cause of new blindness among U.S. adults. Diabetic retinopathy, present after 20

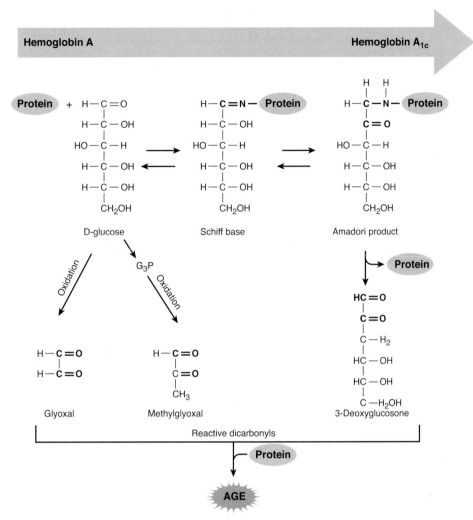

FIGURE 18–10 The formation of advanced glycosylation end-products (AGEs) occurs via multiple pathways. The reversible formation of glycated proteins (Amadori products), such as hemoglobin A_{1c}, through a complex series of chemical reactions, or the direct oxidation of glucose and its metabolites (eg, glyceraldehyde-3 phosphate, G3P), result in the production of reactive dicarbonyls. These moieties react irreversibly with proteins to form AGE.

years in >95% with Type 1 DM and 60% with Type 2 DM, occurs in two distinct stages: nonproliferative and proliferative.

Nonproliferative retinopathy occurs frequently in both Type 1 DM and Type 2 DM. **Microaneurysms** of the retinal capillaries, appearing as tiny red dots, are the earliest clinically detectable sign of diabetic retinopathy (**background retinopathy**). These outpouchings in the capillary wall are thought to be related to loss of the pericytes that surround and support the capillary walls. Vascular permeability is increased. Fat that has leaked from excessively permeable capillary walls appears as shiny yellow spots with distinct borders (**hard exudates**) forming a ring around the area of leakage. The appearance of hard exudates in the area of the macula is often associated with **macular edema,** which is by far the most common cause of visual impairment in Type 2 DM. As retinopathy progresses, signs of ischemia appearing as background retinopathy worsen (**preproliferative stage**). Occlusion of capillaries and terminal arterioles causes areas of retinal ischemia that appear as hazy yellow

areas with indistinct borders (**cotton wool spots** or **soft exudates**) because of the accumulation of axonoplasmic debris at areas of infarction. Retinal hemorrhages can also occur, and retinal veins develop segmental dilation.

Retinopathy can progress to a second, more severe stage characterized by the proliferation of new vessels (**proliferative retinopathy**). Neovascularization is more prevalent in Type 1 DM than in Type 2 DM (25% vs. 15% after 20 years) and is a major cause of blindness. It is hypothesized that retinal ischemia stimulates the release of growth-promoting factors, resulting in new vessel formation. However, these capillaries are abnormal, and traction between new fibrovascular networks and the vitreous can lead to **vitreous hemorrhage** or **retinal detachment,** two potential causes of blindness.

b. Nephropathy—In the United States, more than 50% of end-stage renal disease requiring kidney dialysis or transplantation is due to diabetes. Although end-stage renal disease occurs more frequently in Type 1 DM than in Type 2 DM

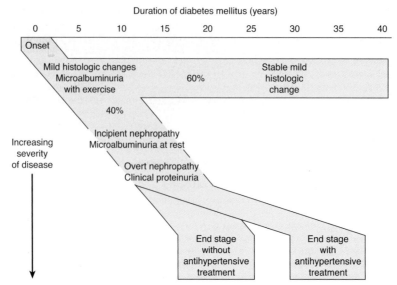

FIGURE 18–11   Development of renal failure in type 1 diabetes.   (Redrawn, with permission, from Omachi R. The pathogenesis and prevention of diabetic nephropathy. West J Med. 1986;145:222. Reproduced with permission from the BMJ Publishing Group.)

(35% vs. 20% after 20 years), Type 2 DM accounts for more than half of the diabetic population with end-stage renal disease because of its greater prevalence. End-stage renal disease also occurs more frequently in Native Americans, African Americans, and Hispanic Americans than in non-Hispanic whites with Type 2 DM.

Diabetic nephropathy results primarily from disordered glomerular function. Histologic changes in glomeruli are indistinguishable in Type 1 DM and Type 2 DM and occur to some degree in the majority of individuals. Basement membranes of the glomerular capillaries are thickened and can obliterate the vessels; the mesangium surrounding the glomerular vessels is increased owing to the deposition of basement membrane-like material and can encroach on the glomerular vessels; and the afferent and efferent glomerular arteries are also sclerosed. **Glomerulosclerosis** is usually diffuse but in 50% of cases is associated with nodular sclerosis. This nodular component, called **Kimmelstiel-Wilson nodules** after the investigators who first described the pathologic changes in diabetic kidneys, is pathognomonic for diabetes.

In Type 1 DM diabetics, glomerular changes are preceded by a phase of **hyperfiltration** resulting from vasodilation of both the afferent and efferent glomerular arterioles, an effect perhaps mediated by two of the counter-regulatory hormones, glucagon and growth hormone, or by hyperglycemia. It is unclear whether this early hyperfiltration phase occurs in Type 2 DM. It has been proposed that the presence of atherosclerotic lesions in older Type 2 diabetics may prevent hyperfiltration and thus account for the lower incidence of overt clinical nephropathy in these individuals.

Early in the course of the disease, the histologic changes in renal glomeruli are accompanied by **microalbuminuria,** a urinary loss of albumin that cannot be detected by routine urinalysis dipstick methods (Figure 18–11). Albuminuria is thought to be due to a decrease in the heparan sulfate content of the thickened glomerular capillary basement membrane. Heparan sulfate, a negatively charged proteoglycan, can inhibit the filtration of other negatively charged proteins, such as albumin, through the basement membrane; its loss, therefore, allows for increased albumin filtration.

If glomerular lesions worsen, **proteinuria** increases and overt nephropathy develops (Figure 18–11). Diabetic nephropathy is defined clinically by the presence of more than 300 mg of urinary protein per day, an amount that can be detected by routine urinalysis. In diabetic nephropathy (unlike other renal diseases), proteinuria continues to increase as renal function decreases. Therefore, end-stage renal disease is preceded by massive, nephrotic-range proteinuria (> 4 g/d). The presence of hypertension speeds this process. Although Type 2 diabetics often already have hypertension at the time of diagnosis, Type 1 patients usually do not develop hypertension until after the onset of nephropathy. In both cases, hypertension worsens as renal function deteriorates. Therefore, control of hypertension is critical in preventing the progression of diabetic nephropathy.

Retinopathy, a process that is also worsened by the presence of hypertension, usually precedes the development of nephropathy. Therefore, other causes of proteinuria should be considered in diabetic individuals who present with proteinuria in the absence of retinopathy.

c. Neuropathy—Neuropathy (Table 18–8) occurs commonly in about 60% of both Type 1 and Type 2 diabetics and is a major cause of morbidity. Diabetic neuropathy can be divided into three major types: (1) a distal, primarily sensory, symmetric polyneuropathy that is by far the most common (50% incidence); (2) an autonomic neuropathy, occurring frequently in individuals with distal polyneuropathy (> 20% incidence); and

(3) much less common, transient asymmetric neuropathies involving specific nerves, nerve roots, or plexuses.

Symmetric distal polyneuropathy—Demyelination of peripheral nerves, which is a hallmark of diabetic polyneuropathy, affects distal nerves preferentially and is usually manifested clinically by a symmetric sensory loss in the distal lower extremities (**stocking distribution**) that is preceded by numbness, tingling, and paresthesias. These symptoms, which begin distally and move proximally, can also occur in the hands (**glove distribution**). Pathologic features of affected peripheral somatic nerves include demyelination and loss of nerve fibers with reduced axonal regeneration accompanied by microvascular lesions, including thickening of basement membranes. Activation of the polyol pathway in nerve cells is thought to play a major role in inducing symmetric distal polyneuropathy in diabetes. In addition, the microvascular disease that accompanies these neural lesions may also contribute to nerve damage. The presence of antibodies to autoantigens in patients with neuropathy also suggests a possible immune component to this disorder. Last, defects in the production or delivery of neurotrophic factors, such as nerve growth factor (NGF), are hypothesized to play a role in the pathogenesis of symmetric distal neuropathy.

Autonomic neuropathy—Autonomic neuropathy often accompanies symmetric peripheral neuropathy, occurs more frequently in Type 1 DM, and can affect all aspects of autonomic functioning, most notably those involving the cardiovascular, genitourinary, and GI systems. Less information is available regarding the morphologic changes occurring in affected autonomic nerves, but similarities to somatic nerve alterations suggest a common pathogenesis.

Fixed, resting **tachycardia** and **orthostatic hypotension** are signs of cardiovascular autonomic nervous system damage that can be easily ascertained on physical examination. Orthostatic hypotension can be quite severe. **Erectile dysfunction** occurs in more than 50% of diabetic men and is due both to neurogenic (parasympathetic control of penile vasodilation) and vascular factors. Sexual dysfunction in diabetic women has not been well studied. Loss of bladder sensation and difficulty emptying the bladder (neurogenic bladder) lead to overflow **incontinence** and an increased risk of urinary tract infections as a result of residual urine. Motor disturbances can occur throughout the GI tract, resulting in delayed gastric emptying (**gastroparesis**), constipation, or diarrhea. Anhidrosis in the lower extremities can lead to excessive sweating in the upper body as a means of dissipating heat, including increased sweating in response to eating (**gustatory sweating**). Autonomic neuropathy can also result in decreased glucagon and epinephrine responses to hypoglycemia.

Mononeuropathy and **mononeuropathy multiplex**—The abrupt, usually painful onset of motor loss in isolated cranial or peripheral nerves (**mononeuropathy**) or in multiple isolated nerves (**mononeuropathy multiplex**) occurs much less frequently than does symmetric polyneuropathy or autonomic neuropathy. Vascular occlusion and ischemia are thought to play a central role in the pathogenesis of these asymmetric focal neuropathies, which are usually of limited duration and occur more frequently in Type 2 DM. The third cranial nerve is the most frequently involved, causing ipsilateral headache followed by ptosis and ophthalmoplegia with sparing of papillary reactivity. In contrast to the rare occurrence of these vascular neuropathies, symptomatic compression by entrapment of peripheral nerves (eg, ulnar nerve at elbow; median nerve at the wrist) occurs in 30% of diabetics and usually involves both the nerve and surrounding tissues.

3. Macrovascular complications—Atherosclerotic macrovascular disease occurs with increased frequency in diabetes, resulting in an increased incidence of myocardial infarction, stroke, and claudication and gangrene of the lower extremities. Although macrovascular disease accounts for significant morbidity and mortality in both types of diabetes, the effects of large-vessel disease are particularly devastating in Type 2 DM and are responsible for approximately 75% of deaths. The protective effect of gender is lost in women with diabetes; their risk of atherosclerosis is equal to that of men (Figure 18–12).

Reasons for the increased risk of **atherosclerosis** in diabetes are threefold: (1) the incidence of traditional risk factors, such as hypertension and hyperlipidemia, is increased (50% and 30% incidence at diagnosis, respectively); (2) diabetes itself is an independent risk factor for atherosclerosis; and (3) diabetes appears to synergize with other known risk factors to increase atherosclerosis. The elimination of other risk factors, therefore, can greatly reduce the risk of atherosclerosis in diabetes (Figure 18–12).

Hypertension occurs with increased frequency in Type 1 DM and Type 2 DM and is associated with an increase in total body extracellular Na^+ content, causing volume expansion and suppression of renin. Despite these similar findings, the epidemiology of hypertension in the two subtypes suggests that different pathophysiologic mechanisms may be operative. In Type 1 DM, hypertension usually occurs after the onset of nephropathy, when renal insufficiency impairs the ability to excrete water and solutes. In Type 2 DM, hypertension is often present at the time of diagnosis in these older, obese, insulin-resistant individuals. Indeed, it has been proposed that insulin resistance and hyperinsulinemia may play a central role both in diabetes and in hypertension. The **metabolic syndrome**, a cluster of metabolic abnormalities in **nondiabetics**—insulin resistance, hyperinsulinemia, glucose intolerance, hypertension, hypertriglyceridemia, low levels of high-density lipoprotein (HDL) cholesterol, and central obesity—is associated with increased cardiovascular risk, in women more than men (relative risk of 3 vs. 2). Insulin resistance is believed to be central to the pathogenesis of this syndrome, whose prevalence, which is 24% in the U.S. population, is increased with age (44% in the age range of 60–69 years), obesity (30–50% in obese adolescents), and certain ethnicities (35% in Hispanic women). Type 2 DM, with its overt hyperglycemia

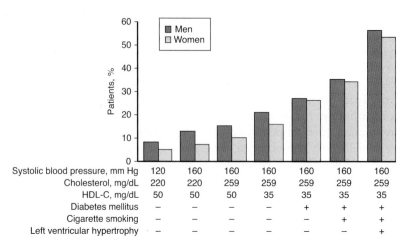

FIGURE 18–12   Estimate of percentage of patients developing coronary artery disease over 10 years based on risk factors. Diabetes equalizes the risk for women and men, which is otherwise lower for women.   (Redrawn, with permission, from Barrett-Conner E et al. Women and heart disease: The role of diabetes and hyperglycemia. Arch Intern Med. 2004;164:934. Copyright © 2004, American Medical Association. All Rights reserved.)

occurring in the setting of these same metabolic abnormalities, may lie at the extreme end of a continuum of metabolic derangements described by this syndrome.

The principal lipid abnormality in poorly controlled Type 1 DM and Type 2 DM is **hypertriglyceridemia,** which is due to increased VLDLs. Hypertriglyceridemia, particularly in Type 2 DM, can also be associated with decreased high-density lipoprotein (HDL) cholesterol. LDL cholesterol may also be elevated both because of increased production (VLDL is catabolized to LDL) and decreased clearance (insulin deficiency may reduce LDL receptor activity). VLDL levels are increased because of insufficient insulin action in adipose tissue. This results in decreased VLDL clearance as a result of decreased lipoprotein lipase activity and in increased VLDL production as a result of increased fatty acid flux from adipose tissue to the liver (ie, increased lipolysis). Hypertriglyceridemia, low HDL cholesterol, and high LDL cholesterol are all risk factors for atherosclerosis. Insulin treatment usually corrects lipoprotein abnormalities in Type 1 DM. In contrast, treatment of hyperglycemia often does not normalize lipid profiles in obese, insulin-resistant individuals with Type 2 DM unless accompanied by weight reduction (ie, by a concomitant reduction in insulin resistance).

Possible reasons why diabetes may be an independent risk factor for atherosclerosis and may also act synergistically with other risk factors include the following: (1) alterations in lipoprotein composition in diabetes that make the particles more atherogenic (ie, increased small dense LDL, increased levels of Lp[a], enhanced oxidation and glycation of lipoproteins); (2) the occurrence of a relative procoagulant state in diabetes, including an increase in certain clotting factors and increased platelet aggregation; (3) proatherogenic alterations in the vessel walls caused either by the direct effects of hyperinsulinemia in Type 2 DM or by boluses of exogenously administered insulin (vs. hepatic first-pass clearance of endogenously secreted insulin) in Type 1 DM,

which include promotion of smooth muscle proliferation, alteration of vasomotor tone, and enhancement of foam cell formation (cholesterol-laden cells that characterize atherogenic lesions); (4) proatherogenic alterations in the vessel walls caused by the direct effects of hyperglycemia, including deposition of glycated proteins, just as occurs in the microvasculature; and (5) the proinflammatory milieu that associated with insulin resistance.

4. Diabetic foot ulcers—Diabetic foot ulcers occur in 15% of diabetics and result in amputations in 2%, an event that is associated with high mortality (50% by 3 years). Risk factors for ulcer development include: (1) increased in insensitive injuries due to symmetric polyneuropathy (present in 75–90% of diabetics with foot ulcers), and manifested clinically by decreased vibratory and cutaneous pressure sensation and absence of ankle reflexes; (2) macrovascular disease (present in 30–40% with foot ulcers) and microvascular disease; (3) infections caused by alterations in neutrophil function and vascular insufficiency; and (4) faulty wound healing caused by unknown factors.

5. Infection—Neutrophil chemotaxis and phagocytosis are defective in poorly controlled diabetes. Cell-mediated immunity may also be abnormal. In addition, vascular lesions can hinder blood flow, preventing inflammatory cells from reaching wounds (eg, foot ulcers) or other possible sites of infection. Therefore, individuals with diabetes are more prone to develop infections and may have more severe infections. As a result, certain common infections (eg, **candidal infections, periodontal disease**) occur more frequently in diabetics. A number of unusual infections also are seen in diabetics (ie, **necrotizing papillitis, mucormycosis** of the nasal sinuses invading the orbit and cranium, and **malignant otitis externa** caused by *Pseudomonas aeruginosa*).

CHECKPOINT

26. How does Type 1 DM result in negative nitrogen balance and protein wasting?

27. What are some acute clinical manifestations of diabetes mellitus?

28. Describe the pathophysiologic mechanisms at work in diabetic ketoacidosis.

29. Explain why ketones may appear to be increasing with appropriate treatment of ketoacidosis.

30. Explain why hyperosmolar coma without ketosis is a more common presentation than ketoacidosis in Type 2 DM.

31. What chronic complication of diabetes mellitus can exacerbate iatrogenic hypoglycemia?

32. What are the most common microvascular and macrovascular complications of long-standing diabetes mellitus, and what are their pathophysiologic mechanisms?

33. What were the major conclusions from DCCT and UKPDS?

34. What pathways activated by oxidative stress are proposed to contribute to the development of complications of diabetes mellitus?

35. What are the characteristics of nonproliferative and proliferative retinopathy in diabetes mellitus?

36. What are the anatomic and physiologic changes observed during the progression of diabetic nephropathy?

37. Does nephropathy usually precede retinopathy in patients with diabetes mellitus?

38. Suggest three reasons for increased risk of atherosclerosis in diabetes mellitus.

39. What are the probable differences in the pathophysiology of hypertension in Type 1 versus Type 2 diabetes mellitus?

40. What three major types of neuropathy are observed in long-standing diabetes mellitus? What are the common symptoms and signs of each?

41. Which types of infections occur with increased frequency in patients with diabetes mellitus, and why?

NEUROENDOCRINE ISLET CELL TUMORS OF THE PANCREAS

While highly prevalent in individuals with multiple endocrine neoplasia type 1 (MEN-1), neuroendocrine tumors arising from the islet cells are otherwise infrequent and account for only 5 % of primary pancreatic neoplasms. However, the clinical manifestations associated with islet cell tumor overproduction of a given hormone are illustrative of their normal physiologic functions (Table 18–9). Those tumors associated with inappropriate secretion of hormones regulating carbohydrate metabolism (insulin, glucagon, somatostatin) are highlighted here.

Insulinoma (β-cell tumor)

A. Clinical Presentation

The occurrence of **fasting hypoglycemia** in an otherwise healthy individual is usually due to an insulin-secreting tumor of the β cells of the islets of Langerhans (**insulinoma;** Table 18–9). Although insulinoma is the most common islet cell tumor, it is still a rare disorder. Insulinomas occur most frequently in the fourth to seventh decades, although they can occur earlier, particularly when associated with multiple endocrine neoplasia type 1 (MEN-1), a neoplastic syndrome characterized by tumors of the parathyroids, pituitary, and endocrine pancreas (see Chapter 17). The diagnosis of hypoglycemia is based on Whipple's triad: (1) symptoms and signs of hypoglycemia, (2) an associated low plasma glucose level, and (3) reversibility of symptoms on administration of glucose.

B. Etiology

In the great majority of cases, insulinomas are benign solitary lesions composed of whorls of insulin-secreting β cells. Multiple tumors, although infrequent (< 10%), are seen most often in patients with MEN-1. Fewer than 10% of the tumors are malignant, as determined by the presence of metastases.

TABLE 18–9 Islet cell tumor syndromes.

Tumor	Major Signs & Symptoms	Malignant (%)	Prevalence in MEN Syndrome[1]
Insulinoma	Fasting hypoglycemia with symptoms of same	10%	10%
Gastrinoma	Enhanced acid secretion with peptic ulcers, esophageal reflux, diarrhea (Zollinger-Ellison syndrome)	40–60%	40%
PPoma	Asymptomatic (watery diarrhea)	40%	10–20%
Glucagonoma	Diabetes, characteristic rash, anorexia, weight loss, anemia, diarrhea	60%	< 2%
Somatostatinoma	Diabetes, cholelithiasis, steatorrhea, weight loss, abdominal pain and fullness	66%	< 2%
VIPoma	Watery diarrhea, hypokalemia, hypochlorhydria	40%	< 2%

[1]MEN, multiple endocrine neoplasia.

C. Pathology and Pathogenesis

Inappropriately high levels of insulin in situations normally characterized by a lowering of insulin secretion (eg, fasting and exercise) result in hypoglycemia. Normally, in the postabsorptive and fasting state, insulin levels decline, leading to an increase in glucagon-stimulated hepatic glucose output and a decrease in insulin-mediated glucose disposal in the periphery, which maintains normal serum glucose levels. With exercise, low insulin allows muscles to use glycogen, glucagon, and other counterregulatory hormones to increase hepatic glucose output and counter-regulatory hormones to mobilize fatty acids for ketogenesis and fatty acid oxidation by muscle. With an insulinoma, insulin levels remain high during fasting or exercise. In this circumstance, glucagon-mediated hepatic glucose output is suppressed while insulin-mediated peripheral glucose uptake continues, and insulin stimulates hepatic fatty acid synthesis and peripheral fatty acid storage while suppressing fatty acid mobilization and hepatic ketogenesis. The result is fasting or exercise-induced hypoglycemia in the absence of ketosis.

D. Clinical Manifestations

Individuals with insulinomas often are symptomatic for years before diagnosis and are self-treated with frequent food intake. Not all patients experience fasting hypoglycemia in the morning (only 30% of insulinoma patients develop hypoglycemia after a diagnostic 12-hour fast). Often they experience late afternoon hypoglycemia, particularly when precipitated by exercise. Because alcohol, like insulin, inhibits gluconeogenesis, alcohol ingestion can also precipitate symptoms. A high percentage of individuals with insulinoma experience neuroglycopenic as well as autonomic symptoms (Table 18–7). Confusion (80%), loss of consciousness (50%), and seizures (10%) often lead to misdiagnoses of psychiatric or neurologic disorders.

Fasting hypoglycemia can be due either to elevated insulin, as occurs in insulinoma, or to non-insulin-mediated effects such as loss of counterregulatory hormones (eg, loss of cortisol in Addison's disease), severe hepatic damage that prevents hepatic glucose production, loss of peripheral stores of substrates for hepatic glucose production (eg, cachexia), or some states of markedly increased glucose utilization (eg, sepsis, cancer). To distinguish **insulin-mediated** from **non-insulin-mediated fasting hypoglycemia,** patients suspected of having insulinoma are subjected to a diagnostic fast during which glucose, insulin, and C peptide levels are measured. An inappropriately elevated insulin level in the setting of hypoglycemia is diagnostic of an insulin-mediated cause of hypoglycemia. Causes of insulin-mediated hypoglycemia other than insulinoma include **surreptitious injection of insulin** or ingestion of oral hypoglycemic medications that stimulate endogenous insulin (**sulfonylureas**) and the presence of **insulin antibodies.** Binding of insulin to the antibodies prevents insulin action, but release of the insulin at an inappropriate time can result in hypoglycemia. Surreptitious insulin administration can be ruled out by C peptide measurements. Because insulin and C peptide are cosecreted, insulinomas will cause elevations in both, whereas elevated levels of exogenous insulin will not be matched by elevations of C peptide in surreptitious injections of insulin. Similarly, insulin antibodies do not result in elevated C peptide levels. Because sulfonylurea drugs stimulate endogenous insulin (and, therefore, C peptide) secretion, insulinoma and inappropriate ingestion of these agents can only be differentiated by measuring drug levels.

Glucagonoma (α-cell tumor)

Glucagonomas are usually diagnosed by the appearance of a characteristic rash in middle-aged individuals, particularly perimenopausal women, with mild diabetes mellitus (Table 18–9). Glucagon levels are usually increased 10-fold relative to normal values but can even be increased 100-fold.

Necrolytic migratory erythema begins as an erythematous rash on the face, abdomen, perineum, or lower extremities. After induration with central blistering develops, the lesions crust over and then resolve, leaving an area of hyperpigmentation. These lesions may be the result of nutritional deficiency, such as the hypoaminoacidemia that occurs from excessive glucagon stimulation of hepatic amino acid uptake and utilization as fuel for gluconeogenesis, rather than the direct effect of glucagon on the skin. Appearance of the rash is a late manifestation of the disease.

Diabetes mellitus or glucose intolerance is present in the vast majority of patients as a result of increased stimulation of hepatic glucose output by the inappropriately high glucagon levels. Insulin levels are secondarily increased. Diabetes is, therefore, mild and is not accompanied by glucagon-stimulated ketosis, because sufficient insulin is present to suppress lipolysis, thus limiting potential substrates for ketogenesis.

Anemia and a variety of nonspecific GI symptoms related to decreased intestinal motility also can accompany glucagonomas.

Although these tumors are solitary and their growth is slow, they are usually large and have often metastasized by the time of diagnosis, making surgical resection difficult. Octreotide, the synthetic somatostatin analogue, can be used to ameliorate symptoms via its suppression of glucagon secretion.

Somatostatinoma (δ-cell tumor)

Somatostatinomas present with a variety of GI symptoms in individuals with mild diabetes. However, these extremely rare tumors are almost uniformly found incidentally during operations for cholelithiasis or other abdominal complaints because the presenting symptoms are both nonspecific and common in an adult population. Documentation of elevated somatostatin levels confirms the diagnosis.

A **classic triad** of symptoms frequently occurs with excessive somatostatin secretion: **diabetes mellitus,** because of its inhibition of insulin and glucagon secretion; **cholelithiasis,** because of its inhibition of gall-bladder motility; and **steator-rhea,** because of its inhibition of pancreatic exocrine function. Hypochlorhydria, diarrhea, and anemia can also occur.

In Type 1 DM and Type 2 DM, the effects of insulin insufficiency are aggravated by the occurrence of elevated glucagon levels. In contrast, with somatostatinomas, both insulin and glucagon are suppressed. Therefore, the hyperglycemia resulting from insulinopenia is tempered by the absence of glucagon stimulation of hepatic glucose output. Although low insulin levels are permissive for lipolysis, glucagon deficiency prevents hepatic ketogenesis. The diabetes associated with somatostatinomas is, therefore, mild and not ketosis prone.

Although the majority of somatostatinomas occur in the pancreas, a significant number are found in the duodenum or jejunum. Like glucagonomas, somatostatinomas are often solitary and large and have frequently metastasized by the time of diagnosis.

CASE STUDIES

Jonathan Fuchs, MD, MPH, & Yeong Kwok, MD

(See Chapter 25, p. 703 for Answers)

CASE 83

A 58-year-old homeless man with long-standing insulin-treated Type 2 diabetes has been diagnosed with right lower extremity cellulitis. He has taken a prescribed oral antibiotic for the past week but has not noticed much improvement. For the last 2 days, he has complained of intermittent fevers and chills, nausea with poor oral intake, and proximally spreading erythema over his right leg. On the evening of admission, a friend notices that he is markedly confused and calls 911. In the emergency room, he is oriented only to his name. The patient is tachypneic, breathing deeply at a rate of 24/min. He is febrile at 38.8 °C. He is normotensive, but his heart rate is elevated at 112 bpm.

On examination, this patient is a delirious, unkempt man with a fruity breath odor. His right lower extremity is markedly erythematous and exquisitely tender to palpation. Serum chemistries reveal a glucose level of 488 mg/dL, potassium of 3.7 mg/dL, and sodium of 132 mEq/L. Urine dipstick is grossly positive for ketones.

Questions

A. Describe the precipitants of ketoacidosis in this diabetic patient.

B. What is the cause of his altered mental status?

C. Describe the patient's respiratory pattern. What is the pathogenetic mechanism?

D. What are important issues to consider in replacing electrolytes in this patient?

CASE 84

A 61-year-old man recently moved to San Francisco and is reestablishing primary care. During a comprehensive review of systems, he reports that he has experienced a 3-year history of "hypoglycemic attacks." These short periods of light-headedness, confusion, palpitations, and tremor occur more frequently in the late afternoon while jogging. His symptoms are relieved after drinking a sugared sports drink. He has no history of diabetes or cancer. His physical examination is unremarkable, and in the clinic a fasting morning glucose level is 93 mg/dL. Suspecting that an insulinoma-induced hypoglycemic state may be responsible for his symptoms, his physician requests a diagnostic fast period during which glucose, insulin, and C peptide levels are measured.

Questions

A. Describe Whipple's triad in the diagnosis of hypoglycemia.

B. What patient history clues suggest insulinoma? Discuss the pathogenesis.

C. How might the tests ordered help identify the cause of the hypoglycemia?

CASE 85

A 52-year-old woman with a 3-year history of diet-controlled diabetes presents to her primary care provider complaining of a "stubborn poison ivy rash" over her legs, which she attributed to a possible exposure to the plant during a recent hike. She presented twice to the urgent care center and received high-potency topical steroid cream for this refractory erythematous rash with central blistering. A review of systems reveals intermittent diarrhea and constipation as well as weight loss. Her serum glucagon level is measured to be 20 times normal.

Questions

A. What is the cause of this patient's rash? What is the proposed mechanism?

B. Describe the proposed pathogenesis of diabetes in this disorder.

C. What is this patient's prognosis for survival?

CASE 86

At the time of an elective laparoscopic cholecystectomy for gallstones, a 44-year-old woman with mild diabetes mellitus and chronic diarrhea is noted to have a 3- × 4-cm solitary mass on the surface of her duodenum. Omental lymphadenopathy is seen. Biopsy demonstrates a high-grade somatostatinoma with lymph node metastasis.

Questions

A. How are patients with somatostatinoma predisposed to cholelithiasis?

B. Why is ketosis an unlikely sequela of somatostatinoma-induced diabetes?

REFERENCES

Diabetes Mellitus

Brownlee M. The pathobiology of diabetic complications: A unifying mechanism. Diabetes. 2005 Jun;54(6):1615–25. [PMID: 15919781]

Cohen P. The twentieth century struggle to decipher insulin signalling. Nat Rev Mol Cell Biol. 2006 Nov;7(11):867–73. [PMID: 17057754]

Cryer PE. Hypoglycemia in diabetes: Pathophysiological mechanisms and diurnal variation. Prog Brain Res. 2006;153:361–5. [PMID: 16876586]

Diabetes Control and Complications Trial Research Group: The effect of intensive treatment of diabetes on the development and progression of long-term complications in insulin-dependent diabetes mellitus. N Engl J Med. 1993 Sep 30;329(14):977–86. [PMID: 8366922]

Dluhy RG et al. Intensive glycemic control in the ACCORD and ADVANCE trials. N Engl J Med. 2008 Jun 12;358(24):2630–3. [PMID: 18539918]

Dunaif A. Insulin resistance in women with polycystic ovary syndrome. Fertil Steril. 2006 Jul;86(Suppl 1):S13–4. [PMID: 16798274]

Freeman H et al. Type-2 diabetes: A cocktail of genetic discovery. Hum Mol Genet. 2006 Oct 15;15 (Spec No 2):R202–9. [PMID: 16987885]

Grundy SM. Metabolic syndrome pandemic. Arterioscler Thromb Vasc Biol. 2008 Apr;28(4):629–36. [PMID: 18174459]

Holst JJ. The physiology of glucagon-like peptide 1. Physiol Rev. 2007 Oct;87(4):1409–39. [PMID: 17928588]

Limbert C et al. Beta-cell replacement and regeneration: Strategies of cell-based therapy for type 1 diabetes mellitus. Diabetes Res Clin Pract. 2008 Mar;79(3):389–99. [PMID: 17854943]

Mazzone T et al. Cardiovascular disease risk in type 2 diabetes mellitus: Insights from mechanistic studies. Lancet. 2008 May 24;371(9626):1800–9. [PMID: 18502305]

Muoio DM, Newgard CB. Mechanisms of disease: Molecular and metabolic mechanisms of insulin resistance and beta-cell failure in type 2 diabetes. Nat Rev Mol Cell Biol. 2008 Mar;9(3):193–205. [PMID: 18200017]

SEARCH for Diabetes in Youth Study Group; Liese D et al. The burden of diabetes mellitus among US youth: Prevalence estimates from the SEARCH for Diabetes in Youth Study. Pediatrics. 2006 Oct;118(4):1510–8. [PMID: 17015542]

UK Prospective Diabetes Study (UKPDS) Group. Intensive blood glucose control with sulphonylureas or insulin compared with conventional treatment and risk of complications in patients with type 2 diabetes (UKPDS 33). Lancet. 1998 Sep 12;352(9131):837–53.

Insulinoma, Glucagonoma, & Somatostatinoma

O'Grady HL et al. Pancreatic neuroendocrine tumours. Eur J Surg Oncol. 2008 Mar;34(3):324–32. [PMID: 17967523]

Disorders of the Hypothalamus & Pituitary Gland

19

Tobias Else, MD, & Gary D. Hammer, MD, PhD

The hypothalamus is the part of the brain where activity of the autonomic nervous system and endocrine glands, which directly control various systems of the body, is integrated with input from other centers that give rise to emotions and behavior. The hypothalamus thus serves to ensure that (1) the organism responds appropriately to deviations from various internal set points (including those for temperature, volume, osmolality, satiety, and body fat content), (2) the responses to such deviations from a set point include coordinated activity of the nervous and endocrine systems, and (3) the emotions and behavior being manifested are appropriate for reflex responses being triggered to correct the deviations from internal set points. The following description outlines the integrative function of the hypothalamus in regard to the coordination of endocrine and CNS responses.

Intravascular volume loss from any cause activates autonomic neural responses, mainly via the sympathetic nervous system to retain fluid and electrolytes, maintain blood pressure through vascular smooth muscle contraction, and maintain cardiac output by increasing heart rate. The effect of these immediate neural responses is reinforced by activation of several hormonal systems. In response to a decrease in intravascular volume, the renin-angiotensin-aldosteronesystem (RAAS) is activated and sodium is retained. Additionally increasing osmolarity triggers thirst and leads to release of vasopressin (antidiuretic hormone [ADH]) from hypothalamic neurons that end in the posterior pituitary, resulting in free water absorption in the kidney. In short, the body maintains intravascular volume by regulating sodium reabsorption through aldosterone, while it regulates osmolarity by increasing fluid intake (thirst) and free water retention by vasopressin.

Emotions interplay with these systems to coordinate appropriate behavioral and hormonal responses. Fear and pain activate limbic, hypothalamic and other centers to coordinate respective defensive (fight or flight) and recuperative stereotypic behaviors. These emotional responses to various stressors (eg, perceived threat to body; fear) also activate the sympathetic nervous system and the hypothalamic-pituitary-adrenal (HPA) axis, which coordinate the mammalian stress response through preparing the body for fight and flight and through mobilization of energy stores. Any kind of stress (eg, physical, mental, metabolic stress) leads to the release of corticotropin-releasing hormone (CRH) from the hypothalamus and consequent adrenocorticotropin (ACTH; pituitary) and cortisol (adrenal cortex) secretion. For example, starvation leads to the activation of the HPA axis and ultimately cortisol-mediated increased gluconeogenesis to maintain basic physiologic functions.

The pituitary gland is the partner of the hypothalamus on the body side of the mind-body interface. Once viewed as the "master gland" in regulation of neuroendocrine systems, the pituitary is now known to be a "middle manager" responding to input from both the brain (via the hypothalamus) and the body (via the various peripheral endocrine glands).

The basic framework for hypothalamic-pituitary function is the **neuroendocrine axis,** a cascade of interacting hormonal products from various regions of the CNS to the hypothalamus, anterior pituitary gland, peripheral endocrine end organs, and peripheral target tissues. Some neuroendocrine axes involve hormones released by the hypothalamus that stimulate cells in the anterior pituitary to secrete other hormones into the systemic circulation. Each of these anterior pituitary hormones travels to a distant endocrine gland to stimulate secretion of yet other hormones that affect various target tissues. Thus, disorders of the hypothalamus and pituitary have important consequences for the pathophysiologic mechanisms of a wide range of disorders involving many different tissues and organs.

This chapter focuses on five clinical entities. The first four reflect the diversity of pituitary disease: pituitary adenomas, panhypopituitarism, vasopressin excess, and vasopressin deficiency. The last, obesity, is one in which the hypothalamus plays a crucial role and which has enormous implications for diseases involving many other organ systems.

NORMAL STRUCTURE & FUNCTION OF THE HYPOTHALAMUS & PITUITARY GLAND

ANATOMY, HISTOLOGY, & CELL BIOLOGY

The hypothalamus is located in the floor and lateral walls of the third ventricle below the hypothalamic sulcus and comprises about 1% of the mass of the brain (Figure 19–1). Hypothalamic nuclei are clusters of neurons whose cell bodies lie in discrete regions (Figure 19–2). From these nuclei, hypothalamic neurons send projections either directly or via neuronal relay to other parts of the central and peripheral nervous systems and secrete hormones that make possible the hierarchical control of various physiologic processes (Table 19–1).

The hypothalamus is connected to the pituitary gland by a stalk, which is composed of axons of some hypothalamic neurons with terminal boutons comprising the posterior pituitary gland (Figure 19–3). The posterior pituitary neurons secrete the peptide hormones oxytocin and vasopressin directly into the systemic circulation. The development of the anterior pituitary from the oral ectoderm is dictated by a tight program of consecutive activation of distinct transcription factors in the differentiating pituitary cell types (Figure 19–4). The pituitary gland is encased in a tough fibrous capsule, positioned in the bony sella turcica. The pituitary gland is bounded above by the optic chiasm and laterally by the cavernous sinus and the structures that traverse it (internal carotid artery, cranial nerves [CN] III and IV, first and second divisions of CN V and VI).

In circumventricular parts of the CNS, the capillaries are fenestrated, allowing neurons to sense various specific chemical stimuli in the bloodstream. These sensory neurons transmit the information regarding changes in stimuli (eg, change in osmolality) to other hypothalamic neurons involved in a variety of specific types of secretory activities.

Other hypothalamic neurons secrete peptide hormones into a specialized capillary bed termed the **pituitary portal system.** Blood in this capillary system flows directly from the median eminence to the anterior pituitary gland, where specific cells that display receptors for the various hypothalamic releasing hormones are found. Binding of hypothalamic hormones to their receptors on cells of the anterior pituitary in turn stimulates the secretion of specific anterior pituitary hormones into the systemic circulation. The portal system allows the cells of the anterior pituitary to be bathed in blood rich in hypothalamic hormones without the dilution that would have occurred in the systemic circulation. This intimate connection between hypothalamus and pituitary has important pathophysiologic consequences (see later).

Once secreted, the anterior pituitary hormones travel via the general bloodstream throughout the body and trigger the release of other hormones from particular endocrine glands.

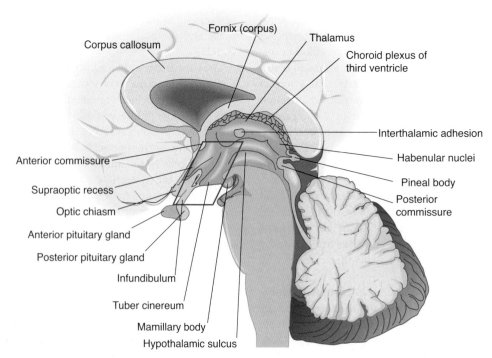

FIGURE 19–1 Sagittal section through the brain showing the diencephalon. (Redrawn, with permission, from Chusid JG. *Correlative Neuroanatomy and Functional Neurology,* 19th ed. Originally published by Lange Medical Publications. Copyright © 1985 by the McGraw-Hill Companies, Inc.)

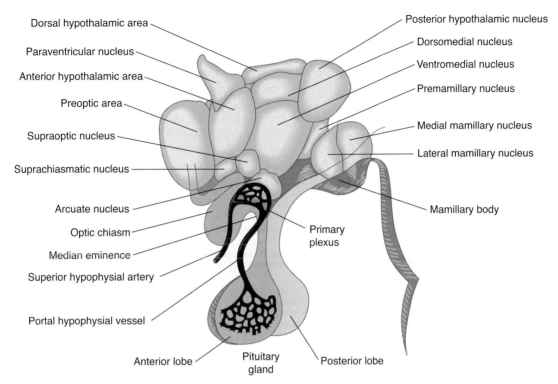

FIGURE 19–2 Human hypothalamus, with a superimposed diagrammatic representation of the portal hypophyseal vessels. (Redrawn, with permission, from Ganong WF. *Review of Medical Physiology*, 20th ed. Originally published by McGraw-Hill. Copyright © 2001 by the McGraw-Hill Companies, Inc.)

These hormones, in turn, have effects on target tissues that influence growth, reproduction, metabolism, and responses to stress. In addition to their effects on target tissues, hormones secreted in response to stimulation by pituitary hormones also feed back and inhibit secretion of the corresponding pituitary and hypothalamic hormones.

The posterior pituitary hormones are involved in a very different type of neuroendocrine axis, one that bypasses secondary endocrine glands and affects peripheral target tissues directly.

Although most peptide factors secreted by the hypothalamus cause release of a pituitary hormone, some are inhibitory factors that block or diminish secretion of particular hormones. There are five main cell types in the anterior pituitary, each of which produces and secretes one of five families of hormones: pro-opiomelanocortin and adrenocorticotropic hormone (ACTH), thyrotropin (TSH), growth hormone (GH), prolactin (PRL), and the gonadotropins, luteinizing hormone (LH), and follicle-stimulating hormone (FSH) (Table 19–2).

In addition to their roles in regulation of neuroendocrine axes, some hypothalamic and pituitary hormones are important, but poorly understood, regulators of immune functions and the inflammatory response. Furthermore, secretion of hypothalamic and pituitary hormones can be significantly influenced by cytokines that regulate the immune response.

CHECKPOINT

1. What is the role of the hypothalamus?
2. What are the neuroendocrine axes, and how do they work?
3. What structures surround the pituitary?
4. Where do the neurons whose axons comprise the posterior pituitary originate?

PHYSIOLOGY OF THE HYPOTHALAMUS & PITUITARY GLAND

ANTERIOR PITUITARY HORMONES

Pro-opiomelanocortin & ACTH

The HPA axis is a major part of the physiologic stress system. A variety of stressors (eg, metabolic, physical, mental stress) result in activation of the HPA axis. The major hypothalamic regulator is the peptide CRH and to a lesser extent arginine vasopressin (AVP), which are produced in the paraventricular and supraoptic nuclei of the hypothalamus and are released into the hypothalamic-pituitary portal system. These hormones trigger synthesis and intracellular transport of a

TABLE 19–1 The hypothalamic nuclei and their main functions.

Nucleus	Location	Major Neurohormones and/or Functions
Supraoptic (SON)	Anterolateral, above the optic tract	ADH: osmoregulation, regulation of ECF volume; OT: regulation of uterine contractions and milk ejection
Paraventricular (PVN)	Dorsal anterior periventricular	Magnacellular PVN
		ADH, OT: same functions as above
		Parvocellular PVN
		TRH: regulation of thyroid function
		CRH: regulation of adrenocortical function, regulation of the sympathetic nervous system and adrenal medulla, regulation of appetite
		ADH: coexpressed with CRH, regulation of adrenocortical function
		VIP: Prolactin-releasing factor (?)
Suprachiasmatic (SCN)	Above the optic chiasm, anteroventral periventricular zone	Regulator of circadian rhythms and pineal function ("Zeitgeber" [pacemaker]): VIP, ADH neurons project mainly to the PVN
Arcuate (ARCN)	Medial basal hypothalamus close to the third ventricle	GHRH: Stimulation of growth hormone
		GnRH: Regulation of pituitary gonadotropins (FSH and LH)
		Dopamine: functions as PIH
		SRIF: Inhibition of GHRH release
		Regulation of appetite (NPY, ART, α-MSH, CART)
Periventricular	Anteroventral	SRIF: Inhibition of growth hormone secretion by direct pituitary action; most abundant SRIF location
Ventromedial (VMN)		GHRH (as above)
		SRIF: Inhibition of GHRH release
		Functions as a satiety center
Dorsomedial (DMN)		Focal point of information processing: receives input from VMN and lateral hypothalamus and projects to the PVN
Lateral hypothalamus		Functions as a hunger center (MCH, orexins)
Preoptic area (POA)		Main regulator of ovulation in rodents. Only a few GnRH neurons in primates
Anterior hypothalamus		Thermoregulation: "cooling center"
		AVOV region: regulation of thirst
Posterior hypothalamus		Thermoregulation: "heating center"

Reproduced, with permission, from Kacsoh B. *Endocrine Physiology*. Originally published by McGraw-Hill. Copyright © 2000 by the McGraw-Hill Companies, Inc.

Abbreviations: ADH, antidiuretic hormone; ECF, extracellular fluid; OT, oxytocin; TRH, thyrotropin-releasing hormone; CRH, corticotropin-releasing hormone; VIP, vasoactive intestinal polypeptide; GHRH, growth hormone releasing hormone; GnRH, gonadotropin-releasing hormone; FSH, follicle stimulating hormone; LH, luteinizing hormone; PIH, prolactin inhibiting hormone; SRIF, somatotropin release-inhibiting factor; NPY, neuropeptide Y; ART, agouti-released transcript; α-MSH, α-melanocyte-stimulating hormone; CART, cocaine and amphetamine-regulated transcript; MCH, melanin concentrating hormone.

large protein termed pro-opiomelanocortin (POMC). POMC is further processed by proteases (prohormone convertases) to release smaller peptides, including a 39-amino-acid-residue peptide, ACTH (Figure 19–5). Although ACTH is the major pituitary hormone that stimulates adrenocortical endocrine function, the amino-terminal part of the POMC peptide (N-POMC) seems to harbor an adrenal growth-promoting function.

ACTH released into the systemic circulation triggers synthesis and secretion of corticosteroids and adrenal androgens. The effect of ACTH on mineralocorticoid synthesis and

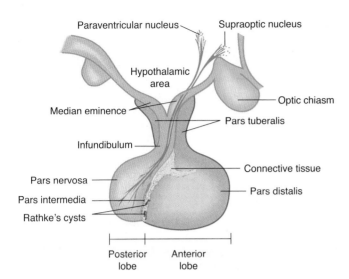

FIGURE 19–3 The component parts of the pituitary and their relationship to the hypothalamus. The pars tuberalis, pars distalis, and pars intermedia, which is rudimentary in humans, form the adenohypophysis. The infundibulum and pars nervosa form the neurohypophysis. (Redrawn and modified, with permission, from the *Ciba Collection of Medical Illustrations,* by Frank H. Netter, MD.)

release is much less pronounced, as it is mainly regulated by the RAAS.

These steroid hormones, in turn, have complex effects on many tissues to protect the animal from stress: They raise blood pressure and blood glucose, alter responsiveness of the immune system, and so on. Glucocorticoids also feed back to the hypothalamus, where they inhibit CRH secretion, and to the pituitary, where they further inhibit ACTH secretion. In the absence of unusual stress, there is a daily diurnal rhythm of CRH, ACTH, and adrenal steroid release.

Pituitary factors (ie, N-POMC, ACTH) are involved in regulating proliferation of adrenal cells and growth of the adrenal layers involved in glucocorticoid and androgen secretion. As a result of chronic activation of the HPA axis, hypertrophy of the target organ (adrenal cortex) occurs. Conversely, conditions that downregulate the HPA axis (eg, exogenous glucocorticoids) result in atrophy of the adrenal cortex. On the other hand, the overall tone of the HPA axis has little or no effect on the growth of the mineralocorticoid-secreting tissues, despite the fact that acute ACTH stimulation triggers the release of mineralocorticoids.

The Glycoprotein Hormones

TSH and the gonadotropins belong to the family of glycoprotein hormones (Table 19–2). The classic glycoprotein hormone family members TSH and the gonadotropins, FSH and LH, as well as the placenta-derived pregnancy hormone human chorionic gonadotropin (hCG) are composed of a common α-glycoprotein subunit (α-GSU) and an individual β-subunit (eg, TSH-β, LH-β). The unique β-subunit of the glycoprotein hormones is responsible for the biologic differences of these hormones. Another member of this family is thyrostimulin, which shares the composition of an α- and β-subunit (α-2, β-5). The physiologic role of this hormone has yet to be determined.

A. Thyrotropin

Thyrotropin is released from specific cells in the pituitary on stimulation by thyrotropin-releasing hormone (TRH) from the hypothalamus. A hypothalamic factor negatively regulating TSH release is somatostatin. TSH, in turn, travels via the systemic bloodstream to the thyroid gland, where it stimulates synthesis and secretion of the thyroid hormones thyroxine and triiodothyronine. Thyroid hormone has effects on nearly

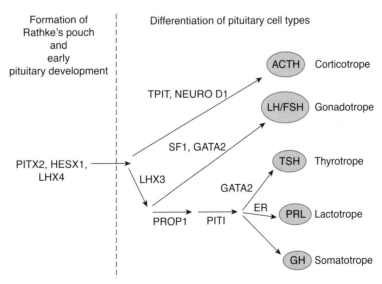

FIGURE 19–4 Diagram of the transcription factors involved in anterior pituitary development. Factors on the left are mainly responsible for Rathke's pouch formation and early pituitary development. On the right side are factors inducing the differentiation into the major five pituitary cell types. Mutations of some of the genes encoding these transcription factors have been shown to result in hypopituitarism.

TABLE 19–2 Pituitary hormones.

	ACTH	GH	Prolactin	TSH	LH	FSH	Thyrostimulin
Peptides	Derived from POMC precursor	Single-chain polypeptide	Single-chain polypeptide	α: α1 β: TSH-β	α: α1 β : LH-β	α: α1 β : FSH-β	α: α2 β:: β 5
Receptor	ACTH-receptor (melanocortin-2-receptor)	GH receptor	Prolactin receptor	TSH receptor	LH receptor	FSH receptor	TSH receptor, ?
Source	Corticotropes (pituitary)	Somatotropes (pituitary)	Lactotropes (pituitary)	Thyrotropes (pituitary)	Gonadotropes (pituitary)	Gonadotropes (pituitary)	Unknown cell type (pituitary)
Hypothalamic releasing hormone	CRH, AVP	GHRH (ghrelin)	TRH	TRH	GnRH	GnRH	?
Hypothalamic inhibiting factors		Somatostatin	Dopamine	Somatostatin, dopamine			
Target	Adrenal gland	Liver (production of IGF-1), peripheral tissue	Mammary gland	Thyroid gland	Ovary (theca cell, granulosa cell, luteal cell)/testis (Leydig cell)	Ovary (granulosa cell)/testis (Sertoli cell)	Unknown
Function	Stimulating cortisol release	Stimulating growth (direct and indirect effect via IGF-1)	Stimulating lactation	Stimulating thyroid hormone release	Stimulating estrogen/testosterone production	Regulating granulosa and Sertoli cell function	Unknown

Key: ACTH, corticotropin; AVP, arginine-vasopressin; CRH, corticotropin-releasing hormone; FSH, follicle-stimulating hormone; GH, growth hormone; GHRH, growth hormone-releasing hormone; GnRH, gonadotropin-releasing hormone; IGF, insulin-like growth factor; LH, luteinizing hormone; POMC, pro-opiomelanocortin; TRH, thyrotropin-releasing hormone; TSH, thyroid-stimulating hormone.

every tissue in the body but especially the cardiovascular, respiratory, skeletal, and central nervous systems. Thyroid hormones are critical at key points in development, and their deficiency during development has effects (eg, severe mental retardation and short stature) that are not fully reversible by subsequent thyroid hormone administration (Chapter 20).

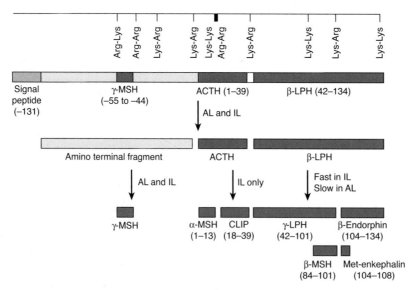

FIGURE 19–5   Schematic representation of the prepro-opiomelanocortin molecule formed in pituitary cells, neurons, and other tissues. The numbers in parentheses identify the amino acid sequences in each of the polypeptide fragments. For convenience, the amino acid sequences are numbered from the amino terminal of corticotrope (ACTH) and read toward the carboxyl terminal portion of the parent molecule, whereas the amino acid sequences in the other portion of the molecule read to the left to –131, the amino terminal of the parent molecule. The locations of Lys-Arg and other pairs of basic amino acid residues are also indicated; these are the sites of proteolytic cleavage in the formation of the smaller fragments of the parent molecule. AL, anterior lobe; IL, intermediate lobe.   (Redrawn, with permission, from Ganong WF. *Review of Medical Physiology*, 22nd ed. McGraw-Hill, 2005.)

Besides its target tissue effects, thyroid hormone feeds back to the pituitary and hypothalamus to inhibit secretion of TSH and TRH. TSH also triggers growth of thyroid tissue, resulting in goiter under conditions of chronic TSH stimulation such as iodine deficiency (see Chapter 20).

B. Gonadotropin

The role of the gonadotropins is to regulate the reproductive system's neuroendocrine axis. Thus, a releasing factor from the hypothalamus termed gonadotropin-releasing hormone (GnRH) stimulates LH and FSH secretion, which stimulates steroidogenesis within the ovaries and testes. Furthermore, the gonadotropins promote Sertoli and theca cell function and gametogenesis. The steroids produced by the ovaries (estrogens) and by the testes (testosterone) inhibit GnRH, LH, and FSH production and have target tissue effects on developing follicles within the ovary itself, on the uterus (controlling the menstrual cycle), on breast development, on spermatogenesis, and on many other tissues and physiologic processes (see Chapters 22 and 23).

As is the case with all neuroendocrine axes, the simple feedback loop is complicated by other inputs (eg, from the CNS) that modify responsiveness (Chapter 7). The discovery that KiSS1-derived peptides (eg, metastin) induce hypothalamic GnRH-release via signaling through a G protein–coupled receptor (GPR54) illustrates this point. A notable feature for many hypothalamic releasing factors, but particularly GnRH, is that secretion occurs in pulsatile fashion and that changes

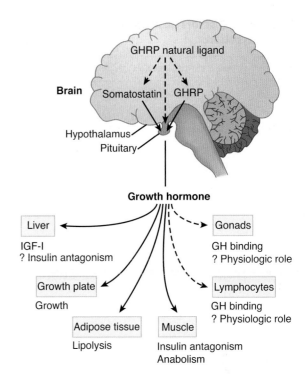

FIGURE 19–7 Schematic representation of multiple sites of growth hormone (GH) action. GHRH, growth hormone–releasing hormone; GHRP, growth hormone–releasing peptide; IGF-I, insulin-like growth factor I. (Redrawn, with permission, from Thorner MO et al. The anterior pituitary. In: *Williams Textbook of Endocrinology,* 9th ed. Wilson JD et al [editors]. Saunders, 1998.)

in the rate and amplitude of secretion result in altered pituitary responsiveness because of downregulation or upregulation of the receptors for the hypothalamic releasing factors found on the surface of the pituitary cells. Not only is the secretion of GnRH episodic, but the secretion of FSH and LH is as well, with a secretory burst every 60 minutes. The gonadotropins follow a typical secretion pattern during the estrus cycle with a midcycle LH surge initiating ovulation.

Growth Hormone & Prolactin

Growth hormone and prolactin are structurally related single-chain polypeptides with different spectrums of action.

A. Growth Hormone

Growth hormone (GH), positively regulated by hypothalamic growth hormone–releasing hormone (GHRH) and inhibited by somatostatin, triggers growth-promoting effects in a wide range of tissues (Figure 19–6). GH has direct (eg, stimulating the growth of cartilage) as well as indirect (eg, via insulin-like growth factor-1 [IGF-1], a polypeptide secreted by the liver and other tissues) actions (Figure 19–7). IGF-1 has insulin-like effects of promoting fuel storage in various tissues. IGF-1 in turn inhibits GHRH and GH secretion. As in the other neuroendocrine feedback axes, the CNS and other factors can significantly influence the simple regulatory axis (Table 19–3). One of these

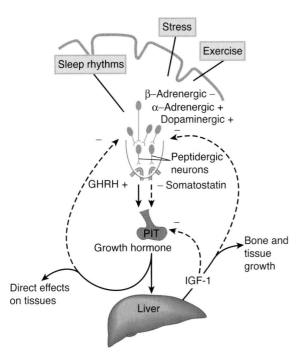

FIGURE 19–6 Schematic diagram of the hypothalamic control of growth hormone secretion. Inhibitory arrows are dashed; stimulating arrows are solid. GHRH, growth hormone–releasing hormone; IGF, insulin-like growth factor. (Redrawn from Reichlin S. Neuroendocrinology. In: *Williams Textbook of Endocrinology,* 9th ed. Wilson JD et al [editors]. Saunders, 1998.)

TABLE 19–3 Factors influencing normal growth hormone secretion.

Factor	Augmented Secretion	Inhibited Secretion
Neurogenic	Stage III and stage IV sleep	REM sleep
	Stress (traumatic, surgical, inflammatory, psychic)	Alpha-adrenergic antagonists
	Alpha-adrenergic agonists	Beta-adrenergic agonists
	Beta-adrenergic antagonists	Acetylcholine antagonists
	Dopamine agonists	
	Acetylcholine agonists	
Metabolic	Hypoglycemia	Hyperglycemia
	Fasting	Rising fatty acid level
	Falling fatty acid level	Obesity
	Amino acids	
	Uncontrolled diabetes mellitus	
	Uremia	
	Hepatic cirrhosis	
Hormonal	GHRH	Somatostatin
	Low insulin-like growth factor	High insulin-like growth factor
	Estrogens	Hypothyroidism
	Glucagon	High glucocorticoid levels
	Arginine vasopressin	
	Ghrelin	

Reproduced, with permission, from Thorner MO et al. The anterior pituitary. In: *Williams Textbook of Endocrinology*, 9th ed. Wilson JD et al (editors). Saunders, 1998.

Key: GHRH, growth hormone–releasing hormone; REM, rapid eye movement.

factors is the gastrointestinal peptide hormone, ghrelin, which acts through the growth hormone–secretagogue receptor to induce GH release. The physiological significance of this process has yet to be determined. Somatostatin inhibits GH release and somatostatin analogues are therefore used to inhibit GH secretion from GH-secreting pituitary tumors.

Some of the actions of GH appear to have a counter-regulatory character in that they raise blood glucose levels and antagonize the action of insulin. In contrast, other actions of GH via IGF-1 are insulin-like. This apparent contradiction makes sense when one considers that promoting growth requires first raising blood levels of substrates and then using them for synthesis. To do the latter without the former would simply make the individual hypoglycemic without promoting long-term growth.

B. Prolactin

The primary role of prolactin in humans is to stimulate breast development and milk synthesis. It is discussed in greater detail in Chapter 22. Prolactin secretion is negatively regulated by the neurotransmitter dopamine from the hypothalamus rather than by a peptide. That is, dopamine acts to inhibit rather than stimulate prolactin secretion. Pathologic processes that result in separation of the pituitary gland from the hypothalamus cause loss of all pituitary hormones except prolactin (**panhypopituitarism** from lack of the hypothalamic releasing hormones). Loss of dopamine results instead in an increase in prolactin secretion from specific anterior pituitary cells now freed of inhibition by dopamine.

Prolactin may also play a role as a regulator of immune functions.

POSTERIOR PITUITARY HORMONES

Vasopressin & Oxytocin

The peptide hormones vasopressin and oxytocin are synthesized in the supraoptic and paraventricular nuclei of the hypothalamus. The axons of the neurons in these nuclei form the posterior pituitary, where these peptide hormones are stored. Thus, there is no need for a separate set of hypothalamic releasing factors to trigger vasopressin or oxytocin release.

A. Vasopressin

In response to a small increase in blood osmolality, the hypothalamic "osmostat" responds by triggering the subjective sense of thirst and at the same time the release of vasopressin. Vasopressin increases the number of active water channels in the cell membranes of renal collecting duct cells, allowing conservation of free water. This increases the concentration of the urine. Conservation of free water and stimulation of thirst have the net effect of correcting the small change in blood osmolality.

Vasopressin binds to at least three classes of receptors. One of these classes of vasopressin receptors (V_{1A}) is found on smooth muscle. Its major effect is to trigger vasoconstriction. V_{1B} receptors are found on corticotropes, and they contribute to increased ACTH secretion. The other class of receptors (V_2) is found in the distal nephrons in the kidneys; its major action is to mediate vasopressin's effects on osmolality. Because of its V2-mediated actions, vasopressin is also known as **antidiuretic hormone** (ADH). The relationship among osmotic forces, volume, and vasopressin secretion is illustrated in Figure 19–8. Although the minute-to-minute function of vasopressin is to maintain blood osmolality, its secretion is also increased by large decreases in intravascular volume. This assists aldosterone in raising intravascular volume, albeit at the expense of lowered osmolality. The combination of ADH-mediated peripheral vasoconstriction and water retention (in the setting of hypotension even with lower

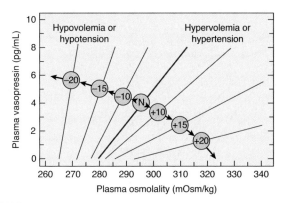

FIGURE 19–8 The influence of hemodynamic status on the os-moregulation of vasopressin in otherwise healthy humans. The numbers in the center circles refer to the percentage change in volume or pressure; N refers to the normovolemic normotensive subject. Note that the hemodynamic status affects both the slope of the relationship between the plasma vasopressin and osmolality and the osmotic threshold for vasopressin release. (Redrawn and adapted from Robertson GL, Shelton RL, Athar S. The osmoregulation of vasopressin. Kidney Int. 1976;10:25. Adapted by Rose BD in: *Clinical Physiology of Acid-Base and Electrolyte Disorders,* 3rd ed. McGraw-Hill, 1989. Reprinted with permission from Kidney International.)

or normal osmolarity) can be understood as a way of helping to maintain perfusion in the face of major intravascular volume deficits, even if the volume and osmolar composition of the perfusing blood are not ideal. In pharmacologic doses,

vasopressin can be used as an adjunct in the treatment of severe hypotensive crises.

B. Oxytocin

Like vasopressin, this peptide is stored in nerve terminals of hypothalamic neurons in the posterior pituitary. It plays an important role in breast and uterine smooth muscle contraction both on a minute-to-minute basis during breast-feeding and in contraction of the uterus during parturition. Besides its function in parturition and lactation, recent research suggests a significant role for oxytocin in the neuropsychological regulation of behavior, such as trust formation and interpersonal bonding (eg, pair and parental attachment).

CHECKPOINT

5. How do neuroendocrine feedback loops of the anterior and posterior pituitary differ?
6. How can two polypeptide hormones whose mature forms have no sequence in common be derived from the same precursor?
7. Describe the distinguishing features of each pituitary neuroendocrine feedback axis.
8. What is the significance of receptor downregulation for hypothalamic control of pituitary function?

PHYSIOLOGY OF THE NEUROENDOCRINE AXIS

A number of features of neuroendocrine axis physiology have important implications for the pathophysiology of disease.

First, the hypothalamic hormones that traverse the pituitary portal system are short-lived. They also have relatively low affinities for their receptors. These properties are generally more characteristic of neurotransmitters in the nervous system than of hormones in the bloodstream. Some of these hormones, and the receptor systems with which they interact, have evolved in ways that take advantage of the unique features of a neuroendocrine axis. For example, in the case of GnRH, secretion is markedly pulsatile in character; a particular rate and amplitude of hypothalamic hormone secretion are crucial for a proper response by the receptor-bearing gonadotropes. If the pulse rate or amplitude is too high, the receptors are downregulated.

Second, for some of the neuroendocrine axes, measurement of a random blood level of the end-organ hormone is not generally clinically useful. A more reliable approach to assessment of neuroendocrine axis function is often to assess the secretory response to a provocative stimulus, or **challenge test.** Thus, an adequate increase in blood cortisol 1 h after an intravenous injection of ACTH provides far more compelling evidence for an intact adrenal gland than does a randomly drawn, unprovoked normal blood level of cortisol.

Finally, besides stimulating end-organ hormone secretion, most of the pituitary hormones exert trophic effects on the hormone-secreting cells of the end organ. Thus, excess of pituitary hormone results in end-organ hypertrophy, and lack of the pituitary hormone results in end-organ atrophy.

PHYSIOLOGY OF BODY WEIGHT CONTROL

Various physiologic control mechanisms integrated by the hypothalamus work to maintain body weight over the short and the long term (Figure 19–9).

The key parameters of short-term regulation of body weight are (1) the amount and composition of food, (2) nutrient absorption and assimilation, and (3) satiety, the sense of having eaten enough food. Satiety is a complex response to food intake that has mechanical, neural, and hormonal components.

A main mechanism by which short-term food intake and satiety are regulated is the communication via the "gut-brain axis." The gut-brain crosstalk uses two main routes of communication, including both neural components, mainly afferent vagal fibers, and hormonal components. Thus, we feel a

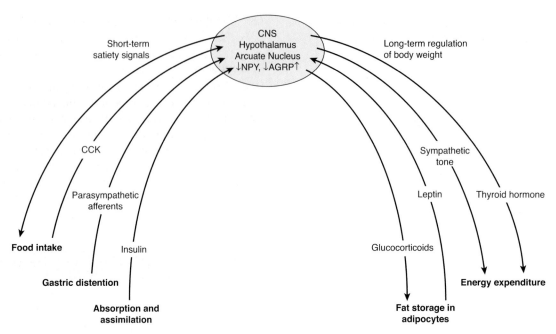

FIGURE 19–9 Physiologic control mechanisms regulating body weight. NPY, neuropeptide Y; AGRP, agouti-related peptide; CCK, cholecystokinin.

sense of fullness in response to mechanical distention of the stomach, which triggers afferent neural pathways to the hypothalamus or via brainstem centers (eg, nucleus of the solitary tract). In addition, hormones are secreted in response to food ingestion and absorption and have direct effects on the hypothalamus to induce satiety. These hormonal signals mainly include anorexigenic satiety signals, such as cholecystokinin (CCK) and glucagon-like peptide-1 (GLP-1), which are released in the gut and directly impact on gastrointestinal mobility and function, but also stimulate gastrointestinal neural signaling to the hypothalamus. Some of these hormones travel directly to the brain and bind to receptors in the hypothalamus or in areas of regulated "open" blood-brain barrier. The only known orexigenic signal arising from the gut is the peptide hormone, ghrelin, suggesting that satiety is more abundantly regulated by the gastrointestinal system than hunger.

In contrast to short-term control of body weight, long-term regulation is largely influenced by the degree of obesity. Fat cells secrete the hormone leptin in proportion to the amount of triglyceride they have stored. Thus, over the long term, excess ingestion of calories resulting in increased fat deposition triggers an increase in leptin secretion. Leptin impinges on its receptors in the hypothalamus so that the individual eats less and, therefore, assimilates fewer calories. Another response to leptin is to increase sympathetic nervous system activity so that more calories are burned.

Conversely, when caloric intake is insufficient to maintain body weight, fat is mobilized, leptin secretion decreases, and set points in the hypothalamus are changed in ways that promote food-seeking behavior, diminish sympathetic neural activity, and generally conserve calories to offset the tendency

toward weight loss. As a result of this feedback loop, further decrease in body weight is resisted. It is likely that this system evolved primarily as a defense against starvation, but it also serves to defend against obesity.

How these signals are normally integrated in the hypothalamus to achieve satiety in the short term and maintain normal body weight in the long term is less clear. The arcuate nucleus of the hypothalamus is the best understood integrator of the regulation of food intake. However, several other hypothalamic nuclei appear to be involved in the control of energy homeostasis and food intake. For example, lesions in the ventromedial region result in obesity, and lesions in the lateral hypothalamus result in weight loss. One hypothesis attempting to integrate current information on the regulation of fuel homeostasis proposes different responses by the body to falling versus rising leptin concentrations, as would be seen in weight loss versus weight gain, respectively. Thus, in response to falling leptin levels, neuropeptide Y is secreted from leptin receptor–bearing cells of the arcuate nucleus in the ventromedial hypothalamus. Neuropeptide Y is believed to mediate hypothalamic responses to starvation.

Another well-described system regulating satiety and food intake within the arcuate nucleus of the hypothalamus is the POMC system. Though the hypothalamic POMC system uses the same peptides for signaling mediators as the pituitary POMC system, they are very different in POMC expression, processing, and receptors. In particular, the main receptor mediating satiety and food intake is a special subtype of melanocortin receptors (MC4-R). In the state of caloric excess, hypothalamic-derived POMC peptides such as melanocyte-stimulating hormone (α-MSH) keep these MC4-R receptors in a tonic activated state. In addition,

TABLE 19–4 Peptides regulating food intake (mainly on the level of the hypothalamus).

Inhibitory	Stimulatory
α-MSH (a product of POMC)	Agouti-related peptide (AGRP)
Leptin	Ghrelin
Cocaine- and amphetamine-related peptide (CART)	Neuropeptide Y
Insulin	MCH
Peptide YY3–36	Orexins
Corticotropin releasing hormone (CRH)	Galanin
Cholecystokinin (CCK)	Endocannabinoids
Glucagon-like peptide-1 (GLP-1)	
Prolactin-releasing peptide	
Insulin-like growth factors I and II	
Calcitonin gene—related peptide (CGRP)	
Somatostatin	
Neuromedin U	
Serotonin	
Bombesin	

hypothalamic POMC neurons are leptin responsive; therefore, these neurons represent an interface between the leptin and the POMC system. As circulating leptin levels parallel the total quantity of fat storage, it makes sense that activa-tion of POMC neurons leads to inhibition of food intake. In the event of caloric restriction, the tonic activation of the MC4-R is reduced by two mechanisms: a decrease in ago-nists (MSH) and, even more important, an increase in avail-ability of antagonists, namely agouti-related peptide (AGRP). These antagonists downregulate not only MSH (agonist driven) but also an intrinsic constitutive activity of the MC4-R. The mode of action of the MC4-R-antagonism by AGRP has been termed "inverse agonism." Furthermore, it is believed that many other neuropeptides, including bombesin, insulin, and a group of peptides termed orexins, have complex effects on the hypothalamus that affect feed-ing, satiety, energy balance, and other parameters relevant for weight control (Table 19–4). The orexins appear to be ligands for previously "orphan" G protein–coupled receptors in the brain. How the effects of these peptides are integrated with those of leptin and neuropeptide Y is a current focus of research. Finally, research strongly implicates leptin in other physiologic functions such as regulating reproductive and immune function as well as bone density.

CHECKPOINT

9. What are the short- and long-term factors involved in normal control of body weight?
10. What is the significance of the short half-life, low affinity, and restricted circulation of most hypothalamic hor-mones?
11. Why are challenge tests particularly important in assess-ing function of a neuroendocrine axis?
12. What happens to an end organ in the absence of the pi-tuitary hormone that normally triggers its secretion?

PATHOPHYSIOLOGY OF SELECTED HYPOTHALAMIC & PITUITARY DISEASES

New studies have implicated the hypothalamus or pituitary gland in the pathophysiology of a variety of complex diseases with major behavioral components. These include anxiety disorders, in which abnormalities of the hypothalamic-pitu-itary-growth hormone axis appear to be a specific pathologic marker; alcoholism, in which neuropeptide Y has been im-plicated in mouse models of this condition; and obesity, in which a host of hypothalamic neuropeptides are affected and, in turn, affect parameters of fuel homeostasis. In most of these disorders, it remains unclear whether hypothalamic and endocrine dysregulation are important causative factors in pathogenesis or epiphenomena mirroring central nervous dysfunction.

OBESITY

Changes in body weight can occur through alteration of sever-al variables, including (1) amount and type of food ingested, (2) central control of satiety, (3) hormonal control of assimi-lation or storage, and (4) physical activity or metabolic rate.

Clinical Presentation & Etiology

Obesity can be defined as excess body weight sufficient to in-crease overall morbidity and mortality. Although extreme obe-sity is associated with dramatically increased mortality, the risks of mild to moderate obesity are less clear. An index of "fatness" is the body mass index (BMI), which equals the weight (in kilo-grams) divided by height (in meters squared). The normal range is 18.5–25 kg/m^2, and clinically significant obesity is a

TABLE 19–5 **Some disorders associated with obesity.**

| Hypertension |
| Diabetes mellitus |
| Coronary artery disease |
| Gallstones |
| Sudden death |
| Cardiomyopathy |
| Sleep apnea |
| Hirsutism |
| Osteoarthritis |
| Gout |
| Stroke |
| Cancer (breast, endometrial, ovarian, cervical, gallbladder in women; prostatic, colorectal in men) |

BMI > 30 kg/m². More than 20% of the U.S. population is obese by this criterion. Individuals with a BMI of 150% of normal have an overall twofold risk of premature death, whereas those who are 200% of normal BMI have a 10-fold risk. Table 19–5 lists some important causes of morbidity and mortality associated with obesity, and Figure 19–10 shows possible pathophysiologic mechanisms involved in their production.

Pathophysiology

Recognition that obesity plays a role in the pathophysiology of disease comes from epidemiologic studies identifying obesity as a risk factor without providing insight into the mechanism of the risk.

Although growing, only a very small number of cases of monogenetic disorders result in obesity in humans. Those syndromes highlight the importance of the aforementioned hypothalamic regulatory systems of body weight control. Several mutations in leptin or the leptin receptor, both resulting in the lack of sufficient leptin effect on the hypothalamus, have been described as a cause of both human and murine

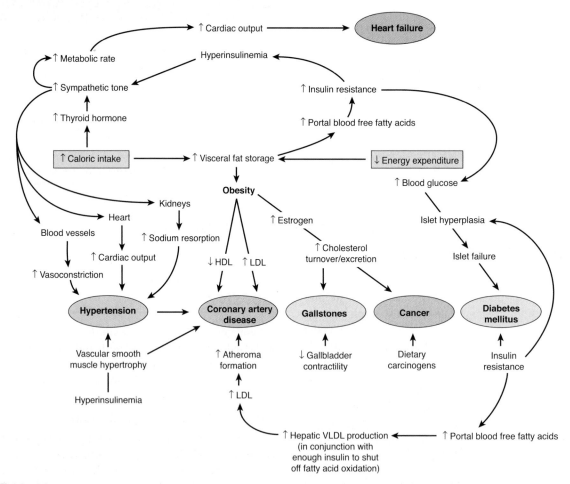

FIGURE 19–10 Role of obesity in the pathophysiology of disease. Some ways by which obesity contributes to disease. Short arrows refer to a change in the indicated parameter, and long arrows indicate a consequence of that change. In some cases, evidence is epidemiologic; in others, it is experimental. HDL, high-density lipoprotein; LDL, low-density lipoprotein; VLDL, very low density lipoproteins. (Redrawn, with permission, from Bray GA. Pathophysiology of obesity. Am J Clin Nutr. 1992;55:488S.)

obesity. Most strikingly, leptin replacement therapy in cases of leptin deficiency leads to complete normalization of body weight. Other mutations have been described in the hypothalamic POMC system. Mutations in the MC4-R as well as mutations in the POMC gene or in POMC-processing proteases, both resulting in reduced MSH levels, lead to severe childhood obesity. Consistent with data describing the involvement of the POMC system in hypothalamic body weight regulation, all mutations within this system result in decreased signaling through the MC4-R and, therefore, increased food intake.

Aside from the monogenic disorders mentioned previously, obesity appears to be the result of multiple mechanisms and many studies have established an imbalance in the neuroendocrine hypothalamic and brain-gut systems. Thus, obesity may be either a cause or a consequence of disease, depending on the disorder. For example, Type 2 diabetes mellitus is sometimes first manifested clinically by sudden weight gain, and this disorder can be difficult to control without weight loss, reflecting the insulin-resistant character of the obese state. Moreover, if the weight can be lost, the diabetes may once again become latent, controlled by diet and exercise alone. In such cases, obesity seems clearly to be an etiologic factor in the development of diabetes mellitus. Yet insulin injections, which may be necessary to control the symptoms of diabetes in such a patient, further exacerbate the weight gain that precipitated the disorder in the first place. Such "chicken-or-egg" relationships make the pathophysiology of obesity particularly difficult to dissect. Nevertheless, important progress has been made toward developing a coherent framework in which to view obesity as both cause and consequence of disease. Some of these observations are noted next.

The number of fat cells in the body is probably established during infancy. One hypothesis is that obesity appearing during adulthood results from enlargement of individual fat cells (hypertrophy) rather than an increased number of fat cells (hyperplasia). Obesity from fat cell hypertrophy appears to be much more easily controlled than obesity from fat cell hyperplasia. Perhaps feedback signals in response to the degree of fat cell hypertrophy are important to the hypothalamic "lipostat."

It now appears that *where* fat is deposited is more important than *how much* is deposited. Thus, so-called visceral or central obesity (omental fat in the distribution of blood flow draining into the portal vein) seems far more important as a risk factor for obesity-related morbidity and mortality than so-called subcutaneous (gynecoid, lower body) or peripheral fat. It appears that visceral fat is more sensitive to catecholamines and less sensitive to insulin, making it a marker of insulin resistance. Consistent with these findings is the observation that obese individuals who engage in vigorous physical activity and whose obesity is largely due to high caloric intake (eg, sumo wrestlers) have subcutaneous rather than visceral fat and do not demonstrate substantial increased insulin resistance. In contrast, the obesity associated with a sedentary lifestyle is believed to be largely visceral obesity and is associated with a greater degree of insulin resistance in patients both

with and without a diagnosis of diabetes mellitus. A parameter reflecting the different kinds of fat distribution is the waist-to-hip ratio, which has been shown to correlate with morbidity.

As mentioned, mutated leptin genes are also associated with obesity in some humans. However, in the vast majority of obese humans, excessive rather than deficient leptin levels are observed. Thus, it appears that the most common form of human obesity involves leptin resistance in the face of high endogenous leptin levels rather than defective leptin secretion as observed in *ob/ob* mice. An animal model for this condition is the obese *db/db* mouse, in which there is a defective leptin receptor. A variety of mechanisms, including diminished signaling through the leptin receptor and diminished transport across the blood-brain barrier, could account for leptin resistance in different individuals.

Psychologic factors also make an important contribution to the development of obesity. For example, obese individuals appear to regulate their desire for food by greater reliance on external cues (eg, time of day, appeal of the food) rather than endogenous signals (eg, feeling hungry).

Last, there is great interest in the development of drugs that alter these pathways (eg, neuropeptide Y and endocannabinoid antagonists) in ways that would promote weight loss as a treatment for obesity. On the contrary, endocannabinoid agonists are used to promote appetite and weight gain in the setting of severe wasting syndrome.

CHECKPOINT

13. Define obesity.
14. What diseases are associated with obesity?
15. Outline several pathophysiologic mechanisms by which obesity contributes to disease.

PITUITARY ADENOMA

An adenoma is a benign tumor of epithelial cell origin. Pituitary adenomas are of particular significance because (1) the pituitary is in an enclosed space with very limited capacity to accommodate an expanding mass and (2) they may arise from cells that secrete hormones, giving rise to hormone overproduction syndromes.

Clinical Presentation

Pituitary adenomas are extremely common and are observed in about one in six autopsies. The majority of pituitary adenomas are clinically inapparent, either because they are nonfunctional or because hormone production does not reach the critical threshold to elicit clinical symptoms. If pituitary adenomas come to medical attention, symptoms and signs are related either to an expanding intracranial mass (headaches, diabetes insipidus, vision changes) or to manifestations of excess or deficiency of one or more pituitary hormones. Hormone deficiency results from destruction of the normal pituitary by the expanding adenoma. Hormone excess occurs when the adenoma secretes a particular hormone. **Microadenomas** (< 10 mm in diameter) are more likely to present with complaints related to hormone excess than to local mass effects because they are small. Conversely, whether or not they secrete hormones, **macroadenomas** (> 10 mm in diameter) can impinge on the optic chiasm above the sella turcica or the cavernous sinuses laterally.

Etiology

Any cell type in the pituitary gland can undergo hyperplasia or give rise to a tumor. Whether the patient with a pituitary tumor presents with a mass effect or symptoms referable to pituitary hormones depends on the size, growth rate, and secretory characteristics of the tumor. Which, if any, hormones the tumor secretes is generally a reflection of the cell type from which the tumor originated. **Gigantism** and **acromegaly** are due to oversecretion of growth hormone. **Cushing's disease** is a syndrome of glucocorticoid excess resulting from oversecretion of ACTH. **Galactorrhea** occurs in patients with prolactin-secreting tumors. Tumors secreting TSH, LH, and FSH are extremely rare and (in accordance with their physiological function) can cause secondary hyperthyroidism, precocious puberty, or ovarian hyperstimulation.

Pathophysiology

Most pituitary adenomas are clonal in origin: A single cell with altered growth control and feedback regulation gives rise to the adenoma. Evidence for the involvement of genetic mutations in the cause of pituitary adenomas comes from the occurrence of familial pituitary tumor syndromes. Mutations in at least three different genes are known to significantly raise the incidence of pituitary tumor formation: *MENIN, CNC,* and *GNAS1.* Mutation of the *MENIN* tumor suppressor gene is the underlying cause of the multiple endocrine neoplasia syndrome type 1 (MEN-1). As is typical for tumor suppressor genes, loss of heterozygosity results in tumor formation. Pituitary tumors as well as tumors of the pancreas and hyperplasia of the parathyroid gland are typical manifestations in MEN-1 patients. Pituitary hyperplasia and microadenomas are also part of Carney's complex (CNC). A subgroup of these patients harbor a mutation in the gene encoding for a protein A kinase subunit, resulting in an altered response to growth regulatory factors. In McCune-Albright syndrome, the *GNAS1* gene, which encodes a G-protein stimulatory subunit, is mutated and renders the protein product constitutively active. Thus, cyclic adenosine monophosphate levels are chronically elevated in these cells, resulting in constitutive hormone gene activation and cell hyperplasia.

Aside from these rare syndromes, the pathogenesis of pituitary adenomas is believed to be a multistep process analogous to the well-described consecutive mutations necessary for the induction of colon carcinomas. Several known or proposed factors have been shown to be part of transformation of pituitary cells (eg, GNAS1, PTTG). Other factors promoting pituitary tumor formation include chromosomal instability, presumably because of an unknown gene mutation, that results in further gene mutations and aneuploidy, altered hypothalamic signaling, and other endocrine and paracrine factors (eg, estrogens, growth factors).

Clinical Manifestations

Clinical manifestations related to mass effects are summarized in Figure 19–11. Bitemporal hemianopia is the classic visual field defect in a patient with an expanding pituitary mass (see Figure 19–11, panel C). It occurs because the crossing fibers of the optic tract, which lie directly above the pituitary gland and innervate the part of the retina responsible for temporal vision, are compressed by the tumor. However, in practice, a wide variety of visual field defects are seen, reflecting the unpredictable nature of the direction and extent of tumor growth as well as anatomic variability. The clinical manifestations of hormone excess are discussed under specific syndromes next.

Regardless of whether a pituitary tumor is producing hormones or not, infarction of or hemorrhage into the expanding mass can destroy the normal pituitary gland. This leaves the patient without one or more of the pituitary hormones. The resulting clinical manifestations are considered later in the discussion of panhypopituitarism.

A. Prolactinoma

Hyperprolactinemia is the most common anterior pituitary disorder and has many causes (Table 19–6). Pathologic hyperprolactinemia, caused by prolactin-secreting adenomas (prolactinomas) or other clinical states that result in elevated prolactin levels such as primary hypothyroidism or dopamine-receptor blocking drug therapy, must be distinguished from the physiologic hyperprolactinemia of pregnancy and lactation. Roughly 40% of tumors found in autopsies are prolactinomas. Most of the patients had no symptoms from microadenomas and died of unrelated causes.

Patients with macroadenomas generally present with mass effect symptoms, whereas those with microadenomas may develop symptoms related to hormonal effects, from either the direct actions of prolactin (galactorrhea in 30–80% of women and up to 33% of men) or prolactin's inhibitory effects on the hypothalamic-pituitary-gonadal axis. The resulting reproductive dysfunction presents variably: amenorrhea, irregular menses, or menses with infertility in women and decreased libido and partial or complete impotence or infertility in men.

Decreased bone density is another common consequence of hyperprolactinemia resulting from hypogonadism and perhaps also poorly understood direct effects of prolactin on bone.

Headaches

A. Stretching of dura by tumor

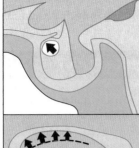

B. Hydrocephalus (rare)

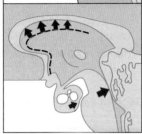

Visual field defects

C. Nasal retinal fibers compressed by tumor

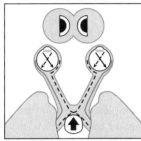

Cranial nerve palsies and temporal lobe epilepsy

D. Lateral extension of tumor

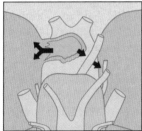

Cerebrospinal fluid rhinorrhea

E. Downward extension of tumor

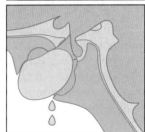

FIGURE 19–11 Various symptoms of pituitary tumor. Headaches are rarely caused by hydrocephalus. Visual field defects caused by extension of the tumor are plotted with the Goldmann perimeter. (Redrawn from Wass JAH. Hypopituitarism. In: *Clinical Endocrinology: An Illustrated Text.* Besser GM et al [editors]. Gower, 1987.)

B. Growth Hormone–Secreting Adenoma

GH-secreting tumors give rise to the syndromes of **gigantism** or **acromegaly** depending on whether they develop before or after closure of the epiphyses. Clinical findings in gigantism and acromegaly are summarized in Table 19–7 and reflect a combination of the insulin-like effects of the hormone, promoting visceromegaly, and the counterregulatory effects, promoting glucose intolerance.

TABLE 19–6 Causes of hyperprolactinemia.

Physiologic causes
Pregnancy
Lactation
Hypothalamic disease
Tumor (eg, metastases, craniopharyngioma, germinoma, cyst, glioma, hamartoma)
Infiltrative disease (eg, sarcoidosis, tuberculosis, histiocytosis X, granuloma)
Pseudotumor cerebri
Cranial radiation
Pituitary disease
Prolactinoma
Acromegaly
Cushing's disease
Pituitary stalk section
Empty sella syndrome
Other tumors (eg, metastases, nonfunctioning adenoma, gonadotrope adenoma, meningioma)
Intrasellar germinoma
Infiltrative disease (eg, sarcoidosis, giant cell granuloma, tuberculosis)
Drugs
Dopamine receptor antagonists (eg, chlorpromazine, fluphenazine, haloperidol, perphenazine, promazine, domperidone, metoclopramide, sulpiride)
Other drugs
Antihypertensives (eg, methyldopa, reserpine, verapamil)
Estrogens
Opioids
Cimetidine
Primary hypothyroidism
Chronic renal failure
Cirrhosis
Neurogenic (eg, breast manipulation, chest wall lesions, spinal cord lesions)
Stress (eg, physical, psychologic)
Idiopathic

Data from Thorner MO et al. The anterior pituitary. In: *Williams Textbook of Endocrinology,* 9th ed. Wilson JD et al (editors). Saunders, 1998.

TABLE 19–7 Clinical and laboratory findings in 57 patients with acromegaly.

Finding	%
Recent acral growth	100
Arthralgias	72
Excessive sweating	91
Weakness	88
Malocclusion	68
New skin tags	58
Hypertension: > 150/90 mm Hg	37
Carpal tunnel syndrome	44
Fasting blood glucose: > 6 mmol/L	30
Abnormal glucose tolerance test: (blood glucose > 6.1 mmol/L [> 110 mg/dL])	68
Heel pad thickness: > 22 mm	91
Serum prolactin: > 25 µg/L	16
Serum phosphorus: > 1.5 mmol/L (> 4.5 mg/dL)	48
Sella volume: > 1300 mm^3	96
Serum T$_4$: < 53 nmol/L (< 3 ng/mL)	0[1]
Serum testosterone (men): < 10 nmol/L (< 3 ng/mL)	23
8:00 AM serum cortisol: < 200 nmol/L (< 8 µg/dL)	4

Modified and reproduced, with permission, from Clemmons DR et al. Evaluation of acromegaly by radioimmunoassay of somatomedin-C. N Engl J Med. 1979;301:1138.

[1]Eleven patients were receiving T$_4$ replacement at the time of the study.

C. ACTH-Secreting Pituitary Adenoma (Cushing's Syndrome)

Secretion of excess cortisol as a result of overproduction of ACTH by a pituitary adenoma is the most common cause of spontaneous Cushing's syndrome (Chapter 21). ACTH-secreting pituitary adenomas are eight times more common in women than in men and must be distinguished from the effects caused by CRH or ACTH arising from outside the hypothalamus and pituitary gland, respectively, and from adrenal adenomas and carcinomas.

The symptoms and signs of ACTH-secreting pituitary adenomas are a consequence of both local mass effects, similar to those discussed previously for other types of pituitary tumors, and effects from overproduction of cortisol by the adrenal gland, as discussed in Chapter 21. **Nelson's syndrome** is the rapid progression of an ACTH-secreting pituitary adenoma, which is often observed after bilateral adrenalectomy to control the symptoms of cortisol excess. With the advent of vigorous glucocorticoid substitution regimens, transsphenoidal pituitary surgery, and radiation therapy, the incidence of this complication has greatly diminished.

HYPOPITUITARISM

Panhypopituitarism is the syndrome resulting from complete loss of all of the hormones secreted by the pituitary gland. Hypopituitarism refers to the loss of one or more pituitary hormones. Causes of hypopituitarism are listed in Table 19-8.

Clinical Presentation

The complex of symptoms in hypopituitarism varies depending on the extent and duration of disease. Regardless of the underlying cause, in non-congenital forms of hypopituitarism, GH deficiency occurs as the earliest hormonal deviance, followed by ACTH and gonadotropin (LH and FSH) deficiencies, and finally, TSH deficiency. In some cases, panhypopituitarism is of sudden onset (eg, caused by pituitary infarction or trauma). These patients may rapidly develop two potentially life-threatening situations as a consequence of loss of ACTH and vasopressin. First, since the patient is unable to mount a stress response because of a lack of ACTH-stimulated glucocorticoid secretion, even relatively mild stress may be lethal. Second, a patient unable to maintain water intake will be unable to compensate for the massive diuresis associated with vasopressin deficiency (**diabetes insipidus**). Thus, the patient will quickly become comatose as a result of profound water loss and the complications of dehydration and hyperosmolarity.

In other cases, pituitary insufficiency develops more insidiously (eg, from progressive destruction of the pituitary gland by a nonsecreting tumor or subsequent to pituitary radiation therapy). In many of these slowly developing cases of panhypopituitarism, the patient comes to medical attention with complaints related to reproductive functions (amenorrhea in women; infertility or erectile dysfunction in men) caused by LH and FSH deficiency. Other patients have nonspecific complaints (eg, lethargy or altered bowel habits), perhaps related to the gradual development of hypothyroidism (from TSH deficiency). Panhypopituitarism may be unmasked only when the patient does poorly during some other unrelated medical emergency because of an inability to mount a protective stress response because of an ACTH and consequent glucocorticoid deficiency.

TABLE 19–8 Causes of hypopituitarism.

Ischemic necrosis of the pituitary
Postpartum necrosis (Sheehan's syndrome)
Head injury
Vascular disease, commonly associated with diabetes mellitus
Neoplasms involving the sella turcica
Nonfunctioning adenoma
Craniopharyngioma
Suprasellar chordoma
Histiocytosis X (eosinophilic granuloma; Hand-Schüller-Christian disease)
Intrasellar cysts
Chronic inflammatory lesions
Tuberculosis, syphilis, sarcoidosis
Infiltrative diseases
Amyloidosis
Hemochromatosis
Mucopolysaccharidoses
Genetic mutations
Part of a syndrome
PITX2, HESX1, LHX3, LHX4
Resulting in combined or isolated hormone deficiency
PROP1, PIT1 (combined pituitary hormone deficiency)
TPIT (ACTH deficiency), *DAX1* (hypogonadotropic hypogonadism)
Hormone genes (eg, POMC, TSH-β)
Prohormone convertases (*PC1*)
Releasing hormone receptor genes (eg, *TRH-R, GnRH-R*)

Modified and reproduced, with permission, from Chandrasoma P, Taylor CR. *Concise Pathology*, 3rd ed. Originally published by Appleton & Lange. Copyright © 1998 by the McGraw-Hill Companies, Inc.

Etiology

Panhypopituitarism of sudden onset is usually due to traumatic disruption of the pituitary stalk, infarction and hemorrhage into a pituitary tumor, or ischemic destruction of the pituitary after systemic hypotension (eg, **Sheehan's syndrome** or postpartum hypopituitarism after massive blood loss in childbirth). A number of rare genetic causes have also been reported (Table 19–8, Figure 19–4). Gradually acquired hypopituitarism is most often due to extension of pituitary tumors or occurs as a complication of radiation therapy for brain tumors.

Pathophysiology

The biochemical hallmark of hypopituitarism is low levels of pituitary hormones in the face of low end-organ products of one or more components of the neuroendocrine axes involving the pituitary. By contrast, primary end-organ failure results in compensatory high levels of the relevant pituitary hormones.

Another biochemical difference between primary end-organ failure and end-organ failure secondary to hypopituitarism is that not all end-organ functions are equally controlled by the pituitary. In the case of the adrenal cortex, for example, although mineralocorticoid secretion can be stimulated by ACTH, it is not dependent on it.

Both of the biochemical distinctions between primary end-organ failure and pituitary failure have important clinical implications. For example, hyperpigmentation occurs in primary adrenal insufficiency because several POMC-derived peptides (MSHs, ACTH) stimulate skin pigmentation via binding to the melanocortin-1 receptor (MC1-R). Because levels of POMC-derived peptides are not elevated in pituitary and hypothalamic insufficiency, hyperpigmentation does not occur. Similarly, the symptoms of adrenal insufficiency secondary to pituitary disease may be more subtle than in the case of primary adrenal failure, because a significant fraction of mineralocorticoid production is preserved even in the absence of ACTH (Chapter 21).

In the case of trauma and pituitary stalk transection, it is notable that hypopituitarism in general and vasopressin deficiency in particular may improve over time as local edema diminishes and some degree of integrity of the pituitary stalk with its connection to the hypothalamus is reestablished. Sometimes, however, these symptoms and signs may worsen over time as the few residual intact cells or connections are lost.

Notably, injuries disconnecting the pituitary from the hypothalamus result in deficiencies of most of the anterior pituitary hormones except prolactin. Indeed, prolactin secretion is usually preserved or elevated because it is the only pituitary hormone regulated by tonic hypothalamic inhibition.

Clinical Manifestations

The symptoms and signs of hypopituitarism depend on the extent and duration of specific pituitary hormone deficiencies and the patient's overall clinical status. Thus, a relative deficiency of vasopressin can be compensated for by increasing water intake; adrenal insufficiency may not be manifest until the patient needs to mount a stress response. Hypothyroidism may become manifest gradually over months because of the relatively long half-life and large reservoir of thyroid hormone normally available in the gland.

The clinical manifestations of hypopituitarism are those of the end-organ deficiency syndromes. Most important are adrenal insufficiency, hypothyroidism, and diabetes insipidus. Less crucial but often the most sensitive clues to the presence of pituitary disease are amenorrhea in women and infertility or impotence in men.

CHECKPOINT

20. What are the most common causes of panhypopituitarism?

21. How do patients with panhypopituitarism come to medical attention?

22. How would you determine what replacement therapy is required for a patient with panhypopituitarism?

DIABETES INSIPIDUS

Diabetes insipidus is a syndrome of polyuria resulting from the inability to concentrate urine and, therefore, to conserve water as a result of lack of vasopressin action.

Clinical Presentation

The initial clinical presentation of diabetes insipidus is polyuria that persists in circumstances that would normally lead to diminished urine output (eg, dehydration), accompanied by thirst. Adults may complain of frequent urination at night (nocturia), and children may present with bed-wetting (enuresis). No further symptoms develop if the patient is able to maintain a water intake commensurate with water loss. The volume of urine produced in the total absence of vasopressin may reach 10–20 L/d. Thus, should the patient's ability to maintain this degree of fluid intake be compromised (eg, damage to hypothalamic thirst regulating centers), dehydration can develop and may rapidly progress to coma.

Etiology

Diabetes insipidus can be due to (1) diseases of the CNS (**central diabetes insipidus**), affecting the synthesis or secretion of vasopressin; (2) diseases of the kidney (**nephrogenic diabetes insipidus**), with loss of the kidney's ability to respond to circulating vasopressin by retaining water; or (3) pregnancy, with probable increased metabolic clearance of vasopressin. In both central and nephrogenic diabetes insipidus, urine is hypotonic. The most common central causes are accidental head trauma, intracranial tumor (eg, craniopharyngioma), and the postintracranial surgery state. Less common causes are listed in Table 19–9. Nephrogenic diabetes insipidus may be familial or caused by renal damage from a variety of drugs. Diabetes insipidus–like syndromes may result from mineralocorticoid excess, pregnancy, and other causes. True nephrogenic diabetes insipidus must be distinguished from an osmotic (and hence vasopressin-resistant) diuresis. Likewise, washout of the medullary interstitial osmotic gradient, which is necessary for the concentration of urine, may occur with prolonged diuresis resulting from any cause and may be confused with true diabetes insipidus. In both cases (osmotic diuresis and medullary washout), the urine is hypertonic or isotonic rather than hypotonic. Finally, extreme primary polydipsia (drinking excessive amounts of water, often because of a psychiatric disorder) results in an appropriately large volume of dilute urine and a low plasma vasopressin level, thus mimicking true diabetes insipidus.

Pathophysiology

A. Central Diabetes Insipidus

Central diabetes insipidus can be either permanent or transient, reflecting the natural history of the underlying disorder (Table 19–9). Only about 15% of the vasopressin-secreting cells of the hypothalamus need to be intact to maintain fluid balance under normal conditions. Simple destruction of the posterior pituitary does not cause sufficient neuronal loss to

TABLE 19–9 Causes of central and nephrogenic diabetes insipidus.

Central diabetes insipidus
Hereditary, familial (autosomal dominant)
Acquired
Idiopathic
Traumatic or postsurgical
Neoplastic disease: craniopharyngioma, lymphoma, meningioma, metastatic carcinoma
Ischemic or hypoxic disorder: Sheehan's syndrome, aneurysms, cardiopulmonary arrest, aortocoronary bypass, shock, brain death
Granulomatous disease: sarcoidosis, histiocytosis X
Infections: viral encephalitis, bacterial meningitis
Autoimmune disorder
Nephrogenic diabetes insipidus
Hereditary, familial (two types)
Acquired
Hypokalemia
Hypercalcemia
Postrenal obstruction
Drugs: lithium, demeclocycline, methoxyflurane
Sickle cell trait or disease
Amyloidosis
Pregnancy

Modified and reproduced, with permission, from Reeves BW, Bichet DG, Andreoli TE. The posterior pituitary and water metabolism. In: *Williams Textbook of Endocrinology*, 9th ed. Wilson JD et al (editors). Saunders, 1998.

result in permanent diabetes insipidus. Rather, destruction of the hypothalamus or at least some of the supraoptic-hypophysial tract must also occur.

A more common finding is transient disease resulting from acute injury with neuronal shock and edema (eg, post-infarction or post-trauma), leading to cessation of vasopressin secretion with subsequent resumption of sufficient vasopressin secretion to resolve symptoms, because of either neuronal recovery or resolution of edema with reestablishment of hypothalamic-pituitary neurovascular integrity.

B. Nephrogenic Diabetes Insipidus

Familial nephrogenic diabetes insipidus is the result of a generalized defect in either the V_2 class of vasopressin receptors or the aquaporin-2 water channel of the renal collecting ducts.

Drug-induced nephrogenic diabetes insipidus appears to result from sensitivity of the vasopressin receptor to lithium, fluoride, and other salts. This occurs in 12–30% of patients treated with these drugs. It is generally reversible on termination of exposure to the offending drug (Table 19–9).

C. Diabetes Insipidus–Like Syndromes

There are several diabetes insipidus–like syndromes. As an example, diabetes insipidus is a rare complication of pregnancy. It appears to be due to excessive vasopressinase in plasma. This enzyme, which selectively degrades vasopressin, is presumably released from the placenta. A hallmark of this entity is that it is reversed by administration of the vasopressin analogue desmopressin acetate, which is resistant to degradation by the enzyme.

Clinical Manifestations

Diabetes insipidus must be distinguished from other causes of polyuria and hypernatremia (Table 19–10). The hallmark of diabetes insipidus is dilute urine, even in the face of hypernatremia. Dipstick testing of the urine for glucose distinguishes diabetes mellitus. Conditions in which **osmotic diuresis** is responsible for polyuria can be distinguished from diabetes insipidus by their normal or elevated urine osmolality. Primary polydipsia is distinguished by the presence of hyponatremia, whereas in diabetes insipidus the serum sodium should be normal or elevated. In primary polydipsia, uncontrolled excess water ingestion drives the polyuria, whereas in diabetes insipidus, hypertonicity stimulates thirst.

Distinguishing central from nephrogenic diabetes insipidus depends ultimately on a determination of responsiveness to injected vasopressin, with a dramatic decrease in urine volume and increase in urine osmolality in the former and little or no change in the latter. In central diabetes insipidus, circulating vasopressin levels are low for a given plasma osmolality, whereas in nephrogenic diabetes insipidus they are high.

Polyuria in nephrogenic diabetes insipidus results from an inability to conserve water in the distal nephron because of a lack of vasopressin-dependent water channels. These chan-

TABLE 19–10   Major causes of hypernatremia.

Impaired thirst
Coma
Essential hypernatremia
Excessive water losses
Renal
Central diabetes insipidus
Nephrogenic diabetes insipidus
Impaired medullary hypertonicity
Extrarenal
Sweating
Osmotic diarrhea
Burns
Solute diuresis
Glucose
Diabetic ketoacidosis
Nonketotic hyperosmolar coma
Other
Mannitol administration
Glycerol administration
Sodium excess
Administration of hypertonic NaCl
Administration of hypertonic $NaHCO_3$

Modified and reproduced, with permission, from Reeves BW, Bichet DG, Andreoli TE. The posterior pituitary and water metabolism. In: *Williams Textbook of Endocrinology*, 9th ed. Wilson JD et al (editors). Saunders, 1998.

nels, which reside within vesicles in the cytoplasm of collecting duct cells, are normally inserted into the apical plasma membrane in response to vasopressin stimulation, permitting increased reabsorption of water. Up to 13% of the volume of the glomerular filtrate can be reclaimed in this manner.

In diabetes insipidus of either central or nephrogenic origin, if the patient is unable to maintain sufficient water intake to offset polyuria, dehydration with consequent hypernatremia develops. Hypernatremia leads to a number of neurologic manifestations, including progressive obtundation (decreased responsiveness to verbal and physical stimuli), myoclonus, seizures, focal deficits, and coma. These neurologic manifestations result from cell shrinkage and volume loss as a result of osmotic forces, sometimes complicated by intracranial hemorrhage because of stretching and rupture of small blood vessels. Barring structural changes such as those leading to hemorrhage, the neurologic consequences of hypernatremia are reversible on resolution of the underlying metabolic disorder.

The time course of hypernatremia is an important variable in the development of neurologic symptoms in that, over time, neurons generate "idiogenic osmoles" (ie, amino acids and other metabolites that serve to raise intracellular osmolality to the level in the blood and thereby minimize fluid shifts out of the cells of the brain). Thus, the more slowly hypernatremia develops, the less likely are neurologic complications resulting from fluid shifts in the brain or from a vascular catastrophe.

CHECKPOINT

23. What clues would suggest diabetes insipidus in a new patient?
24. How would you make a definitive diagnosis of diabetes insipidus?
25. What are the pathophysiologic differences between central and nephrogenic diabetes insipidus?

SYNDROME OF INAPPROPRIATE VASOPRESSIN SECRETION (SIADH)

The syndrome of inappropriate ADH (vasopressin) secretion (SIADH) is one of several causes of a hypotonic state (Table 19–11). SIADH is due to the secretion of vasopressin in excess of what is appropriate for hyperosmolality or intravascular volume depletion.

Clinical Presentation

The cardinal clinical presentation of SIADH is hyponatremia without edema. Depending on the rapidity of onset and the severity, the neurologic consequences of hyponatremia include confusion, lethargy and weakness, myoclonus, asterixis, generalized seizures, and coma.

Etiology

A variety of vasopressin-secreting tumors, CNS disorders, pulmonary disorders, and drugs have been associated with SIADH (Table 19–12). Therefore, it is worth mentioning that the hypothalamic neurons and the posterior pituitary are not always the source of vasopressin secretion. In fact, the hypothalamus and pituitary account for elevated vasopressin levels in only one-third of patients with SIADH, and it is important to regard SIADH as not necessarily a disorder of the hypothalamic-pituitary system. Several metabolic disorders can produce hyponatremia and must be investigated and ruled out before the diagnosis of true SIADH is made. In particular, adrenal insufficiency and hypothyroidism are often associated with hyponatremia. In these conditions, sodium deficiency

TABLE 19–11 The hypotonic syndromes.

Excessive water ingestion
Decreased water excretion
Decreased solute delivery to diluting segments
Starvation
Beer potomania
Vasopressin excess
Syndrome of inappropriate antidiuretic hormone
Drug-induced vasopressin secretion
Vasopressin excess with decreased distal solute delivery
Congestive heart failure
Cirrhosis of the liver
Nephrotic syndrome
Cortisol deficiency
Hypothyroidism
Diuretic use
Renal failure

Modified and reproduced, with permission, from Reeves BW, Bichet DG, Andreoli TE. The posterior pituitary and water metabolism. In: *Williams Textbook of Endocrinology*, 9th ed. Wilson JD et al (editors). Saunders, 1998.

and subsequent volume depletion trigger vasopressin secretion. Hyponatremia accompanying CNS disorders is caused either by SIADH or by cerebral salt wasting (CSW) with an increased release of natriuretic peptides (eg, BNP, ANP). A major difference between these two disorders is in the total extracellular volume, which is increased in SIADH and reduced in CSW.

Pathophysiology

The serum sodium concentration (and hence osmolarity) is normally determined by the balance of water intake, renal solute delivery (a necessary step in water excretion), and vasopressin-mediated distal renal tubular water retention. Disorders in any one of these features of normal sodium balance, or factors controlling them, can result in hyponatremia. Hyponatremia occurs when the magnitude of the disorder exceeds the capacity of homeostatic mechanisms to compensate for dysfunction. Thus, simple excess water ingestion is generally compensated for by renal water diuresis. The exceptions are (1) when water ingestion is extreme (greater than the approximately 18 L daily that can be excreted via the kidney) or (2) when renal solute delivery is limited (eg, in salt depletion), thereby limiting the ability of the kidney to excrete free water.

In hypoadrenal states, renal sodium loss resulting from lack of aldosterone has two consequences. Most importantly,

TABLE 19–12 Causes of SIADH.

Tumors
Bronchial carcinoma (particularly small-cell type)
Other carcinomas: duodenum, pancreas, bladder, ureter, prostate
Leukemia, lymphoma
Thymoma, sarcoma
CNS disorders
Mass lesions: tumors, abscess, hematoma
Infections: encephalitis, meningitis
Cerebrovascular accident
Senile cerebral atrophy
Hydrocephalus
Trauma
Delirium tremens
Acute psychosis
Demyelinating and degenerative disease
Inflammatory disease
Pulmonary disorders
Infections: tuberculosis, pneumonia, abscess
Acute respiratory failure
Positive pressure ventilation
Drugs
Vasopressin, desmopressin acetate
Chlorpropamide
Clofibrate
Carbamazepine
Others: vincristine, vinblastine, tricyclic antidepressants, phenothiazines
Idiopathic
Diagnosis of exclusion

Reproduced, with permission, from Chauvreau ME. Pathology of posterior pituitary. In: *Pathophysiologic Foundations of Critical Care.* Pinsky MR, Dhainaut JA (editors). Williams & Wilkins, 1993.

volume depletion as a consequence of renal sodium loss results in the release of vasopressin; although the primary stimulus for ADH secretion is an elevated plasma osmolarity, ADH release is stimulated by low intravascular volume as well. Second, diminished renal solute delivery impairs the ability of the kidney to excrete a water load, in the case in which ingestion of water exceeds nonrenal water loss.

In hypothyroidism, both renal solute delivery and function of the osmostat to which vasopressin secretion is coupled appear to be impaired, resulting in hyponatremia.

True causes of hyponatremia, including SIADH, must also be distinguished from so-called pseudohyponatremia. **Pseudohyponatremia** occurs in two groups of conditions (Table 19–13). First, there are those in which infusion of hyperosmolar solutions (eg, glucose) pulls water out of cells, thereby diluting the sodium. The key feature of these conditions is hyponatremia without hypo-osmolality. Second, pseudohyponatremia occurs when the nonaqueous fraction of plasma is larger than normal. Sodium only equilibrates with, and is regulated in, the aqueous fraction of plasma, and calculations of serum sodium concentration typically correct for total plasma volume because the nonaqueous fraction of plasma volume is normally negligible. In those relatively rare conditions in which the nonaqueous fraction is significant (eg, severe hyperlipidemic states, multiple myeloma, and other conditions with higher than normal serum lipid or protein concentrations), the calculated sodium concentration will, therefore, be misleadingly low.

The pathophysiologic mechanisms behind most cases of SIADH are not well understood. It has been proposed that baroreceptor input from the lung is impaired in those pulmonary disorders that result in SIADH. CNS lesions causing SIADH are presumed to interrupt the vasopressin-inhibiting neural pathways. Regardless of the mechanism, in most cases the hyponatremia of SIADH is partially limited by secretion of atrial natriuretic peptide. Thus, severe hyponatremia develops only when water intake is relatively increased, and edema formation is rare. The simplest therapy is restriction of free water intake and, in the case of CNS or pulmonary lesions, treatment of the underlying disease.

Clinical Manifestations

The clinical manifestations of SIADH are in part determined by the nature and course of any underlying disorder (eg, CNS

TABLE 19–13 Causes of pseudohyponatremia.

Elevated plasma osmolality
Hyperglycemia
Mannitol administration
Glycerol administration
Normal plasma osmolality
Hyperproteinemia (eg, multiple myeloma)
Hyperlipidemia
Prostate surgery, with use of irrigant fluid containing glycine or sorbitol

Modified and reproduced, with permission, from Reeves BW, Bichet DG, Andreoli TE. The posterior pituitary and water metabolism. In: *Williams Textbook of Endocrinology,* 9th ed. Wilson JD et al (editors). Saunders, 1998.

or pulmonary disease), by the severity of hyponatremia, and by the rapidity with which hyponatremia develops. Regardless of its cause, SIADH can have neurologic manifestations, including confusion, asterixis, myoclonus, generalized seizures, and coma. These occur as a result of osmotic fluid shifts and resulting brain edema and elevated intracranial pressures; brain swelling is limited by the size of the skull. Physiologic mechanisms to counter this swelling include depletion of intracellular osmoles, especially potassium ions. The more rapid the progression of hyponatremia, the more likely it is that brain edema and increased intracranial pressure will develop and that the neurologic complications and herniation will lead to permanent damage. However, even when hyponatremia develops slowly, it can in extreme cases (eg, serum sodium < 110 mEq/L) result in seizures and altered mental status. Central pontine myelinolysis can develop and cause permanent neurologic damage in patients whose hyponatremia is corrected too rapidly.

CHECKPOINT

26. What conditions are associated with SIADH?
27. How would you distinguish SIADH from other causes of hyponatremia?
28. What are the neurologic consequences of SIADH, and how may they be prevented?

CASE STUDIES

Eva M. Aagaard, MD, & Yeong Kwok, MD

(See Chapter 25, p. 704 for Answers)

CASE 87

A 53-year-old woman came to the clinic to get help managing her weight. She has been overweight since childhood and has continued to gain weight throughout her adult life. She has tried numerous diets without lasting success. She initially loses weight, but then regains it after a few months. She is otherwise healthy and is not taking any medications. Other family members are also overweight or obese. She does not do any regular exercise and has a sedentary office job. On examination, she is 5 feet 3 inches tall and 260 pounds, with a body mass index (BMI) of 46.2 (normal < 25).

Questions

A. How is body weight controlled?
B. How is obesity defined?
C. What medical conditions is she at increased risk for due to her obesity?

CASE 88

A 30-year-old woman presents to the emergency department after sideswiping a parked car. She reports that she never saw the car until after she hit it. She denies any trauma to herself but does complain of headache. She states that she has had headaches every day for the last 3 months, and this one is similar to her other headaches. She describes the headache as a frontal throbbing pain that is worse when she lies down and occasionally it wakes her from sleep. She has no significant medical history, takes no medications, and denies alcohol, tobacco, or drug use. On review of systems, she notes irregular menses but denies having other complaints. On examination she appears to be well, with normal vital signs. Her neurologic examination is notable for bitemporal hemianopia. On breast examination, galactorrhea is present but no masses. The remainder of the examination is unremarkable.

Questions

A. What is the likely diagnosis?
B. How did this condition arise?
C. What is the pathogenetic mechanism of her bitemporal hemianopia? Her headaches?
D. What is the cause of her irregular menses? Her galactorrhea?

CASE 89

A 31-year-old woman with a medical history significant for pituitary macroadenoma status post-radiation therapy presents to the clinic with a complaint of amenorrhea. Before the diagnosis of pituitary adenoma, she had irregular menses. This irregularity had persisted, with menses lasting ~3 days, and occurring about once every 1.5–2 months. However, for the last 4 months, she has had no menses. She denies sexual activity. On review of systems, she notes progressive fatigue and 10 pounds of weight gain over several months.

The pituitary macroadenoma was treated with radiation therapy 1 year ago. She has been without medical care since completing therapy because she moved and has not yet found a physician. She is taking no medications. On examination her blood pressure is 100/60 mm Hg and heart rate is 80 beats/min. Neurologic examination is normal except for a slight delay in the relaxation phase of her deep tendon reflexes. On head-neck examination, she has somewhat coarse, brittle brown hair. Neck examination discloses no goiter or masses. Lung, cardiac, and abdominal examinations show no abnormalities. Pelvic examination reveals normal female genitalia without uterine or ovarian masses. Urine pregnancy test is negative.

Questions

A. What is the likely cause of this patient's amenorrhea? Why do you think so?

B. On the basis of her history and physical examination, do you suspect any other hormone deficiencies? Why do you think so?

C. What other hormonal deficiencies should you be concerned about in this patient? Why might they be asymptomatic currently?

CASE 90

A 54-year-old man with a medical history significant for bipolar disease presents to his physician with complaints of polyuria. He states that he must get up three or four times each night to urinate. He also notes frequent thirst. He denies polyphagia, urinary urgency, difficulty initiating urination, and postvoid dribbling. His medical history is notable only for bipolar disease. He has a long-standing history of noncompliance with medications for this disease, with frequent hospitalizations for both mania and depression, but has been stable on lithium for the last 6 months. He denies any symptoms of mania or depression at this time. He takes no other medications. Family history is notable for depression and substance abuse but is otherwise negative. The patient has a history of polysubstance abuse but has been "clean and sober" for the last 6 months.

On examination, the patient's vital signs are within normal limits. Head-neck examination reveals slightly dry mucous membranes. Rectal examination reveals a normal prostate without masses. The remainder of his examination is unremarkable. Urinalysis reveals dilute urine without glucose or other abnormality. Serum electrolytes reveal a mildly increased sodium level. A diagnosis of diabetes insipidus is entertained.

Questions

A. Do you suspect central or nephrogenic diabetes insipidus? Why? How would you confirm the diagnosis?

B. How does lithium cause diabetes insipidus?

C. What is the cause of this patient's polyuria? His thirst?

D. What might occur if this patient were unable to maintain sufficient water intake?

CASE 91

A 75-year-old man with terminal small cell carcinoma of the lung presents to the emergency department with altered mental status. The patient's wife, who cares for him at home, states that he is quite weak at baseline, requiring assistance with all activities of daily living. Over the last few days, he has become progressively more lethargic. She has been careful to adequately hydrate him, waking him every 2 hours to give him water to drink. His appetite has been poor, but he willingly ingests the water, consuming 2–3 quarts per day. He is taking morphine for pain and dyspnea.

On examination, the patient is a cachectic white man in mild respiratory distress. He is lethargic but arousable. He is oriented to person only. Vital signs reveal a temperature of 38 °C, blood pressure of 110/60 mm Hg, heart rate of 88 beats/min, respiratory rate of 18/min, and oxygen saturation of 96% on 3 L of oxygen. On head-neck examination, pupils are 3 mm and reactive, scleras are anicteric, and conjunctivas are pink. Mucous membranes are moist. Neck is supple. There are decreased breath sounds in the left lower posterior lung field and rales in the upper half. Cardiac examination shows a regular heartbeat without murmur, gallop, or rub. Abdomen is benign without masses. Extremities are without edema, cyanosis, or clubbing. Neurologic examination shows only bilateral positive Babinski reflexes and asterixis. Laboratory studies reveal a serum sodium level of 118 mEq/L.

Questions

A. What conditions are associated with SIADH? Which are present in this patient?

B. What pathophysiologic mechanism produces SIADH?

C. What is the cause of this patient's lethargy, confusion, and asterixis?

D. How would you treat this patient's hyponatremia?

REFERENCES

General

Greenspan FS, Gardner DG (editors). *Basic and Clinical Endocrinology,* 8th ed. McGraw-Hill, 2007.

Obesity

Adan RAH et al. Inverse agonism gains weight. Trends Pharmacol Sci. 2003 Jun;24(6):315–21. [PMID: 12823958]

Bates SH et al. The role of leptin receptor in signaling in feeding and neuroendocrine function. Trends Endocrinol Metab. 2003 Dec;14(10):447–52. [PMID: 14643059]

Murphy KG et al. Gut peptides in the regulation of food intake and energy homeostasis. Endocr Rev. 2006 Dec;27(7):719–27. [PMID: 17077190]

Näslund E et al. Appetite signaling: From gut peptides and enteric nerves to brain. Physiol Behav. 2007 Sep 10;92(1-2):256–62. [PMID: 17582445]

O'Rahilly S et al. Human obesity—Lessons from monogenetic disorders. Endocrinology. 2003 Sep;144(9):3757–64. [PMID: 12933645]

Pituitary Adenoma

Daly AF et al. The epidemiology and management of pituitary incidentalomas. Horm Res. 2007;68 (Suppl 5):195–8. [PMID: 18174745]

Mancini T et al. Hyperprolactinemia and prolactinomas. Endocrinol Metab Clin North Am. 2008 Mar;37(1):67–99. [PMID: 18226731]

Melmed S. Mechanisms for pituitary tumorigenesis: The plastic pituitary. J Clin Invest. 2003 Dec;112(11):1603–18. [PMID: 14660734]

Hypopituitarism

Mancini T et al. Hyperprolactinemia and prolactinomas. Endocrinol Metab Clin North Am. 2008 Mar;37(1):67–99. [PMID: 18226731]

Mehta A et al. Developmental disorders of the hypothalamus and pituitary gland associated with congenital hypopituitarism. Best Pract Res Clin Endocrinol Metab. 2008 Feb;22(1):191–206. [PMID: 18279788]

Savage JJ et al. Transcriptional control during mammalian anterior pituitary development. Gene. 2003 Nov 13;319:1–19. [PMID: 14597167]

Toogood AA et al. Hypopituitarism: Clinical features, diagnosis, and management. Endocrinol Metab Clin North Am. 2008 Mar;37(1):235–61. [PMID: 18226739]

Diabetes Insipidus/Oxytocin

Maghnie M. Diabetes insipidus. Horm Res. 2003;59(suppl 1):42–54. [PMID: 12566720]

Marazziti D et al. The role of oxytocin in neuropsychiatric disorders. Curr Med Chem. 2008;15(7):698–704. [PMID: 18336283]

Morello JP et al. Nephrogenic diabetes insipidus. Annu Rev Physiol. 2001;63:607–30. [PMID: 11181969]

Syndrome of Inappropriate ADH Secretion

Adrogué HJ et al. Hyponatremia. N Engl J Med. 2000 May 25;342(21):1581–9. [PMID: 10824078]

Baylis PH. The syndrome of inappropriate antidiuretic hormone secretion. Int J Biochem Cell Biol. 2003 Nov;35(11):1495–9. [PMID: 12824060]

Thyroid Disease

Douglas C. Bauer, MD, & Stephen J. McPhee, MD

20

The thyroid gland synthesizes the hormones **thyroxine** (T_4) and **triiodothyronine** (T_3), iodine-containing amino acids that regulate the body's metabolic rate. Adequate levels of thyroid hormone are necessary in infants for normal development of the CNS, in children for normal skeletal growth and maturation, and in adults for normal function of multiple organ systems. Thyroid dysfunction is one of the most common endocrine disorders encountered in clinical practice. Although abnormally high or low levels of thyroid hormones may be tolerated for long periods of time, usually there are symptoms and signs of overt thyroid dysfunction.

NORMAL STRUCTURE & FUNCTION

ANATOMY

The normal thyroid gland is a firm, reddish brown, smooth gland consisting of two lateral lobes and a connecting central isthmus (Figure 20–1). A pyramidal lobe of variable size may extend upward from the isthmus. The normal weight of the thyroid ranges from 30–40 g. It is surrounded by an adherent fibrous capsule from which multiple fibrous projections extend deeply into its structure, dividing it into many small lobules. The thyroid is highly vascular and has one of the highest rates of blood flow per gram of tissue of any organ.

HISTOLOGY

Histologically, the thyroid gland consists of many closely packed acini, called **follicles,** each surrounded by capillaries and stroma. Each follicle is roughly spherical, lined by a single layer of cuboidal epithelial cells and filled with **colloid,** a proteinaceous material composed mainly of **thyroglobulin** and stored thyroid hormones. When the gland is inactive, the follicles are large, the lining cells are flat, and the colloid is abundant. When the gland is active, the follicles are small, the lining cells are cuboidal or columnar, the colloid is scanty, and its edges are scalloped, forming **reabsorption lacunae** (Figure 20–2). Scattered between follicles are the **parafollicular cells** (**C cells**), which secrete **calcitonin,** a hormone that inhibits bone resorption and lowers the plasma calcium level (see Chapter 17).

The ultrastructure of a follicular epithelial cell is diagrammed in Figure 20–3. The cells vary in appearance with the degree of gland activity. The follicular cell rests on a basal lamina. The nucleus is round and centrally located. The cytoplasm contains mitochondria, rough endoplasmic reticulum, and ribosomes. The apex has a discrete Golgi apparatus, small secretory granules containing thyroglobulin, and abundant lysosomes and phagosomes. At the apex, the cell membrane is folded into microvilli.

PHYSIOLOGY

Formation & Secretion of Thyroid Hormones

A. T_4, T_3, and Thyroglobulin

Thyroid follicular cells have three functions: (1) collect and transport iodine to the colloid; (2) synthesize **thyroglobulin,** a 660,000-Da glycoprotein made up of two subunits and containing many tyrosine residues, and secrete it into the colloid; and (3) release thyroid hormones from thyroglobulin and secrete them into the circulation. The structures of the two thyroid hormones, T_3 and T_4, are shown in Figure 20–4. T_3 and

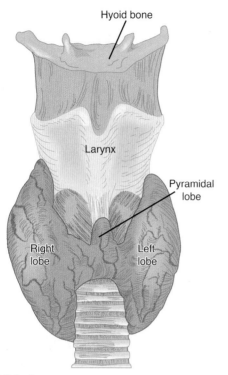

FIGURE 20–1   The human thyroid.   (Redrawn, with permission, from Ganong WF. *Review of Medical Physiology*, 22nd ed. McGraw-Hill, 2005.)

T_4 are synthesized in the colloid by iodination and condensation of tyrosine molecules bound together in thyroglobulin.

B. Iodine Metabolism and Trapping

For normal thyroid hormone synthesis, an adult requires a minimum daily intake of 150 μg of iodine. In the United States, the average intake is about 500 μg/d. Iodine ingested in food is first converted to **iodide,** which is absorbed and taken up by the thyroid. The follicular cells transport iodide from the circulation to the colloid ("iodide trapping" or "iodide pump"). The transporter is a 65-kDa cell membrane protein. This iodide transport is an example of secondary active transport dependent on Na^+-K^+ adenosine triphosphatase (ATPase) for energy; it is stimulated by **thyroid-stimulating hormone** (**TSH, thyrotropin**). At the normal rate of thyroid hormone synthesis, about 120 μg/d of iodide enters the thyroid. About 80 μg/d is secreted in T_3 and T_4, and the rest diffuses into the extracellular fluid and is excreted in the urine.

C. Thyroid Hormone Synthesis and Secretion

Thyroid hormones are synthesized in the colloid, near the apical cell membrane of the follicular cells. Catalyzed by the enzyme thyroidal peroxidase, iodide in the thyroid cell is oxidized to iodine. The iodine enters the colloid and is rapidly bound at the 3 position (Figure 20–4) to tyrosine molecules

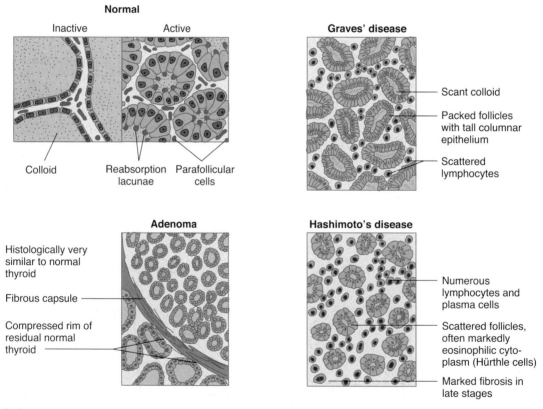

FIGURE 20–2   Normal and abnormal thyroid histology.   (Redrawn, with permission, from Ganong WF. *Review of Medical Physiology*, 22nd ed. McGraw-Hill, 2005; Chandrasoma P, Taylor CE. *Concise Pathology*, 3rd ed. Originally published by Appleton & Lange. Copyright © by the McGraw-Hill Companies, Inc.; Greenspan FS, Gardner DG [editors]: *Basic and Clinical Endocrinology*, 7th ed. McGraw-Hill, 2004.)

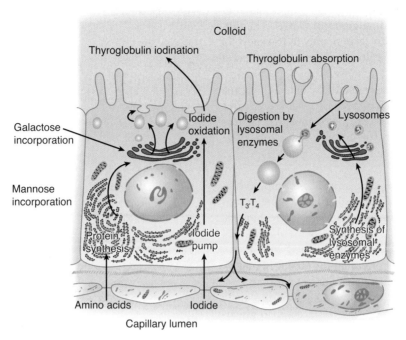

FIGURE 20–3 Thyroid cell ultrastructure (schematic). The processes of synthesis and iodination of thyroglobulin are shown on the left and its reabsorption and digestion on the right. (Redrawn, with permission, from Junqueira LC, Carneiro J, Kelley R. *Basic Histology*, 9th ed. Originally published by Appleton & Lange. Copyright © 1998 by the McGraw-Hill Companies, Inc.)

attached to thyroglobulin, forming **monoiodotyrosine** (**MIT**). MIT is next iodinated at the 5 position, forming **diiodotyrosine** (**DIT**). Two DIT molecules then condense in an oxidative process ("coupling reaction") to form one **thyroxine** (**T$_4$**) molecule. Some **T$_3$** is probably formed within the thyroid gland by condensation of MIT with DIT. A small amount of reverse T$_3$ (rT$_3$) is also formed. Figure 20–4 shows the structures of MIT, DIT, T$_4$, T$_3$, and reverse T$_3$. In the normal thyroid, the average distribution of iodinated compounds is 23% MIT, 33% DIT, 35% T$_4$, 7% T$_3$, and 2% reverse T$_3$.

The thyroid secretes about 80 μg (103 nmol) of T$_4$ and 4 μg (7 nmol) of T$_3$ per day. The folds of the apical cell membrane (lamellipodia) encircle bits of colloid and bring them into the cytoplasm by endocytosis, forming **endosomes.** This process is accelerated by TSH. The endosomes fuse with lysosomes

containing proteases that break peptide bonds between the iodinated residues and thyroglobulin, releasing T$_4$, T$_3$, DIT, and MIT into the cytoplasm. The free T$_4$ and T$_3$ then cross the cell membrane and enter adjacent capillaries. The MIT and DIT are enzymatically degraded in the cell by thyroid deiodinase (iodotyrosine dehalogenase) to iodine and tyrosine, which are reused in colloid synthesis.

D. Thyroid Hormone Transport and Metabolism

The normal plasma level of T$_4$ is approximately 8 μg/dL (103 nmol/L) (range: 5–12 μg/dL or 65–156 nmol/L), and the normal plasma level of T$_3$ is approximately 0.15 μg/dL (2.3 nmol/L) (range: 0.08–0.22 μg/dL or 1.2–3.3 nmol/L). Both hormones are bound to plasma proteins, including albumin,

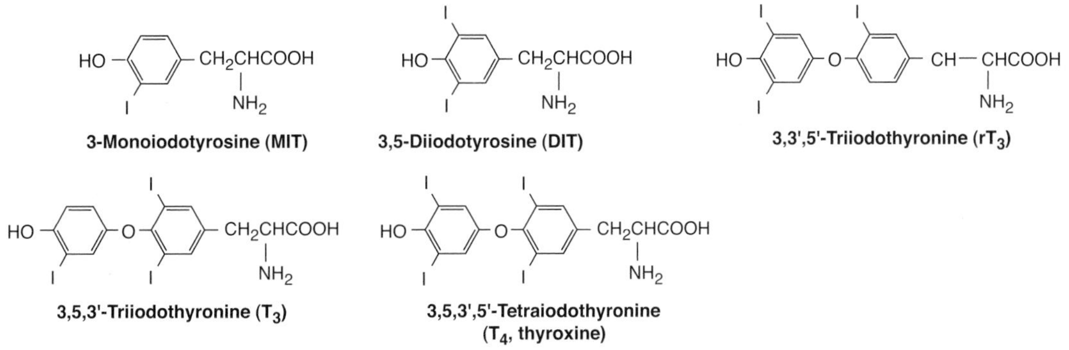

FIGURE 20–4 MIT, DIT, T$_3$, T$_4$, and rT$_3$.

transthyretin (formerly called thyroxine-binding prealbumin [TBPA]), and **thyroxine-binding globulin (TBG)**. The thyroid hormone-binding proteins serve mainly to transport T_4 and T_3 in the serum and to facilitate uniform distribution of hormones within tissues.

Physiologically, it is the free (unbound) T_4 and T_3 in plasma that are active and inhibit pituitary secretion of TSH. The free T_4 and T_3 are in equilibrium with the protein-bound hormones in plasma and tissue and circulate in much lower concentrations. Tissue uptake of the free hormones is proportionate to their plasma concentrations.

Almost all (99.98%) of the circulating T_4 is bound to thyroxine-binding globulin (TBG) and other plasma proteins, so that the free T_4 level is approximately 2 ng/dL. The biologic half-life of T_4 is long (about 6–7 days). Somewhat less T_3 (99.8%) is protein bound. Therefore, compared with T_4, T_3 acts more rapidly and has a shorter half-life (about 30 hours). It is also three to five times more potent on a molar basis.

T_4 and T_3 are metabolized in the liver, kidneys, and many other tissues by deiodination and by conjugation to **glucuronides**. Normally, one third of circulating T_4 is converted to T_3 by 5'-deiodination, and 45% is converted to the metabolically inert **reverse triiodothyronine (rT_3)** by 5-deiodination. About 87% of circulating T_3 derives from peripheral conversion of T_4 to T_3 and only 13% from thyroid secretion. Both T_4 and T_3 are conjugated to glucuronides in the liver and excreted into the bile. On passage into the intestine, the conjugates are hydrolyzed, and small amounts of T_4 and T_3 are reabsorbed (enterohepatic circulation). The rest is excreted in the stool.

Regulation of Thyroid Secretion

Thyroid hormone secretion is stimulated by pituitary **thyroid-stimulating hormone (TSH, thyrotropin)**. Pituitary TSH secretion is, in turn, stimulated by **thyrotropin-releasing hormone (TRH)**, a tripeptide secreted by the hypothalamus that also increases the biologic activity of TSH, by altering its glycosylation.

TSH is a two-subunit glycoprotein containing 211 amino acids. The α-subunit is identical to that of pituitary follicle-stimulating hormone (FSH), luteinizing hormone (LH), and placental human chorionic gonadotropin (hCG). The β-subunit confers the specific binding properties and biologic activity of TSH. The gene encoding the α-subunit is located on chromosome 6, and the gene for the β-subunit is on chromosome 1.

TSH has a biologic half-life of about 60 minutes. The average plasma level of TSH is 2 mU/L (normal range: 0.4–4.8 mU/L). When individuals with autoantibodies, goiter, or a family history of thyroid disease are excluded, the upper limit is somewhat lower, between 2.5–3.0 mU/L. Although the phenomenon is not clinically important, normal TSH secretion exhibits a circadian pattern, rising in the afternoon and evening, peaking after midnight, and declining during the day.

Circulating free T_4 and T_3 inhibit TSH secretion by the pituitary both directly and indirectly by regulating biosynthe-

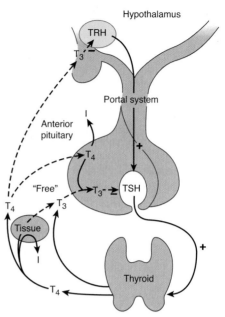

FIGURE 20–5 Hypothalamic-pituitary-thyroid axis. T_4, thyroxine; T_3, triiodothyronine; TRH, thyrotropin-releasing hormone; TSH, thyroid-stimulating hormone. (Redrawn and modified, with permission, from Greenspan FS, Gardner DG [editors]. *Basic and Clinical Endocrinology*, 8th ed. McGraw-Hill, 2007.)

sis of TRH in the hypothalamus. TSH secretion is inhibited by stress, perhaps via glucocorticoid inhibition of TRH secretion. In infants, but not in adults, TSH secretion is increased by cold and inhibited by warmth. Dopamine and somatostatin also inhibit pituitary secretion of TSH. In animals, there is a pituitary-specific form of the thyroid hormone receptor that may be selectively regulated by thyroid hormone. Figure 20–5 illustrates the hypothalamic-pituitary-thyroid axis and various stimulatory and inhibitory factors.

When TSH is secreted or administered, it binds to a specific **TSH receptor (TSH-R)** in the thyroid cell membrane, activating the GTP-binding (G_s) protein-adenylyl cyclase-cyclic adenosine monophosphate (cAMP) cascade. The increase in intracellular cAMP mediates immediate increases in uptake and transport of iodide, iodination of thyroglobulin, and synthesis of iodotyrosines T_3 and T_4. Within a few hours, there is an increase in mRNA for thyroglobulin and thyroidal peroxidase, enhanced lysosomal activity, increased secretion of thyroglobulin into colloid, more endocytosis of colloid, and increased secretion of T_4 and T_3 from the gland. TSH receptor is also expressed in lymphocytes and other tissues, including the pituitary, thymus, kidney, testis, brain, adipocytes, and fibroblasts. TSH-R has also been detected on osteoblast precursors, suggesting that TSH may have a direct effect on bone resorption.

TSH binding to TSH receptor also stimulates membrane phospholipase C, which leads to thyroid cell hypertrophy. With chronic TSH stimulation, the entire gland hypertrophies, increases in vascularity, and becomes a **goiter**.

TSH receptor has been cloned. It is a single-chain glycoprotein composed of 744 amino acids. Two specific amino acid sequences are thought to represent different binding sites for TSH and for the **TSH-R-stimulating antibody (TSH-R [stim] Ab)** found in Graves' disease (see later).

The amount of thyroid hormone needed to maintain normal organ system function in thyroidectomized individuals is defined as the amount necessary to maintain the plasma TSH within the normal range (0.4–4.8 mU/L). About 80% of orally administered levothyroxine is absorbed from the GI tract, and 100–125 μg/d usually maintains a normal plasma TSH in individuals of average size.

Mechanism of Action of Thyroid Hormones

Thyroid hormones enter cells by either passive diffusion or specific transport through the cell membrane and cytoplasm. Within the cell cytoplasm, most of the T_4 is converted to T_3. The nuclear receptor for T_3 has been cloned and found to be similar to the nuclear receptors for glucocorticoids, mineralocorticoids, estrogens, progestins, vitamin D_3, and retinoic acid. For reasons that are unclear, at least two different T_3 receptors, coded by different genes, exist in human tissues. The two biologically active human thyroid hormone receptors (hTR) are labeled hTR-α1 and hTR-β1. The gene for the alpha form is on chromosome 17 and for the beta form on chromosome 3. The two different receptor forms may help to explain both the normal variation in thyroid hormone responsiveness of various organs and the selective tissue abnormalities found in various thyroid resistance syndromes. For example, the brain contains mostly α receptors, the liver contains mostly β receptors, and the heart contains both. Point mutations in the *hTR-β1* gene result in abnormal T_3 receptors and the syndrome of **generalized resistance to thyroid hormone (Refetoff's syndrome)**.

When the T_3 receptor complex binds to DNA, it increases expression of specific genes, with the induction of messenger RNAs. A wide variety of enzymes must be produced to account for the many effects of thyroid hormones on cell function.

Effects of Thyroid Hormones

The effects of thyroid hormones in various organs are summarized in Table 20–1. Thyroid hormones increase the activity of membrane-bound Na^+-K^+ ATPase, increase heat production, and stimulate oxygen consumption (calorigenesis). Thyroid hormones also affect tissue growth and maturation, help regulate lipid metabolism, increase cardiac contractility by stimulating the expression of myosin protein, and increase intestinal absorption of carbohydrates.

The effects of T_4 and T_3 and the catecholamines epinephrine and norepinephrine are closely interrelated. Both increase the metabolic rate and stimulate the nervous system and heart. In humans, the transcriptional effects of T_3 include production of increased β-adrenergic receptors; in animals,

TABLE 20–1 Physiologic effects of thyroid hormones.

Target Tissue	Effect	Mechanism
Heart	Chronotropic	Increase number and affinity of β-adrenergic receptors
	Inotropic	Enhance responses to circulating catecholamines
		Increase proportion of alpha-myosin heavy chain (with higher ATPase activity)
Adipose tissue	Catabolic	Stimulate lipolysis
Muscle	Catabolic	Increase protein breakdown
Bone	Developmental and metabolic	Promote normal growth and skeletal development; accelerate bone turnover
Nervous system	Developmental	Promote normal brain development
Gut	Metabolic	Increase rate of carbohydrate absorption
Lipoprotein	Metabolic	Stimulate formation of LDL receptors
Other	Calorigenic	Stimulate oxygen consumption by metabolically active tissues (exceptions: adult brain, testes, uterus, lymph nodes, spleen, anterior pituitary)
		Increase metabolic rate

Key: ATPase, adenosine triphosphatase; LDL, low-density lipoprotein.

incubation of thyroid cells in a medium containing TSH increases the number of α_1-adrenergic receptors, presumably by inducing their biosynthesis.

CHECKPOINT

1. Describe a thyroid follicle and its change with activity versus inactivity of the gland.
2. What forms of thyroid hormone does the thyroid gland secrete? What are the normal proportions of the different forms? What are the relative potencies of each hormone?
3. To what is thyroid hormone bound during its transport in plasma?
4. How are thyroid hormone levels regulated?
5. What is the mechanism of action of thyroid hormone?
6. What are the most prominent organ system–specific effects of thyroid hormone?

OVERVIEW OF THYROID DISEASE

The symptoms and signs of thyroid disease in humans are predictable consequences of the physiologic effects of thyroid hormones discussed previously. The clinician commonly encounters patients with one of five types of thyroid dysfunction: (1) **hyperthyroidism** (thyrotoxicosis), caused by an excess of thyroid hormones; (2) **hypothyroidism** (myxedema), caused by a deficiency of thyroid hormones; (3) **goiter,** a diffuse enlargement of the thyroid gland, caused by prolonged elevation of TSH; (4) **thyroid nodule,** a focal enlargement of a portion of the gland, caused by a benign or malignant neoplasm; and (5) **abnormal thyroid function tests** in a clinically euthyroid patient.

Several laboratory tests are useful in the initial evaluation of patients suspected of having thyroid dysfunction. The first is plasma TSH measured by a sensitive assay (usually defined by a lower detection limit of 0.1 mU/L or less). TSH is below normal in hyperthyroidism and above normal in hypothyroidism (except in the rare instances of pituitary or hypothalamic disease). The second useful laboratory test is measurement of non-protein-bound thyroxine. Most clinical laboratories are now able to accurately measure free thyroxine (FT_4) directly. Although rarely used today, an estimate of non-protein-bound thyroxine is provided by the free thyroxine index (FT_4I), the product of the total plasma thyroxine (TT_4) and the T_4 resin uptake (RT_4U) (ie, $FT_4I = TT_4 \times RT_4U$). The TT_4 by itself often reflects the functional state of the thyroid hormone–binding proteins. The RT_4U is an indicator of thyroid-binding globulin and serves to correct for alterations in the concentration of binding protein. Some laboratories instead measure T_3 resin uptake (RT_3U).

Although total and free T_3 levels can be measured, they have a short half-life and are technically difficult assays. Under most circumstances, circulating levels of T_3 correlate less well with clinical hyperthyroidism or hypothyroidism.

A variety of thyroid autoantibodies are detectable in patients with thyroid dysfunction, including (1) **thyroidal peroxidase antibody** (**TPO Ab**), formerly termed antimicrosomal antibody; (2) **thyroglobulin antibody** (**Tg Ab**); and (3) **TSH receptor antibody,** either **stimulating** (**TSH-R [stim] Ab**) or **blocking** (**TSH-R [block] Ab**). Thyroglobulin and thyroidal peroxidase antibodies are commonly found in hypothyroidism resulting from Hashimoto's thyroiditis and occasionally in hyperthyroidism from Graves' disease (see later). TSH-R [stim] Ab is present in individuals with hyperthyroidism caused by Graves' disease. Detection of TSH-R [block] Ab in maternal serum is predictive of congenital hypothyroidism in newborns of mothers with autoimmune thyroid disease.

Other procedures such as thyroid scans and the thyrotropin-releasing hormone (TRH) test are discussed later.

PATHOPHYSIOLOGY OF SELECTED THYROID DISEASES

The pathogenesis of the most common thyroid diseases probably involves an autoimmune process with sensitization of the host's own lymphocytes to various thyroidal antigens. Three major thyroidal antigens have been documented: thyroglobulin (Tg), thyroidal peroxidase (TPO), and the TSH receptor. Both environmental factors (eg, viral or bacterial infection or high iodine intake) and genetic factors (eg, defect in suppressor T lymphocytes) may be responsible for initiating autoimmune thyroid disease.

HYPERTHYROIDISM

Etiology

The causes of hyperthyroidism are listed in Table 20–2. Most commonly, thyroid hormone overproduction is due to Graves' disease. In Graves' disease, the TSH receptor autoantibody TSH-R [stim] Ab stimulates the thyroid follicular cells to produce excessive amounts of T_4 and T_3. Less commonly, patients with multinodular goiter may become thyrotoxic without circulating antibodies if given inorganic iodine (eg, potassium iodide) or organic iodine compounds (eg, the antiarrhythmic drug amiodarone, which contains 37% iodine by weight). Multinodular goiters may also develop one or more nodules that become autonomous from TSH regulation and secrete excessive quantities of T_4 or T_3. Patients from regions where goiter is endemic may develop thyrotoxicosis when given iodine supplementation (jod-basedow phenomenon). Large follicular adenomas (> 3 cm in diameter) may produce excessive thyroid hormone.

Occasionally, TSH overproduction (eg, from a pituitary adenoma) or hypothalamic disease may cause excessive thyroid hormone production. The diagnosis is suggested by clinically evident hyperthyroidism with elevated serum T_4 and T_3 and *elevated* serum TSH levels. Neuroradiologic procedures such as computed tomography (CT) scans or magnetic resonance imaging (MRI) of the sella turcica confirm the presence of a pituitary tumor. Even more rarely, hyperthyroidism results from TSH overproduction caused by pituitary (but not peripheral tissue) resistance to the suppressive effects of T_4 and T_3. The diagnosis is suggested by finding elevated serum T_4 and T_3 levels with an inappropriately normal serum TSH level.

Hyperthyroidism may be precipitated by germ cell tumors (choriocarcinoma and hydatidiform mole), which secrete large quantities of human chorionic gonadotropin (hCG). The large

TABLE 20–2 Hyperthyroidism: causes and pathogenetic mechanisms.

Etiologic Classification	Pathogenetic Mechanism
Thyroid hormone overproduction	
Graves' disease	Thyroid-stimulating hormone receptor-stimulating antibody (TSH-R [stim] Ab)
Toxic multinodular goiter	Autonomous hyperfunction
Follicular adenoma	Autonomous hyperfunction
Pituitary adenoma	TSH hypersecretion (rare)
Pituitary insensitivity	Resistance to thyroid hormone (rare)
Hypothalamic disease	Excess TRH production
Germ cell tumors: choriocarcinoma, hydatidiform mole	Human chorionic gonadotropin stimulation
Struma ovarii (ovarian teratoma)	Functioning thyroid elements
Metastatic follicular thyroid carcinoma	Functioning metastases
Thyroid gland destruction	
Lymphocytic thyroiditis	Release of stored hormone
Granulomatous (subacute) thyroiditis	Release of stored hormone
Hashimoto's thyroiditis	Transient release of stored hormone
Drug effect	
Thyrotoxicosis medicamentosa, thyrotoxicosis factitia	Ingestion of excessive exogenous thyroid hormone
Amiodarone	Excess iodine and/or thyroiditis
Interferon alpha	Thyroiditis

quantities of hCG secreted by these tumors bind to the follicular cell TSH receptor and stimulate overproduction of thyroid hormone. Rarely, hyperthyroidism can be produced by ovarian teratomas containing thyroid tissue (struma ovarii). Hyperthyroidism results when this ectopic thyroid tissue begins to function autonomously. Patients with large metastases from follicular thyroid carcinomas may produce excess thyroid hormone, particularly after iodide administration.

Transient hyperthyroidism is occasionally observed in patients with lymphocytic or granulomatous (subacute) thyroiditis (Hashimoto's thyroiditis). In such cases, the hyperthyroidism is due to destruction of the thyroid with release of stored hormone.

Finally, patients who consume excessive amounts of exogenous thyroid hormone (accidentally or deliberately) and those treated with amiodarone or interferon alpha may present with symptoms, signs, and laboratory findings of hyperthyroidism.

Pathogenesis

Whatever the cause of hyperthyroidism, serum thyroid hormones are elevated. Both the free thyroxine (FT_4) and the free thyroxine index (FT_4I) are elevated. In 5–10% of patients, T_4 secretion is normal while T_3 levels are high (so-called **T_3 toxicosis**). Total serum T_4 and T_3 levels are not always definitive because of variations in concentrations of thyroid hormone–binding proteins.

Hyperthyroidism resulting from Graves' disease is characterized by a suppressed serum TSH level as determined by sensitive immunoenzymometric or immunoradiometric assays. However, TSH levels may also be suppressed in some acute psychiatric and other nonthyroidal illnesses. In the rare TSH-secreting pituitary adenomas (so-called **secondary hyperthyroidism**) and in hypothalamic disease with excessive TRH production (so-called **tertiary hyperthyroidism**), hyperthyroidism is accompanied by elevated plasma TSH.

The radioactive iodine (RAI) uptake of the thyroid gland at 4, 6, or 24 hours is increased when the gland produces an excess of hormone (eg, Graves' disease); it is decreased when the gland is leaking stored hormone (eg, thyroiditis), when hormone is produced elsewhere (eg, struma ovarii), and when excessive exogenous thyroid hormone is being ingested (eg, factitious hyperthyroidism). Technetium 99m scanning can provide information similar to that obtained with RAI and is quicker and entails less radiation exposure.

The TRH test is sometimes helpful in diagnosis when patients have confusing results of thyroid function tests. In normal individuals, administration of TRH (500 μg intravenously) produces an increase in serum TSH of at least 6 mU/L within 15–30 minutes. In primary hyperthyroidism, TSH levels are low and TRH administration induces little or no rise in the TSH level.

Graves' Disease

A. Pathology

Graves' disease is the most common cause of hyperthyroidism. In this condition, the thyroid gland is symmetrically enlarged and its vascularity markedly increased. The gland may double or triple in weight. Microscopically, the follicular epithelial cells are columnar in appearance and increased in number and size (Figure 20–2). The follicles are small and closely packed together. The colloid is scanty; the edges are scalloped in appearance secondary to the rapid proteolysis of thyroglobulin. The gland's interstitium is diffusely infiltrated with lymphocytes and may contain lymphoid follicles with germinal centers.

B. Pathogenesis

The serum of more than 90% of patients with Graves' disease contains TSH-R [stim] Ab, an antibody directed against the TSH receptor site in the thyroid follicular epithelial

TABLE 20–3 Autoimmune disorders associated with Graves' disease and Hashimoto's thyroiditis.

Endocrine disorders
Diabetes mellitus
Hypoadrenalism, autoimmune (Addison's disease)
Orchitis or oophoritis, autoimmune
Hypoparathyroidism, idiopathic
Nonendocrine disorders
Pernicious anemia
Vitiligo
Systemic lupus erythematosus
Rheumatoid arthritis
Immune thrombocytopenic purpura
Myasthenia gravis
Sjögren's syndrome
Primary biliary cirrhosis
Chronic active hepatitis

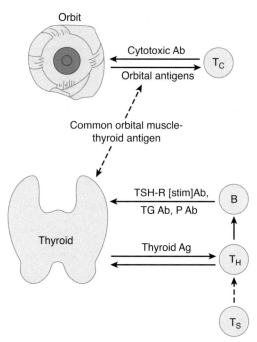

FIGURE 20–6   Proposed pathogenesis of Graves' disease. A defect in suppressor T lymphocytes (T_S) allows helper T lymphocytes (T_H) to stimulate B lymphocytes (B) to synthesize thyroid autoantibodies. The thyroid receptor–stimulating antibody (TSH-R [stim] Ab) is the driving force for thyrotoxicosis. Inflammation of the orbital muscles may be due to sensitization of cytotoxic T lymphocytes (T_C), or killer cells, to orbital antigens linked to an antigen in the thyroid. What triggers this immunologic cascade is not known. Ag, antigen; P Ab, peroxidase or microsomal antibody; Tg Ab, thyroglobulin antibody.   (Redrawn, with permission, from Greenspan FS, Gardner DG. *Basic and Clinical Endocrinology*, 8th ed. McGraw-Hill, 2007.)

membrane. This antibody was formerly called long-acting thyroid stimulator (LATS) or thyroid-stimulating immunoglobulin (TSI). When it binds to the cell membrane TSH receptors, TSH-R [stim] Ab stimulates hormone synthesis and secretion in somewhat the same way as TSH. Although serum levels of TSH-R [stim] Ab correlate poorly with disease severity, its presence can be helpful diagnostically and perhaps prognostically. After discontinuation of antithyroid drug treatment, about 30–50% of patients with Graves' hyperthyroidism relapse. There seems to be a greatly increased recurrence risk if the TSH-R [stim] Ab is still found in plasma at the time of discontinuation of the antithyroid drug treatment, so this test can perhaps be used to predict likely relapse.

The genesis of TSH-R [stim] Ab in patients with Graves' disease is uncertain. However, Graves' disease is familial. A genetic contribution to the development of Graves' disease is suggested by the finding of much higher concordance rates in monozygotic same-sex twin pairs (0.35) than in dizygotic pairs (0.03). In Caucasians, it is associated with the HLA-B8 and HLA-DR3 histocompatibility antigens; in Asians, with HLA-Bw46 and HLA-B5; and in blacks, with HLA-B17. Furthermore, patients with Graves' disease frequently suffer from other autoimmune disorders (Table 20–3). The precipitating cause of this antibody production is unknown, but an immune response against a viral antigen that shares homology with TSH receptor may be responsible. Another theory of the pathogenesis of Graves' disease is a defect of suppressor T

lymphocytes, which allows helper T lymphocytes to stimulate B lymphocytes to secrete antibodies directed against follicular cell membrane antigens, including the TSH receptor (Figure 20–6).

Moderate titers of other autoantibodies (thyroidal peroxidase antibody and TSH-R [block] Ab) can be found in patients with Graves' disease. Their significance is uncertain. In some cases, TSH-R [block] Ab appears after ^{131}I radioiodine therapy of Graves' disease.

Patients with hyperthyroidism from Graves' disease may later develop hypothyroidism by one of several mechanisms: (1) thyroid ablation by surgery or ^{131}I radiation treatment; (2) autoimmune thyroiditis, leading to thyroid destruction; and (3) development of antibodies that block TSH stimulation (TSH-R [block] Ab).

After radioactive iodine therapy, there is often a lag in recovery of thyrotropin (TSH) responsiveness that may last 60–90 days or longer. During this period, decisions regarding further therapy must be based on the patient's clinical status as well as on the serum levels of TSH and thyroid hormones.

Clinical Manifestations

The clinical consequences of thyroid hormone excess (Table 20–4) are exaggerated expressions of the physiologic activity of T_3 and T_4.

An excess of thyroid hormone causes enough extra heat production to result in a slight rise in body temperature and to activate heat-dissipating mechanisms, including cutaneous vasodilation and a decrease in peripheral vascular resistance and increased sweating. The increased basal metabolic rate leads to weight loss, especially in older patients with poor appetite. In younger patients, food intake typically increases, and some patients have seemingly insatiable appetites.

The apparent increased catecholamine effect of hyperthyroidism is probably multifactorial in origin. Thyroid hormones increase β-adrenergic receptors in many tissues, including heart muscle, skeletal muscle, adipose tissue, and lymphocytes. They also decrease α-adrenergic receptors in heart muscle and may amplify catecholamine action at a postreceptor site. Thus, thyrotoxicosis is characterized by an increased metabolic and hemodynamic sensitivity of the tissues to catecholamines. However, circulating catecholamine levels are normal. Drugs that block β-adrenergic receptors reduce or eliminate the tachycardia, arrhythmias, sweating, and tremor of hyperthyroidism. When beta-blockers are used in the treatment of hyperthyroidism, it appears that "nonselective" β-blockers (such as propranolol), which block both β_1 and β_2 receptors, have an advantage over "selective" β_1-blockers (such as metoprolol). The "nonselective" agents appear to reduce the metabolic rate significantly, whereas the "selective" β_1 blockers do not reduce oxygen consumption and provide only symptomatic relief related to the normalization of heart rate.

Thyroid hormone excess causes rapid mentation, nervousness, irritability, emotional lability, restlessness, and even mania and psychosis. Patients complain of poor concentration and reduced performance at work or in school. Tremor is common and deep tendon reflexes are brisk, with a rapid relaxation phase. Muscle weakness and atrophy (**thyrotoxic myopathy**) commonly develop in hyperthyroidism, particularly if severe and prolonged. Proximal muscle weakness may interfere with walking, climbing, rising from a deep knee bend, or weight lift-ing. Such muscle weakness may be due to increased protein catabolism and muscle wasting, decreased muscle efficiency, or changes in myosin. Despite an increased number of β-adrenergic receptors in muscle, the increased proteolysis is apparently not mediated by β receptors, and muscle weakness and wasting are not affected by β-adrenergic blockers. Myasthenia gravis or periodic paralysis may accompany hyperthyroidism.

Vital capacity and respiratory muscle strength are reduced. Extreme muscle weakness may cause respiratory failure.

In hyperthyroidism, cardiac output is increased as a result of increased heart rate and contractility and reduced peripheral vascular resistance. Pulse pressure is increased, and circulation time is shortened in the hyperthyroid state. Tachycardia, usually supraventricular, is frequent and thought to be related to the direct effects of thyroid hormone on the cardiac conducting system. Atrial fibrillation may occur, particularly in elderly patients. Continuous 24-hour electrocardiographic monitoring of thyrotoxic patients shows persistent tachycardia but preservation of the normal circadian rhythm of the heart rate, suggesting that normal adrenergic responsiveness persists.

TABLE 20–4 Clinical findings in hyperthyroidism (thyrotoxicosis).

Symptoms
Alertness, emotional lability, nervousness, irritability
Poor concentration
Muscular weakness, fatigability
Palpitations
Voracious appetite, weight loss
Hyperdefecation (increased frequency of bowel movements)
Heat intolerance
Signs
Hyperkinesia, rapid speech
Proximal muscle (quadriceps) weakness, fine tremor
Fine, moist skin; fine, abundant hair; onycholysis
Lid lag, stare, chemosis, periorbital edema, proptosis
Accentuated first heart sound, tachycardia, atrial fibrillation (resistant to digitalis), widened pulse pressure, dyspnea
Laboratory findings
Suppressed serum TSH level
Elevated serum free thyroxine, elevated serum total T_4, elevated resin T_3 or T_4 uptake, elevated free thyroxine index
Increased radioiodine uptake by thyroid gland (some causes)
Increased basal metabolic rate
Decreased serum cholesterol level

Myocardial calcium uptake is increased in thyrotoxic rats; in humans, calcium channel–blocking agents (eg, diltiazem) can decrease heart rate, number of premature ventricular beats, and number of bouts of supraventricular tachycardia, paroxysmal atrial fibrillation, and ventricular tachycardia. Patients with hyperthyroidism may manifest acute heart failure as a result of left ventricular dysfunction with segmental wall motion abnormalities; its rapid reversibility with treatment suggests that it may be due to myocardial "stunning." Long-standing hyperthyroidism may lead to cardiomegaly and a "high-output" congestive heart failure. Flow murmurs are common and extracardiac sounds occur, generated by the hyperdynamic heart.

Hyperthyroidism leads to increased hepatic gluconeogenesis, enhanced carbohydrate absorption, and increased insulin degradation. In nondiabetic patients, after ingestion of carbohydrate, the blood glucose rises rapidly, sometimes causing glycosuria, and then falls rapidly. There may be an adaptive increase in insulin secretion, perhaps explaining the normal glycemic, glycogenolytic, glycolytic, and ketogenic sensitivity to epinephrine. Diabetic patients have an increased insulin requirement in the hyperthyroid state.

Metabolically, the total plasma cholesterol is usually low, related to an increase in the number of hepatic low-density lipoprotein (LDL) receptors. Lipolysis is increased, and adipocytes show an increase in β-adrenergic receptor density and increased responsiveness to catecholamines. With the rise in metabolic rate, there is also an increased need for vitamins; if dietary sources are inadequate, vitamin deficiency syndromes may occur. Normally, thyroid hormone stimulates osteoblastic production of insulin-like growth factor-I (IGF-I), clearly important for the anabolic effects of thyroid hormone on bone. In hyperthyroid patients, levels of serum IGF-I and several binding proteins (IGFBP-3 and IGFBP-4) are significantly increased before treatment and return to normal after antithyroid drug treatment. In addition, because of enhanced osteoblastic and osteoclastic activity, overtly hyperthyroid patients frequently exhibit accelerated bone turnover and negative calcium and phosphorus balance, resulting in low bone mineral density and increased skeletal fragility. Hypercalciuria and sometimes hypercalcemia can occur. Normalization of thyroid function is associated with a significant attenuation of increased bone turnover followed by an increase in bone mineral density.

There is an increase in frequency of bowel movements (hyperdefecation) as a result of increased GI motility. Accelerated small bowel transit may be caused by increased frequency of bowel contractions and of giant migrating contractions. In severe thyrotoxicosis, abnormal liver function tests may be observed, reflecting malnutrition. Anorexia in untreated hyperthyroidism is associated with older age, anxiety, and abnormal liver function but not with hypercalcemia.

In women, hyperthyroidism may lead to oligomenorrhea and decreased fertility. In the follicular phase of the menstrual cycle, there is an increased basal plasma LH and an increased LH and FSH response to GnRH (Chapter 22). There is an increase in sex hormone–binding globulin, leading to increased levels of total estradiol. In men, hyperthyroidism may cause decreased

fertility and impotence from altered steroid hormone metabolism. Serum levels of total testosterone, total estradiol, sex hormone–binding globulin, LH, and FSH and gonadotropin response to GnRH are significantly greater than normal. However, the ratio of free testosterone to free estradiol is lower than normal. Mean sperm counts are normal, but the percentage of forward progressive sperm motility is lower than normal (Chapter 23). These hormone and semen abnormalities are reversible with successful treatment of the hyperthyroidism. Gynecomastia may occur despite high normal serum testosterone levels secondary to increased peripheral conversion of androgens to estrogens (Chapter 23).

There is an increased plasma concentration of atrial natriuretic peptide (ANP) and its precursors. The plasma ANP concentration correlates with the serum thyroxine level and heart rate and decreases to normal with successful antithyroid therapy.

The wide-eyed stare of hyperthyroid patients may be due to increased sympathetic tone. In addition, proptosis develops in 25–50% of patients with Graves' disease as a result of infiltration of orbital soft tissues and extraocular muscles with lymphocytes, mucopolysaccharides, and edema fluid (Figure 20–7). This may lead to fibrosis of the extraocular muscles, restricted ocular motility, and diplopia. In severe Graves' ophthalmopathy, pressure on the optic nerve or keratitis from corneal exposure may lead to blindness. In patients with Graves' disease, it is clear that thyroid-stimulating antibody is related to Graves' ophthalmopathy. In

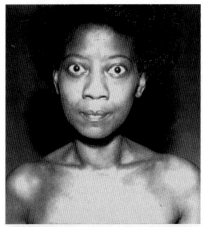
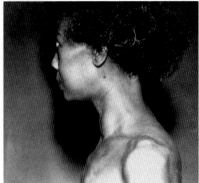

FIGURE 20–7 Graves' disease. (Reproduced with permission of PH Forsham.)

addition, autoantibodies against G2s, a 55-kDa protein found in both thyroid and eye muscle tissue, are definitely associated with Graves' ophthalmopathy. For instance, antibodies reactive with G2s are identified in significantly more patients with active thyroid ophthalmopathy than in patients with Graves' disease without ophthalmopathy, those with Hashimoto's thyroiditis or nonimmunologic thyroid disorders, and those without thyroid disease. The pathogenesis of Graves' ophthalmopathy may involve cytotoxic lymphocytes (killer cells) and cytotoxic antibodies to an antigen common to orbital fibroblasts, orbital muscle, and thyroid tissue (Figure 20–6). It is postulated that cytokines released from these sensitized lymphocytes cause inflammation of orbital tissues, resulting in the proptosis, diplopia, and edema. For unknown reasons, Graves' ophthalmopathy is worse in smokers and may be exacerbated by radioiodine therapy.

The skin is warm, sweaty, and velvety in texture. Hyperpigmentation can be seen on the lower extremities, most strikingly on the shins, the backs of the feet, and the nail beds. The hyperpigmentation is due to basal melanosis and heavy deposition of hemosiderin around dermal capillaries and sweat glands. Its distribution, hemosiderin deposition, and poor response to treatment distinguish it from the hyperpigmentation seen with Addison's disease. There may be onycholysis (ie, retraction of the nail from the nail plate). In Graves' disease, the pretibial skin may become thickened, resembling an orange peel (**pretibial myxedema** or **thyrotoxic dermopathy**). The dermopathy is usually a late manifestation of Graves' disease, and affected patients invariably have ophthalmopathy. The most common form of the dermopathy is nonpitting edema, but nodular, plaque-like, and even polypoid forms also occur. The pathogenesis of thyroid dermopathy may also involve lymphocyte cytokine stimulation of fibroblasts. Thyroid dermopathy is associated with a very high serum titer of TSH-R [stim] Ab.

Untreated hyperthyroidism may decompensate into a state called **thyroid storm.** Patients so affected have tachycardia, fever, agitation, nausea, vomiting, diarrhea, and restlessness or psychosis. The condition is usually precipitated by an intercurrent illness or by a surgical emergency.

CHECKPOINT

12. Describe the physiologic consequences of hyperthyroidism and identify their mechanism (as is best known) on the following systems:

Heart
Liver
Lungs
GI tract
Kidney
Eyes
Skin
Brain
Bone
Reproductive system

HYPOTHYROIDISM

Etiology

The causes of hypothyroidism are listed in Table 20–5. The most common cause is Hashimoto's thyroiditis, which probably results from an autoimmune destruction of the thyroid, although the precipitating cause and exact mechanism of the autoimmunity and subsequent destruction are unknown. Hypothyroidism may also be caused by lymphocytic thyroiditis after a transient period of hyperthyroidism. Thyroid ablation,

TABLE 20–5 Hypothyroidism: causes and pathogenetic mechanisms.

Etiologic Classification	Pathogenetic Mechanism
Congenital	Aplasia or hypoplasia of thyroid gland
	Defects in hormone biosynthesis or action
Acquired	
Hashimoto's thyroiditis	Autoimmune destruction
Severe iodine deficiency	Diminished hormone synthesis, release
Lymphocytic thyroiditis	Diminished hormone synthesis, release
Thyroid ablation	Diminished hormone synthesis, release
Thyroid surgery	
^{131}I radiation treatment of hyperthyroidism	
External beam radiation therapy of head and neck cancer	
Drugs	Diminished hormone synthesis, release
Iodine, inorganic	
Iodine, organic (amiodarone)	
Thioamides (propylthiouracil,[1] methimazole)	
Potassium perchlorate	
Thiocyanate	
Lithium	
Amiodarone	
Sunitinib	
Hypopituitarism	Deficient TSH secretion
Hypothalamic disease	Deficient TRH secretion

[1]Also blocks peripheral conversion of T_4 to T_3.

whether by surgical resection or by therapeutic radiation, commonly results in hypothyroidism.

Congenital hypothyroidism, a preventable cause of mental retardation, occurs in approximately 1 in 4000 births; girls are affected about twice as often as boys. Most cases (85%) are sporadic in distribution, but 15% are hereditary. The most common cause of sporadic congenital hypothyroidism is thyroid dysgenesis, in which hypofunctioning ectopic thyroid tissue is more common than thyroid hypoplasia or aplasia. Although the pathogenesis of thyroid dysgenesis is largely unknown, some cases have been described as resulting from mutations in the transcription factors PAX-8 and TTF-2. The most common problems causing hereditary congenital hypothyroidism are inborn errors of thyroxine (T_4) synthesis. Mutations have been described in the genes coding for the sodium iodide transporter, thyroid peroxidase (TPO), and thyroglobulin. Other cases of congenital hypothyroidism are caused by loss of function mutations in the TSH receptor. Finally, a transient form of familial congenital hypothyroidism is caused by transplacental passage of a maternal TSH receptor blocking antibody (**TSH-R [block] Ab**).

Central hypothyroidism, characterized by insufficient TSH secretion in the presence of low levels of thyroid hormones, is a rare disorder. It is caused by diseases of the pituitary or hypothalamus that result in diminished or abnormal TSH secretion, such as tumors or infiltrative diseases of the hypothalamopituitary area, pituitary atrophy, and inactivating mutations in genes that code for the various proteins involved in regulation of the hypothalamic-pituitary-thyroid axis (Figure 20–5). For example, mutations have been identified in the genes for the TRH receptor, the transcription factors Pit-1 and PROP1, and the TSH β-subunit. Pituitary ("secondary") hypothyroidism is characterized by a diminished number of functioning thyrotropes in the pituitary gland, accounting for a quantitative impairment of TSH secretion. Hypothalamic ("tertiary") hypothyroidism is characterized by normal or sometimes even increased TSH concentrations but qualitative abnormalities of the TSH secreted. These abnormalities cause the circulating TSH to lack biologic activity and to exhibit impaired binding to its receptor. This defect can be reversed by administration of TRH. Thus, TRH may regulate not only the secretion of TSH but also the specific molecular and conformational features that enable it to act at its receptor.

Finally, a variety of drugs, including the thioamide antithyroid medications propylthiouracil and methimazole, may produce hypothyroidism. The thioamides inhibit thyroid peroxidase and block the synthesis of thyroid hormone. In addition, propylthiouracil, but not methimazole, blocks the peripheral conversion of T_4 to T_3. Deiodination of iodine-containing compounds such as amiodarone, releasing large amounts of iodide, may also cause hypothyroidism by blocking iodide organification, an effect known as the Wolff-Chaikoff block. Lithium is concentrated by the thyroid and inhibits the release of hormone from the gland. Most patients treated with lithium compensate by increasing TSH secretion, but some become hypothyroid. Lithium-associated clinical hypothyroidism occurs in about 10% of patients receiving the drug. It occurs more commonly in middle-aged women, particularly during the first 2 years of lithium treatment.

Pathogenesis

Hypothyroidism is characterized by abnormally low serum T_4 and T_3 levels. Free thyroxine levels are always depressed. The serum TSH level is elevated in hypothyroidism (except in cases of pituitary or hypothalamic disease). TSH is the most sensitive test for early hypothyroidism, and marked elevations of serum TSH (> 20 mU/L) are found in frank hypothyroidism. Modest TSH elevations (5–20 mU/L) may be found in euthyroid individuals with normal serum T_4 and T_3 levels and indicate impaired thyroid reserve and incipient hypothyroidism. In patients with primary hypothyroidism (end-organ failure), the nocturnal TSH surge is intact. In patients with central (pituitary or hypothalamic) hypothyroidism, the serum TSH level is low and the normal nocturnal TSH surge is absent.

In hypothyroidism resulting from thyroid gland failure, administration of TRH produces a prompt rise in the TSH level, the magnitude of which is proportionate to the baseline serum TSH level. The hypernormal response is caused by absence of feedback inhibition by T_4 and T_3. However, the TRH test is not usually performed in patients with primary hypothyroidism because the elevated basal serum TSH level suffices to make the diagnosis. The test may be useful in the clinically hypothyroid patient with an unexpectedly low serum TSH level in establishing a central (pituitary or hypothalamic) origin. Pituitary disease is suggested by the failure of TSH to rise after TRH administration; hypothalamic disease is suggested by a delayed TSH response (at 60–120 minutes rather than 15–30 minutes) with a normal increment.

Hashimoto's Thyroiditis

A. Pathology

In the early stages of Hashimoto's thyroiditis, the gland is diffusely enlarged, firm, rubbery, and nodular. As the disease progresses, the gland becomes smaller. In the late stages, the gland is atrophic and fibrotic, weighing as little as 10–20 g. Microscopically, there is destruction of thyroid follicles and lymphocytic infiltration with lymphoid follicles. The surviving thyroid follicular epithelial cells are large, with abundant pink cytoplasm (Hürthle cells). As the disease progresses, there is an increasing amount of fibrosis.

B. Pathogenesis

The pathogenesis of Hashimoto's thyroiditis is unclear. Again, it is possible that a defect in suppressor T lymphocytes allows helper T lymphocytes to interact with specific antigens on the thyroid follicular cell membrane. Once these lymphocytes become sensitized to thyroidal antigens, autoantibodies are formed that react with these antigens. Cytokine release and inflammation then cause glandular destruction. The most important thyroid autoantibodies in Hashimoto's thyroiditis are thyroglobulin antibody (Tg Ab), thyroidal peroxidase antibody (TPO Ab) (formerly termed antimicrosomal antibody), and the TSH receptor blocking antibody (TSH-R [block] Ab). During the early phases, Tg Ab is markedly elevated and TPO Ab only slightly elevated. Later, Tg Ab may disappear, but TPO Ab persists for many years. TSH-R [block] Ab is found in patients with atrophic thyroiditis and myxedema and in mothers who give birth to infants with no detectable thyroid tissue (**athyreotic cretins**). Serum levels of these antibodies do not correlate with the severity of the hypothyroidism, but their presence is helpful in diagnosis. In general, high antibody titers are diagnostic of Hashimoto's thyroiditis; moderate titers are seen in Graves' disease, multinodular goiter, and thyroid neoplasm; and low titers are found in the elderly.

Patients with Hashimoto's thyroiditis have an increased frequency of the HLA-DR5 histocompatibility antigen, and the disease is associated with a host of other autoimmune diseases (Table 20–3). A **polyglandular failure syndrome** has been defined in which two or more endocrine disorders mediated by autoimmune mechanisms occur (Chapter 17). Affected patients frequently have circulating organ- and cell-specific autoantibodies that lead to organ hypofunction.

CHECKPOINT

13. What are some drugs that cause hypothyroidism?
14. What are the most useful initial tests of thyroid function in hypothyroidism? What results would you expect compared with normal?
15. What are the key pathophysiologic findings in Hashimoto's thyroiditis?

Clinical Manifestations

The clinical consequences of thyroid hormone deficiency are summarized in Table 20–6.

Hypothermia is common, and the patient may complain of cold intolerance. The decreased basal metabolic rate leads to weight gain despite reduced food intake.

Thyroid hormones are required for normal development of the nervous system. In hypothyroid infants, synapses develop abnormally, myelination is defective, and mental retardation occurs. Hypothyroid adults have several reversible neurologic abnormalities, including slowed mentation, forgetfulness, decreased hearing, and ataxia. Some patients have severe mental symptoms, including reversible dementia or overt psychosis ("myxedema madness"). The cerebrospinal fluid protein level is abnormally high. However, total cerebral blood flow and oxygen consumption are normal. Deep tendon reflexes are sluggish, with a slowed ("hung-up") relaxation phase. Paresthesias are common, often caused by compression neuropathies resulting from accumulation of myxedema (carpal tunnel syndrome and tarsal tunnel syndrome).

TABLE 20–6 Clinical findings in adult hypothyroidism (myxedema).

Symptoms
Slow thinking
Lethargy, decreased vigor
Dry skin; thickened hair; hair loss; broken nails
Diminished food intake; weight gain
Constipation
Menorrhagia; diminished libido
Cold intolerance
Signs
Round puffy face; slow speech; hoarseness
Hypokinesis; generalized muscle weakness; delayed relaxation of deep tendon reflexes
Cold, dry, thick, scaling skin; dry, coarse, brittle hair; dry, longitudinally ridged nails
Periorbital edema
Normal or faint cardiac impulse; indistinct heart sounds; cardiac enlargement; bradycardia
Ascites; pericardial effusion; ankle edema
Mental clouding, depression
Laboratory findings
Increased serum TSH level
Decreased serum free thyroxine, decreased serum total T_4 and T_3; decreased resin T_3 or T_4 uptake; decreased free thyroxine index
Decreased radioiodine uptake by thyroid gland
Diminished basal metabolic rate
Macrocytic anemia
Elevated serum cholesterol level
Elevated serum CK level
Hyponatremia (from excess secretion of antidiuretic hormone)
Decreased circulation time; low voltage of QRS complex on ECG

Hypothyroidism is associated with muscle weakness, cramps, and stiffness. The serum creatine kinase (CK) level may be elevated. The pathophysiology of the muscle disease in hypothyroidism is poorly understood. Study of the bioenergetic abnormalities in hypothyroid muscle suggests a hormone-dependent, reversible mitochondrial impairment. Changes in energy metabolism are not found in hyperthyroid muscle.

Patients rendered acutely hypothyroid by total thyroidectomy exhibit a decreased cardiac output, decreased stroke volume, decreased diastolic volume at rest, and increased peripheral resistance. However, the pulmonary capillary wedge pressure, right atrial pressure, heart rate, left ventricular ejection fraction, and left ventricular systolic pressure-volume relation (a measure of contractility) are not significantly different from the euthyroid state. Thus, in early hypothyroidism, alterations in cardiac performance are probably primarily related to changes in loading conditions and exercise-related heart rate rather than to changes in myocardial contractility.

In chronic hypothyroidism, echocardiography shows bradycardia and features that suggest cardiomyopathy, including increased thickening of the intraventricular septum and ventricular wall, decreased regional wall motion, and decreased systolic and diastolic global left ventricular function. These changes may be due to deposition of excessive mucopolysaccharides in the interstitium between myocardial fibers, leading to fiber degeneration, decreased contractility, low cardiac output, cardiac enlargement, and congestive heart failure. Pericardial effusion (with high protein content) may lead to findings of decreased electrocardiographic voltage and flattened T waves, but cardiac tamponade is rare.

Hypothyroid patients exhibit decreased ventilatory responses to hypercapnia and hypoxia. There is a high incidence of sleep apnea in untreated hypothyroidism; such patients sometimes demonstrate myopathy of upper airway muscles. Weakness of the diaphragm also occurs frequently and, when severe, can cause chronic alveolar hypoventilation (CO_2 retention). Pleural effusions (with high protein content) may occur.

In hypothyroidism, the plasma cholesterol and triglyceride levels increase, related to decreased lipoprotein lipase activity and decreased formation of hepatic LDL receptors. In hypothyroid children, bone growth is slowed and skeletal maturation (closure of epiphyses) is delayed. Pituitary secretion of growth hormone may also be depressed because thyroid hormone is needed for its synthesis. Hypothyroid animals demonstrate decreased width of epiphysial growth plate and articular cartilage and decreased volume of epiphyseal and metaphyseal trabecular bone. These changes are not solely due to lack of pituitary growth hormone, because administering exogenous growth hormone does not restore normal cartilage morphology or bone remodeling, whereas administering T_4 does. If unrecognized, prolonged juvenile hypothyroidism results in a permanent height deficit.

A normochromic, normocytic anemia may occur as a result of decreased erythropoiesis. Alternatively, a moderate macrocytic anemia can occur as a result of decreased absorption of cyanocobalamin (vitamin B_{12}) from the intestine and diminished bone marrow metabolism. Frank megaloblastic anemia suggests coexistent pernicious anemia.

Constipation is common and reflects decreased GI motility. Achlorhydria occurs when hypothyroidism is associated with pernicious anemia. Ascitic fluid with high protein content may accumulate.

The skin in hypothyroidism is dry and cool. Normally, the skin contains a variety of proteins complexed with polysaccharides, chondroitin sulfuric acid, and hyaluronic acid. In hypothyroid-

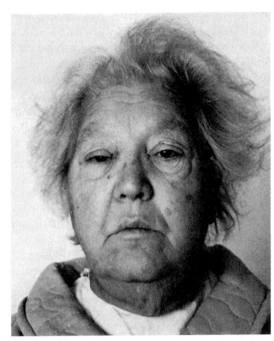

FIGURE 20–8 Myxedema. (Reproduced, with permission, from Greenspan FS, Gardner DG [editors]. *Basic and Clinical Endocrinology*, 7th ed. McGraw-Hill, 2004.)

ism, these complexes accumulate, promoting sodium and water retention and producing a characteristic diffuse, nonpitting puffiness of the skin (myxedema). The patient's face appears puffy, with coarse features (Figure 20–8). Similar accumulation of mucopolysaccharides in the larynx may lead to hoarseness. The hair is brittle and lacking in luster, and there is frequently loss of body hair, particularly over the scalp and lateral eyebrows. If thyroid hormone is administered, the protein complexes are mobilized, a diuresis ensues, and myxedema resolves.

Carotenemia (manifested as yellow-orange discoloration of the skin) may occur in hypothyroidism because thyroid hormones are needed for hepatic conversion of carotene to vitamin A. In the absence of sufficient hormone, carotene accumulates in the bloodstream and skin.

In women, hypothyroidism may lead to menorrhagia from anovulatory cycles. Alternatively, menses may become scanty or disappear secondary to diminished secretion of gonadotropins. Because thyroid hormone normally has an inhibitory effect on prolactin secretion, hypothyroid patients may exhibit hyperprolactinemia, with galactorrhea and amenorrhea. In men, hypothyroidism can cause infertility and gynecomastia from enhanced release of prolactin. Hyperprolactinemia occurs because TRH stimulates prolactin release.

There is reduced renal blood flow and a decreased glomerular filtration rate. The vasoconstriction may be due to decreased concentrations of plasma ANP. The consequent reduced ability to excrete a water load may cause hyponatremia. However, the serum creatinine level is usually normal.

Long-standing severe untreated hypothyroidism may lead to a state called **myxedema coma.** Affected patients have typical myxedematous facies and skin, bradycardia, hypothermia, alveolar hypoventilation, and severe obtundation or coma. This condition is usually precipitated by an intercurrent illness such as an infection or stroke or by a medication such as a sedative-hypnotic. The mortality rate approaches 100% unless myxedema coma is recognized and treated promptly.

CHECKPOINT

16. Describe and explain the physiologic consequence of hypothyroidism (as is best known) on the following:

Nervous system
Muscle
Cardiovascular system
Lungs
Liver
Blood
GI tract
Skin
Reproductive system
Kidney

GOITER

Etiology

Diffuse thyroid enlargement most commonly results from prolonged stimulation by TSH (or a TSH-like agent). Such stimulation may be the result of one of the causes of hypothyroidism (eg, TSH in Hashimoto's thyroiditis) or of hyperthyroidism (eg, TSH-R [stim] Ab in Graves' disease, hCG in germ cell tumors, or TSH in pituitary adenoma). Alternatively, goiter may occur in a clinically euthyroid patient. Table 20–7 lists the causes and pathogenetic mechanisms.

Iodine deficiency is the most common cause of goiter in developing nations. A diet that contains less than 10 μg/d of iodine hinders the synthesis of thyroid hormone, resulting in an elevated TSH level and thyroid hypertrophy. Iodination of salt has eliminated this problem in much of the developed world.

A goiter may also develop from ingestion of **goitrogens** (factors that block thyroid hormone synthesis) either in food or in medication. Dietary goitrogens are found in vegetables of the Brassicaceae family (eg, rutabagas, cabbage, turnips, cassava). A goitrogenic hydrocarbon has been found in the water supply in some locations. Medications that act as goitrogens include thioamides and thiocyanates (eg, propylthiouracil, methimazole, and nitroprusside), sulfonylureas, and lithium. Lithium inhibits thyroid hormone release and perhaps also iodide organification. Most patients remain clinically euthyroid because TSH production increases.

A congenital goiter associated with hypothyroidism (**sporadic cretinism**) may occur as a result of a defect in any of the steps of thyroid hormone synthesis (Table 20–5). All of these defects are rare.

TABLE 20–7 Goiter: causes and pathogenetic mechanisms.

Causes	Pathogenetic Mechanism
I. Goiter associated with hypothyroidism or euthyroidism	
Iodine deficiency	Interferes with hormone biosynthesis
Iodine excess	Blocks secretion of hormone
Goitrogen in diet or drinking water	Interferes with hormone biosynthesis
Goitrogenic medication	Interferes with hormone biosynthesis
Thioamides: propylthiouracil, methimazole, carbimazole	
Thiocyanates: nitroprusside	
Aniline derivatives: sulfonylureas, sulfonamides, aminosalicylic acid, phenylbutazone, aminoglutethimide	
Lithium	Blocks secretion of hormone
Congenital disorders	Various defects in hormone biosynthesis
Defective transport of iodide	
Defective organification of iodide due to absence or reduction of peroxidase or production of an abnormal peroxidase	
Synthesis of an abnormal thyroglobulin	
Abnormal interrelationships of iodotyrosine	
Impaired proteolysis of thyroglobulin	
Defective deiodination of iodotyrosine	
Pituitary and peripheral resistance to thyroid hormone	? Receptor defects
II. Goiter associated with hyperthyroidism	
Graves' disease	TSH-R [stim] Ab stimulation of gland
Toxic multinodular goiter	Autonomous hyperfunction
Germ cell tumor	hCG stimulation of gland
Pituitary adenoma	TSH overproduction
Thyroiditis	Enlargement due to "injury," infiltration, and edema

Goiter with hyperthyroidism is usually due to Graves' disease. In Graves' disease, the gland is diffusely enlarged because of stimulation by TSH-R [stim] Ab and other antibodies rather than by TSH.

Pathogenesis & Pathology

In goiter resulting from impaired thyroid hormone synthesis, there is a progressive fall in serum T_4 and a progressive rise in serum TSH. As the TSH increases, iodine turnover by the gland is accelerated and the ratio of T_3 secretion relative to T_4 secretion is increased. Consequently, the serum T_3 may be normal or increased, and the patient may remain clinically euthyroid. If there is more marked impairment of hormone synthesis, goiter formation is associated with a low T_4, low T_3, and elevated TSH, and the patient becomes clinically hypothyroid.

In the early stages of goiter, there is diffuse enlargement of the gland, with cellular hyperplasia caused by the TSH stimulation. Later, there are enlarged follicles with flattened follicular epithelial cells and accumulation of thyroglobulin. This accumulation occurs particularly in iodine deficiency goiter, perhaps because poorly iodinated thyroglobulin is less easily digested by proteases. As TSH stimulation continues, multiple nodules may develop in some areas and atrophy and fibrosis in others, producing a multinodular goiter (Figure 20–9).

In patients with severe iodine deficiency or inherited metabolic defects, a nontoxic goiter develops because impaired hormone secretion leads to an increase in TSH secretion. The elevation in serum TSH level results in diffuse thyroid hyperplasia. If TSH stimulation is prolonged, the diffuse hyperplasia is followed by focal hyperplasia with necrosis, hemorrhage, and formation of nodules. These nodules often vary from "hot" nodules that can trap iodine and synthesize thyroglobulin to "cold" ones that cannot. In early goiters, the hyperplasia is TSH dependent, but in later stages the nodules become TSH-independent **autonomous nodules.** Thus, over a period of time there may be a transition from a nontoxic, TSH-dependent, diffuse hyperplasia to a toxic or nontoxic, TSH-independent, multinodular goiter.

The exact mechanism underlying this transition to autonomous growth and function is unknown. However, mutations of the *gsp* oncogene have been found in nodules from many patients with multinodular goiter. Such mutations presumably occur during TSH-induced cell division. The *gsp* oncogene is responsible for activation of regulatory GTP-binding (G_s) protein in the follicular cell membrane. Chronic activation of this protein and its effector, adenylyl cyclase, is postulated to result in thyroid cell proliferation, hyperfunction, and independence from TSH.

Clinical Manifestations

With decades of TSH stimulation, enormous hypertrophy and enlargement of the gland can occur. The enlarged gland may weigh 1–5 kg and may produce respiratory difficulties secondary to obstruction of the trachea or dysphagia secondary to obstruction of the esophagus. More modest enlargements pose cosmetic problems.

Some patients with multinodular goiter also develop hyperthyroidism late in life (**Plummer's disease**), particularly after administration of iodide or iodine-containing drugs.

THYROID NODULES & NEOPLASMS

Tumors of the thyroid usually present as a solitary mass in the neck. The most common neoplasm, accounting for 30% of all solitary thyroid nodules, is the **follicular adenoma.** It is a solitary, firm, gray or red nodule, up to 5 cm in diameter, completely surrounded by a fibrous capsule. The surrounding normal thyroid tissue is compressed by the adenoma. Microscopically, the adenoma consists of normal-appearing follicles of varying size, sometimes associated with hemorrhage, fibrosis, calcification, and cystic degeneration. Occasionally, only ribbons of follicular cells are present, without true follicles. Malignant change probably occurs in less than 10% of follicular adenomas.

Thyroid cancers are not common. Most are derived from the follicular epithelium and, depending on their microscopic appearance, are classified as **papillary** or **follicular carcinoma.** The major risk factor predisposing to epithelial thyroid carcinoma is exposure to radiation, but genetic factors have also been recognized. Most papillary and follicular cancers pursue a prolonged clinical course (15–20 years). Papillary carcinoma typically metastasizes to regional lymph nodes in the neck, whereas follicular cancer tends to spread via the bloodstream to distant sites such as bone or lung. **Medullary carcinoma** is an uncommon neoplasm of the C cells (parafollicular cells) of the thyroid that produce calcitonin (see Chapter 17). Approximately 30% of all medullary thyroid carcinomas are a manifestation of multiple endocrine neoplasia type 2 (MEN-2), inherited in an autosomal dominant fashion.

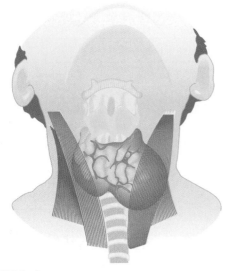

FIGURE 20–9 Multinodular goiter. (Redrawn, with permission, from Greenspan FS, Gardner DG [editors]. *Basic and Clinical Endocrinology*, 8th ed. McGraw-Hill, 2007.)

ABNORMAL THYROID FUNCTION TESTS IN CLINICALLY EUTHYROID INDIVIDUALS

Increases & Decreases in Hormone-Binding Proteins

Sustained increases or decreases in the concentration of TBG and other thyroid-binding proteins in the plasma are produced by several normal and disordered physiologic states and by medications. These are summarized in Table 20–8. For example, TBG levels are elevated during pregnancy and by estrogen and oral contraceptive therapy. TBG levels are depressed in the nephrotic syndrome and by glucocorticoid or androgen therapy.

When a sustained increase in the concentration of TBG and other binding proteins occurs, the concentration of free thyroid hormones falls temporarily. This fall stimulates TSH secretion, which then results in an increase in the production of free hormone. Eventually, a new equilibrium is reached in which the levels of total plasma T_4 and T_3 are elevated, but the concentrations of free hormones, the rate of hormone degradation, and the rate of TSH secretion are normal. Therefore, individuals manifesting sustained increases in TBG and other binding proteins remain euthyroid. When a sustained decrease in the concentration of TBG and other binding proteins occurs, equivalent changes occur in the opposite direction, and again the individuals remain euthyroid.

Abnormal Hormone-Binding Proteins

Changes in serum concentrations of the hormone-binding proteins transthyretin or albumin alone usually do not cause significant changes in thyroid hormone levels. However, several unusual syndromes of **familial euthyroid hyperthyroxinemia** have been described. In the first, a familial syndrome called **euthyroid dysalbuminemic hyperthyroxinemia,** there is abnormal binding of T_4 (but not T_3) to albumin. In the second, there is an increased serum level of transthyretin. In the third, there are alterations in transthyretin, a tetrameric protein that transports 15–20% of circulating T_4. The alterations in transthyretin structure produced by different point mutations can markedly increase its affinity for T_4. In some families, these mutations in transthyretin are transmitted by autosomal dominant inheritance. In all three of these syndromes, total T_4 is elevated, but free T_4 is normal and the patients are euthyroid. A fourth syndrome has also been described in which there is both pituitary and peripheral resistance to thyroid hormone. As noted, this condition may be due to point mutations in the human thyroid receptor (*hTR-β1*) gene, resulting in abnormal nuclear T_3 receptors.

Effects of Nonthyroidal Illness & Drugs

Several nonthyroidal illnesses and various drugs inhibit the 5′-deiodinase that converts T_4 to T_3, resulting in a fall in plasma T_3. Illnesses that depress 5′-deiodinase include severe burns or trauma, surgery, advanced cancer, cirrhosis, renal failure, myocardial infarction, prolonged fever, and caloric deprivation (fasting, anorexia nervosa, malnutrition). The decreased serum T_3 in nonthyroidal illnesses is thought to be an adaptive physiologic change, enabling the sick patient to conserve energy and protein. Drugs that depress 5′-deiodinase include glucocorticoids, propranolol, amiodarone, propylthiouracil, and cholecystography dyes (eg, ipodate, iopanoic acid).

Because T_3 is the major active thyroid hormone at the tissue level, it is surprising that patients with mild to moderate nonthyroidal illness exhibit normal TSH levels despite low T_3 levels and do not appear hypothyroid. However, such patients retain the ability to respond to a further reduction (or to an increase) in serum T_3 by increasing (or decreasing) pituitary TSH secretion. Patients with severe illnesses (eg, those undergoing bone marrow transplantation for leukemia) may manifest impaired TSH secretion.

TABLE 20–8 Effects of normal and disordered physiologic states and medications on plasma thyroid-binding proteins and thyroid hormone levels.

Condition	Concentrations of Binding Proteins	Total Plasma T_4, T_3, RT	Free Plasma T_4, T_3, RT	Plasma TSH	Clinical State
Primary hyperthyroidism	Normal	High	High	Low	Hyperthyroid
Primary hypothyroidism	Normal	Low	Low	High	Hypothyroid
Drugs (estrogens, methadone, heroin, perphenazine, clofibrate), pregnancy, acute and chronic hepatitis, acute intermittent porphyria, estrogen-producing tumors, idiopathic, hereditary	High	High	Normal	Normal	Euthyroid
Drugs (glucocorticoids, androgens, danazol, asparaginase), acromegaly, nephrotic syndrome, hypoproteinemia, chronic liver disease (cirrhosis), testosterone-producing tumors, hereditary	Low	Low	Normal	Normal	Euthyroid

Modified and reproduced, with permission, from Ganong WF. *Review of Medical Physiology,* 22nd ed. McGraw-Hill, 2005.

Most patients with nonthyroidal illnesses have low serum T_3 levels related to the decreased peripheral conversion of T_4 to T_3. However, in some patients, the primary cause of the low serum T_3 is reduced secretion of T_4 by the gland. In others, the binding of T_4 and T_3 by serum thyroid-binding proteins is impaired because of the decreased concentrations of thyroid-binding proteins (Table 20–8) and the presence of circulating inhibitors of binding.

The low T_3 state generally disappears with recovery from the illness or cessation of the drug. Among critically ill patients with low T_3 levels, clinical trials have not demonstrated benefit from T_3 replacement. Because low T_3 levels are difficult to interpret during acute illness, the diagnostic approach should be based primarily on serum TSH levels.

Subclinical Thyroid Disease

With the development of more sensitive tests of thyroid function, it is increasingly recognized that some clinically euthyroid individuals have subclinical thyroid disease, defined as low or high TSH levels but normal circulating T_4 and T_3 levels. Many individuals with subclinical thyroid disease have abnormal TRH stimulation tests, but the clinical significance of these biochemical abnormalities is not known.

Subclinical hypothyroidism is defined as an elevated TSH (> 4.5 mU/L) but normal circulating thyroid hormone levels. In the presence of circulating thyroid autoantibodies, approximately 5% of individuals with subclinical hypothyroidism progress to overt hypothyroidism each year. Subclinical hypothyroidism may be associated with heart failure and subtle neuropsychiatric abnormalities, and some individuals report improved exercise tolerance and an improved sense of well-being when given sufficient thyroxine to normalize serum TSH. Some, but not all, studies suggest that subclinical hypothyroidism may predispose to atherosclerosis and myocardial infarction.

Subclinical hyperthyroidism is defined as a low TSH (< 0.1 mU/L) but normal circulating thyroid hormone levels. Autonomous thyroid nodules are believed to account for many cases.

Several studies have demonstrated subtle abnormalities of cardiac contractility in individuals with subclinical hyperthyroidism, and one prospective study found that individuals older than 65 with TSH < 0.1 mU/L had a threefold greater risk of developing atrial fibrillation than those with normal TSH levels. Subclinical hyperthyroidism may also be associated with bone loss and fracture in postmenopausal women. In a prospective study of women older than 65, the risks of hip and spine fracture were two to three times higher among those with TSH < 0.1 mU/L (mostly from overreplacement with thyroid hormone) compared with those with normal TSH levels. The natural history of subclinical hyperthyroidism is not well known, but in one study of postmenopausal women with endogenous subclinical hyperthyroidism more than 50% had normal TSH levels after 1 year of follow-up.

CHECKPOINT

17. What is a goiter?
18. What are the causes and mechanisms of goiter formation?
19. What is the basis for transition from nontoxic, TSH-dependent diffuse hyperplasia to a toxic or nontoxic TSH-independent multinodular goiter?
20. How large can the thyroid gland become with decades of stimulation?
21. What are the different types of thyroid cancer and their characteristics?
22. What are some physiologic and pathophysiologic conditions in which thyroid metabolism is altered? How and with what effects?
23. What is the overall thyroid status of a patient with a sustained decrease in thyroid-binding globulin?
24. What are some of the factors which depress 5′-deiodinase activity?
25. How does nonthyroidal illness typically affect thyroid hormone levels?

CASE STUDIES

Eva M. Aagaard, MD, & Yeong Kwok, MD

(See Chapter 25, p. 705 for Answers)

CASE 92

A 25-year-old African American woman presents with a complaint of rapid weight loss despite a voracious appetite. Physical examination reveals tachycardia (pulse rate 110 beats/min at rest), fine moist skin, symmetrically enlarged thyroid, mild bilateral quadriceps muscle weakness, and fine tremor. These findings strongly suggest hyperthyroidism.

Questions

A. What other features of the history should be elicited?
B. What other physical findings should be sought?
C. Serum TSH and free thyroxine level are ordered. What results should be anticipated?
D. What are the possible causes of this patient's condition?
E. What is the most common cause of this patient's condition, and what is the pathogenesis of this disorder?
F. What is the pathogenesis of this patient's tachycardia, weight loss, skin changes, goiter, and muscle weakness?

CASE 93

A 45-year-old woman presents complaining of fatigue, 30 pounds of weight gain despite dieting, constipation, and menorrhagia. On physical examination, the thyroid is not palpable; the skin is cool, dry, and rough; the heart sounds are quiet; and the pulse rate is 50 beats/min. The rectal and pelvic examinations show no abnormalities, and the stool is negative for occult blood. The clinical findings suggest hypothyroidism.

Questions

A. What other features of the history should be elicited? What other findings should be sought on physical examination?
B. What is the pathogenesis of this patient's symptoms?
C. What laboratory tests should be ordered, and what results should be anticipated?
D. What are the possible causes of this patient's condition? Which is most likely?
E. What other conditions may be associated with this disorder?

CASE 94

A 40-year-old woman who has recently emigrated from Afghanistan comes to a practice office to establish medical care. She complains only of mild fatigue and depression. Physical examination reveals a prominent, symmetrically enlarged thyroid about twice normal size. The remainder of the examination is unremarkable.

Questions

A. What other features of the history should be elicited?
B. What is the most likely cause of the patient's thyroid enlargement? What is the pathogenetic mechanism of goiter formation in this disease?
C. What laboratory tests should be ordered and why?

CASE 95

A 47-year-old man presents complaining of nervousness, difficulty concentrating, restlessness, and insomnia. He has lost 25 pounds over the past 6 weeks and complains of heat intolerance. Physical examination reveals a 1-cm nodule in the left lobe of the thyroid gland.

Questions

A. What is the most likely explanation for the patient's condition?

B. What laboratory tests should be ordered to confirm the diagnosis? What would you expect the results to be?

C. What further evaluation of the nodule could be undertaken?

D. If a biopsy is done, what can be expected in the pathologist's report?

CASE 96

A 28-year-old woman returns for follow-up after routine laboratory tests show a markedly elevated total T_4 level. The patient is totally asymptomatic, and the physical examination is unremarkable.

Questions

A. What conditions and medications could be responsible for this presentation?

B. What further laboratory tests should be ordered?

C. If the patient is pregnant, how can the elevated total plasma T_4 level be explained?

D. If several asymptomatic family members have been told of similar laboratory test results, what is the most likely explanation of the patient's disorder?

REFERENCES

General

Ai J et al. Autoimmune thyroid diseases: Etiology, pathogenesis, and dermatologic manifestations. J Am Acad Dermatol. 2003 May;48(5):641–59. [PMID: 12734493]

Baloch Z et al; Guidelines Committee, National Academy of Clinical Biochemistry. Laboratory medicine practice guidelines: Laboratory support for the diagnosis and monitoring of thyroid disease. Thyroid. 2003 Jan;13(1):3–126. [PMID: 12625976]

Bassett JH et al. Critical role of the hypothalamic-pituitary-thyroid axis in bone. Bone. 2008 Sep;43(3):418–26. [PMID: 18585995]

Batcher EL et al. Thyroid function abnormalities during amiodarone therapy for persistent atrial fibrillation. Am J Med. 2007 Oct;120(10):880–5. [PMID: 17904459]

Boelaert K et al. Thyroid hormone in health and disease. J Endocrinol. 2005 Oct;187(1):1–15. [PMID: 16214936]

Dayan CM. Interpretation of thyroid function tests. Lancet. 2001 Feb 24;357(9256):619–24. [PMID: 11558500]

Fazio S et al. Effects of thyroid hormone on the cardiovascular system. Recent Prog Horm Res. 2004;59:31–50. [PMID: 14749496]

Greenspan FS. The thyroid gland. In: *Basic and Clinical Endocrinology,* 8th ed. Greenspan FS, Gardner DG (editors). McGraw-Hill, 2007.

Hamilton TE et al. Thyrotropin levels in a population with no clinical, autoantibody, or ultrasonographic evidence of thyroid disease: Implications for the diagnosis of subclinical hypothyroidism. J Clin Endocrinol Metab. 2008 Apr;93(4):1224–30. [PMID: 18230665]

Kahaly GJ et al. Thyroid hormone action in the heart. Endocr Rev. 2005 Aug;26(5):704–28. [PMID: 15632316]

Klein I et al. Thyroid disease and the heart. Circulation. 2007 Oct 9;116(15):1725–35. [PMID: 17923583]

Murphy E et al. The thyroid and the skeleton. Clin Endocrinol (Oxf). 2004 Sep;61(3):285–98. [PMID: 15355444]

Sinclair D: Clinical and laboratory aspects of thyroid autoantibodies. Ann Clin Biochem. 2006 May;43(Pt 3):173–83. [PMID: 16704751]

Squizzato A et al. Clinical review. Thyroid dysfunction and effects on coagulation and fibrinolysis: A systematic review. J Clin Endocrinol Metab. 2007 Jul;92(7):2415–20. [PMID: 17440013]

Tan ZS et al. Thyroid function and the risk of Alzheimer disease: The Framingham Study. Arch Intern Med. 2008 Jul 28;168(14):1514–20. [PMID: 18663163]

Tomer Y, Davies TF. Searching for the autoimmune thyroid disease susceptibility genes: From gene mapping to gene function. Endocr Rev. 2003 Oct;24(5):694–717. [PMID: 14570752]

Hyperthyroidism

Bauer DC et al. Study of Osteoporotic Fractures Research Group. Risk for fracture in women with low serum levels of thyroid-stimulating hormone. Ann Intern Med. 2001 Apr 3;134(7):561–8. [PMID: 12803168]

Bogazzi F et al. Long-term outcome of thyroid function after amiodarone-induced thyrotoxicosis, as compared to subacute thyroiditis. J Endocrinol Invest. 2006 Sep;29(8):694–9. [PMID: 17033257]

.Brennan MD et al. The impact of overt and subclinical hyperthyroidism on skeletal muscle. Thyroid. 2006 Apr;16(4):375–80. [PMID: 16646684]

Cappelli C et al. Prognostic value of thyrotropin receptor antibodies (TRAb) in Graves' disease: A 120 months prospective study. Endocr J. 2007 Dec;54(5):713–20. [PMID: 17675761]

Kavvoura FK et al. Cytotoxic T-lymphocyte associated antigen 4 gene polymorphisms and autoimmune thyroid disease: A meta-analysis. J Clin Endocrinol Metab. 2007 Aug;92(8):3162–70. [PMID: 17504905]

Kim N et al. The role of genetics in Graves' disease and thyroid orbitopathy. Semin Ophthalmol. 2008 Jan-Feb;23(1):67–72. [PMID: 18214794]

Khoo TK et al. Pathogenesis of Graves' opthalmopathy: The role of auto-antibodies. Thyroid. 2007 Oct;17(10):1013–8. [PMID: 17935483]

Nayak B et al. Hyperthyroidism. Endocrinol Metab Clin North Am. 2007 Sep;36(3):617–56. [PMID: 17673122]

Noh JY et al: Thyroid-stimulating antibody is related to Graves' ophthalmopathy, but thyrotropin-binding inhibitor immunoglobulin is related to hyperthyroidism in patients with Graves' disease. Thyroid. 2000 Sep;10(9):809–13. [PMID: 11041459]

Wiersinga WM et al. Pathogenesis of Graves' ophthalmopathy—Current understanding. J Clin Endocrinol Metab. 2001 Feb;86(2):501–3. [PMID: 11157999]

Hypothyroidism

Bayan CM et al. Chronic autoimmune thyroiditis. N Engl J Med. 1996 Jul 11;335(2):99–107. [PMID: 8649497]

Büyükgebiz A. Newborn screening for congenital hypothyroidism. J Pediatr Endocrinol Metab. 2006 Nov;19(11):1291–8. [PMID: 17220056]

Collu R. Genetic aspects of central hypothyroidism. J Endocrinol Invest. 2000 Feb;23(2):125–34. [PMID: 10800768]

Devdhar M et al. Hypothyroidism. Endocrinol Metab Clin North Am. 2007 Sep;36(3):595–615. [PMID: 17673121]

Kavvoura FK et al. Cytotoxic T-lymphocyte associated antigen 4 gene polymorphisms and autoimmune thyroid disease: A meta-analysis. J Clin Endocrinol Metab. 2007 Aug;92(8):3162–70. [PMID: 17504905]

LaFranchi S. Congenital hypothyroidism: Etiologies, diagnosis, and management. Thyroid. 1999 Jul;9(7):735–40. [PMID: 10447022]

Persani L et al. Circulating thyrotropin bioactivity in sporadic central hypothyroidism. J Clin Endocrinol Metab. 2000 Oct;85(10):3631–5. [PMID: 11061514]

Goiter

Hegedüs L et al. Management of simple nodular goiter: Current status and future perspectives. Endocr Rev. 2003 Feb;24(1):102–32. [PMID: 12588812]

Samuels MH. Evaluation and treatment of sporadic nontoxic goiter—Some answers and more questions. J Clin Endocrinol Metab. 2001 Mar;86(3):994–7. [PMID: 11238475]

Thyroid Nodules & Neoplasms

Coltrera MD. Evaluation and imaging of a thyroid nodule. Surg Oncol Clin N Am. 2008 Jan;17(1):37–56. [PMID: 18177799]

Gharib H et al. Thyroid nodules: Clinical importance, assessment, and treatment. Endocrinol Metab Clin North Am. 2007 Sep;36(3):707–35. [PMID: 17673125]

Gimm O. Thyroid cancer. Cancer Lett. 2001 Feb 26;163(2):143–56. [PMID: 11165748]

Moretti F et al. Molecular pathogenesis of thyroid nodules and cancer. Baillieres Best Pract Res Clin Endocrinol Metab. 2000 Dec;14(4):517–39. [PMID: 11289733]

Roman SA. Endocrine tumors: Evaluation of the thyroid nodule. Curr Opin Oncol. 2003 Jan;15(1):66–70. [PMID: 12490764]

Abnormal Thyroid Function Tests in Clinically Euthyroid Individuals

Biondi B et al. The clinical significance of subclinical thyroid dysfunction. Endocr Rev. 2008 Feb;29(1):76–131. [PMID: 17991805]

Cappola AR et al. Thyroid status, cardiovascular risk, and mortality in older adults. JAMA. 2006 Mar 1;295(9):1033–41. [PMID: 16507804]

Chopra IJ. Simultaneous measurement of free thyroxine and free 3,5,3-triiodothyronine in undiluted serum by direct equilibrium dialysis/radioimmunoassay: Evidence that free triiodothyronine and free thyroxine are normal in many patients with the low triiodothyronine syndrome. Thyroid. 1998 Mar;8(3):249–57. [PMID: 9545112]

Chu JW et al. Should mild subclinical hypothyroidism be treated? Am J Med. 2002 Apr 1;112(5):422–3. [PMID: 11904121]

Col NF et al. Subclinical thyroid disease: Clinical applications. JAMA. 2004 Jan 14;291(2):239–43. [PMID: 14722151]

Cooper DS. Clinical practice. Subclinical hypothyroidism. N Engl J Med. 2001 Jul 26;345(4):260–5. [PMID: 11474665]

Cooper DS. Subclinical thyroid disease: Consensus or conundrum? Clin Endocrinol (Oxf). 2004 Apr;60(4):410–2. [PMID: 15049953]

Diez JJ et al. Spontaneous subclinical hypothyroidism in patients older than 55 years: An analysis of natural course and risk factors for the development of overt thyroid failure. J Clin Endocrinol Metab. 2004 Oct;89(10):4890–7. [PMID: 15472181]

Imaizumi M et al. Risk for ischemic heart disease and all-cause mortality in subclinical hypothyroidism. J Clin Endocrinol Metab. 2004 Jul;89(7):3365–70. [PMID: 15240616]

McDermott MT et al. Subclinical hypothyroidism is mild thyroid failure and should be treated. J Clin Endocrinol Metab. 2001 Oct;86(10):4585–90. [PMID: 11600507]

Ochs N et al. Meta-analysis: Subclinical thyroid dysfunction and the risk for coronary heart disease and mortality. Ann Intern Med. 2008 Jun 3;148(11):832–45. [PMID: 18490668]

Papi G et al. Subclinical hypothyroidism. Curr Opin Endocrinol Diabetes Obes. 2007 Jun;14(3):197–208. [PMID: 17940439]

Razvi S et al. The beneficial effect of L-thyroxine on cardiovascular risk factors, endothelial function, and quality of life in subclinical hypothyroidism: Randomized, crossover trial. J Clin Endocrinol Metab. 2007 May;92(5):1715–23. [PMID: 17299073]

Refetoff S. Resistance to thyrotropin. J Endocrinol Invest. 2003 Aug;26(8):770–9. [PMID: 14669836]

Rodondi N et al. Subclinical thyroid dysfunction, cardiac function, and the risk of heart failure. The Cardiovascular Health study. J Am Coll Cardiol. 2008 Sep 30;52(14):1152–9. [PMID: 18804743]

Rodondi N et al. Subclinical hypothyroidism and the risk of heart failure, other cardiovascular events, and death. Arch Intern Med. 2005 Nov 28;165(21):2460–6. [PMID: 16314541]

Surks MI et al. Subclinical thyroid disease: Scientific review and guidelines for diagnosis and management. JAMA. 2004 Jan 14;291(2):228–38. [PMID: 14722150]

21

Disorders of the Adrenal Cortex

Tobias Else, MD, Gary D. Hammer, MD, PhD, & Stephen J. McPhee, MD

The adrenal gland is actually two endocrine organs, one wrapped around the other. The outer **adrenal cortex** secretes many different steroid hormones, including glucocorticoids such as cortisol, mineralocorticoids such as aldosterone, and androgens, chiefly dehydroepiandrosterone (DHEA). The glucocorticoids help to regulate carbohydrate, protein, and fat metabolism. The mineralocorticoids help to regulate Na$^+$ and K$^+$ balance and extracellular fluid volume. The glucocorticoids and mineralocorticoids are essential for survival, but the adrenal androgens have only a minor role in reproductive function. The inner **adrenal medulla,** discussed in Chapter 12, secretes catecholamines (epinephrine, norepinephrine, and dopamine).

Mainly because of their potent immunosuppressive and anti-inflammatory effects, glucocorticoids are used com-monly in pharmacologic doses to treat diseases such as autoimmune disorders. Interestingly, while the deleterious effects of glucocorticoids in states of hypercortisolism and the beneficial effects of their use in pharmacotherapy are rather well understood, the actual role of endogenous glucocorticoids in metabolic homeostasis during times of minimal stress remains somewhat enigmatic.

The major disorders of the adrenal cortex (Table 21–1) are characterized by excessive or deficient secretion of each type of adrenocortical hormone: **hypercortisolism (Cushing's syndrome)**, **adrenal insufficiency (Addison's disease)**, **hyperaldosteronism, hypoaldosteronism,** and **androgen excess (adrenogenital syndrome)**.

NORMAL STRUCTURE & FUNCTION OF THE ADRENAL CORTEX

ANATOMY

The adrenal glands are paired organs located in the retroperitone-al area near the superior poles of the kidneys (Figure 21–1). They are flattened, crescent-shaped structures, which together normal-ly weigh about 8–10 g. Each is covered by tight fibrous capsules and surrounded by fat. The blood flow to the adrenals is copious.

Grossly, each gland consists of two concentric layers: The yellow peripheral layer is the **adrenal cortex,** and the reddish brown central layer is the **adrenal medulla.** Adrenal cortical tissue is sometimes found at other sites, usually near the kid-ney or along the path taken by the gonads during their embryonic descent (Figure 21–1).

HISTOLOGY

The adrenal cortex can be subdivided into three concentric lay-ers: zona glomerulosa, zona fasciculata, and zona reticularis (Figure 21–2). The **zona glomerulosa** is the outermost layer, sit-uated immediately beneath the capsule. Zona glomerulosa cells are columnar or pyramidal in appearance and are arranged in closely packed, rounded, or arched clusters surrounded by cap-illaries. They secrete **mineralocorticoids,** primarily **aldoster-one.** The **zona fasciculata** is the middle layer of the cortex. Zona fasciculata cells are polyhedral in shape and arranged in straight cords or columns, one or two cells thick, running at right angles to the capsule with capillaries between them. The **zona reticu-laris,** the innermost layer of the cortex, lies between the zona fas-ciculata and the adrenal medulla, accounting for only 7% of the mass of the adrenal gland. Zona reticularis cells are smaller than the other two types and are arranged in irregular cords or inter-laced in a network. Zona fasciculata and zona reticularis cells secrete both **glucocorticoids,** primarily **cortisol** and **corticos-terone,** and **androgens** such as **dehydroepiandrosterone.** The ultrastructure of all three types of adrenocortical cells is similar to that of other steroid-synthesizing cells in the body. The steroid hormones produced are low-molecular-weight lipid-soluble molecules able to diffuse freely across cell membranes.

TABLE 21–1 Principal diseases of the adrenal glands.

Hyperfunction of cortex
Bilateral hyperplasia
ACTH excess (affects mainly zona fasciculata and zona reticularis)
Enzyme deficiencies (with ACTH excess)
ACTH-independent macronodular hyperplasia (eg, ectopic receptor expression)
Adenoma
Primary hyperaldosteronism
Hypercortisolism (Cushing's syndrome)
Hyperandrogenism (virilization)
Carcinoma
Cushing's syndrome
Virilization
Feminization (rare)
Hypofunction of cortex
Bilateral adrenal gland destruction (Addison's disease)
Autoimmune
Infection
Ischemia, shock
Hemorrhage, anticoagulation
Metastatic tumor (lung carcinoma, other carcinomas, Kaposi's sarcoma)
Congenital (eg, cytomegalic adrenocortical hypoplasia, *DAX1* mutation)
Hyperfunction of medulla
Pheochromocytoma
Hyperplasia (rare)
Other: ganglioneuroma, neuroblastoma
Hypofunction of medulla

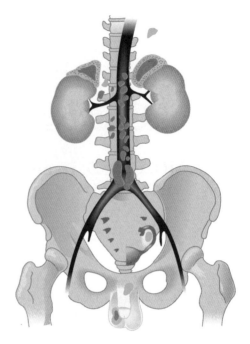

FIGURE 21–1 Human adrenal glands. Note location of adrenal at superior pole of each kidney. Adrenocortical tissue is stippled; adrenal medullary tissue is gray. Also shown (turquoise) are extra-adrenal sites at which cortical and medullary tissues are sometimes found. (Redrawn, with permission, from Forsham PH. The adrenal cortex. In: *Textbook of Endocrinology*, 4th ed. Williams RH [editor]. Saunders, 1968.)

PHYSIOLOGY OF NORMAL ADRENAL CORTEX

1. Glucocorticoids

Glucocorticoid Synthesis, Protein Binding, & Metabolism

Cortisol and corticosterone are referred to as glucocorticoids because they increase hepatic glucose output by stimulating the catabolism of peripheral fat and protein to provide substrate for hepatic gluconeogenesis. The glucocorticoids help

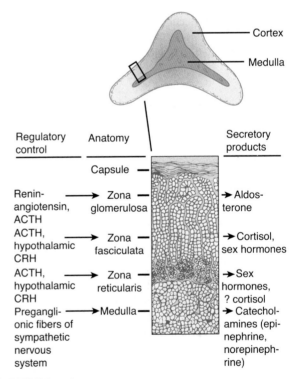

FIGURE 21–2 Anatomy, regulatory control, and secretory products of the adrenal gland. (Redrawn and modified, with permission, from Chandrasoma P, Taylor CE. *Concise Pathology*, 3rd ed. Originally published by Appleton & Lange. Copyright © 1998 by the McGraw-Hill Companies, Inc.)

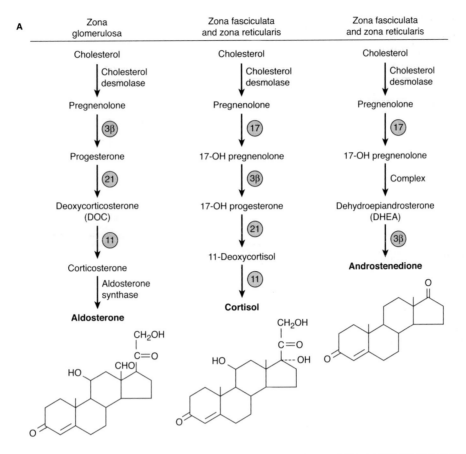

FIGURE 21–3   **A:** Simplified pathways of steroid synthesis in the different zones of the adrenal cortex. Note the differences in the types of enzyme necessary and the different order of enzymatic reactions in the different zones. **B:** Enzymes involved in steroid synthesis. Four of the five enzymes involved are cytochrome P450s and the P450s are commonly known by their cytochrome (CYP) numbers, as shown.

regulate the metabolism of carbohydrates, proteins, and fat. They act on virtually all cells of the body.

A. Synthesis and Binding to Plasma Proteins

The major glucocorticoids secreted by the adrenal cortex are cortisol and corticosterone. Biosynthetic pathways for these hormones are illustrated in Figure 21–3.

Both cortisol and corticosterone are secreted in an unbound state but circulate bound to plasma proteins. They bind mainly to **corticosteroid-binding globulin** (**CBG**) (or **transcortin**) and to a lesser extent to albumin. Protein binding serves mainly to distribute and deliver the hormones to target tissues, but it also delays their metabolic clearance and prevents marked fluctuations of glucocorticoid levels during episodic secretion by the gland.

B. Corticosteroid-Binding Globulin

CBG (molecular weight ~50,000) is an α-globulin synthesized in the liver. Its production is increased by pregnancy, estrogen or oral contraceptive therapy, hyperthyroidism, diabetes, certain hematologic disorders, and familial CBG excess. When the CBG level rises, more cortisol is bound, and the free cortisol level falls temporarily. This fall stimulates pituitary adrenocorticotropic hormone (ACTH) secretion and more adrenal cortisol production. Eventually, the free cortisol level and the ACTH secretion return to normal but with an elevated level of protein-bound cortisol. Similarly, when the CBG level falls, the free cortisol level rises. CBG production is decreased in cirrhosis, nephrotic syndrome, hypothyroidism, multiple myeloma, and familial CBG deficiency.

C. Free and Bound Glucocorticoid—Normally, about 96% of the circulating cortisol is bound to CBG and 4% is free (unbound). The bound hormone is inactive. The free hormone is physiologically active. The normal morning total plasma cortisol level is 5–20 µg/dL (140–550 nmol/L). Because cortisol is protein bound to a greater degree than corticosterone, its half-life in the circulation is longer (~60–90 minutes) than that of corticosterone (~50 minutes).

D. Metabolism—The glucocorticoids are metabolized in the liver and conjugated to glucuronide or sulfate groups. The inactive conjugated metabolites are excreted in the urine and stool. The metabolism of cortisol is decreased in infancy, old age, pregnancy, chronic liver disease, hypothyroidism, anorexia nervosa, surgery, starvation, and other major physiologic stress. Catabolism of cortisol is increased in thyrotoxicosis. Because of its avid protein binding and extensive metabolism before excretion, less than 1% of secreted cortisol appears in the urine as free cortisol.

Regulation of Secretion

A. Adrenocorticotropic Hormone and Corticotropin-Releasing Hormone

—Glucocorticoid secretion is regulated primarily by ACTH, a 39-amino-acid polypeptide secreted by the anterior pituitary. Its half-life in the circulation is very short (~10 minutes). The site of its catabolism is unknown. ACTH regulates both basal secretion of glucocorticoids and increased secretion provoked by stress.

ACTH, in turn, is regulated by hypothalamic corticotropin-releasing hormone (CRH), a 41-amino-acid polypeptide secreted into the median eminence of the hypothalamus. CRH secretion by the hypothalamus is regulated by a variety of neurotransmitters (Figure 21–4) in response to physical and emotional stressors. The hypothalamus is subject to regulatory influences from other parts of the brain, including the limbic system. CRH is transported in the portal-hypophysial vessels to the anterior pituitary (see Chapter 19). There, CRH causes a prompt increase in ACTH secretion. This, in turn, leads to a transient increase in cortisol secretion by the adrenal. Arginine-vasopressin (AVP) is an additional hypothalamic peptide that regulates ACTH release—primarily in response to volume depletion.

The control of ACTH and CRH/AVP secretion involves three components: episodic secretion and diurnal rhythm of ACTH, stress responses of the hypothalamic-pituitary-adrenal axis, and negative feedback inhibition of ACTH secretion by cortisol.

B. Episodic and Diurnal Rhythm of ACTH Secretion

—ACTH is secreted in episodic bursts throughout the day, after a diurnal (circadian) rhythm, with bursts most frequent in the

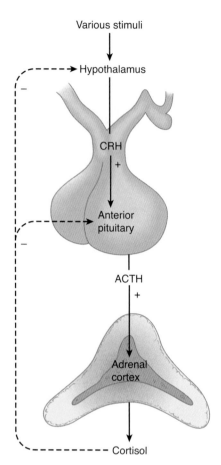

FIGURE 21–4 Feedback mechanism of ACTH-glucocorticoid secretion. Solid arrows indicate stimulation; dashed arrows, inhibition. (Redrawn, with permission, from Junqueira LC, Carneiro J. *Basic Histology*, 10th ed. McGraw-Hill, 2003.)

early morning and least frequent in the evening (Figure 21–5). The peak level of cortisol in the plasma normally occurs between 6:00 and 8:00 AM (during sleep, just before awakening) and the nadir at around 12:00 AM. The diurnal rhythm of ACTH secretion persists in patients with adrenal insufficiency who are receiving maintenance doses of glucocorticoids but is lost in Cushing's syndrome. The diurnal rhythm is altered also by changes in patterns of sleep, light-dark exposure, or food intake; physical stress such as major illness, surgery, trauma, or starvation; psychologic stress, including severe anxiety, depression, and mania; CNS and pituitary disorders; liver disease and other conditions that affect cortisol metabolism; chronic renal failure; alcoholism; and antiserotonergic drugs such as cyproheptadine.

Normally, the morning plasma ACTH concentration is about 25 pg/mL (5.5 pmol/L). Plasma ACTH and cortisol values in various normal and abnormal states are shown in Figure 21–6.

C. Stress Response

—Plasma ACTH and cortisol secretion are also triggered by various forms of stress. Emotional stress (such as fear and anxiety) and bodily injury (such as surgery

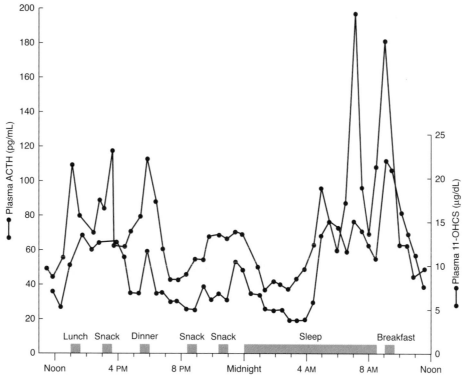

FIGURE 21–5 Fluctuations in plasma ACTH and glucocorticoids (11-OHCS) throughout the day. Note the greater ACTH and glucocorticoid rises in the morning before awakening. (Redrawn, with permission, from Krieger DT et al. Characterization of the normal temporal pattern of plasma corticosteroid levels. J Clin Endocrinol Metab. 1971;32:266.)

or hypoglycemia) release CRH from the hypothalamus. Similarly, vasopressin is released in response to volume depletion. ACTH secretion induced by these hormones, in turn, stimulates a transient increase in cortisol secretion (Figure 21–7). If the stress is prolonged, it may abolish the normal diurnal rhythm of ACTH and cortisol secretion.

D. Negative Feedback—A rising level of plasma cortisol inhibits release of ACTH from the pituitary by both inhibiting CRH release from the hypothalamus and interfering with the stimulatory action of CRH on the pituitary (Figure 21–4). The fall in plasma ACTH leads to a decline in adrenal secretion of cortisol. Conversely, the loss of negative feedback resulting from a drop in plasma cortisol induces a net increase in ACTH secretion. In untreated chronic adrenal insufficiency, there is a marked increase in the rate of ACTH synthesis and secretion.

Condition	Plasma ACTH (pg/mL)	Plasma cortisol (µg/dL)
	0 5 50 500 5000	0 12 25 50 100
Normal, morning		
Normal, evening		
Normal, dexamethasone		
Normal, metyrapone		
Normal, stress		
Addison's disease		
Hypopituitarism		
Congenital adrenal hyperplasia		
Cushing's, hyperplasia		
Cushing's, dexamethasone		
Cushing's, postadrenalectomy		
Cushing's, ectopic ACTH syndrome		
Cushing's, adrenal tumor		
	0 5 50 500 5000	0 12 25 50 100

FIGURE 21–6 Plasma concentrations of ACTH and cortisol in various clinical states. (Redrawn, with permission, from Liddle G. The adrenal cortex. In: *Textbook of Endocrinology*, 5th ed. Williams RH [editor]. Saunders, 1974.)

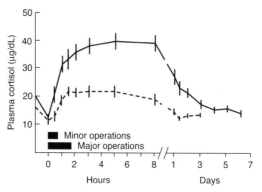

FIGURE 21–7 Plasma cortisol responses to major surgery (continuous line) and minor surgery (broken line) in normal subjects. Mean values and standard errors for 20 patients are shown in each case. (Redrawn, with permission, from Plumpton FS, Besser GM, Cole P. Anesthesia. 1969;24:3.)

ACTH and CRH secretion are also inhibited by chronic pharmacologic treatment with exogenous corticosteroids in proportion to their glucocorticoid potency. When prolonged corticosteroid treatment is stopped, the adrenal is atrophic and unresponsive and the patient is at risk for acute adrenal insufficiency. Chronic suppression of the HPA axis by exogenous glucocorticoids also impacts on hypothalamic CRH and pituitary ACTH secretion and it may take some time to recover after cessation of glucocorticoid treatment. Such adrenal insufficiency after abrupt glucocorticoid withdrawal can be life threatening. The time to recovery to full physiological function of the HPA axis is dependent on duration and dose of glucocorticoid treatment. Moreover, there are significant interindividual differences in these parameters. While there are no useful predictors to facilitate determining which patients are at risk for prolonged adrenal insufficiency, there is some evidence that alternate-day glucocorticoid treatment tends to preserve some adrenal function. Another well-accepted method of preventing long-term suppression of the HPA axis following glucocorticoid therapy is to slowly taper the dosage of exogenous glucocorticoids. Tapering exogenous glucocorticoid has a dual function. A short-term taper (days to a few weeks) of pharmacologic doses of glucocorticoids prevents a rebound flare of the underlying treated disease (eg, autoimmune disorder). A slow taper of exogenous glucocorticoid from physiologic replacement doses to complete discontinuation serves the purpose of allowing the endogenous HPA axis to recover. Such tapering only supports the recovery of HPA-axis function if it is done slowly (weeks to months) with doses below the daily physiologic glucocorticoid equivalent (eg, 5.0–7.5 mg of prednisone).

E. Effects of ACTH on the Adrenal—Circulating ACTH binds to high-affinity receptors (ACTH receptor or MC2 receptor)

on adrenocortical cell membranes, activating adenylyl cyclase, increasing intracellular cyclic adenosine monophosphate (cAMP). There is a dual response to ACTH stimulation: a) immediate production and release of cortisol, and b) induction of steroidogenic enzyme synthesis.

Prolonged hypersecretion or administration of ACTH causes initial hypertrophy followed by hyperplasia of the zona fasciculata and zona reticularis. Growth factors such as additional POMC peptides and insulin-like growth factors play important roles in this process. Conversely, prolonged ACTH deficiency results in adrenocortical atrophy.

Mechanism of Action

The physiologic effects of glucocorticoids in various tissues are the result of their binding to the ubiquitous cytosolic glucocorticoid receptors (GRs) (Figure 21–8). The hormone-GR complexes then enter the nucleus and can act by two main mechanisms: a) **transactivation,** in which the GRs bind to nuclear DNA and promote the transcription of DNA, production of mRNAs, and hence synthesis of proteins; or b) **transrepression**, in which gene transcription is inhibited through interference with other transcription factors.

Effects

The effects of glucocorticoids on target tissues are summarized in Table 21–2. Under physiologic circumstances, the effects of glucocorticoid are not very well understood but appear to be mainly permissive. The effects of glucocorticoids secreted at supraphysiologic levels, however, are well described. In most tissues, glucocorticoids have a catabolic effect, promoting degradation of protein and fat to provide substrate for intermediary metabolism. In the liver, however, glucocorticoids

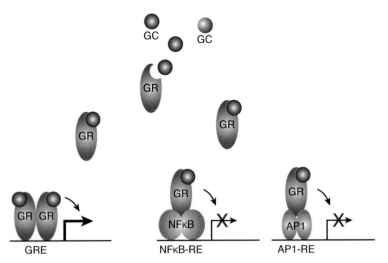

FIGURE 21–8   Mechanism of glucocorticoid action. Glucocorticoid (GC) hormone binds to the cytosolic intracellular glucocorticoid receptor (GR), which dimerizes and then translocates to the nucleus and increases transcription of glucocorticoid responsive target genes (eg, PEPCK, transactivation) or inhibits gene transcription of genes (eg, collagenase, interleukin-2, transrepression) by interference with other transcription factors (eg, nuclear factor kappa-B [NFκB] or activator protein 1 [AP1]). (Arrows depict gene transcription, crossed-out arrows depict inhibited gene transcription; RE, response element).

TABLE 21–2 **Effects of glucocorticoids.**

Target Tissue	Effect	Mechanism
Muscle	Catabolic	Inhibit glucose uptake and metabolism
		Decrease protein synthesis
		Increase release of amino acids, lactate
Fat	Lipolytic	Stimulate lipolysis
		Increase release of FFAs and glycerol
Liver	Synthetic	Increase gluconeogenesis
		Increase glycogen synthesis, storage
		Increase glucose-6-phosphatase activity
		Increase blood glucose
Immune system	Suppression	Reduce number of circulating lymphocytes, monocytes, eosinophils, basophils
		Inhibit T-lymphocyte production of interleukin-2
		Interfere with antigen processing, antibody production and clearance
	Anti-inflammatory	Decrease migration of neutrophils, monocytes, lymphocytes to sites of injury
	Other	Stimulate release of neutrophils from marrow
		Interfere with neutrophil migration out of vascular compartment (produces a relative neutrophilia during glucocorticoid therapy)
Cardiovascular	Increase cardiac output	
	Increase peripheral vascular tone	
Renal	Increase glomerular filtration rate	
	Aid in regulating water, electrolyte balance	
Other	Permissive action	Increase blood glucose
	Resistance to stress	
	Insulin antagonism	

have a synthetic effect, promoting the uptake and use of carbohydrates (in synthesis of glucose and glycogen), amino acids (in synthesis of RNA and protein enzymes), and fatty acids (as an energy source).

During fasting, glucocorticoids help to maintain plasma glucose levels by several mechanisms (Table 21–2). In peripheral tissues, glucocorticoids antagonize the effects of insulin. Glucocorticoids inhibit glucose uptake in muscle and adipose tissue. The brain and heart are spared from this antagonism, and the extra supply of glucose helps these vital organs to cope with stress. In diabetics, the insulin antagonism may worsen control of blood sugar levels, raise plasma lipid levels, and increase the formation of ketone bodies. However, in nondiabetics, the rise in blood glucose levels stimulates a compensatory increase in insulin secretion that prevents these sequelae.

Small amounts of glucocorticoids must be present for other metabolic processes to occur (**permissive action**). For example, glucocorticoids must be present for catecholamines to produce their calorigenic, lipolytic, pressor, and bronchodilator effects and for glucagon to increase hepatic gluconeogenesis.

Glucocorticoids are also required to resist various stresses. Indeed, the increased secretion of pituitary ACTH and consequent increase in circulating glucocorticoids after injury are essential to survival. Hypophysectomized or adrenalectomized individuals treated with only maintenance doses of glucocorticoids may die when exposed to such stress. This underscores the crucial role of glucocorticoids as stress hormones.

2. Mineralocorticoids

Synthesis, Protein Binding, & Metabolism

The primary function of mineralocorticoids is to regulate Na^+ excretion and maintain a normal intra-vascular volume. However, other factors affect Na^+ excretion besides the mineralocorticoids, such as the glomerular filtration rate, atrial natriuretic peptide, presence of an osmotic diuretic, and changes in tubular reabsorption of Na^+ that are not regulated by mineralocorticoid.

A. Synthesis—**Aldosterone** is the principal mineralocorticoid secreted by the adrenal. Deoxycorticosterone also has minor mineralocorticoid activity, as does corticosterone.

B. Protein Binding—Aldosterone is bound to plasma proteins (albumin and corticosteroid-binding globulin) to a lesser extent than glucocorticoids. The amount of aldosterone se-

creted under normal circumstances is small (~0.15 mg/24 h). The normal average plasma concentration of (free and bound) aldosterone is 0.006 µg/dL (0.17 nmol/L). Free (unbound) aldosterone comprises 30–40% of the total.

C. Metabolism—The half-life of aldosterone is short (~20–30 minutes). Aldosterone is catabolized principally in the liver, and its metabolites are excreted in the urine. Less than 1% of secreted aldosterone is excreted in urine in the free form.

Regulation

Aldosterone secretion is regulated primarily by the renin-angiotensin system but also by pituitary ACTH and by the plasma electrolytes, K^+ and, to a lesser extent, Na^+.

A. Regulation by Renin-Angiotensin System—The renin-angiotensin system regulates aldosterone secretion in a feedback fashion (Figure 21–9). **Renin** is a proteolytic enzyme produced from a larger protein, **prorenin.** Renin is excreted by the juxtaglomerular cells of the kidney in response to decreases in renal perfusion pressure and reflex increases in renal nerve discharge. Once in the circulation, renin acts on **angiotensinogen,** to form **angiotensin I,** a decapeptide. In the lung and elsewhere, angiotensin I is converted by **angiotensin-converting enzyme** (ACE) to **angiotensin II,** an octapeptide. Angiotensin II binds to zona glomerulosa cell membrane receptors and stimulates synthesis and secretion of aldosterone. Aldosterone promotes Na^+ and water retention, causing plasma volume expansion, which then shuts off renin secretion. In the supine state, there is a diurnal rhythm of aldosterone and renin secretion; the highest values are in the early morning before awakening.

The physiologic stimuli for the renin-angiotensin system to increase aldosterone secretion include factors that reduce renal perfusion such as extracellular fluid volume depletion, dietary Na^+ restriction, and decreases in intra-arterial vascular

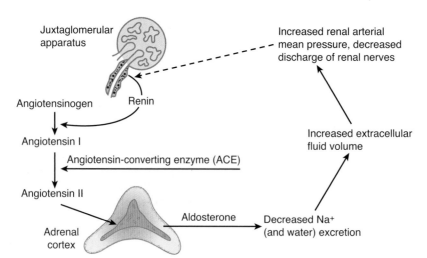

FIGURE 21–9   Feedback mechanism regulating aldosterone secretion. The dashed arrow indicates inhibition.   (Redrawn, with permission, from Ganong WF. *Review of Medical Physiology,* 22nd ed. McGraw-Hill, 2005.)

pressure (eg, resulting from hemorrhage or upright posture). Other disease states that cause reduced renal perfusion include renal artery stenosis, salt-losing disorders, congestive heart failure, and hypoproteinemic states (cirrhosis of the liver, or nephrotic syndrome). These disorders increase renin secretion, producing **secondary hyperaldosteronism.**

B. Regulation by ACTH—ACTH also stimulates mineralocorticoid output. More ACTH is needed to stimulate mineralocorticoid than glucocorticoid secretion, but the amount required is still within the range of normal ACTH secretion. The effect of ACTH on aldosterone secretion is transient, however. Even if ACTH secretion remains elevated, aldosterone production declines to normal within 48 hours, perhaps because renin secretion decreases in response to hypervolemia.

C. Regulation by Plasma Electrolytes—An increase in plasma K^+ concentration—or a fall in plasma Na^+—stimulates aldosterone release. Although minor changes of plasma K^+ (≤ 1 mEq/L) have an effect, major changes in plasma Na^+ (drops of about 20 mEq/L) are needed to stimulate aldosterone secretion. Na^+ depletion increases the affinity and number of angiotensin II receptors on adrenocortical cells.

Mechanism of Action

Aldosterone, like other steroid hormones, acts by binding to a mineralocorticoid receptor (MR) in the cytosol. The expression of the MR is restricted to a small number of tissues, such as the kidney. Interestingly, glucocorticoids also have a high affinity to the MR, but usually do not exert mineralocorticoid effects because mineralocorticoid-sensitive tissues express the enzyme 11-hydroxysteroid dehydrogenase type 2, which metabolizes and inactivates glucocorticoids before it can bind to the MR. The aldosterone-MR complex moves into the nucleus of the target cell and increases transcription of DNA, induction of mRNA, and stimulation of protein synthesis by ribosomes. The aldosterone-stimulated proteins have two effects: a rapid effect to increase the activity of epithelial sodium channels (ENaCs) by increasing the insertion of ENaCs into the cell membrane from a cytosolic pool, and a slower effect to increase the synthesis of ENaCs. One of the genes activated by aldosterone is the gene for serum- and glucocorticoid-regulated kinase (sgk), a serine-threonine protein kinase. The *sgk* gene product increases ENaC activity (Figure 21–10). Aldosterone also increases the mRNAs for the three subunits that comprise the ENaCs.

The fact that the principal effect of aldosterone on Na^+ transport takes 10–30 minutes to develop and even longer to peak indicates that it depends on the synthesis of new proteins by the genomic mechanism. However, aldosterone also binds directly to distinct membrane receptors with a high affinity for aldosterone, and, by a rapid nongenomic action, increases the activity of membrane Na^+-K^+ exchangers to increase intracellular Na^+.

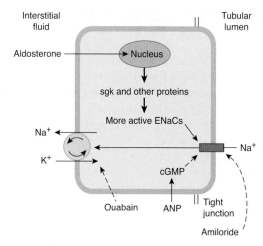

FIGURE 21–10 Mechanism of action of aldosterone in an epithelial cell of the renal tubule's collecting duct. In the kidney, aldosterone acts primarily on the principal cell of the collecting ducts. Under the influence of aldosterone, increased amounts of Na^+ are exchanged for K^+ and H^+ in the renal tubules, producing a K^+ diuresis and an increase in urine acidity. Na^+ enters via the epithelial sodium channels (ENaCs) in the apical membrane and is pumped into the interstitial fluid by Na^+-K^+ ATPases in the basolateral membrane. Aldosterone activates the genome to produce sgk and other proteins, and the number of active ENaCs is increased. (Redrawn and modified, with permission, from Ganong WF. *Review of Medical Physiology*, 22nd ed. McGraw-Hill, 2005.)

Effects

The target organs for the mineralocorticoids include the kidney, colon, duodenum, salivary glands, and sweat glands. In the distal renal tubules and collecting ducts, aldosterone acts to promote the exchange of Na^+ for K^+ and H^+, causing Na^+ retention, K^+ diuresis, and increased urine acidity. Elsewhere, it acts to increase the reabsorption of Na^+ from the colonic fluid, saliva, and sweat. The mineralocorticoids may also increase K^+ and decrease Na^+ concentrations in muscle and brain cells. Aldosterone action on epithelial cells of the choroid plexus alters the composition of cerebrospinal fluid in a fashion thought to contribute to blood-pressure regulation. In the heart, aldosterone has been shown to induce heart remodeling and interstitial and perivascular fibrosis of the myocardium.

CHECKPOINT

9. How is aldosterone secretion regulated?
10. How does the effect of ACTH on aldosterone secretion differ from the effect on glucocorticoid secretion?
11. What are the overall effects of aldosterone?

PATHOPHYSIOLOGY OF SELECTED ADRENOCORTICAL DISORDERS

Characteristic syndromes are produced by excessive or deficient secretion of each type of adrenal hormone. Excessive glucocorticoid secretion (**Cushing's syndrome**) results in a moon-faced, plethoric appearance, with truncal obesity, purple abdominal striae, hypertension, osteoporosis, mental aberrations, protein depletion, and glucose intolerance or frank diabetes mellitus.

Excessive mineralocorticoid secretion **hyperaldosteronism** leads to Na$^+$ retention, usually without edema, and K$^+$ depletion, resulting in hypertension, muscle weakness, polyuria, hypokalemia, metabolic alkalosis, and sometimes hypocalcemia and tetany.

Excessive androgen secretion causes masculinization (**adrenogenital syndrome**) and precocious pseudopuberty or female pseudohermaphroditism.

Deficient glucocorticoid secretion resulting from autoimmune or other destruction of the adrenal glands (**Addison's disease**) causes symptoms of weakness, fatigue, malaise, anorexia, nausea and vomiting, weight loss, hypotension, hypoglycemia, and marked intolerance of physiologic stress (eg, infection). Elevation of plasma ACTH may produce hyperpigmentation.

Associated mineralocorticoid deficiency leads to renal Na$^+$ wasting and K$^+$ retention and can produce manifestations of severe dehydration, hypotension, decreased cardiac size, hyponatremia, hyperkalemia, and metabolic acidosis. Deficient mineralocorticoid secretion also occurs in patients with renal disease and low circulating renin levels (**hyporeninemic hypoaldosteronism**).

CUSHING'S SYNDROME

Cushing's syndrome is the clinical condition resulting from chronic exposure to excessive circulating levels of glucocorticoids (Figure 21–11). It is also called **hyperadrenocorticalism** and **hypercortisolism.** The most common cause of the syndrome is excess secretion of ACTH from the anterior pituitary gland (**Cushing's disease**).

Etiology

Cushing's syndrome may occur either spontaneously or as the result of chronic glucocorticoid administration (iatrogenic

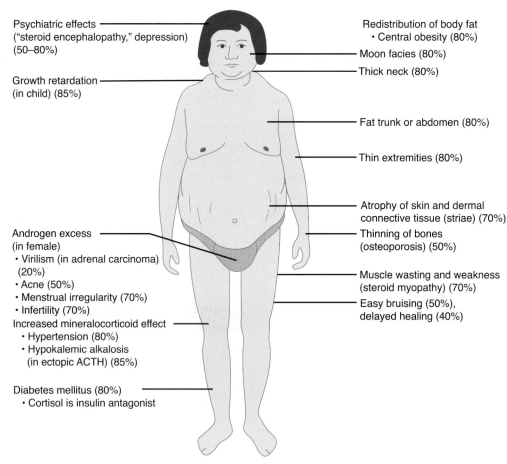

Psychiatric effects
("steroid encephalopathy," depression)
(50–80%)

Growth retardation
(in child) (85%)

Androgen excess
(in female)
• Virilism (in adrenal carcinoma)
  (20%)
• Acne (50%)
• Menstrual irregularity (70%)
• Infertility (70%)
Increased mineralocorticoid effect
  • Hypertension (80%)
  • Hypokalemic alkalosis
    (in ectopic ACTH) (85%)

Diabetes mellitus (80%)
• Cortisol is insulin antagonist

Redistribution of body fat
• Central obesity (80%)
Moon facies (80%)
Thick neck (80%)

Fat trunk or abdomen (80%)

Thin extremities (80%)

Atrophy of skin and dermal
connective tissue (striae) (70%)
Thinning of bones
(osteoporosis) (50%)

Muscle wasting and weakness
(steroid myopathy) (70%)
Easy bruising (50%),
delayed healing (40%)

FIGURE 21–11 Typical findings in Cushing's syndrome.

Cushing's syndrome). The overall incidence of spontaneous Cushing's syndrome is approximately two to four cases per million population. It is nine times more common in women than in men. The major causes of Cushing's syndrome are summarized in Table 21–3.

A. Hypothalamic CRH Hypersecretion

Uncommonly, patients with Cushing's syndrome have **diffuse hyperplasia of pituitary corticotroph cells** responsible for ACTH hypersecretion. The hyperplasia is probably due to hypersecretion of CRH by the hypothalamus or nonhypothalamic tumors that secret ectopic CRH. Chronic CRH hypersecretion does not cause pituitary adenomas.

B. Pituitary Cushing's Disease

Cushing's disease is the most common cause of noniatrogenic hypercortisolism. It is four to six times more prevalent in women than in men. Patients with Cushing's disease have a pituitary adenoma causing excessive secretion of ACTH (Figure 21–12). Such adenomas are located in the anterior pituitary, are usually less than 10 mm in diameter (**microadenomas**), and are composed of basophilic corticotroph cells containing ACTH in secretory granules. **Macroadenomas** are less common and carcinomas extremely rare. Pituitary adenomas are common, found in 10–25% of unselected autopsy series, and in about 10% of asymptomatic individuals subjected to magnetic resonance imaging (MRI). Use of molecular biology techniques to determine the clonal origin of corticotroph tumors has shown that ACTH-secreting pituitary adenomas are monoclonal, arising from a single progenitor cell. Presumably, somatic mutations are required for tumorigenesis.

In Cushing's disease, the chronic ACTH hypersecretion causes bilateral hyperplasia of the adrenal cortex. Combined adrenal weights (normal: 8–10 g) range from 12 g to 24 g. The adrenal hyperplasia is most typically micronodular, but in some patients, particularly those with long-standing Cushing's disease, macronodular hyperplasia develops.

C. Ectopic ACTH Syndrome

In the **ectopic ACTH syndrome,** a nonpituitary tumor synthesizes and hypersecretes biologically active ACTH or an ACTH-like peptide (Figure 21–12). The neoplasms most frequently responsible are small cell carcinomas of the lung and bronchial carcinoid tumors. Ectopic ACTH hypersecretion is more common in men, largely owing to the more frequent occurrence of these lung tumors in men. Other associated tumors are listed in Table 21–3. Chronic ACTH hypersecretion causes marked bilateral adrenocortical hyperplasia, with combined adrenal weights ranging from 24–50 g or more. The ACTH secreted by the nonpituitary tumor causes adrenal hyperfunction, and the high circulating cortisol levels suppress hypothalamic secretion of CRH and the pituitary secretion of ACTH. Pituitary corticotroph cells have a decreased ACTH content.

TABLE 21–3 Major causes of Cushing's syndrome.

NONIATROGENIC
ACTH dependent
1. Cushing's disease (ACTH-secreting pituitary adenoma):
• *Epidemiology:* 68% of cases of noniatrogenic Cushing's syndrome. More common in women (F-M ratio of approximately 8:1). Age at diagnosis usually 20–40 years.
• *Clinical features:* Hyperpigmentation and hypokalemic alkalosis are rare; androgenic manifestations limited to acne and hirsutism. Secretion of cortisol and adrenal androgens is only moderately increased.
• *Course:* Slow progression over several years.
2. Ectopic ACTH syndrome:
• *Epidemiology:* 15% of cases of spontaneous Cushing's syndrome. More common in men (M-F ratio of approximately 3:1). Age at diagnosis usually 40–60 years. Occurs most commonly in patients with small cell carcinoma of lung and bronchial carcinoid tumors. Rarely, other tumors secrete ACTH; these include carcinoid tumors of the thymus, gut, pancreas, or ovary; pancreatic islet cell tumors; ovarian cancer; medullary thyroid carcinoma; pheochromocytoma; small cell carcinoma of vagina or uterine cervix.
• *Clinical features:* Frequently limited to weakness, hypertension, and glucose intolerance, resulting from the rapid onset of hypercortisolism. Weight loss and anemia are common effects of malignancy. Primary tumor usually apparent. Hyperpigmentation, hypokalemia, and alkalosis may occur from the mineralocorticoid effects of cortisol and other steroids secreted.
• *Course:* With underlying carcinoma, hypercortisolism is of rapid onset, steroid hypersecretion is frequently severe, with equally elevated levels of glucocorticoids, androgens, and deoxycorticosterone. With underlying benign tumor, more slowly progressive course.
ACTH independent
3. Functioning adrenocortical tumor:
• *Epidemiology:* 17% of cases of Cushing's syndrome. Adrenal adenoma in 9%, adrenal carcinoma in 8%. More common in women. Adrenal carcinoma occurs in about 2 per million population per year. Age at diagnosis usually 35–40 years.
• *Clinical features and course:* Adenoma: Onset is gradual. Usually secretes only cortisol. Hypercortisolism is mild to moderate. Androgenic effects absent. Carcinoma: Rapid onset, rapidly progressive. Marked elevations of glucocorticoids, androgens, and mineralocorticoids. Hypokalemia, abdominal pain, abdominal masses, hepatic and pulmonary metastases.
IATROGENIC
4. Exogenous glucocorticoid administration:
• Glucocorticoid administered in high doses in the treatment of nonendocrine disorders.

D. Ectopic CRH Syndrome

The ectopic CRH syndrome is a rare cause of Cushing's syndrome (see Figure 21–12). Most cases have been associated with bronchial carcinoid tumors.

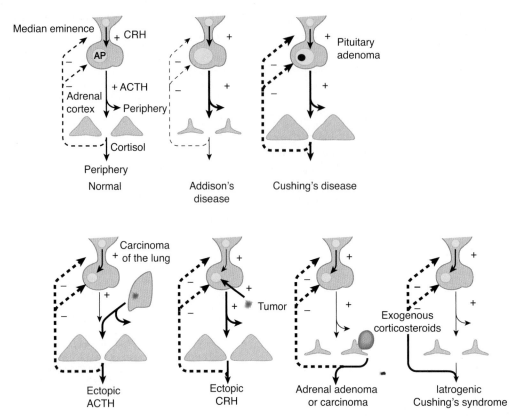

FIGURE 21–12 Hypothalamic, pituitary, and adrenal cortical relationships. Solid arrows indicate stimulation; dashed arrows, inhibition. **Normal:** Corticotropin-releasing hormone (CRH) elaborated by the median eminence of the hypothalamus stimulates secretion of adrenocorticotropic hormone (ACTH) by the anterior pituitary (AP). ACTH triggers the synthesis and release of cortisol, the principal glucocorticoid of the adrenal cortex. A rising level of cortisol inhibits the stimulatory action of CRH on ACTH release (or cortisol may inhibit CRH release), completing a negative feedback loop. **Addison's disease:** In primary destructive disease of the adrenal cortex, the level of plasma cortisol is very low, and the effect of CRH on the anterior pituitary proceeds without inhibition, causing a marked increase in the secretion of ACTH. High levels of ACTH produce characteristic skin pigmentary changes. **Cushing's disease:** The primary lesion may be at the level of the pituitary or hypothalamus. In either case, production of ACTH and cortisol is excessive. The former causes bilateral adrenal hyperplasia and the latter causes clinical manifestations of hypercortisolism. Cells of the anterior pituitary are relatively resistant to the high levels of circulating cortisol. **Ectopic ACTH:** In this syndrome, ACTH or an ACTH-like peptide is elaborated by a tumor such as carcinoma of the lung. The adrenals are stimulated, circulating cortisol is increased, and pituitary ACTH secretion is inhibited. **Ectopic CRH:** In this rare syndrome, CRH is elaborated by a tumor such as a bronchial carcinoid. The pituitary is stimulated, and there is elaboration of excess ACTH. The adrenals are stimulated, and circulating cortisol is increased. The hypercortisolism causes diminished hypothalamic CRH production; however, the negative feedback on the pituitary production of ACTH is overcome by the ectopic CRH. **Adrenal adenoma or carcinoma:** An adenoma or carcinoma of the adrenal cortex may produce cortisol autonomously. When the rate of production exceeds physiologic quantities, Cushing's syndrome results; the effect of CRH on the anterior pituitary is inhibited by the high levels of circulating cortisol, with resultant diminished ACTH secretion and atrophy of normal adrenal tissue. **Iatrogenic Cushing's syndrome:** Exogenous corticosteroid administration in excess of physiologic quantities of cortisol leads directly to peripheral manifestations of hypercortisolism and inhibits the effect of CRH on the anterior pituitary, with resultant diminished ACTH secretion, diminished cortisol production, and atrophy of normal adrenal tissue. (Redrawn and modified, with permission, from Burns TW, Carlson HE. Endocrinology. In: *Pathologic Physiology: Mechanisms of Disease.* Sodeman WA, Sodeman TM [editors]. Saunders, 1985.)

E. Functioning Adrenocortical Tumors

Both **adrenocortical adenomas** and **carcinomas** may cause Cushing's syndrome by elaborating cortisol autonomously (Figure 21–12). Adenomas are usually 1–6 cm in diameter, weigh 10–70 g, are encapsulated, and consist predominantly of zona fasciculata cells. They are relatively inefficient in cortisol synthesis. Adrenal carcinomas are usually large, weighing 100 g to several kilograms, and are often palpable as an abdominal mass by the time Cushing's syndrome becomes clinically manifest. Grossly, they are highly vascular, with areas of necrosis, hemorrhage, cystic degeneration, and calcification. They are highly malignant lesions, tending to invade adrenal capsule, neighboring organs and blood vessels and metastasize to the liver and lungs.

F. Adrenal Micronodular Hyperplasia

ACTH-independent adrenal micronodular hyperplasia is a rare cause of Cushing's syndrome. Pathologically, it is characterized by multiple small, pigmented, usually bilateral cortisol-secreting adenomas. About half of cases occur sporadically in children and young adults. The remainder occur as an autosomal dominant disorder in association with blue nevi; pigmented lentigines (freckles) of the skin and mucosal surfaces of the head and face; cutaneous, mammary, and atrial myxomas; pituitary somatotroph adenomas; and tumors of peripheral nerves, testes, and other endocrine glands (Carney complex).

G. Adrenal Macronodular Hyperplasia

Another rare cause of Cushing's syndrome is bilateral adrenal macronodular hyperplasia. In this condition, both glands are markedly enlarged, with bulging nodules found at cut section. Microscopically, the nodules reveal a variegated histologic pattern characterized by trabecular, adenoid, and zona glomerulosa–like structures. Occasionally, the hyperplasia may be unilateral. Some patients with macronodular hyperplasia do not show typical cushingoid features. In these cases, the macronodular hyperplasia is most often discovered incidentally on ultrasound or computed tomography (CT) examination of the abdomen and can be considered benign.

Pathophysiology

The various causes of Cushing's syndrome can be divided into two categories: ACTH dependent and ACTH independent. The causes of ACTH-dependent Cushing's syndrome include Cushing's disease (80% of ACTH-dependent cases), ectopic ACTH hypersecretion (20%), and ectopic CRH secretion (rare), all of which are characterized by chronic ACTH hypersecretion and increased secretion of cortisol. Causes of ACTH-independent Cushing's syndrome include glucocorticoid-secreting adrenocortical adenomas and carcinomas and adrenal micronodular and macronodular hyperplasia, all of which are characterized by autonomous secretion of cortisol and suppression of pituitary ACTH (Figures 21–12 and 21–13).

A. Cushing's Disease

In Cushing's disease, there is a persistent overproduction of ACTH by the pituitary adenoma. The ACTH hypersecretion is disorderly, episodic, and random; the normal diurnal rhythm of ACTH and cortisol secretion is usually absent. Plasma levels of ACTH and cortisol vary and may at times be within the normal range (Figure 21–13). However, a **24-hour urine free cortisol** measurement confirms hypercortisolism. The excessive cortisol does not suppress ACTH secretion by the pituitary adenoma.

Most (90%) patients with Cushing's disease have exaggerated plasma ACTH and cortisol responses to CRH stimulation and incompletely suppressed secretion of ACTH and cortisol by exogenous glucocorticoids (eg, dexamethasone). Although these findings suggest that the pituitary adenoma cells are unusually sensitive to CRH and relatively resistant to glucocorticoids, the findings may simply be due to the increased number of ACTH-secreting cells. About 10% of patients with pituitary microadenomas do not exhibit major increases in plasma ACTH in response to CRH. Presumably,

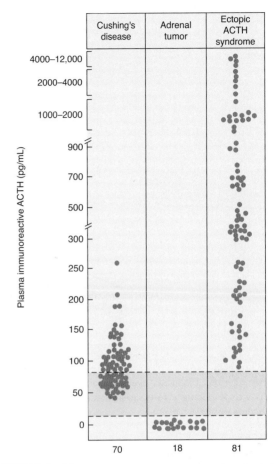

FIGURE 21–13 Basal plasma ACTH concentrations in patients with various types of noniatrogenic Cushing's syndrome. The colored zone represents the normal range. (Redrawn, with permission, from Scott AP et al. Pituitary adrenocorticotropin and the melanocyte stimulating hormones. In: *Peptide Hormones.* Parsons JA [editor]. University Park Press, 1979.)

the clonal cells of such patients have a receptor or postreceptor defect.

Despite ACTH hypersecretion, the pituitary and adrenals fail to respond normally to stress. Stimuli such as hypoglycemia or surgery fail to increase ACTH and cortisol secretion, probably because chronic hypercortisolism has suppressed CRH secretion by the hypothalamus. Hypercortisolism also inhibits other normal pituitary and hypothalamic functions, affecting thyrotropin, growth hormone, and gonadotropin release. Surgical removal of the ACTH-producing pituitary adenoma reverses these abnormalities.

B. Ectopic ACTH Syndrome

In the ectopic ACTH syndrome, hypersecretion of ACTH and cortisol is random and episodic and quantitatively greater than in patients with Cushing's disease (Figure 21–13). Indeed, plasma levels and urinary excretion of cortisol, adrenal androgens, and other steroids are often markedly elevated. Ectopic ACTH secretion by tumors is usually not suppressible by exogenous glucocorticoids such as dexamethasone (Figure 21–14).

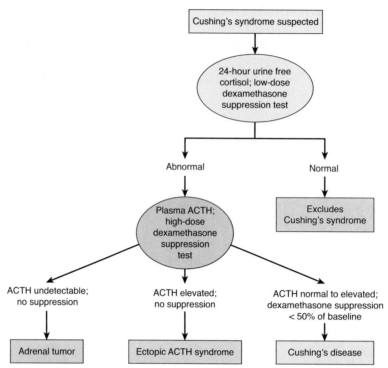

FIGURE 21–14 Diagnostic evaluation of Cushing's syndrome and procedures for determining the cause. Boxes enclose clinical diagnoses, and ovals enclose diagnostic tests. (Redrawn, with permission, from Baxter JD, Tyrrell JB. The adrenal cortex. In: *Endocrinology and Metabolism,* 2nd ed. Felig P, Baxter JD [editors]. McGraw-Hill, 1987.)

C. Ectopic CRH Syndrome

Clinically, the ectopic CRH syndrome is indistinguishable from the ectopic ACTH syndrome. Biochemically, however, plasma CRH concentrations are elevated (not suppressed), and CRH-stimulated secretion of ACTH is suppressible with high doses of dexamethasone (not so in the ectopic ACTH syndrome). Sometimes, nonpituitary tumors produce both CRH and ACTH ectopically.

D. Adrenal Tumors

Primary adrenal adenomas and carcinomas are not under hypothalamic-pituitary control and thus autonomously hypersecrete cortisol. The hypercortisolism suppresses pituitary ACTH production, resulting in atrophy of the uninvolved adrenal cortex (Figure 21–12). Steroid secretion is random and episodic and not usually suppressible by dexamethasone. With adrenal carcinomas, overproduction of androgenic precursors is common, resulting in hirsutism or virilization of adult women or children of either sex. On the other hand, with adrenal adenomas, production of androgenic precursors is relatively limited. Thus, their clinical manifestations are chiefly those of cortisol excess.

It is not known why adrenal adenomas develop, but activating mutations of receptors for corticotropic factors have been found. Although structural mutations of the ACTH receptor gene have not been detected, some tumors have been found to have aberrant expression of receptors for a variety of hormones (eg, GI inhibitory peptide, luteinizing

hormone [LH]/human chorionic gonadotropin [hCG], and somatostatin receptors), neuropeptides (vasopressin, serotonin [5-HT], and γ-adrenergic receptors), cytokines (interleukin [IL]-1 receptors), and possibly leptin. For example, patients with food-induced ACTH-independent Cushing's syndrome have been identified. In these patients, cortisol secretion by a unilateral adrenal adenoma or by bilateral macronodular adrenal hyperplasia is stimulated by the gut hormone GI inhibitory peptide (GIP). Abnormal expression of GIP receptors on the adrenal tumor cells allows them to respond to food intake with an increase in cAMP and subsequent cortisol production.

E. Bilateral Micronodular Hyperplasia

ACTH levels are low, and cortisol is not suppressed by high doses of dexamethasone.

F. Bilateral Macronodular Hyperplasia

Again, hypercortisolism, low plasma ACTH, loss of diurnal rhythm of ACTH, and lack of suppression with high doses of dexamethasone are found. Patients with bilateral ACTH-independent macro-nodular adrenal hyperplasia have been found to have abnormal adrenal receptors, including those for gastric inhibitory polypeptide (food-induced hypercortisolism), vasopressin, β-adrenergic agonists, LH/hCG (hypertension during pregnancy and after menopause), or serotonin (5-HT).

G. Subclinical Cushing's Syndrome

With routine use of ultrasound and CT imaging studies, adrenal masses are being detected with increased frequency in asymptomatic patients. Termed "incidentalomas" (see later discussion), a substantial percentage are hormonally active. From 5% to 20% produce glucocorticoids. Such autonomous glucocorticoid production without specific symptoms and signs of Cushing's syndrome is termed subclinical Cushing's syndrome. With an estimated prevalence of 79 cases per 100,000 persons, subclinical Cushing's syndrome is much more common than classic Cushing's syndrome. Depending on the amount of glucocorticoid secreted by the tumor, the clinical spectrum ranges from slightly attenuated diurnal cortisol rhythm to complete atrophy of the contralateral adrenal gland with lasting adrenal insufficiency after unilateral adrenalectomy.

Clinical Manifestations

Glucocorticoid excess leads to glucose intolerance in several ways. First, cortisol excess promotes synthesis of glucose in the liver from amino acids liberated by protein catabolism. The increased hepatic gluconeogenesis occurs via stimulation of the enzymes glucose-6-phosphatase and phosphoenolpyruvate carboxykinase. Second, there is an increase in hepatic synthesis of glycogen and ketone bodies. Third, cortisol antagonizes the action of insulin in peripheral glucose utilization, perhaps by inhibiting glucose phosphorylation. The glucose intolerance and hyperglycemia are signaled by thirst and polyuria. Overt diabetes mellitus occurs in 10–15% of patients with Cushing's syndrome. The diabetes is characterized by insulin resistance, ketosis, and hyperlipidemia, but acidosis and microvascular complications are rare.

With chronic cortisol excess, muscle wasting occurs as a result of excess protein catabolism, decreased muscle protein synthesis, and induction of insulin resistance in muscle via a postinsulin receptor defect. Proximal muscle weakness occurs in about 60% of cases. It is usually manifested by difficulty in climbing stairs or rising from a chair or bed without use of the arms. Fatigue when combing or drying the hair is also seen.

Obesity and redistribution of body fat are probably the most recognizable features of Cushing's syndrome. Weight gain is often the initial symptom. The obesity is centralized, with relative sparing of the extremities. The redistribution of adipose tissue affects mainly the face, neck, trunk, and abdomen. Thickening of facial fat rounds the facial contour, producing the "moon facies." An enlarged dorsocervical fat pad ("buffalo hump") can occur with weight gain from any cause; increased fat pads that fill and bulge above the supraclavicular fossae are more specific for Cushing's syndrome. Abdominal fat deposition results in centripetal obesity, with an elevated waist-to-hip circumference ratio (> 1.0 in men and > 0.8 in women) in 50% of patients with Cushing's syndrome. This fat deposition occurs both subcutaneously and intra-abdominally, most prominently around the viscera, perhaps because intra-abdominal fat appears to have a higher density of glucocorticoid receptors than other fat tissue.

The reason for the abnormal fat distribution is unknown. However, plasma leptin levels are significantly elevated in patients with Cushing's syndrome compared with both nonobese healthy individuals and obese individuals with a similar percentage of body fat but no endocrine or metabolic disorder. Leptin, the obese (*ob*) gene product, is an adipocyte-derived satiety factor that helps to regulate appetite and body weight. The elevated leptin in patients with Cushing's syndrome is probably a result of the visceral obesity. Glucocorticoids may act, at least in part directly, on adipose tissue to increase leptin synthesis and secretion. Chronic hypercortisolism may also have an indirect effect via the associated hyperinsulinemia or insulin resistance.

Given the known lipolytic effects of glucocorticoids, the increased fat deposition caused by glucocorticoid excess seems paradoxical. It may be explained by the increase in appetite or by the lipogenic effects of the hyperinsulinemia that the cortisol excess causes.

Glucocorticoid excess inhibits fibroblasts, leading to loss of collagen and connective tissue. Thinning of the skin, abdominal striae, easy bruisability, poor wound healing, and frequent skin infections are the result. Atrophy leads to a translucent appearance of the skin. Cutaneous atrophy is best appreciated as a fine "cigarette paper" wrinkling or tenting of the skin over the dorsum of the hand or over the elbow.

On the face, corticosteroid excess causes perioral dermatitis, characterized by small follicular papules on an erythematous base around the mouth, and a rosacea-like eruption, characterized by central facial erythema. Facial telangiectases and plethora over the cheeks may result from loss of subcutaneous tissue with hypercortisolism. Steroid acne, characterized by numerous pustular lesions reflecting androgenic effects or papular lesions reflecting glucocorticoid effects, sometimes occurs on the face, chest, or back. **Acanthosis nigricans,** a dark, soft, velvety skin with fine folds and papillae, may occur in intertriginous areas, such as under the breasts and in the groin, or at sites of friction, such as the neck or belt line. Acanthosis nigricans is thought to result from two changes in the skin's extracellular matrix: decreased viscosity caused by altered glycosaminoglycan formation and abnormal deposition of the extracellular matrix in papillae that protrude from the dermis.

Prominent reddish purple **striae** occur in 50–70% of patients, most commonly over the abdominal wall, breasts, hips, buttocks, thighs, and axillae. The striae result from increased subcutaneous fat deposition, which stretches the thin skin and ruptures the subdermal tissues. These striae are depressed below the skin surface because of loss of underlying connective tissue and are wider (not infrequently 0.5–2.0 cm) than the pinkish-white striae of pregnancy or rapid weight gain. Easy bruisability occurs in about 40% of cases. Ecchymoses occur after minimal trauma, resulting in purpura. Wound healing is delayed, and surgical incisions sometimes undergo dehiscence. Fungal infections of the skin and mucous membranes are frequent, including tinea versicolor, seborrheic dermatitis, onychomycosis, and oral candidiasis.

In the ectopic ACTH syndrome, hyperpigmentation of the skin may occur owing to the markedly elevated level of circulating ACTH, which has some melanocyte-stimulating hormone (MSH)-like activity. However, hyperpigmentation is rare in Cushing's disease or adrenal tumors except after total adrenalectomy (Nelson's syndrome).

In about 80% of female patients, hirsutism from increased secretion of adrenal androgens occurs over the face, abdomen, breasts, chest, and upper thighs. Acne often accompanies the hirsutism.

Although the physiologic role of glucocorticoids in bone and Ca^{2+} metabolism is not well understood, excessive glucocorticoid production inhibits bone formation and accelerates bone resorption (see Chapter 17). Glucocorticoids exert direct effects on the main cell types that regulate bone metabolism. They inhibit osteoblast differentiation, inducing osteoblast and osteocyte apoptosis while at the same time prolonging osteoclast survival.

As mentioned earlier, hypercortisolism also leads to a state of hypogonadism (due to inhibition of hypothalamic GnRH) in both males and females and therefore reduces the beneficial effect of sex hormones on bone strength.

Furthermore, glucocorticoid excess decreases intestinal Ca^{2+} absorption and increases urinary Ca^{2+} excretion (hypercalciuria), resulting in a negative Ca^{2+} balance. Glucocorticoids impair intestinal absorption and renal tubular reabsorption of Ca^{2+} by inhibiting the effects of vitamin D on the intestine and renal tubules as well as hydroxylation of vitamin D in the liver. There is a secondary increase in PTH secretion, accelerating bone resorption.

As a result of the hypercalciuria, kidney stones occur in about 15% of patients. Such patients may present with renal colic. Glucocorticoids also reduce the renal tubular reabsorption of phosphate, leading to phosphaturia and reduced serum phosphorus concentrations.

The combination of decreased bone formation and increased bone resorption ultimately leads to a generalized loss in bone mass (**osteoporosis**) and an increased risk of bony fracture. The fracture risk is potentiated by accompanying myopathy that predisposes to falls. Osteoporosis is present in most patients; back pain is an initial complaint in 58% of cases. X-ray films frequently reveal vertebral compression fractures (16–22% of cases), rib fractures, and sometimes multiple stress fractures. For unknown reasons, avascular (aseptic) necrosis of bone (usually of the femur or humerus) occurs sometimes with exogenous (iatrogenic) corticosteroids but is rare with endogenous hypercortisolemia.

Glucocorticoid excess alters the normal inflammatory response to infection or injury by several mechanisms. On the molecular level, glucocorticoids exert their effect by activating the GR which in turn interferes with other transcription factors (eg, nuclear factor kappa-B [NFκB], activator protein [AP1]) necessary for transcription of proinflammatory genes and immune mediators. Generally glucocorticoids decrease the number of CD_4 T lymphocytes and more potently inhibit TH_1-associated cytokines (eg, interleukin 2). They also inhibit fibroblastic activity, preventing the walling off of bacterial and other infections. Therefore, patients with hypercortisolism are more prone to diseases that require a cell-mediated immune response, such as tuberculosis, fungal or *Pneumocystis* infections.

Glucocorticoids induce lipocortins, which in turn inhibit the action of phospholipase A_2 in releasing arachidonic acid from tissue phospholipids, thereby reducing formation of leukotrienes, which are powerful mediators of inflammation; they also decrease formation of thromboxanes, prostaglandins, and prostacyclin. They inhibit the accumulation and migration of polymorphonuclear neutrophils to sites of inflammation. In addition, they decrease local swelling and block the systemic effects of bacterial toxins.

Glucocorticoid excess also suppresses manifestations of allergic disorders that are due to the release of histamine from tissues.

Hypertension occurs in 75–85% of patients with spontaneous Cushing's syndrome. The exact pathogenesis of the hypertension is unclear. It may be related to salt and water retention from the mineralocorticoid effects of the excess glucocorticoid which in high concentrations escape the inactivation by 11β-hydroxysteroid dehydrogenase type 2. Alternatively, it may be due to increased secretion of angiotensinogen. Whereas plasma renin activity and concentrations are generally normal or suppressed in Cushing's syndrome, angiotensinogen levels are elevated to approximately twice normal because of a direct effect of glucocorticoids on its hepatic synthesis, and angiotensin II levels are increased by about 40%. Administration of the angiotensin II antagonist saralasin to patients with Cushing's syndrome causes a prompt 8- to 10-mm Hg drop in systolic and diastolic blood pressure. Studies in experimental animals have demonstrated that glucocorticoids exert permissive effects on vascular tone by a variety of mechanisms. Some involve vascular smooth muscle cells, including an increased secretion of the vasoconstrictor endothelin, an increase in Ca^{2+} uptake and Ca^{2+} channel antagonist binding, and an increase of α_{1B}-adrenergic receptors. In addition, glucocorticoids cause a decrease in atrial natriuretic peptide (ANP)-mediated cyclic guanosine monophosphate formation, leading to decreased vasodilation by ANP. Glucocorticoids inhibit nitric oxide synthase in vascular endothelial cells, predisposing to vasoconstriction. Glucocorticoids also sensitize arterioles to the pressor effects of catecholamines.

Gonadal dysfunction occurs commonly in Cushing's syndrome and is the result of increased secretion of adrenal androgens (in females) and cortisol (in males and females) from the adrenal cortex. In premenopausal women, the androgens may cause hirsutism, acne, amenorrhea, and infertility. Hypercortisolism appears to affect the hypothalamic gonadotropin-releasing hormone (GnRH) pulse generator to inhibit normal LH and follicle-stimulating hormone (FSH) pulsatility and pituitary responsiveness to GnRH. The high levels of cortisol can thus suppress pituitary LH secretion. In women, this results in menstrual irregularities, including amenorrhea, oligomenorrhea, and polymenorrhea. In men, this results in decreased testosterone secretion by the testis, for which the increased adrenal secretion of weak androgens does not compensate. Decreased libido, loss of body hair, small and soft testes, and impotence ensue.

Excess glucocorticoids frequently produce mental symptoms, including euphoria, increased appetite, irritability, emotional lability, and decreased libido. Many patients experience impaired cognitive function, with poor concentration and poor memory, and disordered sleep, with decreased rapid eye movement sleep and early morning awakening. Glucocorticoid excess also accelerates the basic electroencephalographic rhythm. Significant psychiatric illness—mainly depression but also anxiety, psychosis with delusions or hallucinations, paranoia, or hyperkinetic (even manic) behavior—occurs in 51–81% of patients with Cushing's syndrome. The pathogenesis of these CNS effects is not well understood.

Glucocorticoid excess inhibits growth in children, in part by directly inhibiting bone cells and by decreasing growth hormone and thyroid-stimulating hormone (TSH) secretion and somatomedin generation. Glucocorticoids suppress growth also by exerting direct effects on the growth plate, including inhibition of mucopolysaccharide production, resulting in reduced cartilaginous bone matrix and epiphyseal proliferation.

With long-standing hypercortisolism, there may be mild to moderate elevations of intraocular pressure and glaucoma, perhaps related to swelling of collagen strands in the trabecular meshwork, which interferes with aqueous humor drainage. Posterior subcapsular cataracts may develop. About half of patients will develop exophthalmos, which is often asymptomatic. Visual field defects occur in 40% of patients with pituitary macroadenomas related to pressure on the optic chiasm; field defects do not occur with microadenomas.

Routine laboratory tests in Cushing's syndrome usually demonstrate a high normal hemoglobin, hematocrit, and red blood cell number. Polycythemia occurs rarely, secondary to androgen excess. The total white blood cell count is usually normal; however, the percentages of lymphocytes and eosinophils and the total lymphocyte and eosinophil counts are frequently subnormal.

Serum electrolytes are usually normal. Hypokalemic metabolic alkalosis sometimes occurs as a result of mineralocorticoid hypersecretion in patients with ectopic ACTH syndrome or adrenocortical carcinoma. Fasting hyperglycemia occurs in about 10–15% of patients; postprandial hyperglycemia and glucosuria are more common. Most patients with Cushing's syndrome have secondary hyperinsulinemia and abnormal glucose tolerance tests. The serum Ca^{2+} is generally normal; the serum phosphorus is low normal or slightly low. Hypercalciuria can be demonstrated in 40% of cases.

Routine x-ray films may reveal cardiomegaly resulting from hypertensive or atherosclerotic heart disease, vertebral compression fractures, rib fractures, and renal calculi.

The ECG may show left ventricular hypertrophy (LVH) from hypertension, ischemia, or ST-T wave changes from electrolyte disturbances (eg, flattening of T waves from hypokalemia).

Patients with subclinical Cushing's syndrome lack the classic stigmas of hypercortisolism but frequently have obesity, hypertension, and Type 2 diabetes mellitus.

Diagnosis

Suspected hypercortisolism can be investigated by several approaches (Figure 21–14). Current recommendations involve a stepwise approach to diagnostic evaluation. The first step is to demonstrate pathologic hypercortisolemia and confirm the diagnosis of Cushing's syndrome. The second step is to distinguish ACTH-independent disease from ACTH-dependent disease, followed by either adrenal or pituitary imaging. For patients with ACTH-dependent disease, the final step is to determine the anatomic localization of the ACTH source, by MRI or, if equivocal, by inferior petrosal sinus sampling (IPSS) or cavernous sinus sampling (CSS).

Measurement of free cortisol in a 24-hour urine specimen collected on an outpatient basis demonstrates excessive excretion of cortisol (24-hour urinary free cortisol levels > 100 μg/24 hours). Urinary free cortisol values are rarely normal in Cushing's syndrome. Urinary free cortisol measurement is the most sensitive and specific test to screen for and confirm the presence of Cushing's syndrome.

Performance of an overnight 1-mg dexamethasone suppression test will demonstrate lack of the normal suppression of adrenal cortisol production by exogenous corticosteroid (dexamethasone). The overnight dexamethasone suppression test is accomplished by prescribing 1 mg of dexamethasone at 11:00 PM, and then obtaining a plasma cortisol level the next morning at 8:00 AM. In normal individuals, the dexamethasone suppresses the early morning surge in cortisol, resulting in plasma cortisol levels of < 2 μg/dL (56 nmol/L); in Cushing's syndrome, cortisol secretion is not suppressed to as great a degree, and values are often > 10 μg/dL (280 nmol/L).

If the overnight dexamethasone suppression test is normal, the diagnosis is very unlikely; if the urine free cortisol is also normal, Cushing's syndrome is excluded. If the results of both tests are abnormal, hypercortisolism is present and the diagnosis of Cushing's syndrome can be considered established if conditions causing false-positive results (pseudo-Cushing's syndrome) are excluded (acute or chronic illness, obesity, high-estrogen states, drugs, alcoholism, and depression). The CRH test is a useful adjunct in patients with borderline elevated urinary cortisol levels resulting from probable pseudo-Cushing's state.

In patients with equivocal or borderline results, a 2-day low-dose dexamethasone suppression test is often performed (0.5 mg every 6 hours for eight doses). Normal responses to this test exclude the diagnosis of Cushing's syndrome. Normal responses are an 8:00 AM plasma cortisol less than 2 μg/dL (56 nmol/L); a 24-hour urinary free cortisol less than 10 μg/24 h (< 28 μmol/24 h); and a 24-hour urinary 17-hydroxycorticosteroid level less than 2.5 mg/24 h (6.9 μmol/24 h) or 1 mg/g creatinine (0.3 mmol/mol creatinine).

Confirmation of the diagnosis of Cushing's syndrome entails measurement of plasma ACTH level and a high-dose dexamethasone suppression test (Figure 21–14). Assay of the plasma ACTH level helps to differentiate ACTH-dependent from ACTH-independent causes of Cushing's syndrome. The high-dose dexamethasone suppression test is useful for differentiating pituitary from ectopic ACTH secretion. These tests are then followed by imaging procedures (eg, thin-section CT scan or MRI) to determine the location of a suspected pituitary, adrenal, lung, or other tumor.

With adrenal carcinomas, CT typically demonstrates an inhomogeneous adrenal mass with irregular margins and variable contrast enhancement of solid components. MRI can also detect these tumors and can assess invasion into large vessels.

CLINICALLY INAPPARENT ADRENAL MASS (INCIDENTALOMA)

Adrenal masses are common. Routine autopsy studies find an adrenal mass in at least 3% of persons older than 50 years. Most of these pose no threat to health, but a small proportion cause endocrinologic problems. Approximately 1 in 4000 adrenal tumors is malignant.

Incidentalomas are clinically inapparent masses discovered incidentally in the course of diagnostic testing or treatment for other clinical conditions (excluding patients undergoing imaging for cancer). Estimated prevalence of incidentaloma ranges from 0.1% of patients undergoing routine screening with ultrasonography to 0.42% of patients being evaluated for nonendocrinologic complaints to 4.3% of patients with a previous diagnosis of cancer. The prevalence rises with age from < 1% for persons younger than 30 years to 7% for those 70 years or older.

Pathologically, clinically inapparent adrenal masses can be either benign (adenomas, some pheochromocytomas, myelolipomas, ganglioneuromas, adrenal cysts, hematomas) or malignant (adrenocortical carcinomas, some pheochromocytomas, metastases from other cancers). Adrenocortical carcinoma occurs with an estimated prevalence of 1–2 per 1 million persons. Adrenocortical carcinoma is more likely if the adrenal tumor is large (> 4 cm).

Diagnostic evaluation is typically performed to determine whether the lesion is hormonally active or nonfunctioning and whether it is likely to be malignant or benign.

In unselected patients and those without endocrinologic symptoms, most adrenal incidentalomas (> 70%) are nonfunctioning tumors. However, up to 20% of patients have subclinical hormonal overproduction; such patients may be at risk for metabolic or cardiovascular disorders. Most common (~5–10%) is cortisol overproduction, sometimes termed subclinical Cushing's syndrome. Less common are catecholamine excess from pheochromocytomas, aldosterone excess from adenomas, and sex hormone excess from virilizing or feminizing tumors. Experts recommend that all patients have a 1-mg dexamethasone suppression test and measurement of plasma (or urinary) free metanephrines, and hypertensive patients should have determinations of serum potassium and plasma aldosterone concentration–plasma renin activity ratio.

Patients with subclinical autonomous glucocorticoid hypersecretion may progress to develop metabolic disorders, such as insulin resistance, or full-blown Cushing's syndrome.

The size and appearance of the mass on CT or MRI can help in distinguishing malignant from benign tumors. For example, > 60% of incidentalomas smaller than 4 cm are benign adenomas and < 2% are adrenocortical carcinomas. By contrast, for lesions larger than 6 cm, 25% are carcinomas and < 15% are benign adenomas. In addition, if a CT scan reveals a smooth-bordered, homogeneous mass with a low value on a standardized measure of x-ray absorption (CT attenuation value of < 10 Hounsfield units [HU]), the mass is likely a benign adenoma. Utility of radionuclide scintigraphy and positron emission tomography scanning is unclear. CT-guided fine-needle aspiration biopsy can be helpful in the diagnosis of patients with a history of cancer and a heterogeneous adrenal mass with a high CT attenuation value of > 20 HU.

Surgery is usually recommended for patients with unilateral incidentalomas found on history, physical examination, and laboratory studies to have symptoms, signs, and biochemical evidence of glucocorticoid, mineralocorticoid, catecholamine, or sex hormone excess. Surgery is also recommended for all patients with biochemical evidence of pheochromocytomas, whether symptomatic or not. Management of patients with subclinical hyperfunctioning adrenal cortical adenomas is more controversial; both surgical and nonsurgical approaches are used.

Recommended monitoring consists of a second imaging study 6–12 months later and follow-up endocrinologic studies to exclude hormonal hypersecretion for at least 4 years. No further monitoring is recommended for patients with nonsecreting tumors that remain stable in size. Follow-up of patients with nonfunctioning masses shows that the vast majority of incidentalomas remain stable in size: About 5–25% increase in size by ≥ 1 cm, and 3–4% decrease in size. Overall, ≤ 20% of nonfunctioning tumors develop hormone overproduction (usually cortisol, rarely catecholamine or aldosterone, hypersecretion) when monitored for up to 10 years. Tumors ≥ 3 cm are more likely to develop hyperfunction than smaller masses.

CHECKPOINT

12. What are the symptoms and signs of excess of each class of adrenal steroids?

13. What are the major causes of Cushing's syndrome?

14. How is the regulation of glucocorticoid secretion altered in patients with Cushing's disease? With ectopic ACTH secretion? With autonomous adrenal tumors?

15. What are the symptoms and signs of glucocorticoid excess?

16. Name some different ways to make the diagnosis of Cushing's disease in a patient with suggestive symptoms and signs.

ADRENOCORTICAL INSUFFICIENCY

Adrenocortical insufficiency generally occurs because of either destruction or dysfunction of the adrenal cortex (**primary adrenocortical insufficiency**) or deficient pituitary ACTH or hypothalamic CRH secretion (**secondary adrenocortical insufficiency**). However, congenital defects in any one of several enzymes occurring as "inborn errors of metabolism" can lead to deficient cortisol secretion. Enzyme deficiencies can also result from treatment with various drugs, such as metyrapone, amphenone, and mitotane.

The causes of adrenocortical insufficiency are shown in Table 21–4. No matter what the origin, the clinical manifestations of primary adrenocortical insufficiency are a consequence of deficiencies of cortisol, aldosterone, and, in women, androgenic steroids. Secondary adrenal insufficiency results in a selective cortisol (and androgen) deficiency.

Etiology

A. Primary Adrenocortical Insufficiency

Primary adrenocortical insufficiency (Addison's disease) is most often due to autoimmune destruction of the adrenal cortex (~80% of cases). In the past, tuberculosis involving the adrenals was the most common cause, but it now accounts for about 20% of cases. Less common causes include other granulomatous diseases such as histoplasmosis, adrenal hemorrhage or infarction, metastatic carcinoma, and AIDS-related (cytomegalovirus) adrenalitis.

Primary adrenal insufficiency is rare, with reported prevalence rates of 39–60 cases per 1 million population. However, as the number of patients with AIDS increases and as patients with malignancies live longer, more cases of adrenocortical insufficiency may be encountered. Addison's disease is somewhat more common in women, with a female-to-male ratio of 1.25:1. It usually occurs in the third to fifth decades.

1. Autoimmune adrenocortical insufficiency—Autoimmune destruction of the adrenal glands is thought to be related to generation of **antiadrenal antibodies.** Circulating adrenal autoantibodies can be detected in more than 80% of patients with autoimmune adrenal insufficiency, either isolated or associated with autoimmune polyglandular syndrome type 1 or type 2 (see later discussion). These adrenal autoantibodies are of at least two types: adrenal cortex antibodies (ACA) and antibodies to the steroid 21-hydroxylase enzyme (cytochrome P450c21). The 21-hydroxylase antibodies are highly specific for Addison's disease. In asymptomatic patients, these antibodies may also be important predictors for the subsequent development of adrenal insufficiency. When adrenal autoantibodies are present, 41% of patients develop adrenal insufficiency within 3 years. In adults with other organ-specific autoimmune disorders (eg, premature ovarian failure), researchers have found that detection of adrenal cortex or 21-hydroxylase antibodies was associated with progression to

TABLE 21–4 Causes of adrenocortical insufficiency.

Primary adrenocortical insufficiency (Addison's disease)
Autoimmune (about 80%)
Tuberculosis
Adrenal hemorrhage and infarction
Histoplasmosis and other granulomatous infections
Metastatic carcinoma and lymphoma (non-Hodgkin's)
HIV, AIDS-related opportunistic infection
Amyloidosis
Sarcoidosis
Hemochromatosis
Radiation therapy
Antiphospholipid syndrome
Surgical adrenalectomy
Enzyme inhibitors (metyrapone, aminoglutethimide, trilostane, ketoconazole)
Cytotoxic and chemotherapeutic agents (mitotane, megestrol)
Congenital defects (X-linked adrenoleukodystrophy, enzyme defects, adrenal hypoplasia, familial glucocorticoid deficiency)
Secondary adrenocortical insufficiency
Chronic exogenous glucocorticoid therapy
Pituitary tumor
Hypothalamic tumor
Acquired hypothalamic isolated CRH deficiency

Modified and reproduced, with permission, from Greenspan FS, Strewler GJ (editors). *Basic and Clinical Endocrinology*, 5th ed. Originally published by Appleton & Lange. Copyright © 1997 by the McGraw-Hill Companies, Inc.

overt Addison's disease in 21% and to subclinical hypoadrenalism in 29%. In children, the risk was even higher: In those with other organ-specific autoimmune diseases (eg, hypoparathyroidism), detection of adrenal autoantibodies was associated with a 90% risk of overt Addison's disease and a 10% risk of subclinical hypoadrenalism. In patients with subclinical adrenal insufficiency and positive ACA and 21-hydroxylase autoantibodies, corticosteroid treatment can lead to disappearance of autoantibodies and recovery of normal adrenocortical function.

Autoantibodies to other tissue antigens are frequently found in patients with autoimmune adrenocortical insufficiency as well. Thyroid antibodies have been found in 45%, gastric parietal cell antibodies in 30%, intrinsic factor antibodies in 9%, parathyroid antibodies in 26%, gonadal antibodies in 17%, and islet cell antibodies in 8%.

It is not surprising, therefore, that autoimmune adrenal insufficiency is frequently associated with other autoimmune endocrine disorders. Two distinct polyglandular syndromes involving the adrenal glands have been described. **Autoimmune polyendocrine syndrome type I (APS-I)** is a rare autosomal recessive disorder caused by a mutation in the autoimmune regulator (*AIRE*) with onset in childhood. The diagnosis requires at least two of the following: adrenal insufficiency, hypoparathyroidism, and mucocutaneous candidiasis. Other endocrine disorders are sometimes associated, including gonadal failure and type 1 diabetes mellitus. There is also an increased incidence of other nonendocrine immunologic disorders, including alopecia, vitiligo, pernicious anemia, chronic hepatitis, and GI malabsorption. The autoimmune pathogenesis of this condition involves antibody formation against cytochrome P450 cholesterol–side chain cleavage enzyme (P450scc). This enzyme converts cholesterol to pregnenolone, an initial step in cortisol synthesis (see Figure 21–3). P450scc is found in both the adrenal glands and gonads but not in other tissues involved in APS-1.

Autoimmune polyendocrine syndrome type II (APS-II) consists of adrenal insufficiency, Hashimoto's thyroiditis, and type 1 diabetes mellitus. It is associated with the haplotypes HLA-B8 (DW3) and -DR3. Its pathogenesis involves antibody formation against the 21-OH enzyme mentioned previously. Other autoimmune complications such as vitiligo, pernicious anemia, celiac disease, and myasthenia gravis are present in a subset of patients.

Pathologically, the adrenal glands are small and atrophic, and the capsule is thickened. There is an intense lymphocytic infiltration of the adrenal cortex. Cortical cells are absent or degenerating, surrounded by fibrous stroma and lymphocytes. The adrenal medulla is preserved.

2. Adrenal tuberculosis—Tuberculosis causes adrenal failure by total or near-total destruction of both glands. Such destruction usually occurs gradually and produces a picture of chronic adrenal insufficiency. Adrenal tuberculosis usually results from hematogenous spread of systemic tuberculous infection (lung, GI tract, or kidney) to the adrenal cortex. Pathologically, the adrenal is replaced with caseous necrosis; both cortical and medullary tissue is destroyed. Calcification of the adrenals can be detected radiographically in about 50% of cases.

3. Bilateral adrenal hemorrhage—Bilateral adrenal hemorrhage leads to rapid destruction of the adrenals and precipitates acute adrenal insufficiency. In children, hemorrhage is usually related to fulminant meningococcal septicemia (**Waterhouse-Friderichsen syndrome**) or pseudomonas septicemia. In adults, hemorrhage is related to anticoagulant therapy of other disorders in one third of cases. Other causes in adults include sepsis, coagulation disorders (eg, antiphospholipid syndrome), adrenal vein thrombosis, adrenal metastases, traumatic shock, severe burns, abdominal surgery, and obstetric complications.

Pathologically, the adrenal glands are often massively enlarged. The inner cortex and medulla are almost entirely replaced by hematomas. There is ischemic necrosis of the outer cortex, and only a thin rim of subcapsular cortical cells survives. There is often thrombosis of the adrenal veins.

The pathogenesis of such acute adrenal insufficiency is thought to be related to a stress-induced increase in ACTH levels, which markedly increases adrenal blood flow to such a degree that it exceeds the capacity for adrenal venous drainage. Thrombosis may then lead to hemorrhage. In surviving patients, the hematomas may later calcify.

4. Adrenal metastases—Metastases to the adrenals occur frequently from lung, breast, and stomach carcinomas, melanoma, lymphoma, and many other malignancies. However, metastatic disease seldom produces adrenal insufficiency because more than 90% of both adrenals must be destroyed before overt adrenal insufficiency develops. On pathologic examination, the adrenal glands are often massively enlarged.

5. AIDS-related adrenal insufficiency—Adrenal insufficiency in AIDS usually occurs in the late stages of HIV infection. The adrenal gland is commonly affected by opportunistic infection (especially cytomegalovirus, disseminated *Mycobacterium avium-intracellulare*, *M tuberculosis*, *Cryptococcus neoformans*, *Pneumocystis jirovecii*, and *Toxoplasma gondii*) or by neoplasms such as Kaposi's sarcoma. Although pathologic involvement of the adrenal glands is frequent, clinical adrenal insufficiency is uncommon. More than half of patients with AIDS have necrotizing adrenalitis (most commonly resulting from cytomegalovirus infection), but it is usually limited in extent to less than 50–70% of the gland. Because adrenal insufficiency does not occur until more than 90% of the gland is destroyed, clinical adrenal insufficiency occurs in less than 5% of patients with AIDS.

In addition, medications used by AIDS patients can alter steroid secretion and metabolism. Ketoconazole interferes with steroid synthesis by the adrenals and gonads. Rifampin, phenytoin, and opioids increase steroid metabolism.

All AIDS patients should be considered to be at high risk for primary or secondary adrenal insufficiency. As patients with AIDS live longer because of improved treatment, subclinical abnormalities may progress to clinically significant adrenal insufficiency.

6. Genetic disorders of adrenal insufficiency—These disorders can be subclassified into three categories: 1) congenital adrenal hyperplasia (see disorders of adrenal androgen synthesis below), 2) adrenal hypoplasia congenita with cytomegaly, and 3) adrenal hypoplasia congenita without cytomegaly.

Mutation of the *DAX1* gene causes X-linked adrenal hypoplasia congenita with delayed-onset adrenal insufficiency and hypogonadotropic hypogonadism. The adrenal cortex in this disorder consists of peculiarly shaped, large adrenal cells with large nuclei, which leads to the name, cytomegaly.

Adrenal hypoplasia congenita without cytomegaly mainly comprises the **ACTH insensitivity syndromes,** a group of rare diseases in which resistance to ACTH is either the sole feature or associated with other symptoms. In **familial glucocorticoid deficiency** (**FGD**), adrenocortical unresponsiveness to ACTH causes both decreased adrenal secretion of glucocorticoids and androgens and increased pituitary secretion of ACTH. Responsiveness to angiotensin II is normal. Affected infants and young children come to medical attention because of symptoms of cortisol deficiency, especially cutaneous hyperpigmentation, growth retardation, recurrent hypoglycemia, and recurrent infections. Older children may later manifest tall stature related to advanced bone age. The diagnosis is suggested when cortisol secretion does not respond to either endogenous or exogenous ACTH stimulation. On histologic examination, there is preservation of the zona glomerulosa but degeneration of the zona fasciculata and zona reticularis.

To date, there are two genes known to cause the classical disorder of **FGD**. In FGD1, the resistance to ACTH is caused by one of several missense mutations within the coding region of the ACTH receptor (*MC2R*). In FGD2, the ACTH receptor accessory protein (*MRAP*), which ensures localization of the ACTH receptor in the plasma membrane has been shown to be mutated and dysfunctional.

B. Secondary Adrenocortical Insufficiency

Secondary adrenocortical insufficiency most commonly results from ACTH deficiency caused by chronic exogenous glucocorticoid therapy. Rarely, ACTH deficiency results from pituitary or hypothalamic tumors or from isolated CRH deficiency. Genetic disorders leading to secondary adrenal insufficiency have also been described (eg, *TPIT, POMC* mutations).

Pathophysiology

A. Primary Adrenocortical Insufficiency

Gradual adrenocortical destruction, such as occurs in the autoimmune, tuberculous, and other infiltrative diseases, results initially in a decreased adrenal glucocorticoid reserve. Basal glucocorticoid secretion is normal but does not increase in response to stress and surgery; trauma or infection can precipitate acute adrenal crisis. With further loss of cortical tissue, even basal secretion of glucocorticoids and mineralocorticoids becomes deficient, leading to the clinical manifestations of chronic adrenal insufficiency. The fall in plasma cortisol reduces the feedback inhibition of pituitary ACTH secretion (Figure 21–12), and the plasma level of ACTH rises (Figure 21–15).

Rapid adrenocortical destruction such as occurs in septicemia or adrenal hemorrhage results in sudden loss of both glucocorticoid and mineralocorticoid secretion, leading to acute adrenal crisis.

B. Secondary Adrenocortical Insufficiency

Secondary adrenocortical insufficiency occurs when large doses of glucocorticoids are given for their anti-inflammatory

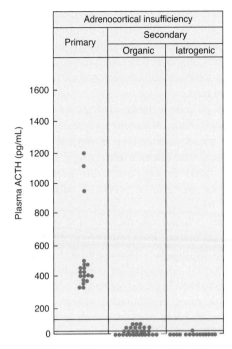

FIGURE 21–15 Basal plasma ACTH levels in primary and secondary adrenocortical insufficiency. (Data from Besser GM, et al. Immunoreactive corticotropin levels in adrenocortical insufficiency. Br Med J. 1971;1:374–376.)

and immunosuppressive effects in treatment of asthma, rheumatoid arthritis, ulcerative colitis, and other diseases. If such treatment is extended beyond 4–5 weeks, it produces prolonged suppression of CRH, ACTH, and endogenous cortisol secretion (Figure 21–12). Should the exogenous steroid treatment be abruptly discontinued, the hypothalamus and pituitary are unable to respond normally to the reduction in level of circulating glucocorticoid. The patient may develop symptoms and signs of chronic adrenocortical insufficiency or, if subjected to stress, acute adrenal crisis. Prolonged suppression of the hypothalamic-pituitary-adrenal axis can be avoided by using alternate-day steroid regimens whenever possible.

ACTH deficiency is the primary problem in secondary adrenocortical insufficiency. The ACTH deficiency leads to diminished cortisol and adrenal androgen secretion, but aldosterone secretion generally remains normal. In the early stages, there is a decreased pituitary ACTH reserve. Basal ACTH and cortisol secretion may be normal but does not increase in response to stress. With progression, there is further loss of ACTH secretion, atrophy of the adrenal cortex, and decreased basal cortisol secretion. At this stage, there is decreased responsiveness not only of pituitary ACTH to stress but also of adrenal cortisol to stimulation with exogenous ACTH.

Clinical Manifestations

The clinical manifestations of glucocorticoid deficiency are nonspecific symptoms: weakness, lethargy, easy fatigability, anorexia, nausea, and occasionally vomiting. Hypoglycemia occurs occasionally. In primary adrenal insufficiency, hyperpigmentation of skin and mucous membranes also occurs. In secondary adrenal insufficiency, hyperpigmentation does not occur, but arthralgias and myalgias may occur. Other clinical features of adrenocortical insufficiency are listed in Table 21–5 and detailed next.

Impaired gluconeogenesis predisposes to hypoglycemia. Severe hypoglycemia may occur spontaneously in children. In adults, the blood glucose level is normal provided there is adequate intake of calories, but fasting causes severe (and potentially fatal) hypoglycemia. In acute adrenal crisis, hypoglycemia may also be provoked by fever, infection, or nausea and vomiting.

In primary adrenal insufficiency, the persistently low or absent plasma cortisol level results in marked hypersecretion of ACTH by the pituitary. Because ACTH has intrinsic MSH activity, a variety of pigmentary changes can occur. These include generalized hyperpigmentation (diffuse darkening of the skin); increased pigmentation of skin creases, nail beds, nipples, areolae, pressure points (such as the knuckles, toes, elbows, and knees), and scars formed after the onset of ACTH

TABLE 21–5 Clinical features of adrenocortical insufficiency.

Primary and secondary adrenal insufficiency
Tiredness, weakness, mental depression
Anorexia, weight loss
Dizziness, orthostatic hypotension
Nausea, vomiting, abdominal cramps, diarrhea
Hyponatremia
Hypoglycemia
Normocytic anemia, lymphocytosis, eosinophilia
Primary adrenal insufficiency
Hyperpigmentation of skin, mucosa
Salt craving
Hyperkalemia
Secondary adrenal insufficiency
Pallor
Amenorrhea, decreased libido, impotence
Scanty axillary and pubic hair
Small testes
Prepubertal growth deficit, delayed puberty
Headache, visual symptoms

Modified and reproduced, with permission, from Oelkers W. Current concepts: Adrenal insufficiency. N Engl J Med. 1996;335:1206.

excess; increased tanning and freckling of sun-exposed areas; and hyperpigmentation of the buccal mucosa, gums, and perivaginal and perianal areas. These changes do not occur in secondary adrenal insufficiency because ACTH secretion is low, not high, in this condition.

Vitiligo occurs in 4–17% of patients with the autoimmune form of adrenal insufficiency but is rare in insufficiency from other causes.

In primary adrenal insufficiency, aldosterone deficiency results in renal loss of Na^+ and retention of K^+, causing hypovolemia and hyperkalemia. The hypovolemia, in turn, leads to prerenal azotemia and hypotension. Salt craving has been documented in about 20% of patients with adrenal insufficiency.

Patients may also be unable to excrete a water load. Hyponatremia may develop, reflecting retention of water in excess of Na^+. The defective water excretion is probably related to increases in posterior pituitary vasopressin secretion; these can be reduced by glucocorticoid administration. In addition, the glomerular filtration rate (GFR) is low. Treatment with mineralocorticoids raises the GFR by restoring plasma volume, and treatment with glucocorticoids improves the GFR even further.

The inability to excrete a water load may predispose to water intoxication. A dramatic example of this sometimes occurs when untreated patients with adrenal insufficiency are given a glucose infusion and subsequently develop high fever ("**glucose fever**"), collapse, and die. The pathogenesis of this condition is related to metabolism of the glucose, leaving free water to dilute the extracellular fluid. This dilution results in an osmotic gradient between the interstitial fluid and cells of the hypothalamic thermoregulatory center, which causes cells to swell and malfunction.

In secondary adrenal insufficiency, aldosterone secretion by the zona glomerulosa is usually preserved. Thus, clinical manifestations of mineralocorticoid deficiency, such as volume depletion, dehydration, hypotension, and electrolyte abnormalities, generally do not occur. Hyponatremia may occur as a result of inability to excrete a water load but is not accompanied by hyperkalemia.

Hypotension occurs in about 90% of patients. It frequently causes orthostatic symptoms and occasionally syncope or recumbent hypotension. Hyperkalemia may cause cardiac arrhythmias, which are sometimes lethal. Refractory shock may occur in glucocorticoid-deficient individuals who are subjected to stress. Vascular smooth muscle becomes less responsive to circulating epinephrine and norepinephrine, and capillaries dilate and become permeable. These effects impair vascular compensation for hypovolemia and promote vascular collapse. A reversible cardiomyopathy has been described.

Cortisol deficiency commonly results in loss of appetite, weight loss, and GI disturbances. Weight loss is common and, in chronic cases, may be profound (15 kg or more). Nausea and vomiting occur in most patients; diarrhea is less frequent. Such GI symptoms often intensify during acute adrenal crisis.

In women with adrenal insufficiency, loss of pubic and axillary hair may occur as a result of decreased secretion of adrenal androgens. Amenorrhea occurs commonly, in most cases related to weight loss and chronic illness but sometimes as a result of ovarian failure or hyperprolactinemia.

CNS consequences of adrenal insufficiency include personality changes (irritability, apprehension, inability to concentrate, and emotional lability), increased sensitivity to olfactory and gustatory stimuli, and the appearance of electroencephalographic waves slower than the normal alpha rhythm.

Patients with **acute adrenal crisis** have symptoms of high fever, weakness, apathy, and confusion. Anorexia, nausea, and vomiting may lead to volume depletion and dehydration. Abdominal pain may mimic that of an acute abdominal process. Evidence suggests that the symptoms of acute glucocorticoid deficiency are mediated by significantly elevated plasma levels of cytokines, particularly IL-6 and, to a lesser extent, IL-1 and TNF. Hyponatremia, hyperkalemia, lymphocytosis, eosinophilia, and hypoglycemia occur frequently. Acute adrenal crisis can occur in patients with undiagnosed ACTH deficiency and in patients receiving corticosteroids who are not given increased steroid dosage during periods of stress. Precipitants include infection, trauma, surgery, and dehydration. If unrecognized and untreated, coma, severe hypotension, or shock unresponsive to vasopressors may rapidly lead to death.

Laboratory findings in primary adrenocortical insufficiency include hyponatremia, hyperkalemia, occasional hypoglycemia, and mild azotemia (Table 21–6). The hyponatremia and hyperkalemia are manifestations of mineralocorticoid deficiency. The azotemia, with elevations of blood urea nitrogen (BUN) and serum creatinine, is due to volume depletion and dehydration. Mild acidosis is frequently present. Hypercalcemia of mild to moderate degree occurs infrequently.

In secondary adrenocortical insufficiency, mineralocorticoid secretion is usually normal. Thus, serum Na^+, K^+, creatinine, bicarbonate, and BUN are usually normal. Plasma glucose may be low, although severe hypoglycemia is unusual.

Hematologic manifestations of adrenal insufficiency include normocytic, normochromic anemia, neutropenia, lymphocytosis, monocytosis, and eosinophilia. Hyperprolactinemia occurs

when serum cortisol levels are low. Abdominal x-ray films demonstrate adrenal calcification in about 50% of patients with Addison's disease caused by adrenal tuberculosis and in a smaller percentage of patients with bilateral adrenal hemorrhage. CT scans detect adrenal calcification even more frequently in such cases and may also reveal bilateral adrenal enlargement in cases of adrenal hemorrhage; tuberculous, fungal, or cytomegalovirus infection; metastases; and other infiltrative diseases. Electrocardiographic findings include low voltage, a vertical QRS axis, and nonspecific ST wave changes related to electrolyte abnormalities (eg, peak T waves from hyperkalemia).

Diagnosis

A. Primary Adrenal Insufficiency

To establish the diagnosis of fully developed primary adrenal insufficiency, the physician must demonstrate an inability of the adrenal glands to respond normally to ACTH stimulation. This is usually done by performing an ACTH stimulation test (Figure 21–16). To do so, the physician obtains an 8:00 AM plasma cortisol, then administers 250 μg of synthetic ACTH (cosyntropin) intravenously or intramuscularly. Repeat plasma cortisol levels are obtained 30 and 60 minutes later. Normal individuals have a normal 8:00 AM plasma cortisol and usually a twofold or greater increase in plasma cortisol following cosyntropin. Patients with Addison's disease have a low 8:00 AM plasma cortisol and virtually no increase in plasma cortisol after cosyntropin. At a specificity of 95%, the sensitivity 250-μg cosyntropin stimulation test is 97% for primary adrenal insufficiency.

B. Secondary Adrenocortical Insufficiency

The diagnosis of ACTH deficiency from exogenous glucocorticoids is suggested by obtaining a history of chronic glucocorticoid therapy or by finding cushingoid features on physical examination. Hypothalamic or pituitary tumors leading to ACTH deficiency usually produce symptoms and signs of other endocrinopathies. Deficient secretion of other pituitary hormones such as LH and FSH or TSH may produce hypogonadism or hypothyroidism (see Chapter 19). Excessive secretion of growth hormone or prolactin from a pituitary adenoma may produce acromegaly or amenorrhea and galactorrhea. Unfortunately, the conventional ACTH stimulation test uses a dose (250 μg ACTH) that is supraphysiologic and capable of transiently stimulating the adrenal cortex in some patients with secondary (pituitary or hypothalamic) adrenal insufficiency. Therefore, at a specificity of 95%, the sensitivity of the 250-μg cosyntropin stimulation test is only 57% for secondary adrenal insufficiency. Thus, in evaluating patients with suspected central causes, some experts now recommend using a much lower dose (1 μg) of ACTH in the ACTH stimulation test. However, the test sensitivity for the 1-μg cosyntropin stimulation test is only 61%. Consequently, for patients in whom the pretest probability of secondary adrenal insufficiency

TABLE 21–6 Typical plasma electrolyte levels in normal humans and in patients with adrenocortical diseases.

	Na^+ (mEq/L)	K^+ (mEq/L)	Cl^- (mEq/L)	HCO_3^- (mEq/L)
Normal	142	4.5	105	25
Adrenal insufficiency	120	6.7	85	45
Primary hyperaldosteronism	145	2.4	96	41
Hypoaldosteronism	145	6.7	105	25

Modified and reproduced, with permission, from Ganong WF. *Review of Medical Physiology*, 22nd ed. McGraw-Hill, 2005.

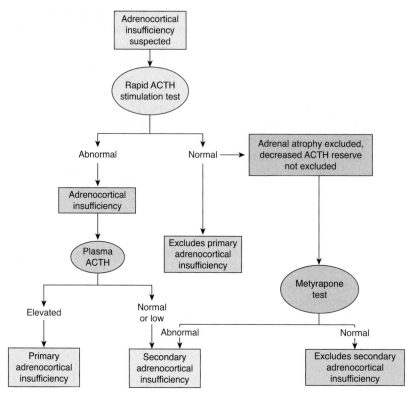

FIGURE 21–16   Diagnostic evaluation of suspected primary or secondary adrenocortical insufficiency. Boxes enclose clinical diagnoses, and ovals enclose diagnostic tests.   (Redrawn, with permission, from Miller WL, Tyrrell JB. The adrenal cortex. In: *Endocrinology and Metabolism,* 3rd ed. Felig P, Baxter JD, Frohman LA [editors]. McGraw-Hill, 1995.)

is high, tests involving stimulation of the hypothalamus (ie, hypoglycemia following insulin injection) are recommended.

HYPERALDOSTERONISM (EXCESSIVE PRODUCTION OF MINERALOCORTICOIDS)

Primary hyperaldosteronism occurs because of excessive unregulated secretion of aldosterone by the adrenal cortex. It is now thought to be the most common potentially curable and specifically treatable cause of hypertension. **Secondary hyperaldosteronism** occurs because aldosterone secretion is stimu-

lated by excessive secretion of renin by the juxtaglomerular apparatus of the kidney.

The clinical features of hyperaldosteronism may also be due to non-aldosterone-mediated mineralocorticoid excess. Causes include Cushing's syndrome; congenital adrenal hyperplasia resulting from 11β-hydroxylase deficiency or 17α-hydroxylase deficiency; the syndrome of apparent mineralocorticoid excess resulting from 11β-hydroxysteroid dehydrogenase (11β-HSD) deficiency; primary glucocorticoid resistance; and Liddle's syndrome resulting from activating mutations of the gene encoding for β- and γ-subunits of the renal epithelial sodium channel.

Etiology

The causes of hyperaldosteronism are listed in Table 21–7.

A. Primary Hyperaldosteronism

Primary hyperaldosteronism usually results from an aldosterone-secreting tumor of the adrenal cortex, most often a solitary **adenoma** (Figure 21–17). Bilateral tumors are unusual. Small satellite adenomas are sometimes found. Adenomas are readily identified by their characteristic golden yellow color. The adjacent adrenal cortex may be compressed. Adenomas producing excessive aldosterone are indistinguishable from those producing excessive cortisol except that they tend to be smaller (usually < 2 cm in diameter). Primary hyperaldosteronism was

TABLE 21–7 Causes of hyperaldosteronism.

Primary hyperaldosteronism
Aldosterone-secreting adrenocortical adenoma
Bilateral hyperplasia of zona glomerulosa
Glucocorticoid-remediable hyperaldosteronism
Aldosterone-secreting adrenocortical carcinoma (rare)
Idiopathic
Secondary hyperaldosteronism
Renal ischemia
Renal artery stenosis
Malignant hypertension
Decreased intravascular volume
Congestive heart failure
Chronic diuretic or laxative use
Hypoproteinemic states (cirrhosis, nephrotic syndrome)
Sodium-wasting disorders
Chronic renal failure
Renal tubular acidosis
Juxtaglomerular cell hyperplasia (Bartter's syndrome)
Surreptitious vomiting or diuretic ingestion (pseudo-Bartter's syndrome)
Oral contraceptives
Renin-secreting tumors (rare)

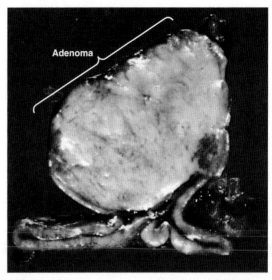

FIGURE 21–17 Cross section of adrenal, showing an adrenocortical adenoma in a patient with primary hyperaldosteronism. The gross and microscopic features do not permit differentiation of aldosterone- and cortisol-secreting adenomas in most cases. (Reproduced, with permission, from Chandrasoma P, Taylor CE. *Concise Pathology*, 3rd ed. Originally published by Appleton & Lange. Copyright © 1998 by the McGraw-Hill Companies, Inc.)

traditionally regarded as a rare cause of hypertension and not worth looking for in the absence of hypokalemia. However, the development and application of the ratio of plasma aldosterone concentration to plasma renin activity as a screening test to the population of hypertensives has resulted in a marked increase in detection rate, suggesting that primary hyperaldosteronism is actually quite common in patients with hypertension; most have normal serum potassium levels. Up to 15% of patients diagnosed as having essential hypertension have primary hyperaldosteronism.

Bilateral adrenal hyperplasia accounts for most of the remaining cases of primary hyperaldosteronism (idiopathic hyperaldosteronism). Affected patients have bilateral nonadenomatous hyperplasia of the zona glomerulosa. Selective adrenal vein sampling looking for lateralized aldosterone secretion is the most reliable means of differentiating a unilateral aldosterone-producing adenoma from bilateral adrenal hyperplasia.

Unilateral adrenal hyperplasia is a rare cause of hyperaldosteronism. Selective adrenal-vein sampling to determine plasma aldosterone concentrations can help to define unilaterality of disease.

Adrenocortical carcinomas producing only aldosterone are extremely rare. Such tumors are generally large.

A dominantly inherited form of hyperaldosteronism—**glucocorticoid-remediable aldosteronism** (GRA)—has been identified. As noted in Chapter 11, affected patients have a "hybrid" 11β-hydroxylase-aldosterone synthase gene in which the 11β-hydroxylase gene's regulatory elements are fused to the coding region of the aldosterone synthase gene. Therefore, ACTH stimulates aldosterone synthase activity. The hybrid *CYP11B1/CYP11B2* gene arises from an unequal crossing over between the two *CYP11B* genes during meiosis. The hybrid gene can be detected in peripheral blood leukocyte DNA by Southern blot or polymerase chain reaction methods. The clinical phenotype varies from severe early-onset hypertension to much milder blood pressure elevation; hypokalemia is usually mild. Affected individuals apparently have an increased risk of premature stroke. Because expression of the hybrid gene is stimulated by ACTH, leading to increased production of aldosterone and other steroids, the hyperaldosteronism is glucocorticoid suppressible. Treatment with low doses of dexamethasone inhibits ACTH.

B. Secondary Hyperaldosteronism

Secondary hyperaldosteronism is common. It results from excessive renin production by the juxtaglomerular apparatus of the kidney. The high renin output occurs in response to (1) renal ischemia (eg, renal artery stenosis or malignant hypertension), (2) decreased intravascular volume (eg, congestive heart failure, cirrhosis, nephrotic syndrome, laxative or diuretic abuse), (3) Na^+-wasting disorders (eg, chronic renal failure or renal tubular acidosis), (4) hyperplasia of the juxtaglomerular apparatus (Bartter's syndrome), or (5) renin-secreting tumors. In these states, stimulation of the zona glomerulosa by the renin-angiotensin system leads to increased aldosterone production.

Pathologically, in secondary hyperaldosteronism, the adrenals may appear grossly normal, but microscopically there may be hyperplasia of the zona glomerulosa.

Pathophysiology

In primary hyperaldosteronism, there is a primary (autonomous) increase in aldosterone production by the abnormal zona glomerulosa tissue (adenoma or hyperplasia). However, circulating levels of aldosterone are still modulated to some extent by variations in ACTH secretion. The chronic aldosterone excess results in expansion of the extracellular fluid volume and plasma volume. In turn, this expansion is registered by stretch receptors of the juxtaglomerular apparatus and Na^+ flux at the macula densa, leading to suppression of renin production and low circulating plasma renin activity.

Patients with secondary hyperaldosteronism also produce excessively large amounts of aldosterone but, in contrast to patients with primary hyperaldosteronism, have elevated plasma renin activity.

Clinical Consequences of Mineralocorticoid Excess

The major consequences of chronic aldosterone excess are Na^+ retention and K^+ and H^+ wasting by the kidney.

The excess aldosterone initially stimulates Na^+ reabsorption by the renal collecting and distal tubules, causing the extracellular fluid volume to expand and the blood pressure to rise. When the extracellular fluid expansion reaches a certain point, however, Na^+ excretion resumes despite the continued action of aldosterone on the renal tubule. This **"escape" phenomenon** is probably due to increased secretion of **atrial natriuretic peptide.** Because the escape phenomenon causes the excretion of excess salt, affected patients are not edematous. Such escape from the action of aldosterone does not occur in the distal tubules. There, the elevated aldosterone levels promote continued exchange of Na^+ for K^+ and H^+, causing K^+ depletion and alkalosis. Affected patients are not markedly hypernatremic because water is retained along with the Na^+.

The chronic aldosterone excess also produces a prolonged K^+ diuresis. Total body K^+ stores are depleted, and hypokalemia develops. Patients may complain of tiredness, loss of stamina, weakness, nocturia, and lassitude, all symptoms of K^+ depletion. Prolonged K^+ depletion damages the kidneys (**hypokalemic nephropathy**), causing resistance to ADH (vasopressin). The resultant loss of concentrating ability causes thirst and polyuria (especially nocturnal).

When the K^+ loss is marked, intracellular K^+ is replaced by Na^+ and H^+. The intracellular movement of H^+, along with increased renal secretion of H^+, causes metabolic alkalosis to develop.

Hypertension—related to Na^+ retention and expansion of plasma volume—is a characteristic finding. Hypertension can range from borderline to severe but is usually mild or moderate. Accelerated (malignant) hypertension is extremely rare. Because the hypertension is sustained, however, it may produce retinopathy, renal damage, or left ventricular hypertrophy. For example, patients with primary hyperaldosteronism resulting from aldosterone-producing adenomas have increased wall thickness and mass and decreased early diastolic filling of the left ventricle compared with patients who have essential hypertension. Thus, the chance of curing hypertension with resection of an adrenal adenoma is less predictable than the likelihood of correcting the related biochemical abnormalities. Only 50% of patients with adenomas are normotensive 5 years after adrenalectomy; old patients in particular are more likely to require postoperative antihypertensive medications. Patients with no family history of hypertension and who required two or fewer antihypertensive agents preoperatively are more likely to resolve their hypertension after removal of an adrenal tumor.

The heart may be mildly enlarged as a result of plasma volume expansion and left ventricular hypertrophy. Severely K^+-depleted patients may develop blunting of baroreceptor function, manifested by postural falls in blood pressure without reflex tachycardia, or even malignant arrhythmias and sudden cardiac death.

The K^+ depletion causes a minor but detectable degree of carbohydrate intolerance (demonstrated by an abnormal glucose tolerance test). This may be due to impaired pancreatic insulin release and reduction in insulin sensitivity related to the hypokalemia. The decrease in glucose tolerance is corrected after K^+ repletion.

In addition, the alkalosis accompanying severe K^+ depletion may lower the plasma Ca^{2+} to the point at which latent or frank tetany occurs (see Chapter 17). The hypokalemia may cause severe muscle weakness, muscle cramps, and intestinal atony. Paresthesias may develop as a result of the hypokalemia and alkalosis. A positive Trousseau's or Chvostek's sign is suggestive of alkalosis and hypocalcemia (see Chapter 17).

Laboratory findings in hyperaldosteronism include hypokalemia and alkalosis (Table 21–6). Typically, the serum K^+ is below 3.6 mEq/L (3.6 mmol/L), serum Na^+ is normal or slightly elevated, serum HCO_3^- is increased, and serum Cl^- is decreased (hypokalemic, hypochloremic metabolic alkalosis). There is an inappropriately large amount of K^+ in the urine.

The hematocrit may be reduced because of hemodilution by the expanded plasma volume. Affected patients may fail to concentrate urine and may have abnormal glucose tolerance tests.

The plasma renin level is suppressed in primary hyperaldosteronism and elevated in secondary hyperaldosteronism. Adrenal cortisol production is normal or low.

The ECG may show changes of modest left ventricular hypertrophy and K^+ depletion (flattening of T waves and appearance of U waves).

Diagnosis of Hyperaldosteronism

A. Primary Hyperaldosteronism

In the past, the diagnosis of primary hyperaldosteronism was usually suggested by finding hypokalemia in an untreated patient with hypertension (ie, one not taking diuretics) (Table 21–6). However, a low-Na^+ intake, by diminishing renal K^+ loss, may mask total body K^+ depletion. In patients with normal renal function, dietary salt loading will unmask hypokalemia as a manifestation of total body K^+ depletion. Thus, finding a low serum K^+ in a hypertensive patient on a high-salt intake and not receiving diuretics warrants further evaluation for hyperaldosteronism. Currently, the best screening test for primary hyperaldosteronism involves determinations of plasma aldosterone concentration (normal: 1–16 ng/dL) and plasma renin activity (normal: 1–2.5 ng/mL/h), and calculation of the plasma aldosterone-renin ratio (normal: < 25). Patients with aldosterone-renin ratios of ≥ 25 require further evaluation.

Subsequent workup entails measuring the 24-hour urinary aldosterone excretion and the plasma aldosterone level with the patient on a diet containing more than 120 mEq of Na^+ per day. The urinary aldosterone excretion exceeds 14 μg/d, and the plasma aldosterone is usually greater than 90 pg/mL in primary hyperaldosteronism.

High-resolution CT or MRI of the adrenal glands may help to differentiate between **adrenal adenoma** and bilateral **adrenal hyperplasia**. The gold standard for diagnosis is bilateral adrenal venous sampling, which is more sensitive and specific than imaging, to identify a unilateral cause of primary hyperaldosteronism.

B. Secondary Hyperaldosteronism

Patients with secondary hyperaldosteronism due to malignant hypertension, renal artery stenosis, or chronic renal disease also excrete large amounts of aldosterone but, in contrast to primary hyperaldosteronism, have elevated plasma renin activity.

CHECKPOINT

22. What are the causes of hyperaldosteronism?
23. What are the presenting symptoms and signs of hyperaldosteronism?
24. How is the diagnosis of hyperaldosteronism made?

HYPOALDOSTERONISM: DEFICIENT MINERALOCORTICOID PRODUCTION OR ACTION

Primary mineralocorticoid deficiency (hypoaldosteronism) may result from destruction of adrenocortical tissue, defects in adrenal synthesis of aldosterone, inadequate stimulation of aldosterone secretion (hyporeninemic hypoaldosteronism), or resistance to the ion transport effects of aldosterone, such as are seen in pseudohypoaldosteronism. Hypoaldosteronism is characterized by Na^+ loss, with hyponatremia, hypovolemia, and hypotension, and impaired secretion of both K^+ and H^+ in the renal tubules, resulting in hyperkalemia and metabolic acidosis. Renin activity is typically increased.

A **secondary deficiency** of endogenous mineralocorticoids may occur when renin production is suppressed or deficient. Renin production may be suppressed by the Na^+ retention and volume expansion resulting from exogenous mineralocorticoids (fludrocortisone acetate) or mineralocorticoid-like substances (licorice or carbenoxolone). When this happens, hypertension, hypokalemia, and metabolic alkalosis result. When renin production is deficient and unable to stimulate mineralocorticoid production, Na^+ loss, hyperkalemia, and metabolic acidosis occur.

Etiology

Acute and chronic adrenocortical insufficiency were discussed previously. In long-standing **hypopituitarism,** atrophy of the zona glomerulosa occurs, and the increase in aldosterone secretion normally produced by surgery or other stress is absent. **Hyporeninemic hypoaldosteronism (type IV renal tubular acidosis)** is a disorder characterized by hyperkalemia and acidosis in association with (usually mild) chronic renal insufficiency. Typically, affected individuals are men in the fifth to seventh decades of life who have underlying pyelonephritis, diabetes mellitus, gout, or nephrotic syndrome. The chronic renal insufficiency is usually not severe enough to account for the hyperkalemia. Plasma and urinary aldosterone levels and plasma renin activity are consistently low and unresponsive to stimulation by upright posture, dietary Na^+ restriction, or furosemide administration. The syndrome is thought to be due to impairment of the juxtaglomerular apparatus associated with the underlying renal disease. Hyporeninemic hypoaldosteronism also has been described transiently in critically ill patients, such as those with septic shock. Two genetic disorders may produce the symptoms and signs of hypoaldosteronism. In **congenital adrenal hyperplasia,** there are enzymatic abnormalities in mineralocorticoid biosynthesis (see below). Mutations in the *CYP11B2* gene for 11-hydroxylase cause aldosterone synthase deficiency, an isolated defect of aldosterone biosynthesis. Aldosterone levels are low. In **pseudohypoaldosteronism,** there is renal tubular resistance to mineralocorticoid hormones. Affected patients manifest symptoms and signs of hypoaldosteronism, but aldosterone levels are high. **Pseudohypoaldosteronism type 1** is frequently due to mutations involving the amiloride-sensitive epithelial sodium channel. Gordon's syndrome (**pseudohypoaldosteronism type 2**), characterized by hypertension, hyperchloremic acidemia, hyperkalemia, and intact renal function, is due to resistance to the kaliuretic but not sodium reabsorptive effects of aldosterone. The genetic basis of this condition is still unknown.

Clinical Consequences of Mineralocorticoid Deficiency

Patients undergoing bilateral adrenalectomy, if not given mineralocorticoid replacement therapy, will develop profound urinary Na^+ losses resulting in hypovolemia, hypotension, and, eventually, shock and death. In adrenal insufficiency, these changes can be delayed by increasing the dietary salt intake. However, the amount of dietary salt needed to prevent them entirely is so large that collapse and death are inevitable unless mineralocorticoid treatment with fludrocortisone acetate is also initiated. Secretion of both K^+ and H^+ is impaired in the renal tubule, resulting in hyperkalemia and metabolic acidosis.

DISORDERS OF ADRENAL ANDROGEN PRODUCTION

The adrenal cortex also secretes androgens, principally **androstenedione, dehydroepiandrosterone** (DHEA), and **dehydroepiandrosterone sulfate** (DHEAS). In general, the secretion of adrenal androgens parallels that of cortisol. ACTH is the major factor regulating androgen production by the adrenal cortex. The adrenal androgens are secreted in an unbound state but circulate weakly bound to plasma proteins, chiefly albumin. They are metabolized either by degradation and inactivation or by peripheral conversion to the more potent androgens testosterone and dihydrotestosterone. The androgen metabolites are conjugated either as glucuronides or sulfates and excreted in the urine.

DHEA has both masculinizing and anabolic effects. However, it is less than one fifth as potent as the androgens produced by the testis. Consequently, it has very little physiologic effect under normal conditions. In women, the androgenic steroids (adrenal and ovarian) are thought to be required for the maintenance of libido and the capacity to achieve orgasm, perhaps through a trophic action on the clitoris.

Excessive secretion of adrenal androgens may occur as an associated phenomenon with Cushing's syndrome, particularly that resulting from adrenocortical neoplasms (particularly carcinomas). Excessive production of adrenal androgens has little effect in mature males but may cause hirsutism in mature females. It may result in precocious pseudopuberty in prepubertal boys and in masculinization in prepubertal girls.

Excessive secretion of adrenal androgens may also be congenital, resulting from one of several enzymatic defects in steroid metabolism in **congenital adrenal hyperplasia** (CAH). CAH occurs in both sexes and it is the most common cause of ambiguous genitalia. It is a relatively common disease, occurring in 1 in 5000 to 1 in 15,000 births.

CAH is actually a group of autosomal recessive disorders, in each of which, because of an enzyme defect, the bulk of steroid hormone production by the adrenal cortex shifts from corticosteroids to androgens. Congenital adrenal hyperplasia is caused by mutations in the *CYP21*, *CYP11B1*, *CYP17*, and *3βHSD* genes that encode steroidogenic enzymes and by mutations in

the gene encoding the intracellular cholesterol transport protein, steroidogenic acute regulatory protein (StAR). Each of these defects causes different biochemical and clinical consequences. The name of the syndrome derives from the fact that all of the biochemical defects lead to impaired cortisol secretion, resulting in compensatory hypersecretion of ACTH and consequent hyperplasia of the adrenal cortex. The two most frequent causes of congenital adrenal hyperplasia are 21β-hydroxylase or 11β-hydroxylase deficiency (Figure 21–3). More than 90% of cases are due to deficiency of the enzyme steroid 21β-hydroxylase. The 21β-hydroxylase enzyme (cytochrome P450c21) is encoded by the gene *CYP21A2*. More than 50 different *CYP21A2* mutations have been reported, perhaps accounting for a wide range of congenital adrenal hyperplasia phenotypes. Most are spontaneous mutations, including point mutations, small deletions or insertions, or complete gene deletions. However, 15 mutations, which constitute 90–95% of alleles, derive from intergenic recombination of DNA sequences between the *CYP21A2* gene and a neighboring pseudogene (an inactive gene that is transcribed but not translated). These intergenic *CYP21A2* mutations are caused by conversion of a portion of the active *CYP21A2* gene sequence into a pseudogene sequence, resulting in a less active or inactive gene (gene conversion).

Other cases of congenital adrenal hyperplasia are related to steroid 11β-hydroxylase (cytochrome P450c11) deficiency. Deletion hybrid genes, because of unequal crossing over between *CYP11B1* (11β-hydroxylase) and *CYP11B2* (aldosterone synthase), are associated with this form of congenital adrenal hyperplasia. *CYP11B1*, the gene encoding 11β-hydroxylase, is expressed in high levels in the zona fasciculata and is regulated by ACTH. *CYP11B2*, the gene encoding aldosterone synthase, is expressed in the zona glomerulosa and is primarily regulated by the renin-angiotensin system.

Impaired *CYP21A2* or *CYP11B1* activity causes deficient production of both cortisol and aldosterone. The low serum cortisol stimulates ACTH production; adrenal hyperplasia occurs, and precursor steroids—in particular 17-hydroxyprogesterone—accumulate. The accumulated precursors cannot enter the cortisol synthesis pathway and thus spill over into the androgen synthesis pathway, forming androstenedione and DHEA. Prenatal exposure to excessive androgens results in masculinization of the female fetus, leading to ambiguous genitalia at birth. Newborn males have normal genitalia.

During the newborn period, there are two classic presentations of congenital adrenal hyperplasia resulting from classic 21β-hydroxylase deficiency: salt wasting and non-salt wasting (also called "simple virilizing"). Neonates with the salt-wasting form have severe cortisol and aldosterone deficiencies and, if undiagnosed and untreated, will develop potentially lethal adrenal crisis and salt wasting at 2–3 weeks of age. Those with the simple virilizing form have sufficient cortisol and aldosterone production to avoid both adrenal crisis and salt wasting and are usually diagnosed because of virilization between birth and 5 years of age. Postnatally, both sexes present with virilization, reflecting the continuing androgen excess. The excess androgens during childhood can produce pseudoprecocious puberty, premature growth acceleration, early epiphyseal fusion, and adult short stature. Variability in the phenotype occurs, depending on the severity of the 21β-hydroxylase deficiency.

The diagnosis of 21β-hydroxylase-deficient nonclassic adrenal hyperplasia (NCAH) is suggested by finding a morning plasma level of the cortisol precursor 17-hydroxyprogesterone > 4 ng/mL (12.0 nmol/L) (obtained in women during the follicular phase) or > 10 ng/mL (30.3 nmol/L) after ACTH stimulation (see Figure 21–3). Diagnosis of specific defects is confirmed by genotyping of the relevant genes.

Analysis of DNA obtained by chorionic villus sampling in early pregnancy permits prenatal diagnosis. Administration of dexamethasone to the mother of an affected female fetus can prevent genital ambiguity. Postnatally, lifelong hormonal replacement with hydrocortisone (glucocorticoid) and fludrocortisone (mineralocorticoid) can ensure normal puberty and fertility. Antiandrogen therapy (with flutamide) plus inhibition of androgen-to-estrogen conversion (with testolactone) permits reduction in the dose of hydrocortisone sometimes required to suppress androgen levels.

Deficiency of adrenal sex hormones usually has little effect in the presence of normal testes or ovaries. In mature women, minor menstrual abnormalities may occur.

CHECKPOINT

25. What are the causes of hypoaldosteronism?
26. What are the clinical manifestations of hypoaldosteronism?
27. What is the effect of excess or deficiency of adrenal androgens on otherwise normal adult men and women (ie, individuals with normal gonads)?

CASE STUDIES

Eva M. Aagaard, MD, & Yeong Kwok, MD

(See Chapter 25, p. 707 for Answers)

CASE 97

A 35-year-old woman has hypertension of recent onset. Review of systems reveals several months of weight gain and menstrual irregularity. On examination she is obese, with a plethoric appearance. The blood pressure is 165/98 mm Hg. There are prominent purplish striae over the abdomen and multiple bruises over both lower legs. The patient's physician entertains a diagnosis of hypercortisolism (Cushing's syndrome).

Questions

A. What other features of the history and physical examination should be sought?
B. Assuming that the diagnosis of hypercortisolism is correct, what is the underlying pathogenesis of this patient's hypertension, weight gain, and skin striae?
C. List four causes of Cushing's syndrome and discuss the relationships among the hypothalamus, pituitary, and adrenal in each case. Which is the most likely cause in this patient?
D. How can the diagnosis of hypercortisolism be established in this patient?

CASE 98

A 56-year-old man undergoes an abdominal computed tomography (CT) scan in the evaluation of abdominal pain. The scan is unremarkable except for the finding of a 3-cm mass in the right adrenal gland. The mass is homogeneous and smooth, and it has low x-ray absorption on the CT scan. The patient has a normal examination and feels well otherwise.

Questions

A. What are the possible diagnoses of this mass, and what should be the next step in the evaluation?
B. What follow-up needs to be pursued and why?

CASE 99

A 38-year-old woman presents for annual follow-up of previously diagnosed Hashimoto's thyroiditis, for which she has been receiving thyroid replacement therapy (levothyroxine, 0.15 mg/d). She reports a gradual onset of weakness, lethargy, and easy fatigability over the last 3 months. Review of systems reveals only recent menstrual irregularity, with no menses in 2.5 months. Blood pressure is 90/50 mm Hg (compared with previous readings of 110/75 and 120/80 mm Hg), and her weight is down 13 pounds since her last visit 11 months ago. The skin appears to be tanned, but the patient denies sun exposure. The physician seeing her wonders whether she has now developed adrenal insufficiency (Addison's disease).

Questions

A. What other features of the history and physical examination should be sought?

B. If Addison's disease has developed, what should the serum electrolytes show, and why?

C. How can the diagnosis of adrenal insufficiency be established in this patient?

D. What is the pathogenesis of the hypotension, weight loss, and skin hyperpigmentation?

CASE 100

A 42-year-old man presents for evaluation of newly diagnosed hypertension. He is currently taking no medications and offers no complaints. A careful review of systems reveals symptoms of fatigue, loss of stamina, and frequent urination, particularly at night. Physical examination is normal except for a blood pressure of 168/100 mm Hg. Serum electrolytes are reported as follows: sodium, 152 mEq/L; potassium, 3.2 mEq/L; bicarbonate, 32 mEq/L; chloride, 112 mEq/L. The clinical picture is consistent with a diagnosis of primary hyperaldosteronism.

Questions

A. What is the mechanism by which primary hyperaldosteronism causes the history, physical examination, and laboratory findings in this patient?

B. What should the urinalysis and measurement of urine electrolytes show, and why?

C. How can the diagnosis of hyperaldosteronism be established in this patient?

CASE 101

A 64-year-old man with a long history of gout and type 2 diabetes mellitus comes in for a routine checkup. Serum chemistries are as follows: sodium, 140 mEq/L; potassium, 6.3 mEq/L; bicarbonate, 18 mEq/L; BUN, 43 mg/dL; creatinine, 2.9 mg/dL; glucose, 198 mg/dL. Chart review shows previous potassium values of 5.3 mEq/L and 5.7 mEq/L. The patient is currently taking only colchicine, 0.5 mg daily, and glyburide, 5 mg twice daily.

Questions

A. What is the most likely cause of this patient's hyperkalemia, and what is its pathogenesis?

B. What are other possible causes of hypoaldosteronism?

C. Plasma renin activity and aldosterone levels are sent to the laboratory. What results should be anticipated?

REFERENCES

General

Aron DC et al. Glucocorticoids and adrenal androgens. In: *Basic and Clinical Endocrinology*, 8th ed. Greenspan FS, Gardner DG (editors). McGraw-Hill, 2007.

Cushing's Syndrome

Allolio B et al. Clinical review: Adrenocortical carcinoma: Clinical update. J Clin Endocrinol Metab. 2006 Jun;91(6):2027–37. [PMID: 16551738]

Elamin MB et al. Accuracy of diagnostic tests for Cushing's syndrome: A systematic review and metaanalyses. J Clin Endocrinol Metab. 2008 May;93(5):1553–62. [PMID: 18334594]

Lacroix A et al. Ectopic and abnormal hormone receptors in adrenal Cushing's syndrome. Endocr Rev. 2001 Feb;22(1):75–110. [PMID: 11159817]

Morris DG et al. Dynamic test in the diagnosis and differential diagnosis of Cushing's syndrome. J Endocrinol Invest. 2003;26(7 Suppl):64–73. [PMID: 14604068]

Clinically Inapparent Adrenal Mass ("Incidentaloma")

National Institutes of Health. NIH state of the science statement on the management of the clinically inapparent adrenal mass ("incidentaloma"). NIH Consens State Sci Statements. 2002 Feb 4-6;19(2):1–25. [PMID: 14768652]

Reincke M. Subclinical Cushing's syndrome. Endocrinol Metab Clin North Am. 2000 Mar;29(1):43–56. [PMID: 10732263]

Adrenocortical Insufficiency

Else T et al. Genetic analysis of adrenal absence: Agenesis and aplasia. Trends Endocrinol Metab. 2005 Dec;16(10):458-68. [PMID: 16275119]

Hahner S et al. Management of adrenal insufficiency in different clinical settings. Expert Opin Pharmacother. 2005 Nov;6(14):2407–17. [PMID: 16259572]

Nieman LK. Dynamic evaluation of adrenal hypofunction. J Endocrinol Invest. 2003;26(7 Suppl):74–82. [PMID: 14604069]

Hyperaldosteronism

Giacchetti G et al. Primary aldosteronism, a major form of low renin hypertension: From screening to diagnosis. Trends Endocrinol Metab. 2008 Apr;19(3):104–8. [PMID: 18313325]

McMahon GT et al. Glucocorticoid-remediable aldosteronism. Cardiol Rev. 2004 Jan-Feb;12(1):44–8. [PMID: 14667264]

Rossi GP et al. Primary aldosteronism: Cardiovascular, renal and metabolic implications. Trends Endocrinol Metab. 2008 Apr;19(3):88–90. [PMID: 18314347]

Young WF Jr. Minireview: Primary aldosteronism—Changing concepts in diagnosis and treatment. Endocrinology. 2003 Jun;144(6):2208–13. [PMID: 12746276]

Hypoaldosteronism

White PC. Aldosterone synthase deficiency and related disorders. Mol Cell Endocrinol. 2004 Mar 31;217(1-2):81–87. [PMID: 15134805]

Disorders of Adrenal Androgen Production (Congenital Adrenal Hyperplasia)

Arlt W et al. Adult consequences of congenital adrenal hyperplasia. Horm Res. 2007;68 (Suppl 5):158–64. [PMID: 18174737]

Riepe FG et al. Recent advances in diagnosis, treatment, and outcome of congenital adrenal hyperplasia due to 21-hydroxylase deficiency. Rev Endocr Metab Disord. 2007 Dec;8(4):349–63. [PMID: 17885806]

Speiser PW. Prenatal and neonatal diagnosis and treatment of congenital adrenal hyperplasia. Horm Res. 2007;68 (Suppl 5):90–2. [PMID: 18174718]

Disorders of the Female Reproductive Tract

22

Karen J. Purcell, MD, PhD, & Robert N. Taylor, MD, PhD

Disorders of the female reproductive system can occur as a result of disease in one of the many varied reproductive organs: the ovaries, the fallopian tubes, the uterus, the cervix, the vagina, or the breast. During the reproductive years, these disorders often present as **altered menstruation, pelvic pain,** or **infertility.** Cancers arising in these tissues occur more often in the late reproductive or menopausal years. Unfortunately, for several reasons, they often have high mortality rates and a high incidence of metastases when they are diagnosed. Some organs are located deep and are relatively inaccessible to palpation (ovaries). Others have few sensory nerves (ovary, fallopian tubes) and hence remain asymptomatic. Additionally, the breasts have large amounts of adipose tissue, which can make early detection of breast cancer difficult. The one exception is the uterine cervix. It has easy access to surveillance with use of the Papanicolaou smear and human papillomavirus (HPV) screening, which have led to a dramatically reduced mortality rate of cervical cancer.

Disorders of the female reproductive system can also occur as a result of disease in other organs whose function affects reproductive organs (eg, the brain, hypothalamus, pituitary, thyroid, adrenals, kidney, and liver). Presentation of these disorders is typically painless.

Alternatively, disorders of the reproductive system can cause disorders in other tissues. Ovarian hormones are necessary for the maintenance and health of most tissues in women. Alterations in these hormones can lead to **osteoporosis** (loss of bone mass), atrophy and inflammation of estrogen-deprived tissues (eg, atrophic vaginitis), atherogenesis and alterations in cardiovascular compliance, and an increased risk of some forms of cancer (eg, endometrial carcinoma as a consequence of estrogen excess). Dysfunction of the reproductive system also can contribute to unique variants of systemic disorders, such as gestational diabetes and the hypertensive syndrome of **preeclampsia-eclampsia.**

CHECKPOINT

1. How do female reproductive system disorders present during the reproductive years?
2. To what might you ascribe the lack of reduction in mortality rate from ovarian cancer in contrast to cervical cancer?
3. What are some consequences of reproductive system dysfunction?

NORMAL STRUCTURE & FUNCTION OF THE FEMALE REPRODUCTIVE TRACT

ANATOMY

The reproductive pelvic organs include the vagina, cervix, uterus, fallopian tubes, and ovaries (Figure 22–1). The two **ovaries** contain thousands of **follicles,** each with an **oocyte** and surrounding **granulosa cells,** which are embedded in a matrix of thecal cells. These supporting cells produce steroids and paracrine products important in follicular maturation and coordination of events in reproduction (Table 22–1). The **fallopian tubes,** which are open to the peritoneal space, connect the ovaries to the uterus. The **uterus** contains an internal hormone-sensitive lining, termed the endometrium. During nonpregnant cycles, menstrual bleeding occurs as the monthly culmination of endometrial growth, development, and sloughing in response to changes in blood levels of estrogen and progesterone (Figure 22–2). During pregnancy, the

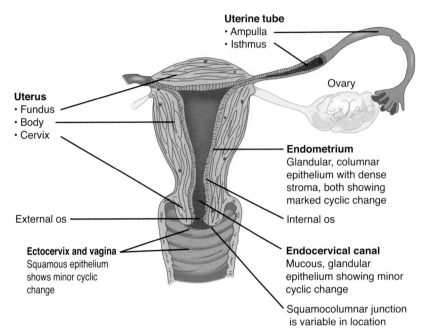

FIGURE 22–1   Anatomic landmarks of the uterus and adjacent organs.   (Redrawn, with permission, from Chandrasoma P, Taylor CE. *Concise Pathology*, 3rd ed. Originally published by Appleton & Lange. Copyright © 1998 by the McGraw-Hill Companies, Inc.)

endometrium produces of a wide variety of endocrine and paracrine products, which promote embryonic implantation (Table 22–2). Surrounding the endometrium is the muscle layer of the uterus, termed the myometrium. Contractions of the myometrium lead to menstrual cramps or expel the fetus at parturition. The cervix is attached to the uterus and allows passage of menses or the fetus into the **vagina,** the muscular tube opening into the vulva.

The **breasts** (Figure 22–3) produce, store, and eject milk upon appropriate hormonal and physical stimulation.

SEXUAL DIFFERENTIATION & MATURATION OF ESTROGEN-DEPENDENT TISSUES

Embryonic Sexual Differentiation

During embryonic development, the primordial gametes originate in the endoderm of the yolk sac, allantois, and hindgut and migrate to the genital ridge by week 5 or 6 of gestation. Once at the genital ridge, they multiply and induce male or female gonads depending on the identity of the sex chromosomes. In the male, the *SRY* gene of the Y sex chromosome directs development of male gonads (testes). In the absence of this gene, the gonads develop into female gonads (ovaries). The presence of testes versus ovaries, normally a consequence of the chromosomal sex, determines the **gonadal sex** of the individual.

Until week 8 of gestation, the sex of the embryo cannot be determined morphologically; therefore, this period is termed the **indifferent phase** of sexual development. After this time, differentiation of the internal and external genitalia occurs,

determining the **phenotypic sex** of the individual, which becomes fully developed after puberty. During embryogenesis, the internal genitalia are formed from a dual genital duct system within the urogenital ridge. The first to form is the wolffian duct, followed by the müllerian duct, which is dependent on prior wolffian duct development. After 8 weeks of gestation, production of **müllerian inhibitory substance** (MIS) by Sertoli cells in the fetal testes leads to regression of the müllerian ducts, whereas production of **testosterone** by the Leydig cells leads to persistence of the wolffian duct and subsequent development of the prostate, epididymis, and seminal vesicles. In the absence of these secretions, female internal reproductive organs are formed from the müllerian ducts, and the wolffian structures degenerate. Similarly, the external genitalia of males develop in the presence of dihydrotestosterone; in the absence of this hormone, the common embryologic structures give rise to female external genitalia. Exposure to androgens can result in virilization of the external genitalia of female embryos, whereas androgen deficiency results in defective male development (Figure 22–4). Therefore, the male phenotype is induced while no ovarian secretions are necessary for expression of the female phenotype.

During development, the female ovaries contain about 7 million oogonia by 24 weeks of gestation. The majority of these cells die during intrauterine life, leaving only about 1 million primary oocytes at birth. This decreases to about 400,000 by puberty. The surviving oogonia are arrested at the prophase of meiosis I. Completion of the first meiotic division does not occur until the time of ovulation, and the second meiosis is completed with fertilization. Only about 400 of these oocytes mature and are released by ovulation during a woman's lifetime; the others undergo **atresia** at various stages of development.

TABLE 22–1 Endocrine and paracrine products of the ovary in addition to steroids.

Products	Compartment	Regulatory Factors
Inhibin	Granulosa, theca, corpus luteum	FSH, EGF, IGF-1, GnRH, VIP, TGF
Activin	Granulosa	FSH
Anti-müllerian hormone	Granulosa, cumulus oophorus	LH, FSH
Follistatin	Follicles	LH, FSH
Relaxin	Corpus luteum, theca	n.d.
	Placenta, uterus	?PRL, LH, oxytocin, PGs
Oocyte meiosis inhibitor	Follicular fluid	n.d.
Follicle regulatory protein	Follicular fluid, granulosa, luteal	FSH, GnRH
Plasminogen activator	Granulosa	n.d.
Extracellular membrane proteins	Granulosa, follicular fluid	FSH, GnRH
Insulin-like growth factor-1	Granulosa	LH, FSH, GH, EGF, TGF, PDGF, estrogen
Epidermal growth factor-like	Granulosa, theca	Gonadotropins
Transforming growth factor-α	Theca, interstitial	FSH
Basic fibroblast growth factor	Corpus luteum	n.d.
Transforming growth factor-β	Theca, interstitial, granulosa	Fibronectin, FSH, TGF-β
Platelet-derived growth factor	Granulosa	n.d.
Nerve growth factor	Ovary	n.d.
Pro-opiomelanocortin	Corpus luteum, interstitial, luteal, granulosa	n.d.
Enkephalin	Ovary	n.d.
Dynorphin	Ovary	n.d.
Gonadotropin-releasing hormone	Ovary, follicular fluid, granulosa	n.d.
Oxytocin	Corpus luteum, granulosa	LH, FSH, PGF$_{2\alpha}$
Vasopressin	Ovary, follicular fluid	n.d.
Renin	Follicular fluid, theca, luteal	LH, FSH
Angiotensin II	Follicular fluid	n.d.
Atrial natriuretic factor	Corpus luteum, ovary, follicular fluid	n.d.
Luteinization inhibitor and luteinization stimulator	Follicular fluid	n.d.
Gonadotropin surge-inhibiting factor	Granulosa	n.d.
Luteinizing hormone receptor-binding inhibitor	Corpus luteum	n.d.
Neuropeptide Y, calcitonin gene-related peptide, substance P, peptide histidine methionine, somatostatin	Nerve fibers	n.d.
Vasoactive intestinal peptide	Nerve fibers	n.d.
c-mos	Oocytes	Developmental

Key: EGF, epidermal growth factor; FSH, follicle-stimulating hormone; GH, growth hormone; GnRH, gonadotropin-releasing hormone; IGF, insulin-like growth factor; LH, luteinizing hormone; n.d., not determined; PDGF, platelet-derived growth factor; PG, prostaglandin; PGF, prostaglandin F; PRL, prolactin; TGF, transforming growth factor; VIP, vasoactive intestinal peptide.

Modified and reproduced, with permission, from Ackland JF et al. Nonsteroidal signals originating in the gonads. Physiol Rev. 1992;72:731.

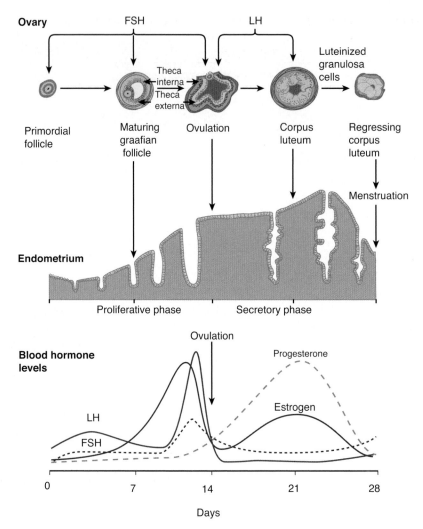

FIGURE 22–2   Changes in the ovary, endometrium, and blood hormone levels during the menstrual cycle. FSH, follicle-stimulating hormone; LH, luteinizing hormone.   (Redrawn, with permission, from Chandrasoma P, Taylor CR. *Concise Pathology*, 3rd ed. Originally published by Appleton & Lange. Copyright © 1998 by the McGraw-Hill Companies, Inc.)

PUBERTY

Secondary sexual characteristics develop at puberty, when maturation of the capacity for adult reproductive function occurs. The changes that occur in the brain and hypothalamus that initiate the onset of puberty to result in the establishment of sleep-dependent (first) and the later truly pulsatile release of gonadotropin-releasing hormone (GnRH) from the hypothalamus have eluded researchers for decades. However, the recent discovery of the hypothalamic kisspeptin/GPR54 ligand/receptor pair as the key mediators of the onset of puberty has been hailed as a major breakthrough in the field that already has clinical implications for diagnosis and treatment of pubertal disorders and infertility.

The increase in GnRH leads to an increase in and a pulsatile pattern of luteinizing hormone (LH) and then follicle-stimulating hormone (FSH) secretion, hormones collectively termed gonadotropins. Before about age 10 years in girls, gonadotropin secretion is at low levels and does not display a pulsatile character. After this age, pulsatile release of GnRH begins and initiates folliculogenesis, leading to cyclic changes in estrogen and progesterone production. These changes allow estrogen-dependent tissues, such as the breasts and the endometrium, to complete their maturation. The appearance of the first menstrual period is termed **menarche.**

CHECKPOINT

4. What is the difference between the chromosomal, gonadal, and phenotypic sex of an individual?

5. Approximately what percentage of the total number of oocytes present in the ovaries of a female at birth completes their maturation and is released upon ovulation over the course of her reproductive life?

6. Describe some changes that occur in the female with the onset of puberty.

TABLE 22–2 Endocrine and paracrine products of the endometrium.

Lipids	Cytokines	Peptides
Prostaglandins	Interleukin-1α	Prolactin
Thromboxanes	Interleukin-1β	Relaxin
Leukotrienes	Interleukin-6	Renin
	Interferon-γ	Endorphin
	Colony-stimulating factor-1	Epidermal growth factor
		Insulin-like growth factors (IGFs)
	Vascular endothelial growth factor (VEGF)	Fibroblast growth factor
		Platelet-derived growth factor
		Transforming growth factor
		IGF-binding proteins
		Glycodelin
		Tumor necrosis factor
		Parathyroid hormone–like peptide

Modified and reproduced, with permission, from Speroff L, Glass RH, Kase NG. *Clinical Gynecologic Endocrinology and Infertility*, 6th ed. Lippincott Williams & Wilkins, 1999.

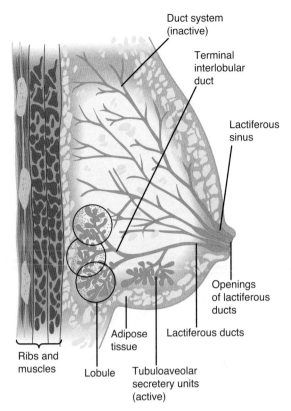

FIGURE 22–3 Schematic drawing of female breast showing the mammary glands with ducts that open in the nipple. The outlines of the lobules do not exist in vivo but are shown for instructional purposes. The stippling indicates the loose intralobular connective tissue. (Redrawn, with permission, from Junqueira LC, Carneiro J. *Basic Histology*, 10th ed. McGraw-Hill, 2003.)

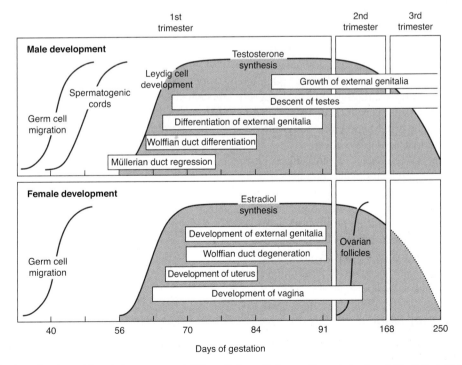

FIGURE 22–4 Timing of male and female human sexual differentiation. (Redrawn, with permission, from Griffin JE, Ojeda SR. *Textbook of Endocrine Physiology*, 2nd ed. Oxford University Press, 1992.)

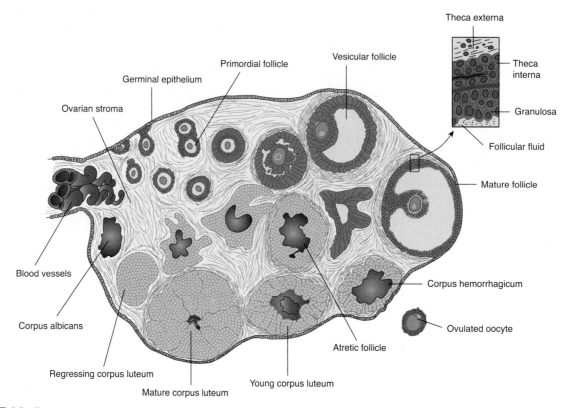

FIGURE 22–5 Diagram of the mammalian ovary, showing the sequential development of a follicle and the formation of a corpus luteum. An atretic follicle is shown in the center, and the structure of the wall of the mature follicle is detailed at the upper right. (Redrawn, with permission, from Gorbman A, Bern H. *Textbook of Comparative Endocrinology.* Wiley, 1962.)

THE MENSTRUAL CYCLE

Normal female reproductive function involves coordinated interaction between the brain and ovaries under the influence of other organs such as the liver (which metabolizes hormones and makes steroid-binding globulins), adrenals, and thyroid glands. With this coordination, cyclic changes during the course of the menstrual cycle allow the reproductive organs to perform specific functions at different points in time to optimize the chances for successful reproduction. When these mechanisms malfunction, the result may be infertility, altered menstrual bleeding, amenorrhea, or even cancer.

The menstrual cycle has three phases. The **follicular** phase typically lasts 14 days and culminates in the production of a mature oocyte. Initially, a cohort of follicles begins to grow, but ultimately a single dominant follicle is selected and the rest undergo a process of degeneration and apoptotic death, termed **atresia** (Figure 22–5). The follicular phase is followed by **ovulation,** in which the dominant follicle releases its mature oocyte to be transported through the uterine tubes for fertilization and subsequent implantation in a receptive uterus. The third, **luteal,** phase also averages 14 days and is characterized by luteinization of the ruptured follicle to produce the corpus luteum. The physiology of each of these phases in the menstrual cycle is best understood by considering three compartments: neuroendocrine, ovarian, and uterine (Figure 22–6).

The neuroendocrine axis involves the hypothalamus, the pituitary, and the ovary. Neurons within the hypothalamus synthesize the peptide **GnRH,** and its secretion is modulated by endogenous opioids and corticotropin-releasing hormone (CRH). GnRH is secreted directly into the portal circulation of the pituitary in a pulsatile fashion. This pulsatility is required for proper activation of its receptor located on the **gonadotropes,** which are cells located in the anterior pituitary. In response, the gonadotropes secrete the polypeptides **FSH** and **LH,** collectively called gonadotropins, which stimulate the ovary to produce estrogen and inhibin. Inhibin feeds back to

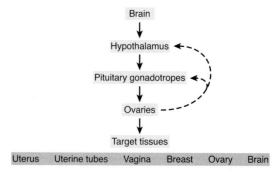

FIGURE 22–6 Female reproductive neuroendocrine feedback axis. Solid arrows indicate stimulation; dashed arrows indicate inhibition.

suppress FSH secretion but has no effect on LH. Estrogen also affects the pituitary by increasing the number of GnRH receptors and its sensitivity to GnRH stimulation. With continued estrogen production by the ovaries, a critical concentration is reached for a sufficient time to lead to a midcycle LH surge and subsequent ovulation. After this surge, high levels of progesterone produced by the corpus luteum suppress gonadotropin release for the duration of the luteal phase.

Within the ovary, LH and FSH lead to the synthesis and secretion of steroid hormones and paracrine/autocrine proteins (Table 22–1), directing the maturation of a single oocyte for ovulation. During the early follicular phase, FSH stimulates growth of a cohort of follicles and increases the production of inhibin and activin in granulosa cells. Activin acts in the ovary to augment the effect of FSH: increasing aromatase activity and increasing production of FSH and LH receptors. LH stimulates the production of androgens in the thecal cells, which is augmented by inhibin. Androgens diffuse into the granulosa cells to be converted to estrogen through the enzymatic reaction of aromatization. As the follicular phase progresses, inhibin production comes under the control of LH, and the increasing amounts of inhibin lead to further conversion of androgens to produce the high levels of estrogen needed for the LH surge.

The midcycle LH surge triggers the final steps of oocyte maturation and resumption of meiosis within the dominant follicle. Changes in follicular prostaglandins and proteases allow digestion of the follicular wall leading to oocyte extrusion and ovulation. The follicular cells remaining after ovulation develop into a structure termed the **corpus luteum,** which synthesizes and releases large amounts of both estrogen and progesterone. Continued secretion from the corpus luteum requires LH stimulation; in its absence, degeneration occurs.

The uterine compartment reacts to the steroids produced from the ovaries throughout the menstrual cycle. During the follicular phase, the endometrium proliferates under the influence of estrogen, creating straight glands with thin secretions and microvascular proliferation. During the luteal phase, the high levels of estrogen and progesterone promote maturation of the endometrium, which develops tortuous glands engorged with thick secretions and proteins (Figure 22–2). Additionally, the endometrium secretes a number of endocrine and paracrine factors (Table 22–2). These changes are optimal for implantation. In the absence of implantation, the corpus luteum cannot sustain the high levels of progesterone production and the endometrial vasculature cannot be maintained. This leads to sloughing of the endometrium and the onset of menstruation, which marks the nadir of estrogen and progesterone levels, ending the cycle (Figure 22–2).

Contraception

Birth control pills are a pharmacologic means of preventing pregnancy by disrupting the precise timing of hormone-directed events necessary for reproduction. Current formulations include progestins alone as well as combinations of estrogens and progestins. Most preparations of estrogen and progestin block the LH surge at midcycle, thereby preventing ovulation. However, other contraceptive actions include effects on estrogen- and progesterone-sensitive tissues, such as inducing changes in cervical mucus and the endometrial lining that are unfavorable to sperm transport and embryonic implantation, respectively.

In order to mitigate the unpleasant side effects of nausea and bloating, as well as the dangerous side effect of thrombosis, the doses of estrogen and progestin have been decreased over the years. Other nonoral formulations also have been developed. A transdermal patch allows absorption of estrogen and progestin without "first-pass" metabolism in the liver. Transvaginal absorption is also available with a soft ring placed monthly in the vagina. Both of these formulations provide similar contraceptive efficacy to the oral contraceptive pills.

PHYSIOLOGY OF OVARIAN STEROIDS

Like the adrenal gland, the ovary is a steroid factory. The ovary secretes three types of steroids: **progesterone,** containing 21 carbons; **androgens,** containing 19 carbons; and **estrogens,** containing 18 carbons. Steroid synthesis occurs by conversion from cholesterol in a series of biochemical reactions catalyzed by enzymes in the mitochondria and the endoplasmic reticulum (see Chapter 21). Generally, the rate-limiting step in steroid production is side chain cleavage of cholesterol within the mitochondrion by the enzyme cytochrome P450, family 11, subfamily A, polypeptide 1 (CYP11A1) to generate the basic steroid nucleus. This nucleus is further modified in the endoplasmic reticulum to generate the various steroid hormones. Because steroids are synthesized by a cascade of enzyme reactions in various pathways, a block in one step (eg, resulting from a congenital enzyme defect or inhibition by certain drugs) can result in lack of synthesis of one steroid and "spillover" of precursors into another. Such defects are the hallmark of congenital adrenal hyperplasia (discussed in Chapter 21).

The major mechanism of steroid hormone action involves diffusion across the plasma membrane, binding of the steroid to receptor proteins in the cytoplasm or nucleus, and, after movement to the nucleus, if necessary, activation of transcription of certain genes by binding of the steroid-receptor complex to specific regions of DNA. In this way, the pattern of gene expression is changed in the various steroid-responsive tissues (ie, those that contain steroid receptors). Membrane-bound steroid receptors also have been shown to activate phosphorylation cascades typically regulated by growth factors.

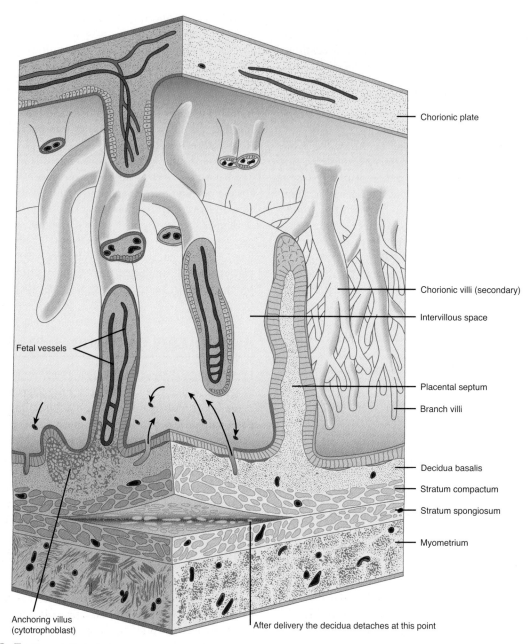

FIGURE 22–7   Placental anatomy. (Redrawn, with permission, from Copenhaver WM, Kelly DE, Wood RL. *Bailey's Textbook of Histology,* 17th ed. Williams & Wilkins, 1978.)

CHECKPOINT

7. What are the primary target tissues for GnRH? For go-nadotropins? For ovarian steroids?

8. Why is pulsatile secretion of GnRH important?

9. What are some specialized features of GnRH action?

10. What are the specific effects of gonadotropins on the ovary?

11. How does the structure of the uterine lining differ in the midproliferative versus the late secretory stages, and for what reproduction-related events is each stage optimized?

12. What products are made by a granulosa cell in the dominant follicle over the course of its lifetime?

PREGNANCY

Prerequisites for a Successful Pregnancy

A number of changes must occur in reproductive and other organs for establishment and successful completion of a pregnancy. Fertilization requires successful ovulation, capture of the mature oocyte by the fibriae of the fallopian tubes, and transport of the zygote to the uterus. Because fertilization usually occurs in the ampulla, it also requires effective transport of viable sperm into the distal tube.

After implantation, a placenta forms consisting of two functional layers, the cytotrophoblast and the syncytiotrophoblast, as well as an adjacent maternal layer, the endometrial decidua with the underlying mesenchymal core (Figure 22–7). The placenta

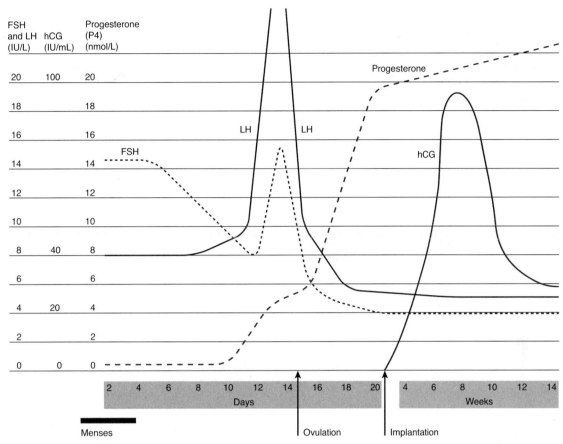

FIGURE 22–8 Hormone production during pregnancy. (FSH, follicle-stimulating hormone; LH, luteinizing hormone; hCG, human chorionic gonadotropin.) (Redrawn and modified, with permission, from Speroff L, Glass RH, Kase NG. *Clinical Gynecologic Endocrinology and Infertility,* 7th ed. Lippincott Williams & Wilkins, 2005.)

allows intimate apposition of maternal and fetal circulations for exchange of nutrients, oxygen, and waste products. In addition, the placenta secretes a variety of important hormones, including an LH-like hormone termed **human chorionic gonadotropin (hCG)**. Unlike LH secretion by the gonadotrophs of the anterior pituitary, placental secretion of hCG is not inhibited by the high levels of estrogen and progesterone. The hCG maintains the corpus luteum for a period of 8–10 weeks until the full progesterone-producing capacity of the placenta has developed. At that point, hCG levels fall and the mature placenta produces progesterone from the maternal supply of cholesterol (Figure 22–8). Other factors produced by the placenta include placental growth hormone (GH-P), and a growth hormone–like protein termed **human chorionic somatomammotropin (hCS)**, also known as **placental lactogen (hPL)** (Table 22–3).

During most of pregnancy, the fetus provides the placenta with androgens, which are used to make estrogens secreted into the maternal circulation (Figure 22–9). This reflects the action of a special zone in the fetal adrenal cortex engaged in androgen production. Toward the end of pregnancy, the increasing ACTH secretion by the fetal pituitary triggers the fetal adrenal to produce cortisol in addition to androgen. This switch may play a role in triggering the onset of labor.

In addition to the changes in organs with pregnancy-specific functions, physiologic changes occur in essentially every maternal organ system. These include increased blood volume (increased by more than 40% by the middle of the third trimester), increased total body water (increased by 6–8 L), and increased cardiac output because of increased stroke volume (increased by 30%) and heart rate (increased by 15%). A striking increase in minute ventilation (increased by 50% compared with nonpregnant state) without any change in respiratory rate is observed as a result of increased tidal volume (Chapter 9). Dramatic increases in renal blood flow and glomerular filtration rate (increased by 40%) are also seen. Most of these alterations are related in complex ways to the effects of steroid hormones produced in pregnancy.

Role of Steroids in Pregnancy

The precise role of various steroids in pregnancy is incompletely understood. The demonstrated and proposed roles of progesterone in pregnancy include (1) promotion of implantation; (2) suppression of the maternal immune response to fetal antigens, thus preventing rejection of the fetus; (3) cardiovascular compliance; (4) provision of substrate for manufacture by the fetal adrenal of glucocorticoids and

TABLE 22–3 Endocrine and paracrine products in pregnancy other than steroids.

Fetal Compartment	Placental Compartment	Maternal Compartment
Alpha-fetoprotein	Hypothalamic-like hormones	Decidual proteins
	GnRH	Prolactin
	CRH	Fibronectin
	TRH	VEGF
	Somatostatin	Relaxin
	Pituitary-like hormones	IGFBP-1
	hCG	Interleukin-1
	hCS	Colony-stimulating factor-1
	GH-P	Glycodelin (progesterone-associated endometrial protein)
	ACTH	
	Growth factors	Corpus luteum proteins
	IGF-1	Relaxin
	Epidermal growth factor	Prorenin
	Platelet-derived growth factor	
	Fibroblast growth factor	
	Transforming growth factor-β	
	Inhibin Activin	
	Cytokines	
	Interleukin-1	
	Interleukin-6	
	Colony-stimulating factor	
	Other	
	Opioids	
	Prorenin	
	Pregnancy-specific β-glycoprotein	
	Pregnancy associated plasma protein A	

Data from Cowan BD, Morrison JC. Management of abnormal genital bleeding in girls and women. (Current concepts.) N Engl J Med. 1991;324:1710.

mineralocorticoids; (5) maintenance of uterine quiescence through gestation; and (6) a role in parturition. Estrogens contribute to (1) volume expansion; (2) cardiac remodeling; and (3) preparative production of clotting factors, anticipating blood loss that commonly follows delivery.

Human Chorionic Somatomammotropin & Fuel Homeostasis in Pregnancy

Another example of fetal-placental-maternal interactions is seen in the actions of hCS (Figure 22–10). This "counterregulatory" hormone (ie, a hormone whose actions oppose those of insulin) appears to serve as a defense against fetal hypoglycemia. From a metabolic standpoint, pregnancy is a form of "accelerated starvation" characterized by fasting hypoglycemia, as fuel substrates produced by the mother are consumed by the growing fetus. The hCS produced by the placenta in response to hypoglycemia serves to increase lipolysis, thereby raising maternal free fatty acid levels and ultimately blood glucose and ketone levels. This "diabetogenic" role of hCS is a major additional burden on the maternal compartment and contributes to the tendency for diabetes mellitus to emerge in susceptible individuals during pregnancy. Normally, glucose is the major fuel source for the fetus. However, in the event of glucose deprivation, ketones provide a ready emergency fuel supply (as they do in starvation) for both the mother and, via the placenta, for the fetus.

CHECKPOINT

13. How is the corpus luteum maintained until the placenta has developed adequately?
14. What are some possible roles of steroids during pregnancy?
15. Why is new-onset diabetes mellitus a common complication of pregnancy?

LACTATION

Breast Structure & Development

The rudiments for breast development are established during embryonic development. During puberty, rising estrogen levels stimulate breast growth as one of a number of female secondary sexual characteristics. Breast growth involves both proliferation and branching of lactiferous ducts as well as accumulation of adipose and connective tissue. In the mature breast, each terminal lactiferous duct drains clusters of tubuloalveolar secretory units lined by milk-secreting epithelial cells and is suspended in connective and adipose tissue well populated with lymphocytes. The mature female breast consists of a cluster of 15–25 lactiferous ducts, each emerging independently at the nipple (Figure 22–3). Both the pubertal and pregnant phases of breast growth require the permissive

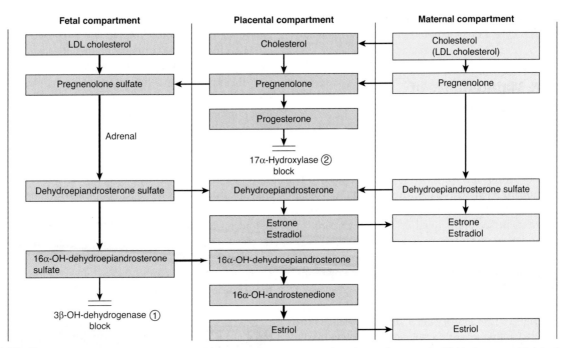

FIGURE 22–9 Fetal-placental-maternal cooperation in steroidogenesis. LDL, low-density lipoprotein; 3β-Hydroxysteroid dehydrogenase, hydroxy-Δ-5-steroid dehydrogenase, 3 β- and steroid Δ-isomerase (HSD3β); 17α-Hydroxylase, 17α-hydroxylase activity of cytochrome P450, family 17, subfamily A, polypeptide 1 (CYP17A1). (Data from Speroff L et al. Regulation of the menstrual cycle. In: *Clinical Gynecologic Endocrinology and Infertility,* 6th ed. Lippincott Williams & Wilkins, 1999.)

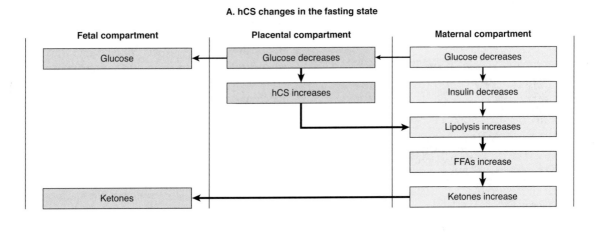

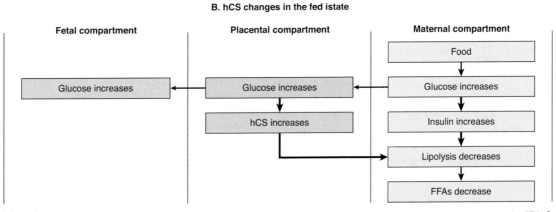

FIGURE 22–10 Fetal-placental-maternal cooperation in fuel homeostasis. hCS, human chorionic somatomammotropin; FFA, free fatty acids. (Data from Speroff L, Glass RH, Kase NG. *Clinical Gynecologic Endocrinology and Infertility,* 6th ed. Lipppincott Williams & Wilkins, 1999.)

influence of glucocorticoids, thyroxine, and insulin for full development, and their actions are potentiated by estrogen and progesterone.

Initiation & Maintenance of Milk Synthesis & Secretion

During pregnancy, prolactin, progesterone, and hCS play a dominant role in stimulating breast growth and the capacity for milk production. Actual lactation, or milk release, however, is inhibited by the high levels of estrogen and progesterone present before birth. After delivery of the placenta, estrogen and progesterone levels fall dramatically, removing this block. Maintenance of milk secretion requires the joint action of both anterior and posterior pituitary factors (Figure 22–11) as well as interaction between the mother and infant. Suckling stimulates afferent neural pathways that suppress dopamine levels in the hypothalamus, thereby maintaining high levels of prolactin necessary for milk synthesis. At the same time, suckling, by triggering afferent sensory nerve fibers (as well as other stimuli such as the infant's cry), stimulates synthesis, transport, and secretion of oxytocin from the posterior pituitary. Oxytocin promotes contraction of mammary myoepithelial cells, thereby triggering ejection of milk from the mammary epithelial alveoli and out the nipple.

Toward the end of pregnancy, there is an increase in the lymphocyte population in the vasculature and connective tissue of the breast. These lymphocytes secrete immunoglobulin

A (IgA) into the local bloodstream, from which it is taken up by the mammary epithelial cells. By the process of transcytosis, IgA crosses the mammary epithelial cells to be deposited into the luminal secretion (milk). This mechanism, coupled with the transplacental transport of maternal IgG, is responsible for conferring passive immunity on the newborn. The earliest mammary gland secretion after birth, termed colostrum, has particularly high immunoglobulin content.

The high level of prolactin maintained during lactation also has a contraceptive effect, primarily by inhibition of pulsatile secretion of GnRH. The precise mechanism is not known but may involve a short feedback loop by which prolactin stimulates dopamine release, which, in turn, elevates endogenous opioid release and inhibits GnRH secretion. There may also be effects of prolactin directly on the ovary that contribute to lactational anovulation and amenorrhea. However, it should be noted that the contraceptive effect of prolactin is only moderate and, therefore, of low reliability.

CHECKPOINT

16. Which hormones are involved in breast development?
17. Why is milk rarely secreted before parturition?
18. What is the probable mechanism of lactational amenorrhea?

Menopause

Menopause is the point in a woman's life when, as a result of exhaustion of the supply of functioning ovarian follicles, menstrual cycles cease. Ten years before menopause, at approximately age 40 years, reproductive function starts to diminish. This is manifested as a decreased frequency of ovulation and alterations in menstrual patterns. During this time, despite increased GnRH-stimulated LH and FSH secretion, less estrogen is produced because of the relative paucity and insensitivity of remaining follicles. This transitory period of diminishing reproductive function approaching menopause is termed the **climacteric.**

During the climacteric transition, the hormonal status of women changes from a cyclic high-estrogen state to a steady-state low-estrogen postmenopausal state. This leads to **vasomotor symptoms** such as hot flushes ("hot flashes"), sweating, and chills. Psychologic symptoms such as irritability, tension, anxiety, and depression may also be observed. After menopause, other more gradual changes can appear. In addition to atrophy of estrogen-dependent tissues such as the vaginal epithelium, a gradual loss in bone density leading to **osteoporosis** can occur.

A modest degree of androgen production from thecal cells of the residual ovarian stroma continues even in the absence of follicular growth. In postmenopausal women, ovarian and adrenal androgens continue to be aromatized into estrogens by the enzyme aromatase (cytochrome P450, family 19, subfamily A, polypeptide 1, or CYP19A1) in adipose tissue and

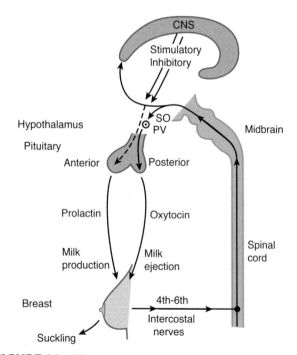

FIGURE 22–11 The role of anterior and posterior pituitary factors in milk synthesis and secretion. SO, supraoptic nucleus; PV, paraventricular nucleus. (Redrawn, with permission, from Rebar RW. The breast and physiology of lactation. In: *Maternal-Fetal Medicine: Principles and Practice.* Creasy RK, Resnick R [editors]. Saunders, 1984.)

hair follicles. The significance of peripheral aromatization in relation to severity of symptoms of menopause varies in different individuals.

In the medical literature, menopause was often viewed as an "endocrinopathy," specifically as a disorder of estrogen deficiency. To treat the vasomotor symptoms and osteoporosis, hormone replacement therapy (HRT) was often prescribed. Given the interaction of estrogen on the cardiovascular system, HRT had also been thought to improve cardiovascular events, and several trials suggested its usefulness in primary and secondary prevention of coronary heart disease. Results of prospective studies, however, showed no benefit in cardiovascular protection with HRT. The Women's Health Initiative showed that the increased risk of thromboembolic disease and invasive breast cancer associated with estrogen and progesterone replacement outweighed the benefit of fewer events of colon cancer and hip fractures. Treatment with estrogen replacement therapy without progesterone in women who had undergone hysterectomy did not show any increase in breast cancer but instead suggested possible breast cancer prevention. The other risks and benefits were similar. From these studies, it is recognized that HRT should not be used for cardiovascular prevention or initiated in women older than 60 years. Use for symptomatic relief of menopausal symptoms is still appropriate after counseling the patient about the global risks and benefits of treatment.

CHECKPOINT

19. What are the symptoms of menopause?
20. What is the primary source of the estrogen found in the bloodstream of postmenopausal women not on estrogen replacement therapy?
21. Compare LH and FSH levels before puberty, during the reproductive years, and after the menopause.

OVERVIEW OF FEMALE REPRODUCTIVE TRACT DISORDERS

Many female reproductive disorders can be traced to a particular level of the neuroendocrine feedback axis and thus can be categorized as resulting from central (pituitary, hypothalamus, or other brain centers which influence the hypothalamus) or end-organ (ovarian or target tissue, eg, uterine) dysfunction.

DISORDERS OF CENTRAL HYPOTHALAMIC-PITUITARY FUNCTION

Any change in the precise rate or amplitude of GnRH secretion by the hypothalamus can result in altered pituitary responsiveness (eg, downregulation of GnRH receptors or altered gonadotropin secretion). This altered pituitary function, in turn, results in disordered ovarian function (eg, inadequate steroidogenesis with or without anovulation) and altered target tissue response (eg, endometrial atrophy and menstrual abnormalities). Many central (eg, psychic stress) and peripheral (eg, body fat content) inputs affecting pulsatile GnRH release are integrated in the hypothalamus. Thus, altered GnRH release from the hypothalamus is a common cause of amenorrhea (eg, in athletic young women).

DISORDERS OF THE OVARY

Proper ovarian function involves responsiveness to gonadotropins, intrinsic viability of follicles, and a host of paracrine interactions within and between individual follicles. Polycystic ovarian syndrome (PCOS) is an example of ovarian dysfunction resulting from a self-perpetuating cycle of altered feedback relationships (see later discussion). Polycystic ovarian syndrome is manifested by anovulation, hirsutism, infertility, dyslipidemia, and either abnormal uterine bleeding or amenorrhea.

DISORDERS OF THE UTERUS, FALLOPIAN TUBES, & VAGINA

Because normal menstrual bleeding is most directly a function of the growth state of the uterine endometrium, disorders of the uterus, including hormonal dysfunction, myomas (fibroids, benign tumors of the underlying myometrium), and cancer of the endometrium itself, often present with abnormal vaginal bleeding.

Pelvic infections can produce adhesions and scarring of the uterus or fallopian tubes that result in infertility. The initial presentation typically includes abdominal and pelvic (cervical and adnexal) pain and with either fever, an elevated white blood cell count, or a positive endocervical culture. Common infectious agents include gonorrhea, anaerobic bacteria, and *Chlamydia*. Multiple organisms are usually involved. Prompt and aggressive antibiotic therapy is important in treating these infections to limit permanent damage to sensitive reproductive structures. Pelvic infections can develop into tubo-ovarian abscesses requiring surgical drainage.

DISORDERS OF PREGNANCY

The normal events of pregnancy potentially set the stage for a wide array of localized and systemic disorders. Abnormalities in the process of implantation, for example, appear to predispose to recurrent miscarriage and preeclampsia-eclampsia (see later). In addition, genetic predisposition to disease that might otherwise remain latent for decades may be manifested first—often transiently—during pregnancy.

A good example of the latter is the genetic predisposition to development of diabetes mellitus. As discussed, pregnancy is a counterregulatory state, with elevation of multiple blood glucose-elevating hormones, especially hCS. Because of the insulin-resistant features of pregnancy, blood glucose control in diabetics who become pregnant is more difficult. Nondiabetic patients can also develop diabetes transiently during pregnancy (gestational diabetes mellitus). Gestational diabetes mellitus is common and involves 2–5% of all pregnancies in the United States. Many of these individuals go on to manifest Type 2 diabetes mellitus later in life.

Poor control of blood glucose during pregnancy has effects on the mother, on the course of the pregnancy, and on the fetus. Maternal retinopathy and nephropathy may appear during the course of the pregnancy, although the long-term severity of the mother's disease is probably not altered by pregnancy. There is a higher incidence of acute complications of diabetes, including ketoacidosis, hypoglycemia, and infections during pregnancy. Patients with gestational and pregestational diabetes mellitus are at greater risk for preeclampsia-eclampsia. Poor glucose control also increases the rate and risk of cesarean section with associated anesthetic and surgical morbidity.

The effects of poor glucose control on the fetus are even more profound. Unexplained fetal deaths, spontaneous abortions, and **congenital anomalies** are increased. Just how gestational diabetes increases the risk of congenital anomalies is not well understood. Some studies have implicated altered myoinositol and prostaglandin metabolism. Other studies have demonstrated embryopathic effects of oxygen free radicals generated at elevated levels in diabetic pregnancies.

Fetal **macrosomia** (large body size) is increased in poorly controlled diabetics. High maternal blood glucose triggers increased fetal insulin secretion and, therefore, results in a larger fetus. As the fetus becomes larger, the risk of fetopelvic disproportion increases, which contributes to traumatic vaginal deliveries or an increased frequency of cesarean section. Neonatal hypoglycemia, hypocalcemia, polycythemia, and hyperbilirubinemia also may occur.

The high levels of steroids and other products in the pregnant state can lead to a range of other serious medical complications. Pregnancy is paradoxically associated with both

TABLE 22–4 Factors predisposing to thrombosis in pregnancy.

Factor	Mechanism
Estrogen effects	Alterations in blood flow resulting in increased hemostasis
	Increased blood viscosity due to impaired erythrocyte deformability
	Activation of coagulation due to elevated factors I (fibrinogen), VII, VIII, IX, X, and XII and decreased antithrombin
Nonestrogen effect	Depressed fibrinolytic activity

hemorrhage and thrombosis (Table 22–4). Both are related to the special functions of the placenta and its adaptations in the course of mammalian evolution.

Separation of the placenta from the wall of the uterus at birth poses a threat of massive, life-threatening hemorrhage given the intimate apposition of the placenta and the maternal blood supply, 10% of which is funneled to the uterus. As an adaptation to this risk, pregnancy is a hypercoagulable state established in part by estrogen stimulation of hepatic coagulation proteins. Physiologically, this increased tendency toward coagulation and decreased activity of the fibrinolytic system may serve to control postpartum hemorrhage. Pathologically, these same factors pose a risk of inappropriate thrombosis. It has been calculated that the risk of thrombophlebitis is increased nearly 50 times in the first month postpartum compared with the nonpregnant state. When thrombosis does occur, therapy is complicated by the teratogenic risks associated with the standard treatment with warfarin. Therefore, pregnant patients with thrombosis are given subcutaneous heparin therapy.

Miscarriage, Ectopic Pregnancy, & Placental Disorders

At least 15% of all pregnancies terminate in a spontaneous abortion as a result of genetic or environmental factors before the period when extrauterine life is possible (about 24 weeks of gestation and 750 g body weight). Inevitable abortion presents with heavy bleeding, pain, and dilation of the internal os. Threatened abortion is considered when painless uterine bleeding occurs with a closed, uneffaced cervix.

For patients presenting with vaginal bleeding and pain in the first trimester, miscarriage must be distinguished from molar pregnancy and ectopic pregnancy. Ectopic pregnancy results from implantation of the blastocyst into the lining of the tube rather than the endometrium. Damaged or scarred fallopian tubes, from previous pelvic infections or endometriosis, impede transit of the mature ovum or zygote, leading to a predisposition for ectopic pregnancies. In this location, the embryo is not viable but growth of the embryo results in rupture and potentially life-threatening hemorrhage unless it is surgically or medically eliminated. Diagnosis is made by a failure of serum β-hCG to rise appropriately in the first several weeks of pregnancy and by failure to localize an intrauterine pregnancy by ultrasonography.

Third-trimester bleeding is typically associated with **placenta previa** (placental obstruction of all or part of the internal cervical os) or **placental abruption** (premature separation of a normally implanted placenta after the first trimester). Women who have had multiple prior pregnancies are at increased risk of placenta previa, which is believed to be due to scar tissue formation from previous implantations. Placental abruption is due to hemorrhage into the decidual plate secondary to vascular rupture and is associated with hypertension, smoking, and multiple pregnancies, all of which would be expected to affect the condition of the placental vasculature. Hemorrhage can be massive and life threatening.

TROPHOBLASTIC DISEASES

Molar pregnancies are abnormal growths resulting from trophoblastic proliferation (**hydatidiform mole**). Rarely, they coexist with a fetus (**partial mole**). The prevalence in the United States is approximately 1 per 1500 pregnancies, but in certain areas of Asia it is as high as 1 per 125 pregnancies. The tissue in complete moles has higher malignant potential and is purely of paternal origin, whereas that of partial moles is usually benign and typically contains an extra set of paternal chromosomes (triploidy). Most moles present with vaginal bleeding and are diagnosed during evaluation of threatened abortion by (1) lack of a fetus and (2) presence of hydropic trophoblastic tissue on ultrasound imaging. Particularly severe nausea of pregnancy, a uterus larger than expected for gestational age, and an extremely elevated hCG level are suggestive, but not diagnostic, of molar pregnancy.

The complications of hydatidiform mole include high risks of (1) **choriocarcinoma,** a malignant, trophoblastic neoplasm with high potential for metastasis, especially to lung and brain; (2) hyperthyroidism with added risk of thyroid storm during induction of anesthesia; and (3) severe hemorrhage or trophoblastic tissue pulmonary embolism during suction curettage procedure to remove the molar products. The extremely high levels of hCG that occur with molar pregnancy and choriocarcinoma can result in cross-activation of the thyroid-stimulating hormone (TSH) receptor and trigger hyperthyroidism in some patients. Approximately 5% of women with hydatidiform mole subsequently develop choriocarcinoma. The serum β-hCG can be used as a sensitive test to detect the continued presence of malignant tissue. The exquisite sensitivity of choriocarcinoma to chemotherapy has made it a readily curable malignancy if detected early.

DISORDERS OF THE BREAST

Intrinsic disorders of the breast are either malignant (breast cancer) or benign (eg, fibrocystic disease). Breast disease also can occur as a result of the effects of other disorders or drug therapy, as in galactorrhea. In women, the breast, like other estrogen- and progesterone-responsive tissues, displays cyclic changes in concert with alterations in the level of ovarian steroids through the menstrual cycle. Subtle imbalances in the relative levels of estrogen and progesterone may be the cause of so-called **benign breast disease.** This term refers to abnormalities ranging from normal premenstrual breast tenderness relieved with menstruation at one extreme to so-called fibrocystic disease at the other. In fibrocystic disease, breast fibrosis and cysts are associated with mammary epithelial hyperplasia. Normal breast tissue may have either fibrosis or cysts but not epithelial cell hyperplasia. True fibrocystic disease with epithelial cell hyperplasia is a risk factor for breast cancer in much the same way that endometrial hyperplasia resulting from unopposed estrogen action is a risk factor for endometrial cancer.

CHECKPOINT

22. What are some central causes of menstrual disorders?
23. Why might you suspect some patients with choriocarcinoma to develop hyperthyroidism?
24. Are fibrocystic changes a risk factor for breast cancer?

DISORDERS OF SEXUAL DIFFERENTIATION

Under certain circumstances, aberrations can occur during embryogenesis that alter the normal course of events in chromosomal, gonadal, or phenotypic sexual development. An example of such an aberration in chromosomal sex is **Turner's syndrome** (45, X). Individuals with Turner's syndrome are phenotypic females with primary amenorrhea, absent secondary sexual characteristics, short stature, multiple congenital anomalies, and bilateral streak gonads.

An example of altered gonadal sex is the syndrome of pure **gonadal dysgenesis.** Affected individuals have bilateral streak gonads and an immature female phenotype, but unlike those with Turner's syndrome they are of normal height, have no associated somatic defects, and have a normal female karyotype.

Disorders of phenotypic sex include female and male **pseudohermaphroditism.** These syndromes result from exposure of female embryos to excessive maternal or exogenous androgens during sexual differentiation or from defects in androgen synthesis or tissue sensitivity in the embryo (eg, congenital adrenal hyperplasia).

PATHOPHYSIOLOGY OF SELECTED FEMALE REPRODUCTIVE TRACT DISORDERS

MENSTRUAL DISORDERS

Disorders of the menstrual cycle include (1) **amenorrhea** (lack of menstrual bleeding), which may be primary amenorrhea (ie, the failure of onset of menstrual periods by age 16) or secondary amenorrhea (ie, the lack of menstrual periods for 6 months in a previously menstruating woman); (2) **dysmenorrhea** (pain and other symptoms accompanying menstruation); or (3) **menorrhagia** (excessive vaginal bleeding) or **metrorrhagia** (irregular or abnormally protracted vaginal bleeding).

Etiology

A. Amenorrhea

The cause of amenorrhea can be traced to one of four broad categories of conditions (Table 22–5):

1. Normal physiologic processes such as pregnancy and menopause.
2. Disorders of the uterus or the pathway of menstrual flow such as destruction of the endometrium after curettage coupled with infection, which can cause scarring and adhesion formation within the uterus (**Asherman's syndrome**).
3. Disorders of the ovary such as gonadal failure resulting from a range of chromosomal, developmental, and structural abnormalities, autoimmune disorders, premature loss of follicles, and poorly understood syndromes in which ovaries with follicles are resistant to gonadotropin stimulation.
4. Disorders of the hypothalamus or pituitary resulting in either lack of or disordered GnRH secretion and, as a consequence, insufficient gonadotropin secretion to maintain ovarian steroid production. The causes of hypothalamic and pituitary dysfunction include prolactin-secreting tumors of the pituitary gland, hypothyroidism, excessive stress and exercise, and weight loss.

Within these categories, amenorrhea can have very diverse specific causes.

B. Dysmenorrhea

Dysmenorrhea is pain, typically cramping in character and lower abdominal in location, occurring in the days just before

TABLE 22–5 Causes of amenorrhea.

Category	Common Causes	Pathophysiologic Mechanisms	How to Make a Diagnosis	Intervention
Normal physiologic processes	Pregnancy	Sustained high estrogen and progesterone	Serum β-hCG, history	Prenatal care
	Menopause	Lack of estrogen	Clinical diagnosis	Recommendations for osteoporosis prevention
Disorders of the uterus and outflow tract	Disorders of sexual development	Excessive androgen exposure	Physical examination	Surgical treatment
	Congenital anomalies (eg, imperforate hymen)		Physical examination	Surgical treatment
	Asherman's syndrome	Endometrial destruction (eg, by vigorous curettage)	Lack of response to estrogen-progestin trial; direct visualization of scant endometrium	
Disorders of the ovary	Gonadal dysgenesis	Deletion of genetic material from the X chromosome	Karyotype	Remove streak gonads if Y chromosome is present in view of high risk of germ cell cancer
	Premature ovarian failure	Lack of viable follicles	Check gonadotropins	
	Polycystic ovary disease	Altered intraovarian hormone relationships	Clinical diagnosis in patients with chronic anovulation and androgen excess	Decrease ovarian androgen secretion (wedge resection, oral contraceptives); increase FSH secretion
Disorders of the hypothalamus or pituitary	Stress, athletic endeavor, underweight	Altered GnRH pulses	Check serum TSH, PRL, gonadotropins	Replacement if deficient; search for tumor if excessive

Key: hCG, human chorionic gonadotropin; FSH, follicle-stimulating hormone; GnRH, gonadotropin-releasing hormone; TSH, thyroid-stimulating hormone; PRL, prolactin.

TABLE 22-6 Categories of dysmenorrhea.

Categories	Etiology	Distinguishing Features
Primary dysmenorrhea	Prostaglandins	Lack of organic pelvic disease
Secondary dysmenorrhea		
Endometriosis	Ectopic endometrium, including intramyometrial endometrial tissue	Finding of endometriosis lesions on laparoscopy
Pelvic inflammatory disease	Infection	Positive culture
Anatomic lesions (imperforate hymen, intrauterine adhesions, leiomyomas, polyps)	Congenital, inflammatory, or neoplastic	Findings on physical examination, ultrasound
Premenstrual syndrome (PMS)	Unknown	Association with emotional, behavioral, and other symptoms

TABLE 22-7 Causes of abnormal vaginal bleeding.

Childhood	
Genital lesions	Endocrine changes
Vaginitis	Estrogen ingestion
Foreign body	Precocious puberty
Trauma	Ovarian tumors
Tumors	
Adolescents and adults	
Dysfunctional uterine bleeding	Malignant diseases
Estrogen breakthrough	Endometrial cancer
Estrogen withdrawal	Cervical cancer
Diseases of the genital tract	Vaginal cancer
Benign conditions	Pregnancy
Uterine leiomyoma	Ectopic pregnancy
Cervical polyp	Threatened abortion
Endometrial polyp	Miscarriage
Genital laceration	Other causes
Endometrial hyperplasia	Thyroid disease
	von Willebrand's disease
	Thrombocytopenia

and during menstrual flow. Dysmenorrhea can occur as a primary disorder in the absence of identifiable pelvic disease or may be secondary to underlying pelvic disease such as endometriosis (Table 22–6).

C. Abnormal Vaginal Bleeding

Vaginal bleeding is abnormal if it occurs (1) prepubertally, (2) at the time of usual menses but is of longer than usual duration, (3) at the time of usual menses but is heavier than usual, (4) between menstrual periods, or (5) after menopause in the absence of pharmacologic treatment with estrogen and progesterone (postmenopausal bleeding). The categories of abnormal vaginal bleeding and some specific causes are presented in Table 22–7.

Pathology & Pathogenesis

A. Amenorrhea

The pathogenesis of amenorrhea depends on the level of the neuroendocrine reproductive axis from which the disorder stems and, at each level of the axis, whether it is due to a structural problem or to a functional problem of hormonal control. In a previously menstruating patient presenting with amenorrhea, it is important first to rule out pregnancy and then to assess thyroid function (serum TSH level) and pituitary function (serum prolactin level) before approaching the workup of amenorrhea, compartment by compartment.

1. **Uterine disorders**—Scarring and damage to the underlying stem cells from which the endometrium proliferates will lead to amenorrhea. In most cases, this occurs in the setting of endometritis after **curettage** (scraping of the en-

dometrium) either for postpartum bleeding or dysfunctional uterine bleeding.

To determine the presence of a functional endometrium, an amenorrheic patient is given either progesterone alone or the sequential combination of estrogen and progesterone. Renewed vaginal bleeding after cessation of the hormonal therapy suggests that the endometrium is intact. This response also indicates that the cause of amenorrhea lies elsewhere (ie, is due to an endocrine defect causing lack or insufficiency of cyclic estrogen and progesterone stimulation).

2. **Ovarian failure**—Amenorrhea resulting from ovarian failure can be either primary or secondary to dysfunction higher in the female neuroendocrine reproductive axis. Primary ovarian failure occurs with a premature loss of all follicles. This can result from genetic disorders (chromosomal aberrations), autoimmune disorders (lymphocytic oophoritis), metabolic problems (galactosemia) or exogenous insults such as chemotherapy, toxins, or radiation. Secondary ovarian failure is caused by a lack of gonadotropin stimulation of otherwise normal ovaries, resulting in failure to produce the estrogen and progesterone needed for menstrual cycles.

   a. **Genetic causes**—Genetic causes of ovarian failure include Turner's syndrome (abnormality in or absence of an X chromosome) and mosaicism (multiple cell lines of varying sex chromosome composition). Approximately 40% of patients who appear to have Turner's syndrome (short stature, webbed neck, shield chest, and hypergonadotropic hypoestrogenic amenorrhea) prove to be mosaics. The presence of any Y chromosome in the karyotype of these individuals carries a high risk for gonadal germ cell tumors and is an indication for gonadectomy. Thus, a karyotype should be performed on any amenorrheic individual younger than 30 with high FSH and LH levels.

b. **Premature ovarian failure**—Premature ovarian failure occurs when atresia of follicles is accelerated in an ovary of a woman of reproductive age. It presents with symptoms and signs of menopause resulting from estrogen deficiency at an inappropriately young age. LH and FSH levels are elevated. There is a lack of estrogen production and an absence of viable follicles. In some instances, premature ovarian failure is just one manifestation of an autoimmune polyglandular failure syndrome in which autoantibodies destroy a number of different tissues, including the ovary. These patients also may have associated hypothyroidism, adrenal insufficiency, or pernicious anemia (Chapters 13, 20, and 21).

c. **Chronic anovulation**—Other patients are found to have adequate numbers of follicles, but these fail to

TABLE 22–8 **Causes and mechanisms of chronic anovulation.**

Causes	Mechanisms
Thyroid disease	Altered estrogen clearance
Hyperthyroidism	Decreased androgen clearance with resulting increased peripheral aromatization to estrogen
Hypothyroidism	
Hyperprolactinemia	Altered gonadotropin-releasing hormone (GnRH) pulses
Obesity	Increased peripheral aromatization of androgens to estrogens
	Decreased steroid hormone-binding globulin, resulting in increased free estrogen and testosterone
	Increased insulin resistance, resulting in increased secretion of insulin, which increases ovarian stromal production of androgens
Primary ovarian failure	Genetic disorders (eg, Turner's syndrome)
Secondary ovarian failure	Cytotoxic drugs
	Irradiation
	Autoimmune disorders

Data from Speroff L, Glass RH, Kase NG. *Clinical Gynecologic Endocrinology and Infertility*, 6th ed. Lippincott Williams & Wilkins, 1999.

TABLE 22–9 **Clinical consequences of chronic anovulation.**

Infertility
Menstrual dysfunction (either amenorrhea or dysfunctional uterine bleeding)
Hirsutism and acne (androgen excess state)
Increased risk of endometrial cancer
Possible increased risk of breast cancer
Increased risk of cardiovascular disease
Increased risk of diabetes mellitus (hyperinsulinemia)

Data from Speroff L, Glass RH, Kase NG. *Clinical Gynecologic Endocrinology and Infertility*, 6th ed. Lippincott Williams & Wilkins, 1999.

mature and ovulate. This condition is known as **chronic anovulation** and is manifested as amenorrhea with intermittent bleeding (caused by uncoordinated overgrowth of the endometrium in response to stimulation by estrogen alone). Left untreated, the high estrogen level places these women at increased risk for endometrial carcinoma. Among the causes of chronic anovulation is thyroid dysfunction (Table 22–8). Both hyperthyroidism and hypothyroidism can alter ovarian function and the metabolism of androgens and estrogens, resulting in a variety of menstrual disorders. Another cause of chronic anovulation is hyperprolactinemia. It has been proposed that progressively more severe hyperprolactinemia presents first as an inadequate luteal phase with recurrent abortion, then as anovulation with intermittent bleeding, and finally as amenorrhea. Clinical consequences of chronic anovulation are summarized in Table 22–9.

d. **Hormonal feedback disorders**—Disruption of the coordinated cyclical interaction between the ovary and the brain can also lead to anovulation. This occurs in patients with **polycystic ovarian syndrome** (**PCOS**), which affects 2–5% of reproductive age women who present with amenorrhea and hirsutism (Table 22–10). Patients are often obese with hyperinsulinemia with insulin resistance and dyslipidemia. In addition, they have elevated plasma androgens, together with elevated plasma estrogens that are predominantly estrone derived from peripheral aromatization of adrenal androgens in the granulosa cell by the enzyme aromatase (cytochrome P450, family 19, subfamily A, polypeptide 1, or CYP19A1).

The hyperinsulinemia is believed to be a key etiologic factor. Insulin results in decreased hepatic synthesis of steroid hormone-binding globulin (SHBG) and insulin-like growth factor binding protein-1 (IGFBP-1) (Figure 22–12). The decreased levels of binding proteins results in an increase in free androgens,

TABLE 22–10 **Manifestations of polycystic ovary syndrome.**[1]

Hirsutism	95%
Large ovaries	95%
Infertility	75%
Amenorrhea	55%
Insulin resistance	50%
Obesity	40%
Dysmenorrhea	28%
Persistent anovulation	20%

Modified, with permission, from Baulieu EE, Kelly PA (editors). *Hormones: From Molecules to Disease.* Chapman & Hall, 1990.

[1]Figures are percentage of patients with syndrome manifesting each symptom or sign.

estrogens, and IGF-1. IGF-1 and high levels of insulin stimulate the IGF-1 receptor, leading to increased thecal androgen production in response to LH, contributing to the hyperandrogenemic state. The high androgens favor atresia of developing follicles and disrupt the feedback relationships that normally result in selection of a dominant follicle for ovulation (Figure 22–12). The resulting anovulation is associated with amenorrhea and estrogen-induced endometrial hyperplasia with breakthrough bleeding. The elevated estrogen levels also are implicated in the development of endometrial cancer. Thus, events occurring in the brain, ovary, and bloodstream of these patients work together to constitute a vicious cycle that maintains the aberrant feedback relationships.

The high levels of androgens in the bloodstream are responsible for hirsutism. Patients with elevated androgens from totally different causes (eg, Cushing's disease and congenital adrenal hyperplasia) also display amenorrhea associated with polycystic ovaries, suggesting that the structural changes in the ovaries are secondary to the disordered feedback.

e. **Pituitary disorders**—Head trauma resulting in pituitary stalk transection with loss of hypothalamic-pituitary communication should be considered in patients with new-onset infertility with amenorrhea. The same is true of vascular accidents such as **Sheehan's syndrome,** in which postpartum hemorrhage causes hypotension and consequent ischemic necrosis of the pituitary. Enlargement of the anterior pituitary during pregnancy may predispose to ischemia under conditions of hypotension. The pituitary approximately doubles in size during normal pregnancy, largely as a result of hypertrophy and hyperplasia of prolactin-secreting lactotrophs.

f. **Hypothalamic disorders**—Inputs from various central pathways impinge on the mediobasal portion of the hypothalamus, including the arcuate nucleus, from which GnRH pulses originate. Medications and illicit drugs that affect the neurotransmitters used in these

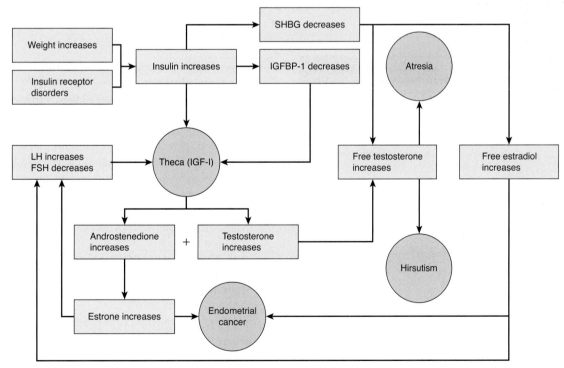

FIGURE 22–12 Pathogenesis of the various clinical manifestations of the polycystic ovary syndrome. SHBG, steroid hormone-binding globulin; IGFBP-1, insulin-like growth factor binding protein-1; IGF, insulin-like growth factor; FSH, follicle-stimulating hormone; LH, luteinizing hormone. (Redrawn, with permission, from Barnes HV. *Clinical Medicine: Selected Problems with Pathophysiologic Correlations.* Year Book Medical Publishers, 1988.)

pathways (opioids, dopamine, and norepinephrine) can, therefore, affect GnRH secretion as well. This underscores the importance of a taking a detailed medication and social history in the workup of amenorrhea.

Also important is a detailed history of behavioral patterns or any recent life changes. Psychic stress (eg, that associated with moving to a different country) can lead to altered GnRH secretion and subsequent amenorrhea that lasts up to 1 year. Vigorous exercise and excessive weight loss can also lead to impaired GnRH pulsatility, accounting for the amenorrhea seen in competitive athletes and in women with **anorexia nervosa.**

Thus, a wide range of factors that alter pulsatile release of GnRH can influence female reproductive physiology. Lack of menstrual periods because of a change in one of these factors is termed **hypothalamic amenorrhea** and is a common cause of infertility. Correction of the underlying cause often leads to a return of normal cyclic ovulation. If not, pulsatile GnRH therapy can reestablish the normal patterns of pituitary stimulation, receptor-mediated responsiveness, and feedback, restoring fertility.

g. **Indirect influences**—In addition to factors that work directly on the GnRH-secreting neurons, indirect influences must be considered. Primary hypothyroidism, as well as primary or secondary hyperprolactinemia, can result in altered GnRH pulse frequency and amplitude. The subsequent diminished gonadotropin secretion produces a secondary ovarian failure and amenorrhea. Examples of conditions that result in secondary hyperprolactinemia include lactation and treatment with drugs that have dopamine-blocking effects (eg, antipsychotic agents).

CHECKPOINT

25. Name four kinds of stress that can cause hypothalamic amenorrhea.
26. What are the consequences of untreated amenorrhea?

B. Dysmenorrhea

Primary dysmenorrhea is due to disordered or excessive prostaglandin production by the secretory endometrium of the uterus in the absence of a structural lesion. Prostaglandin F2α (PGF2α) stimulates myometrial contractions of the nonpregnant uterus, whereas prostaglandins of the E series inhibit its contraction. It appears that patients with severe dysmenorrhea generally have excessive production of PGF2α rather than increased sensitivity to this prostaglandin as a cause of excessive myometrial contraction. Excessive contractions of the myometrium result in ischemia of uterine muscle, which stimulates uterine pain fibers of the autonomic nervous system. Anxiety, fear, and stress may lower the pain threshold and thereby exaggerate the prominence of these symptoms from one patient to another and over time in a given patient.

Among the secondary causes of dysmenorrhea is **endometriosis,** a disorder in which implants of ectopic endometrial tissue respond cyclically to estrogen and progesterone (Table 22–6). This is a common disorder affecting 10–25% of women of reproductive age. The presenting symptoms of patients with endometriosis can range from pain and cramping during menstruation to adhesions with frank bowel obstruction in severe cases. Typical locations for ectopic endometrial tissue include the pelvic portion of the peritoneal cavity and ovaries. Establishment of endometrial tissue in these locations is believed to occur by either or both of two mechanisms: (1) transport of sloughed endometrial tissue by retrograde menstruation through the uterine tubes or (2) metaplasia of undifferentiated celomic epithelial mesenchyme in the peritoneum, perhaps under the influence of growth factors present in retrograde menstrual efflux. Research findings support the hypothesis of a vicious cycle involving peritoneal inflammation with elevated cytokines in peritoneal fluid and secretion of angiogenic factors that maintain ectopic endometrial tissue. A characteristic feature of endometriosis is amelioration after pregnancy and after menopause. This observation provides a therapeutic rationale for the most common modes of medical therapy, which include birth control pills; synthetic progestins (medroxyprogesterone acetate) or androgens (danazol), which block the midcycle LH surge; and long-acting GnRH analogues that down-regulate the reproductive neuroendocrine axis. Some of these drugs may also work by downregulation of cytokine production. It is unclear how endometriosis causes infertility, although inflammatory cytokines have been invoked.

C. Abnormal Vaginal Bleeding

The pathogenesis of abnormal vaginal bleeding depends on its cause, as outlined next.

1. **Functional disorders**—Depending on individual endocrine variables as described previously, the disorder results in altered amounts and timing of genital tract flow rather than a complete cessation of menses.
2. **Structural lesions**—Structural lesions that alter the contour of the endometrial cavity often lead to dysfunctional uterine bleeding. Endometrial polyps present with premenstrual or intermenstrual spotting. Fibroids, however, more often lead to menometrorrhagia. When these benign tumors are located within the endometrial cavity or within the wall of the uterus, they can disrupt the regulation of the endometrial vasculature. Therefore, very heavy prolonged or sporadic bleeding can occur.
3. **Malignancy**—Both precancerous and cancerous lesions of the uterus or cervix can produce abnormal vaginal bleeding. Endometrial hyperplasia is often the consequence of excessive estrogen stimulation or estrogen stimulation without progestin exposure. It can progress to endometrial cancer with continued estrogen excess. Unopposed estrogen stimulation can occur because of 1) an ovarian disorder (eg, chronic anovulation), 2) enhanced

peripheral aromatization of adrenal androgens by cytochrome P450, family 19, subfamily A, polypeptide 1 (CYP19A1), or 3) estrogen therapy without progestin (eg, "natural estrogen" supplementation for perimenopausal symptoms). Endometrial cancer is largely a peri- and postmenopausal disease; only 5% of cases occur during the reproductive years. Endometrial cancer spreads by direct involvement of lymphatics with distant metastases to the lung, brain, skeleton, and abdominal organs. Patients with endometrial cancer typically present with abnormal vaginal bleeding. As with ovarian cancer, ascites, bowel obstruction, and associated pleural effusions occur in widespread disease.

Dysplasia of the cervix and cervical cancer can also present with abnormal vaginal bleeding. Carcinogens in tobacco as well as persistent infection with certain subtypes of human papillomavirus (HPV) have been shown to increase the risk of cervical cancer. If untreated, cervical cancer spreads directly to the other pelvic organs; death often occurs through hemorrhage, infection, or renal failure secondary to ureteral obstruction. Currently, the American College of Obstetricians and Gynecologists recommends that uninfected girls and women between the ages of 9 and 26 years be vaccinated against HPV in order to prevent cervical cancer.

4. **Systemic conditions with altered coagulation**—Normal blood clotting involves both coagulation factors and platelets. Disorders affecting the production, quality, and survival of either clotting factors or platelets can cause abnormal vaginal bleeding (Table 22–11).

TABLE 22–11 Disorders of coagulation.

Disorders resulting in thrombocytopenia
Suppressed platelet production
von Willebrand disease
Splenic sequestration
Accelerated platelet destruction
Nonimmunologic (eg, prosthetic valves)
Immunologic
Viral and bacterial infections
Drugs
Autoimmune mechanisms (eg, idiopathic thrombocytopenic purpura)
Disorders resulting in clotting factor deficiency
Congenital disorders of coagulation
Acquired disorders of coagulation
Vitamin K deficiency
Liver disease
Disseminated intravascular coagulation

Data from Handin RI. Disorders of the platelet and vessel wall. In: *Harrison's Principles of Internal Medicine*, 14th ed. Fauci A et al (editors). McGraw-Hill, 1998.

CHECKPOINT

27. What are effective medical therapies for endometriosis, and how do they work?
28. What factors predispose to cervical cancer?

Clinical Manifestations

A. Amenorrhea

The clinical symptoms and signs that accompany amenorrhea depend on its category (Table 22–5). In genetic disorders, particularly disorders of sexual development, various degrees of delayed puberty, such as lack of breast development and absence of pubic hair, may accompany amenorrhea. In outflow tract disorders (eg, imperforate hymen), pain from occult, obstructed menstruation may occur on a cyclic basis. Generally, disorders of the uterus and the hypothalamic-pituitary axis that result in amenorrhea are painless. Secondary ovarian failure resulting in amenorrhea is often preceded by symptoms referable to decreased estrogen and progesterone production. These include hot flushes and other vasomotor symptoms.

The most common complication in the nonpregnant patient with amenorrhea is infertility. Additional complications depend on the specific cause of lack of menstruation. Osteoporosis is a major potential long-term complication of inadequate estrogen production. Inadequate estrogen can also be associated with thinning of estrogen-dependent epithelia, such as that of the vagina, resulting in atrophic vaginitis. This symptom usually responds to topical estrogen creams. In the case of inadequate progesterone production—typically associated with irregular vaginal bleeding but seen also in some cases of amenorrhea—the risk of endometrial cancer is greatly increased. Endometrial cancer is the most common cancer of the female genital tract; 34,000 new cases are identified annually in the United States. Risk factors for endometrial cancer include early menarche, late menopause, nulliparity, obesity, hypertension, and diabetes mellitus.

B. Dysmenorrhea

Dysmenorrhea may be accompanied by a variable constellation of symptoms, including sweating, weakness and fatigue, insomnia, nausea, vomiting, diarrhea, back pain, headache (including both migraine and tension headaches; see Chapter 7), dizziness, and even syncope. Prostaglandin synthesis inhibitors (nonsteroidal anti-inflammatory agents) often alleviate many of these symptoms if treatment is started early enough to avert the cascade of events that occur with production of prostaglandins.

With **premenstrual syndrome,** dysmenorrhea is accompanied by additional symptoms, including a sensation of bloating, weight gain, edema of the hands and feet, breast tenderness, acne, anxiety, aggression, mood irritability, food cravings, and change in libido. An initial approach should be to encourage changes in lifestyle if indicated by the history (eg, more sleep, exercise, improved diet, and less tobacco, alcohol, and caffeine). Pharmacologic therapy with serotonin-reuptake inhibitors (SSRIs) has proven beneficial in addition to behavioral modification.

C. Abnormal Vaginal Bleeding

The symptoms and signs that accompany abnormal vaginal bleeding vary with the cause. In children, vulvovaginitis is the most frequent disorder, accompanied by a mucopurulent discharge that may become bloody with mucosal erosion. Other prominent causes, including foreign objects and tumors, can be assessed by physical examination. In adolescents and adults, dysfunctional uterine bleeding is most common, but other causes must be considered, including pregnancy (assessed by serial serum β-hCG determinations and ultrasound examination), trauma (by history and physical examination), cancer (by colposcopy and hysteroscopy), and systemic disorders such as a hemorrhagic diathesis (by platelet, prothrombin, and partial thromboplastin time determinations) and thyroid disease (by serum TSH, total and free thyroxine determinations). In postmenopausal women, one fifth of cases of vaginal bleeding prove to be endometrial cancer.

INFERTILITY

Infertility is defined as the absence of conception after at least 1 year of regular sexual intercourse without contraception.

Etiology

In approximately 30% of cases, infertility is due to male factors (eg, inadequate sperm count) (see Chapter 23). For female infertility, about 40% of cases are due to ovulatory failure, about 40% are due to endometrial or tubal disease, about 10% are due to rarer causes (eg, thyroid disease or hyperprolactinemia), and about 10% remain undefined after full workup (Table 22–12).

Pathology & Pathogenesis

A. Ovulatory Causes

Infertility referable to ovarian dysfunction can result from disorders of the hypothalamus or pituitary, resulting in inadequate gonadotropic stimulation of the ovary; from ovarian disorders, resulting either in inadequate secretory products or failure to ovulate; or from both types of disorders occurring at the same time. Correction of the underlying cause will often restore fertility. In many cases, exogenous administration of gonadotropins will stimulate the ovaries to produce follicular

TABLE 22–12 Causes of female infertility.[1]

Cause	Patients with Infertility
Ovulatory dysfunction	40%
Diminished ovarian reserve	
Oligo-ovulation or amenorrhea	
PCOS	
Hypothalamic amenorrhea	
Other	
Tubal or pelvic pathology	40%
Endometriosis	
Scarring and adhesions (from pelvic inflammatory disease, chronic infection, tubal surgery, ectopic pregnancy, or ruptured appendix)	
Miscellaneous	10%
Thyroid disease	
Pituitary disease (hyperprolactinemia)	
Unexplained	10%

Data from Speroff L, Glass RH, Kase NG. *Clinical Gynecologic Endocrinology and Infertility,* 6th ed. Lippincott Williams & Wilkins, 1999.

[1]In infertile couples, problems in the male account for 30% of the total.

growth. The oocytes can then be released in vivo and fertilized by intercourse or by artificial insemination. Alternatively, the mature oocytes can be removed from the woman to be used in in vitro fertilization (IVF), where fertilization occurs within the laboratory and embryos are returned to the uterus.

One of the most common ovarian disorders, called diminished ovarian reserve, is age related and can involve both the oocytes themselves and the secretory products of the ovary. There is accelerated loss of follicles with the approach of menopause. With follicular depletion, FSH levels tend to rise, reflecting inadequate production of inhibin. This could result from an inadequate number of follicles, diminished competence of the remaining follicles, diminished steroidogenesis by the aging ovary, or some combination of these factors. Regardless of the specific reason, the net effect is a shortened follicular phase and is associated with increased rates of infertility. Treatment with clomiphene citrate, a weak estrogen antagonist, is a means of diminishing negative feedback and increasing gonadotropin stimulation of the ovary and restoring ovulation.

Other etiologies of ovulation dysfunction include conditions that alter the coordination between ovary and hypothalamus, such as PCOS and hypothalamic amenorrhea. In these scenarios, the oocytes do not undergo the appropriate development and maturation to lead to regular ovulation and subsequently cause infertility.

B. Tubal and Pelvic Causes

Given normal follicles and reproductive neuroendocrine axis function, the major cause of infertility is abnormality of the endometrium or fallopian tubes. Prior or ongoing pelvic infections, with adhesions or inflammation, can result in failure of sperm or egg transport, failure of implantation, or implantation in an inappropriate location (ectopic pregnancy).

Endometriosis, presumably occurring due to the cyclic proliferation and sloughing of ectopic endometrial tissue, results in inflammation, scarring, and adhesion formation. New data suggest that endometriosis may arise from a circulating endometrial stem cell population. This condition should be suspected when infertility is associated with severe dysmenorrhea. Surgical and medical therapies are efficacious in the reduction of endometriosis-associated pain. The effects of endometriosis treatment on infertility remain controversial.

C. Other Causes of Female Infertility

Most of the less common causes of infertility can be grouped into those disorders that affect the production of GnRH by the hypothalamus or the hormone's effect on the pituitary (eg, thyroid disease and hyperprolactinemia).

CHECKPOINT

29. What are the most common causes of infertility in couples?
30. How do postcoital high-dose estrogens work as a contraceptive?
31. What feature of the history suggests a tubal or uterine cause of infertility?

PREECLAMPSIA-ECLAMPSIA

Pregnancy is associated with a host of medical complications in which clinical management requires an understanding of both the underlying physiology of pregnancy and the pathophysiology of the particular disorder. The syndrome of preeclampsia-eclampsia, characterized by hypertension, proteinuria, and edema, is chosen for focus for several reasons. First, preeclampsia-eclampsia is one of the most common causes of maternal death in the United States and the developed world. Second, it illustrates how pathophysiologic mechanisms in pregnancy may be far more complex—and the clinical consequences far more serious—than would have been expected from a simple consideration of each of the presenting symptoms in isolation. Third, advances have significantly altered current thinking about the pathogenesis of this disorder.

Clinical Presentation

Hypertension can develop during pregnancy as an isolated finding, **pregnancy-induced hypertension** (PIH), or as a component of a dangerous disorder, **preeclampsia-eclampsia.**

Treatment guidelines for PIH are different than those for essential hypertension in the nonpregnant patient; elevated maternal blood pressure is often left untreated unless symptomatic or if severe hypertension develops. Because placental perfusion is dependent on a pressure difference between the maternal and fetal circulations, decreases in maternal blood pressure can lead to underperfusion of the placenta. This can result in **placental insufficiency** and fetal distress.

The hypertension seen in preeclampsia is associated with proteinuria and edema. This syndrome occurs in approximately 5% of pregnancies in the United States. Eclampsia, the superimposition of generalized tonic-clonic seizures on pregnancy-induced hypertension, can occur as the initial presenting sign of this syndrome or during its progression. Table 22–13 summarizes the symptoms and signs of preeclampsia-eclampsia.

Etiology

Preeclampsia-eclampsia is thought to derive from faulty implantation, resulting in a systemic disorder of endothelial cell activation (see later discussion). Predisposing factors for the development of preeclampsia include first pregnancy, obesity,

TABLE 22–13 Symptoms and signs of preeclampsia-eclampsia.

Maternal syndrome
Pregnancy-induced hypertension
Excessive weight gain (> 1 kg/wk)
Generalized edema
Ascites
Hyperuricemia
Proteinuria
Hypocalciuria
Increased plasma von Willebrand factor concentration
Increased plasma cellular fibronectin
Reduced plasma antithrombin concentration
Reduced angiogenic activity
Thrombocytopenia
Increased packed cell volume
Increased serum liver enzyme levels
Fetal syndrome
Intrauterine growth retardation
Intrauterine hypoxemia

Data from Roberts JM, Redman CWG. Preeclampsia: More than pregnancy-induced hypertension. Lancet. 1993;341:1447.

preexisting diabetes or hypertension, hydatidiform mole, malnutrition, and a family history of preeclampsia.

Pathology & Pathogenesis

The placenta of preeclamptic patients shows signs of premature aging, including degeneration, hyaline deposition, calcification, and congestion. The maternal decidua also shows hemorrhage and necrosis with thrombosis of spiral arteries and diffuse infarcts.

Normally, blood vessels of the uterine wall undergo striking morphologic changes at the site of implantation, facilitating placental perfusion. The diameters of the spiral arteries increase and the muscular and elastic components are lost. However, for unknown (perhaps immune-mediated) reasons, these early angiogenic changes of implantation do not occur—or at least not fully—in patients who will develop preeclampsia-eclampsia later in gestation. As a result, a condition of relative placental ischemia is established, with the release of lipid and protein factors that damage the maternal vascular endothelium, at first within the decidua and later systemically. Oxidative injury is believed to work with maternal factors (eg, obesity, diabetes, diet, genes) to cause generalized endothelial cell damage.

Endothelial activation has two important pathophysiologic consequences. First, the balance between vasodilation and vasoconstriction is altered, specifically by diminished production of vasodilator products such as prostacyclin and nitric oxide, increased production of vasoconstrictive thromboxane, endothelin and platelet-derived growth factor. As a result, there is increased vasoconstriction of small placental bed arterioles, with hypoperfusion and ischemia of downstream tissues and systemic hypertension. Second, the endothelial cell barrier between platelets and the collagen of basement membranes is breached.

As a result of the latter changes, additional events are set in motion, including platelet aggregation, activation of the clotting cascade, and production of vasoactive substances causing capillary leak. This results in further tissue hypoperfusion, edema formation, and proteinuria, the hallmarks of preeclampsia-eclampsia. Because these processes result in further vascular endothelial damage, a vicious circle is established.

Interesting speculation has centered on the potential of serotonin to modulate vasodilation and angiogenic growth factors. New data also invoke a role for agonistic autoantibodies directed against the second extracellular loop of the angiotensin II AT1 receptor, resulting in the vasospasm associated with preeclampsia.

Clinical Manifestations

Preeclampsia has a plethora of manifestations (Table 22–13). Beyond the presenting symptoms of hypertension, edema, and proteinuria, patients also can have increased deep tendon reflexes, or placental abruption. Hepatic periportal congestion, hemorrhage, and necrosis can lead to elevated liver func-

TABLE 22–14 Complications of preeclampsia-eclampsia.

Cerebral hemorrhage
Cortical blindness
Retinal detachment
HELLP syndrome (*hemolysis, elevated liver enzymes, low platelets*)
Hepatic rupture
Disseminated intravascular coagulation (DIC)
Pulmonary edema
Laryngeal edema
Acute renal cortical necrosis
Acute renal tubular necrosis
Abruptio placentae
Intrauterine fetal asphyxia and death

Data from Roberts JM, Redman CWG. Pre-eclampsia: More than pregnancy-induced hypertension. Lancet. 1993;341:1447.

tion tests and ultimate rupture of the hepatic capsule. Severe preeclampsia also can produce renal changes, including glomerular endothelial cell swelling, mesangial proliferation, and marked narrowing of glomerular capillary lumens. The renal cortex displays significant cortical ischemia that may progress to frank necrosis and acute renal failure. Thrombocytopenia and disseminated intravascular coagulopathy (DIC) as well as cerebral vascular accidents also may occur (Table 22–14). Eclampsia, or maternal seizure resulting from cerebral ischemia and petechial hemorrhage, can occur in this setting or can appear as the first manifestation of this disease. Preeclampsia-eclampsia also carries risks for the fetus. Placental deterioration and insufficiency can result in intrauterine growth restriction (IUGR) and fetal hypoxia. Delivery of the fetus and placenta is the only definitive cure for this syndrome, which carries a high mortality rate for mother and child (Table 22–14).

CHECKPOINT

32. What are the hallmarks of preeclampsia-eclampsia?
33. What are the risks to the fetus of untreated maternal hypertension?
34. What are some of the maternal sequelae of preeclampsia-eclampsia?

CASE STUDIES

Eva M. Aagaard, MD, & Yeong Kwok, MD

(See Chapter 25, p. 709 for Answers)

CASE 102

A 24-year-old woman presents to the clinic complaining of painful menses. She states that for the last several years she has had cramping pain in the days preceding her menses as well as during her menses. In addition, she notes bloating and weight gain in the week before her menses, with swelling of her hands and feet. She has irritability and severe mood swings during that time such that she cries easily and for no reason seems to become enraged at her family or boyfriend. On review of systems she denies urinary symptoms, vaginal discharge, or GI symptoms. She has no significant medical history. She has never been pregnant. She has never had a sexually transmitted disease. She is sexually active only with her long-standing boyfriend and states that they always use condoms. She takes no medications. Her physical examination is unremarkable.

Questions

A. What are some possible causes of this woman's dysmenorrhea? Which do you think is most likely? Why?

B. What is the pathophysiologic mechanism responsible for her dysmenorrhea?

C. How would you treat her symptoms?

CASE 103

A 28-year-old woman presents to the clinic with a complaint of infertility. She states that she and her husband have been trying to get pregnant for approximately 1 year without success. She had menarche at age 14 years. Since that time, she has had regular menses lasting 5 days, without significant dysmenorrhea or abnormal bleeding. She has never been pregnant. Medical history is notable for gonorrhea and trichomoniasis at age 18. In addition, she has had an abnormal Pap smear consistent with human papillomavirus at age 20 years, with normal Pap smears since that time. She takes no medications. She has been married for 2 years and is sexually active only with her husband. Before her marriage she had approximately 25 sexual partners, most during her college years. Her physical examination is unremarkable.

Questions

A. What are the most common causes of female infertility?

B. What do you suspect is the cause of this patient's infertility? Why?

CASE 104

A 28-year-old woman presents to her obstetrician for her regularly scheduled prenatal examination. She is 30 weeks pregnant. She has noted some swelling of her hands and feet in the last 2 weeks that seems to be getting progressively worse, such that she is no longer able to wear her rings and can only wear open-heeled shoes. She is otherwise without complaints. She has no past medical problems. This is her first pregnancy. She has had regular prenatal care and, thus far, with no complications. She is taking only prenatal multivitamins. Family history is notable for maternal hypertension and diabetes. She is married and works as a schoolteacher. She denies alcohol, tobacco, and drug use. On examination she appears to be well, with blood pressure of 152/95 mm Hg. Fundal height is consistent with gestational age. Fetal heart rate is 140 beats/min. Extremities have 1+ lower extremity edema to the knees and trace edema of the hands. Urine dipstick reveals 3+ protein.

Questions

A. What is the likely diagnosis?

B. What are some risk factors for developing this condition?

C. How does this condition develop? How does it result in maternal hypertension, edema, and proteinuria?

D. What are the risks to the fetus if this condition is left untreated?

E. What are the maternal sequelae of leaving this condition untreated? What is the treatment?

REFERENCES

General

Ault KA. Human papillomavirus vaccines: An update for gynecologists. Clin Obstet Gynecol. 2008 Sep;51(3):527–32. [PMID: 18677145]

Buchanan TA et al. Gestational diabetes mellitus. J Clin Invest. 2005 Mar;115(3):485–91. [PMID: 15765129]

Chang RJ. The reproductive phenotype in polycystic ovary syndrome. Nat Clin Pract Endocrinol Metab. 2007 Oct;3(10):688–95. [PMID: 17893687]

Diamond J. Unwritten knowledge. Nature. 2001 Mar 29;410(6828):521. [PMID: 11279469]

ESHRE Capri Workshop Group. Genetic aspects of female reproduction. Hum Reprod Update. 2008 Jul-Aug;14(4):293–307. [PMID: 18385259]

Lam C et al. Circulating angiogenic factors in the pathogenesis and prediction of preeclampsia. Hypertension. 2005 Nov;46(5):1077–85. [PMID: 16230516]

Lingappa VR, Farey K. *Physiological Medicine.* McGraw-Hill, 2000.

Menon R et al. Ethnic differences in key candidate genes for spontaneous preterm birth: TNF-alpha and its receptors. Hum Hered. 2006;62(2):107–18. [PMID: 17047334]

Newton ER. Preterm labor, preterm premature rupture of membranes, and chorioamnionitis. Clin Perinatol. 2005 Sep;32(3):571–600. [PMID: 16085021]

Schmitz T et al. Selective use of fetal fibronectin detection after cervical length measurement to predict spontaneous preterm delivery in women with preterm labor. Am J Obstet Gynecol. 2006 Jan;194(1):138–43. [PMID: 16389023]

Sibai B et al. Pre-eclampsia. Lancet. 2005 Feb 26-Mar 4;365(9461):785–99. [PMID: 15733721]

Speroff L, Fritz MA. *Clinical Gynecologic Endocrinology and Infertility,* 7th ed. Lippincott Williams & Wilkins, 2004.

Strauss JF, Barbieri RL. Disorders of pregnancy. In: *Yen and Jaffe's Reproductive Endocrinology,* 5th ed. Elsevier Saunders, 2004.

Vohr BR et al. Gestational diabetes: The forerunner for the development of maternal and childhood obesity and metabolic syndrome? J Matern Fetal Neonatal Med. 2008 Mar;21(3):149–57. [PMID: 18297569]

Xia Y et al. Angiotensin receptors, autoimmunity, and preeclampsia. J Immunol. 2007 Sep 15;179(6):3391–5. [PMID: 17785770]

Menstrual Disorders

Berga SL et al. Use of cognitive behavior therapy for functional hypothalamic amenorrhea. Ann N Y Acad Sci. 2006 Dec;1092:114–29. [PMID: 17308138]

Davis JR. Prolactin and reproductive medicine. Curr Opin Obstet Gynecol. 2004 Aug;16(4):331–7. [PMID: 15232488]

Deligeoroglou E et al. Menstrual disorders during adolescence. Pediatr Endocrinol Rev. 2006;3 Suppl 1:150.

Guzick DS. Polycystic ovary syndrome. Pediatr Endocrinol Rev. 2006 Jan;3 Suppl 1:150–9. [PMID: 16641850]

Poppe K et al. Female infertility and the thyroid. Best Pract Res Clin Endocrinol Metab. 2004 Jun;18(2):153–65. [PMID: 15157833]

Rigon F et al. Menstrual disorders in adolescence. Minerva Pediatr. 2006 Jun;58(3):227–46. [PMID: 16832328]

Infertility

Mårdh PA. Tubal factor infertility, with special regard to chlamydial salpingitis. Curr Opin Infect Dis. 2004 Feb;17(1):49–52. [PMID: 15090891]

Patel SS et al. Oocyte quality in adult polycystic ovary syndrome. Semin Reprod Med. 2008 Mar;26(2):196–203. [PMID: 18302111]

Sasson IE et al. Stem cells and the pathogenesis of endometriosis. Ann N Y Acad Sci. 2008 Apr;1127:106–15. [PMID: 18443337]

Toniolo D et al. X chromosome and ovarian failure. Semin Reprod Med. 2007 Jul;25(4):264–71. [PMID: 17594607]

Disorders of the Male Reproductive Tract

Mikkel Fode, Jens Sønksen, MD, PhD,
Stephen J. McPhee, MD, & Dana A. Ohl, MD

Male reproductive tract functions include androgen homeostasis, spermatogenesis, sperm transport and storage, and normal erectile and ejaculatory function ability. The control of these functions involves the pituitary gland, central and peripheral nervous systems, and genitalia. This chapter considers two common disorders of the male reproductive tract: male infertility and benign prostatic hyperplasia.

NORMAL STRUCTURE & FUNCTION OF THE MALE REPRODUCTIVE TRACT

ANATOMY & PHYSIOLOGY

The male reproductive tract is composed of the testes, genital ducts, accessory glands, and penis (Figure 23–1).

The testes are responsible for the production of testosterone and spermatozoa. Each testis is approximately 4 cm in length and 20 mL in volume. The testis is divided into lobules consisting of seminiferous tubules (inside which sperm are produced) and intertubular connective tissue (Figure 23–2). The seminiferous tubules converge to form another network of tubules called the rete testis through which the fluid secreted by the seminiferous tubules is delivered to the ductal system of the epididymis.

The seminiferous tubules are surrounded by a basal membrane and a specialized spermatogenic epithelium, consisting of Sertoli cells providing mechanical support, protection, and nourishment to the developing germ cells. At puberty, tight junctions between the Sertoli cells form an impermeable lining within the tubular wall called the blood-testis barrier. The blood-testis barrier divides the seminiferous tubules into a basal compartment and an adlumenal compartment, separating more advanced germ cells from the immune system. This separation is necessary because mature sperm are potentially antigenic since they are not present before puberty when much of the individual's central immune tolerance is established. The Leydig cells in the intertubular connective tissue produce testosterone.

Both testosterone production and spermatogenesis are controlled by the hypothalamic-pituitary-gonadal axis. The hypothalamus produces gonadotropin-releasing hormone (GnRH) in a pulsatile fashion. GnRH courses through the hypothalamic-pituitary portal system to stimulate the anterior pituitary to secrete (also in a pulsatile fashion) the two gonadotropins, luteinizing hormone (LH) and follicle-stimulating hormone (FSH). FSH stimulates the Sertoli cells to produce paracrine growth factors and other products supporting spermatogenesis. FSH also stimulates the production of inhibin in response to active spermatogenesis and androgen-binding globulin (ABP).

Under the influence of LH, the Leydig cells produce testosterone. Concentrations of testosterone in the seminiferous tubules are 80–100 times greater than in the general circulation. Androgens act on spermatogenesis via the Sertoli cells, and high testicular levels of androgens are essential for spermatogenesis. Circulating testosterone provides negative feedback on secretion of GnRH, LH, and FSH.

Inhibin exerts negative feedback on FSH secretion by the pituitary, while testosterone exerts negative feedback on LH secretion by both the hypothalamus and the pituitary.

During spermatogenesis, primitive germ cells develop into mature spermatozoa as they move from the basement membrane to the lumen of the tubules. The immature germ cells near the basement membrane are called spermatogonia and have the normal diploid number of 46 chromosomes. Beginning

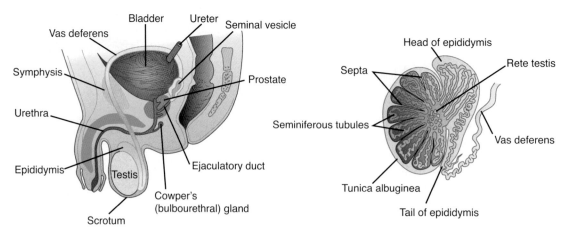

FIGURE 23–1   Anatomy of male reproductive system (left) and duct system of testis (right).   (Redrawn, with permission, from Ganong WF. *Review of Medical Physiology*, 22nd ed. McGraw-Hill, 2005.)

at puberty and continuing throughout life, the spermatogonia divide mitotically, maintaining the population. Some of the spermatogonia differentiate into primary spermatocytes and enter the first meiotic division. During the prophase of the first meiotic division, duplication of DNA, pairing of homologous chromosomes, and crossing over take place and the spermatocytes develop a duplicated set of 46 chromosomes. The spermatocytes (now called secondary spermatocytes) then undergo the second meiotic division producing spermatids, which have a haploid number of unduplicated chromosomes. In this way, four spermatids are produced from each spermatogonium. Spermatids then undergo a maturation process called spermiogenesis to form spermatozoa. In this

process, condensation of the nuclear chromatin takes place and the enzyme-filled acrosome cap is formed. The spermatids also elongate and develop flagella. Spermiogenesis ends with the spermatozoa being released from the germinal epithelium. The process in which the primary spermatogonia divide and develop into mature spermatozoa takes about 74 days.

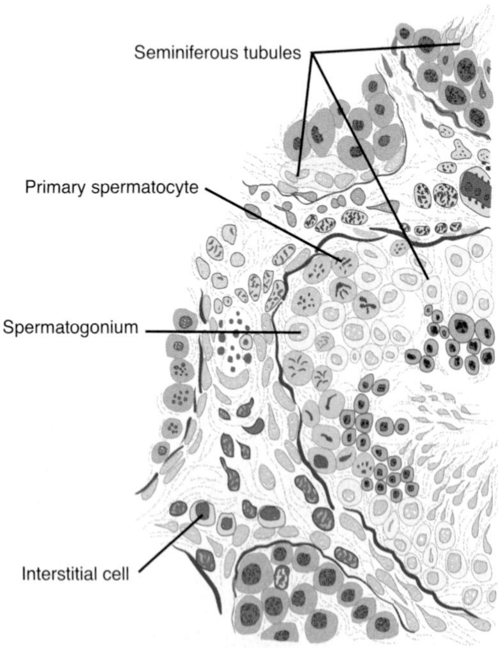

After spermiogenesis, spermatozoa are released into the lumen of the seminiferous tubule, then course through the rete testis into the epididymis. Epididymal transit takes 5–14 days, and during transit, the spermatozoa mature and become capable of progressive movement in a process involving changes in membrane, metabolism, and morphology. Sperm are stored in the cauda epididymis until the time of ejaculation. During ejaculation, they travel through the vas deferens via the inguinal canal, and medially to the posterior and inferior part of the urinary bladder to fuse with the duct of the seminal vesicle forming the combined ejaculatory duct. The ejaculatory ducts run through the prostate entering the prostatic portion of the urethra at the verumontanum distal to the internal bladder sphincter (Figure 23–3).

During normal erection, parasympathetic fibers travel from S2-S4 through the pelvic nerve and the pelvic plexus to the cavernous nerve where they release acetylcholine (ACh) and nitric oxide (NO). Their release causes relaxation of the smooth muscles of the penile corpora, which in turn leads to increased blood flow and blood trapping, resulting in erection.

The ejaculatory reflex is initiated by cerebral perception of erotic stimuli and afferent input from genital tactile sensation via the dorsal nerves of the penis. Seminal emission refers to the transport of ejaculate from the ampulla of the vas deferens into the posterior urethra and is the result of peristaltic contractions of smooth muscle cells in the epididymis, vas deferens, and accessory sex glands under sympathetic control from the fibers arising from T10-T12. Following the initial emission of semen into the posterior urethra, sympathetic contraction (T10-T12) of the posterior urethra and closure of the bladder neck (preventing retrograde ejaculation into the

FIGURE 23–2   Schematic section of testis.   (Redrawn, with permission, from Ganong WF. *Review of Medical Physiology*, 22nd ed. McGraw-Hill, 2005.)

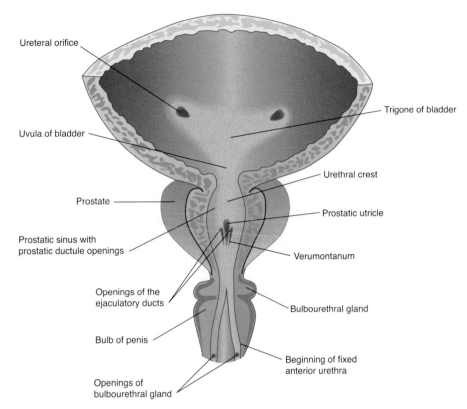

FIGURE 23–3 Anatomic relationships of the prostate. (Redrawn, with permission, from Lindner HH. *Clinical Anatomy.* Originally published by Appleton & Lange. Copyright © 1989 by the McGraw-Hill Companies, Inc.)

bladder) are initiated and the external urethral sphincter relaxes. The projectile phase of the ejaculation is a spinal cord reflex mediated by the somatic fibers from S2 to S4 running through the pudendal nerve causing rhythmic contractions of the periurethral and pelvic floor muscles.

In the female reproductive tract, the spermatozoa must migrate through the cervical mucus and then undergo several functional and structural changes collectively termed capacitation. These changes are necessary for the spermatozoa's ability to fertilize the oocyte as they facilitate the acrosome reaction, during which the sperm plasma membrane fuses with the outer acrosomal membrane. This exposes the contents of the acrosome, such as acrosin and hyaluronidase, allowing penetration of the oocyte. Capacitation can also be induced by incubation in suitable laboratory medium.

Sperm cells only make up 1–2% of the semen volume. The rest of the seminal plasma is produced in the accessory male sex glands. The seminal vesicles produce two-thirds of the ejaculate volume and provide fructose as an energy source, as well as seminogellin, which contributes to seminal coagulation. The prostate supplies about one-third of the ejaculate and this includes prostate-specific antigen, a proteolytic enzyme that cleaves seminogellin, effecting liquefaction. Finally, the bulbourethral glands contribute a small amount of clear mucoid discharge, released mainly during sexual stimulation before ejaculation.

PHYSIOLOGY

Androgen Synthesis, Protein Binding, & Metabolism

The testes secrete two steroid hormones that are essential to male reproductive function: testosterone and dihydrotestosterone. The pathways for testicular androgen biosynthesis are illustrated in Figure 23–4.

Testosterone, a C_{19} steroid, is synthesized from cholesterol by the interstitial (Leydig) cells of the testes and from androstenedione secreted by the adrenal cortex. The majority of circulating testosterone is bound to sex-hormone–binding globulin (SHBG) and is unavailable for biological activity.

The remainder is loosely bound to albumin and is available for target tissue action. Only about 2% is unbound in circulation. The albumin-bound and free fractions make up the "bioavailable" testosterone in circulation. SHBG is synthesized in the liver and may be increased in certain clinical conditions. The effect of increasing SHBG in circulation is to lower the bioavailable fraction, so that while the serum total testosterone level is normal, hypogonadism occurs at the tissue level because of protein binding. The most common causes of increased SHBG are liver dysfunction, hyperestrogenemia, obesity, and aging. Testosterone levels through the lifespan are characterized in Figure 23–5. The negative feedback control mechanisms for testosterone are depicted in Figure 23–6.

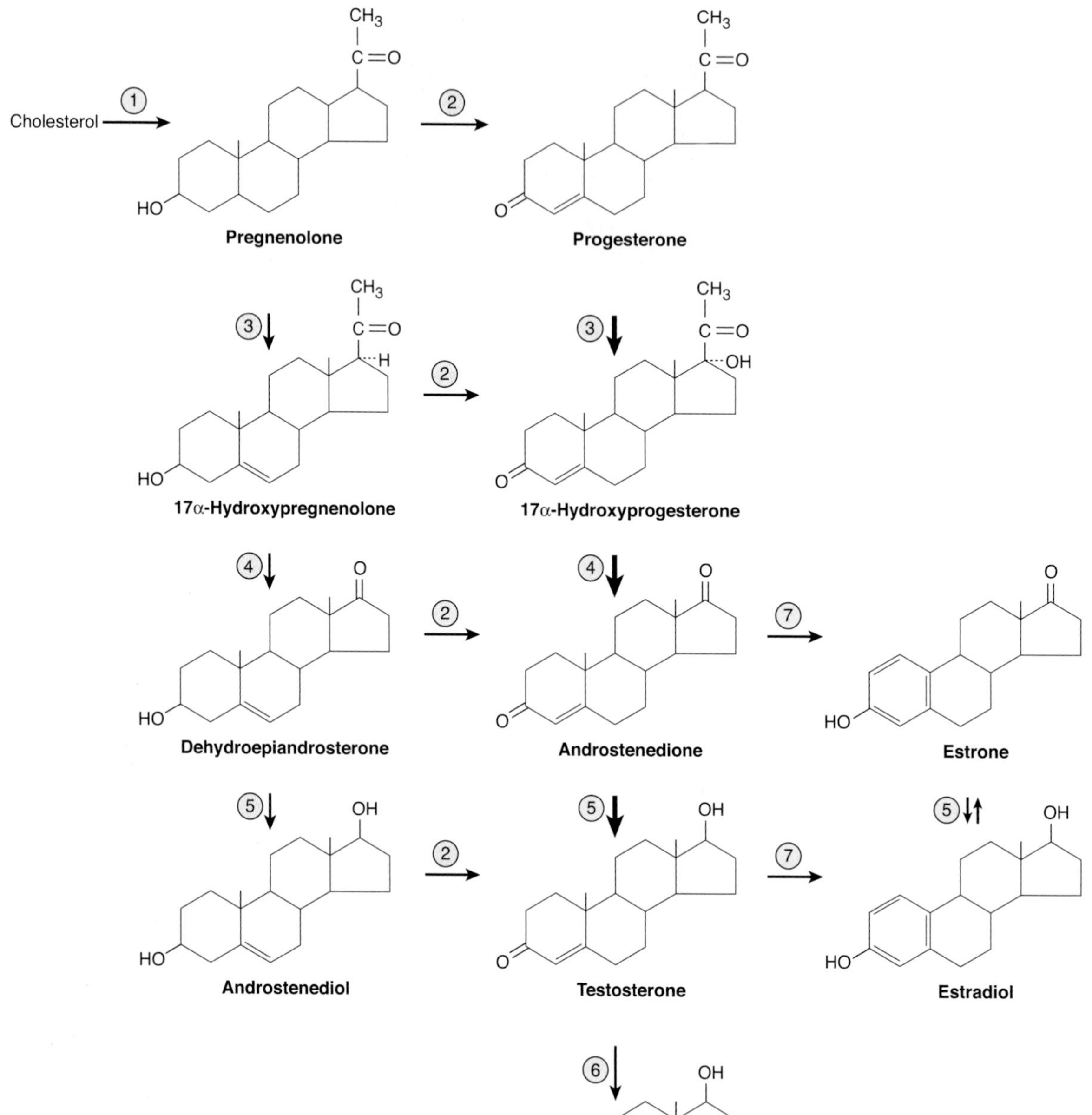

FIGURE 23–4 Biosynthesis and metabolism of testosterone. Heavy arrows indicate major pathways. Circled numbers represent enzymes as follows: ① cytochrome P450, family 11, subfamily A, polypeptide 1 (CYP11A1); ② hydroxy-Δ-5-steroid dehydrogenase, 3β- and steroid Δ-isomerase (HSD3β); ③ 17α-hydroxylase activity of cytochrome P450, family 17, subfamily A, polypeptide 1 (CYP17A1); ④ 17,20-lyase activity of cytochrome P450, family 17, subfamily A, polypeptide 1 (CYP17A1); ⑤ hydroxysteroid (17β) dehydrogenase (HSD17β); ⑥ steroid-5α-reductase, α polypeptide 2 (3-oxo-5 α-steroid Δ4-dehydrogenase α) (SRD5A); ⑦ cytochrome P450, family 19, subfamily A, polypeptide 1 (CYP19A1). (Redrawn, with permission, from Greenspan FS, Gardner DG [editors]. *Basic and Clinical Endocrinology,* 8th ed. McGraw-Hill, 2007.)

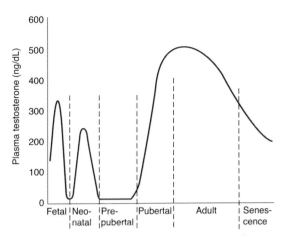

FIGURE 23–5 Plasma testosterone levels at various ages in males. (Redrawn, with permission, from Ganong WF. *Review of Medical Physiology*, 22nd ed. McGraw-Hill, 2005.)

Dihydrotestosterone (DHT) is derived both from direct secretion by the testes (about 20%) and from conversion in peripheral tissues (about 80%) of testosterone and other androgen (and estrogen) precursors secreted by the testes and adrenals. DHT circulates in the bloodstream. The normal plasma DHT level for the adult male is 27–75 ng/dL (0.9–2.6 nmol/L) (Table 23–1).

Estradiol is produced by aromatization of testosterone in the peripheral circulation. The aromatase enzyme is present in abundant amounts in fatty tissue. Thus, obesity can increase conversion of testosterone, with resultant hyperestrogenemia, down-regulation of the hypothalamic-pituitary-gonadal axis, and hypogonadism.

Effects of Androgens

Circulating testosterone or DHT crosses the membrane of the target cell and enter the cytoplasm. Testosterone may be converted to the more potent DHT inside the target cell. Testosterone or DHT binds to the androgen receptor, and the complex is then transported to the cell's nucleus, where it binds to DNA and initiates mRNA synthesis. The resultant proteins synthesized account for the subsequent androgenic changes that occur (Figure 23–7).

In the fetus, androgens are necessary for normal differentiation and development of the internal and external male genitalia. During puberty, androgens are needed for normal growth of the male genital structures, including the scrotum, epididymis, vas deferens, seminal vesicles, prostate, and penis. During adolescence, androgens and estrogens cause rapid growth of skeletal muscle and bone. Androgens are also responsible for development of the secondary sex characteristics summarized in Table 23–2. During adult life, androgens are necessary for normal male reproductive function. Specifically, androgens stimulate erythropoiesis, preserve bone structure and muscle mass, and maintain libido and erectile function.

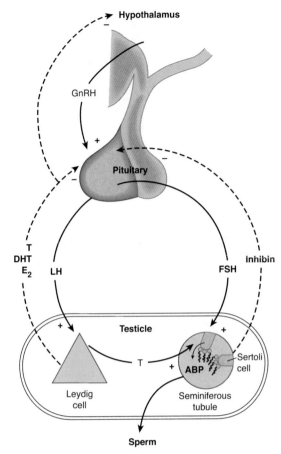

FIGURE 23–6 Endocrine control of male reproductive system. ABP, androgen-binding protein; GnRH, gonadotropin-releasing hormone; T, testosterone; E_2, estradiol; DHT, dihydrotestosterone. (Redrawn and modified, with permission, from Greenspan FS, Gardner DG [editors]. *Basic and Clinical Endocrinology*, 8th ed. McGraw-Hill, 2007.)

TABLE 23–1 Normal plasma level for pituitary and gonadal hormones in men.

Hormone	Conventional Units	SI Units
Testosterone, total	260–1000 ng/dL	9.0–34.7 nmol/L
Testosterone, free	50–210 pg/mL	173–729 pmol/L
Dihydrotestosterone	27–75 ng/dL	0.9–2.6 nmol/L
Androstenedione	50–200 ng/dL	1.7–6.9 nmol/L
Estradiol	15–40 pg/mL	55–150 pmol/L
Estrone	15–65 pg/mL	55.5–240 pmol/L
FSH	2–15 mIU/mL	2–15 U/L
LH	2–15 mIU/mL	2–15 units/L
PRL	1.6–18.8 ng/mL	0.07–0.8 nmol/L

Key: FSH, follicle-stimulating hormone; LH, luteinizing hormone; PRL, prolactin.

Data from Gardner DG, Shoback D (editors). *Greenspan's Basic and Clinical Endocrinology*, 8th ed. McGraw Hill, 2007.

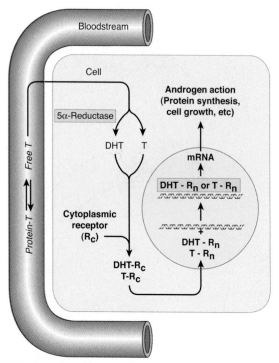

FIGURE 23–7   Mechanism of androgen action. DHT, dihydrotestosterone; T, testosterone; R_c, cytoplasmic receptor, which becomes the nuclear receptor, R_n, in the nucleus. (Redrawn, with permission, from Greenspan FS, Gardner DG [editors]. *Basic and Clinical Endocrinology*, 8th ed. McGraw-Hill, 2007.)

TABLE 23–2   Pubertal development of male secondary sex characteristics.

External genitalia	Penis increases in length and width; scrotum becomes pigmented and rugose
Internal genitalia	Seminal vesicles enlarge and secrete
Larynx	Larynx enlarges, vocal cords increase in length and thickness, voice deepens
Hair	Beard appears; scalp hairline recedes anterolaterally; pubic hair appears with male pattern (triangle with apex up); axillary, chest, and perianal hair appears
Musculoskeletal	Shoulders broaden; skeletal muscles enlarge
Skin	Sebaceous gland secretions increase and thicken
Mental	More aggressive, active attitude appears; libido develops

Modified from Ganong WF. *Review of Medical Physiology,* 22nd ed. McGraw-Hill, 2005.

CHECKPOINT

1. What is the purpose of seminiferous tubule tight junctions?
2. What are the roles of the two major cell populations in the testis, the Leydig cells and the Sertoli cells?
3. How is testosterone secretion regulated?
4. What are the target cells of LH and FSH?
5. What are the relative concentrations of testosterone in the peripheral circulation and the testicular tissue?
6. Describe the sequence of events leading up to and during ejaculation.
7. How is estradiol created in men?
8. What are the effects of androgens?

PATHOPHYSIOLOGY OF SELECTED MALE REPRODUCTIVE TRACT DISORDERS

MALE INFERTILITY

For conception to occur, the following conditions must be met: (1) The testes must have normal spermatogenesis; (2) the spermatozoa must complete their maturation; (3) the ducts for sperm transport must be patent; (4) the prostate and seminal vesicles must supply adequate amounts of seminal fluid; (5) the coital technique must enable the male partner to deposit his semen near the female's cervix; (6) the spermatozoa must be able to penetrate the cervical mucus and reach the uterine tubes; and (7) the spermatozoa must undergo capacitation and the acrosome reaction, fuse with the oolemma, and

be incorporated into the ooplasm. Any defect in this pathway can result in infertility.

Infertility is defined as the inability of a couple to achieve pregnancy despite unprotected intercourse for a period of more than 12 months. About 15% of all couples are infertile and it is estimated that a male factor plays a role in about half of the cases. In spite of this, the evaluation of the male partner is often neglected, mainly because of the high pregnancy rates that can be achieved by assisted reproductive techniques (ART). This practice is unfortunate since male infertility can often be cured, sparing the female partner the extensive treatment and cost of ART. Furthermore, evidence suggests that ART procedures can be associated with increased risks for

TABLE 23–3 Etiology of male infertility.

Pretesticular	Testicular	Posttesticular
Hypothalamic-pituitary disorders	Varicocele	Ductular obstruction, scarring
Panhypopituitarism	Trauma	Pelvic, retroperitoneal, inguinal, or scrotal surgery (eg, retroperitoneal lymphadenectomy, herniorrhaphy, Y-V plasty, transurethral resection of prostate, vasectomy)
Gonadotropin deficiency	Testicular torsion	
Isolated LH deficiency (fertile eunuch)	Orchiopexy	
Biologically inactive LH	Infection	Genital tract infections (eg, venereal disease, prostatitis, tuberculosis)
Combined LH and FSH deficiency (eg, Kallmann's syndrome)	Mumps orchitis	Cystic fibrosis
Prader-Willi syndrome	Drugs and toxins	Retrograde ejaculation (eg, diabetic autonomic neuropathy, postsurgical, medications)
Laurence-Moon-Biedl syndrome	Medications (eg, sulfasalazine, cimetidine, nitrofurantoin, cyclophosphamide, chlorambucil, vincristine, methotrexate, procarbazine)	Antibodies to sperm or seminal plasma
Cerebellar ataxia	Ingestants (eg, alcohol, marijuana)	Developmental abnormalities
Pituitary tumors (eg, prolactinoma)	Environmental exposures (eg, pesticides, radiation, thermal exposure)	Penile anatomic defects (eg, hypospadias, epispadias, chordee)
Systemic illness (eg, cirrhosis, uremia)	Chromosomal abnormalities (eg, Klinefelter's syndrome [XXY seminiferous tubule dysgenesis], Y chromosome microdeletions)	Congenital absence (bilateral or unilateral) of the vas deferens; bilateral ejaculatory duct obstruction; or bilateral obstructions within the epididymides—all associated with mutations in the cystic fibrosis transmembrane conductance regulator (CFTR) gene
Thyroid disorders (eg, hyperthyroidism, hypothyroidism)	Developmental abnormalities	
Adrenal disorders (eg, adrenal insufficiency, congenital adrenal hyperplasia)	Cryptorchidism	Androgen insensitivity (eg, androgen receptor deficiency, testicular feminization syndrome)
Drugs (eg, phenytoin, androgens)	Congenital absence of vas deferens, seminal vesicles	Poor coital technique
	Immotile cilia syndrome	Sexual dysfunction, impotence
	Bilateral anorchia (vanishing testes syndrome)	Idiopathic
	Leydig cell aplasia	
	Noonan's syndrome (male Turner's syndrome)	
	Myotonic dystrophy	
	Defective androgen biosynthesis (eg, 5α-reductase deficiency)	

Key: LH, luteinizing hormone.

both mother and child. Finally, neglecting to examine the infertile man properly risks overlooking serious conditions such as testicular cancer that may coexist with infertility.

Male infertility can be divided into pretesticular, testicular, and posttesticular forms. A comprehensive list of etiologies is noted in Table 23–3, genetic male infertility causes are listed in Table 23–4, and causes of testicular atrophy in Table 23–5.

A. Pretesticular Causes

The pretesticular causes of infertility are disorders of the hypothalamic-pituitary-gonadal axis. They can originate on either the hypothalamic level (gonadotropin-releasing hormone) or the pituitary level (luteinizing hormone and

FSH). These endocrinopathies are most often caused by mutations in genes involved in the biosynthesis of the hormones, growth factors or receptors, and associated signal transduction pathways. These endocrinopathies are collectively referred to as **hypogonadotropic hypogonadism** with low LH and FSH. These deficiencies result in a loss of intratesticular testosterone production and cessation of spermatogenesis.

Hypogonadotropic hypogonadism is an uncommon cause of male infertility but important to recognize, since replacement therapy can be initiated. The condition is characterized either by decreased output of gonadotropin-releasing hormone (GnRH), causing circulating levels of FSH and LH to diminish, or by rare disorders of the pituitary (with normal GnRH) that

TABLE 23–4 Chromosomal and genetic disorders causing male infertility.

Disorder	Cause of Infertility	Defect
Chromosomal		
Klinefelter's syndrome	Oligoazoospermia, hyalinization of seminiferous tubules	47,XXY or 46,XY/47,XXY mosaic karyotype
XX male syndrome	SCOS	46,XX SRY translocation to short arm of X
XYY male syndrome		47,XYY karyotype
Genetic		
Disorders of GnRH secretion		
Kallmann's syndrome		
GnRH receptor defects		
Prader-Willi syndrome	Decreased GnRH secretion	*KAL* gene mutation
Congenital adrenal hypoplasia	Defects in G protein coupled for GnRH	*GNRHR* gene mutation
		15q11q13 mutation
Idiopathic	Decreased GnRH secretion	*DAX1* gene mutation
hypogonadotropic	Decreased GnRH secretion	Prohormone convertase-1 (*PC1*) gene mutation
hypogonadism	Decreased GnRH secretion	
Disorders of androgen function	Excessive androgens inhibit pituitary secretion of gonadotropins	Steroidogenic enzyme mutations
Congenital adrenal hyperplasia		
Androgen insensitivity syndromes (Reifenstein's syndrome, testicular feminization, Lub's syndrome, Rosewater's syndrome)	Androgen insensitivity	AR gene mutation
Kennedy's syndrome		
5α-reductase deficiency		Expansion of polyglutamine tract in the AR transactivation domain
		5α-reductase gene mutations
Y chromosome microdeletions		
AZFa		*DBY*, *USP9Y* gene defect
Complete deletion	SCOS	
Partial deletion	Variable phenotype: ligozoospermia to SCOS	
AZFb		*RBMY1* gene defect
Complete deletion	Spermatogenic arrest	
Partial deletion	Variable phenotype: oligozoospermia to SCOS	
AZFc		*DAZ* gene defect
Complete or partial deletion	Variable phenotype: oligozoospermia to SCOS	
Yq complete deletion	Azoospermia	
Cystic fibrosis	Congenital absence of vas deferens	*CFTR* gene defect

Key: SCOS, Sertoli-cell–only syndrome; GnRH, gonadotropin-releasing hormone; AR, androgen receptor.

TABLE 23–5 Causes of testicular atrophy.

Trauma
Testicular torsion
Hypopituitarism
Cryptorchidism
Klinefelter's syndrome (47,XXY)
Alcoholism and cirrhosis
Infection (eg, mumps orchitis, gonococcal epididymitis)
Malnutrition and cachexia
Radiation
Obstruction to outflow of semen
Aging
Drugs (eg, estrogen therapy for prostatic cancer)

Modified, with permission, from Chandrasoma P, Taylor CR. *Concise Pathology*, 3rd ed. Originally published by Appleton & Lange. Copyright © 1998 by the McGraw-Hill Companies, Inc.

result in primary deficiencies of FSH and/or LH. These defects result in deficient androgen secretion and spermatogenesis.

Disorders resulting in abnormal synthesis and release of GnRH are most often caused by mutations, small deletions, or polymorphic expansions within genes involved in the endocrine or humoral regulation of sexual development and function. Disorders of GnRH synthesis and release can also be caused by hypothalamic tumors. Disorders without a known cause are termed idiopathic hypogonadotropic hypogonadism. Men suffering from GnRH deficiencies have firm prepubertal-sized testes and a small penis.

Kallmann's syndrome is caused by a deficiency in GnRH secretion from the hypothalamus due to mutation in the *KALIG-1* gene on Xp22.3. This gene codes for a protein necessary in olfactory and in GnRH axonal migration from the olfactory placode to the septal preoptic nuclei. Patients with Kallmann's syndrome are typically tall and anosmic, and often present with failure of pubertal initiation. Patients may also have congenital deafness, asymmetry of the cranium and face, cleft palate, cerebellar dysfunction, cryptorchidism, or renal abnormalities. Some men with Kallmann's syndrome suffer only from infertility due to an isolated gonadotropin deficiency and have no other phenotypic abnormalities.

Other causes of pubertal failure include mutations in the recently discovered hypothalamic kisspeptin peptide or its cognate receptor GPR54. This ligand/receptor pair has proven to be one of the key mediators of pubertal onset, with clinical implications for diagnosis and treatment of infertility and related disorders.

Mutations in *Dax1*, another X chromosome gene, cause hypogonadotropic hypogonadism in association with congeni-

tal adrenal hypoplasia. *Dax1* encodes an orphan nuclear hormone receptor that has a critical role in the development of the hypothalamus, pituitary, adrenal, and gonads and in the maintenance of testicular epithelial integrity and spermatogenesis.

GnRH receptor mutations are also associated with hypogonadotropic hypogonadism. The GnRH receptor is a G-protein–coupled receptor for the GnRH ligand. Patients with GnRH mutations have a spectrum of reproductive dysfunction from partial to complete hypogonadism.

The *PC1* or convertase-1 gene is believed to have a role in GnRH secretion and release of the precursor molecule in the hypothalamus; mutation of this gene causes hypogonadotropic hypogonadism in conjunction with obesity and diabetes mellitus.

Prader-Willi syndrome is caused either by mutations or deletions of a specific locus within paternal chromosome 15 or, less commonly, when maternal uniparental disomy (2 maternal copies) of this locus occur. The predominant features of this syndrome are obesity, mild or moderate mental retardation, and infantile hypotonia. Usually, hypogonadotropic hypogonadism is also present, compromising fertility.

Hemochromatosis is associated with treatable hypogonadotropic hypogonadism; some men with hemochromatosis develop primary testicular failure.

Genetic mutations can result in **biologically inactive LH or FSH** by altering FSH or LH structure or FSH or LH receptor activity. These abnormalities result in a spectrum of dysfunction from complete virilization failure to less severe hypogonadism.

Pituitary mass lesions are an uncommon, but recognized, cause of hypogonadotropic hypogonadism and male infertility. Such lesions interfere with the release of LH and FSH, either by direct compression of the portal system or by decreasing secretion of these gonadotropins.

In **hyperprolactinemia,** the elevated serum prolactin level causes hypogonadism because it interferes with the normal pulsatile release of GnRH. Adenomas of the pituitary can cause hyperprolactinemia, in combination with headaches and visual field impairment because of direct compression on the optic chiasm. Selective serotonin reuptake inhibitors can also cause hyperprolactinemia.

Spermatogenesis is dependent on a high androgen concentration. Genetic steroidogenic enzyme defects can cause failure of any one of the chemical conversions involved in the production of testosterone together with cortisol and aldosterone. This can lead to **congenital adrenal hyperplasia,** with impaired corticosteroid and androgenic steroid syntheses. The resulting androgen deficiency causes phenotypic abnormalities ranging from incomplete virilization to completely feminized genitalia and cryptorchid testes.

The androgen receptor (*AR*) gene is a nuclear steroid receptor (transcription factor) encoded by a single copy gene on the X chromosome. **Androgen insensitivity syndromes** result from abnormalities in this gene and are manifested by defects in AR structure and/or function. Mutations that completely disrupt AR function result in feminization of 46 XY individuals. In less severe cases, phenotypes range in a spectrum from simple male infertility to ambiguous genitalia and hypospadias. In severe cases, since a portion of testosterone is converted to estradiol by aromatization, estradiol levels are usually elevated and feminization occurs in a similar fashion to normal XX females at the time of puberty. An androgen receptor abnormality should be suspected in a patient with a family history of intersex disorders in one or more maternal uncles.

Anabolic steroid abuse results in negative feedback at the level of the hypothalamus and pituitary, and LH and FSH release is reduced. This in turn disables endogenous testosterone production and spermatogenesis since normal spermatogenesis requires both FSH and adequate intratesticular testosterone. Decreased testicular size and gynecomastia can also be seen in association with long-time anabolic steroid abuse. The extent and reversibility of these detrimental effects depend on dose and duration of use. Normal hormonal function usually returns after these agents are discontinued.

B. Testicular Causes

Overall, these conditions damage spermatogenic potential by direct effects on the testicles.

Varicoceles are considered the most common cause of subfertility in men. The term **varicocele** refers to abnormally dilated scrotal veins. A varicocele is present in about 15% of the normal male population, but in approximately 40% of men presenting with infertility.

Possible pathogenic mechanisms in varicocele formation include the anatomical configuration of the left internal spermatic vein, incompetent or absent valves, and potential for a partial left renal vein compression between the aorta and the superior mesenteric artery (the "nutcracker" phenomenon). An acute varicocele can also be caused by retroperitoneal malignancies with arteriovenous shunting into the venous system.

Varicoceles are associated with impaired spermatogenesis by one of several mechanisms: increased scrotal temperatures, alterations in testicular blood flow, reduced testicular size, overproduction of adrenal steroid metabolites, increased oxidative stress, which may damage cell membrane integrity or cause DNA damage, and alterations in the hypothalamic-pituitary-gonadal axis, leading to decreased serum testosterone levels. The pathophysiology of the impaired spermatogenesis is likely multifactorial in many cases.

Several studies have shown decreased semen quality and increased sperm DNA damage in varicocele patients compared to normal controls. However, the evidence for a clinical benefit of varicocele repair in improving fertility is not incontrovertible.

Genetic disorders are characterized as of entire chromosomes (abnormalities of the karyotype), as deletions of specific areas of chromosomes, or as specific mutations within genes. These disorders can alter spermatogenesis and impair normal development of the genital tract, thus decreasing fertilization capacity.

Chromosome defects are categorized as either numerical or structural. Numerical chromosome abnormalities include deletion or duplication of whole chromosomes. Structural chromosome abnormalities include deletion, inversion, or duplication of a portion of a chromosome, or translocation of part of one chromosome to another chromosome. Both autosomal and sex chromosomes may be affected. Such abnormalities occur with much greater frequency in infertile men than in the general population. About 1 in 20 infertile men has a chromosomal abnormality and most of these cases involve a sex chromosome. Usually these men are azoospermic or severely oligospermic.

Klinefelter's syndrome (47,XXY) is the most common chromosomal disorder associated with infertility. Patients with Klinefelter's syndrome are severely oligospermic or azoospermic. The phenotype of men with Klinefelter's syndrome varies but can include increased height, female hair distribution, gynecomastia, decreased level of intelligence, diabetes mellitus, obesity, increased incidence of leukemia and nonseminomatous extragonadal germ cell tumors, small firm testes, and infertility. Laboratory studies show increased serum FSH, normal or increased serum estradiol, and normal or low serum testosterone (with a tendency to decrease with age). Leydig cell function is commonly impaired in men with Klinefelter's syndrome. Patients with Klinefelter's syndrome who are mosaics with 46,XY/47,XXY have a less severe phenotype, including a variable presence of germ cells and sperm production.

There are other less common whole chromosome defects. Most patients with **mixed gonadal dysgenesis** have a mosaic karyotype of 45,X/46,XY, but others have a normal 46,XY. Affected individuals can have male, female, or ambiguous genitalia, streak gonads, or normal testes. The **XX male syndrome** (46,XX) is caused by translocation of the *SRY* sex-determination gene from the paternal Y chromosome to the paternal X of the offspring, resulting in "normal" development of testes in the XX fetus, but lack of all spermatogenic genes normally found on the Y chromosome. The **XYY male syndrome** (47,XYY) is characterized by decreased intelligence, antisocial behavior, an increased incidence of leukemia, and impairment of spermatogenesis.

Microdeletions of the Y chromosome have been shown to be of great importance in male infertility. The long arm of the Y chromosome contains genes that are critical for spermatogenesis (Figure 23–8). The genes most often causing defective spermatogenesis are found in the azoospermia factor region (AZF) where three nonoverlapping intervals (AZFa, AZFb, and AZFc) exist. Y chromosome microdeletions are detected by polymerase chain reaction–based mapping of molecular markers and genes. The most frequently deleted region is AZFc (approximately 60% of Y chromosome deletions), followed by AZFb (35%) and AZFa (5%). There can also be large deletions that span more than one region.

Microdeletions in the AZF region are responsible for azoospermia or severe oligozoospermia (sperm concentrations of less than 5 million/mL). Such AZF microdeletions are estimated to account for about 7–10% of male factor infertility. Affected men do not have other phenotypic abnormalities.

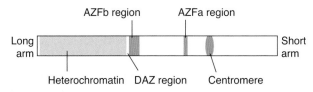

FIGURE 23–8 Diagrammatic representation of areas responsible for male infertility on long arm of Y chromosome (Yq). (Redrawn, with permission, from Iammarrone E et al. Male infertility. Best Pract Res Clin Obstet Gynaecol. 2003;17:211.)

Among men with microdeletions in the AZFc region of the Y chromosome, 70% still have sufficient sperm production to allow sperm extraction via testis biopsy. If spermatozoa are obtained from patients with the Y deletion, they are functionally competent to achieve fertilization in vitro, but transmit the deletion and associated infertility to any male offspring. Among men with microdeletions in the AZFb and AZFa regions, none have sperm on testicular biopsy.

Cryptorchidism is the term used if testicular descent does not proceed normally during development and the testis remains in the abdominal cavity or groin. The prevalence of cryptorchidism is approximately 3% in full-term newborns, but only 1–2% by age 6 months. About 85% of all cases of cryptorchidism are unilateral.

Failure of normal testicular descent can result in impaired spermatogenesis. About 50–70% of unilaterally cryptorchid men are oligospermic or azoospermic and almost 100% of bilaterally cryptorchid men are azoospermic.

Exposure to testicular toxins is clearly a significant cause of defects in spermatogenesis. Numerous substances and occupations have been implicated, but these potential gonadotoxins have been difficult to study because of inadequate study sample size and because of confounding factors that are difficult to control.

The different germ cell populations each display their own sensitivity to different toxins. Spermatogonia are located outside the blood-testis barrier and are exposed to any toxin entering the interstitial fluid. Conversely, spermatocytes and spermatids are located within the adluminal compartment and are, at least partly, protected by the blood-testis barrier. Injury to the Sertoli cells can impair spermatogenesis, whereas injury to the Leydig cells can cause disturbances in hormone balance. Toxins may also interfere with hormone balance by causing alterations in androgen or gonadotropin receptor binding, alterations in circulating gonadotropin levels, and alterations in the metabolism of androgens. The effects of gonadotoxins may be reversible if the offending agent is removed before azoospermia occurs.

Cigarette smoking has been associated with an overall reduction in semen quality, and specifically a reduction in sperm count and motility and an increase in abnormal forms. Cigarette smoking can also cause damage to sperm DNA. A meta-analysis of 21 studies of the effect of cigarette smoking on semen quality revealed that smoking lowered sperm con-

centration by 13–17% in 7 studies and no effect in 14 studies. However, it remains controversial whether smoking actually decreases male fertility rates.

Also controversial is whether second-hand smoke from a male partner can affect female fertility. There is, however, some evidence that maternal smoking may be related to decreased sperm counts in the offspring. Finally, the risk of developing erectile dysfunction is almost doubled for smokers compared to nonsmokers, and this can limit male fertility.

Testicular temperatures are approximately 2 °C below core body temperature and spermatogenesis is dependent on this cooler temperature. Factors such as clothing, lifestyle, season, and fever can cause increases in scrotal temperature. Increases in scrotal temperature reduce sperm quantity and quality.

Chemotherapy and radiation therapy, used in men with testicular cancer, Hodgkin's disease, or leukemia, are potent **gonadotoxins**. For example, both radiation therapy and chemotherapy can cause permanent damage to the germinal epithelium with variable recovery of spermatogenesis. Therefore, it is recommended that patients bank their semen before such therapy is initiated. Specimens with high sperm concentration and motility and low levels of DNA damage can be preserved in relatively large aliquots suitable for intrauterine insemination (IUI). If only a single specimen is available, this should be preserved in small aliquots and be used for in vitro fertilization (IVF) or intracytoplasmic sperm injection (ICSI).

If patients receiving chemotherapy remain azoospermic after recovery from their cancers, there is still a significant chance (41% in one study) that sperm can be obtained with testicular sperm extraction for IVF or ICSI.

Testicular or epididymal infections may lead to infertility. For example, although in children mumps is generally a self-limited disease, in postpubertal males, mumps may result in orchitis. Necrosis from acute swelling and increased intratesticular pressure can cause permanent testicular atrophy and infertility.

Epididymitis can lead to scarring of the tubules and obstruction of sperm flow.

Torsion of the spermatic cord with interruption of testicular blood flow results in acute, intense testicular pain. If untreated, the absence of blood flow after 4–6 hours of torsion causes irreparable damage. Torsion may also induce sperm autoimmunity due to a breakdown of the blood testis barrier during the ischemic event.

Testicular trauma can lead to scrotal or testicular edema, hematoma, hematocele, hydrocele, torsion, fracture, or rupture. These may result in testicular atrophy as well as the development of antisperm antibodies. In both testicular torsion and trauma, early surgery can result in testicular salvage. If an operation is performed in the initial 72 hours after injury, the testicle can be salvaged in up to 90% of patients.

C. Posttesticular Causes

Ductal obstruction can occur anywhere along the male reproductive system and results of semen analysis vary with the site of obstruction. Complete obstruction of the ejaculatory duct results in a low-volume, acidic, fructose-negative ejaculate. Obstruction of the vasa or epididymides results in a normal-volume, alkaline, fructose-positive ejaculate. Men with ductal obstruction as the only cause for their infertility have normal serum testosterone and FSH levels.

Obstruction is either congenital or acquired. Congenital causes include congenital atresia or stenosis of the ejaculatory ducts and utricular, or Müllerian and Wolffian duct cysts. Acquired vasal obstruction may be caused by inguinal or pelvic surgery, but is most commonly the result of a **vasectomy**. Epididymal obstruction may be caused by scrotal surgery and epididymitis. Epididymitis can result from a number of genitourinary infections, including the sexually transmitted diseases chlamydia and gonorrhea. Finally, **ejaculatory duct obstruction** may be due to genitourinary infections, pelvic surgery, urethral trauma, chronic prostatitis, and calcifications and cysts in the prostate or seminal vesicles.

Congenital bilateral absence of the vas deferens (CBAVD) is part of the phenotypic spectrum of cystic fibrosis (CF). CF is an autosomal recessive disease and about 1 in 25 Caucasians are carriers for it. Mutations of the cystic fibrosis transmembrane conductance regulator (*CFTR*) gene cause the disease; more than 500 such mutations have been identified. CBAVD occurs in 1–2% of infertile men, making it the most common congenital abnormality of the Wolffian duct system. While most patients with classic CF carry severe mutations on both CFTR gene loci, patients with CBAVD can have a severe mutation in only one CFTR gene coupled with a minor mutation in the other or minor mutations on both loci. Men with CBAVD also have hypoplastic, nonfunctional seminal vesicles and ejaculatory ducts, and epididymal remnants, frequently composed of only the caput regions that are firm and distended. Other manifestations of the disease of CF such as pulmonary, pancreatic, and gastrointestinal dysfunction are usually absent.

However, spermatogenesis is not impaired in these patients and they can undergo sperm-retrieval procedures and have their semen used in ART. To diminish the possibility of classic CF in the offspring, men with CBAVD and their wives should be screened for *CFTR* mutations and referred to genetic counseling before sperm retrieval and in vitro fertilization.

Men with idiopathic epididymal obstruction have also been found to have an increased incidence of CF mutations and probably simply represent a variant phenotype from the patient with classic CBAVD. These men should also undergo CF testing before epididymal sperm aspiration or reconstruction surgery. Finally, patients presenting with unilateral absence of the vas deferens are also considered at risk and should undergo analysis of the *CFTR* gene.

Ejaculatory duct obstruction is an uncommon cause of male infertility, representing about 1% of cases. Most cases are bilateral because of the close proximity of the ostia of both ejaculatory ducts anatomically. The condition may be congenital or acquired. Occasionally, congenital isolated ejaculatory duct obstruction may be associated with *CFTR* mutations, and genetic screening is appropriate. Acquired cases may be due to prostatic nodule formation or inspissated secretions in the ejaculatory ducts causing calculi. Utricular cysts may also obstruct the ejaculatory ducts.

Symptoms from ejaculatory duct obstruction include infertility, decreased ejaculate volume, reduced ejaculatory force, hematospermia, pain with ejaculation, and dysuria. Occasionally, patients with ejaculatory duct obstruction will have a palpable seminal vesicle or mass on rectal examination, or prostatic or epididymal tenderness, but usually they have normal physical examinations and normal hormonal profiles.

Clinically, ejaculatory duct obstruction must be considered in patients with azoospermia, low ejaculate volume, absence of fructose in the ejaculate, and normal serum gonadotropin and testosterone levels. Transrectal ultrasonography (TRUS) has also led to the identification of patients with seminal vesicle dilation or genitourinary cysts causing oligospermia or azoospermia, decreased motility, and reduced ejaculatory volume.

Partial obstruction of the ejaculatory duct has also been recognized. Affected patients have low-volume ejaculate and variable semen quality. Unfortunately, semen quality may worsen after attempting corrective surgery. Seminal vesicle aspiration after ejaculation may aid in diagnosing partial ejaculatory duct obstruction.

Immunologic infertility may result from a breach in the blood-testis barrier, exposing the mature spermatozoa to the immune system with the formation of antisperm antibodies. **Antisperm antibodies** may be present in the blood or in reproductive tract secretions. Risk factors for the formation of antisperm antibodies in men include trauma to the testes, epididymitis, congenital absence of the vas deferens, or vasectomy. It may also be caused by dysregulation of normal immunosuppressive activities within the male reproductive tract. Antisperm antibodies are found in 5–10% of infertile couples but are also present in 1–2.5% of fertile men. Antisperm antibodies react with all of the major regions of sperm and can impair sperm motility, sperm penetration through the cervical mucus, acrosome reaction, and sperm-oocyte interactions and fertilization.

High levels of circulating antisperm antibodies may reduce successful outcomes from treatment by intercourse, IUI, or IVF. However, if intracytoplasmic sperm injection (ICSI) is used in conjunction with IVF, antisperm antibodies do not have a negative effect on the outcome of the procedure.

Disorders of ejaculation are uncommon but important causes of male infertility. The disorders can be divided into premature ejaculation, anejaculation, and retrograde ejaculation.

Premature ejaculation is the inability to control ejaculation for a satisfactory length of time during intercourse. The condition has been reported to affect up to 31% of men 18 to 59 years of age. **Premature ejaculation** causes distress as a sexual dysfunction for both partners but seldom leads to infertility, as ejaculation usually occurs intravaginally.

Anejaculation describes the complete absence of seminal emission into the posterior urethra. True anejaculation is always connected with central or peripheral nervous system dysfunction or with drugs. Orgasm (climax) may or may not be achieved. **Spinal cord injury** is the most common neurological cause of anejaculation even though many men with spinal cord injury do have reflex erections and some capability for vaginal intercourse. Congenital spinal abnormalities, such as spina bifida, and other neurological conditions that affect spinal cord function or its sympathetic outflow (multiple sclerosis, transverse myelitis, and vascular spine injuries) can also impair ejaculation. These disorders resemble the spinal cord injury group in their dysfunction. Periaortic or pelvic surgery including retroperitoneal lymph node dissection can damage the nerves and cause ejaculatory dysfunction. Finally, men with diabetes mellitus are at risk for complications such as vasculopathy and neuropathy, which can affect ejaculatory function. Typically, men with diabetic neuropathy develop ejaculatory dysfunction in a slowly progressive fashion, going from a decreased amount of ejaculate to retrograde ejaculation to anejaculation. As with other long-term complications of diabetes, this condition is related to poor control of the patient's blood sugar. Several classes of drugs are also potentially responsible for anejaculation: alpha-adrenergic blockers, antipsychotics, and antidepressants. Anejaculation can also be psychogenic or idiopathic.

Retrograde ejaculation accounts for 0.3–2% of cases of male infertility. It is caused by a dysfunction in bladder neck closure that results in a total or partial absence of antegrade ejaculation. In this condition, with ejaculation, the ejaculate flows into the bladder, the path of least resistance. Since bladder neck closure is controlled by alpha-adrenergic neurons of the sympathetic nervous system, the condition can be caused by the same conditions as neurogenic anejaculation: retroperitoneal lymph node dissection, diabetes mellitus, Y-V plasty and other bladder neck surgery, transurethral resection of the prostate, and idiopathic. Drug causes included α_1-adrenoreceptor antagonists, antipsychotics, and antidepressants.

Retrograde ejaculation is diagnosed when, after absent or intermittent emission of ejaculate during ejaculation, sperm is found in the bladder urine, which may be cloudy. Patients experience a normal or decreased orgasm but may note a "dry" ejaculation.

Epididymitis refers to inflammation due most commonly to infection of epididymis arising from a sexually transmitted disease or a urinary tract infection. In men younger than 35 years, the most common sexually transmitted pathogens are *Chlamydia trachomatis* and *Neisseria gonorrhoeae*. In young children and in men older than 35 years, the most common urinary tract pathogen is *E coli*. Epididymitis in a child mandates exclusion of a urinary tract anomaly.

In the absence of ductal obstruction, however, the role of infection in causing infertility is controversial. Potential deleterious effects of infection on male fertility include decreased spermatogenesis, breaches in the blood-testis barrier leading to sperm autoimmunity, and seminal oxidative stress due to an increase in seminal fluid oxidant levels or a decrease in seminal fluid antioxidant levels.

D. Idiopathic Oligospermia

It appears that there is a genetic basis for male infertility, which is currently classified as idiopathic in many men (dis-

cussed later). However, despite advances in molecular diagnostics, the pathophysiology of spermatogenic failure in a majority of infertile men remains unknown. Assisted reproductive techniques are the best treatment option for patients with idiopathic oligospermia.

Pathology

Percutaneous or open testicular biopsy specimens may show any of several lesions involving the entire testes or only portions. The most common lesion is "**maturation arrest,**" defined as failure to complete spermatogenesis beyond a particular stage. There can be early- or late-arrest patterns, with cessation of development at either the primary spermatocyte or the spermatogonial stage of the spermatogenic cycle. The second most common and least severe lesion is "**hypospermatogenesis,**" in which all stages of spermatogenesis are present but there is a reduction in the number of germinal epithelial cells per seminiferous tubule. Peritubular fibrosis may be present. "**Germ cell aplasia**" is a more severe lesion characterized by complete absence of germ cells, with only Sertoli cells lining the seminiferous tubules (**Sertoli-cell–only** syndrome [SCOS]). The most severe lesion (eg, in Klinefelter's syndrome) is hyalinization, fibrosis, and sclerosis of the tubules. These findings usually indicate irreversible damage.

CHECKPOINT

9. What are the major categories of causes of male infertility? Name several specific causes in each category.

10. From the perspective of the male reproductive system, what are the steps that must occur for conception?

11. What is the value of testing for a CFTR mutation or Y-chromosome microdeletion?

12. What is the most common cause of obstructive azoospermia in the population?

Clinical Manifestations

A. Symptoms and Signs

A couple attempting to conceive should have an evaluation for infertility if pregnancy fails to occur within one year of regular unprotected intercourse. Evaluation should be done before one year if there are risk factors for infertility either in the male or in the female or if the couple is worried about infertility. Also, an evaluation can be initiated sooner if the couple has a good understanding of ovulation timing, and they have had more than simple random attempts at pregnancy. The reason for initiating an examination sooner rather than later is that the longer a couple remains subfertile, the less chance they have for an effective cure.

The evaluation should attempt to identify an underlying cause of the infertility in order to either initiate treatment or ART or to recommend donor insemination or adoption. The evaluation should also identify underlying pathology that requires medical attention. If the patient is to undergo ART, a genetic evaluation of the infertile man is important in order to avoid transferring possible abnormalities to the child.

The full evaluation of the infertile man should consist of a history, physical examination, and laboratory tests, including both semen analysis and endocrine evaluation.

History—This includes both a complete general medical history and a comprehensive reproductive evaluation.

In the reproductive evaluation, the duration of infertility and information on coital technique, frequency, and timing are assessed. Because sperm survival in the female reproductive tract is about 2–5 days, the most effective time of intercourse is in the 48 hours after the ovulation. Pregnancy rates are highest with daily intercourse around this time. The history should inquire about use of lubricants since many of these are spermicidal. The patient is also asked about general sexual function including erectile and ejaculatory function.

The evaluation must also include developmental history and childhood illnesses, including congenital abnormalities and pubertal development. Treatment for delayed puberty is obviously salient.

Information on systemic medical illnesses, prior surgeries, urogenital traumas, and genitourinary infections, including mumps orchitis should be noted. Respiratory problems are especially important, as there is a correlation between sinopulmonary conditions and infertility.

Past surgeries may impact fertility. Any pelvic surgery can interrupt the vas deferens or cause neurogenic erectile or ejaculatory dysfunction. Retroperitoneal surgery can impair seminal emission due to injury to the sympathetic nervous system. Hernia repair can cause an iatrogenic injury to the vas deferens.

Current, as well as past, medications should be listed. Of particular interest are antihypertensives, alpha blockers, antidepressants, and anabolic steroids such as testosterone and others contained in dietary supplements. Possible gonadotoxin exposure must be assessed. The patient should be asked specific questions regarding cigarette smoking, marijuana use, and excessive alcohol intake, which can all suppress spermatogenesis. The family history should include questions regarding reproduction, hypogonadism, cryptorchidism, congenital defects, and cystic fibrosis.

Physical Examination—The physical examination should include a general evaluation, but it should also focus on the secondary sex characteristics and genitalia.

Androgen status is evaluated by assessing the secondary sex characteristics, including body habitus, virilization, body hair, and gynecomastia. The penis should be examined to look for the location of the urethral meatus and penile curvature or angulation.

Examination of the genitalia includes palpation of the testes with the patient standing. Testicular size is measured (by means of calipers, orchidometer, or ultrasound). The normal adult testis is ovoid, measuring 4–5 cm in length and 2–3 cm in both transverse and anteroposterior dimensions, and has a mean volume of at least 20 mL. Small testes most likely indicate impaired spermatogenesis since the seminiferous tubules form over 90% of the testis. Abnormal testicular dimensions are present in about two-thirds of men with infertility. In men with severe spermatogenic defects, such as those with Klinefelter's syndrome or Y-chromosome microdeletions, the testicular size is that of a prepubertal male.

The examination should also identify the presence of a hydrocele, spermatocele, varicocele, or hernia. The vas deferens and epididymis should be examined for evidence of obstruction, manifested by induration and enlargement of these structures. Physical examination may reveal absence of the vas deferens and epididymis. Renal ultrasound should be performed on individuals with unilateral or bilateral vasal agenesis because these abnormalities can be associated with renal anomalies.

Varicocele examination should be done in a warm room to allow for complete relaxation of the scrotal wall. The patient needs to be examined standing at rest, and again with Valsalva maneuver. Approximately 90% of varicoceles are left sided. Varicoceles are graded from 1 to 3. With the patient standing, a grade 3 varicocele is readily visible; a grade 2 varicocele is palpable without employing the Valsalva maneuver; and a grade 1 varicocele is palpable only with the Valsalva maneuver. The patient should also be examined in the lying position, to ensure that the dilated veins collapse. If they remain dilated after assuming the recumbent position, there is a higher likelihood of retroperitoneal pathology as the source of the varicocele, and an imaging study is indicated. Also, a large difference in spermatic cord diameter between standing and recumbent positions may be an indication that a varicocele is present.

Semen Analysis—Semen collection should be done in a glass container since plastic may contain spermatocidal chemicals. The preferred method is by masturbation. Standard instructions for semen collection include a defined period of abstinence of 2–3 days. Longer periods of abstinence lead to decreased sperm motility, and shorter periods result in low semen volume and sperm concentration.

Semen analysis provides information on semen volume, and sperm concentration, motility, and morphology. This information helps to define the severity of the male factor in infertility in a couple. Semen analysis also includes examination of the spermatozoa and the seminal fluid. In normal men, the ejaculate volume is 1.5–5 mL, and the normal semen pH is slightly alkaline (range 7.2–8.0). The normal sperm parameters include sperm concentration $\geq$ 20 million sperm/mL, motility $\geq$ 50% motile sperm, and normal morphology $\geq$ 30%. Sperm motility is defined as the percentage of sperm moving in 10 random high-power fields. The quality of motile sperm can then be observed by the degree and pattern of forward progression displayed by the majority of motile spermatozoa. Sperm morphology is evaluated by Kruger's strict criteria, which divides sperm into normal and abnormal morphology on the basis of a normal range of >14%. Standard semen analysis criteria are shown in Table 23–6.

TABLE 23–6 Semen analysis: normal values and definitions.

Characteristic	Reference Standard
Ejaculate volume	> 2 mL
pH	7.2–7.8
Sperm concentration	≥ 20 million/mL
Sperm count	≥ 40 million/mL
Sperm motility	≥ 50% with normal motility
Sperm morphology	≥ 15%[1]–30% with normal forms

Term	Definition
Normospermia	Normal ejaculate (as defined by reference standards above)
Oligozoospermia	Sperm concentration < 20 million/mL
Asthenozoospermia	< 50% of spermatozoa with forward progression of < 25% with rapid progression
Azoospermia	No spermatozoa in ejaculate
Aspermia	No ejaculate

Data from World Health Organization. Reference values of semen variables. In: *WHO Laboratory Manual for the Examination of Human Semen and Sperm-Cervical Mucus Interaction*, 4th ed. Cambridge University Press, 1999.

[1]Strict criterion.

Semen analysis will diagnose 9 out of 10 men with reduced semen quality. However, because semen can vary over time and is often affected by exogenous factors, a single semen analysis has a low specificity. Therefore, two to three tests at least one month apart are recommended.

If sperm are absent in a routine semen analysis, the specimen should be centrifuged to assess for very low sperm numbers. The finding of any sperm rules out complete ductal obstruction or complete absence of spermatogenesis. If persistent low volume is seen, examination of the post-orgasm urine should be undertaken to exclude retrograde ejaculation.

Evidence of sperm agglutination should be noted; increased clumping is suggestive of inflammatory or immunologic processes. Testing for antisperm antibodies testing would be indicated in such cases.

About 25% of men with sperm concentrations below 12.5 million/mL can father a child through spontaneous conception; conversely, 10% of men with a normal female partner cannot contribute to pregnancy despite a sperm concentration of up to 25 million/mL. This indicates that a small proportion of men with normal semen parameters have dysfunctional sperm. In other words, the normal ranges for the semen analysis give an indication of a man's fertility, but its values are not absolute. In such men, a number of specialized tests can be used to provide a clue as to the reason for infertility.

Additional tests of the ejaculate can also be important. Absent or low-volume ejaculate suggests retrograde ejaculation, lack of emission, ejaculatory duct obstruction, hypogonadism, or CBAVD. With low semen volumes (< 1 mL) and azoospermia, the seminal pH and fructose content are determined. If both are low, it suggests agenesis, decreased function, or obstruction of the seminal vesicles.

Patients with partial ejaculatory duct obstruction often present with low-volume semen, oligoasthenospermia and poor forward progression of sperm (see the section on **Posttesticular causes**).

Endocrine Evaluation—An endocrine evaluation of the hypothalamic-pituitary-testicular axis should be performed if oligospermia or azoospermia is present. Spermatogenesis is evaluated by serum FSH and inhibin, while the Leydig cell function is evaluated by serum LH, testosterone, sex hormone–binding globulin (SHBG), and free testosterone. A single measurement is usually sufficient to determine a patient's clinical endocrine status even though gonadotropins are secreted in a pulsatile manner. The relationship of testosterone, LH, FSH, and prolactin helps to identify the clinical condition.

Men with azoospermia caused by nonexistent sperm production produce very low levels of inhibin, leading to high FSH levels. Normal FSH and inhibin levels in an azoospermic man suggest normal spermatogenesis with obstruction. In men with spermatogenic arrest, normal values of FSH and inhibin can be found, especially if maturation arrest is present, since there may be enough spermatogenic progress to allow inhibin secretion. A combination of both inhibin and FSH levels has been shown to have a better diagnostic value than either one alone.

Nonmeasurable levels of FSH and LH are found in patients with pituitary or hypothalamic hypogonadism and in patients with hCG-producing testicular tumors. They are also seen in patients with a history of anabolic steroid abuse, and these synthetic substances are not measurable by standard testosterone assays.

Combined elevation of FSH and LH levels is seen in association with severe testicular damage and reflects a decline in both Sertoli cell and Leydig cell function.

Men with clinical hypogonadotropic hypogonadism should have MRI of the pituitary gland and the hypothalamus to evaluate the possibility of a pituitary tumor. If the serum gonadotropin levels are low and the serum testosterone level is half the lower limit of normal, further evaluation of the remaining pituitary hormones should also be performed. This includes assessment of other pituitary–end-organ axes, to exclude panhypopituitarism. The thyroid axis is most commonly checked by obtaining serum thyroid-stimulating hormone (TSH) and free T_4 levels. A serum prolactin should be measured to exclude a prolactin-secreting adenoma. Finally, if the hypogonadotropic hypogonadism remains unexplained, serum iron, total iron-binding capacity, and ferritin levels should be performed to exclude hemochromatosis.

Fructose is produced in the seminal vesicles, and its absence in the semen implies obstruction of the ejaculatory ducts. This test is currently used sparingly, as more emphasis is placed on low semen volume as a screening test, and **transrectal ultrasound of the prostate** as a confirmatory test. Obstruction of the ejaculatory ducts is strongly suggested by a seminal vesicle anteroposterior diameter of ≥ 1.5 cm on ultrasound.

Leukospermia (excessive numbers of leukocytes in the semen) may adversely affect sperm movement and fertilization ability, perhaps because of excessive generation of reactive oxygen species by the leukocytes. Also, with active prostatic infection, swelling of the prostate can lead to a functional obstruction of the ejaculatory ducts. The finding of leukospermia should prompt further investigations to exclude a genital tract infection.

A variety of in vitro tests have been developed to assess sperm function in an attempt to explain previously hidden male factors in couples with unexplained infertility. These couples have significantly lower in vitro fertilization rates compared with those in whom simple uterine tubal problems can be identified. These tests are designed to uncover defects in sperm capacitation and motion, in binding to the zona pellucida, in acrosome reaction, and in ability to penetrate the oocyte. The in vitro **sperm mucus-penetration test** assesses the capacity of spermatozoa to move through a column of midcycle cervical mucus and aids in detection of impaired motility caused by antibodies.

In the optimized **sperm penetration assay,** the infertile man's sperm are placed in egg yolk buffer, cooled, and stored at cold temperature overnight, then subjected to rapid heating in the morning, and incubated with hamster oocytes that have had the zona pellucida removed enzymatically to allow penetration. Results are reported as either the percentage of ova that have been penetrated (normal is 100% of the oocytes penetrated) or as the number of sperm penetrations per ovum, termed the sperm capacitation index (normal is > 5).

The **hemizona assay** assesses the fertilizing capability of sperm using the zona pellucida from a nonfertilizable, nonliving human oocyte. The zona is divided in half. One half is incubated with the infertile man's sperm, and the other half is incubated with sperm from a known fertile donor. The number of sperm binding to the zona is compared and expressed as a ratio. However, a major problem with this assay is the limited availability of human ova. The identification of zona pellucida glycoprotein 3 (ZP3) as the primary determinant of sperm-zona binding has led to exploring use of recombinant human ZP3 rather than the zona itself for testing sperm-zona interactions.

High-resolution **transrectal US** can be used to evaluate the seminal vesicles for dysplasia or obstruction; the ejaculatory ducts for scarring, cysts, or calcifications; and the prostate for calcifications.

Internal spermatic venography is occasionally used to demonstrate testicular venous reflux in a man with a suspected varicocele when the physical examination is difficult or in a man with a suspected recurrence after surgical repair.

Testicular biopsy is useful in azoospermic men to distinguish intrinsic testicular abnormalities from ductal obstruction. Testicular biopsy can recover some spermatozoa for ICSI in nearly all men with azoospermia due to obstruction, and in 40–75% of men with nonobstructive azoospermia, depending on the reason for the poor production. The best yield of operative sperm retrieval is in men with hypospermatogenesis, followed by those with germinal aplasia (due to presence of patchy normal sperm production). The prognosis is worst in men with maturation arrest, in whom a probable genetic "block" of advanced sperm production is a likely cause.

A suggested algorithm for the evaluation and treatment of male infertility is shown in Figure 23–9.

BENIGN PROSTATIC HYPERPLASIA

Benign prostatic hyperplasia (BPH) is nonmalignant growth of the prostate stroma and epithelial glands that causes enlargement of the prostate gland. Growing slowly over decades, the gland can eventually reach up to 10 times the normal adult prostate size in severe cases. Benign prostatic hyperplasia is a common age-related disorder. Most men are asymptomatic, but clinical symptoms and signs occur in up to one third of men older than 65, and each year more than 400,000 men in the United States undergo TURP.

Etiology

The cause of benign prostatic hyperplasia is unknown. However, aging and hormonal factors are both clearly important. Age-related increases in prostate size are evident at autopsy, and the development of symptoms is age related. Data from autopsy studies show pathologic evidence of benign prostatic hyperplasia in less than 10% of men in their 30s, in 40% of men in their 50s, more than 70% of men in their 60s, and almost 90% of men in their 80s. Clinical symptoms of bladder outlet obstruction are seldom found in men younger than 40 years but are found in about one-third of men older than 65 years and in up to three-fourths of men at age 80 years. Prostatic androgen levels, particularly DHT levels, play an important role in development of the disorder. These factors are discussed next.

Pathology

The normal prostate is composed of both stromal (smooth muscle) and epithelial (glandular) elements. Each of these elements—alone or in combination—can cause hyperplastic nodules and ultimately the symptoms of benign prostatic hyperplasia. Pathologically, the hyperplastic gland is enlarged, with a firm, rubbery consistency. Although small nodules are often present throughout the gland, benign prostatic hyperplasia arises most commonly in the periurethral and transition zones of the gland (Figure 23–10). With advancing age, there

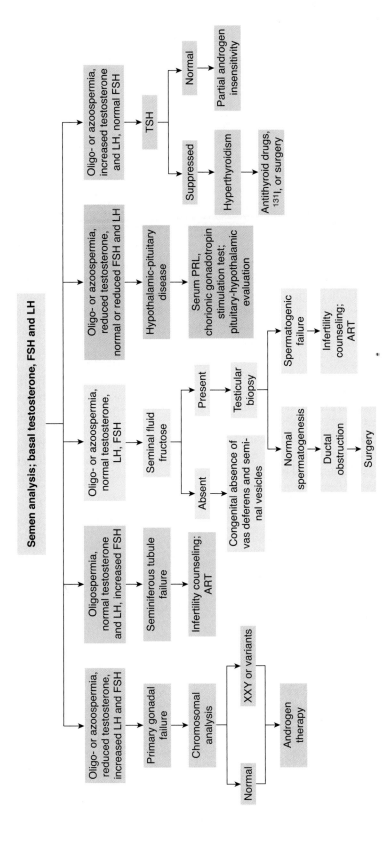

FIGURE 23–9   Approach to diagnosis of male infertility. ART, assisted reproductive technologies; FSH, follicle-stimulating hormone; LH, luteinizing hormone; TSH, thyroid-stimulating hormone; PRL, prolactin. (Redrawn, with permission, from Greenspan FS, Gardner DG [editors]. *Basic and Clinical Endocrinology,* 8th ed. McGraw Hill, 2007.)

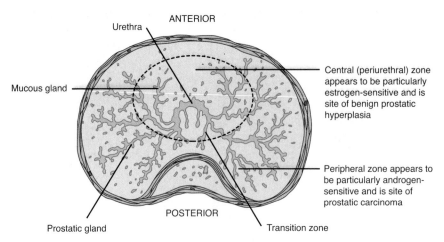

FIGURE 23–10   Structure of the prostate. (Redrawn, with permission, from Chandrasoma P, Taylor CE. *Concise Pathology*, 3rd ed. Originally published by Appleton & Lange. Copyright © 1998 by the McGraw-Hill Companies, Inc.)

is an increase in the overall size of the transition zone as well as an increase in the number—and later the size—of nodules. The urethra is compressed and has a slit-like appearance.

Histologically, benign prostatic hyperplasia is a true hyperplastic process because studies document an increase in prostatic cell number. The prostatic nodules are composed of both hyperplastic glands and hyperplastic stromal muscle. Most periurethral nodules are stromal in character, but transition zone nodules are most often glandular tissue. The glands become larger than normal, with stromal muscle between the proliferative glands. Perhaps as much as 40% of the hyperplastic prostate is smooth muscle. The cellular proliferation leads to a tight packing of glands within a given area. There is an increase in the height of the lining epithelium, and the epithelium often shows papillary projections (Figure 23–11). There is also some hypertrophy of individual epithelial cells.

In men with benign prostatic hyperplasia, the bladder shows both detrusor (bladder wall) smooth muscle hypertrophy and trabeculation associated with an increase in collagen deposition.

Pathogenesis

Although the actual cause of benign prostatic hyperplasia is undefined, several factors are known to be involved in the pathogenesis. These include age-related prostatic growth, prostatic capsule, androgenic hormones and their receptors, prostatic smooth muscle and adrenergic receptors, stromal-epithelial interactions and growth factors, and detrusor responses.

A. Age-Related Prostatic Growth

The size of the prostate does not always correlate with the degree of obstruction. The amount of periurethral and transition zone tissue may relate more to the degree of obstruction than the overall prostate size. However, the idea that the clinical symptoms of benign prostatic hyperplasia are due simply to a mass-related increase in urethral resistance is probably too sim-

plistic. Instead, some of its symptoms may be due to obstruction-induced detrusor dysfunction and neural alterations in the bladder and prostate. This has been demonstrated in men with lower urinary tract symptoms undergoing urodynamic testing, which measures perfusion pressure of the urethra.

B. Prostatic Capsule

The presence of a capsule around the prostate is thought to play a role in development of obstructive symptoms. Besides man, the dog is the only animal known to develop benign prostatic hyperplasia. However, the canine prostate lacks a capsule, and dogs do not develop obstructive symptoms. In men, the capsule presumably causes the "pressure" created by the expanded periurethral-transition zone tissue to be trans-

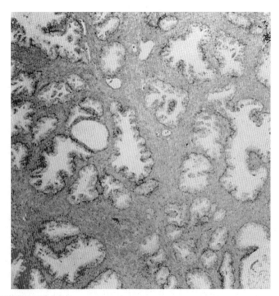

FIGURE 23–11   Benign prostatic hyperplasia. (Reproduced, with permission, from Chandrasoma P, Taylor CE. *Concise Pathology*, 3rd ed. Originally published by Appleton & Lange. Copyright © 1998 by the McGraw-Hill Companies, Inc.)

TABLE 23–7 Mechanisms and side effects of antiandrogenic treatment for benign prostatic hyperplasia.

Agent	Mechanism	Side Effects[1]
Androgen ablation		
GnRH agonists (eg, nafarelin, leuprolide, buserelin, goserelin)	Inhibits pituitary LH secretion, decreases T and DHT. Reduces prostate volume by ≈ 35%.	Hot flushes, loss of libido, impotence, gynecomastia.
True antiandrogens		
(eg, flutamide, bicalutamide)	Androgen receptor inhibition.	Gynecomastia or nipple tenderness, no significant incidence of impotence.
5α-Reductase inhibitors[2]		
(eg, finasteride, dutasteride)	Decreases DHT, no alteration in T or LH. Reduces prostate volume by ≈ 20%.	3% to 4% incidence of impotence and decreased libido.
Mixed mechanism of action		
Progestins (eg, megestrol acetate, hydroxyprogesterone caproate, medrogestone)	Inhibits pituitary LH secretion, decreases T and DHT, androgen receptor inhibition.	Loss of libido, impotence, heat intolerance.
Cyproterone acetate	Androgen receptor inhibition, inhibits pituitary LH secretion, variable decreases in T and DHT.	Loss of libido, impotence (variable).

Modified and reproduced, with permission, from McConnell JD. Benign prostatic hyperplasia: Hormonal treatment. Urol Clin North Am. 1995;22:387.

Key: GnRH, gonadotropin-releasing hormone; LH, luteinizing hormone; T, testosterone; DHT, dihydrotestosterone.

[1]Other than GI, hematologic, and CNS reactions.

[2]5α-Reductase: steroid-5α-reductase, α polypeptide 2 (3-oxo-5 α-steroid Δ4-dehydrogenase α) or SRD5A.

mitted to the urethra, leading to an increase in urethral resistance. Surgical incision of the prostatic capsule or removal of the obstructing portion of the prostate, whether by transurethral resection or by open prostatectomy, is effective in relieving symptoms.

C. Hormonal Regulation of Prostatic Growth

Development of benign prostatic hyperplasia requires testicular androgens as well as aging. There are several lines of evidence for this relationship. First, men who are castrated before puberty or who have disorders of impaired androgen production or action do not develop benign prostatic hyperplasia. Second, the prostate, unlike other androgen-dependent organs, maintains its ability to respond to androgens throughout life. Androgens are required for normal cell proliferation and differentiation in the prostate. They may also actively inhibit cell turnover and death. Finally, androgen deprivation at various levels of the hypothalamic-pituitary-testicular axis can reduce prostate size and improve obstructive symptoms (Table 23–7).

Although androgenic hormones are clearly required for the development of benign prostatic hyperplasia, testosterone is not the major androgen in the prostate. Instead, 80–90% of prostatic testosterone is converted to the more active metabolite DHT by the enzyme 5α-reductase. Two subtypes of 5α-reductase (type 1 and type 2) have been described. Both type 1 and type 2 isoenzymes are found in skin and liver, but only the type 2 isoenzyme is found in the fetal and adult urogenital tract, including both basal epithelial cells and stromal cells in the prostate. Two 5α-reductase inhibitor drugs are used clinically:

Finasteride inhibits only the type 2 isoenzyme, and dutasteride inhibits both the type 1 and 2 isoenzymes (see later). In the prostate, it appears that DHT synthesis largely depends on the type 2 enzyme and that, once it is synthesized, the DHT acts in a paracrine fashion on androgen-dependent epithelial cells. The nuclei of these cells contain large numbers of androgen receptors (Figure 23–12). DHT levels are the same in hyperplastic and normal glands. However, prostatic levels of DHT remain high with aging even though peripheral levels of testosterone decrease. These decreases in plasma androgen levels are further amplified by an age-related increase in the plasma SHBG level, resulting in relatively greater decreases in free testosterone than in total testosterone levels.

Suppression of androgens leads to reduction in prostate size and relief of symptoms of bladder outlet obstruction. True antiandrogens, which block the action of testosterone and DHT in the prostate, should be distinguished from agents that impair androgen production (Table 23–7). GnRH agonists work by paradoxically downregulating GnRH receptors in the pituitary, producing a transient increase and subsequent long-term reduction in concentrations of LH. A variety of antiandrogen treatment approaches have been used clinically, including GnRH agonists (nafarelin, leuprolide, buserelin), androgen receptor inhibitors (cyproterone acetate, flutamide), progestogens, and 5α-reductase inhibitors (finasteride, dutasteride) (Figure 23–13). Complete suppression of androgen action can lead to intolerable adverse effects, such as erectile dysfunction, flushing, and loss of libido. However, the 5α-reductase inhibitors finasteride and dutasteride suppress both

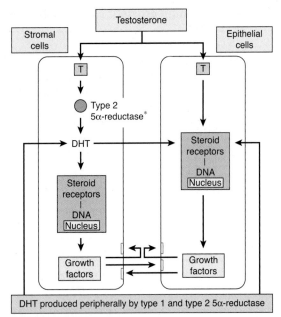

FIGURE 23–12 Mechanism of androgen action on prostatic stromal and epithelial cells. After testosterone (T) diffuses into the cell, it can interact directly with the androgen (steroid) receptors bound to the promoter region of androgen-related genes. In the stromal cell, a majority of T is converted into dihydrotestosterone (DHT), which acts in an autocrine fashion in the stromal cell and in a paracrine fashion after diffusing into nearby epithelial cells. DHT produced peripherally in skin and liver can also diffuse into the prostate and act in an endocrine fashion. *5α-Reductase: steroid-5α-reductase, α polypeptide 2 (3-oxo-5 α-steroid Δ4-dehydrogenase α) or SRD5A.

plasma and prostatic DHT levels by approximately 65–95%. Treatment with these agents has been shown to induce significant decreases in the size of the prostate as a whole and in the size of the periurethral zone. The 5α-reductase inhibitors must be given for at least 6–12 months to have beneficial

effects and must be continued indefinitely thereafter. Both GnRH agonists and 5α-reductase inhibitors have been shown to be effective in improving symptoms and urinary flow rates in patients with benign prostatic hyperplasia, particularly in men with larger (> 40 g) prostates. The 5α-reductase inhibitors are less effective than GnRH agonists in reducing the size of the prostate but cause fewer side effects. Because of the adverse side effects produced by total androgen deprivation with GnRH agonists, and because the 5α-reductase inhibitors are effective without these side effects, GnRH agonists have a minor role in the everyday treatment of symptoms from BPH.

Androgen receptor levels remain high with aging, thus maintaining the mechanism for androgen-dependent cell growth. Nuclear androgen receptor levels have been found to be higher in prostatic tissue from men with benign prostatic hyperplasia than in that from normal controls. The regulation of androgen receptor expression in benign prostatic hyperplasia is now being studied at the transcriptional level.

Finally, androgens are not the only important hormones contributing to the development of benign prostatic hyperplasia. Estrogens appear to be involved in induction of the androgen receptor. Serum estrogen levels increase in men with age, absolutely or relative to testosterone levels. Age-related increases in estrogens may thus increase androgen receptor expression in the prostate, leading to increases in cell growth (or decreases in cell death). Intraprostatic levels of estrogen are increased in men with benign prostatic hyperplasia. Patients with benign prostatic hyperplasia who have larger prostatic volumes tend to have higher plasma levels of estradiol. Studies of prostatic specimen tissue have documented an accumulation of DHT, estradiol, and estrone that correlates with patient age. The results show a dramatic increase of the estrogen-androgen ratio with increasing age, particularly in the stroma of prostatic tissue.

Investigations have suggested a role for estradiol in particular, demonstrating powerful cell-specific, nontranscriptional

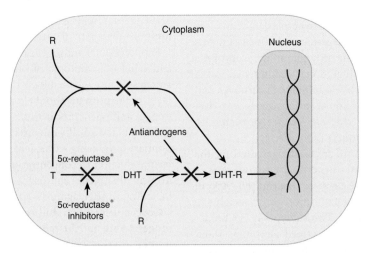

FIGURE 23–13 Site of action of antiandrogens and 5α-reductase inhibitors. X, site of blockade. *5α-Reductase: steroid-5α-reductase, α polypeptide 2 (3-oxo-5 α-steroid Δ4-dehydrogenase α) or SRD5A. (Redrawn, with permission, from Oesterling JE. Endocrine therapies for symptomatic benign prostatic hyperplasia. Urology. 1994;3[2 suppl]:7.)

effects of estradiol on the human prostate. Estradiol, acting in concert with SHBG, has been found to produce an eightfold increase in intracellular cAMP in hyperplastic prostatic tissue. This increase in cAMP does not occur with estrogens such as diethylstilbestrol, which do not bind to SHBG, and is not blocked by the antiestrogen tamoxifen. Both of these findings suggest that the classic estrogen receptor is not involved. On the other hand, DHT, which blocks the binding of estradiol to SHBG, completely negates the effect of estradiol on cAMP. Finally, the SHBG-estradiol-responsive second-messenger system has been primarily localized to the prostatic stromal cells and not to the epithelial cells.

Thus, estrogens may be causally linked to the onset of benign prostatic hyperplasia and may have an important supportive role in its maintenance. Aromatase inhibitors such as atamestane can produce marked reductions in both serum levels and intraprostatic concentrations of estrogens, including estradiol and estrone. However, to date, clinical trials with aromatase inhibitors for benign prostatic hyperplasia have been disappointing.

D. Growth Factors

Evidence suggests that prostatic growth is under the direct control of specific growth factors and only indirectly modulated by androgens. According to this evidence, growth factors from both the fibroblast growth factor (FGF) family and the transforming growth factor (TGF) "superfamily" act together to regulate growth. These growth factors are polypeptides that modulate cell proliferation. The FGF family stimulates cell division and growth: Basic fibroblast growth factor (bFGF) stimulates both growth of stroma and blood vessels (angiogenesis), and fibroblast growth factor 7 (FGF7; also known as keratinocyte growth factor [KGF]) stimulates growth of epithelial cells. On the other hand, members of the transforming growth factor-β (TGF-β) family inhibit cell division. TGF-β_1 primarily inhibits growth of stroma and TGF-β_2 growth of epithelial cells. In the normal prostate, the rate of cell death is equaled by the rate of cell production. It is hypothesized that a balance exists in the stroma between the stimulatory effects of bFGF and the inhibitory effects of TGF-β_1 and in the epithelial glands between FGF7 stimulation and TGF-β_2 inhibition. In benign prostatic hyperplasia, when excess growth of stroma predominates, bFGF is overproduced relative to its regulator TGF-β_1; when excess growth of epithelial glands occurs, FGF7 is overproduced relative to TGF-β_2.

Other growth factors, including epidermal growth factor and insulin-like growth factors (IGF-I and IGF-II), are also known to stimulate prostatic tissue growth. The IGF axis has been implicated in the pathogenesis of benign prostatic hyperplasia via the paracrine action of IGFs and IGF-binding proteins (IGFBPs). It is hypothesized that DHT may increase IGF-II activity, mainly in the periurethral region, which, in turn, induces benign proliferation of both epithelial and stromal cells, characteristic of benign prostatic hyperplasia. It is also hypothesized that, in normal prostatic stromal cells,

TGF-β_1 exerts its antiproliferative effects by stimulating the production of IGFBP-3, which acts as an inhibitory factor for cell growth, either indirectly, by inhibiting IGFs, or directly, by interacting with cells. In cells cultured from hyperplastic prostatic tissue, prostatic stromal cells have a reduced IGFBP-3 response to TGF-β_1 and demonstrate decreased TGF-β_1-induced growth inhibition relative to normal prostatic stromal cells. Growth factors undoubtedly also play a role in the development of bladder hypertrophy in response to outflow obstruction (see later). TGF-β is known to stimulate collagen synthesis and deposition in the bladder.

Targeting peptide growth factors offers a potential means of regulating prostatic enlargement and relieving symptoms associated with benign prostatic hyperplasia. Preliminary clinical trials of growth factor antagonists have led to significant improvements in urinary symptoms, maximal flow rates, and residual volumes.

E. Prostatic Smooth Muscle and Adrenergic Receptors

Prostatic smooth muscle represents a significant proportion of the gland. Urethral elasticity and the degree of bladder outlet obstruction are undoubtedly influenced by the relative content of smooth muscle within the prostate in patients with benign prostatic hyperplasia. Undoubtedly, both resting and dynamic prostatic smooth muscle tone play a major role in the pathophysiology of benign prostatic hyperplasia. Smooth muscle cells in the prostate—at the bladder neck and in the prostatic capsule—are richly populated with α-adrenergic receptors. Contraction of the prostate and bladder neck are mediated by α_1-adrenergic receptors. Stimulation of these receptors results in a dynamic increase in prostatic urethral resistance. Alpha$_1$-adrenergic receptor blockade clearly diminishes this response and has been found to improve symptoms, urinary flow rates, and residual urine volumes in patients with benign prostatic hyperplasia within 2–4 weeks after start of therapy. The selective α_1-blockers prazosin, terazosin, doxazosin, and alfuzosin have been extensively studied and found to be effective (Table 23–8).

TABLE 23–8 Alpha-receptor blockade for benign prostatic hyperplasia.

Agent	Site and Mechanism of Action	Side Effects
Phenoxybenzamine	Presynaptic and postsynaptic α_1, α_2 blockade	Hypotension
Prazosin	Postsynaptic α_1 blockade	Hypotension (especially postural hypotension leading to syncope)
Terazosin		
Doxazosin		
Alfuzosin		
Tamsulosin	Postsynaptic α_{1a}	

Because the bladder's smooth muscle cells do not contain a significant number of α_1 receptors, alpha-blocker therapy can selectively diminish urethral resistance without affecting detrusor smooth muscle contractility.

Studies have suggested that the α_1 receptors involved in the contraction of prostate smooth muscle appear to be α_{1a} receptors (previously called α_{1c} receptors). Clinical studies have established the efficacy of the subtype-selective α_{1a} antagonist, tamsulosin.

Contractile protein gene expression in stromal smooth muscle cells is significantly altered after alpha blockade. This suggests that alpha-blocking agents may work not only by the simple relaxation of muscle tone but also by affecting the phenotypic expression of contractile proteins in prostatic smooth muscle cells.

Alpha-blockers may also work by changing the balance between prostate cell growth and death. Some investigators hypothesize that benign prostatic hyperplasia occurs as a result of a decrease in apoptosis (programmed cell death), allowing more cells to accumulate in the prostate, hence causing its enlargement. The alpha-blockers doxazosin and terazosin have been shown to induce apoptosis in the stroma of the prostate.

F. Possible Mechanisms of Bladder Outlet Obstruction

There are several ways in which benign prostatic hyperplasia might cause obstruction of the bladder neck. The prominent median lobe may simply act as a ball valve, restriction may occur from the nondistensible capsule, static obstruction may result from the enlarged prostate surrounding the prostatic urethra, and dynamic obstruction may occur from inability to relax prostatic smooth muscle. In fact, clinical data support a role for each of these proposed factors. For example, TURP frequently relieves obstructive symptoms, as does simple surgical incision of the prostatic capsule. Medications that shrink the prostate or relax smooth muscle also relieve bladder outlet obstruction and increase urinary flow rates.

Various thermal therapies have been investigated as less invasive surgical procedures than TURP for benign prostatic hyperplasia, including transurethral microwave, high-intensity focused US, laser-delivered interstitial thermal therapies, and transurethral needle ablation of the prostate (TUNA). These procedures use different forms of energy such as microwave, US, laser, and radiofrequency to produce the thermal injury. It is unclear whether these procedures work by anatomic shrinkage or debulking of the obstructing enlarged prostate or by physiologic alteration of voiding function. In pathologic studies of TUNA, for example, coagulative necrosis gradually changes to retractile fibrous scar. This could cause a decrease in the volume of the treated area even without a significant decrease in prostatic volume. Alternatively, severe thermal damage to intraprostatic nerve fibers may reduce the dynamic component of the bladder outlet obstruction by denervation of receptors or sensory nerves.

G. Bladder Response to Obstruction

Many of the clinical symptoms of benign prostatic hyperplasia are related to obstruction-induced changes in bladder function rather than to outflow obstruction per se. Thus, one third of men continue to have significant voiding problems even after surgical relief of obstruction. Obstruction-induced changes in bladder function are of two basic types. First, there are changes that lead to **detrusor overactivity** (**instability**). These are clinically manifested by frequency and urgency. These two symptoms cause much of the distress related to BPH and are sometimes quite out of proportion to the degree of obstruction. Thus, treatment of the bladder overactivity may have more impact than treatment of the obstruction. Second, there are changes that lead to **decreased detrusor contractility.** These are clinically manifested by symptoms of decreased force of the urinary stream, hesitancy, intermittency, increased residual urine, and, in a minority of cases, **detrusor failure.**

The bladder's response to obstruction is largely adaptive (Figure 23–14). The initial response is the development of detrusor smooth muscle hypertrophy. It is hypothesized that this increase in muscle mass, although an adaptive response to increased intravesical pressure and one that maintains urinary outflow, is associated with significant intracellular and extracellular changes in smooth muscle cells that predispose to detrusor instability. In experimental animal models, unrelieved obstruction results in significant increases in detrusor extracellular matrix (collagen).

In addition to obstruction-induced changes in the smooth muscle cells and extracellular matrix of the bladder, there is increasing evidence that chronic obstruction in patients with untreated benign prostatic hyperplasia may alter neural responses as well, occasionally predisposing to detrusor failure.

Traditional therapies for symptoms associated with bladder obstruction have been directed toward relief of bladder outflow resistance. New treatments of obstructive detrusor instability have been suggested using drugs that are autonomically

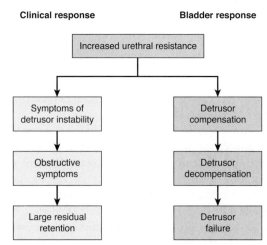

FIGURE 23–14 Schematic of natural history of benign prostatic hyperplasia. (Redrawn, with permission, from McConnell JD. The pathophysiology of benign prostatic hyperplasia. J Androl. 1991;11:356.)

active (such as α_1 antagonists) and drugs that stabilize muscle cell membranes (such as anticholinergic agents). In the past, anticholinergic drugs were avoided because of fear that inhibiting bladder activity would lead to acute urinary retention, but that fear has not been substantiated in recent studies.

The effects of chronic obstruction on the bladder are still not well understood. Future studies must examine the importance of changes in receptor density, affinity, and distribution as well as agonist release and degradation that occur during chronic obstruction and the ultrastructural and physiologic changes that occur with relief of obstruction.

Clinical Manifestations

A. Symptoms and Signs

Obstruction to urinary outflow and bladder dysfunction are responsible for the major symptoms and signs of benign prostatic hyperplasia. Prostatic enlargement may cause either acute or chronic urinary retention. With **acute urinary retention,** there is painful dilation of the bladder, with inability to void. Acute urinary retention is often precipitated by swelling of the prostate caused by infarction of a nodule or by certain medications. With **chronic urinary retention,** there are both obstructive and irritative voiding symptoms. Occasionally, a patient presents with marked urinary retention, yet few if any symptoms.

There are two types of symptoms: irritative, which are related to bladder filling, and obstructive, which are related to bladder emptying. **Irritative symptoms** occur as a consequence of bladder hypertrophy and dysfunction and include urinary frequency, nocturia, and urgency. The patient commonly complains of difficulty initiating urination and decreased flow, causing decreased caliber and force of the urinary stream. These observations may be more related to the bladder's response to the obstruction, rather than to direct effects of the obstruction itself. **Obstructive symptoms** result from distortion and narrowing of the bladder neck and prostatic urethra, leading to incomplete emptying of the bladder. Obstructive symptoms include difficulty initiating urination, decreased force and caliber of the urinary stream, intermittency of the urinary stream, urinary hesitancy, and dribbling.

To evaluate objectively the severity and complexity of symptoms in benign prostatic hyperplasia, a symptom index has been developed by the American Urologic Association. The self-administered questionnaire evaluates patient symptoms, such as bladder emptying, frequency, intermittency, urgency, and nocturia, and quality of life. The symptom index has been validated and found to have good test-retest reliability and to discriminate well between affected patients and controls. In clinical trials, there have been good correlations between urinary symptoms and the total score, and the instrument has proved useful to describe changes in symptoms over time and after treatment.

Complications of the chronic bladder dilation include hypertrophy of the bladder wall musculature and development of diverticula; urinary tract infection of the stagnant bladder urine; hematuria, particularly with infarction of a prostatic nodule; and chronic renal failure and azotemia from bilateral hydroureter and hydronephrosis. The most troublesome symptom that patients may experience from chronic bladder dilation is the inability to urinate on command. This can be treated by teaching the patient the technique of intermittent self-catheterization to empty the bladder about every 4 hours.

Digital rectal examination may reveal either focal or diffuse enlargement of the prostate. However, the size of the prostate as estimated by digital rectal examination does not correlate well with either the symptoms or signs of benign prostatic hyperplasia or the need for treatment. Examination of the lower abdomen may reveal a distended bladder, consistent with urinary retention, which may occur silently in the absence of severe symptoms.

B. Laboratory Tests and Evaluation

Laboratory tests performed to evaluate patients with benign prostatic hyperplasia include blood urea nitrogen and serum creatinine to exclude renal failure and urinalysis and urine culture to exclude urinary tract infection. Elevations of blood urea nitrogen (BUN) or serum creatinine from BPH occur only rarely. Intravenous pyelography (IVP) or US is usually not performed in patients with normal findings on these simple laboratory tests. Instead, it is generally reserved for patients with hematuria or suspected hydronephrosis. When an IVP or US is done in men with benign prostatic hyperplasia, it typically shows elevation of the bladder base by the enlarged prostate; trabeculation, thickening, and diverticula of the bladder wall; elevation of the ureters; and poor emptying of the bladder. Uncommonly, in a neglected patient, the IVP or US shows hydronephrosis, putting him at risk for acute kidney failure.

The most useful technique for assessing the significance of benign prostatic hyperplasia is urodynamic evaluation with uroflowmetry and cystometry. In these tests, the patient voids and various measurements are made. In uroflowmetry, the maximal urinary flow rate is recorded. If the peak flow rate is less than 10 mL/s, the patient is considered to have significant bladder outlet obstruction. However, the patient must void at least 150 mL for the measurement to be considered reliable. Pressure-flow studies are simultaneous recordings of urinary bladder pressure and urinary flow rates, which provide information about urethral resistance. These pressure flow studies can help in finding which patients are less likely to benefit from prostatic surgery by providing information on detrusor function. Cystourethroscopy is usually reserved for patients who have hematuria that remains unexplained despite an IVP or US or preoperatively for patients who require TURP. Validated symptom scores, estimation of prostate volume, and determination of serum prostate-specific antigen can help to predict the progression of benign prostatic hyperplasia. New ultrasound techniques also hold promise.

CHECKPOINT

13. Which is the major androgen controlling prostate size?
14. What are some of the different ways in which androgens can be suppressed to decrease prostate size and obtain at least temporary relief of obstructive symptoms?
15. What are the effects of antiestrogen treatment on males with benign prostatic hyperplasia?
16. What is the role of α_1-adrenergic receptors in benign prostatic hyperplasia?
17. What are some bladder changes that occur in patients with benign prostatic hyperplasia?
18. What are some symptoms and signs of benign prostatic hyperplasia?
19. How is the diagnosis of benign prostatic hyperplasia made?

CASE STUDIES

Eva M. Aagaard, MD, & Yeong Kwok, MD

(See Chapter 25, p. 710 for Answers)

CASE 105

A married couple presents to a primary care physician with a complaint of infertility. They have been trying to get pregnant for approximately 1 year. During that time they have had intercourse approximately three or four times a week without birth control. This is the woman's second marriage. She has a normal 3-year-old child from her prior marriage. The man has never had a child to his knowledge. He denies sexual dysfunction. He has had both gonorrhea and chlamydial infection in his early 20s, with one episode of prostatitis for which he was treated. His medical history is otherwise unremarkable. He takes no medications. He denies tobacco or drug use and drinks only rarely. On examination, his testes are approximately $4.5 \times 3 \times 2.5$ cm bilaterally. The epididymis is irregular to palpation bilaterally. There are no varicoceles or hernias. The vas deferens is present and without abnormality. The prostate is of normal size and without bogginess or tenderness. The penis is without fibrosis or angulation. The urethral meatus is appropriately situated.

Questions

A. What are the categories of male infertility? Give the major causes in each category.

B. What do you suspect is the likely cause of infertility in this patient? Why?

C. Given the likely diagnosis, what would you expect to find on semen analysis? Why? What would you expect the serum testosterone, LH, and FSH to be? Why?

D. What other tests may be helpful in confirming the diagnosis?

CASE 106

A 68-year-old man presents to the physician with a complaint of urinary frequency. He states that he has noted increased urgency and frequency for approximately 1 year, but his symptoms have become progressively worse. He states that currently he seems to have to urinate "all the time" and often feels as if he has not completely emptied his bladder. He must get up to urinate three or four times each night. In addition, in the last month, he sometimes has postvoid dribbling. He denies fevers, weight loss, or bone pain. His medical history is notable only for hypertension. His medications include atenolol and aspirin. The family history is negative for malignancy.

On examination, he appears healthy. His vital signs are notable for a blood pressure of 154/92 mm Hg. Prostate is diffusely enlarged without focal nodule or tenderness. Benign prostatic hyperplasia is suspected.

Questions

A. How would you make the diagnosis of benign prostatic hyperplasia?

B. What factors are known to be responsible for the pathogenesis of this disorder?

C. How would you classify this patient's symptoms? What is the mechanism by which benign prostatic hyperplasia causes these symptoms?

REFERENCES

General

Ganong WF. *Review of Medical Physiology,* 22nd ed. McGraw-Hill, 2005.

Kronenberg HM et al. *Williams Textbook of Endocrinology,* 11th ed. Saunders Elsevier, 2008.

Kumar V et al. *Robbins and Cotran Pathologic Basic of Disease,* 7th ed. Saunders Elsevier, 2005.

Lee DK et al. Endocrine mechanisms of disease. Expression and degradation of androgen receptor: Mechanism and clinical implication. J Clin Endocrinol Metab. 2003 Sep;88(9):4043–54. [PMID: 12970260]

Mruk DD et al. Sertoli–Sertoli and Sertoli–germ cell interactions and their significance in germ cell movement in the seminiferous epithelium during spermatogenesis. Endocr Rev. 2004 Oct;25(5):747–806. [PMID: 15466940]

Male Infertility

Beranova M et al. Prevalence, phenotypic spectrum, and modes of inheritance of gonadotropin-releasing hormone receptor mutations in idiopathic hypogonadotropic hypogonadism. J Clin Endocrinol Metab. 2001 Apr;86(4):1580–8. [PMID: 11297587]

Bhasin S. Approach to the infertile man. J Clin Endocrinol Metab. 2007 Jun;92(6):1995–2004. [PMID: 17554051]

Brugh VM III et al. Male factor infertility: Evaluation and management. Med Clin North Am. 2004 Mar;88(2):367–85. [PMID: 15049583]

Creasy DM. Pathogenesis of male reproductive toxicity. Toxicol Pathol. 2001 Jan-Feb;29(1):64–76. [PMID: 11215686]

Cuppens H et al. CFTR mutations and polymorphisms in male infertility. Int J Androl. 2004 Oct;27(5):251–6. [PMID: 15379964]

Guzick DS et al. National Cooperative Reproductive Medicine Network. Sperm morphology, motility, and concentration in fertile and infertile men. N Engl J Med. 2001 Nov 8;345(19):1388–93. [PMID: 11794171]

Jarow JP. Endocrine causes of male infertility. Urol Clin North Am. 2003 Feb;30(1):83–90. [PMID: 12580560]

Krausz C et al. Genetic risk factors in male infertility. Arch Androl. 2007 May-Jun;53(3):125–33. [PMID: 17612870]

Nudell DM et al. Common medications and drugs: How they affect male fertility. Urol Clin North Am. 2002 Nov;29(4):965–73. [PMID: 12516765]

Ohl DA et al. Anejaculation and retrograde ejaculation. Urol Clin North Am. 2008 May;35(2):211–20. [PMID: 18423241]

Sigman M et al. Male infertility. In: *Campbell-Walsh Urology,* 9th Ed. Wein AJ et al. (editors). Saunders, 2007.

Simoni M et al. EAA/EMQN best practice guidelines for molecular diagnosis of Y-chromosomal microdeletions. State of the art 2004. Int J Androl. 2004 Aug;27(4):240–9. [PMID: 15271204]

Skaletsky H et al. The male-specific region of the Y chromosome is a mosaic of discrete sequence classes. Nature. 2003 Jun 19;423(6942):825–37. [PMID: 12815422]

Benign Prostatic Hyperplasia

Cohen P et al. Transforming growth factor-beta induces growth inhibition and IGF-binding protein-3 production in prostatic stromal cells: Abnormalities in cells cultured from benign prostatic hyperplasia tissues. J Endocrinol. 2000 Feb;164(2):215–23. [PMID: 10657857]

Djavan B et al. The pathophysiology of benign prostatic hyperplasia. Drugs Today (Barc). 2002 Dec;38(12):867–76. [PMID: 12582474]

Eaton CL. Aetiology and pathogenesis of benign prostatic hyperplasia. Curr Opin Urol. 2003 Jan;13(1):7–10. [PMID: 12490809]

Foster CS. Pathology of benign prostatic hyperplasia. Prostate. 2000;9(Suppl):4–14. [PMID: 11056496]

Lam JS et al. Changing aspects in the evaluation and treatment of patients with benign prostatic hyperplasia. Med Clin North Am. 2004 Mar;88(2):281–308. [PMID: 15049579]

Lepor H. The pathophysiology of lower urinary tract symptoms in the ageing male population. Br J Urol. 1998 Mar;81 Suppl 1:29–33. [PMID: 9589015]

Lin VK et al. Alpha-blockade downregulates myosin heavy chain gene expression in human benign prostatic hyperplasia. Urology. 2001 Jan;57(1):170–5. [PMID: 11164176]

Roehrborn CG et al. Alpha$_1$-adrenergic receptors and their inhibitors in lower urinary tract symptoms and benign prostatic hyperplasia. J Urol. 2004 Mar;171(3):1029–35. [PMID: 14767264]

Rosenberg MT et al. A practical guide to the evaluation and treatment of male lower urinary tract symptoms in the primary care setting. Int J Clin Pract. 2007 Sep;61(9):1535–46. [PMID: 17627768]

Thorpe A et al. Benign prostatic hyperplasia. Lancet. 2003 Apr 19;361(9366):1359–67. [PMID: 12711484]

Inflammatory Rheumatic Diseases

24

Allan C. Gelber, MD, MPH, PhD,
Stuart M. Levine, MD, &
Antony Rosen, MB, ChB, BSc

The inflammatory rheumatic diseases form a group of disorders that are highly variable in their phenotypic expression. However, they have in common the presence of localized and/or systemic inflammation, which results in characteristic connective tissue and internal organ damage. Among these diseases, the specific clinical and pathologic features of each disorder likely reflect the initiating and propagating stimuli that determine the specific tissues targeted, and the inflammatory effector mechanisms that predominate.

Although the spectrum of inflammatory rheumatic diseases is broad, some general principles provide a framework within which to discuss the pathophysiology of all. One of the most useful constructs is a kinetic one, which focuses on disease initiation, propagation and flares, and it is useful for discussion of both acute and chronic diseases. Understanding the stimuli and mechanisms responsible for each of these phases among the different diseases permits a deeper insight into these fascinating and complex syndromes.

OVERVIEW OF INFLAMMATORY RHEUMATIC DISEASES

ACUTE DISEASES

The initiating force of acute diseases (eg, gout, immune complex vasculitis) is often exogenous and clearly recognizable (eg, crystal deposition, new medication, systemic bacterial, or viral infection). The disease is self-limited due to the success of the inflammatory response in removing the offending initiating stimulus (eg, crystals in gout; bacterial antigen or drug in immune complex vasculitis; Figure 24–1). Despite resolution of the acute episode, flares may occur on reexposure to the initiating stimulus.

CHRONIC DISEASES

The initiating force in chronic diseases (eg, systemic lupus erythematosus [SLE], rheumatoid arthritis) is often remote and

no longer recognizable once the unique disease phenotype becomes fully established and the diagnosis clear. Propagation of the disease typically occurs as a result of an autoimmune response, inducing a self-amplifying cycle of damage. Conditions leading to the initiation of chronic autoimmune diseases occur rarely, but once a disease is established flares are frequent. This circumstance probably reflects the abundant capacity of the immune system to "remember" previously encountered antigens and to respond to them with greater vigor when encountered again, even at lower concentrations (Figure 24–1).

Different tissues are affected in various diseases (eg, specific synovial joints in gout and rheumatoid arthritis; skin, joints, kidney, serosal surfaces, nervous system, and blood cell lines in SLE).

PATHOGENESIS OF INFLAMMATION

The nature of tissue damage and joint injury is determined in part by the inflammatory and immune effector functions that predominate. Additionally, the pathologic features of the

chronic inflammatory disorders reflect the combination of inflammatory damage and the consequences of healing.

Acute diseases

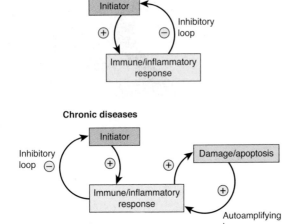

FIGURE 24–1   Kinetics of acute and chronic inflammatory rheumatic diseases.

ENDOTHELIAL ACTIVATION

Recruitment and activation of specific subsets of inflammatory and immune cells are essential determinants of the pathologic features. In this regard, the role of activation of regional blood vessel endothelium by proinflammatory cytokines (eg, tumor necrosis factor [TNF], interleukin [IL]-1) must be emphasized. Several cytokines induce the expression on endothelial cells of ligands for the adhesion-promoting receptors of inflammatory cells (integrins and selectins) and allow neutrophils and monocytes to adhere to the vessel wall in the inflamed area and migrate into the underlying tissues.

CYTOKINES

Distinct classes of immune effector function are activated depending on the pattern of cytokines that predominate during initiation of the inflammatory response. For example, some cytokines (eg, IL-12) produced by infected monocyte-macrophages skew the lymphocyte response toward T_H1 cells (which generate the T_H1 cytokines IL-2, interferon-γ, and TNF) that are associated with activation of macrophage killing functions and protection against invading intracellular pathogens. In contrast, the presence of IL-4 during the initial response induces the differentiation of T_H2 lymphocytes, which generate T_H2 cytokines (eg, IL-4, IL-5, IL-6, and IL-10). These cytokines have their predominant function in the activation of B cells and antibody generation. A new subset of helper T cells that develop in the presence of the cytokines TGF-β and IL-6 has recently been described. These cells are termed T_H17 cells because of their characteristic secretion of IL-17. They appear to be critically involved in granulocyte recruitment, protection against certain types of bacteria, and generation of chronic inflammation and autoimmunity.

Although significant overlap exists, specific pathologic features tend to accompany the different cytokine patterns (eg, granulomas for T_H1 versus immune complex disease for T_H2). In addition, significant recent data point to an important role for type I interferons (IFN-α and -β) in inducing novel pathways of monocyte differentiation in patients with SLE that enhance responses to self-antigens.

COMPLEMENT PATHWAY

The classical complement pathway is activated when antibody binds to its specific antigen. Activation of the complement cascade induces inflammatory cell recruitment and activation (with all the consequences mentioned later) as well as other features of the acute inflammatory response (eg, increased capillary permeability).

MYELOMONOCYTIC CELLS AND IMMUNE COMPLEX FORMATION

Although myelomonocytic cells (neutrophils and macrophages) have numerous effector pathways that function to rid the host of foreign invaders, some of these effector mechanisms can damage healthy tissue if released in large amounts. These include free radical species generated during the respiratory burst as well as a variety of secretory products contained in the granules of these inflammatory cells. Important granule contents include a variety of proteases such as cathepsins, elastase, and collagenase. These products are liberated into the extracellular medium in the inflammatory locus, where they accumulate and may have damaging effects on normal connective tissue. In addition, numerous proinflammatory mediators released in this environment (including TNF, IL-1, IL-6, prostaglandins, and leukotrienes) attract further inflammatory cells to the area and amplify the potential to generate tissue damage if the inflammatory response is not adequately quenched.

Numerous studies have emphasized the roles of the complement pathway and immunoglobulin Fc gamma receptors (FcγR) in the activation of myelomonocytic cell effector function that result in tissue damage. For example, Fc receptors play a critical role in generating the pathologic picture characteristic of immune complex–mediated diseases (see below). Clinical conditions in which this situation might arise include drug reactions, serum sickness, and infections (infective endocarditis, streptococcal skin and pharyngeal infections, and others). Autoimmune diseases are characteristically antigen driven, but in this case the humoral response is directed against self-antigens (eg, nucleosomes in SLE). Under conditions leading to the liberation of significant amounts of self-antigen from host tissue (cell damage or death), immune complex formation, Fc receptor binding, and complement activation may result.

The consequences of immune complex formation and deposition are similar whether caused by foreign antigens or self-antigens. Notably, immune complex–mediated renal disease and vasculitis that occur in several murine models of SLE are completely absent in the FcγR knockout mouse.

CELLULAR CYTOTOXICITY

Lymphocyte-Mediated Cytotoxicity

Certain T lymphocytes (ie, CD8+ T cells) are capable of killing target cells. When target cell destruction exceeds the capacity for renewal, impaired tissue function can result. As with other lymphocyte functions, this effector function is activated only on ligation of the T-cell receptor by a specific peptide (bound within the cleft of a major histocompatibility complex [MHC] molecule). On recognition of antigen on the surface of a target cell, cytotoxic T lymphocytes induce the death of those cells, using several distinct mechanisms. One prominent mechanism involves the Fas-Fas-ligand (FasL) pathway, whereby FasL present on activated lymphocytes binds to the Fas receptor on target cells and activates target cell apoptosis. The second prominent mechanism involves the release of cytotoxic T-lymphocyte secretory granules. These granules contain at least two distinct classes of proteins. One, called **perforin**, allows water, salt, and proteins (including the second class of granule protein, the granzymes) to enter the target cell cytoplasm through mechanisms that still remain unclear. The **granzymes,** a family comprising several proteases, target a number of critical cellular substrates and activate the process of apoptosis (programmed cell death) within the target cell.

Antibody-Dependent Cellular Cytotoxicity

The destruction of antibody-coated target cells by natural killer cells is called antibody-dependent cellular cytotoxicity (ADCC) and occurs when the Fc receptor of a natural killer (NK) cell binds to the Fc portion of the surface-bound anti-body. The cytotoxic mechanism involves the release of cytoplasmic granules containing perforin and granzymes into the cytoplasm of the antibody-coated cell (similar to cytotoxic T lymphocyte–mediated killing, described previously).

This mechanism has been implicated in autoantibody-mediated syndromes, in which the autoantigen resides at the cell surface or relocates to this site after an insult. An example of this is the photosensitive skin disease that occurs in patients with SLE who possess the Ro autoantibody. On exposure to ultraviolet light, the Ro antigen is released from keratinocytes and binds to their surface. Circulating Ro antibodies bind the antigen at this site, with induction of FcR-mediated effector pathways.

HOST TISSUE DIFFERENTIATION

In response to inflammatory mediators (including cytokines) and T cells, cells in tissues ordinarily unrelated to the immune response can alter their form and function to support (and in some cases drive) a chronic inflammatory response. This mechanism has been recently described in myositis (see below), where the inflammatory and autoimmune response is focused to areas of ongoing damage and regeneration.

CHECKPOINT

1. What is the hallmark of the rheumatic diseases?
2. What three kinetic features account for the specific clinical and pathologic characteristics of the different rheumatic diseases?
3. What six inflammatory effector mechanisms account for the inflammation seen in the rheumatic diseases? Give an example of a disease that illustrates each principle.

PATHOPHYSIOLOGY OF SELECTED RHEUMATIC DISEASES

GOUT

Clinical Presentation

Gout is the classic example of crystal-induced inflammation of synovial joints. It is a common condition, presenting in 1–4% of adult men. Deposition of monosodium urate crystals in the joint space leads to episodes of severe acute joint pain and swelling (particularly in the great toe, midfoot, ankle, and knee). These episodes tend to resolve completely and spontaneously within a week even in the absence of therapy. If not properly treated, however, this acute, self-limited form of the disease can evolve over many years into a chronic, destructive pattern resulting in more frequent and sustained periods of pain and resultant joint deformity. Accumulations of urate crystals elsewhere in the body can lead to subcutaneous deposits called tophi.

Etiology

The critical initiating factor in gout is the precipitation of monosodium urate crystals in synovial joints. This occurs when body fluids become supersaturated with uric acid (generally at serum levels > 7 mg/dL). Indeed, the degree of hyperuricemia correlates well with the development of gout, with annual incidence rates of about 5% for serum uric acid levels > 9 mg/dL. Increased levels of serum uric acid result either from underexcretion (90% of patients) or overproduction (10%) of

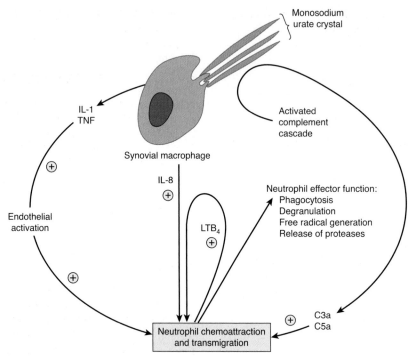

FIGURE 24–2   Mechanisms in initiation and amplification of the acute inflammatory response in gout involve both cytokines and humoral mediators.

uric acid. A decreased glomerular filtration rate is the most frequent cause of decreased excretion of uric acid and may be due to numerous causes (see Chapter 16). Diuretic administration is also a frequent cause of decreased excretion of uric acid. Overproduction defects can result from primary defects in the purine salvage pathway (eg, hypoxanthine phosphoribosyl transferase deficiency), leading to an increase in de novo purine synthesis and high flux through the purine breakdown pathway. Diseases causing increased cell turnover (eg, myeloproliferative disorders, psoriasis) and DNA degradation (eg, tumor lysis syndrome) are secondary causes of hyperuricemia.

Pathophysiology

Although the concentration of monosodium urate in joint fluid slowly equilibrates with that in the serum, formation of crystals is markedly influenced by physical factors such as temperature and blood flow. The propensity for gout to involve distal joints (eg, great toes and ankles), which are cooler than other body parts, probably reflects the presence of local physical conditions at these sites remote from the body core that favor crystal formation.

Monosodium urate crystals are not biologically inert. Their highly negatively charged surfaces function as efficient initiators of the acute inflammatory response. The crystals are potent activators of the classic complement pathway, generating complement cleavage products (eg, C3a, C5a) that are strong chemoattractants for neutrophil influx (Figure 24–2). The crystals also activate the kinin system and in that way induce local vasodilation, pain, and swelling. Phagocytosis of

crystals by synovial macrophages activates the inflammasome (a complex of proteins that sense certain intracellular stressors and activate IL-1 maturation) and stimulates the release of proinflammatory cytokines (eg, IL-1, TNF, IL-8, PGE$_2$). These products increase adhesion molecule expression on local vessel endothelium to facilitate neutrophil adhesion and migration and are also potent chemoattractants for neutrophils. Neutrophils also amplify their own recruitment by releasing leukotriene LTB$_4$ upon phagocytosis of urate crystals (Figure 24–2).

The intense inflammatory response in gout typically resolves spontaneously and completely over the course of several days, even without therapy. This down-modulation of the inflammatory response is a typical feature of acute inflammation, whereby the inflammatory response itself successfully removes the proinflammatory stimulus (Table 24–1). Numerous mechanisms appear to be responsible: (1) efficient phagocytosis of crystals, preventing activation of newly recruited inflammatory cells; (2) increased heat and fluid influx, altering local physical and chemical conditions to favor crystal solubilization; (3) coating of crystals with serum proteins, rendering the surface of the crystals less inflammatory; (4) secretion of a variety of anti-inflammatory cytokines (eg, TGF-β) by activated joint macrophages; and (5) phagocytosis of previously activated apoptotic neutrophils by macrophages in the joint, altering the balance of cytokines secreted by these macrophages in such a way that secretion of proinflammatory cytokines is inhibited while anti-inflammatory cytokine secretion is enhanced.

Thus, gout represents an excellent example of an acute inflammatory response initiated by a proinflammatory force.

TABLE 24–1 Mechanisms causing down-modulation of the inflammatory response in gout.

Efficient phagocytosis of crystals
Increased heat and fluid influx, favoring solubilization
Coating of crystals with serum proteins, shielding their pro-inflammatory surfaces
Secretion of anti-inflammatory cytokines (eg, TGF-β) by activated joint macrophages
Phagocytosis of apoptotic neutrophils, enhancing anti-inflammatory effects

The response is acute, highly focused, and self-limited rather than self-sustaining and associated with little tissue destruction in the acute phase. Flares of disease represent recurrence of crystals in a proinflammatory form in the joints. Myelomonocytic cells and humoral factors (eg, cytokines and the complement and kinin cascades) are critical mediators of the acute syndrome.

Clinical Manifestations

A. Podagra and Episodic Oligoarticular Arthritis

Podagra—severe inflammatory arthritis at the first metatarsophalangeal joint—is the most frequent manifestation of gout. Patients typically describe waking in the middle of the night with dramatic pain, redness, swelling, and warmth of the area. Flares of gout typically produce one of the most intense forms of inflammatory arthritis. The toes and, to a lesser extent, the midfoot, ankles and knees are the most common sites for gout flares. Gout flares frequently occur in circumstances that increase serum uric acid levels, such as metabolic stressors leading to increased DNA or adenosine triphosphate (ATP) turnover (eg, sepsis or surgery) or dehydration. Agents that reduce prostaglandin synthesis (eg, nonsteroidal anti-inflammatory drugs), reduce neutrophil migration into the joints (eg, colchicine), or decrease the activation of myelomonocytic cells (eg, corticosteroids) reduce the duration of a gouty flare.

Gouty arthritis can be diagnosed by examination of synovial fluid from an actively inflamed joint under a polarizing microscope. Monosodium urate crystals can be seen as negatively birefringent needle-like structures that extend across the diameter of and are engulfed by polymorphonuclear neutrophils.

B. Formation of Tophi

Firm, irregular subcutaneous deposits of monosodium urate crystals may occur in patients with chronic gout and are referred to as tophi. Tophi most often form along tendinous tissues on the extensor surfaces of joints and tendons as well as on the outer helix of the ear. Such tophi may extrude chalky material, containing urate crystals, onto the skin surface and can be viewed for diagnostic purposes under polarized microscopy.

C. Chronic Erosive Polyarthritis

In some patients, the total body burden of uric acid increases greatly over years; deposits of monosodium urate crystals occur at multiple joint sites. This may result in a persistent but more indolent inflammatory arthritis associated with remodeling of the thin synovial membrane into a thickened inflammatory tissue. Destructive and irreversible joint deformities resulting from bone and cartilage erosions often develop in this circumstance. Renal tubular injury and nephrolithiasis can also develop under these conditions.

Treatment

Therapy for acute gouty arthritis consists of agents that decrease inflammatory cell recruitment and activation to the involved joints. In contrast, prevention or prophylaxis of recurrent attacks of gouty arthritis requires chronic therapy to decrease serum uric acid levels into the normal range, where dissolution of crystals is favored. Several agents are available that can accomplish this purpose. These include uricosuric agents (eg, probenecid), which enhance excretion of uric acid into the urine, and allopurinol, which inhibits uric acid synthesis by inhibition of xanthine oxidase (a critical enzyme in the uric acid synthetic pathway). Xanthine oxidase inhibitors are conceptually appropriate for treatment of uric acid overproducers (10% of patients), and uricosuric agents for treating uric acid underexcretors (90% of patients). However, agents that decrease uric acid production can be used for therapy of hyperuricemia irrespective of cause and are often more convenient in terms of dosage regimens. Several newer recombinant molecule therapies, including an enzyme called uricase that directly breaks down uric acid, and a soluble IL-1 receptor antagonist, have shown promising early results in the treatment of refractory gout.

CHECKPOINT

4. What physical factors other than uric acid concentration influence crystal formation in gout?

5. What are some proinflammatory products released by synovial macrophages upon phagocytosis of urate crystals?

6. Suggest five reasons why the intense acute inflammatory response in gout typically resolves spontaneously over the course of several days even in the absence of therapy.

7. What are three metabolic conditions that can precipitate a gout flare?

8. Name three chronic sequelae of recurrent gout flares.

IMMUNE COMPLEX VASCULITIS

Clinical Presentation

Immune complex vasculitis is an acute inflammatory disease of small blood vessels that occurs in the setting of ongoing antigen load and an established humoral (antibody) immune response. Tissues affected include the skin (leukocytoclastic vasculitic rash), joints (inflammatory arthritis of small and medium-sized synovial joints), and kidney (immune complex–mediated glomerulonephritis).

Etiology

Antigens are frequently derived from exogenous sources, including infections (eg, streptococcal skin infections) and numerous drugs (especially antibiotics). An intense inflammatory response to such antigens accounts for one of the names ("hypersensitivity vasculitis") given to this disorder. Release of endogenous antigens in the setting of an autoimmune response (eg, SLE; see later discussion) may similarly initiate the vasculitic process.

Pathophysiology

Any antigen that elicits a humoral immune response may give rise to circulating immune complexes if the antigen remains present in abundant quantities once antibody is generated. Immune complexes are efficiently cleared in most circumstances by the reticuloendothelial system and are rarely pathogenic. Their pathogenic potential is realized when circulating immune complexes are deposited in the subendothelium, where they set in motion the complement cascade and activate myelomonocytic cells. The propensity for immune complexes to deposit is a function of the relative amounts of antigen and antibody and of the intrinsic features of the complex (ie, composition, size, and solubility). The solubility of immune complexes is not a fixed property, because it is profoundly influenced by the relative concentrations of antigen and antibody, which generally change as an immune response evolves. For physicochemical reasons, soluble immune complexes formed at slight antigen excess are not effectively cleared by the reticuloendothelial system and are of a size that allows them to gain access to and be deposited at subendothelial and extravascular sites (Figure 24–3). When antibody is present in excess, immune complexes are rapidly cleared by the reticuloendothelial system and deposition does not occur.

Thus, if foreign antigens (eg, drugs or infectious organisms) induce an antibody response in the setting of antigen excess, significant numbers of immune complexes of the appropriate size are formed and they may then be deposited in small vessels in various target organs (in skin, joints, kidney, blood vessel walls) where they activate several effector pathways (eg, FcR receptor, classic complement cascade) and where they may lead to the characteristic skin rashes (eg, palpable purpura), arthritis, and glomerulonephritis, which are the hallmarks of small-vessel vasculitis. As the immune response progresses and titers of specific antibody rise, or as the offending agent is removed, complexes are more effectively cleared, leading to resolution of the vasculitis.

A classic example of the altered pathogenicity of immune complexes at various antigen-antibody ratios is serum sickness. (Penicillin-induced hypersensitivity vasculitis represents a similar example.) When serum products from animals (eg, horses) are injected into humans for a therapeutic purpose (eg, as once was used for passive immunization against snake venom), the foreign serum proteins stimulate an immune response, with antibodies first appearing approximately 1 week after injection. Soon thereafter, immune complexes appear, followed by the development of fever, arthritis, rash, and glomerulonephritis, consistent with deposition of soluble immune complexes and myelomonocytic cell activation at multiple tissue sites. As the antibody titers rise, immune complexes are no

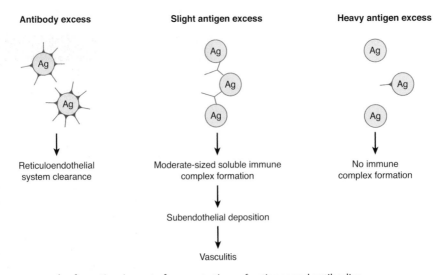

FIGURE 24–3   Immune complex formation. Impact of concentrations of antigens and antibodies.

longer formed at great antigen excess but approach the zone of equivalence and then the zone of antibody excess. The latter complexes are effectively cleared and thus lose their pathogenicity as the immune response evolves. Provided that antigen administration is not sustained, the inflammatory disease will resolve spontaneously as those immune complexes that were deposited early (during the soluble phase) are cleared. Such significant clinical effects of immune complexes usually occur only when the initial antigen load is great (eg, a large bacterial load or drug administration).

Clinical Manifestations of Immune Complex Vasculitis

Affected tissues are all highly enriched in small blood vessels, which are the target of injury in this syndrome.

A. Cutaneous Small-Vessel (Leukocytoclastic) Vasculitis

A common clinical presentation of immune complex–induced vasculitis in the skin is palpable purpura, which appears as red or violaceous papules. Cutaneous immune complex vasculitis seldom causes severe pain or tissue breakdown and only rarely leads to long-term injury (see Chapter 8).

B. Polyarthritis

The most common pattern of joint involvement with immune complex disease is that of a severe, rapid-onset and self-limited symmetric polyarthritis. As the immune complexes are phagocytosed and cleared, the immune response remits unless further waves of immune complexes are deposited.

C. Glomerulonephritis

Glomeruli are beds of small blood vessels in the kidney where immune complexes are likely to be deposited. Acute immune complex glomerulonephritis causes proteinuria, hematuria, and formation of red blood cell casts, due to disruption of the glomerular basement membrane caused by subendothelial complex deposition. In cases of extensive immune complex–mediated injury, immune complex vasculitis can cause oliguria and acute renal failure.

The most effective treatment for immune complex vasculitis is elimination of the inciting antigen (eg, by discontinuation of an offending drug). Medications that reduce the degree of activation of myelomonocytic cells (eg, corticosteroids) are also helpful.

Contrast between Immune Complex Vasculitis, Wegener's Granulomatosis, & Polyarteritis Nodosa

The vasculitides are a diverse group of inflammatory syndromes characterized by inflammatory destruction of blood vessels. However, not all forms of vasculitis are caused by im-

TABLE 24–2 Classification of vasculitic syndromes based on vessel size.

Vessel Size	Examples	Epidemiology and Demographics
Small vessel	Immune complex mediated; Henoch-Schönlein purpura	Common, evanescent. Predominantly in children, relatively common compared with other autoimmune conditions
Medium vessel	Polyarteritis nodosa	Rare; about 5 cases per million
Large vessel	Giant cell arteritis	Only in patients older than 50 years; about 100 cases per million

mune complex deposition. This fact is highlighted by the current classification system for the systemic vasculitides, which segregates diseases on the basis of the size of the blood vessel involved, by the presence of circulating autoantibodies, and by the histologic presence or absence of immune complexes (Table 24–2).

It is useful to contrast the clinical and pathophysiologic features of immune complex vasculitis (see prior discussion) with those of the "pauci-immune" vasculitic processes, which include Wegener's granulomatosis and polyarteritis nodosa. The clinical hallmarks of Wegener's granulomatosis include granulomatous inflammation of the upper airway (eg, sinusitis) and lower airway and lungs, as well as a necrotizing vasculitis involving the kidneys and many other organs. Although immune complex deposition is not a prominent feature in the pathophysiology of Wegener's granulomatosis, a specific group of antibodies highly specific to this disease may play an important propagating role. These "ANCA" antibodies [antineutrophil cytoplasmic antibodies], directed against components situated within neutrophil cytoplasmic granules, may bind to and activate neutrophils at the interface of the plasma and vessel wall and cause them to degranulate and damage the vascular wall at these sites.

In contrast, neither ANCA antibodies nor immune complex deposition plays a central role in the pathogenesis of polyarteritis nodosa, a vasculitis affecting medium-sized muscular arteries and arterioles. In this condition, the pathologic hallmark is an intense and destructive myelomonocytic cellular infiltrate in the blood vessel wall (called *fibrinoid necrosis*), leading to vessel occlusion, marked luminal narrowing and obsolescence. The dominant pathologic features of this disease, therefore, are organ and tissue dysfunction related to decreased perfusion and subsequent impaired oxygen delivery from severely damaged medium-sized vessels. Common manifestations of this condition include infarction of nerve trunks (eg, mononeuritis multiplex), bowel ischemia (eg, mesenteric insufficiency causing abdominal angina), kidney ischemia (eg, renal insufficiency), and deep cutaneous ulcerations. The different vasculitic syndromes, therefore, express unique phenotypes, clinical symptoms and signs, and pathologic features reflecting their distinct underlying pathophysiologic mechanisms.

SYSTEMIC LUPUS ERYTHEMATOSUS

Clinical Presentation

SLE is the prototypic systemic autoimmune rheumatic disease, characterized by chronic inflammatory injury to, and subsequent damage of, multiple organ systems. A key feature of this disease is the unique adaptive immune response, driven by antigens contained in self tissues, which is apparently responsible for much of the widespread pathologic consequences of the disease. Clinically, SLE is episodic in nature, with a course characterized by flares and remissions. It is also highly variable in severity, ranging from mild to life threatening. Tissues frequently affected include the skin, joints, kidneys, blood cell lines, serosal surfaces, and brain.

Epidemiology

The prevalence of SLE is approximately 30 cases per 100,000 in the general population in the United States. It occurs about nine times more frequently in women than in men and is most prevalent in blacks. Prevalence estimates rise to approximately 1 in 250 young African American women.

Etiology

SLE is a complex disease because of an interplay between inherited susceptibilities (more than 20 different genetic loci are implicated) and poorly defined environmental factors. Genetic deficiencies of the proximal components of the classic complement pathway (eg, C1q, C1r, C1s, C4), although rare in most populations, are the strongest known risk factors defined for the development of lupus. Studies have demonstrated that the classic complement pathway is required for the efficient noninflammatory clearance of apoptotic cells by macrophages. The development of lupus in individuals with these deficiencies may relate to impaired clearance of apoptotic cells

TABLE 24–3 Autoantigens in systemic lupus erythematosus.

Nuclear	Nucleosomes (dsDNA and histone core)
	Ribonucleoprotein complexes
	Sm
	nRNP
	Ro (60 kDa)
	La
Cytoplasmic	Ribosomal protein P
	Ro (52 kDa)
Membrane associated	Anionic phospholipids or phospholipid-binding proteins

in this setting, with proinflammatory consequences (see later discussion). The mechanisms whereby environmental factors (eg, drugs, viral infections) function to initiate or propagate SLE are not yet well understood.

Pathophysiology

It is useful to view the pathogenesis of SLE in discrete phases even though these phases are not clearly separable clinically. Indeed, it is likely that events underlying initiation occur before the onset of clinically defined disease, which requires chronic amplification of the propagation phase to become clinically apparent.

A. Initiation

The exuberant autoantibody response in lupus targets a highly specific group of self-antigens (Table 24–3). Although this group of autoantigens does not share common features (eg, structure, distribution, or function) in healthy cells, these molecules are unified during apoptotic cell death, when they become clustered and structurally modified in apoptotic surface blebs (Figure 24–4). Indeed, studies suggest that the initiating event in lupus is a unique form of apoptotic cell death that occurs in a proimmune context (eg, viral infection). Several environmental exposures have been persuasively associated with disease initiation in SLE. These include sunlight exposure (associated with both disease onset and flares), viral infection (Epstein-Barr virus exposure is strongly associated with SLE in children), and certain drugs. These are agents to which humans are commonly exposed, suggesting that those individuals who develop SLE have underlying abnormalities that render them particularly susceptible to disease initiation.

A critical susceptibility defect for the development and propagation of SLE appears to be impairment of normal clearance of apoptotic cells in tissues. Thus, in normal individuals, the fate of most apoptotic cells is rapid and efficient phagocytosis by macrophages, and antigens ingested in this way are

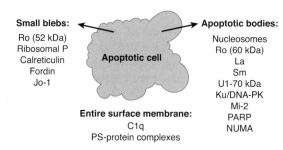

Small blebs:
Ro (52 kDa)
Ribosomal P
Calreticulin
Fordin
Jo-1

Apoptotic cell

Apoptotic bodies:
Nucleosomes
Ro (60 kDa)
La
Sm
U1-70 kDa
Ku/DNA-PK
Mi-2
PARP
NUMA

Entire surface membrane:
C1q
PS-protein complexes

FIGURE 24–4 Although sharing no features in healthy cells, autoantigens become unified in apoptotic cells. Here, they become clustered at the surface of the apoptotic cells, and this structure is modified.

rapidly degraded. Furthermore, phagocytosis of apoptotic cells inhibits secretion of proinflammatory cytokines from macrophages and induces secretion of several anti-inflammatory cytokines, contributing to the impaired ability of apoptotic cells to initiate a primary immune response. Last, the avid phagocytosis of apoptotic cells by normal macrophages prevents significant numbers from accessing dendritic cell populations, which are highly efficient initiators of primary immune responses. Together, these factors ensure that normal individuals do not efficiently immunize themselves with apoptotic material derived from their own tissues. In contrast, impaired clearance of apoptotic cells is observed in a subgroup of patients with SLE. Under conditions in which apoptotic material is not efficiently cleared by macrophages (eg, in C1q deficiency), suprathreshold amounts of this material may gain access to potent antigen-presenting cell populations under proimmune conditions and initiate a response to molecules whose structure has been modified during delayed apoptotic cell death.

B. Propagation

Autoantibodies in lupus can cause tissue injury by a variety of mechanisms:

1. The most common pathogenic mechanism is generation and deposition of immune complexes, in which antigen is derived from damaged and dying cells. When the concentration and size of the relevant complexes favor subendothelial deposition, these markedly proinflammatory complexes initiate inflammatory effector functions that result in tissue damage (see prior discussion). Of particular importance is the ability of immune complexes to ligate the Fcγ receptor, which activates myelomonocytic cell effector functions. The deposition of immune complexes in the kidney, joints, and skin underlies several of the central clinical features of SLE.

2. Autoantibodies bind to extracellular molecules in the target organs and activate inflammatory effector functions at that site, with consequent tissue damage. Examples of this phenomenon include autoimmune hemolytic anemia and thrombocytopenia as well as the photosensitive skin disease of the neonatal lupus syndrome (see later discussion).

3. Autoantibodies directly induce cell death by ligating cell surface molecules or by penetrating into living cells and exerting functional effects.

It is important to note that the intracellular antigens that drive the immune response in SLE can be derived from damaged or apoptotic cells. Such damage or apoptosis occurs commonly in the course of immune effector pathways. Thus, these effector pathways can generate additional antigen, further stimulating the immune system and generating still more antigen. This autoamplification is a central feature of the propagation phase of lupus.

Type I interferons have recently been shown to play a central role in amplification pathways in SLE, with clear evidence of increased type I interferon activity during active disease. Type I interferons induce the differentiation of monocytes into potent antigen-presenting dendritic cells. Additionally, type I interferons enhance signaling through toll-like receptors (TLRs), specifically increasing the pro-inflammatory signaling of SLE antigens containing nucleic acids through TLR 3, 7, and 9. Additionally, type I interferons sensitize target cells to death through various inflammatory effector pathways, increasing the antigen load presented to the immune system.

C. Flares

One of the characteristic features of an immune response is the establishment of immunologic memory, so that when the organism again encounters the antigen the immune system responds more rapidly and vigorously to lower concentrations than were required to elicit the primary response. Flares in SLE appear to reflect immunologic memory, occurring in response to rechallenge of the primed immune system with antigen. Apoptosis not only occurs during cell development and homeostasis (particularly of hematopoietic and epithelial cells) but also in many disease states. Thus, numerous stimuli (eg, ultraviolet light exposure, viral infection, endometrial and breast epithelial involution) may conceivably provoke disease flares.

Clinical Manifestations

SLE is a multisystem autoimmune disease that affects predominantly women during the childbearing years (mean age at diagnosis is 30 years). It is characterized clinically by periodicity, and the numerous exacerbations that occur over the years are termed flares. The symptoms are highly variable but tend to be stereotyped in a given individual (ie, the prominent clinical features often remain constant over years). Production of specific autoantibodies is a universal feature. Several organ systems are frequently affected. Prominent among these is the skin, in which photosensitivity and a variety of SLE-specific skin rashes (including a rash over the malar region, discoid pigmentary changes to the external ear, and erythema over the dorsum of fingers) are common. Like those who have other immune complex–mediated diseases, patients with SLE may manifest a nonerosive symmetric polyarthritis. Renal disease, which takes the form of a spectrum of glomerulonephritides, is a frequent major cause of morbidity and mortality. Patients may manifest a variety of hematologic symptoms (including hemolytic anemia, thrombocytopenia, and leukopenia), inflammation of serosal surfaces (including pleuritic and pericarditic chest pain), as well as several neurologic syndromes (eg, seizures, organic brain syndrome).

An intriguing neonatal SLE syndrome occurs in the offspring of mothers who have antibodies directed against the Ro, La, or U1-RNP proteins. In this condition, passive transfer of maternal autoantibodies across the placenta results in congenital heart block and photosensitivity in the neonate as a result of antibody-associated destruction of developing tissues such as cardiac conduction system and skin cells that transiently express these antigens.

SJÖGREN'S SYNDROME

Clinical Presentation

Sjögren's syndrome is a prevalent and slowly progressive autoimmune rheumatic disorder in which the exocrine glands are the primary target tissue. Affected individuals frequently manifest intense dryness of their eyes (xerophthalmia) and mouth (xerostomia), giving rise to the alternate name keratoconjunctivitis sicca. Histologically, an intense mononuclear inflammatory infiltrate is observed in affected lacrimal and salivary glands. Like other autoimmune rheumatic diseases, prominent polyclonal hypergammaglobulinemia and high-titer levels of characteristic autoantibodies are frequent features of the syndrome.

Epidemiology

Sjögren's syndrome occurs in approximately 1–3% of the adult population. As with SLE, the prevalence is about nine times more frequent in women than men. The prototypic affected individual is a woman in the fourth or fifth decade of life. Sjögren's syndrome occurs as both a primary disorder and as a secondary process, in the context of another well-defined autoimmune rheumatic disorder (especially SLE and rheumatoid arthritis).

Etiology

Viruses have been implicated in the development of Sjögren's syndrome but conclusive data are lacking. Epithelial cells in salivary glands can be infected by a number of viral pathogens (including Epstein-Barr virus, cytomegalovirus, hepatitis C, HIV, and coxsackievirus). In an autoimmune mouse model, CMV infection leads to initial infection of salivary glands, followed later by autoimmune salivary gland inflammation. Whether a similar process occurs during initiation of the human disease is not yet known.

Pathophysiology

Although the cause of Sjögren's syndrome remains unclear, several pathways have been implicated in pathogenesis. Central among these is autoimmunity to epithelial tissues, with an immune response directed against several ubiquitously expressed antigens (eg, Fodrin, Ro, and La) as well as to some antigens expressed specifically in secretory epithelial cells (eg, type 3 muscarinic acetylcholine receptors [M3R]). The antibodies to M3R are believed to prevent stimulated secretion of saliva and tears and may be important generators of the hyposecretion that characterizes the disease. In addition, exocrine tissues are also infiltrated with activated cytotoxic lymphocytes, which induce death of duct and acinar epithelium, with progressive loss of functioning salivary tissue. The enrichment of HLA-DR3 in patients with Sjögren's syndrome may reflect the enhanced ability of these molecules to present peptides contained within the pathogenic autoantigens.

Clinical Manifestations

The most prominent presenting symptoms in Sjögren's syndrome are ocular and oral dryness. Intense xerophthalmia (ocular dryness) may express itself as eye irritation, with a foreign body sensation or with pain. Such impairment in tear production heightens the risk for corneal ulcer or perforation.

Impaired production of saliva, at rest and with stimulation when eating, contributes to the prominent symptom of xerostomia (dry mouth). Affected persons often relate difficulty in swallowing dry foods or in speaking at length. An altered sensation of taste or of oral burning may occur. Characteristically, individuals affected by Sjögren's syndrome are susceptible to new-onset and severe dental caries at the gum line in mid-adult life. This reflects the loss of the essential antibacterial functions of saliva, with consequent excessive concentration of bacteria at dental surfaces.

Other epithelial surfaces may be similarly affected by diminished secretions and contribute to dryness. For example, patients may complain of skin and vaginal dryness. Dryness in the respiratory tract may give rise to hoarseness and recurrent bronchitis. (It is noteworthy that when immune activation is severe, patients experience systemic symptoms, including fatigue, arthralgia, myalgia, and low-grade fever.) Other potentially affected organ systems include the kidneys, lungs, joints, and liver (resulting in interstitial nephritis, interstitial pneumonitis, nonerosive polyarthritis, and intrahepatic bile duct inflammation). As many as half of the affected individuals experience autoimmune thyroid disease. Those patients with particularly severe disease are at increased risk for cutaneous vasculitis (including palpable purpura and skin ulceration) and lymphoproliferative disorders.

Treatment

Current therapy is aimed primarily at symptomatic improvement. Available agents include artificial tears, which serve as topical lubricants to aid with eye dryness. Maintaining oral hydration, with access to a regular supply of beverages, is encouraged. Use of sugar-free gum and lozenges may stimulate salivary flow. More recently, new cholinergic agonists have come to market aimed at improving oral hydration by stimulating increased salivary production, via muscarinic receptors, in affected submandibular salivary glands. Effective anti-inflammatory and immunosuppressive treatment for Sjögren's syndrome has not yet been found, indicating that the components of the critical amplification loops have not yet been discovered. For those affected by severe disease sequelae (including systemic vasculitis and mononeuritis multiplex), administration of systemic immunosuppression is necessary.

INFLAMMATORY MYOSITIS

Clinical Presentation

The inflammatory myopathies—polymyositis and dermatomyositis—are characterized by the gradual development of progressive motor weakness affecting the arms and legs, as well as the trunk, in association with histologic evidence of muscle inflammation. While such inflammation predominantly involves striated muscle, it is important to recognize that smooth muscle and even cardiac muscle may similarly, though less commonly, be affected. Often, the afflicted patient experiences increasing difficulty when rising from a seated position, in getting out of bed, or in ascending a flight of stairs. It may become increasingly difficult to reach up and lift dishes from an upper shelf or to even brush one's hair.

At the most severe end of the disease spectrum, affected persons may develop profound impairment in swallowing solid foods and in full lung expansion, arising from pathologic involvement of visceral muscle affecting the esophageal and diaphragmatic muscle tissues, respectively. These disease manifestations may result in nasal regurgitation of swallowed liquid beverages and in profound respiratory compromise. There is also a predilection for extramuscular involvement to occur, including of the lung parenchyma (interstitial pulmonary fibrosis) and peripheral joints (inflammatory polyarthritis), and in those with dermatomyositis, mild, moderate, or even severe inflammation of the integument. At the same time, diplopia (double vision, resulting from a paretic ocular muscle) is distinctly uncommon in these two myositis disorders.

Epidemiology

The inflammatory myopathies are relatively rare disorders. Polymyositis has been estimated to occur with an annual incidence rate of approximately 5 cases per million. Women are affected twice as often as men. Interestingly, dermatomyositis has a bimodal distribution in terms of age at onset; the first peak occurs in childhood, and the second peak occurs in mid and late adult life. Of note, polymyositis may clearly occur as a primary disorder in and of itself. However, the polymyositis phenotype may also occur as a secondary process, but when present in the context of another well-defined autoimmune rheumatic disorder, such as systemic lupus erythematosus, it is otherwise clinically and histologically indistinguishable.

Etiology

Autoantibodies are present in approximately 60% of all patients with an inflammatory myositis. Two best examples are both anti Jo-1 antibodies (that target histidyl tRNA synthetase), which are found in approximately 20% of all patients with myositis and in approximately 70% of patients with a myositis/interstitial lung disease overlap syndrome, and anti-Mi-2 antibodies (that target CHD4, a DNA binding protein), which are specific to dermatomyositis. Since both nuclear and cytoplasmic antigens are targeted for an immune response in these diseases, both antinuclear antibodies (ANA) and anticytoplasmic antibodies (ANCA) can be found.

Recent studies suggest that one source of these autoantigens is the regenerating muscle cell itself, which expresses higher levels of myositis autoantigens than its normal counterpart. Some tumor cells also express these same antigens at high levels. An intriguing pathophysiologic hypothesis is that the immune response that targets similar antigens in both tumor and inflamed muscle cells might be responsible for the link between inflammatory myositis and malignancy.

Pathophysiology

Polymyositis and dermatomyositis share several similar pathologic features but possess distinct ones as well. These include patchy involvement, presence of inflammatory infiltrates, and areas of muscle damage and regeneration. In polymyositis, inflammation is located around individual muscle fibers ("perimysial"), and the infiltrate is T-cell (CD8+>CD4+) and macrophage predominant. It has been suggested that the inflammation seen in polymyositis is driven by autoantigens expressed in the muscle environment, given the restricted T-cell repertoire in both circulating and muscle-infiltrating lymphocytes. Proinflammatory cytokines may induce a striking upregulation of MHC class I molecules seen on affected muscle cells but not adjacent normal myocytes. This MHC class I upregulation may lead to muscle damage through antigen-specific interactions with infiltrating CD8+ T cells, or through indirect mechanisms, by triggering a cell-damaging unfolded protein response ("UPR" or "ER stress") in the muscle itself. Further damage occurs when infiltrating T cells degranulate and release perforin and proteolytic granzymes at specific sites of contact within the affected muscle.

In dermatomyositis, the pathology looks quite different, although the outcome—profound muscle weakness—is the same. The major pathologic hallmarks of this condition include atrophy at the periphery of muscle bundles ("perifascicular atrophy"), and a predominantly B-cell and CD4+ T-cell infiltrate localized to the perifascicular space and surrounding capillaries (which are reduced in number). Activation of the complement cascade is seen as well. Major involvement of the capillaries has led many experts to suggest that the primary disorder in dermatomyositis is a small-vessel vasculitis, with myositis occurring later as a result of tissue ischemia and repair. The characteristic skin and nailfold capillary changes seen in patients with dermatomyositis lend support to this notion.

Clinical Manifestations

The inflammatory myopathies characteristically begin over a number of weeks to a few months. The hallmark symptom of both polymyositis and dermatomyositis is weakness. This characteristically involves the upper and lower extremities and is predominantly proximal rather than distal in location. While muscle pain or myalgia may be present, weakness is the predominant symptom. Routine daily activities that one might otherwise take for granted can become quite a chore, or even an impossible ordeal, to perform. Examples include standing up from a chair or toilet seat. In addition, the cutaneous features of dermatomyositis can be quite debilitating and include a painful, burning sensation of affected skin, as well as skin cracking and even breakdown with open ulceration.

There are four characteristic criteria for the diagnosis of polymyositis, which are: (1) weakness, (2) elevated laboratory parameters of muscle tissue (eg, creatine phosphokinase or aldolase), (3) an irritable electromyogram upon electrodiagnostic evaluation (producing sharp waves, spontaneous discharges), and (4) an inflammatory infiltrate upon histologic evaluation. In patients with dermatomyositis, a fifth criterion is a characteristic skin rash. Erythematous and/or violaceous discoloration may occur periorbitally or in a V-neck distribution on the trunk. These prototypic skin changes are termed periorbital heliotrope and shawl signs, respectively. Erythematous scaly eruptions may also occur over the extensor surface of the metacarpophalangeal (MCP) and proximal interphalangeal (PIP) joints and are termed Gottron's sign. Extensive sheets of muscle and soft tissue calcification may occur in children beset with dermatomyositis. Though recent efforts to modify the original diagnostic criteria, by integration of newer imaging modalities, including magnetic resonance imaging, or use of newer autoantibodies with specificities for the inflammatory myopathies have been proposed, the original criteria remain the foundation for these two muscle disorders.

An important additional clinical feature of the inflammatory myopathies has been the finding of an association with cancer in multiple demographic groups and among diverse populations. In adult patients, the new diagnosis of an inflammatory myopathy not infrequently heralds the co-occurrence or subsequent development within 1–5 years of a malignancy. The veracity of this observation has been confirmed in several population-based studies that link the diagnoses of dermatomyositis and polymyositis with cancer in cancer registries. A diagnosis of dermatomyositis carries a 2-fold greater risk of incident malignancy, particularly stomach, lung, breast, colon, and ovarian cancers.

Treatment

Corticosteroids are the front-line therapy for the inflammatory myopathies and are often required in high doses, for an ex-

tended period of time, to bring the marked inflammation in affected muscle tissues under control and to restore the patient's full functional capacity. Therefore, careful review of the clinical and histologic evidence supporting the diagnosis of an inflammatory myopathy is indicated in order to be confident that the potential drug-associated toxicity to which the patient is being exposed is warranted. In addition, the clinician also must recognize that a subset of treatment-refractory patients with presumed polymyositis may in fact be cases of a toxic myopathy (ie, related to the use of colchicines or a statin) or be attributable to a different myopathy (eg, inclusion body myositis). Second-line immunosuppressive agents integrated into treatment algorithms for the inflammatory myopathies include methotrexate, mycophenolate mofetil, intravenous immunoglobulin, and rituximab.

RHEUMATOID ARTHRITIS

Clinical Presentation

Rheumatoid arthritis is a chronic systemic inflammatory disease characterized by persistent symmetric inflammation of multiple peripheral joints. It is one of the most common inflammatory rheumatic diseases and is characterized by the development of a chronic inflammatory proliferation of the synovial linings of diarthrodial joints, which leads to aggressive cartilage destruction and progressive bony erosions. Untreated, rheumatoid arthritis often leads to progressive joint destruction, disability, and premature death.

Epidemiology

The prevalence of rheumatoid arthritis in the United States is approximately 1% in the general population; similar prevalence rates have been observed worldwide. The disorder occurs approximately three times more frequently in women than in men and has its peak onset in the fifth to sixth decade of life.

Etiology

Like SLE, rheumatoid arthritis is a systemic autoimmune disease in which abnormal activation of B cells, T cells, and innate immune effectors occurs. In contrast to SLE, the majority of inflammatory activity in rheumatoid arthritis occurs in the joint synovium. Although the cause of rheumatoid arthritis is unknown, a complex set of genetic and environmental factors appears to contribute to disease susceptibility. Because the incidence of rheumatoid arthritis has been observed to be similar in many cultures and geographic regions across the globe, it is assumed that the environmental exposures that provoke rheumatoid arthritis must be widely distributed. Early rheumatoid arthritis is closely mimicked by transient inflammatory arthritis provoked by several microbial pathogens. Thus, although a role for infection in the development of rheumatoid arthritis has long been postulated, it is not yet satisfactorily proven. Specific class II MHC alleles (HLA-DR4), sharing a consensus QKRAA motif in the peptide-binding groove, have been highly related to disease susceptibility and to greater severity of rheumatoid arthritis.

Pathophysiology

Much of the pathologic damage that characterizes rheumatoid arthritis is centered around the synovial linings of joints. Normal synovium is composed of a thin cellular lining (one to three cell layers thick) and an underlying interstitium, which contains blood vessels but few cells. The synovium normally provides nutrients and lubrication to adjacent articular cartilage. Rheumatoid arthritis synovium, in contrast, is markedly abnormal, with a greatly expanded lining layer (8–10 cells thick) composed of activated cells and a highly inflammatory interstitium replete with B cells, T cells, and macrophages and vascular changes (including thrombosis and neovascularization). At sites where synovium and articular cartilage are contiguous, rheumatoid arthritis synovial tissue (called pannus) invades and destroys adjacent cartilage and bone.

Although the causes of rheumatoid arthritis remain unclear, several important components of pathogenesis have been identified. As discussed previously, it is useful to separate the initiating and propagating phases of the disease and to recognize that the established rheumatoid arthritis phenotype reflects a self-sustaining and amplified inflammatory state.

A. Genetic Factors

Concordance rates in twins vary between 15% and 35%, implicating genetic factors in the pathogenesis of rheumatoid arthritis. The most striking of these genetic factors defined to date involves a specific subset of MHC class II alleles whose presence appears to predominantly determine disease severity (patients homozygous for disease-associated alleles have the most severe disease). These MHC molecules function as antigen-presenting scaffolds, which present peptides to CD4 T cells. Disease-associated alleles (belonging to HLA-DR4/DR1 serotypes) share a sequence along their antigen-presenting groove, termed the "shared epitope." It has been postulated that these alleles present critical antigens to the T cells, which play a role in initiating and driving progression of this disease. However, no specific antigens have yet been identified. Recent high-throughput genomewide genetic association studies have identified several new genetic risk factors for the development of RA. These genes (ie, *PADI4*, *PTPN22*, *CTLA4*, *STAT4*, and others) are involved in generating and propagating inflammatory responses and possibly autoantibody production as well.

B. Nongenetic Factors

1. **Environmental and infectious factors**—Although numerous bacterial and viral pathogens have been investigated as perhaps having a role in the initiation of rheumatoid arthritis, scrutiny has failed to identify a role for any specific infectious cause. It is conceivable that any of several different infectious agents might be able to induce non-pathogen-specific changes in the joint that are associated with disease initiation in susceptible individuals.

2. **Autoimmunity**—There is significant evidence supporting a role for autoimmunity in generating the rheumatoid arthritis phenotype, including the presence of antigen-driven autoantibodies such as IgG rheumatoid factors and anti-cyclic citrullinated peptide (anti-CCP) antibodies. Anti-CCP antibodies, in particular, are highly specific for RA and, as with the autoantibodies seen in SLE, can appear several years prior to the onset of disease. They appear to be a marker of a more destructive and aggressive RA phenotype, and their titers may be modulated by disease activity. The reasons these citrullinated peptides are targeted in RA are unknown, but potential explanations include an increase in a member of the peptidyl arginine deiminase family of enzymes (PADI, the enzymes that mediate the conversion of arginine to citrulline) activity in synovial tissue or altered activity of these enzymes due to genetic polymorphisms.

Cytokine elaboration in rheumatoid arthritis is markedly T_H1 biased. Although the cytokine profile in rheumatoid arthritis synovium is highly complex, with numerous proinflammatory and anti-inflammatory cytokines expressed simultaneously (eg, TNF, IL-1, IL-6, granulocyte-macrophage colony-stimulating factor [GM-CSF]), studies have persuasively demonstrated that TNF is an important upstream principle in the propagation of the rheumatoid arthritis inflammatory lesion (see later). Thus, when pathways downstream of TNF are inhibited with soluble TNF receptors or monoclonal antibodies to TNF, a rapid and markedly beneficial effect on the inflammatory synovitis and overall state of well-being is noted in many patients. Interestingly, the effects of anti-TNF therapy were limited to the duration of therapy, and symptoms and signs of inflammation returned rapidly on discontinuation of therapy. Recent data also implicate T_H17 cells in the pathogenesis of RA.

Clinical Manifestations

Rheumatoid arthritis is most typically a persistent, progressive disease presenting in women in the middle years of life. Fatigue and joint inflammation, characterized by pain, swelling, warmth, and morning stiffness, are hallmarks of the disease. Almost invariably, multiple small and large synovial joints are affected on both the right and left sides of the body in a symmetric distribution. Involvement of the small joints of the hands, wrists, and feet as well as the larger peripheral joints, including the hips, knees, shoulders, and elbows, is typical. Involved joints are demineralized, and joint cartilage and juxtaarticular bone are eroded by the synovial inflammation, inducing joint deformities. Although the lower spine is spared, cervical involvement can also occur, potentially leading to spinal instability. In highly active cases, extra-articular manifestations can occur. These include lung nodules, subcutaneous "rheumatoid" nodules (typically present over extensor surfaces), ocular inflammation (including scleritis), or small-vessel vasculitis.

Treatment

Prompt and aggressive treatment to control inflammation in rheumatoid arthritis can slow or even stop progressive joint erosion. A number of immunomodulatory medications have shown benefit in treating rheumatoid arthritis. The primary pathway through which methotrexate—the drug most commonly used as single-agent therapy for rheumatoid arthritis—acts to diminish joint inflammation is still debated. One hypothesis suggests that methotrexate induces increased local release of adenosine, a short-acting anti-inflammatory mediator.

Rheumatoid arthritis is one of the first conditions in which biologic modifiers of defined pathogenic pathways such as anti-TNF therapy have been used successfully to treat disease. Inhibitors of TNF (etanercept, infliximab, and adalimumab) act by sequestering TNF, either to a recombinant soluble form of the TNF receptor (etanercept) or to monoclonal antibodies to TNF (infliximab, adalimumab). Although these agents have a high likelihood of achieving benefit in patients with rheumatoid arthritis, their use is still limited by their high cost and the potential risks of drug-associated toxicity (including susceptibility to life-threatening infections and induction of other autoimmune syndromes). Furthermore, although they are among the most potent agents yet described for the control of rheumatoid arthritis, there remain patients who fail to experience disease remission when treated only with TNF blockade. As a general principle of therapy in rheumatoid arthritis, it appears that using multiple agents with (presumably) different and complementary mechanisms of action can lead to additional benefit. T-cell–B-cell–APC interactions clearly play important roles in the propagation phase of RA, and it is therefore not surprising that additional biological agents have also shown efficacy in the treatment of RA, including agents that inhibit B cells (eg, rituximab) and costimulation (eg, CTLA4-Ig).

CHECKPOINT

14. What are the antigens against which antibodies are directed in SLE?
15. How many different genetic loci are believed to confer susceptibility to SLE? Which are the strongest ones?
16. What is believed to be the relationship of apoptosis to the initiation of SLE?
17. What prevents normal individuals from being immunized to apoptotic cell debris, and why does this host defense break down in patients with SLE?
18. What are three stimuli that typically provoke SLE flares?
19. What are the most prominently affected organ systems in SLE?

CASE STUDIES

Jonathan Fuchs, MD, MPH, & Yeong Kwok, MD

(See Chapter 25, p. 711 for Answers)

CASE 107

A 58-year-old man with a long history of treated essential hypertension and mild renal insufficiency presents to the urgent care clinic complaining of pain in the right knee. His primary care provider saw him 1 week ago and added a thiazide diuretic to improve his blood pressure control. He had been feeling well until the night before the clinic visit, when he noted some redness and slight swelling of his knee. He went to sleep and was awakened early by significant swelling and pain. He was able to walk only with assistance. He has no history of knee trauma.

Physical examination confirmed the presence of a swollen right knee, which was erythematous and warm. Joint aspiration recovered copious dark yellow, cloudy synovial fluid. Microscopic analysis demonstrated 30,000 leukocytes/μL, a negative Gram stain, and many needle-like, negatively birefringent crystals consistent with acute gout.

Questions

A. What factors may have precipitated this gout flare?
B. Describe the inflammatory pathways involved in acute gout.
C. What agents should the urgent care physician consider in treating this gout flare? What are their mechanisms of action?

CASE 108

A 24-year-old man presents with a worsening rash. One week ago, he had been at an urgent care center with a sore throat and was diagnosed with "strep throat." He was prescribed penicillin and had been getting better. The day before presentation, he noted the development of a pink rash on his trunk, and on the day of his evaluation, it spread to his arms and legs. On examination, the patient has a symmetric maculopapular rash covering his extremities and trunk. Some of the lesions on his legs are palpable.

Questions

A. What is the likely cause of this patient's rash?

B. What is the underlying pathophysiology in this case?

C. What other organs can this disorder affect and why?

CASE 109

A 28-year-old nursery school teacher developed a marked change in the color of her urine ("cola-colored") 1 week after she contracted impetigo from one of her students. She also complained of new onset of global headaches and retention of fluid in her legs. Examination revealed a blood pressure of 158/92, resolving honey-crusted pustules over her right face and neck, 1+ pitting edema of her ankles, and no cardiac murmur. Urinalysis revealed 2+ protein and numerous red cells and red cell casts. Her serum creatinine was elevated at 1.9 mg/dL. Serum complement levels (CH50, C3, and C4) were low. She was diagnosed with poststreptococcal glomerulonephritis.

Questions

A. What is the relationship between her skin infection and the subsequent development of glomerulonephritis?

B. Describe the pathogenesis of this disorder.

C. What is the natural history of this form of immune complex vasculitis?

CASE 110

A 22-year-old African-American woman with a family history of SLE reports intermittent arthralgias in her knees. She denies any facial rash, photosensitivity, chest pain, or shortness of breath. She is convinced she has lupus and requests confirmatory blood tests.

Questions

A. What additional history may be helpful in supporting the diagnosis of lupus as the cause of this patient's arthralgias?

B. Why is it essential to elicit a medication history when considering this diagnosis?

C. Describe three possible mechanisms of autoantibody-induced tissue injury in SLE.

D. Describe the natural history of the disease. Which stimuli have been implicated in the exacerbations that punctuate its course?

CASE 111

A 47-year-old woman presents to the clinic with a four-week history of fatigue, bilateral hand pain and stiffness, and hand and wrist joint swelling. About a month before presentation, she noticed that her hands were stiffer in the morning, but thought that it was due to too much typing. However, the stiffness has worsened, and she now needs about an hour each morning to "loosen up" her hands. As the day goes on, the stiffness improves, although it does not go away entirely. She has also noticed that her knuckles and wrists are swollen and feel somewhat warm. Physical examination reveals warm, erythematous wrists and metacarpal joints bilaterally. Hand x-ray films show periarticular demineralization and erosions, and blood test results are significant for a mild anemia, elevated sedimentation rate, and a positive rheumatoid factor. The patient is diagnosed with rheumatoid arthritis.

Questions

A. What is the basic pathogenic process in rheumatoid arthritis?
B. Describe the interplay between genetic and environmental factors that leads to the pathogenic process.
C. How are novel treatments being used to treat this condition?

REFERENCES

General

Duan-Porter WD et al. Autoantigens: The critical partner in initiating and propagating systemic autoimmunity. Ann N Y Acad Sci. 2005;1062:127–36. [PMID: 16461795]

Lanzavecchia A. How can cryptic epitopes trigger autoimmunity? J Exp Med. 1995 Jun 1;181(6):1945–8. [PMID: 7539032]

Ryan JG et al. The spectrum of autoinflammatory diseases: Recent bench to bedside observations. Curr Opin Rheumatol. 2008 Jan;20(1):66–75. [PMID: 18281860]

Sercarz EE et al. Dominance and crypticity of T cell antigenic determinants. Annu Rev Immunol. 1993;11:729–66. [PMID: 7682817]

Gout

Bieber JD, Terkeltaub RA: Gout: On the brink of novel therapeutic options for an ancient disease. Arthritis Rheum. 2004 Aug;50(8):2400–14. [PMID: 15334451]

Ellman MH et al. Crystal-induced arthropathies: Recent investigative advances. Curr Opin Rheumatol. 2006 May;18(3):249–55. [PMID: 16582687]

Pascual E et al. Therapeutic advances in gout. Curr Opin Rheumatol. 2007 Mar;19(2):122–7. [PMID: 17278926]

Vitart V et al. *SLC2A9* is a newly identified urate transporter influencing serum urate concentration, urate excretion and gout. Nat Genet. 2008 Apr;40(4):437–42. [PMID: 18327257]

Vasculitis

Bosch X et al. Treatment of antineutrophil cytoplasmic antibody associated vasculitis: A systematic review. JAMA. 2007 Aug 8;298(6):655–69. [PMID: 17684188]

Jennette JC et al. New insight into the pathogenesis of vasculitis associated with antineutrophil cytoplasmic autoantibodies. Curr Opin Rheumatol. 2008 Jan;20(1):55–60. [PMID: 18281858]

Seo P, Stone JH. Large vessel vasculitis. Arthritis Rheum. 2004 Feb 15;51(1):128–39. [PMID: 14872466]

Seo P et al. Small-vessel and medium-vessel vasculitis. Arthritis Rheum. 2007 Dec 15;57(8):1552–9. [PMID 18050229]

Systemic Lupus Erythematosus

Botto M et al. Homozygous C1q deficiency causes glomerulonephritis associated with multiple apoptotic bodies. Nat Genet. 1998 May;19(1):56–9. [PMID: 9590289]

Rosen A et al. Clearing the way to mechanisms of autoimmunity. Nat Med. 2001 Jun;7(6):664—5. [PMID: 11385500]

Sjögren's Syndrome

Gottenberg JE et al. Activation of IFN pathways and plasmacytoid dendritic cell recruitment in target organs of primary Sjögren's syndrome. Proc Natl Acad Sci U S A. 2006 Feb 21;103(8):2770–5. [PMID: 16477017]

Larché MJ. A short review of the pathogenesis of Sjögren's syndrome. Autoimmun Rev. 2006 Feb;5(2):132–5. [PMID: 16431344]

Inflammatory Myositis

Bohan A et al. Polymyositis and dermatomyositis (first of two parts). N Engl J Med. 1975 Feb 13;292(7):344–7. [PMID: 1090839]

Bohan A et al. Polymyositis and dermatomyositis (second of two parts). N Engl J Med. 1975 Feb 20;292(8):403–7. [PMID: 1089199]

Casciola-Rosen L et al. Enhanced autoantigen expression in regenerating muscle cells in idiopathic inflammatory myopathy. J Exp Med. 2005 Feb 21;201(4):591–601. [PMID: 15728237]

Grundtman C et al. Immune mechanisms in the pathogenesis of idiopathic inflammatory myopathies. Arthritis Res Ther. 2007;9(2):208. [PMID: 17389031]

Levine SM. Cancer and myositis: New insights into an old association. Curr Opin Rheumatol. 2006 Nov;18(6):620–4. [PMID: 17053509]

Rheumatoid Arthritis

Feldmann M et al. Anti-TNF alpha therapy of rheumatoid arthritis: What have we learned? Annu Rev Immunol. 2001;19:163–96. [PMID: 11244034]

Smolen JS et al. New therapies for treatment of rheumatoid arthritis. Lancet. 2007 Dec 1;370(9602):1861–74. [PMID: 17570481]

Case Study Answers

Yeong Kwok, MD, Eva M. Aagaard, MD,
& Jonathan D. Fuchs, MD, MPH

C H A P T E R

25

CASE 1

A. The four types of osteogenesis imperfecta are type I (mild), type II (perinatal, lethal), type III (progressive, deforming), and type IV (deforming with normal scleras). All forms of osteogenesis imperfecta are characterized by increased susceptibility to fractures ("brittle bones"), but there is considerable phenotypic heterogeneity, even within individual subtypes. Approximately one fourth of the cases of type I or type IV osteogenesis imperfecta represent new mutations; in the remainder, the history and examination of other family members reveal findings consistent with autosomal dominant inheritance. Type III is also transmitted as an autosomal dominant trait, although type III can occasionally be transmitted in an autosomal recessive manner. Type II, the most severe form, generally occurs as a result of a sporadic dominant mutation.

B. Type II osteogenesis imperfecta presents at birth (or even in utero) with multiple fractures and bony deformities, resulting in death in infancy and, therefore, not likely to be seen in a child 4 years of age. Type III presents at birth or in early infancy with multiple fractures—often prenatal—and progressive bony deformities. The absence of prenatal fractures and early deformities in this patient's history is most suggestive of type I or type IV osteogenesis imperfecta. These individuals generally present in early childhood with one or a few fractures of long bones in response to minimal or no trauma, as seen in this case. Type I and type IV osteogenesis imperfecta are differentiated by their clinical severity and scleral hue. Type I tends to be less severe, with 10–20 fractures during childhood plus short stature but few or no deformities. These patients tend to have blue scleras. Patients with type IV osteogenesis imperfecta tend to have more fractures, resulting in significant short stature and mild to moderate deformities. Their scleras are normal or gray.

C. In patients with type I osteogenesis imperfecta, the fracture incidence decreases after puberty and the main features in

adult life are mild short stature, conductive hearing loss, and occasionally dentinogenesis imperfecta (defective dentin formation in tooth development).

D. The fundamental defect in most individuals with type I osteogenesis imperfecta is reduced synthesis of type I collagen resulting from loss-of-function mutations in *COL1A1*. Several potential molecular defects are responsible for *COL1A1* mutations in type I osteogenesis imperfecta, including alterations in a regulatory region leading to reduced transcription, splicing abnormalities leading to reduced steady-state levels of RNA, and deletion of the entire *COL1A1* gene. However, in many cases, the underlying defect is a single base pair change that creates a premature stop codon (also known as a "**nonsense mutation**") in exons 6–49. In a process referred to as "nonsense-mediated decay," partially synthesized mRNA precursors that carry the nonsense codon are recognized and degraded by the cell. Each of these mutations gives rise to greatly reduced (partial loss-of-function) or no (complete loss-of-function) mRNA. Because the nonmutant *COL1A1* allele continues to produce mRNA at a normal rate (ie, there is no dosage compensation), heterozygosity for a complete loss-of-function mutation results in a 50% reduction in the total rate of $pro\alpha1(I)$ mRNA synthesis, whereas heterozygosity for a partial loss-of-function mutation results in a less severe reduction. A reduced concentration of pro1(I) chains limits the production of type I procollagen, leading to both a reduced amount of structurally normal type I collagen and an excess of unassembled $pro\alpha2(I)$ chains, which are degraded inside the cell. This ultimately results in fragile bones.

CASE 2

A. The primary metabolic defect in phenylketonuria (PKU) is the inability to hydroxylate phenylalanine, an essential step in the conversion of phenylalanine to tyrosine and the synthesis of protein. This condition is most commonly due to a defect in phenylalanine hydroxylase, the responsible enzyme, or less commonly, to a defect in the metabolism of tetrahydrobiopterin (BH_4), an essential co-factor in the hydroxylation of phenylalanine. This leads to the accumulation of phenylalanine and its metabolites.

B. The accumulation of phenylalanine and its metabolites, especially phenylpyruvate, directly reduces energy production and protein synthesis, and affects neurotransmitter homeostasis in the developing brain, since many neurotransmitters are derived from amino acids. Elevated levels of phenylalanine also inhibit amino acid transport across the blood-brain barrier, causing an amino acid deficit in the cerebrospinal fluid. All these effects combine to cause mental retardation, developmental delay, and seizures. Affected individuals also suffer from eczema, the mechanism of which is not well understood, and have hypopigmentation due to inhibition of melanocytes from the excess phenylalanine. Most, if not all, of the above consequences of PKU can be prevented by strict dietary management to ensure that excessive serum phenylalanine concentrations do not occur.

C. PKU is inherited as an autosomal recessive trait. The reproductive fitness of affected untreated individuals is poor, meaning that they are unlikely to produce offspring. Theories have been proposed about why the trait has persisted at a relatively high rate in the population. It is known that the rate of spontaneous PKU mutation is low. Two potential explanations for the high rate of the defective gene are the founder effect and heterozygote advantage. The founder effect occurs when a population founded by a small number of ancestors has by chance a high frequency of a deleterious gene. Heterozygote advantage refers to the fact that certain genes may actually confer a benefit in the heterozygote state even though the homozygote state is disadvantageous. This is the case for the genetic defect in sickle cell disease, in which heterozygote carriers have a relative resistance to malaria.

CASE 3

A. Fragile X-associated mental retardation is a syndrome caused by a genetic mutation of the X chromosome. The mutation leads to failure of the region between bands Xq27 and Xq28 to condense at metaphase, thereby increasing the "fragility" of the region. The mutation appears as an amplification of a $(CGG)_n$ repeat within the untranslated region of a gene named *FMR1*. The *FMR1* gene encodes an RNA-binding protein named FMR1. However, in affected individuals, amplification of the gene results in methylation of an area known as the CpG island, located at Xq27.3. This methylation prevents expression of the FMR1 protein.

The FMR1 protein is normally expressed in brain and testes. This protein resembles a group of proteins named hnRNPs (heterogeneous nuclear RNA-binding proteins) that function in the processing or transport of nuclear mRNA precursors. It is believed that the FMR1 protein plays a general role in the cellular metabolism of nuclear RNA but only in the tissues in which it is primarily expressed (ie, the CNS and testes). This would explain in part the symptoms of mental retardation and enlarged testes. It is not known why the absence of *FMR1* expression leads to joint laxity and hyperextensibility and facial abnormalities.

B. Fragile X-associated mental retardation is an X-linked disease. Given that a male child inherits his X chromosome from his mother, she is clearly the carrier of the mutation.

The boy's mother and grandparents do not demonstrate the phenotype of fragile X-associated mental retardation because of the processes of premutation and parental imprinting. As mentioned, the mutation in fragile X is associated with amplification of a segment of DNA containing the sequence $(CGG)_n$. This segment is highly variable in length. In individuals who are neither carriers nor affected, the number of repeats is generally less than 50. In transmitting males and unaffected carrier females, the number of repeats is usually between 70 and 100. Alleles with 55 or more repeats are unstable and often exhibit expansion after maternal transmission; these individuals are generally considered to carry the premutation. They are unaffected phenotypically, but the regions are unstable and when transmitted from generation to generation tend to undergo amplification into a full mutation. Although premutation carriers do not develop a typical FMR syndrome, recent studies indicate that female premutation carriers exhibit a 20% incidence of premature ovarian failure, whereas male premutation carriers are at increased risk for a tremor-ataxia syndrome. In both cases, the mechanism is likely to be explained by somatic expansion of the premutation. Full mutations, observed in all affected individuals, always have more than 200 amplifications.

The most important determinant of whether a premutation allele is subject to amplification is the sex of the parent who transmits the premutation allele. A premutation allele transmitted by a female expands to a full mutation with a likelihood proportionate to the length of the premutation. In contrast, a premutation allele transmitted by a male rarely expands to a full mutation regardless of the length of the premutation. This process is called parental imprinting. Thus, it is likely that the boy's mother and grandfather are carriers of a premutation allele and are, therefore, unaffected and that this gene amplified to a full mutation on transmission to the boy.

C. The chance that her unborn child will be affected depends on its gender. If it is a boy, the chance that it will be affected is approximately 80%, whereas if it is a girl the chance is only 32%.

CASE 4

A. Leber's hereditary optic neuropathy (LHON) arises from a mutation in mitochondrial DNA (mtDNA). The mtDNA encodes protein components of the electron transport chain involved in the generation of adenosine triphosphate (ATP). Mutations in the mtDNA can result in the inability to generate ATP. This defect especially affects tissues with intensive ATP use such as the skeletal muscle and the central nervous system. It is not understood why the defect in LHON is largely confined to the optic nerve and the retina. Other mitochondrial disorders do affect skeletal muscle, most notably, mitochondrial encephalomyopathy with ragged red fibers (MERRF).

B. LHON is inherited through mtDNA mutations. All the mtDNA in our bodies comes exclusively from the egg. The sperm makes no contribution of mtDNA. Therefore, LHON is inherited only from the mother. In addition, a typical cell carries 10–100 separate mtDNA molecules, only a fraction of which carry the mutation. This is known as **heteroplasmy.** Within any one affected woman, the level of mutant DNA in different eggs may vary from 10% to 90%. Thus, some offspring may be severely affected while others may not show any signs. Furthermore, within any given offspring, the level of mutant mtDNA will vary from tissue to tissue and from cell to cell.

C. LHON affects males 4 to 5 times more often than females. This difference is thought to be due to a factor on the X chromosome that modifies the severity of a mitochondrial mutation. Even though mtDNA encodes essential components of the electron transport chain, there are copies for most mitochondrial components also encoded on the nuclear genome.

CASE 5

A. Down syndrome occurs approximately once in every 700 live births. Common features include developmental delay, growth retardation, congenital heart disease (50%), immunodeficiency, and characteristic major and minor facial and dysmorphic features, including upslanting palpebral fissures (82%), excess skin on the back of the neck (81%), brachycephaly (75%), hyperextensible joints (75%), flat nasal bridge (68%), epicanthal folds (59%), small ears (50%), and transverse palmar creases (53%).

B. There are two major genetic abnormalities associated with Down syndrome. The most common abnormality occurs in children born to parents with normal karyotypes. It is caused by nondisjunction of chromosome 21 during meiotic segregation, resulting in one extra chromosome 21 or in trisomy 21 with 47 chromosomes on karyotyping. Alternatively, Down syndrome can be caused by DNA rearrangement resulting in fusion of chromosome 21 to another acrocentric chromosome via its centromere. This abnormal chromosome is called a robertsonian translocation chromosome. Unlike those with trisomy 21, these individuals have 46 chromosomes on karyotyping. This type of translocation can sometimes be inherited from a carrier parent.

Both of these genetic abnormalities result in a 50% increase in gene dosage for nearly all genes on chromosome 21. In other words, the amount of protein produced by all or nearly all genes on chromosome 21 is approximately 150% of normal in Down syndrome. The genes that have been shown to contribute to the Down syndrome phenotype include the gene that encodes the amyloid protein found in the senile plaques of Alzheimer's disease and the one that encodes the cytoplasmic form of superoxide dismutase, which plays an important role in free radical metabolism.

C. It is not known why advanced maternal age is associated with an increased risk of Down syndrome. One theory suggests that biochemical abnormalities affect the ability of paired chromosomes to disjoin and that these abnormalities accumulate over time. Because germ cell development is completed in females before birth, these biochemical abnormalities are able to accumulate within the egg cells as the mother ages, thereby increasing the risk of nondisjunction. Another hypothesis is that structural, hormonal, and immunologic changes occur in the uterus as the woman ages, producing an environment less able to reject a developmentally abnormal embryo. Therefore, an older uterus would be more likely to support a trisomy 21 conceptus to term. Alternatively, it is possible that a combination of these and other genetic factors may contribute to the relationship between advanced maternal age and an increased incidence of Down syndrome.

CASE 6

A. The overall risk of phenylketonuria is approximately 1:10,000, although there is great geographic and ethnic variability. The highest risk occurs among Yemenite Jews (incidence of 1:5000), whereas Northern Europeans develop the disease at a rate of 1:10,000 and African Americans at a rate of 1:50,000.

B. The primary defect in phenylketonuria is a defect in phenylalanine hydroxylase. This enzyme is responsible for converting phenylalanine into tyrosine, a nonessential amino acid. Tyrosine is then used in multiple biosynthetic processes, including protein synthesis and metabolism, and the products of these processes, fumarate and acetoacetate, are used in gluconeogenesis. When hydroxylation of phenylalanine does not occur, phenylalanine accumulates and is transaminated to form phenylpyruvate and subsequently phenylacetate, both of which are detected in increased amounts in the blood and urine in individuals with phenylketonuria.

C. The primary manifestations of phenylketonuria are moderate to severe mental retardation, seizures, growth retardation, hypopigmentation, and eczematous skin.
Elevated phenylalanine levels have a direct effect on energy production, protein synthesis, and neurotransmitter homeostasis in the developing brain. Phenylalanine can also inhibit

the transport of neutral amino acids across the blood-brain barrier, leading to a selective amino acid deficiency in the cerebrospinal fluid. These general effects on CNS metabolism lead to the neurologic manifestations of phenylketonuria.

The hypopigmentation in phenylketonuria is probably caused by an inhibitory effect of excess phenylalanine on the production of dopaquinone in melanocytes, the rate-limiting step in melanin production.

The pathophysiology of eczema is not well understood, but the disorder is seen in several other inborn errors of metabolism in which plasma concentrations of branched-chain amino acids are elevated.

D. Phenylketonuria is generally treated with a phenylalanine-restricted diet. This diet begins at birth with the use of a semisynthetic formula low in phenylalanine, combined with breast milk, and empirically titrated to a plasma phenylalanine level of ≤ 1 mmol/L. The diet must be continued indefinitely. Because this treatment results in persistent subtle neuropsychologic defects, researchers are examining alternative options, including somatic gene therapy.

E. When this child is herself of childbearing age, she must be counseled about the risks of maternal phenylketonuria. The syndrome, caused by in utero exposure to maternal hyperphenylalaninemia, is manifested by microcephaly, growth retardation, congenital heart disease, and severe developmental delay, regardless of fetal genotype. The incidence can be reduced by rigorous control of maternal phenylalanine concentrations from before conception until birth to levels much lower than generally required for postpartum management of phenylketonuria-affected individuals.

CASE 7

A. The most likely cause of this child's recurrent infections is severe combined immunodeficiency disease (SCID). These patients have complete or near-complete failure of development of both cellular and humoral components of the immune system. Placental transfer of maternal immunoglobulin is insufficient to protect these children from infection, and for that reason they present at a very early age with severe infections.

B. SCID is a heterogeneous group of genetic and cellular disorders characterized by a failure in the cellular maturation of lymphoid stem cells, resulting in reduced numbers and function of both B and T lymphocytes and hypogammaglobulinemia. The genetic and cellular defects can occur at many different levels, starting with surface membrane receptors, but also including deficiencies in signal transduction or metabolic biochemical pathways. Although the different molecular defects may cause clinically indistinguishable phenotypes, identification of specific mutations allows for improved genetic counseling, prenatal diagnosis, and carrier detection.

The most common genetic defect is an X-linked form of SCID in which the maturation defect is mainly in the T-lymphocyte lineage and is due to a point mutation in the γ chain of the IL-2 receptor. This defective γ chain is shared by the receptors for IL-4, IL-7, IL-9, and IL-15, leading to dysfunction of all of these cytokine receptors. Defective signaling through the IL-7 receptor appears to block normal maturation of T lymphocytes. Defective IL-2 responses inhibit proliferation of T, B, and NK cells, explaining the combined immune defects seen in XSCID patients.

Several autosomally inherited defects have also been identified. A defect in the α chain of the IL-7 receptor can lead to an autosomal recessive form of SCID through mechanisms similar to XSCID but with intact NK cells.

About 20% of SCID cases are caused by a deficiency of adenosine deaminase (ADA), which is an enzyme in the purine salvage pathway, responsible for the metabolism of adenosine. Absence of the ADA enzyme results in an accumulation of toxic adenosine metabolites within the cells. These metabolites inhibit normal lymphocyte proliferation and lead to extreme cytopenia of both B and T lymphocytes. The combined immunologic deficiency and clinical presentation of this disorder, known as SCID-ADA, is identical to that of the other forms of SCID. Skeletal abnormalities and neurologic abnormalities may be associated with this disease.

An alternate autosomally recessive form of SCID is a deficiency of ZAP-70, a tyrosine kinase important in normal T-lymphocyte function. Deficiency of this tyrosine kinase results in total absence of CD8 T lymphocytes and functionally defective CD4 T lymphocytes, but normal B-lymphocyte and NK activity. Deficiencies of both p56^{kk} and Jak3 (Janus kinase 3) can also lead to SCID through defective signal transduction; p56^{kk} is a T-cell receptor–associated tyrosine kinase that is essential for T-cell differentiation, activation, and proliferation. Jak3 is a cytokine receptor-associated signaling molecule. Finally, patients have been identified with defective recombination activating gene (*RAG-1* and *RAG-2*) products. RAG-1 and RAG-2 initiate recombination of antigen-binding proteins, immunoglobulins and T-cell receptors. The defect leads to both quantitative and qualitative (functional) deficiencies of T and B lymphocytes.

C. Without treatment, most patients with SCID die within the first 1–2 years.

CASE 8

A. This child has X-linked agammaglobinemia, formerly called Bruton's agammaglobinemia. The history of multiple infections occurring after the age of 6 months, the family history of a maternal uncle with lethal infection, the severe current infection with *Streptococcus pneumoniae*, and the absence of circulating B lymphocytes are characteristic of this disorder.

B. The main defect is a mutation in the *BTK* (Bruton's tyrosine kinase) gene, which is located on the X chromosome. This gene's product is a B-cell–specific signaling protein necessary for normal B-cell maturation. The mutation affects the catalytic domain of the protein, halting B-cell maturation. This, in turn, leads to absence or greatly reduced levels of the immunoglobulins IgA, IgG, and IgM. Their absence or reduction is a particular problem with fighting infections from encapsulated bacteria because these bacteria require antibody binding for efficient opsonization. Therefore, patients are particularly susceptible to infections with bacteria such as *Haemophilus influenzae* and *S pneumoniae*. Because they cannot mount an antibody response, they also develop very little immunity to these infections and are thus susceptible to repeated infections with the same organism.

C. The affected child is relatively protected by circulating maternal antibodies until 4–6 months of age. The child's immune system is otherwise unaffected, but as the levels of maternal antibodies decrease, the child becomes increasingly susceptible to infection, particularly from encapsulated bacteria.

CASE 9

A. Individuals with common variable immunodeficiency (CVI) commonly develop recurrent sinopulmonary infections such as sinusitis, otitis media, bronchitis, and pneumonia. Bronchiectasis may develop as a result of these recurrent infections. They may also develop GI malabsorption from bacterial overgrowth or chronic *Giardia* infection in the small bowel.

B. CVI is a heterogeneous disorder in which the primary immunologic abnormality is a marked reduction in antibody production, with normal or reduced numbers of circulating B cells. This is most commonly caused by a defect in the terminal differentiation of B lymphocytes in response to T-lymphocyte–dependent and T-lymphocyte–independent stimuli. However, defects in B-lymphocyte development have been shown to occur at any stage of the maturation pathway.

In approximately 80% of patients, the defect is intrinsic to the B-lymphocyte population. In the rest, a variety of T-cell abnormalities lead to immune defects with subsequent impairment of B-cell differentiation. T-lymphocyte dysfunction can be manifested as increased suppressor T-lymphocyte activity, decreased cytokine production, defective synthesis of B-lymphocyte growth factors, defective cytokine gene expression in T cells, decreased T-cell mitogenesis, and deficient lymphokine activated killer cell function.

C. Individuals with CVI are at increased risk of autoimmune disorders and malignancies. The autoimmune disorders most commonly seen in association with CVI include immune thrombocytopenic purpura, hemolytic anemia, and symmetric seronegative arthritis. The malignancies associated with CVI include lymphomas, gastric carcinoma, and skin cancers.

D. Treatment is mainly symptomatic along with replacement of immune globulin with monthly infusions of IVIG.

CASE 10

A. Pneumocystis pneumonia is commonly seen in AIDS. An HIV-1 antibody test should be obtained whenever the diagnosis of *Pneumocystis jiroveci* is suspected.

B. AIDS is the consequence of infection with HIV-1, a retrovirus, which infects multiple cell lines, including lymphocytes, monocytes, macrophages, and dendritic cells. With HIV infection, there is an absolute reduction of CD4 T lymphocytes, an accompanying deficit in CD4 T-lymphocyte function, and an associated increase in CD8 cytotoxic T lymphocytes (CTLs). In addition to the cell-mediated immune defects, B-lymphocyte function is altered such that many infected individuals have marked hypergammaglobulinemia but impaired specific antibody responses. The resultant immunosuppression predisposes patients to the constellation of opportunistic infections that characterizes AIDS.

The loss of CD4 cells seen in HIV infection is the result of multiple mechanisms, including (1) autoimmune destruction, (2) direct viral infection and destruction, (3) fusion and formation into multinucleated giant cells, (4) toxicity of viral proteins to CD4 T lymphocytes and hematopoietic precursors, and (5) apoptosis (programmed cell death).

C. The clinical manifestations of HIV infection and AIDS are the direct consequence of progressive and severe immunosuppression and can be correlated with the degree of CD4 T-lymphocyte destruction. HIV infection may present as an acute, self-limited febrile syndrome. This is often followed by a long, clinically silent period, sometimes associated with generalized lymphadenopathy. The time course of disease progression may vary; the majority of individuals remain asymptomatic for 5–10 years. Approximately 70% of HIV-infected individuals will develop AIDS after a decade of infection. Approximately 10% of those infected manifest rapid progression to AIDS within 5 years after infection. A minority of individuals are "long-term nonprogressors." Genetic factors, host cytotoxic immune responses, and viral load and virulence all appear to impact susceptibility to infection and the rate of disease progression. Multidrug antiretroviral therapy has dramatically changed this natural history and markedly prolonged survival.

As the CD4 count declines, the incidence of infection increases. At CD4 counts between 200/μL and 500/μL, patients are at an increased risk for bacterial infections, including pneumonia and sinusitis. As CD4 counts continue to drop—generally below 250/μL—they are at high risk for opportunistic infections such as pneumocystic pneumonia, candidiasis, toxoplasmosis, cryptococcal meningitis, cytomegalovirus (CMV) retinitis, and *Mycobacterium avium* complex infection. HIV-infected individuals are also at increased risk for certain malignancies, including Kaposi's sarcoma, non-Hodgkin's lymphoma, primary CNS lymphoma, invasive cervical carcinoma, and anal squamous cell carcinoma. Other manifestations of AIDS include AIDS dementia complex, peripheral neuropathy, monoarticular and polyarticular arthritides, unexplained fevers, and weight loss.

CASE 11

A. This patient's presentation is characteristic of untreated infective endocarditis, an infection of the cardiac valves. The most common predisposing factor is the presence of abnormal cardiac valves related to rheumatic heart disease, mitral valve prolapse with an audible murmur, congenital heart disease, prosthetic valve, or prior endocarditis. Injection drug use is also an important risk factor for this disease. The patient's history of significant illness as a child after a sore throat suggests the possibility of rheumatic heart disease.

B. The most common infectious agents causing native valve endocarditis are gram-positive bacteria, including viridans streptococci, *S aureus,* and enterococci. Given the history of recent dental work, the most likely pathogen in this patient would be viridans streptococci, which are normal mouth flora that can become transiently bloodborne after dental work.

C. The hemodynamic factors that predispose patients to the development of endocarditis include (1) a high-velocity jet stream causing turbulent flow, (2) flow from a high- to a low-pressure chamber, and (3) a comparatively narrow orifice separating two chambers that creates a pressure gradient. The lesions of endocarditis tend to form on the surface of the valve in the lower pressure cardiac chamber. The predisposed, damaged endothelium of an abnormal valve—or jet stream–damaged endothelium—promotes the deposition of fibrin and platelets, forming sterile vegetations. When bacteremia occurs, such as after dental work, microorganisms can be deposited on these sterile vegetations (Figure 4–5). Once infected, the lesions continue to grow through further deposition of platelets and fibrin. These vegetations act as a sanctuary from host defense mechanisms such as phagocytosis and complement-mediated lysis. It is for this reason that prolonged administration of bactericidal antibiotics and possible operative intervention are required for cure.

D. The painful papules found on the pads of this man's fingers and toes are Osler's nodes. They are thought to be caused by deposition of immune complexes in the skin. The painless hemorrhagic macules (Janeway lesions) and splinter hemorrhages are thought to result from microembolization of the cardiac vegetations.

E. In addition to the symptoms described in this man (fever, chills, night sweats, malaise, Roth spots, Janeway lesions, splinter hemorrhages, and Osler nodes), patients with infective en-

docarditis can develop multisystem complaints, including headaches, back pain, focal neurologic symptoms, shortness of breath, pulmonary edema, chest pain, cough, decreased urine output, hematuria, flank pain, abdominal pain, and others. These symptoms and signs reflect (1) hemodynamic changes from valvular damage, (2) end-organ damage by septic emboli (right-sided endocarditis causes emboli to the lungs; left-sided endocarditis causes emboli to the brain, spleen, kidney, GI tract, and extremities), (3) immune complex deposition causing acute glomerulonephritis, and (4) persistent bacteremia and distal seeding of infection, resulting in abscess formation.

Death is usually caused by hemodynamic collapse after rupture of the aortic or mitral valves or by septic emboli to the CNS, resulting in brain abscesses or mycotic aneurysms with resultant intracranial hemorrhage. Risk factors for a fatal outcome include left-sided cardiac involvement, bacterial cause other than *S viridans,* medical comorbidities, complications from endocarditis (congestive heart failure, valve ring abscess, or embolic disease), and, in one study, medical management without valvular surgery.

CASE 12

A. The most likely diagnosis in this patient is meningitis. The acuity and severity of presentation are most consistent with a pyogenic bacterial cause, although viral, mycobacterial, and fungal causes should be considered as well. In adults, the most likely bacterial pathogens are *Neisseria meningitidis* and *Streptococcus pneumoniae.* In newborns younger than 3 months, the most common pathogens are those to which the infant is exposed in the maternal genitourinary canal, including *E coli* and other gram-negative bacilli, group B and other streptococci, and *Listeria monocytogenes.* Between the ages of 3 months and 15 years, *N meningitidis* and *S pneumoniae* are the most common pathogens. *H influenzae,* previously the most common cause of meningitis in this age group, is now primarily a concern in the unimmunized child.

B. Most cases of bacterial meningitis begin with colonization of the host's nasopharynx (Figure 4–7, panel A). This is followed by local invasion of the mucosal epithelium and subsequent bacteremia (Figure 4–7, panel B). Cerebral endothelial cell injury follows and results in increased blood-brain barrier permeability, facilitating meningeal invasion (Figure 4–7, panel C). The resultant inflammatory response in the subarachnoid space causes cerebral edema, vasculitis, and infarction, ultimately leading to decreased cerebrospinal fluid flow, hydrocephalus, worsening cerebral edema, increased intracranial pressure, and decreased cerebral blood flow (Figure 4–8).

Bacterial pathogens responsible for meningitis possess several characteristics that facilitate the steps just listed. Nasal colonization is facilitated by pili on the bacterial surface of *N meningitidis* that assist in mucosal attachment. *N meningitidis, H influenzae,* and *S pneumoniae* also produce IgA proteases that cleave IgA, the antibody commonly responsible for inhibiting adherence of pathogens to the mucosal surface. By cleaving the antibody, the bacteria are able to evade this important host defense mechanism. In addition, *N meningitidis, H influenzae,* and *S pneumoniae* are often encapsulated, which can assist in nasopharyngeal colonization as well as systemic invasion. The capsule inhibits neutrophil phagocytosis and resists classic complement-mediated bactericidal activity, enhancing bacterial survival and replication.

It remains unclear how bacterial pathogens gain access to the CNS. It is thought that cells of the choroid plexus may contain receptors for them, facilitating movement into the subarachnoid space. Once the bacterial pathogen is in the subarachnoid space, host defense mechanisms are inadequate to control the infection. Subcapsular surface components of the bacteria, such as the cell wall and lipopolysaccharide, induce a marked inflammatory response mediated by IL-1, IL-6, matrix metalloproteinases, and TNF. Despite the induction of a marked inflammatory response and leukocytosis, there is a relative lack of opsonization and bactericidal activity such that the bacteria are poorly cleared from the cerebrospinal fluid. The host inflammatory response, with cytokine and proteolytic enzyme release, leads to loss of membrane integrity, with resultant cellular swelling and cerebral edema, contributing to many of the pathophysiologic consequences of this disease.

C. Cerebral edema may be vasogenic, cytotoxic, or interstitial in origin. Vasogenic cerebral edema is principally caused by the increase in the blood-brain barrier permeability that occurs when the bacteria invade the cerebrospinal fluid. Cytotoxic cerebral edema results from swelling of the cellular elements of the brain. This occurs because of toxic factors released by the bacteria and neutrophils. Interstitial edema is due to obstruction of cerebrospinal fluid flow.

D. Any patient suspected of having bacterial meningitis should have emergent lumbar puncture with Gram stain and culture of the cerebrospinal fluid. If there is concern about a focal neurologic problem—such as may occur with abscess—CT or MRI of the brain may be performed before lumbar puncture.

Antibiotics should be started immediately, without waiting for imaging study or lumbar puncture if delay is anticipated in these procedures. The importance of the immune response in triggering cerebral edema has led researchers to study the role of adjuvant anti-inflammatory medications for bacterial meningitis. The use of corticosteroids has been shown to decrease the risk of sensorineural hearing loss among children with *H influenzae* meningitis and mortality among adults with pneumococcal meningitis, and these agents are routinely given at the time of initial antibiotic therapy.

CASE 13

A. The patient described in this case has a moderately severe infection and an underlying diagnosis of COPD, requiring hospitalization but not ICU admission. The most likely pathogens are *S pneumoniae, H influenzae,* and *Moraxella catarrhalis.* Other potential pathogens include *Mycoplasma pneumoniae, Chlamydophila pneumoniae, Legionella pneumophila,* and respiratory viruses (Tables 4–8 and 4–9). Tuberculosis and fungi should also be considered, although these are less likely in this patient with such an acute presentation. Anaerobes are also unlikely without a history of substance abuse or recent depressed mental status. If this patient required ICU admission, the atypical pathogens, *M pneumoniae* and *C pneumoniae,* are much less likely, and *S aureus* and *Pseudomonas aeruginosa* should be added to the differential diagnosis, particularly if the patient had been recently hospitalized.

B. Pulmonary pathogens reach the lungs by one of four routes: (1) inhalation, (2) aspiration of upper airway contents, (3) spread along the mucosal membrane surface, and (4) hematogenous spread.

C. Normal pulmonary antimicrobial defense mechanisms (Figure 4–9) include the following: (1) aerodynamic filtration by subjection of incoming air to turbulence in the nasal passages and then abrupt changes in the direction of the airstream as it moves through the pharynx and tracheobronchial tree; (2) the cough reflex to remove aspirated material, excess secretions, and foreign bodies; (3) the mucociliary transport system, moving the mucous layer upward to the larynx; (4) phagocytic cells, including alveolar macrophages and PMNs, as well as humoral and cellular immune responses, which help to eliminate the pathogens; and (5) pulmonary secretions containing surfactant, lysozyme, and iron-binding proteins, which further aid in bacterial killing.

D. Common host risk factors include the following: (1) an immunocompromised state, resulting in immune dysfunction and increased risk of infection; (2) chronic lung disease, resulting in decreased mucociliary clearance; (3) alcoholism or other reduction of the level of consciousness, which increases the risk of aspiration; (4) injection drug abuse, which increases the risk of hematogenous spread of pathogens; (5) environmental or animal exposure, resulting in inhalation of specific pathogens; (6) residence in an institution, with its associated risk of microaspirations, and exposure via instrumentation (catheters and intubation); and (7) recent influenza infection, leading to disruption of respiratory epithelium, ciliary dysfunction, and inhibition of PMNs. This patient has a history of chronic lung disease, increasing his risk of pneumonia, and he is immunocompromised by the use of corticosteroids for his COPD.

CASE 14

A. There are three primary modes of transmission of pathogens causing infectious diarrhea. Pathogens such as *Vibrio cholerae* are water-borne and transmitted via a contaminated water supply. Several pathogens, including *S aureus* and *Bacillus cereus,* are transmitted by contaminated food. Finally, some pathogens, such as *Shigella* and *Rotavirus,* are transmitted by person-to-person spread and are, therefore, commonly seen in institutional settings such as child care centers.

B. The description of this patient's diarrhea as profuse and watery suggests a small bowel site of infection. The small bowel is the site of significant electrolyte and fluid transportation. Disruption of this process leads to the production of profuse watery diarrhea, as seen in this patient.

C. The most likely cause of diarrhea in this patient, who has recently returned from Mexico, is enterotoxigenic *E coli* (ETEC), which is the most common cause of traveler's diarrhea. Diarrhea results from the production of two enterotoxins that "poison" the cells of the small intestine, causing watery diarrhea. ETEC produces both a heat-labile and a heat-stable enterotoxin. The heat-labile enterotoxin activates adenylyl cyclase and formation of cAMP, which stimulates water and electrolyte secretion by intestinal endothelial cells. The heat-stable toxin produced by ETEC results in guanylyl cyclase activation, also causing watery diarrhea.

CASE 15

A. Factors that contribute to hospital-related sepsis are invasive monitoring devices, indwelling catheters, extensive surgical procedures, and the increased numbers of immunocompromised patients.

B. Sepsis generally starts with a localized infection. Bacteria may then invade the bloodstream directly (leading to bacteremia and positive blood cultures) or may proliferate locally and release toxins into the bloodstream. Gram-negative bacteria contain an endotoxin, the lipid A component of the lipopolysaccharide-phospholipid-protein complex present in the outer cell membrane. Endotoxin activates the coagulation cascade, the complement system, and the kinin system as well as the release of several host mediators such as cytokines, platelet-activating factor, endorphins, endothelium-derived relaxing factor, arachidonic acid metabolites, myocardial depressant factors, nitric oxide, and others. As sepsis persists, host immunosuppression plays a critical role. Specific stimuli such as organism, inoculum, and site of infection stimulate **CD4 T cells** to secrete cytokines with either inflammatory (type 1 helper T cell) or anti-inflammatory (type 2 helper T cell) properties (Figure 4–11). Among patients who die of sepsis, there is significant loss of cells essential for the adaptive immune response (B lymphocytes, CD4 T cells, dendritic cells). **Apoptosis** is thought to play a key role in the decrease in these cell lines, and downregulates the surviving immune cells.

C. A hyperdynamic circulatory state, described as **distributive shock** to emphasize the maldistribution of blood flow to various tissues, is the common hemodynamic finding in sepsis.

The release of vasoactive substances (including nitric oxide) results in loss of normal mechanisms of vascular autoregulation, producing imbalances in blood flow with regional shunting and relative hypoperfusion of some organs. Myocardial depression also occurs, with reduction in both the left and the right ventricular ejection fractions and increases in end-diastolic and end-systolic volumes. This myocardial depression has been attributed to direct toxic effects of nitric oxide, TNF, and IL-1. Refractory hypotension can ensue, resulting in end-organ hypoperfusion and injury.

D. Organ failure results from a combination of decreased perfusion and microvascular injury induced by local and systemic inflammatory responses to infection. Maldistribution of blood flow is accentuated by impaired erythrocyte deformability, with microvascular obstruction. Aggregation of neutrophils and platelets may also reduce blood flow. Demargination of neutrophils from vascular endothelium results in further release of inflammatory mediators and subsequent migration of neutrophils into tissues. Components of the complement system are activated, attracting more neutrophils and releasing locally active substances such as prostaglandins and leukotrienes. The net result of all of these changes is microvascular collapse and, ultimately, organ failure.

E. The outcome in sepsis depends on the number of organs that fail, with a mortality rate of 70% in patients who develop failure of three or more organ systems.

CASE 16

A. Carcinoid tumors arise from neuroendocrine tissue, specifically the enterochromaffin cells. These cells migrate during embryogenesis to the submucosal layer of the intestines and the pulmonary bronchi. Therefore, carcinoid tumors are most commonly found in the intestines and lungs.

B. Since carcinoid tumors are derived from neuroendocrine tissue, they can secrete many peptides that have systemic effects. This secretion is due to the inappropriate activation of latent synthetic ability that all neuroendocrine cells possess. Many of the peptides are vasoactive and can cause vasodilation, resulting in flushing. They can also cause wheezing, diarrhea, excessive salivation, or fibrosis of the heart valves or other tissues.

C. Serotonin production is characteristic of gut carcinoid tumors. Serotonin is metabolized to 5-HIAA. Therefore, finding high levels of 5-HIAA in a 24-hour urine collection in a patient with flushing or other symptoms is highly suggestive of the diagnosis. Bronchial carcinoids rarely produce 5-HIAA and, therefore, rarely present with carcinoid syndrome; instead, they often produce ectopic ACTH, resulting in Cushing's syndrome.

CASE 17

A. Adenomas are thought to be related to colorectal carcinoma by means of stepwise genetic alterations (or hits), with adenomas representing a precancerous lesion that may ultimately progress to cancer. It is believed that stepwise genetic alterations, including both oncogene activation and tumor suppressor gene inactivation, result in phenotypic changes that progress to neoplasia.

B. Two principal lines of evidence support the model of stepwise genetic alterations in colon cancer: (1) Familial colon cancer syndromes are known to result from germline mutations, implicating a genomic cause. Familial adenomatous polyposis is the result of a mutation in the *APC* gene, whereas hereditary nonpolyposis colorectal carcinoma is associated with mutations in the DNA repair genes *hMSH2* and *hMLH1*. (2) Several factors linked to an increased risk of colon cancer are known to be carcinogenic. Substances derived from bacterial colonic flora, foods, or endogenous metabolites are known to be mutagenic. Levels of these substances can be decreased by taking a low-fat, high-fiber diet. Epidemiologic studies suggest that such a change in diet might reduce the risk of colon cancer.

C. The earliest molecular defect in the pathogenesis of colon cancer is the acquisition of somatic mutations in the *APC* gene in the normal colonic mucosa. This defect causes abnormal regulation of β-catenin, which leads to abnormal cell proliferation and the initial steps in tumor formation. Subsequent defects in the TGF-β signaling pathway inactivate this important growth inhibitory pathway and lead to further tumor mucosal proliferation and the development of small adenomas. Mutational activation of the *K-ras* gene leads to constitutive activation of an important proliferative signaling pathway and is common at these stages. It further increases the proliferative potential of the adenomatous tumor cells. Deletion or loss of expression of the *DCC* gene is common in the progression to invasive colon cancers. The DCC protein is a transmembrane protein of the immunoglobulin superfamily and may be a receptor for certain extracellular molecules that guide cell growth or apoptosis. Mutational inactivation of *p53* is also a commonly observed step in the development of invasive colon cancer, seen in late adenomas and early invasive cancers, and leads to loss of an important cell cycle checkpoint and inability to activate the p53-dependent apoptotic pathways. In parallel to these sequential abnormalities in the regulation of cell proliferation, colon cancers also acquire defects in mechanisms that protect genomic stability. These generally involve mutations in mismatch repair genes or genes that prevent chromosomal instability, including *MSH2, MLH1, PMS1,* and *PMS2*. Germline mutations in these genes cause the hereditary nonpolyposis colorectal cancer (HNPCC) syndrome. Nonhereditary colon cancers develop genomic instability through defects in the chromosomal instability (CIN) genes. Defects in these genes lead to the gain or loss of large segments or entire chromosomes during replication, leading to aneuploidy.

D. Early in the progression of dysplasia, disrupted architecture results in the formation of fragile new blood vessels and destruction of existing blood vessels. These changes often occur before invasion of the basement membrane and, therefore, before progression to true cancer formation. These friable vessels can cause microscopic bleeding. This can be tested for by fecal occult blood testing, an important tool in the early detection of precancerous and cancerous colonic lesions.

CASE 18

A. Linkage analysis has identified genetic markers that are known to confer a high risk of developing breast cancer. Two such genes in particular have been found, *BRCA1* and *BRCA2*. Both are involved in repair of DNA. Inherited mutations of *BRCA1* or *BRCA2* are associated with a lifetime risk of developing breast cancer of up to 80%. Mutations in these genes are also associated with a high incidence of ovarian cancer and can lead to increased incidences of prostate cancer, melanoma, and breast cancer in males.

B. There are two major subtypes of breast cancer. Ductal carcinomas arise from the collecting ducts in the breast glandular tissue. Lobular carcinomas arise from the terminal lobules of the glands.

C. While it is still contained by the basement membrane, the tumor is called carcinoma in situ. Invasive carcinoma occurs when tumor cells breach the basement membrane. Both ductal and lobular carcinomas may be either in situ or invasive. By definition, an in situ tumor does not carry a risk of spreading to the lymph nodes or of creating distant metastases. Finding an in situ tumor raises the affected individual's risk of developing a subsequent breast cancer, in either breast, and one of either subtype. Therefore, carcinoma in situ is a marker of heightened susceptibility to developing invasive breast cancer.

D. There are specific therapies that target receptors present in breast cancer. The amount of estrogen exposure is correlated with breast cancer risk. Antiestrogen therapy has long been used with success in patients with estrogen receptor–positive breast cancer, although half of patients diagnosed with breast cancer are estrogen receptor–negative. More recently, antibodies that target the HER2 receptor, a tyrosine kinase growth factor receptor, are used in tumors with an overexpression of the HER2 receptor.

CASE 19

A. Testicular cancer arises from germinal elements within the testes. Germ cells give rise to spermatozoa and thus can theoretically retain the ability to differentiate into any cell type. The pluripotent nature of these cells is witnessed in the production of mature teratomas. These benign tumors often contain mature elements of all three germ cell layers, including hair and teeth.

B. During early embryogenesis, germline epithelium migrates along the midline of the embryo. This migration is followed by formation of the urogenital ridge and ultimately the aggregation of germline cells to form the testes and ovaries. The pattern of migration of the germline epithelium predicts the location of extragonadal testicular neoplasms. These neoplasms are found in the midline axis of the lower cranium, mediastinum, and retroperitoneum.

C. One can monitor the serum concentrations of proteins expressed during embryonic or trophoblastic development to monitor tumor progression and response to therapy. These proteins include alpha-fetoprotein and human chorionic gonadotropin.

CASE 20

A. Sarcomas arise from mesenchymal tissue. These include myocytes, adipocytes, osteoblasts, chondrocytes, fibroblasts, endothelial cells, and synovial cells.

B. Many sarcomas are more common in younger people. This is thought to be because the cells of origin such as chondrocytes or osteoblasts are dividing more rapidly in childhood and adolescence than in adulthood.

C. Because osteosarcomas arise from osteoblasts, they retain their ability to produce a bone matrix of calcium and phosphorus within the tumor.

CASE 21

A. The theory that chronic immune stimulation or modulation may play an early role in the formation of lymphoma is supported by several observations. Iatrogenic immunosuppression, as seen in this patient and in other transplant patients, can increase the risk of B-cell lymphoma, possibly associated with Epstein-Barr virus infection. An increased risk of lymphoma is also seen in other immunosuppressed patients, such as those with AIDS and autoimmune diseases.

B. This patient has been diagnosed with a follicular cleaved cell lymphoma, a well-differentiated or low-grade lymphoma. Low-grade lymphomas retain the morphology and patterns of gene expression of mature lymphocytes, including cell surface markers such as immunoglobulin in the case of B lymphocytes. Their clinical course is generally more favorable, being

characterized by a slow growth rate. Paradoxically, however, these lymphomas tend to present at a more advanced stage, as in this case.

C. Follicular lymphomas arise from lymphoblasts of the B-cell lineage. Common chromosomal abnormalities include translocations of chromosome 14, including t(14;18), t(11;14), and t(14;19). The t(14;18) translocation results in a fusion gene known as IgH; *bcl-2*, which juxtaposes the immunoglobulin heavy chain enhancer on chromosome 14 in front of the *bcl-2* gene on chromosome 18. This results in enhanced expression of an inner mitochondrial protein encoded by *bcl-2*, which has been found to inhibit the natural process of cell death, or apoptosis. Apoptosis is required to remove certain lymphoid clones whose function is not needed. Inhibition of this process probably contributes to proliferation of lymphoma cells.

D. This patient's symptoms of fever and weight loss are known as B symptoms. They are thought to be mediated by a variety of cytokines produced by lymphoma cells or may occur as a reaction of normal immune cells to the lymphoma. Two commonly implicated cytokines are IL-1 and TNF.

CASE 22

A. Like all neoplasms, leukemias are classified by their cell of origin. The first branch point is whether the malignant cell is of myeloid or lymphoid lineage, resulting in either a myeloid or lymphocytic leukemia. All types can be acute, presenting with more than 20% blasts on bone marrow biopsy, or chronic, presenting in a more indolent fashion with a usually slowly progressive course of many years. Lymphocytic leukemias are further divided into T-cell or B-cell leukemias depending on the type of lymphoid cell of origin. This type can be distinguished by the cluster of differentiation (CD) antigens found on the surface of the tumor cells. Myeloid leukemias are also divided into subtypes depending on the type of myeloid cell from which the leukemia arises. AML types M1–M3 arise from myeloblasts. Types M4 and M5 arise from monocytes. Type M6 arises from erythrocyte precursors, called normoblasts. Type M7 arises from platelet precursors, called megakaryoblasts.

B. Acute leukemias typically present with pancytopenia, or a decrease in the counts of all of the normal blood cells, including the normal white cells (the leukemic cells accounting for almost all of the high total WBCs), red blood cells, and platelets. This is caused by the crowding out of normal precursors in the bone marrow by the abnormally dividing blast cells, and by the inhibition of normal hematopoiesis due to secretion of cytokines and inhibitory substances. The patient's presenting symptoms are directly related to the blood abnormalities. The fatigue and pallor are due to the anemia (lack of red blood cells) and the resulting reduced oxygen-carrying capacity. The petechiae and bleeding are from the lack of platelets, inhibiting the ability of the blood to clot. Patients with leukemia are susceptible to serious infections due to the lack of normal WBCs. Finally, the markedly elevated numbers of leukemic cells can clog small blood vessels and result in strokes, retinal vein occlusion, and pulmonary infarction.

C. Chromosomal deletions, duplications, and translocations have been identified in leukemias. One such genetic abnormality is the so-called Philadelphia chromosome, a balanced translocation of chromosomes 9 and 22, that is commonly found in chronic myelogenous leukemia (CML). This translocation results in a fusion gene, *bcr-abl*, which encodes a kinase that phosphorylates key proteins involved in cell growth. A therapeutic agent, imatinib mesylate, blocks the bcr-abl kinase by competing with the ATP binding site and can induce remissions in patients suffering from CML.

CASE 23

A. Paraneoplastic syndromes are defined as bodily effects produced by a tumor at distant targets. There are many well-described syndromes that result from the inappropriate production of a hormone, cytokine, or other signaling peptide by the tumor. The peptides produced by certain tumor types often do not reflect the tissue of origin of the tumor cell and are the result of activation of latent genes not normally expressed by mature tissue. These products are secreted into the bloodstream by the tumor and circulate to distant tissues where they may exert their effects.

B. The patient is suffering from the syndrome of inappropriate antidiuretic hormone (SIADH). Small cell lung cancers can produce ADH, which causes excess retention of free water. This, in turn, causes lowering of the sodium concentration, leading to swelling in the tissues, including the brain, causing altered consciousness, coma, and potentially even death.

C. Small cell lung cancers can also produce ACTH, which stimulates excess cortisol production by the adrenals. This can lead to Cushing's syndrome with symptoms and signs of weight gain, myopathy, easy bruising, and hypertension. Hypercalcemia can also occur in lung cancers as well as in many other types of tumors. This results from activation of the parathyroid hormone–related protein (PTHrP) gene as well as local effects on bone, which raise the serum calcium level.

CASE 24

A. The most likely cause of anemia in this patient is iron deficiency. Iron deficiency anemia is the most common form of anemia. In developed nations, it is primarily the result of iron loss, almost always through blood loss. In men and in postmenopausal women, blood is most commonly lost from the

GI tract, as in this case. In premenopausal women, menstrual blood loss is the major cause of iron deficiency.

In this man, there are no symptoms of significant bleeding from the gut as would be manifested by gross blood (hematochezia) or metabolized blood in the stool (melena, usually described as black-colored stool), and he has no GI complaints. This makes some of the benign GI disorders such as peptic ulcer, arteriovenous malformations, and angiodysplasias less likely. He has no symptoms of inflammatory bowel disease such as diarrhea or abdominal pain. Concern is thus aroused about possible malignancy, particularly colon cancer.

B. Blood loss results in anemia via a reduction in heme synthesis. With loss of blood comes loss of iron, the central ion in the oxygen-carrying molecule, heme. When there is iron deficiency, the final step in heme synthesis, during which ferrous iron is inserted into protoporphyrin IX, is interrupted, resulting in inadequate heme synthesis. Globin biosynthesis is inhibited by heme deficiency through a **heme-regulated translational inhibitor** (**HRI**). Elevated HRI activity (a result of heme deficiency) inhibits a key transcription initiation factor for heme synthesis, eIF2. Thus, there are both less heme and fewer globin chains available in each red cell precursor. This directly causes anemia, a decrease in the hemoglobin concentration of the blood.

C. In this man, because he is symptomatic, the peripheral blood smear is likely to be significantly abnormal. As the hemoglobin concentration of individual red blood cells falls, the cells take on the classic picture of microcytic (small), hypochromic (pale) erythrocytes. There is also apt to be anisocytosis (variation in size) and poikilocytosis (variation in shape), with target cells. The target cells occur because of the relative excess of red cell membrane compared with the amount of hemoglobin within the cell, leading to "bunching up" of the membrane in the center.

D. Laboratory tests may be ordered to confirm the diagnosis. The most commonly ordered test is serum ferritin, which, if low, is diagnostic of iron deficiency. Results may be misleading, however, in acute or chronic inflammation and severe illness. Because ferritin is an acute-phase reactant, it can rise in these conditions, resulting in a normal ferritin level. Serum iron and transferrin levels can also be misleading because these levels can fall not only in anemia but also in many other illnesses. Typically in iron deficiency, however, serum iron levels are low, whereas total iron-binding capacity (TIBC) is elevated. The ratio of serum iron to TIBC is less than 20% in uncomplicated iron deficiency. Serum (soluble) transferrin receptor (TfR), released by erythroid precursors, is elevated in iron deficiency. A high ratio of TfR to ferritin may predict iron deficiency when ferritin is not diagnostically low.

Occasionally, when blood tests are misleading, a bone marrow biopsy is performed to examine for iron stores. Iron is normally stored as ferritin in the macrophages of the bone marrow and is stained blue by Prussian blue stain. A decrease in the amount of iron stores on bone marrow biopsy is diagnostic of iron deficiency. More commonly, however, the response to an empiric trial of iron supplementation is used to determine the presence of iron deficiency in complicated cases.

E. Fatigue, weakness, and shortness of breath are the direct results of decreased oxygen-carrying capacity, which leads to decreased oxygen delivery to metabolically active tissues, causing this patient's symptoms. He is pale because there is less oxygenated hemoglobin per unit of blood, and oxygenated hemoglobin is red, giving color to the skin. Pallor results also from a compensatory mechanism whereby superficial blood vessels constrict, diverting blood to more vital structures.

CASE 25

A. The probable cause of this woman's anemia is vitamin B_{12} (cobalamin) deficiency, which is characterized by anemia, glossitis, and neurologic impairment. Vitamin B_{12} deficiency results in anemia via effects on DNA synthesis. Cobalamin is a crucial cofactor in the synthesis of deoxythymidine from deoxyuridine. Cobalamin accepts a methyl group from methyltetrahydrofolate, leading to the formation of methylcobalamin and reduced tetrahydrofolate. Methylcobalamin is required for the production of the amino acid methionine from homocysteine. Reduced tetrahydrofolate is required as the single-carbon donor in purine synthesis. Thus, cobalamin deficiency depletes stores of tetrahydrofolate, lowering purine production and impairing DNA synthesis. Impaired DNA synthesis results in decreased production of red blood cells. It also causes megaloblastic changes in the blood cells in the bone marrow. These cells are subsequently destroyed in large numbers by intramedullary hemolysis. Both processes result in anemia.

B. The peripheral blood smear varies depending on the duration of cobalamin deficiency. In this patient, because she is profoundly symptomatic, we would expect a full-blown megaloblastic anemia. The peripheral smear would have significant anisocytosis and poikilocytosis of the red cells as well as hypersegmentation of the neutrophils. In severe cases, morphologic changes in peripheral blood cells may be difficult to differentiate from those seen in leukemia.

Other laboratory tests that may be ordered include a lactate dehydrogenase (LDH) level and indirect bilirubin determination. Both should be elevated in cobalamin deficiency, reflecting the intramedullary hemolysis that occurs in vitamin B_{12} deficiency. Serum vitamin B_{12} would be expected to be low. Antibodies to intrinsic factor are usually detectable. Concurrent elevations of both serum methylmalonic acid and serum homocysteine are highly predictive of B_{12} deficiency.

The various causes of megaloblastic anemia can often be differentiated by a Schilling test. This test measures the oral absorption of radioactively labeled vitamin B_{12} with and without added intrinsic factor, thereby directly evaluating the mecha-

nism of the vitamin deficiency. It must be performed after cobalamin stores have been replenished.

C. Pernicious anemia is caused by autoimmune destruction of the gastric parietal cells, which are responsible for production of stomach acid and intrinsic factor. Autoimmune destruction of these cells leads to achlorhydria (loss of stomach acid), which is required for release of cobalamin from foodstuffs. The production of intrinsic factor decreases. Intrinsic factor is required for the effective absorption of cobalamin by the terminal ileum. Together these mechanisms result in vitamin B_{12} deficiency.

The evidence that parietal cell destruction is autoimmune in nature is strong. Pathologically, patients with pernicious anemia demonstrate gastric mucosal atrophy with infiltrating lymphocytes, predominantly antibody-producing B cells. Furthermore, more than 90% of patients with this disease demonstrate antibodies to parietal cell membrane proteins, primarily to the proton pump. More than half of patients also have antibodies to intrinsic factor or to the intrinsic factor-cobalamin complex. These patients also have an increased risk of other autoimmune diseases.

D. The patient's tachycardia is probably a reflection of profound anemia. Unlike many other causes of anemia, pernicious anemia often leads to very severe decreases in the hemoglobin concentration. This results in a marked decrease in the oxygen-carrying capacity of the blood. The only way to increase oxygenation to metabolically active tissues is to increase cardiac output. This is accomplished by raising the heart rate. Over time, the stresses this puts on the heart can result in high-output congestive heart failure.

The neurologic manifestations—paresthesias and impaired proprioception—seen in this patient are caused by demyelination of the peripheral nerves and posterolateral spinal columns, respectively. The lack of methionine caused by vitamin B_{12} deficiency appears to be at least partly responsible for this demyelination, but the exact mechanism is unknown. Demyelination eventually results in neuronal cell death. Therefore, neurologic symptoms may not be improved by treatment of the vitamin B_{12} deficiency.

CASE 26

A. Classic, childhood-onset cyclic neutropenia results from mutations in the gene for a single enzyme, neutrophil elastase. Most cases reflect an autosomal dominant inheritance; however, sporadic adult cases also occur, and these are associated with neutrophil elastase mutations as well.

Studies of neutrophil kinetics in affected patients reveal that the gene defect results in abnormal production—rather than abnormal disposition—of neutrophils. In cyclic neutropenia, it is hypothesized that the mutant neutrophil elastase may have an overly inhibitory effect, causing prolonged trough periods and inadequate storage pools to maintain a normal peripheral neutrophil count. This production defect affects other cell lines as well, resulting in cyclic depletion of all storage pools. Because development of neutrophils from progenitor stage to maturity takes 2 weeks and the life span is only 12 days, depletion of the neutrophil cell line becomes clinically apparent. The other cell lines have longer life spans, and although they too undergo cyclic decreases in production, these decreases do not become clinically apparent.

The exact cause of the relationship between the cyclic waves of maturation and the neutrophil elastase mutation is not known. Because multiple cell lines are seen to cycle, it is believed that neutrophil elastase mutations accelerate the process of **apoptosis** (programmed cell death) in early progenitor cells unless they are "rescued" by granulocyte colony-stimulating factor (G-CSF). Some evidence suggests that neutrophil elastase can antagonize G-CSF action, but the relationship of mutated neutrophil elastase to G-CSF action in cyclic neutropenia is not well understood.

Clinically, administration of pharmacologic doses of G-CSF (filgrastim) to affected individuals has three interesting effects that partially overcome the condition. First, although cycling continues, mean neutrophil counts increase at each point in the cycle, such that patients are rarely neutropenic. Second, cycling periodicity decreases immediately from 21 days to 14 days. Third, other cell line fluctuations change in parallel; their cycle periodicity also decreases to 14 days, suggesting that an early progenitor cell is indeed at the center of this illness. However, the fact that cycling does not disappear demonstrates that there are other abnormalities yet to be discovered. It also suggests that there may be an inherent cycling of all stem cells in normal individuals, which is modulated by multiple cytokines in the marrow.

B. The periodic neutropenia with spontaneous remission seen in this patient is characteristic of cyclic neutropenia. In this disease, patients develop a drop in neutrophil count approximately every 3 weeks (19–22 days), with nadirs (low neutrophil counts) lasting 3–5 days. Patients are generally well during periods when the neutrophil cell count is normal and become symptomatic as the counts drop below 250/μL. Neutrophils are responsible for a significant portion of the immune system's response to both bacterial and fungal infections. Thus, the primary clinical manifestation of cyclic neutropenia is recurrent infection. Each nadir is usually characterized by symptoms of fever and malaise. Cervical lymphadenopathy and oral ulcers, as seen in this patient, are also common. Life-threatening bacterial and fungal infections are uncommon but can occur, particularly as a result of infection from endogenous gut flora. More commonly, however, patients develop skin infections and chronic gingivitis.

C. The peripheral blood smear should be normal except for a paucity of neutrophils. Those neutrophils present would be normal in appearance. The bone marrow, however, would be expected to show increased numbers of myeloid precursors such as promyelocytes and myelocytes. Mature neutrophils would be

rare. If marrow examination were repeated in 2 weeks—after neutrophil counts have improved—the results would be normal.

CASE 27

A. The most likely diagnosis in this patient is drug-associated immune thrombocytopenia. Many drugs—but most commonly heparin—have been associated with this phenomenon.

B. Heparin leads to thrombocytopenia via two distinct mechanisms, both involving antibodies. It appears that heparin can bind to a platelet-produced protein, platelet factor 4 (PF4), which is released by platelets in response to activation. The heparin-PF4 complex acts as an antigenic stimulus, provoking the production of IgG. IgG can then bind to the complex, forming IgG-heparin-PF4. The new complex can bind to platelets via the Fc receptor of the IgG molecule or via the PF4 receptor. This binding can lead to two distinct phenomena. The first is platelet destruction by the spleen. Antibody adherence to the platelets changes their shape, causing the spleen to recognize them as abnormal and destroy them. This leads to simple thrombocytopenia, with few sequelae.

The second phenomenon is platelet activation, which can lead to more significant sequelae. After formation of an IgG-heparin-PF4 complex, both IgG and PF4 can bind to platelets. The platelets can become cross-linked, leading to platelet aggregation. This decreases the number of circulating platelets, leading to thrombocytopenia. However, it may also lead to the formation of thrombus, or "white clot."

C. Even though the platelet count in drug-associated immune thrombocytopenia may be very low, significant bleeding is unusual. Most commonly, the primary manifestation is easy bruising, and, at platelet counts less than 5000/μL, petechiae may be seen on the skin or mucous membranes. When actual bleeding does occur, it is generally mucosal in origin, such as nosebleed, gingival bleeding, or GI blood loss.

As noted, when thrombocytopenia is due to heparin, paradoxical clotting may occur instead of bleeding. Thrombus formation often occurs at the site of previous vascular injury or abnormality and can present as either arterial or venous thrombosis.

CASE 28

A. Virchow's triad consists of three possible contributors to the formation of a clot: decreased blood flow, blood vessel injury or inflammation, and changes in the intrinsic properties of the blood. This patient has no history of immobility or other cause of decreased blood flow. She does, however, have a history of blood vessel injury (ie, deep vein thrombosis). Despite the absence of symptoms of a lower extremity thrombosis, this is still the most likely site of origin of the pulmonary embolus. Finally, the recurrence now of thrombus formation along with the family history of clots is suggestive of a change in the intrinsic properties of the blood, as seen in the inherited hypercoagulable states.

B. The most common hypercoagulable states include activated protein C resistance (factor V Leiden), protein C deficiency, protein S deficiency, antithrombin III deficiency, and hyperprothrombinemia (prothrombin gene mutation). Except for hyperprothrombinemia, each of these results in clot formation because of a lack of adequate anticoagulation rather than overproduction of procoagulant activity; hyperprothrombinemia is caused by excess thrombin generation.

The most common site of the problem in the coagulation cascade is at factor Va, which is required for activation of factor X, the central factor in the entire coagulation cascade. Protein C is the major inhibitor of factor Va. It acts by cleaving factor V into an inactive form, thereby slowing the activation of factor X. The negative effect of protein C is enhanced by protein S. Quantitative or qualitative reduction in either of these two proteins thus results in the unregulated procoagulant action of factor Xa.

Activated protein C resistance is the most common inherited hypercoagulable state. It results from a mutation in the factor V gene. This mutation alters the three-dimensional conformation of the cleavage site within factor Va, where protein C usually binds. Protein C is then unable to bind to factor Va and is, therefore, unable to inactivate it. Coagulation is not inhibited.

Antithrombin inhibits the coagulation cascade at an alternative site. It inhibits the serine proteases: factors II, IX, X, XI, and XII. Deficiency of antithrombin results in an inability to inactivate these factors, allowing the coagulation cascade to proceed unrestrained at multiple coagulation steps.

Hyperprothrombinemia is the second most common hereditary hypercoagulable state and the only one so far recognized as being due to overproduction of procoagulant factors. It is caused by a mutation of the prothrombin gene that leads to elevated prothrombin levels. The increased risk of thrombosis is thought to be due to excess thrombin generation when the Xa-Va-Ca^{2+}-PL complex is activated.

C. This patient may be evaluated by various laboratory tests for the presence of an inherited hypercoagulable state. Quantitative evaluation of the relative amounts of protein C, protein S, and antithrombin can be performed. Qualitative tests that assess the ability of these proteins to inhibit the coagulation cascade can be measured via clotting assays. The presence of the specific mutation in factor V Leiden can be assessed via polymerase chain reaction testing.

CASE 29

A. This patient has parkinsonism. The resting tremor (which improves with activity), "cog-wheeling" rigidity, and difficulty with gait (especially with initiation of walking and with changing direction) are all characteristic of parkinsonism. While there are many causes of parkinsonism, including toxins, head trauma, drugs, encephalitis, and other degenerative diseases, the most common cause is Parkinson disease, an idiopathic degenerative neurological disorder.

B. Parkinson disease results from selective degeneration of the monoamine-containing neurons in the basal ganglia and brainstem, particularly the pigmented dopaminergic neurons of the substantia nigra. This region is involved in regulation of movement, particularly in initiating and stopping actions. In addition to the degeneration of the dopaminergic neurons, scattered neurons elsewhere contain eosinophilic cytoplasmic inclusion bodies, called Lewy bodies.

C. Through studies of familial cases of Parkinson disease as well as parkinsonism produced by toxins, some of the molecular processes involved have been discovered. One cause of parkinsonism is 1-methyl-4-phenyl-1,2,3,6-tetrahydropyridine (MPTP), a neurotoxin that was once a contaminant in illicit opioid drugs. It caused parkinsonism by being metabolized to *N*-methyl-4-phenylpyridinium (MPP+), which was taken up through dopamine uptake sites on dopamine nerve terminals and concentrated in mitochondria. This led to disturbed mitochondrial function and ultimately to cell death. In familial cases of Parkinson disease, there have been several mutations identified involving genes encoding several proteins: parkin, alpha-synuclein, DJ-1, ubiquitin, and PTEN-induced kinase. Leucine-rich repeat kinase 2 (LRRK2) mutation is a recently discovered genetic cause of Parkinson disease and accounts for 4% of familial cases. These mutations are being studied to find clues about the molecular mechanisms involved in the pathogenesis of Parkinson disease.

CASE 30

A. The most likely diagnosis in this patient is myasthenia gravis, a disease characterized by fluctuating fatigue and weakness of muscles with small motor units, particularly the ocular muscles. Myasthenia gravis is an autoimmune disorder resulting in simplification of the postsynaptic region of the neuromuscular end plate. Patients with this disease have lymphocytic infiltration at the end plate plus antibody and complement deposition along the postsynaptic membrane. Circulating antibodies to the receptor are present in 90% of patients, blocking acetylcholine binding and activation. The antibodies can cross-link the receptor molecules, leading to receptor internalization and degradation. They also activate complement-mediated destruction of the postsynaptic region, resulting in simplification of the end plate. Many patients who lack antibodies to the acetylcholine receptor instead have autoantibodies against the muscle-specific receptor tyrosine kinase, which is an important mediator of acetylcholine receptor clustering at the end plate. These antibodies inhibit clustering of receptors in muscle cell culture. Thus, patients with myasthenia gravis have impaired ability to respond to acetylcholine release from the presynaptic membrane.

B. Muscles with small motor units are most affected in myasthenia gravis. The ocular muscles are most frequently affected; oropharyngeal muscles, flexors and extensors of the neck and proximal limbs, and erector spinae muscles are next most commonly involved. In severe cases and without treatment, the disease can progress to involve all muscles, including the diaphragm and intercostal muscles, resulting in respiratory failure.

C. Normally, the number of quanta of acetylcholine released from the nerve terminal decreases with repetitive stimuli. There are usually no clinical consequences of this decrease because a sufficient number of acetylcholine receptor channels are opened despite the reduced amount of neurotransmitter. In myasthenia gravis, however, there is a deficiency in the number of acetylcholine receptors. Therefore, as the number of quanta released decreases, there is a decremental decline in neurotransmission at the neuromuscular junction. This is manifested clinically as muscle fatigue with sustained or repeated activity.

D. Myasthenia gravis is associated both with a family history of autoimmune disease and with the presence of coexisting autoimmune diseases. Hyperthyroidism, rheumatoid arthritis, systemic lupus erythematosus, and polymyositis are all seen with increased frequency in these patients. These patients also have a high incidence of thymic disease; most demonstrate thymic hyperplasia and 10–15% have thymomas.

E. There are two basic strategies for treating this disease: decreasing the immune-mediated destruction of the acetylcholine receptors and increasing the amount of acetylcholine available at the neuromuscular junction. As noted previously, many patients with myasthenia gravis demonstrate disease of the thymus gland. The thymus is thought to play a role in the pathogenesis of myasthenia gravis by supplying helper T cells that are sensitized to thymic nicotinic receptors. Removal of the thymus in patients with generalized myasthenia gravis can improve symptoms and even induce remission. Plasmapheresis, corticosteroids, and immunosuppressant drugs can all be used to reduce the levels of antibody to acetylcholine receptors, thereby suppressing disease. Increasing the amount of acetylcholine available at the neuromuscular junction is accomplished by the use of cholinesterase inhibitors. Cholinesterase is responsible for the breakdown of acetylcholine at the neuromuscular junction. By inhibiting the breakdown of acetylcholine, cholinesterase inhibitors can compensate for the normal decline in released neurotransmitter during repeated stimulation and thus decrease symptoms.

CASE 31

A. The characteristic pathologic finding in Alzheimer's disease (AD) is the finding of neuritic plaques, made of a dense amyloid core surrounded by dystrophic neuritis, reactive astrocytes, and microglia. There are also neurofibrillary tangles, synaptic loss, and neuronal loss. Interestingly, the severity of disease does not correlate with plaque number.

B. In neurological disorders, the location of the lesion predicts what function will be affected. In AD, the neuritic plaques are most prominent in the hippocampus, entorhinal cortex, association cortex, and basal forebrain. These are areas involved in memory and higher order cortical functions such as judgment and insight. This explains why memory loss, poor judgment, and denial are such common presenting symptoms. In contrast, the motor and sensory cortexes are not prominently affected, and thus loss of motor and sensory function is not present until much later in the course of the disease.

C. The major protein in neuritic plaques is amyloid beta-peptide. This is a protein derived from beta-amyloid precursor protein (APP) that is encoded by a gene on chromosome 21. Increased production of APP results in increased amyloid beta-peptide, which is known to be toxic to cultured neurons. Individuals who produce excess APP, such as people with trisomy 21 or families with inherited mutations of the APP gene, develop early onset AD.

D. Currently, there is no role for genetic testing for AD. Only about 10% of the cases of AD are familial, and in these cases, several different mutations have been identified in affected families. It has also been recognized that individuals with a subtype 4 of apolipoprotein E have an increased risk of developing AD. However, 15% of the population carries this subtype, and most cases of AD develop in people who do not carry this subtype. Even among carriers, many never develop AD. Therefore, testing for it is not recommended.

CASE 32

A. Generalized tonic-clonic seizures are characterized by sudden loss of consciousness followed rapidly by tonic contraction of the muscles, causing extension of the limbs and arching of the back. This phase lasts approximately 10–30 seconds and is followed by a clonic phase of limb jerking. The jerking builds in frequency, peaking after 15–30 seconds, and then gradually slows over another 15–30 seconds. The patient may remain unconscious for several minutes after the seizure. This is generally followed by a period of confusion lasting minutes to hours.

B. Recurrent seizures are in many cases idiopathic, particularly those seen in children. Seizures may also be due to brain injury from trauma, stroke, mass lesion, or infection. Finally, one must consider metabolic causes such as hypoglycemia, electrolyte abnormalities, and alcohol withdrawal. The cause of this patient's seizure is unknown because of the lack of an available history.

However, because he has focal neurologic findings, with decreased movement of his left side, one must suspect an underlying brain lesion in the right cerebral hemisphere.

C. Seizures occur when neurons are activated synchronously. The kind of seizure depends on the location of the abnormal activity and the pattern of spread to different parts of the brain. The formation of a seizure focus in the brain may result from disruption of normal inhibitory circuits. This disruption may occur because of alterations in ion channels or from injury to inhibitory neurons and synapses. Alternatively, a seizure focus may be formed when groups of neurons become synchronized by reorganization of neural networks after brain injury. After formation of a seizure focus, local discharge may then spread. This spread occurs by a combination of mechanisms. After synchronous depolarization of abnormally excitable neurons—known as the paroxysmal depolarizing shift—extracellular potassium accumulates, depolarizing nearby neurons. Increased frequency of depolarization then leads to increased calcium influx into nerve terminals. This increases neurotransmitter release at excitatory synapses by a process known as posttetanic potentiation, whereby normally quiescent voltage-gated and *N*-methyl-D-aspartate (NMDA) receptor-gated excitatory synaptic neurotransmission is increased and inhibitory synaptic neurotransmission is decreased. The net effect of these changes is recruitment of neighboring neurons into a synchronous discharge, causing a seizure.

CASE 33

A. The diagnosis in this patient is stroke, characterized by the sudden onset of focal neurologic deficits that persist for at least 24 hours. The focal symptoms and signs that result from stroke correlate with the area of the brain supplied by the affected blood vessel. In this case, the patient has weakness and sensory loss on the right side. These symptoms suggest involvement of the left middle cerebral artery or at least its associated vascular territory. The vascular territory supplied by the middle cerebral artery includes the lateral frontal, parietal, lateral occipital, and anterior and superior temporal cortex and adjacent white matter as well as the caudate, putamen, and internal capsule.

B. Risk factors for stroke include age, male sex, hypertension, hypercholesterolemia, diabetes, smoking, heavy alcohol consumption, and oral contraceptives.

C. Stroke is classified as either ischemic or hemorrhagic in origin. Ischemic stroke may result from thrombotic or embolic occlusion of the vessel. Hemorrhagic stroke may result from intraparenchymal hemorrhage, subarachnoid hemorrhage, subdural hemorrhage, epidural hemorrhage, or hemorrhage within an ischemic infarction. Given the CT scan result, it is likely that this man has sustained an ischemic rather than a

hemorrhagic stroke. Hemorrhagic and ischemic strokes can be difficult to differentiate on clinical grounds, but the former often produce a less predictable pattern of neurologic deficits. This is because the neurologic deficits in hemorrhagic stroke depend both on the location of the bleed and on factors that affect brain function at a distance from the hemorrhage, including increased intracranial pressure, edema, compression of neighboring brain tissue, and rupture of blood into the ventricles or subarachnoid space.

D. The most likely underlying cause of stroke in this patient is atherosclerosis. Atherosclerosis arises from vascular endothelial cell injury, often caused by chronic hypertension or hypercholesterolemia, both present in this man. Endothelial injury stimulates attachment of circulating monocytes and lymphocytes that migrate into the vessel wall and stimulate proliferation of smooth muscle cells and fibroblasts. This results in plaque formation. Damaged endothelium also serves as a nidus of platelet aggregation that further stimulates proliferation of smooth muscle and fibroblasts. The plaques formed may enlarge and occlude the vessel, leading to thrombotic stroke, or may rupture, releasing emboli and causing embolic stroke.

CASE 34

A. The lesions described are characteristic of psoriasis vulgaris. Psoriasis is both a genetic and an environmental disorder. A genetic origin is supported by several lines of evidence. There is a high rate of concordance for psoriasis in monozygotic twins and an increased incidence of psoriasis in the relatives of affected individuals. Furthermore, overexpression of gene products of class I alleles of the major histocompatibility complex (MHC) is seen in patients with psoriasis. However, psoriasis is not likely to be completely genetic in nature. Individuals with a genetic predisposition to the disorder appear to require environmental triggers, at least in some cases, such as trauma, cold weather, infections, and various medications.

B. In psoriasis, there is shortening of the usual duration of the keratinocyte cell cycle and doubling of the proliferative cell population. This excessive epidermatopoiesis results in skin thickening and plaque formation. In addition to skin thickening, truncation of the cell cycle leads to an accumulation of cells within the cornified layer with retained nuclei. This pattern is known as parakeratosis and results in neutrophil migration into the cornified layer. Together these form the silvery scale characteristic of psoriasis. Finally, psoriasis induces endothelial cell proliferation, resulting in pronounced dilation, tortuosity, and increased permeability of the capillaries in the superficial dermis and causing erythema.

C. Many immunologic abnormalities have been implicated in psoriasis, but the exact pathophysiologic mechanism remains unclear. As mentioned, psoriasis is associated with overexpression of MHC class I gene products. This suggests that CD8 T lymphocytes are involved, because the complex of MHC class I protein and antigen is the ligand of the T-cell receptor of CD8 cells. Also seen in psoriasis is overexpression of a large number of cytokines, particularly IL-2.

CASE 35

A. The lesions described are characteristic of the "pruritic polygonal purple papules" of lichen planus. Although the triggers of lichen planus are often obscure, several drugs have been implicated. Antimalarial agents (eg, chloroquine) and therapeutic gold are the drugs most closely linked to this phenomenon. It is believed that these agents and other unknown triggers result in a cell-mediated autoimmune reaction leading to damage of the basal keratinocytes of the epidermis.

B. As mentioned, the triggers leading to lichen planus formation are often idiopathic. However, it appears that some form of antigenic stimulation leads to infiltration and activation of CD4 T lymphocytes. These stimulated CD4 cells elaborate cytokines, leading to the recruitment of cytotoxic T lymphocytes. Cell-mediated cytotoxicity, cytokines, interferon-γ, and tumor necrosis factor combine to injure keratinocytes and contribute to vacuolization and necrosis of these cells. Injured, enucleated keratinocytes coalesce to form colloid bodies. Melanocytes are destroyed as "innocent bystanders," and melanin is phagocytosed by macrophages.

C. The appearance of the lichen planus papules is a direct reflection of the underlying histopathologic features. The dense array of lymphocytes in the superficial dermis yields the elevated, flat-topped appearance of the papule. The whitish coloration—Wickham's striae—results from chronic inflammation and hyperkeratosis of the cornified layer of the epidermis. The purple hue of the lesions is caused by the macrophage phagocytosis of the released melanin to form melanocytes. Although the melanin is brown-black, the melanophages are embedded in a colloid matrix. This causes extensive scattering of light by an effect known as the Tyndall effect, resulting in interpretation of the lesion as dusky or violaceous by the human eye.

CASE 36

A. The lesions described are characteristic of erythema multiforme. The lack of mucosal involvement suggests erythema multiforme minor.

B. Erythema multiforme is similar to lichen planus in that both are interface dermatitides and both are caused by some inciting agent that results in lymphocyte migration to the epidermis and papillary dermis. Cytotoxic T cells then combine with elaborated cytokines, interferon-γ, and tumor necrosis

factor to kill keratinocytes, resulting in enucleation, vacuolization, and coalescence to form colloid bodies.

Unlike lichen planus, with its dense dermal inflammatory infiltrate, the dermal infiltrate of lymphocytes in erythema multiforme is sparse. Thus, the vacuolated keratinocytes widely distributed in the epidermal basal layer are more conspicuous.

C. Many cases of erythema multiforme minor are triggered by herpes simplex virus (HSV), as seen in this patient. The evidence to support this association derives from both clinical and molecular data. Clinically, it has long been documented that erythema multiforme is often preceded by herpes simplex infection. Furthermore, antiherpetic agents such as acyclovir can suppress the development of erythema multiforme in some individuals. Molecular studies have confirmed the presence of herpes simplex DNA within skin from erythema multiforme lesions. HSV DNA is also present in the peripheral blood lymphocytes and lesional skin after resolution of the rash but is not found in nonlesional skin.

D. The target-like lesions seen in erythema multiforme reflect zonal differences in the inflammatory response and its deleterious effects. At the periphery of the lesion, inflammation and vacuolization are sparse, resulting in the erythematous halo. The dusky bull's eye in the center, on the other hand, is an area of dense epidermal vacuolization and necrosis.

CASE 37

A. The major alternative diagnoses to consider are bullous pemphigoid and pemphigus, although other blistering diseases such as erythema multiforme and dermatitis herpetiformis should be considered as well. Bullous pemphigoid is characterized by subepidermal and pemphigus by intraepidermal vesiculation. The distinction is important because bullous pemphigoid has a more favorable prognosis.

B. Microscopically, bullous pemphigoid lesions show a subepidermal cleft containing lymphocytes, eosinophils, neutrophils, and eosinophilic material, representing extravasated macromolecules such as fibrin. An inflammatory infiltrate of eosinophils, neutrophils, and lymphocytes is also present in the dermis beneath the cleft.

C. Direct immunofluorescence microscopy demonstrates IgG and C3 bound in a linear distribution along the epidermal-dermal junction. These autoantibodies are bound to a 230-kDa protein within the lamina lucida, known as the "bullous pemphigoid antigen." This antigen has been localized to the hemidesmosomal complex of the epidermal basal cell. Its role is not established.

D. Blister formation is believed to begin with the binding of IgG to the bullous pemphigoid antigen, activating the complement cascade. Complement fragments then induce mast cell degranulation and attract neutrophils and eosinophils. The granulocytes and mast cells release multiple enzymes, resulting in enzymatic digestion of the epidermal-dermal junction and separation of the layers. It is also possible that the bullous pemphigoid antigen plays a vital structural role that is compromised when the autoantibodies bind, leading to cleavage of the epidermal-dermal junction.

CASE 38

A. Palpable purpura over the distal lower extremities or other dependent areas—recurring over a period of months—and histologic study revealing fibrinoid necrosis are most consistent with leukocytoclastic vasculitis. Common precipitants include infections and medications. Bacterial, mycobacterial, and viral infections can all trigger leukocytoclastic vasculitis; *Streptococcus* and *Staphylococcus* are the most common infectious precipitants. *S pneumoniae* is the most common cause of pneumonia in this age group and may have been the precipitant in this man. Hepatitis C is also associated with leukocytoclastic vasculitis. Many drugs have been associated with this disorder, including antibiotics, thiazides, and nonsteroidal anti-inflammatory drugs (NSAIDs). Of the antibiotics, penicillins, such as the amoxicillin given to this man, are the most common offenders.

B. Eliciting factors such as microbial antigens or medications trigger the formation of immune complexes, consisting of antibodies bound to the exogenous antigen. For reasons not yet clear, these complexes are preferentially deposited in the small cutaneous vessels (venules). After becoming trapped in the tissue of the venules, the immune complexes activate the complement cascade, and localized production of chemotactic fragments and vasoactive molecules ensues. This attracts neutrophils, which release enzymes, resulting in destruction of the immune complexes, neutrophils, and vessels. Ultimately, erythrocytes and fibrin are able to exude through the vessel wall and enter the surrounding dermis, resulting in the classic finding of palpable purpura.

C. Leukocytoclastic vasculitis lesions are raised and papular because lesional skin is altered and expanded by an intense vasocentric infiltrate containing numerous neutrophils. The lesions are purpuric or erythematous because of the extravasated red blood cells that accumulate in the dermis.

D. Leukocytoclastic vasculitis may also involve small vessels in other portions of the body, including the joint capsules, soft tissues, kidneys, liver, and GI tract. The most common systemic symptoms include arthralgias, myalgias, and abdominal pain. It would be important to evaluate for these symptoms and order laboratory tests to assess liver or renal involvement.

CASE 39

A. The diagnosis is likely to be *Rhus* dermatitis (poison ivy and oak), a form of allergic contact dermatitis. The history of hiking in a heavily wooded area 2 days before onset of the rash is a helpful clue. However, the finding on physical examination of blisters arranged in straight lines helps make the diagnosis. Straight lines and angles suggest an exogenous cause for a skin eruption. In this case, poison ivy leaves traced a line across the skin as the patient walked through the brush, and she developed an allergic contact dermatitis in the pattern of the exposure.

B. A common misconception regarding *Rhus* dermatitis is that blister fluid from broken blisters (or even touching the blistered area) causes the eruption to spread. In fact, once the eruption has developed, the allergen has been irreversibly bound to other proteins or has been so degraded that it cannot be transferred to other sites. In this case, the patient developed large blisters or bullae in response to the contactant at the original sites of contact, the legs. This means that she had a severe reaction to the allergen. Intense inflammation such as this can result in the autosensitization phenomenon, which in this case explains the development of ill-defined erythematous plaques with small papules and vesicles within the plaques seen on this patient's arms and trunk. Alternatively, inadvertent contact with contaminated clothes or other surfaces can induce new areas of dermatitis. The *Rhus* allergen is tremendously stable and can persist on unwashed clothing and remain capable of inducing allergic contact dermatitis for up to 1 year.

C. If the allergen exposure is transient, the first exposure to a *Rhus* antigen often does not result in a reaction at the exposure site. However, a contingent of "armed and ready" memory T cells is now policing the skin, waiting for the allergen to reappear. The individual is said to be sensitized. When the person is exposed to the antigen again, the elicitation phase begins. Langerhans' cells process antigen and migrate to lymph nodes, but presentation and T-cell proliferation also occur at the site of contact with the allergen. Nonspecific T cells in the vicinity are recruited and stimulated by the inflammatory cytokines released by the specifically reactive T cells, and an amplification loop ensues, eventuating in clinically recognizable dermatitis. This complex series of events takes time to develop, resulting in the 24- to 48-hour delay between reexposure and rash eruption.

CASE 40

A. The probable diagnosis is erythema nodosum (EN), given their appearance as tender ill-defined nodules. The anterior lower legs are the most common locations for such lesions to develop. The patient probably has subclinical streptococcal pharyngitis. The fact that the patient herself had symptoms of pharyngitis, which were alleviated with antibiotics, is helpful. However, because the antibiotics course was much shorter than required (2 days vs. the standard 10), she must be suspected of having a partially treated (subclinical) infection. Until the infection is adequately treated, the patient will continue to manifest EN as a hypersensitivity response. Once the infection has been eradicated, the skin lesions should subside within several weeks. Persistent EN should prompt a thorough search for an alternate cause.

B. Common causes of EN include streptococcal pharyngitis, many different medications (including sulfa drugs), estrogen-containing oral contraceptives or pregnancy, and inflammatory bowel disease. There are numerous other possible causes.

C. Erythema nodosum is thought to represent a systemic delayed-type hypersensitivity reaction that localizes to the subcutis for unknown reasons.

D. In erythema nodosum, the inflammatory response consists of lymphocytes, histiocytes, neutrophils, and eosinophils scattered throughout the septal compartment of the subcutis with frequent multinucleated histiocytes. The septa are thickened and may become fibrotic, depending on the density of the infiltrate and the duration of the reaction. Even though the infiltrate is largely confined to subcutaneous septa, there is commonly an element of fat necrosis at the edges of the subcutaneous lobules in erythema nodosum. Evidence of fat necrosis may be seen in the form of an infiltrate of "foamy" (lipid-laden) macrophages at the periphery of subcutaneous lobules or in the form of small stellate clefts within multinucleate macrophages, indicating an element of lipomembranous fat necrosis.

CASE 41

A. The likely diagnosis is sarcoidosis. Because sarcoidosis is a diagnosis of exclusion, a thorough workup for specific causes is warranted. A skin biopsy should demonstrate changes typical for sarcoidosis with negative histochemical stains for mycobacterial and fungal organisms. Additionally, tissue culture performed on affected skin should be negative. Chest x-ray film is helpful to rule out tuberculosis and to investigate the presence of hilar adenopathy. Bone films may demonstrate characteristic findings as well.

B. This patient has sarcoidal papules around the edges of the nostrils, a finding known as lupus pernio or nasal rim sarcoidosis. This finding indicates that this patient is at high risk for significant involvement of the tracheobronchial tree or lung parenchyma. The complaint of chronic cough should also suggest lung involvement. Regardless of symptoms and dermatologic presentation, the possibility of pulmonary involvement

should always be investigated in all cases of sarcoidosis because it is quite common and sometimes asymptomatic.

C. Sarcoidosis is a nodular dermatitis with histiocytic granulomas situated within the dermis. There are few lymphocytes present in and around the granulomas. Multinucleated histiocytes are frequently present.

D. Sarcoidosis is seen clinically as an elevation (papule, plaque, or nodule) caused by the expansion of the dermis by the infiltrate. There is no scale overlying the lesions because the epidermis is not affected.

CASE 42

A. Contrary to popular perception, acne is not caused by dirt clogging the pores. In fact, "blackheads" (open comedones) are black because of oxidation of the keratinaceous debris within the dilated follicles, not because of "dirt" at all. However, some exogenous substances such as oily cosmetics or petrolatum-based hair care products may promote comedone formation and thus exacerbate acne. Cleansing does not affect any of the four steps essential to the development of acne, because all of these steps occur within the follicles. Cleansing merely removes surface debris and oil. The patient should be advised to use a gentle soap or nonsoap cleanser designed for the face and to avoid scrubbing the skin with rough cloths, towels, or scrubbing pads, which is not helpful in ameliorating acne and may cause secondary irritation, making topical treatments less tolerable. She should also be advised to use nongreasy cosmetics, usually those labeled as "noncomedogenic," as well as hair care products without petrolatum.

B. Keratinocytes fail to slough from the follicles as they should. As a result, the follicle becomes plugged (a comedo). The buildup of sebum behind the plug expands the follicle. *Propionibacterium acnes* overgrowth in the follicle breaks down sebum. Bacterial factors and sebum breakdown products attract neutrophils to the follicle, thus forming a pustule. Follicular rupture induces an intense inflammatory response in the dermis seen clinically as an inflammatory papule or pustule. Scarring may be the end result.

C. Follicular plugging may be corrected with retinoids (vitamin A analogues) either topically or, if the condition is severe enough, orally. Retinoids promote the proper desquamation of keratinocytes. Bacteria are controlled with topical or oral antibiotics. Some common topical antibiotic agents include benzoyl peroxide and clindamycin. Oral antibiotics such as erythromycin or tetracycline are frequently used in addition to topical antibiotics. These agents are not merely antibacterial but are known to have anti-inflammatory properties independent of their antibacterial action. Last, sebum production may be decreased through the use of retinoids, again topically or orally, although oral therapy is much more effective for this purpose, or with antiandrogen medications such as spironolactone and oral contraceptives.

CASE 43

A. Asthma can be induced by many provocative agents. These can be broadly categorized as (1) physiologic or pharmacologic mediators of normal smooth muscle contraction, such as histamine; (2) physicochemical agents, such as cold or exercise; and (3) allergens, such as pollen. This patient's history (seasonal predilection) is most consistent with allergen-induced asthma. The worsening symptoms in the last few months may be due to an allergic reaction to the roommate's cat.

B. The earliest events in asthma are the activation of local inflammatory cells, primarily mast cells and eosinophils, by the provocative agents described previously. This can occur by specific IgE-dependent mechanisms or indirectly by chemical irritant exposure or osmotic stimuli. Acute-acting mediators, including leukotrienes, prostaglandins, and histamine, induce smooth muscle contraction, mucus hypersecretion, and vasodilation with endothelial leakage and local edema formation. Epithelial cells also participate, releasing leukotrienes, prostaglandins, and inflammatory cytokines. Additional inflammatory cells, including neutrophils and eosinophils, are recruited to the airway mucosa. In addition, the cell cytokines released promote growth of mast cells and eosinophils, the influx and proliferation of T cells, and the differentiation of B lymphocytes into IgE- and IgA-producing plasma cells. Ultimately, this ongoing inflammation results in injury to epithelial cells, denudation of the airway, greater exposure of afferent sensory nerves, and subsequent smooth muscle hyperresponsiveness, chronic inflammation, submucosal gland hypersecretion, and increased mucus volume.

C. Wheezing is caused by a combination of smooth muscle contraction and mucus hypersecretion and retention, resulting in airway caliber reduction and prolonged turbulent airflow. The sensations of shortness of breath and chest tightness are also the result of a number of concerted changes. These include the detection by spindle cell stretch receptors of the greater muscular effort required to overcome the increased airway resistance as well as detection of thoracic distention resulting from chest hyperinflation, decreased lung compliance, and increased work of breathing. These are sensed by the chest wall nerves and manifested as chest tightness and shortness of breath. As obstruction worsens, hypoxemia and CO_2 retention occur, further perpetuating the sensation of dyspnea (shortness of breath).

D. This patient's symptoms are relatively mild, occurring only intermittently. In between exacerbations, her pulmonary function tests may be normal. During an attack, all indices of expiratory airflow may be reduced, including FEV_1, FEV_1/FVC, and peak expiratory flow rate. FVC may also be reduced as a result of premature airway closure. Total lung capacity, functional residual capacity, and residual volume may be increased as a consequence of airflow obstruction and incomplete emptying of lung units. DLCO may be increased because of increased lung and capillary blood volume.

CASE 44

A. Although the primary insult and specific events in disease initiation remain unknown in idiopathic pulmonary fibrosis, a common series of cellular events that mediate and regulate the inflammatory process and fibrotic response have been described. This set of events includes (1) initial tissue injury; (2) vascular injury and activation, with increased permeability, exudation of plasma proteins into the extravascular space, and variable thrombosis and thrombolysis; (3) epithelial injury and activation, with loss of barrier integrity and release of proinflammatory mediators; (4) increased leukocyte adherence to activated endothelium, with transit of activated leukocytes into the interstitium; and (5) continued injury and repair processes characterized by alterations in cell populations and increased matrix production.

B. Chronic cough results from the chronic irritation of airways produced by the bronchial and bronchiolar distortion that accompanies fibrotic damage to terminal respiratory units. Multiple factors contribute to the symptom of dyspnea. The fibrosis of lung parenchyma and decrease in normal surfactant cells in idiopathic pulmonary fibrosis lead to a need for greater distending pressure for inspiration. This is sensed by the C fibers in fibrotic alveolar walls or the stretch receptors in the chest wall, causing the sensation of dyspnea. In severe disease, altered gas exchange with mismatching can cause significant hypoxia. Hypoxia contributes to both the sensation of dyspnea and the tachypnea noted on examination. The diffuse inspiratory crackles reflect the successive opening on inspiration of respiratory units that are collapsed owing to the fibrosis and the loss of normal surfactant. The cause of digital clubbing is not known.

C. Chest x-ray film may show small lung volumes; increased densities are more prominent in the lung periphery. In more advanced disease, honeycombing may be seen, reflecting fibrosis surrounding expanded small airspaces.

Pulmonary fibrosis produces a restrictive pattern on pulmonary function tests. This is manifested as reductions in TLC, FEV_1, and FVC, with preservation of or increases in FEV_1/FVC and expiratory flow rates. DLCO decreases progressively as fibrosis continues and lung capillaries are obliterated.

CASE 45

A. In general, heart failure can be caused by (1) inappropriate workloads placed on the heart, such as volume or pressure overload; (2) restricted filling of the heart; (3) myocyte loss; or

(4) decreased myocyte contractility. This patient's history of prior myocardial infarction has caused myocyte loss and is a likely cause of this man's heart failure. In addition, he has a long-standing history of hypertension and possible recent ischemia, both of which can cause decreased myocardial contractility and, therefore, heart failure.

B. Cardiogenic pulmonary edema, as is present in this patient, results from a net increase in transmural pressure (hydrostatic or oncotic). Increased transmural pressure may result from increased pulmonary venous pressure (causing increased capillary hydrostatic pressure), increased alveolar surface tension (thereby lowering interstitial hydrostatic pressure), or decreased capillary colloid osmotic pressure. When the rate of ultrafiltration rises beyond the capacity of the pericapillary lymphatics to remove it, interstitial fluid accumulates. If formation exceeds lymphatic clearance, alveolar flooding results.

CASE 46

A. Thromboemboli almost never originate in the pulmonary circulation. More than 95% of pulmonary thromboemboli arise from the deep veins of the lower extremity: the popliteal, femoral, and iliac veins. The findings of right lower extremity warmth, erythema, and swelling—along with a positive Homans' sign—in this patient support the view that this is very likely the site of origin of thromboembolism. It is important to note, however, that the absence of such lower extremity findings does not exclude the diagnosis of thrombus from the lower extremity, because findings are insensitive.

B. This patient has multiple risk factors for pulmonary embolism, and he was at high risk for such an event. He is older than 40 years, was anesthetized for more than 30 minutes for his total knee replacement, and underwent orthopedic surgery (risk imposed by immobilization). His risk for calf vein thrombosis is as high as 84%, and the risk of fatal pulmonary embolism is approximately 5%. All such patients should receive prophylactic therapy with anticoagulants postoperatively.

C. All patients with pulmonary emboli have some degree of mechanical obstruction. The effect depends on the proportion of the pulmonary circulation obstructed (how large the pulmonary embolus is) and the severity of preexisting cardiopulmonary disease. As the degree of obstruction of pulmonary circulation increases, pulmonary artery pressures rise, ultimately leading to right ventricular strain. In severe pulmonary embolism, occlusion of the pulmonary outflow tract may occur, severely reducing cardiac output and causing cardiovascular collapse and death.

D. Pulmonary embolism decreases or eliminates perfusion distal to the site of the occlusion. Initially, ventilation remains unchanged or even increased, resulting in lung segments with high $\dot{V}/\dot{Q}$ ratios. If there is complete obstruction of perfusion, alveolar dead space accumulates, resulting in impaired carbon dioxide excretion. After several hours, hypoperfusion reduces production of surfactant by type II alveolar cells, resulting in edema, alveolar collapse, and atelectasis. These latter changes may cause decreased ventilation. If perfusion to these areas increases, areas of low $\dot{V}/\dot{Q}$ ratios will occur. Such areas result in true shunting. An increase in the A-a ΔPO_2 is seen in more than two-thirds of cases, and hypoxemia is a common, though nonspecific, finding.

CASE 47

A. In acute respiratory distress syndrome (ARDS), the main pathophysiologic mechanism is the loss of integrity of the alveolar and/or the capillary epithelium. Normally, the alveolar epithelium is nearly impermeable to proteins, creating an osmotic gradient that keeps fluid from entering the alveoli. However, in ARDS, the alveolar and/or the capillary epithelium is injured, causing leakage of proteins and other osmotically active solutes into the interstitial space or into the alveoli themselves. The influx of solutes then draws in fluid and results in pulmonary edema. In addition, the protein products in the alveoli, particularly the fibrinogen and fibrin degradation products, inactivate surfactant, decreasing lung compliance and increasing alveolar collapse and causing atelectasis.

B. ARDS has many causes. ARDS can result from an inhalational injury that damages the alveolar epithelium directly. Possible causes include aspiration of acidic gastric contents, near drowning, inhalation of smoke, toxic gases, or chemicals, or high-pressure mechanical ventilation. ARDS can also result from circulatory factors that damage the capillary epithelium, such as circulating toxins in bacteremia, lung damage from severe hypotension, disseminated intravascular coagulation, high-altitude pulmonary edema, or pneumonia.

C. The severe hypoxia found in ARDS is due to several factors. First, alveolar atelectasis and edema reduce the number of alveoli available for gas exchange. Compounding the problem is that these nonventilated areas continue to be perfused, resulting in ventilation/perfusion ($\dot{V}/\dot{Q}$) mismatch and shunting. Also the lungs lose their compliance due to the accumulation of fluid, atelectasis, and loss of surfactant. This necessitates increasing the pressure of the mechanical ventilation, which often worsens the problem. The areas that are relatively normal are overventilated and overdistended by the high-pressure ventilation, leading to decreased perfusion and gas exchange, compounding the $\dot{V}/\dot{Q}$ mismatch.

CASE 48

A. The three most common causes of aortic stenosis are congenital abnormalities (unicuspid, bicuspid, or fused leaflets), rheumatic heart disease, and degenerative valve disease resulting from calcium deposition. The most likely cause in this patient is rheumatic heart disease. Congenital aortic stenosis generally presents before age 30 years, whereas degenerative aortic stenosis is the most common cause in persons older than 70 years. Furthermore, this patient has a history of recurrent streptococcal sore throat, suggesting the possibility of rheumatic heart disease.

B. Syncope in aortic stenosis is usually due to decreased cerebral perfusion from the fixed obstruction, but it may also occur because of transient atrial arrhythmias with loss of effective atrial contribution to ventricular filling. Arrhythmias arising from ventricular tissue are also more common in patients with aortic stenosis and can result in syncope.

C. Angina can be caused by a number of different mechanisms. Approximately half of all patients have comorbid significant coronary artery disease, which can lead to angina. Even without coronary artery disease, aortic stenosis causes compensatory ventricular hypertrophy. Ventricular hypertrophy causes an increase in oxygen demand as well as compression of the vessels traversing the cardiac muscle, resulting in decreased oxygen supply. The result is relative ischemia of the myocytes. Finally, in the case of calcified aortic valves, calcium emboli can cause coronary artery obstruction, although this is rare.

D. Carotid upstroke is decreased (pulsus parvus) and late (pulsus tardus) because of the fixed obstruction to flow. Left ventricular hypertrophy causes the apical impulse to be displaced laterally and to become sustained. The increased dependence on atrial contraction is responsible for the prominent S_4. Flow through the restricted aortic orifice results in the midsystolic murmur, whereas regurgitant flow causes the diastolic murmur.

E. Once symptoms occur in aortic stenosis, without treatment the prognosis is poor. Life expectancy is 2 years if angina is due to aortic stenosis and 3 years if aortic stenosis is the cause of syncope.

CASE 49

A. The fundamental problem in aortic regurgitation is volume overload of the left ventricle during diastole. In aortic regurgitation, blood enters the left ventricle both from the pulmonary veins and from the aorta (through the leaky aortic valve). The left ventricular stroke volume can increase dramatically, although the effective stroke volume may be minimally changed since much of the increase in stroke volume leaks back into the left ventricle. If the regurgitation develops slowly, the heart responds to the increased diastolic volume by elongation of the sarcomeres (dilation) and thickening of the wall (hypertrophy). This can result in an enlarged heart that is displaced to the left. All of these changes are characteristic of slowly progressive aortic regurgitation. However, if the condition develops quickly, over a few days, such as during destruction of the

aortic valve from infective endocarditis, these compensatory mechanisms do not have a chance to develop.

B. In aortic regurgitation, the pulse pressure is widened both because of an increase in systolic pressure and a falling diastolic pressure. The systolic pressure is increased due to the increased stroke volume. The diastolic pressure is decreased due to the regurgitant flow back into the left ventricle and the increased compliance of the great vessels. This large difference between systolic and diastolic pressures is readily felt in the peripheral pulse as a sudden rise, then drop, in pressure. There are many physical signs resulting from this phenomenon, including the so-called water-hammer pulse (Corrigan's pulse), head bobbing (de Musset's sign), pulsation of the uvula (Müller's sign), and arterial pulsations of the nailbeds (Quincke's pulse).

C. The high-pitched diastolic murmur at the left lower sternal border is from the regurgitant flow through the leaky aortic valve. The diastolic rumbling at the apex, also known as the Austin Flint murmur, is from the regurgitant flow impinging on the anterior leaflet of the mitral valve, causing a functional mitral stenosis. The systolic murmur at the left upper sternal border is from the increased stroke volume flowing across the aortic valve during systole.

D. Early in aortic regurgitation, there is no congestive heart failure because the left ventricle adapts to the increased volume by enlarging and thickening. However, at some point the compensatory mechanisms fail, and the end-diastolic pressure in the left ventricle rises. This rise in end-diastolic pressure is transmitted through the pulmonary veins to the lungs where it results in pulmonary edema due to increases in hydrostatic pressure. This buildup of fluid in the alveoli causes impaired oxygenation, leading to shortness of breath. In milder cases, the shortness of breath may only become evident when there is increased demand or, in severe cases, may manifest at rest. For example, increased demand can occur during exertion. It may also occur during sleep, when the supine position allows the interstitial fluid from dependent tissues to reenter the circulation, causing an increased intravascular volume.

CASE 50

A. The likely diagnosis in this patient is mitral stenosis. The history of a long illness following a sore throat in childhood is suggestive of acute rheumatic fever, the most common cause of mitral stenosis. The diastolic murmur results from the impaired blood flow across the narrowed mitral valve. The irregularly irregular rhythm is due to atrial fibrillation, and the shortness of breath and rales are due to the congestive heart failure of advanced mitral stenosis.

B. The normal mitral valve area is 5–6 cm^2. When it becomes narrowed to less than 1 cm^2, the flow of blood from the left atrium to the left ventricle is compromised enough to result elevated left atrial pressure and volume. These elevations cause the left atrium to dilate, disrupting the orderly initiation of each heartbeat. Chaotic electrical activity replaces the usual control of the heart rhythm by the sinoatrial node, and atrial fibrillation ensues. The elevated left atrial pressure is also transmitted to the pulmonary veins and capillaries resulting in congestive heart failure, pulmonary edema, and hemoptysis from leakage of engorged pulmonary veins.

C. The blood in the dilated left atrium is relatively static, and clots can form there in approximately 20% of patients with mitral stenosis. If these thrombi enter the left ventricle, they can be pumped out to the systemic circulation causing a sudden arterial blockage, such as a stroke.

CASE 51

A. The patient's decompensation was likely triggered by the development of acute mitral regurgitation. The leaflets of the mitral valve are tethered by chordae tendineae, which are in turn attached to the ventricular wall by papillary muscles. The papillary muscles derive their blood supply from the left circumflex coronary artery and can become ischemic and even rupture if the blood supply is interrupted. When this happens, the leaflet is no longer tethered, and the valve no longer closes with systole, resulting in the sudden development of acute mitral regurgitation.

B. In mitral regurgitation, blood regurgitates into the left atrium from the left ventricle during systole. This leads to both volume and pressure overload of the left atrium, which in turn is transmitted to the pulmonary vasculature. It can also lead to dilation of the atrium and disruption of the heart's electrical system, causing arrhythmias such as atrial fibrillation. The increased pulmonary pressures can lead to congestive heart failure. Also, in contrast to mitral stenosis, there is also an element of volume overload on the left ventricle, as the regurgitant blood from the left atrium goes back into the left ventricle during diastole.

C. If mitral regurgitation develops more slowly, the heart has a chance to adapt to the increased volume. The left ventricle, in particular, can dilate and hypertrophy in response to the increased stroke volume (though usually not to the extent that this LV dilation and hypertrophy happens in aortic regurgitation). As a result, the apical impulse becomes displaced to the left.

CASE 52

A. The most likely diagnosis in this patient is coronary artery disease, specifically angina pectoris. Because the symptoms are exertional only and have been stable for several months, this patient would be classified as having stable angina. If the pain occurred at rest, with less and less activity, or more frequently or for a longer duration despite similar activity levels, he would be classified as having unstable angina.

B. By far the most common cause of coronary artery disease is atherosclerosis of the large epicardial arteries, and this is the most likely cause in this patient. A less common cause is coronary artery vasospasm, found most often in Japanese individuals. Vasospastic angina is most often nonexertional. Rare causes include emboli and congenital abnormalities.

C. This patient has several cardiac risk factors, including male gender, a family history of coronary artery disease, hyperlipidemia, smoking, and hypertension.

D. The mechanism by which atherosclerotic plaques form remains unclear and is the subject of much debate. It appears that atherosclerosis starts early in life, when the endothelial linings of the blood vessels are exposed to shear stress. The injury that results causes the endothelial cells to release vascular cell adhesion molecules to which monocytes become attached and enter the subendothelium, where they engulf oxidized LDL, forming foam cells. The injured endothelium, in combination with the foam cells, forms the fatty streak characteristic of atherosclerosis. Oxidized LDL causes the release of cytokines and inhibition of NO. Vascular smooth muscle moves from the media to the intima, where they proliferate, laying down collagen and matrix and taking up oxidized LDL to form more foam cells. T cells also accumulate in the growing plaque. T cells, smooth muscle cells, and endothelial cells produce various cytokines and growth factors responsible for further cell migration and proliferation. Ultimately, the thickened and distorted artery wall takes up calcium, creating a brittle plaque.

E. Chest pain is due to myocardial ischemia, which occurs when cardiac oxygen demand exceeds supply. In the case of stable angina, fixed narrowing of one or more coronary arteries by atherosclerotic plaque occurs. When the patient exercises, cardiac oxygen demand increases. However, because of the decreased diameter of the coronary arteries, insufficient blood flow, and, therefore, insufficient oxygen, is supplied to the heart. Chest pain has been attributed to this ischemia; however, it has been shown that up to 80% of all ischemic episodes are asymptomatic. When present, chest pain is thought to be triggered by adenosine release, causing stimulation of the sympathetic afferent fibers that innervate the atrium and ventricle. These fibers then traverse the sympathetic ganglia and five upper thoracic dorsal roots of the spinal cord. These fibers converge with fibers from other structures in the spinal cord, which accounts for the frequent sensation of pain in the chest wall, back, and arm.

CASE 53

A. The probable diagnosis in this patient is pericarditis.

B. The most common cause of pericarditis is infection. Although bacteria, protozoa, and fungi can all cause pericarditis, viruses are most common offender, in particular the coxsackieviruses. Coxsackievirus infection is the most likely cause in this patient given his young age, absence of underlying diseases, and viral prodrome. Pericarditis also occurs after injury (eg, myocardial infarction, thoracotomy, chest trauma, or radiation therapy). Less common causes include collagen-vascular diseases (lupus erythematosus, scleroderma, rheumatoid arthritis), neoplasms, and renal failure.

C. Chest pain is probably due to pericardial inflammation. The pleuritic nature of the chest pain may be due to inflammation of the adjacent pleura.

D. The sound heard on cardiac examination is characteristic of a pericardial friction rub, which is pathognomonic for pericarditis. It is believed to be caused by friction between the visceral and parietal pericardial surfaces. The three components are attributable to the rapid movements of the cardiac chambers. The systolic component is related to ventricular contraction and is the one most commonly heard. There are two diastolic components: one in early diastole resulting from rapid ventricular filling and one late in diastole caused by atrial contraction. The two diastolic components frequently merge, so that a two-component rub is most often heard.

E. One complication of pericarditis is pericardial effusion. Sudden onset of pericardial effusion may lead to tamponade. This sudden addition of fluid increases pericardial pressure to the level of right atrial and ventricular pressures, causing chamber collapse and inadequate filling. Physical findings consistent with tamponade include elevated jugular venous pressure, hypotension, paradoxical pulse, and muffled heart sounds.

A second complication of pericarditis is fibrosis resulting in constrictive pericarditis. In constrictive pericarditis, early diastolic filling is normal, but the filling is suddenly stopped by the nonelastic fibrotic pericardium. This cessation of filling is probably responsible for the diastolic knock classically heard in this disease. In addition, because of the limited flow into the heart, systemic and, therefore, jugular venous pressures are elevated. Kussmaul's sign may also be present (ie, inappropriate increase in jugular venous pressure with inspiration). Finally, elevated systemic venous pressures can lead to accumulation of fluid in the liver and intraperitoneal space, resulting in hepatomegaly and ascites.

CASE 54

A. Hypertension is generally defined as a blood pressure greater than 140/90 mm Hg on three consecutive doctor's office visits, and prehypertension as blood pressures of 120–139/80–89 mm Hg. Although this patient would certainly be considered to have high blood pressure on this visit, he would not yet be diagnosed with hypertension.

B. In long-standing severe hypertension, one may note hypertensive retinopathy, including narrowed arterioles or even retinal hemorrhages and exudates. Cardiac enlargement resulting from hypertrophy may be noted as a displaced and prominent point of maximal impulse on cardiac palpation. An S_4 may be heard on cardiac auscultation.

C. Complications of hypertension include accelerated atherosclerosis resulting in ischemic heart disease, thrombotic strokes, cerebral hemorrhages, and renal failure. In severe hypertension, encephalopathy may occur.

D. By far the most common cause of hypertension is essential hypertension, and that is probably the cause in this patient. Because the patient is black, salt sensitivity may be a contributory factor. Other relatively common causes are diffuse renal disease, medications, renal arterial disease, and neurologic disorders. Less commonly, coarctation of the aorta, mineralocorticoid excess, glucocorticoid excess, and catecholamine excess can cause hypertension.

CASE 55

A. The four major pathophysiologic types of shock are hypovolemic, distributive, cardiogenic, and obstructive. Given the patient's age, history of severe trauma, and physical findings, the most likely type in this case is hypovolemic shock.

B. In hypovolemic shock, decreased blood volume leads to inadequate perfusion of the tissues. This results in increased anaerobic glycolysis and production of lactic acid. Lactic acidosis depresses the myocardium, decreases peripheral vascular responsiveness to catecholamines, and may cause coma. Decreased mean arterial blood pressure decreases arterial baroreceptor firing, resulting in increased vasomotor discharge. This causes generalized vasoconstriction. Vasoconstriction in the skin causes coolness and pallor.

C. There are five causes of hypovolemic shock: hemorrhage, trauma, surgery, burns, and fluid loss resulting from vomiting or diarrhea. This patient was in a motor vehicle accident, resulting in traumatic shock. This was caused by blood loss into the abdomen, as suggested by the physical examination.

CASE 56

A. Other historical features to be elicited include chest pain (12%), flushing (14%), excessive sweating (50%), fainting (40%), and GI symptoms such as nausea or vomiting (19%), abdominal pain (14%), and diarrhea (6%).

In addition, a medical history or family history of genetic diseases increasing the risk of pheochromocytoma should be elicited, as should a family history of pheochromocytoma independent of other genetic syndromes. Approximately 20–30% of pheochromocytomas are familial. About half of all familial cases are caused by one of three syndromes: neurofibromatosis type 1, von Hippel–Lindau syndrome, and multiple endocrine neoplasia type 2 (MEN-2). The remainder appear to be due to germline mutations in several genes, including *RET*, *VHL*, *SDHB*, and *SDHD*.

B. Pheochromocytoma is usually diagnosed by demonstrating abnormally high concentrations of catecholamines or their breakdown products in the urine or plasma. Increases in plasma metanephrine concentrations are greater and more consistent than increases in plasma catecholamines or urinary metanephrines. A reliable assay showing increased plasma or urine levels of metanephrines is usually sufficient to establish the diagnosis. If the patient has paroxysmal symptoms, sampling of blood or timed urine collections during an episode may be needed to establish the diagnosis. Administration of clonidine, 0.3 mg orally, can also be used to differentiate patients with pheochromocytoma from those with essential hypertension. Clonidine normally suppresses sympathetic nervous system activity and substantially lowers plasma norepinephrine levels, reducing blood pressure. However, in patients with pheochromocytoma, clonidine has little or no effect on the blood pressure or plasma catecholamine level because these tumors behave autonomously.

C. As a tumor of adrenal medullary tissue, pheochromocytoma produces symptoms of catecholamine excess. Anxiety, headache, and palpitations are direct effects of catecholamine discharge; the weight loss is secondary to one of the metabolic effects of excessive circulating catecholamines. These include an increase in basal metabolic rate and an increase in glycolysis and glycogenolysis, leading to hyperglycemia and glycosuria.

CASE 57

A. This patient likely has achalasia, a condition where the lower esophageal sphincter fails to relax properly. Under normal circumstances, the lower esophageal sphincter is a 3–4 cm ring of smooth muscle that is contracted, under stimulation by vagal cholinergic inputs. When a swallow is initiated, vagal inhibitory fibers allow the sphincter to relax so that the bolus of food can pass into the stomach. In achalasia, there is degeneration of the myenteric plexus and loss of the inhibitory neurons that allow this relaxation. Therefore, the sphincter remains tightly closed. The neural dysfunction can also extend further up the esophagus as well, and effective esophageal peristalsis is also often lost.

B. Injection of botulinum toxin into the lower esophageal sphincter in patients with achalasia diminishes the excitatory pathways responsible for the tonic contraction of the sphincter and allows its partial relaxation.

C. The tight closure of the lower esophageal sphincter in achalasia can result in a dilation of the lower portion of the esophagus and storage of up to 1 L of material there. This material can become infected and aspirated into the lungs. It can also cause esophageal mucosal ulceration and even perforation or rupture.

CASE 58

A. This patient appears to suffer from reflux esophagitis. Normally, the tonically contracted lower esophageal sphincter provides an effective barrier to reflux of acid from the stomach back into the esophagus. This is reinforced by secondary esophageal peristaltic waves in response to transient lower esophageal sphincter relaxation. Effectiveness of that barrier can be altered by loss of lower esophageal sphincter tone, increased frequency of transient relaxations, loss of secondary peristalsis after a transient relaxation, increased stomach volume or pressure, or increased production of acid, all of which can make more likely reflux of acidic stomach contents sufficient to cause pain or erosion. Recurrent reflux can damage the mucosa, resulting in inflammation, hence the term "reflux esophagitis." Recurrent reflux itself predisposes to further reflux because the scarring that occurs with healing of the inflamed epithelium renders the lower esophageal sphincter progressively less competent as a barrier.

B. Many factors such as her food choices (eg, chocolate), medications such as benzodiazepines, and smoking decrease lower esophageal sphincter tone, resulting in reflux of acid-rich gastric contents into the esophageal lumen. This process is exacerbated at night when she lies down to sleep.

C. The most common complication is the development of stricture in the distal esophagus. Progressive obstruction, initially to solid food and later to liquid, presents as dysphagia. Other complications of recurrent reflux include hemorrhage or perforation; hoarseness, coughing, or wheezing; and pneumonia as a result of aspiration of gastric contents into the lungs, particularly during sleep. Epidemiologic studies suggest that cigarette smoking and alcohol abuse associated with recurrent reflux result in a change in the esophageal epithelium from squamous to columnar histology, termed **Barrett's esophagus.** In 2–5% of cases, Barrett's esophagus leads to the development of esophageal adenocarcinoma.

CASE 59

A. Excessive acid secretion or diminished mucosal defenses predispose to the development of acid-peptic disease, specifically gastric ulcer. Most gastric ulcers are believed to be related to impaired mucosal defenses, because the acid and pepsin secretory capacity of some affected patients is normal or even below normal. Motility defects have been proposed to contribute to development of gastric ulcer in at least three ways: (1) by a tendency of duodenal contents to reflux back through an incompetent pyloric sphincter (bile acids in the duodenal reflux material act as an irritant and may be an important contributor to a diminished mucosal barrier against acid and pepsin); (2) by delayed emptying of gastric contents, including reflux material, into the duodenum; and (3) by delayed gastric emptying and hence food retention, resulting in increased gastrin secretion and gastric acid production. It is not known whether these motility defects are a cause or a consequence of gastric ulcer formation. Mucosal ischemia may also play a role in the development of a gastric ulcer (see Answer B following). Subsets of gastric ulcer patients with each of these defects have been identified. Thus, the risk factors (NSAID ingestion, smoking, psychologic stress, *H pylori* infection) that have been associated with gastric ulcer probably act by diminishing one or more mucosal defense mechanisms.

B. Prostaglandins are known to increase mucosal blood flow as well as bicarbonate and mucus secretion and to stimulate mucosal cell repair and renewal. Thus, their deficiency, resulting from NSAID ingestion or other insults, may predispose to gastritis and gastric ulcer, as might diminished bicarbonate or mucus secretion due to other causes.

C. *H pylori* can cause acid-peptic disease by multiple mechanisms, including altered signal transduction, resulting in increased inflammation, increased acid secretion, and diminished mucosal defenses. It may also affect apoptosis in the GI tract. Despite the high rate of association of inflammation with *H pylori* infection, the important role of other factors is indicated by the fact that only about 15% of *H pylori*–infected individuals ever develop a clinically significant ulcer. These other factors (both genetic and environmental, such as cigarette smoking) must account for the individual variations and are pathophysiologically important. Nevertheless, the role of *H pylori* is of particular clinical importance because, of patients who do develop acid-peptic disease, almost all have *H pylori* infection. Furthermore, treatment that does not eradicate *H pylori* is associated with rapid recurrence of acid-peptic disease in most patients. Recent studies have also associated different strains of *H pylori* with different forms and degrees of acid-peptic disease and implicated *H pylori* infection in the development of GI tract cancers. Cornerstones of therapy for this patient include discontinuation of ibuprofen, proton pump inhibitors to decrease acid production, and antibiotics to treat the *H pylori* infection.

CASE 60

A. Normal gastric emptying is influenced in part by the intrinsic enteric nervous system and its autonomic control. These systems are compromised by long-standing diabetes and its associated autonomic neuropathy.

It is likely that this patient's elevated fingerstick glucose is due to poor adherence to the medical regimen. This is supported by 6 months of worsening peripheral neuropathy. The newly diagnosed gastroparesis may, however, complicate attempts at improved glucose control.

B. His diarrhea may be multifactorial. Poorly coordinated pyloric contractions may result in entry into the duodenum of too large a bolus of chyme, which is ineffectively handled by the small intestine. Malabsorption results, leading to diarrhea. This malabsorption also predisposes to bacterial overgrowth, which may further exacerbate his diarrhea.

CASE 61

A. There are many factors involved in gallstone formation, but they can be divided into factors affecting bile composition and factors affecting gallbladder motility. Factors affecting the lithogenicity of bile include the cholesterol content, the presence of nucleating factors, prostaglandins, and estrogen, the rate of bile formation, and the rate of water and electrolyte absorption. Gallbladder motility also plays a major factor. Usually, bile does not stay in the gallbladder long enough to form a gallstone, but it may happen if stasis occurs.

B. In premenopausal women, high levels of serum estrogens promote gallstone formation in two ways: Estrogens both increase cholesterol concentration of bile and decrease gallbladder motility. Bile stasis and elevation of its cholesterol concentration enable gallstone formation.

C. A gallstone may become lodged in the cystic duct, obstructing the emptying of the gallbladder. This can lead to inflammation (cholecystitis) and infection of the static contents (empyema) of the gallbladder. If untreated, such inflammation and infection can lead to necrosis of the gallbladder and sepsis. If a gallstone becomes lodged in the common bile duct, it can cause obstructive jaundice with elevation in serum bilirubin levels. If it lodges further along the common bile duct and blocks the pancreatic duct near the sphincter of Oddi, it can cause acute pancreatitis, perhaps because the digestive enzymes of the pancreas are trapped in the pancreatic duct and cause inflammation of the pancreas.

CASE 62

A. As the name suggests, enterotoxigenic *E coli* produces toxins that cause hypersecretion of fluids and electrolytes into the small intestinal lumen through activation of adenylyl cyclase and the formation of cAMP. This is a secretory diarrhea.

B. Unlike an osmotic or malabsorptive diarrhea, the passengers' secretory diarrhea continues despite poor oral intake. The absence of bloody stool makes inflammatory diarrhea less likely.

C. In most cases of traveler's diarrhea caused by pathogenic *E coli*, symptoms are self-limited. Preventing dehydration is essential, and persistent or particularly severe cases may be treated with antibiotics.

CASE 63

A. Crohn's disease is a regional enteritis that primarily affects the distal ileum and colon but may affect the GI tract from mouth to anus as evidenced by the significant oral aphthous ulcers seen in this patient.

B. The pathogenesis of Crohn's disease remains unclear. Many factors have been speculated to contribute to the development of Crohn's disease, including microorganisms (bacteria and viruses), dietary factors, genetic factors, defective immune responses, and psychosocial factors. The association of Crohn's disease with other known hereditary disorders, such as cystic fibrosis and ankylosing spondylitis, is indirect evidence of a genetic component. The normal gut is able to modulate frank inflammatory responses to its constant bombardment with dietary and microbial antigens in the lumen. This modulation may be defective in Crohn's disease, resulting in uncontrolled inflammation. There has been considerable recent interest in the role of cytokines, such as interleukins and tumor necrosis factor (TNF), in Crohn's disease. Cytokine profiles of the T_H1 category have been implicated in Crohn's disease. Mice lacking interleukin-10 have a T_H1 cytokine profile and develop a Crohn's disease–like inflammation of the intestine. Monoclonal antibodies to TNF reduce inflammation in affected animals and humans.

C. Acute and chronic inflammation cause a relapsing and remitting clinical course. Complications such as small bowel obstruction can occur as a result of active inflammation or, more commonly, from chronic fibrotic stricturing. Fistulization, abscesses, perianal disease, carcinoma, and malabsorption are other known complications of Crohn's disease.

D. Extraintestinal manifestations include migratory arthritis, inflammatory disorders of the skin, eye, and mucous membranes, gallstones from malabsorption of bile salts from the terminal ileum, and nephrolithiasis from increased oxalate absorption. Amyloidosis is a serious complication of Crohn's disease, as is thromboembolic disease.

CASE 64

A. Diverticular disease (diverticulosis) commonly affects older patients and is caused by herniation of mucosa and submucosa through the muscularis layer of the colon. There are both structural and functional abnormalities that contribute to its development. The structural integrity of the muscularis layer may be compromised by abnormal connective tissue. The functional abnormality may involve the development of a pressure gradient between the colonic lumen and the peritoneal space, which results from vigorous wall contractions needed to propel stool through the colon. Higher pressures are created to compensate for poor dietary fiber intake affecting normal stool bulk. Epidemiologic data support this assertion because the incidence of diverticular disease has increased with our society's reliance on fiber-poor foods and consequent constipation.

B. Opioids for abdominal pain control should be avoided because they directly raise intraluminal pressure and may increase the risk of perforation.

C. There are two important complications of diverticulosis. Diverticular bleeding from intramural arteries that rupture into the diverticula is a common cause of lower GI tract bleeding in the elderly. Diverticulitis, as seen in this patient, is due to a focal area of inflammation in the wall of a diverticulum in response to irritation from retained fecal material. Fever, abdominal pain, and diarrhea or constipation are typically present. The local infection may progress to an abscess with or without perforation, requiring surgical intervention.

CASE 65

A. This patient likely has irritable bowel syndrome. She has the three classic symptoms of irritable bowel syndrome: crampy abdominal pain, alternating constipation and diarrhea, and bloating. She also has normal laboratory and colonoscopy results. The onset of irritable bowel syndrome after a gastroenteritis is not unusual.

B. Irritable bowel syndrome is a complex and not well understood condition. Affected patients have decreased intestinal motility along with increased intestinal pain sensitivity, also known as visceral hyperalgesia. Both of these can result from alterations in the intrinsic and extrinsic nervous systems of the intestine. One hypothesis is that intestinal inflammation from an infection or other insult results in these intestinal nervous system changes, which in turn lead to altered intestinal motility, secretion, and sensation.

CASE 66

A. Acute hepatitis is an inflammatory process, causing liver cell death, which can be initiated by viral infection or, in this case, by toxic exposure. Prescription and nonprescription drugs are common inciters of acute hepatic injury and can be divided into predictable, dose-related toxicity (eg, acetaminophen) and unpredictable, idiosyncratic reactions such as with isoniazid. Isoniazid is an infrequent but important cause of acute hepatitis and may in susceptible individuals be due to a genetic predisposition to certain pathways of drug metabolism that create toxic intermediates. Synergistic reactions between drugs have also been implicated in acute liver failure. Recovery of normal hepatic function typically follows prompt discontinuation of the offending agent.

B. Histologic findings in acute hepatitis include focal liver cell degeneration and necrosis, portal inflammation with mononuclear cell infiltration, bile duct prominence, and cholestasis. Less commonly, acute hepatitis may result in bridging hepatic necrosis. Normal lobular architecture is largely restored in the recovery phase.

C. Jaundiced skin and icteric scleras on physical examination suggest hyperbilirubinemia from intrahepatic cholestasis caused by the acute hepatic injury. As a result, conjugated bilirubin is inadequately excreted into the bile, explaining the appearance of clay-colored stools. Conjugated bilirubin is also extruded from hepatocytes into the bloodstream, and its water-soluble metabolites are excreted by the kidneys, darkening the urine. These changes in stool and urine often precede clinically evident jaundice. Yellowing of the skin reflects the accumulation of water-insoluble metabolites of bilirubin and is usually not appreciated on examination until the serum bilirubin rises above 2.5 mg/dL.

CASE 67

A. This patient has chronic hepatitis B infection. The absence of recurrent acute episodes and extrahepatic involvement suggests chronic persistent infection. Further histologic, serologic, and autoimmune markers are helpful to determine more precisely whether hepatitis B infection is a chronic persistent or chronic active infection.

B. Approximately 5% of patients acutely infected with hepatitis B will mount an immune response that fails to clear the liver of virus, resulting in a chronic carrier state. Two thirds of these patients will develop chronic persistent infection characterized by a relatively benign course and rare progression to cirrhosis. One third will develop chronic active disease marked by histologic changes such as piecemeal necrosis, portal inflammation, distorted lobular architecture, and fibrosis. Chronic active hepatitis patients are at greater risk of progression to cirrhosis, and, independently of this risk, are predisposed to hepatocellular carcinoma.

C. Hepatitis D superinfection increases the likelihood of chronic active hepatitis beyond that which usually follows isolated hepatitis B infection. Coinfection is associated with a high incidence of fulminant hepatic failure.

D. Immune-mediated damage is supported by liver biopsy results demonstrating inflammation with lymphocytic infiltration. Viral DNA integrates itself into the genome of the infected cell, and viral antigens are expressed on the surface associated with class I HLA determinants, resulting in lymphocytic cytotoxicity. The degree of injury is largely related to viral replication and the host's immune response.

CASE 68

A. The exact mechanism of alcohol-induced injury to the liver is unknown; however, it is thought that the marked distortion of hepatic architecture, fibrous tissue deposition and scarring, and regenerative nodule formation result from multiple processes. Chronic alcohol use has been associated with impaired protein synthesis, lipid peroxidation, and the formation of acetaldehyde, which may interfere with membrane lipid integrity and disrupt cellular functions. Local hypoxia, as well as cell-mediated and antibody-mediated cytotoxicity, have also been implicated.

B. Portal hypertension is in part responsible for many of the complications of cirrhosis, including clinically apparent ascites, a sign of liver disease associated with poor long-term survival. Although no single hypothesis can explain its pathogenesis, portal hypertension and inappropriate renal retention of sodium are important elements of any theory. Portal hypertension changes the hepatocellular architecture, resulting in increased intrahepatic vascular resistance. This elevates the sinusoidal pressures transmitted to the portal vein and other vascular beds. Splenomegaly and portal-to-systemic shunting result. Vasodilators such as nitric oxide are shunted away from the liver and not cleared from the circulation, resulting in peripheral arteriolar vasodilation. Decreased renal artery perfusion from this vasodilation is perceived as an intravascular volume deficit by the kidney, encouraging sodium and water resorption. By overwhelming oncotic pressure, increased hydrostatic pressure from fluid retention in the portal vein results in ascites formation. Exceeding lymphatic drainage capacity, ascites accumulates in the peritoneum.

C. Splenomegaly and hypersplenism are a direct consequence of elevated portal venous pressure. Thrombocytopenia and hemolytic anemia occur as a result of both sequestration of these formed elements by the spleen and the depressive effect of alcohol on the bone marrow. The frequent bruising and the elevated prothrombin time in this patient highlight the coagulopathy seen in cirrhosis and chronic liver disease. As a result of inadequate bile excretion, there is impaired absorption of the fat-soluble vitamin K, a vitamin necessary for the activation of specific clotting factors. In addition, inadequate hepatic synthesis of other clotting factors causes a coagulopathy.

CASE 69

A. Biliary tract disease is a common cause of acute pancreatitis. It is hypothesized that the inciting event is obstruction of the common bile and main pancreatic ducts by a gallstone lodged in the ampulla of Vater. Parenchymal injury may be caused by the local reflux of bile or duodenal contents. It has also been proposed that inflammation is caused by bacterial toxins or free bile acids transported from the gallbladder to the pancreas through lymphatics.

B. Although choledocholithiasis appears to be the most likely cause of this patient's acute pancreatitis, other causes should be considered, for example, alcohol use, infection (viral, bacterial, and parasitic), concomitant drugs, recent surgeries, comorbid rheumatologic disease, and a family history of pancreatitis. Laboratory studies such as a serum calcium and lipid panel, including triglycerides, would be helpful in ruling out important metabolic causes of pancreatitis. Of note, however, the cause of the pancreatitis remains unclear despite workup in approximately 15–25% of cases. To help guide prognosis, Ranson's criteria require an assessment of the white blood cell count, serum glucose, LDH, and AST.

C. Acute respiratory distress syndrome (ARDS) may be caused, in part, by activated pancreatic enzymes such as circulating phospholipases, which are released systemically and interfere with the normal function of pulmonary surfactant. In addition, the systemic release of both the CC and CXC families of cytokines and endotoxin, beginning shortly after pain onset and peaking 36–48 hours later, corresponds temporally with the profound clinical decline observed. In particular, substance P, neurokinin-1, and platelet activating factor (PAF) are involved in the proinflammatory responses seen in pancreatitis-associated acute lung injury.

CASE 70

A. Alcoholism is the most common cause of chronic pancreatitis, accounting for 70–80% of cases. The risk is directly related to the duration and amount of alcohol consumed, but in fact, only 5–10% of heavy drinkers actually develop the disease.

B. It is thought that ethanol causes secretion of insoluble pancreatic proteins that calcify and occlude the pancreatic duct. This results in progressive fibrosis and subsequent destruction of glandular tissue. In addition, deficiencies of dietary antioxidants such as zinc and selenium may lead to the buildup of toxic free radicals. Unlike other forms of chronic pancreatitis, alcohol-related chronic disease may evolve from multiple episodes of severe acute pancreatitis.

C. Fat malabsorption is a hallmark of severe pancreatic insufficiency. The long-standing inflammation and fibrosis of chronic pancreatitis destroy exocrine tissue and lead to inadequate delivery of digestive enzymes to the duodenum in both prandial and postprandial states. Decreased bicarbonate delivery fails to inhibit gastric acid inactivation of enzymes and bile acids. As a result, bile salts precipitate and micelle formation, required for intestinal fat absorption, is impaired. In addition, chronic alcohol intake may independently reduce exocrine pancreatic function by directly inhibiting the cholinergic and cholecystokinin pathways.

D. Proton pump inhibitors may be helpful adjuvant therapy along with pancreatic enzyme replacement by decreasing postprandial gastric acid secretion, commonly seen in patients with severe pancreatic insufficiency.

CASE 71

A. Courvoisier's law distinguishes the causes of the gallbladder findings on physical examination. A palpable gallbladder makes gallstones of the common bile duct less likely than carcinoma of the pancreas because gallstones typically result in inflammation and subsequent scarring, resulting in a shrunken, and not a distended, gallbladder.

B. Adenocarcinomas of the pancreas may present with anemia, migratory thromboembolic disease, or disseminated intravascular coagulation. The coagulopathies may be related to thromboplastins released within the mucinous secretions of the adenocarcinoma.

C. Clinical prognostic factors include tumor size, site, clinical stage, lymph node metastasis, type of surgery, anemia requiring blood transfusion, performance status, and adjuvant radiation therapy. The poor overall prognosis (< 5% 5-year survival, and only 15–20% of patients undergoing curative tumor resections live > 5 years) can be attributed primarily to the advanced stage of the disease by the time it presents clinically, rapid rate of local tumor expansion, and early systemic dissemination.

CASE 72

A. The clinical summary and the elevated creatine kinase suggest rhabdomyolysis-induced acute tubular necrosis (ATN). Crush injuries release myoglobin into the bloodstream that precipitates in the renal tubules, causing intrarenal toxicity and subsequent failure. With this underlying defect, antibiotic therapy may exacerbate the situation or may induce a separate inflammatory interstitial nephritis. The absence of documented hypotension makes ischemia-mediated ATN less likely.

B. The fractional excretion of sodium, FE_{Na+}, derived from measurement of the urine and plasma sodium and creatinine, reflects the ability of the kidney to generate a concentrated urine. This function is essentially lost in the setting of acute tubular necrosis, and the patient's urine osmolarity is probably less than 350 mOsm/L. More commonly in the setting of myoglobinuria-induced ATN, her FE_{Na+} would be greater than 2%; however the FE_{Na+} has been noted to be less than 1% in some cases of rhabdomyolysis.

C. Mainstays of treatment involve maintenance of a vigorous alkaline diuresis to prevent myoglobin precipitation in the tubules and adjusting renally cleared antibiotics to prevent further nephrotoxicity.

CASE 73

A. This patient probably suffers from osteoporosis, accelerated by her underlying renal failure. The pathogenesis of bone disease is multifactorial. Calcium is poorly absorbed from the gut because of decreased renally generated vitamin 1,25-$(OH)_2D_3$ levels. Hypocalcemia results and is further exacerbated by high serum phosphate levels from impaired phosphate excretion by the kidney. Low serum calcium and hyperphosphatemia trigger PTH secretion, which depletes bone calcium and contributes to osteomalacia and osteoporosis. Also implicated are the diminished responsiveness of bone to vitamin D_3 and chronic metabolic acidosis.

B. Easy fatigability is often attributable to a worsening normochromic, normocytic anemia seen in chronic renal failure. This occurs primarily because of impaired synthesis of erythropoietin by the kidney and a loss of its stimulatory effect on the bone marrow. To improve symptoms, exogenous erythropoietin is started to raise the hematocrit of 25–28% typically seen in chronic renal failure patients.

C. A pericardial friction rub suggests uremia-related pericarditis. This is thought to occur from uremic toxins that irritate and inflame the pericardium. The absence of this finding, lack of asterixis, and clear mentation suggest that despite underlying chronic renal failure the patient does not exhibit evidence of uremia at this time.

CASE 74

A. Peripheral edema is essential to the diagnosis of nephrotic syndrome and occurs when the serum albumin falls below 3 mg/dL. The edema, however, is primarily a direct consequence of sodium retention resulting from a fall in GFR from renal disease rather than from arterial underfilling from low plasma oncotic pressure in the setting of hypoalbuminemia.

B. Minimal change disease, as the name suggests, is associated with few or no changes apparent on light microscopy, as opposed to other subtypes of glomerulonephritis associated with varying degrees of segmental sclerosis or basement membrane thickening. Immunofluorescence staining is generally unremarkable, whereas membranous glomerulonephritis is characterized by IgG and C3 deposited uniformly along capillary loops. However, the pathologic changes are most evident on electron microscopy, which reveals obliteration of epithelial foot processes. Minimal change disease is typically seen in children, but when found in adults it can be idiopathic or can follow upper respiratory tract infection, be associated with tumors such as Hodgkin's disease, or be related to hypersensitivity reactions.

C. Nephrotic syndrome is associated with a hypercoagulable state resulting from loss of other proteins besides albumin that are involved in normal coagulation such as antithrombin and proteins C and S. Immobilization from a prolonged hospital stay puts this patient at additional risk for deep venous thrombosis.

CASE 75

A. This patient is presenting with his first episode of renal stone disease. Most commonly, stones are calcium containing and reflect idiopathic hypocalciuria. Hyperparathyroidism and hyperuricosuria are other important causes of calcium stones. If the patient is able to collect a passed stone, analysis of its composition would be helpful in diagnosis of the subtype and in tailoring treatment.

B. After effective pain control is achieved, the patient may return home, and adequate hydration with 2 L/day should be reinforced. Hydration may dilute unknown substances that predispose to stone formation and minimize the likelihood of Ca^{2+} precipitation in the nephron. High-protein diets in known stone formers predispose to recurrent calcium nephrolithiasis. This results from a transient increase in calcium resorption from bone and increased filtration through the nephron in response to a protein load that stimulates the GFR. A high-sodium diet should be avoided because Na^+ predisposes to Ca^{2+} excretion and increases the saturation of monosodium urate, which acts as a nidus for calcium oxalate stone formation. Finally, citrate supplementation may be considered because of its ability to chelate calcium in solution, forming soluble complexes as opposed to calcium oxalate or phosphate.

C. Fragments of renal pelvis stones that break off and travel down the ureter produce the pain syndrome known as colic. Distention at the level of the renal pelvis, ureter, or renal capsule can produce pain that can become quite significant in the setting of acute obstruction.

CASE 76

A. Primary hyperparathyroidism accounts for most cases of hypercalcemia in the outpatient setting. Given the chronic nature of this woman's symptoms and the history of recurrent renal stones, this is the most likely diagnosis. However, particularly in older individuals, hypercalcemia of malignancy is another important cause to consider. Medications, particularly lithium and the thiazide diuretics, also cause hypercalcemia. Other causes include familial hypocalciuric hypercalcemia, thyrotoxicosis, granulomatous diseases, milk-alkali syndrome, and adrenal insufficiency.

B. In primary hyperparathyroidism there is excessive secretion of PTH in relation to the serum calcium. This is due both to an increase in parathyroid cell mass and to a reduced sensitivity to serum calcium levels, resulting in a qualitative regulatory defect in serum PTH secretion.

The *PRAD1* gene, which produces D1 cyclin, has been implicated in the pathogenesis of primary hyperparathyroidism. Cyclins are cell cycle regulatory proteins. *PRAD1* and the gene encoding PTH are both located on the long arm of chromosome 11. An inversion event occurs leading to juxtaposition of the 5′-regulatory domain of the PTH gene upstream to the *PRAD1* gene. This leads to abnormally regulated transcription of the *PRAD1* gene in a parathyroid-specific manner. Overproduction of the *PRAD1* gene product, D1 cyclin, increases cell proliferation.

The *MEN1* gene, also on chromosome 11, has been implicated in both MEN-1 kindreds and in up to 25% of people with nonfamilial benign primary hyperparathyroidism. *MEN1* appears to be a tumor suppressor gene. The hyperparathyroidism in MEN-2a and MEN-2b appears to be caused by mutations in the RET protein.

C. The diagnosis of primary hyperparathyroidism is confirmed by at least two simultaneous measurements of serum calcium and intact PTH. An elevated or normal PTH in the setting of hypercalcemia confirms the diagnosis.

CASE 77

A. The likely diagnosis in this patient is familial hypocalciuric hypercalcemia (FHH). The diagnosis is suggested by the findings of an elevated serum calcium level with normal levels of intact parathyroid hormone (PTH) and 1,25-OH vitamin D. It is also possible that the patient has mild primary hyperparathyroidism as well, but the low urinary calcium excretion strongly suggests FHH rather than hyperparathyroidism.

B. This condition results from a defect in the CaSR, a member of the G protein receptor family. CaSR is highly expressed in the kidney and parathyroid glands. In the kidney, CaSR detects the serum calcium concentration and adjusts the urinary calcium excretion accordingly. In the parathyroid glands, CaSR regulates the secretion of PTH. If CaSR is defective, it misreads the serum calcium concentration as inappropriately low and causes the kidneys to retain calcium and the parathyroid glands to secrete excess PTH. Fortunately, in FHH, the elevation in serum

calcium tends to be mild, and most patients are clinically asymptomatic. A rare, severe form that manifests in infancy is called neonatal severe primary hyperparathyroidism. Although this is a genetic disorder with an autosomal dominant mode of inheritance, there is no genetic testing available for the condition because the various responsible mutations are dispersed over the large gene encoding the calcium receptor.

CASE 78

A. Hypercalcemia is most commonly seen in solid tumors, primarily squamous cell carcinomas, renal cell carcinoma, and breast carcinoma. It also occurs frequently in multiple myeloma. It occurs less commonly in lymphomas and leukemias. Given this patient's long-standing smoking history and abnormal lung examination, the most likely diagnosis is squamous cell carcinoma of the lung.

B. Serum PTH should be undetectable, and PTHrP should be elevated. This is due to the fact that 70–80% of malignancy-induced hypercalcemia is caused by tumor secretion of PTHrP. This is true of squamous cell carcinoma–induced hypercalcemia.

C. PTHrP is homologous with PTH at its amino terminal and is recognized by the type 1 PTH receptor. Therefore, it has effects on bone and kidney similar to those of PTH, including increasing bone resorption, increasing phosphate excretion, and decreasing renal calcium excretion.

CASE 79

A. The parathyroid glands lie in close proximity to the thyroid gland and are, therefore, at risk of trauma, devascularization, or removal during thyroid surgery. Damage to the parathyroid glands results in decreased PTH release, with resultant inability to maintain serum calcium concentrations. Because PTH is required to stimulate the renal production of 1,25-(OH)$_2$D, levels of 1,25-(OH)$_2$D are low in patients with hypoparathyroidism. This leads to reduced intestinal calcium absorption. In the absence of adequate PTH and 1,25-(OH)$_2$D, the mobilization of calcium from bone is abnormal. Furthermore, because less PTH is available to act in the distal nephron, urinary calcium excretion may be high. A combination of these mechanisms is responsible for the hypocalcemia seen in hypoparathyroidism.

There may be a prolonged latent period before symptomatic hypocalcemia develops. Hypoparathyroidism may vary in severity. In this case, it is likely that the patient has decreased parathyroid reserve only. The increased stress on her parathyroid glands because of her pregnancy has probably precipitated her symptomatic hypocalcemia.

B. Chvostek's sign is elicited by tapping on the facial nerve anterior to the ear. Twitching of the ipsilateral facial muscles is a positive test. A positive Trousseau sign is demonstrated by inflating the sphygmomanometer above the systolic blood pressure for 3 min. Painful carpal muscle contractions and spasms signify a positive test. Both signs indicate latent tetany secondary to hypocalcemia.

C. Serum phosphate is often but not invariably elevated in hypoparathyroidism. Hyperphosphatemia occurs because the proximal tubular effect of PTH to promote phosphate excretion is lost.

CASE 80

A. Medullary carcinoma of the thyroid is a C-cell neoplasm. Because C cells are neuroendocrine cells, they have the capacity to release several hormones. The secretion of serotonin, prostaglandins, or calcitonin probably causes the watery (secretory) diarrhea this patient has. Flushing is generally caused by tumor production either of substance P or of calcitonin gene-related peptide, both of which are vasodilators.

B. The diagnosis would be made most efficiently by fine-needle aspiration of the thyroid nodules. They should demonstrate the characteristic C-cell lesion with positive immunostaining for calcitonin. A serum calcitonin level would also be beneficial, because it is typically elevated in medullary carcinoma and correlates with extent of tumor burden. Calcitonin levels may be monitored during treatment to assess response.

C. As noted, serum calcitonin levels are a useful means of assessing tumor burden and for monitoring disease progression during and after treatment. Serum carcinoembryonic antigen (CEA) is also frequently elevated in patients with medullary carcinoma and present at all stages of the disease. Rapid increases in CEA predict a worse clinical course.

All patients with medullary carcinoma of the thyroid should be tested for the *RET* oncogene. Although this patient denies a family history of MEN, she is young (< 40 years) and has a bilateral tumor, both of which are concerning for hereditary forms of medullary carcinoma and the MEN syndromes. More than 90% of patients with MEN-2 harbor *RET* mutations. Even sporadic cases of medullary carcinoma should be tested for *RET* mutations, because new mutations in the *RET* gene are frequently present, and family members can then be screened for these mutations.

If MEN-2 syndrome is detected in this patient, she should be tested for pheochromocytoma before undergoing thyroid surgery by determinations of plasma or urinary metanephrines and by adrenal CT scanning.

CASE 81

A. Genetics are very important in determining peak bone mass and loss. However, a number of hormonal and environmental factors can reduce the genetically determined peak bone mass or hasten the loss of bone mineral and thus present important risk factors for osteoporosis. The most important etiologic factor in osteoporosis is sex steroid deficiency, either estrogen in the case of postmenopausal women or testosterone in hypogonadal men. Another important cause is excess cortisol either in the form of exogenous corticosteroid use or endogenous excess in Cushing's syndrome. Other medications such as heparin, thyroid hormone, and anticonvulsants can also cause osteoporosis. Immobilization, alcohol abuse, and smoking are also important risk factors. Diet in the form of adequate calcium and vitamin D intake and weight-bearing exercise are also vital because they are necessary to build peak bone mass and minimize loss. Many additional disorders affecting the GI, hematologic, and connective tissue systems can contribute to the development of osteoporosis (Table 17–10).

B. This patient likely has a combination of post-menopausal and age-related osteoporosis. Postmenopausal osteoporosis is caused by accelerated bone resorption. Although bone formation is also increased, it is insufficient to fully counteract bone resorption and net bone loss occurs. The cellular basis for the activation of bone resorption in postmenopausal osteoporosis is somewhat unclear. Osteoclasts have estrogen receptors, and this may account at least in part for their activation during estrogen deficiency. There is also evidence that osteoclast-stimulating cytokines, such as interleukin-6, are released from other bone cells after menopause.

The pathogenesis of age-related or senile osteoporosis is even less clear. Again, there is an uncoupling of bone resorption and bone formation, such that bone formation does not keep pace with resorption. Deficiency of dietary calcium and 1,25-$(OH)_2D$ is one important pathogenic factor. As people age, intestinal calcium absorption is decreased while renal calcium loss is preserved, resulting in an increased need for dietary calcium. This occurs at a time when most people reduce their calcium intake.

In addition, some older individuals may be deficient in vitamin D, further impairing their ability to absorb calcium. Particularly in northern climates, where sunlight exposure is reduced in the winter months, borderline low levels of 1,25-$(OH)_2D$ and mild secondary hyperparathyroidism are evident by the end of winter.

Secondary hyperparathyroidism may also occur in the aged as a result of decreased renal function. As renal function decreases, so may renal production of 1,25-$(OH)_2D$, thereby increasing PTH secretion. Reduced 1,25-$(OH)_2D$ secretion also results in decreased calcium absorption, exacerbating the intrinsic inability of the aging intestine to absorb calcium. Because the responsiveness of the parathyroid gland to calcium seems to be reduced in aging, the hyperparathyroidism seen in aging seems to be the result of the combined effects of aging on the kidney, intestine, and parathyroid gland.

C. There are three major risk factors for fractures in osteoporosis: decreased bone density, poor bone quality, and falls. For every standard deviation below the mean bone density for age, there is a twofold to threefold increased risk for fracture. The microarchitecture of bone also determines its mechanical strength and its ability to withstand stress. Finally, fractures rarely occur unless people fall or otherwise sustain trauma. Muscle weakness, impaired vision, impaired balance, sedative use, and environmental factors (eg, stairs, carpeting) are all important risk factors for falls and, therefore, fractures.

D. The 6-month mortality rate for hip fracture is approximately 20%, much of it resulting from the complications of immobilizing a frail person in a hospital bed. The complications include pulmonary embolus and pneumonia. About half of elderly people with a hip fracture will never walk freely again.

E. Treatments for reduced bone mass include calcium and vitamin D supplementation, estrogen replacement therapy with hormone replacement therapy or raloxifene, antiresorptive agents, such as the bisphosphonates and calcitonin, and PTH.

CASE 82

A. Osteomalacia can result from vitamin D deficiency, phosphate deficiency, hypophosphatasia, and several toxic substances (fluoride, aluminum, and phosphate-binding agents) with effects on bone. Vitamin D deficiency is the likely cause in this patient. She is homebound and bed-bound in a basement apartment, preventing adequate sunlight exposure. She is a strict vegetarian, even refraining from eating dairy products, so she has limited to no exposure to dietary supplementation. Finally, the x-ray evidence of pseudofracture of the pubic rami is strongly indicative of vitamin D-deficient osteomalacia.

B. Vitamin D deficiency produces osteomalacia in two stages. Initially, decreased vitamin D leads to decreased intestinal calcium absorption and secondary hyperparathyroidism. Serum calcium is maintained at the expense of increased renal phosphate excretion and hypophosphatemia. Ultimately, however, hypocalcemia ensues. Poor delivery of calcium and phosphate to bone results in impaired mineralization of the matrix. Osteoid or unmineralized matrix, therefore, accumulates at the bone-forming surfaces.

C. If bone undergoes biopsy for quantitative histomorphometry, osteoid seams and a reduction in the mineralization rate are found.

CASE 83

A. Ketoacidosis is caused by a severe lack of insulin seen most commonly in patients with type 1 diabetes mellitus. It may be the initial presentation of this disorder. However, in this patient with a long-standing history of type 2 diabetes and resultant insulin resistance and true insulinopenia, ketosis was precipitated by acute infection. In this case, severe cellulitis induced counterregulatory hormone production, which inhibits insulin's action. Thus, in the effective absence of insulin, lipolysis generates fatty acids that are preferentially converted to ketone bodies by the liver, resulting in ketoacidosis.

B. Altered mental status in diabetic ketoacidosis, as in hyperosmolar coma, most closely correlates with the degree of hyperosmolality induced by hyperglycemia and the associated osmotic diuresis. Profound intracellular dehydration is seen in the brain as fluid shifts in response to elevated plasma osmolality. The effective osmolality in this patient is calculated as follows: $2(132 + 3.7) + 488/18 = 298.5$. Coma occurs when the effective plasma osmolality reaches 340 mOsm/L. Although alterations in mental status can occur as plasma osmolality rises above the upper limit of normal (295 mOsm/L), patients usually do not exhibit anything more than mild to moderate drowsiness at the level of osmolarity seen in this patient. Therefore, other possible causes of altered mental status should be considered, including stroke, infection, and drugs.

C. This patient exhibits Kussmaul breathing (hyperpnea that effectively drops the PCO_2 to partially compensate for the underlying metabolic acidosis). This respiratory pattern is commonly seen with a blood pH less than 7.20. In addition, the fruity odor detected on his breath is due to the keto acid acetone produced in this disorder.

D. Mainstays of treatment for diabetic ketoacidosis include concomitant insulin therapy and free water and electrolyte replacement. The osmotic diuresis results in significant free water loss and total body potassium depletion. However, the serum potassium appears normal because of the shift of K^+ out of cells and into the extracellular space—induced by acidosis, hyperglycemia, and insulinopenia. Correction of the acidosis and hyperglycemia with insulin therapy shifts potassium back into cells. Unless carefully monitored and replete, serum K^+ levels can drop dangerously low, leading to potentially fatal cardiac arrhythmias. Phosphate depletion can also be seen, but replacement is considered only in severe cases because of the risks of intravenous phosphate repletion.

CASE 84

A. Whipple's triad sets forth the diagnostic criteria for hypoglycemia: (1) symptoms and signs of hypoglycemia, (2) an associated low plasma glucose level, and (3) improvement in symptoms with the administration of glucose. This patient's self-diagnosis of hypoglycemic attacks meets these criteria.

B. The patient's age and the fasting hypoglycemia are suggestive of insulinoma, an insulin-secreting tumor of the B cells of the islets of Langerhans. Normally during exercise, insulin levels decline, allowing for significant glycogen uptake in the periphery. In addition, glucagon-stimulated hepatic glucose output increases so as to maintain adequate serum glucose levels, and counterregulatory hormones mobilize fatty acids for ketogenesis and fatty acid oxidation by muscle. However, during exercise, an elevated insulin level secreted by an insulinoma suppresses the glucagon-mediated glucose output while insulin-induced peripheral glucose uptake continues. Thus, the patient becomes hypoglycemic and his symptoms recur.

C. Hypoglycemia in the setting of an elevated serum insulin level essentially rules out examples of non-insulin-mediated causes of hypoglycemia such as Addison's disease, sepsis, and severe hepatic injury. The differential diagnosis of insulin-mediated hypoglycemia includes surreptitious insulin injection, oral hypoglycemic use (stimulating endogenous insulin production), and the presence of insulin antibodies. In this patient, a C peptide measurement was elevated, suggesting that this was not due to surreptitious injections or to antibodies. A greater challenge is to distinguish insulinoma from oral hypoglycemic use, both of which show an elevated C peptide and, therefore, require the direct measurement of serum levels of oral hypoglycemic agents to confirm the latter diagnosis.

CASE 85

A. Necrolytic migratory erythema is typically a late manifestation of glucagonoma and may be the result of hypoaminoacidemia stemming from excessive glucagon-mediated hepatic uptake of amino acids. This nutritional deficiency, rather than a direct effect of glucagon itself, is linked to the dermatologic manifestations.

B. Diabetes or glucose intolerance is usually mild, seen in response to hyperstimulation of hepatic glucose output by supranormal glucagon levels. Subsequently, serum insulin is increased, which prevents lipolysis and an associated ketotic state.

C. Glucagonomas are usually malignant, and weight loss and liver metastasis are commonly seen at the time of diagnosis; surgical resection is rarely pursued. Once diagnosed, the median survival is typically less than 3 years.

CASE 86

A. Somatostatinomas are very rare tumors, typically associated with a triad of findings, including diabetes, steatorrhea, and cholelithiasis. The latter finding is thought to be due to somatostatin-induced gallbladder hypomotility.

B. Because somatostatin suppresses both insulin and glucagon secretion, the resulting hyperglycemic state is mild and not accompanied by glucagon-mediated hepatic ketogenesis.

CASE 87

A. Body weight is controlled by a complex interaction of hormones that act on the hypothalamus. They can inhibit food intake and/or increase metabolism (the action of leptin), thereby promoting weight loss in the face of excess weight gain. They can also stimulate appetite (the action of ghrelin) and decrease metabolism. There have been many other peptides identified that take part in the regulation of body weight.

B. Body mass index (BMI) is the most commonly used index of overweight and obesity. The BMI is calculated as the patient's body weight (in kilograms) divided by the height (in meters squared). The normal range is defined as a BMI of 18.5–25, overweight is defined as a BMI of 25.1–30, and obesity is defined as a BMI of > 30.

C. Obesity increases the risk of developing many medical conditions. Obesity increases insulin resistance and can lead to the development of type 2 diabetes. Obese people have increased vascular tone and sodium retention, leading to hypertension. These two risk factors, as well as decreases in high-density lipoprotein cholesterol and increases in low-density lipoprotein cholesterol, in obese persons can lead to coronary artery disease or stroke. The excess soft tissue in the head and neck can lead to obstructive sleep apnea. Increases in serum estrogen and cholesterol levels in obese individuals can lead to gallstones. The excess wear and tear on joints can lead to osteoarthritis. Also, obese individuals have an increased risk of several cancers.

CASE 88

A. The likely diagnosis is pituitary adenoma.

B. The pituitary adenoma probably developed from a single cell with altered growth control and feedback regulation. Mutations in at least three different genes are known to significantly raise the incidence of pituitary tumor formation and are implicated in the familial causes of pituitary adenomas: *MENIN, CNC,* and *GNAS1*. In this patient, a multistep process of genetic alterations and local cell reactions likely led to the formation of the adenoma. There are several known or proposed factors that have been shown to be part of transformation of pituitary cells (eg, GNAS1, PTTG). Other factors promoting pituitary tumor formation include chromosomal instability, presumably because of an unknown gene mutation, which results in further gene mutations and aneuploidy, altered hypothalamic signaling, and other endocrine and paracrine factors (eg, estrogens, growth factors).

C. Both this patient's bitemporal hemianopia and her headaches are symptoms of the mass effect of the pituitary adenoma. The bitemporal hemianopia occurs because the crossing fibers of the optic tract, which lie directly above the pituitary gland and innervate the part of the retina responsible for temporal vision, are compressed by the tumor. Her headaches are caused by stretching of the dura by the tumor.

D. Irregular menses and galactorrhea are symptoms of prolactin excess. Galactorrhea occurs because of the direct effect of prolactin, and irregular menses are due to the indirect effect of prolactin of suppressing gonadal function.

CASE 89

A. This patient probably suffers from amenorrhea resulting from hypopituitarism. Her history of pituitary radiation is strongly suggestive of this cause. Radiation therapy frequently results in progressive destruction of the pituitary gland. This results in LH and FSH deficiency, causing menstrual irregularity and ultimately amenorrhea.

B. The patient's history of fatigue and weight gain, in conjunction with the physical examination findings of dry brittle hair and delayed relaxation phase of her deep tendon reflexes, suggests the diagnosis of hypothyroidism. Again, given her history of pituitary radiation, TSH deficiency is the probable cause.

C. One should be concerned about the diagnosis of panhypopituitarism in this patient. In addition to LH, FSH, and TSH deficiency, she may also have deficiencies of ACTH and vasopressin. Because mineralocorticoid secretion is only partially controlled by ACTH, sufficient glucocorticoid may be present even in the absence of ACTH. Adrenal insufficiency may go unnoticed until another unrelated medical emergency occurs and the patient is unable to mount a normal protective stress response. Vasopressin deficiency may go unnoticed so long as the patient is able to maintain adequate intake of fluids to compensate for the inability to concentrate urine.

CASE 90

A. Both central and nephrogenic diabetes insipidus result in the same symptoms: polyuria, polydipsia, hypotonic urine, and hypernatremia. The history of lithium use, however, is suggestive of nephrogenic diabetes insipidus. To confirm the diagnosis, one must assess responsiveness to injected vasopressin. In central diabetes insipidus, vasopressin causes a dramatic decrease in urine volume and an increase in urine osmolarity. This occurs because the basic defect in central diabetes insipidus is a lack of vasopressin. In nephrogenic diabetes insipidus, injected vasopressin has little or no effect because the kidneys are unable to respond to the circulating vasopressin.

B. Vasopressin receptors in the kidney appear to be sensitive to lithium and other salts, preventing vasopressin binding and, therefore, disabling the kidney's ability to retain water.

C. Polyuria in nephrogenic diabetes insipidus results from inability to conserve water in the distal nephron because of a lack of vasopressin-dependent water channels. These channels are normally inserted into the apical plasma membrane in response to vasopressin stimulation, resulting in water conservation. In nephrogenic diabetes insipidus, the kidneys are resistant to circulating vasopressin and unable to respond to it. Thirst results from the hypertonicity brought on by the inability to concentrate the urine.

D. If the patient is unable to maintain sufficient water intake for any reason, dehydration and hypernatremia result. This can lead to progressive obtundation, myoclonus, seizures, and ultimately coma.

CASE 91

A. SIADH is caused by a variety of vasopressin-secreting tumors, CNS disorders, pulmonary disorders, and drugs. Small cell bronchial carcinoma is an important cause of SIADH and present in this patient. His lung examination and fever suggest the possibility of pneumonia, another cause of SIADH. Although this patient is not currently undergoing therapy for lung cancer, several chemotherapeutic agents can cause SIADH, including vincristine and vinblastine, and it would be important to determine whether the patient was given either of these drugs during his therapy.

B. SIADH is due to secretion of vasopressin in excess of what is appropriate for hyperosmolarity or intravascular volume depletion. The pathophysiologic mechanisms behind most cases of SIADH are poorly understood. However, in this patient, the most likely cause is small cell lung cancer, which is probably secreting vasopressin.

C. The patient's neurologic symptoms are the result of osmotic fluid shifts causing brain edema and elevated intracranial pressures. These are the result of hyponatremia.

D. Hyponatremia resulting from SIADH is treated with simple water restriction. Treatment of the underlying disease can help as well.

CASE 92

A. Other historical features to be elicited include heat intolerance, excessive sweating, nervousness, irritability, emotional lability, restlessness, poor concentration, muscle weakness, palpitations, and increased frequency of bowel movements.

B. The examiner should evaluate the eyes for stare, lid lag, proptosis, and abnormal eye movements; the heart for irregular rhythm, flow murmur, and congestive failure; the breasts for gynecomastia; the nails for onycholysis; the pretibial area for dermopathy; and the deep tendon reflexes for a rapid relaxation phase.

C. The free thyroxine (free T_4) should be high; the TSH level should be low. Rarely, hyperthyroidism is caused by secondary or tertiary hyperthyroidism as a result of excessive TSH or TRH production, respectively. In these cases, TSH would be elevated.

D. Possible causes of this patient's condition include thyroid hormone overproduction (in Graves' disease, toxic multinodular goiter, autonomous hyperfunctioning follicular adenoma), thyroid gland destruction with release of stored hormone (in thyroiditis), or ingestion of excessive exogenous thyroid hormone.

E. Graves' disease is the most common cause of hyperthyroidism. In Graves' disease, TSH receptor autoantibodies, TSH-R [stim] Ab, are present in the circulation. These are autoantibodies of the IgG class, directed against TSH receptors on the follicular cell membrane. When they bind to the cell membrane TSH receptors, they stimulate the thyroid follicular cells to produce excessive amounts of T_4 and T_3, causing hyperthyroidism. The precipitating cause of this antibody production is unknown, but an immune response against a viral antigen that shares homology with TSH-R may be responsible. Another theory of the pathogenesis of Graves' disease is a defect of suppressor T lymphocytes, which allows helper T lymphocytes to stimulate B lymphocytes to secrete antibodies directed against follicular cell membrane antigens, including the TSH receptor.

F. Tachycardia is thought to be related to direct effects of excess thyroid hormone on the cardiac conducting system. Weight loss results from an increase in the basal metabolic rate. Autoantibodies have been identified that stimulate the growth of thyroid epithelial cells and produce the goiter of Graves' disease. The muscle weakness is related to increased protein catabolism and muscle wasting, decreased muscle efficiency, and changes in myosin.

CASE 93

A. Other features to be elicited in the history include cold intolerance, mental slowing, forgetfulness, lethargy, muscle weakness or cramps, and hair loss. The examiner should also evaluate the body temperature, the musculature for weakness, the face and skin for puffiness and carotenemia, the extremities for edema, and the deep tendon reflexes for sluggishness and a slowed ("hung-up") relaxation phase.

B. Weight gain is related to a decrease in the basal metabolic rate. Constipation is caused by decreased GI motility. Menorrhagia results from anovulatory menstrual cycles. Thyroid atrophy and fibrosis may result from lymphocytic infiltration and destruction of thyroid follicles, destruction of the thyroid by surgery or radiation, or atrophy as a result of diminished TSH secretion. The skin changes of hypothyroidism are the result of accumulation of polysaccharides in the dermis.

The quiet heart sounds may be related to development of pericardial effusion or of cardiomyopathy caused by deposi-

tion of mucopolysaccharides in the interstitium between myocardial fibers.

C. Serum TSH is the most sensitive test for detecting hypothyroidism. TSH is elevated in almost all cases of hypothyroidism, with the rare exceptions of pituitary and hypothalamic disease. Free thyroxine levels should be low.

D. In the adult, hypothyroidism may result from Hashimoto's (autoimmune) thyroiditis, lymphocytic thyroiditis, thyroid ablation (via surgery or radiation), hypopituitarism or hypothalamic disease, and drugs. The most likely cause of this patient's hypothyroidism is Hashimoto's thyroiditis both because it is the most common cause and because of the atrophic thyroid gland on examination.

E. Other autoimmune disorders, including endocrine disorders such as diabetes mellitus and hypoadrenalism, and nonendocrine disorders such as pernicious anemia, systemic lupus erythematosus, and myasthenia gravis are all seen with increased frequency in patients with Hashimoto's thyroiditis.

CASE 94

A. The physician should ask about causes of goiter such as increased intake of foods containing goitrogens (eg, rutabagas, cabbage, turnips, cassava), diminished intake of foods containing iodine (eg, fish), and use of medications associated with goiter (eg, propylthiouracil, methimazole, nitroprusside, sulfonylureas, lithium). Symptoms of thyroid encroachment on surrounding structures such as respiratory or swallowing difficulties should be elicited. Because of this patient's fatigue and depression, the physician should also probe for other symptoms of hypothyroidism.

B. The most common cause of goiter in developing nations is dietary iodine deficiency. Because this patient is 40 years of age and recently emigrated from Afghanistan, iodine deficiency would be the most likely cause. A diet low in iodine (< 10 μg/d) hinders the synthesis of thyroid hormone, resulting in decreased thyroid hormone secretions and an elevated TSH level. The elevation in serum TSH level results in diffuse thyroid hyperplasia. If TSH stimulation is prolonged, the diffuse hyperplasia is followed by focal hyperplasia with necrosis, hemorrhage, and formation of nodules.

C. The serum TSH should be determined to exclude hypothyroidism.

CASE 95

A. Primarily on the basis of the history consistent with hyperthyroidism and the presence of a single thyroid nodule palpable on examination, this patient most likely has hyperthyroidism resulting from an autonomous hyperfunctioning follicular adenoma.

B. A serum TSH should be ordered and possibly a free thyroxine index. The free thyroxine index will be elevated and the serum TSH suppressed if the patient is truly hyperthyroid.

C. A radioactive iodine scan could be performed to confirm the diagnosis. Radioactive iodine uptake will be elevated in the region of the nodule and suppressed elsewhere. Thyroid scan will show a "hot" nodule.

D. Biopsy of the nodule will show normal follicles of varying size. Excisional biopsy will show compression of surrounding normal thyroid and areas of hemorrhage, fibrosis, and calcification or cystic degeneration. Biopsy is important to rule out the diagnosis of thyroid cancer, although given the patient's symptoms of hyperthyroidism, this is less likely.

CASE 96

A. Although this patient has an elevated total T_4 level, she has no symptoms or signs of hyperthyroidism. An elevated total T_4 level in clinically euthyroid individuals may be idiopathic or may be due to pregnancy, acute or chronic hepatitis, acute intermittent porphyria, estrogen-producing tumors, and hereditary disorders. Drugs that may cause elevated total T_4 levels are estrogens (including oral contraceptives), methadone, heroin, perphenazine, and clofibrate.

B. The resin uptake of T_4 or T_3 (RT_4U or RT_3U) should be determined and the free thyroxine index calculated. The serum TSH level should be normal if the patient is euthyroid.

C. Elevated TBG levels in pregnancy lead to increased binding of free T_4. When the free T_4 falls, the pituitary secretes more TSH. This, in turn, leads to increased T_4 production by the gland and equilibration at a new level at which the total T_4 level is elevated but the free T_4 level is again normal.

D. A syndrome of familial euthyroid hyperthyroxinemia is most likely. These inherited syndromes may be caused by several mechanisms, including abnormal binding of T_4 (but not T_3) to albumin, an increased serum level of transthyretin, altered affinity of transthyretin for T_4, or pituitary and peripheral resistance to thyroid hormone.

CASE 97

A. Additional features of Cushing's syndrome include hirsutism (82%), muscular weakness (58%) and muscular atrophy (70%), back pain (58%), acne (40%), psychologic symptoms (40%), edema (18%), headache (14%), polyuria and polydipsia (10%), and hyperpigmentation (6%).

B. The exact cause of hypertension in hypercortisolism remains unclear. It may be related to salt and water retention from the mineralocorticoid effects of the excess glucocorticoid, to increased secretion of angiotensinogen or deoxycorticosterone, or to a direct effect of glucocorticoids on blood vessels.

The cause of the obesity and redistribution of body fat seen in Cushing's syndrome is also somewhat unclear. It may be explained by the increase in appetite or by the lipogenic effects of hyperinsulinemia caused by cortisol excess. The striae result from increased sub-cutaneous fat deposition, which stretches the thin skin and ruptures the subdermal tissues. These striae are depressed below the skin surface because of loss of underlying connective tissue.

C. Major causes of Cushing's syndrome include Cushing's disease (ACTH-secreting pituitary adenoma), ectopic ACTH syndrome, functioning adrenocortical adenoma or carcinoma, and long-term high-dose exogenous glucocorticoid intake (iatrogenic Cushing's syndrome).

In Cushing's disease and in ectopic ACTH syndrome, production of both ACTH and cortisol is excessive. Adrenocortical adenomas or carcinomas are characterized by autonomous secretion of cortisol and suppression of pituitary ACTH. The most likely cause in this patient, a 38-year-old woman with gradual onset of symptoms, is Cushing's disease (ACTH-secreting pituitary adenoma).

D. Current recommendations involve a stepwise approach to diagnostic evaluation. The first step is to demonstrate pathologic hypercortisolemia and confirm the diagnosis of Cushing's syndrome. Measurement of free cortisol in a 24-hour urine specimen collected on an outpatient basis demonstrates excessive excretion of cortisol (24-hour urinary free cortisol levels > 150 μg/24 h) and is the most sensitive and specific screening test for Cushing's syndrome. Urinary free cortisol values are rarely normal in Cushing's syndrome. Performance of an overnight 1-mg dexamethasone suppression test will demonstrate lack of the normal suppression by exogenous corticosteroid (dexamethasone) of adrenal cortisol production. The overnight dexamethasone suppression test is accomplished by prescribing 1 mg of dexamethasone at 11:00 PM and then obtaining a plasma cortisol level the following morning at 8:00 AM. In normal individuals, the dexamethasone suppresses the early morning surge in cortisol, resulting in plasma cortisol levels of < 5 μg/dL (0.14 μmol/L); in Cushing's syndrome, cortisol secretion is not suppressed to as great a degree, and values are > 10 μg/dL (0.28 μmol/ L). If the overnight dexamethasone suppression test result is normal, the diagnosis is very unlikely; if the urine free cortisol level is also normal, Cushing's syndrome is excluded. If both test results are abnormal, hypercortisolism is present and the diagnosis of Cushing's syndrome can be considered established provided that conditions causing false-positive results (pseudo-Cushing's syndrome) are excluded (acute or chronic illness, obesity, high-estrogen states, drugs, alcoholism, and depression). The CRH test is a useful adjunct in patients with borderline elevated urinary cortisol levels resulting from probable pseudo-Cushing's state. In patients with equivocal or borderline results, a 2-day low-dose dexamethasone suppression test is often performed (0.5 mg every 6 hours for eight doses). Normal responses to this test exclude the diagnosis of Cushing's syndrome. Normal responses are an 8:00 AM plasma cortisol < 5 µg/dL (138 nmol/L); a 24-hour urinary free cortisol < 10 µg/24 h (< 28 µmol/24 h); and a 24-hour urinary 17-hydroxycorticosteroid level < 2.5 mg/24 h (6.9 µmol/24 h) or 1 mg/g creatinine (0.3 mmol/mol creatinine).

The second step is to distinguish ACTH-independent disease from ACTH-dependent disease (Figure 21–14) with assay of the plasma ACTH level. The high-dose dexamethasone suppression test is useful for differentiating pituitary from ectopic ACTH secretion.

The final step for patients with ACTH-dependent disease is to determine the anatomic localization of the ACTH source by MRI or thin-section CT (pituitary, adrenal, lung, or other) or, if equivocal, by inferior petrosal sinus sampling (IPSS) or cavernous sinus sampling (CSS).

CASE 98

A. An incidentally found adrenal mass is often referred to as an adrenal incidentaloma. The mass could be an adrenal adenoma or a non-adenoma, which could be a malignancy (primary adrenocortical carcinoma, pheochromocytoma, or a metastatic cancer from a different source), infiltrating process, hemorrhage, or cyst. The evaluation of an adrenal mass requires both a functional and an anatomic workup. The functional evaluation is to determine whether the mass is producing excess adrenal hormone by performing a dexamethasone suppression test (or 24-hour urine free cortisol) to exclude hypercortisolism, by measuring the plasma or urinary metanephrines to exclude pheochromocytoma, and by measuring the serum potassium and aldosterone-to-renin ratio to exclude hyperaldosteronism.

B. Anatomically, the lesion needs to be evaluated to determine level of concern for malignancy. Lesions like the one in this patient that are small (< 3 cm) and homogenous and low in signal intensity (< 10 HU) are likely benign, lipid-rich adenomas. Lesions that are large (> 6 cm), heterogenous and not low in signal intensity can be malignant. Lesions that are functional and those that do not fulfill the criteria for benignity are usually removed. A mass that is not removed is followed up with one surveillance CT scan 6–12 months later to ensure that it is not enlarging, which would suggest malignancy. Clinical and/or hormonal reevaluation can be repeated periodically if the patient develops symptoms consistent with a hyperfunctional adrenal tumor since nonfunctioning adenomas may (rarely) develop hormone overproduction at a later time.

CASE 99

A. Other symptoms of chronic adrenal insufficiency include anorexia, nausea, vomiting, hypoglycemia, and personality changes. The examiner should look also for orthostatic changes in blood pressure and pulse, hyperpigmentation of the mucous membranes and other areas, vitiligo, and loss of axillary and pubic hair.

B. The serum sodium is typically low and the serum potassium high. In Addison's disease, the deficiency of cortisol is associated with a deficiency of aldosterone, resulting in unregulated renal loss of sodium and retention of potassium. Additional blood chemistry findings suggesting Addison's disease include mild acidosis, azotemia, and hypoglycemia.

C. The diagnosis of hypoadrenocorticism can be established by performing an ACTH stimulation test. In Addison's disease, there is a low 8:00 AM plasma cortisol and virtually no increase in plasma cortisol 30 minutes and 60 minutes after administration of 250 µg of synthetic ACTH (cosyntropin) intravenously or intramuscularly. At a specificity of 95%, the sensitivity of the 250-µg cosyntropin stimulation test is 97% for primary adrenal insufficiency.

D. Hypotension, including recumbent hypotension, occurs in about 90% of patients with Addison's disease and may cause orthostatic symptoms and syncope. These symptoms are related to the volume contraction resulting from unregulated renal losses of sodium.

Cortisol deficiency commonly results in loss of appetite and in GI disturbances, including nausea and vomiting. Weight loss is common and, in chronic cases, may be profound (15 kg or more).

In primary adrenal insufficiency, the persistently low or absent plasma cortisol level results in marked hypersecretion of ACTH by the pituitary. ACTH has intrinsic melanocyte-stimulating hormone activity, causing a variety of pigmentary changes in the skin, including generalized hyperpigmentation.

CASE 100

A. The major consequences of chronic aldosterone excess are sodium retention and potassium and hydrogen ion wasting by the kidney. Aldosterone binds to a mineralocorticoid receptor in the cytosol. The steroid-receptor complex then moves into the nucleus of the target cell and increases transcription of DNA, induction of mRNA, and stimulation of protein synthesis by ribosomes. The aldosterone-stimulated proteins have two effects: a rapid effect, to increase the activity of epithelial sodium channels (ENaCs) by increasing the insertion of ENaCs into the cell membrane from a cytosolic pool, and a slower effect to increase the synthesis of ENaCs. One of the genes activated by aldosterone is the gene for serum- and glucocorticoid-regulated kinase (sgk), a serine-threonine protein kinase. The *sgk* gene product increases ENaC activity (Figure

21–10). Aldosterone also increases the mRNAs for the three subunits that comprise the ENaCs. Aldosterone also binds directly to distinct membrane receptors with a high affinity for aldosterone and, by a rapid, nongenomic action, increases the activity of membrane Na^+-K^+ exchangers to increase intracellular Na^+. In the distal renal tubules and collecting ducts, aldosterone acts to promote the exchange of Na^+ for K^+ and H^+, causing Na^+ retention, K^+ diuresis, and increased urine acidity. Elsewhere, it acts to increase the reabsorption of Na^+ from the colonic fluid, saliva, and sweat. Increased sodium is associated with fluid retention, blunting the hypernatremia. The net effect in hyperaldosteronism is the mild hypernatremia, hypokalemia, and acidosis seen is this patient.

Hypertension results from this underlying sodium retention and subsequent expansion of plasma volume. The prolonged potassium diuresis produces symptoms of potassium depletion, including muscle weakness, muscle cramps, nocturia (frequent nighttime urination), and lassitude. Blunting of baroreceptor function, manifested by postural falls in blood pressure without reflex tachycardia, may develop.

B. Prolonged potassium depletion damages the kidney (hypokalemic nephropathy), causing resistance to antidiuretic hormone (vasopressin). Patients may be unable to concentrate urine (nephrogenic diabetes insipidus), resulting in symptoms of thirst and polyuria and the finding of a low urine specific gravity (< 1.010). Urinary electrolytes show an inappropriately large amount of potassium in the urine.

C. The diagnosis of primary hyperaldosteronism is already suggested by finding hypokalemia in an untreated patient with hypertension. Currently, the best screening test for primary hyperaldosteronism involves determinations of plasma aldosterone concentration (normal: 1–16 ng/dL) and plasma renin activity (normal: 1–2.5 ng/mL/h), and calculation of the plasma aldosterone-renin ratio (normal: < 25). Patients with aldosterone-renin ratios of ≥ 25 require further evaluation.

Subsequent workup entails measuring the 24-hour urinary aldosterone excretion and the plasma aldosterone level with the patient on a diet containing more than 120 mEq of Na^+ per day. The urinary aldosterone excretion exceeds 14 µg/d, and the plasma aldosterone is usually > 90 pg/mL in primary hyperaldosteronism. High-resolution CT or MRI of the adrenal glands can also help to differentiate between **adrenal adenoma** and bilateral **adrenal hyperplasia.** The gold standard for diagnosis is bilateral adrenal venous sampling, which is more sensitive and specific than imaging, to identify a unilateral cause, namely, an adrenal adenoma causing the primary hyperaldosteronism.

CASE 101

A. This patient probably has hyporeninemic hypoaldosteronism (type IV renal tubular acidosis), a disorder characterized by hyperkalemia and acidosis in association with (usually mild) chronic renal insufficiency. The syndrome is thought to be due to impairment of renin production by the juxtaglomerular apparatus, associated with underlying renal disease. Chronic renal insufficiency is usually not severe enough by itself to account for the hyperkalemia. Impaired secretion of both potassium and hydrogen ion in the renal tubule causes the observed hyperkalemia and metabolic acidosis.

B. Other causes of hypoaldosteronism include (1) bilateral adrenalectomy; (2) acute or chronic adrenocortical insufficiency; (3) ingestion of exogenous mineralocorticoids (fludrocortisone) or inhibitors of the 11β-hydroxysteroid dehydrogenase type 2 enzyme (licorice), leading to sodium retention, volume expansion, and suppression of renin production; (4) long-standing hypopituitarism, resulting in atrophy of the zona glomerulosa; (5) congenital adrenal hypoplasia, caused by one or more enzymatic abnormalities in mineralocorticoid biosynthesis; and (6) pseudohypoaldosteronism, in which there is renal tubular resistance to mineralocorticoid hormones, presumably because of a deficiency of mineralocorticoid hormone receptors.

C. Plasma and urinary aldosterone levels and plasma renin activity are consistently low and unresponsive to stimulation by ACTH administration, upright posture, dietary sodium restriction, or furosemide administration.

CASE 102

A. Dysmenorrhea may be a primary disorder in which no identifiable pelvic disease is present, or it may be secondary to an underlying pelvic disease. Among the most common causes are endometriosis, chronic pelvic infections, and adhesions from prior infections or ectopic pregnancies. Finally, dysmenorrhea may occur as a part of premenstrual syndrome, in which it is associated with other symptoms, including bloating, weight gain, edema, irritability, mood swings, and acne. This patient's constellation of symptoms in combination with her lack of prior medical problems and normal physical examination makes premenstrual syndrome the most likely diagnosis.

B. Dysmenorrhea in premenstrual syndrome and in primary dysmenorrhea is due to disordered or excessive prostaglandin production by the secretory endometrium of the uterus. Patients with dysmenorrhea have excessive production of prostaglandin $F_{2\alpha}$, which stimulates myometrial contractions of the uterus. Excessive contractions of the myometrium cause ischemia of the uterine muscle, thereby stimulating uterine pain fibers. Anxiety, fear, and stress may lower the pain threshold and thereby exaggerate the prominence of these symptoms from one patient to another and over time in a given patient.

C. The first step in treating patients with premenstrual syndrome is to encourage lifestyle changes such as more sleep, exercise, improved diet, and discontinuation or decreased use of tobacco, alcohol, and caffeine. Pharmacologic therapy with serotonin-reuptake inhibitors (SSRIs) has proven beneficial in addition to behavioral modification. Additionally, pain may be treated with monthly pharmacotherapy with prostaglandin synthesis inhibitors such as NSAIDs.

CASE 103

A. Infertility is due to female factors about 70% of the time. In about 40% of these cases, it is due to ovulatory failure, as occurs in hypothalamic, pituitary, and ovarian disorders. Another 40% are due to endometrial or tubal disease, as occurs with pelvic infections and endometriosis. Ten percent are due to less common causes such as those that affect the production of GnRH by the hypothalamus or the hormone's effect on the pituitary (thyroid disease, hyperprolactinemia) and those that affect ovarian feedback (hypergonadism, polycystic ovary disease). The final 10% are of unknown cause.

B. The most likely cause of this patient's infertility is endometrial and tubal scarring as a result of her prior sexually transmitted diseases. Infections such as gonorrhea and the often asymptomatic chlamydial infections can cause scarring and adhesions. This scarring may impede sperm or egg transport and implantation. Her history of regular menses and her normal examination argue against the other causes of female infertility (other than idiopathic). Finally, it is possible that the infertility results from her husband (male factor infertility) and not the patient herself.

CASE 104

A. The most likely diagnosis is preeclampsia-eclampsia. Although preeclampsia can be difficult to differentiate from essential hypertension developing during pregnancy, the fact that her hypertension developed after week 20 and was associated with edema and proteinuria strongly suggests a diagnosis of preeclampsia.

B. Predisposing factors for the development of preeclampsia include first pregnancy, multiple previous pregnancies, preexisting diabetes or hypertension, hydatidiform mole, malnutrition, and a family history of preeclampsia.

C. For unclear (perhaps immune-mediated) reasons, changes that normally occur in the blood vessels of the uterine wall early in implantation do not occur in patients with preeclampsia-eclampsia. A condition of relative placental ischemia is established. Undetermined factors are released that cause damage to vascular endothelium. This damage occurs first within the placenta and later throughout the body. Endothelial damage alters the balance between vasodilation and vasoconstriction, with increased vasoconstriction of small blood vessels and resultant hypoperfusion and ischemia of downstream tissues and systemic hypertension. The endothelial cell barrier between platelets and the collagen of basement membranes is breached. As a result of these changes, there is increased platelet aggregation, activation

of the clotting cascade, and production of vasoactive substances causing capillary leak. Further tissue hypoperfusion, edema formation, and proteinuria result. These processes all cause further endothelial damage, thus establishing a vicious circle. Interesting recent speculation has centered on the potential of serotonin to modulate vasodilation or vasoconstriction, respectively, via the 5-HT$_1$ or 5-HT$_2$ serotonin receptors. New data also invoke a role for agonistic autoantibodies directed against the second extracellular loop of the angiotensin II AT1 receptor, resulting in the vasospasm associated with preeclampsia.

D. The risks to the fetus of preeclampsia-eclampsia are the consequence of placental deterioration and insufficiency and include intrauterine growth retardation and hypoxia.

E. Patients can develop multiple complications as a result of preeclampsia-eclampsia, including malignant hypertension, hepatic damage (periportal necrosis, congestion, and hemorrhage can lead to elevated liver function tests and ultimately rupture of the hepatic capsule), renal changes (glomerular endothelial cell swelling, mesangial proliferation, marked narrowing of glomerular capillary lumens, and cortical ischemia that may progress to frank necrosis and acute renal failure), thrombocytopenia, disseminated intravascular coagulopathy (DIC), and cerebrovascular accidents. Eclampsia, or maternal seizures resulting from cerebral ischemia and petechial hemorrhage, can occur in this setting or can appear as the first manifestation of this disease. Delivery of the fetus is the only definitive cure for this syndrome, which carries a high mortality rate for mother and child.

CASE 105

A. About 15% of all couples are infertile and it is estimated that a male factor plays a role in about half of the cases. Of these, approximately 50% are potentially treatable. Identifiable causes of male infertility are classified into three major categories: (1) pretesticular causes, (2) testicular causes, and (3) posttesticular causes. Pretesticular causes are generally hormonal in nature and include hypothalamic-pituitary disorders, thyroid disorders, adrenal disorders, and drugs that can affect hormonal secretion or action. Testicular causes may be chromosomal (Klinefelter's syndrome) or developmental (cryptorchidism) or may result from varicocele, trauma, infection (mumps), or drugs and toxins. Posttesticular causes include ductule obstruction and scarring, retrograde ejaculation, antibodies to sperm or seminal plasma, developmental abnormalities (penile anatomic defects), androgen insensitivity, poor coital technique, and sexual dysfunction. Despite evaluation, the majority of cases of male infertility are idiopathic in nature, without a currently identifiable cause.

B. Considering the history of sexually transmitted diseases and the physical examination findings of epididymal irregularity, the most likely diagnosis is bilateral obstruction to sperm outflow.

C. Semen analysis should reveal oligospermia (< 20 million sperm/mL semen) or, more likely, azoospermia (absence of sperm). These abnormalities would be expected because the epididymal abnormalities on examination suggest bilateral obstruction to the outflow of sperm. LH, FSH, and testosterone should all be normal because no defects are present in the hypothalamic-pituitary axis or in the testes themselves.

D. Testing of fructose in the seminal fluid was once performed because fructose is produced in the seminal vesicles, and its absence in the semen implies obstruction of the ejaculatory ducts. This test is currently used sparingly, and more emphasis is placed on low semen volume as a screening test and transrectal ultrasound of the prostate as a confirmatory test. Obstruction of the ejaculatory ducts is strongly suggested by a seminal vesicle anteroposterior diameter of > 1.5 cm on ultrasound. Testicular biopsy may also be helpful in distinguishing intrinsic testicular pathology from ductal obstruction.

CASE 106

A. The diagnosis of benign prostatic hyperplasia is suspected based on the history and physical examination. A symptom index questionnaire may be administered to the patient to objectively evaluate the severity and complexity of symptoms. Digital rectal examination reveals the enlarged prostate seen here. Prostatic enlargement may be focal or diffuse, and the degree of enlargement does not necessarily correlate with the degree of symptoms. Serum urea nitrogen and creatinine are measured to exclude renal failure, and urinalysis is performed to rule out infection. In most patients, this is enough to make the diagnosis of benign prostatic hyperplasia. A urodynamic evaluation with uroflowmetry and cystometry may be undertaken to assess the significance of the disorder. These pressure-flow studies can help in determining which patients are less likely to benefit from prostatic surgery by providing information on detrusor function. Renal ultrasonography or intravenous urography may be performed on patients with hematuria or suspected hydronephrosis. Ultrasonography of the prostate with possible biopsy may be necessary to exclude prostate cancer as the cause of symptoms.

B. Although the actual cause of benign prostatic hyperplasia is unclear, several factors have been identified as contributing factors. These include age-related growth of the prostate, the presence of a prostatic capsule, androgenic hormones and their receptors (especially dihydrotestosterone), stromal-epithelial interactions and growth factors (FGF, TGF), and detrusor responses.

C. This patient has both irritative symptoms and obstructive symptoms. His irritative symptoms include urinary frequency, nocturia, and urgency. These occur as the result of bladder hypertrophy and dysfunction. His obstructive symptoms include incomplete emptying and postvoid dribbling. These are caused by distortion and narrowing of the bladder neck and prostatic urethra, leading to incomplete emptying of the bladder.

CASE 107

A. Gout flares are typically precipitated by a combination of metabolic and physical stressors in the setting of either urate underexcretion, seen in the vast majority of cases, or urate overproduction. The mild renal insufficiency may be associated with a decreased glomerular filtration rate and thus poor urate excretion. The recent addition of a diuretic further exacerbated this underlying impairment.

B. Multiple inflammatory pathways are invoked by the negatively charged urate crystals. For example, they activate the classic complement pathway whose cleavage products serve as effective neutrophil chemoattractants. The kinin system is stimulated by crystals as well, contributing to the inflammatory signs seen on examination such as tenderness and erythema from local vasodilation. In addition, macrophages phagocytose urate crystals, initiating the release of proinflammatory cytokines (eg, IL-1 and TNF), which activate the vascular endothelium, encouraging neutrophil adhesion and migration. Neutrophils are able to simulate their own recruitment by releasing leukotriene B4 in response to urate crystal phagocytosis.

C. Therapy for an acute gouty flare should target the proinflammatory mediators described previously. NSAIDs such as ibuprofen reduce prostaglandin synthesis, colchicine impairs the migration of neutrophils into the joints, and corticosteroids deactivate myelomonocytic cells responsible for crystal phagocytosis and subsequent cytokine release. Because gouty flares are typically self-limited events, treatment is offered to alleviate symptoms and reduce the duration of the flare. On the other hand, uricosuric agents, such as probenecid, and xanthine oxidase inhibitors, such as allopurinol, are typically reserved for the prevention of future attacks.

CASE 108

A. This patient likely has an immune complex vasculitis. When it manifests itself in the skin, it is also called cutaneous small vessel or leukocytoclastic vasculitis.

B. Immune complexes are generated by the combination of an antigen and an antibody. In this case, the antigen is the penicillin that the person has been taking regularly for a week. The penicillin stimulated an antibody response, leading to antibody production against, and then binding to, the penicillin. The antigen-antibody complexes are soluble and they are deposited in the subendothelial space, in this case, in the small vessels of the skin. There, they trigger an inflammatory response, which causes a rash. If the supply of new antigen is cut off (eg, by stopping the medication), the immune complexes are cleared by the immune system and the process resolves.

C. The same process can also affect the joints and the kidneys, both areas rich in small blood vessels. The specific organ(s) affected depend on the solubility of the specific antigen-antibody complex.

CASE 109

A. Poststreptococcal glomerulonephritis results from a skin infection with a nephritogenic strain of group A (β-hemolytic) streptococci such as type 12. The abrupt onset of hematuria ("cola"-colored urine), edema, and variable degrees of hypertension most commonly occur 7–14 days after streptococcal pharyngitis or impetigo and can occur sporadically or in clusters. Significant glomerular damage can lead to rapid progression to oliguria and acute renal failure.

B. Bacterial infections can cause glomerular damage through the deposition of antibody-antigen complexes. Vasculitis does not occur, however, in the setting of all infections. Rather, subendothelial deposition of immune complexes is required to damage highly vascularized nephrons by fixing complement (this explains the serum levels measured) and by activating myelomonocytic cells. Deposition of these complexes can only occur in the presence of excess antigens to make the complexes soluble, permitting them access to the subendothelial space and enabling them to cause injury.

C. This disorder is usually self-limited; 95% of individuals recover normal renal function within 2 months after onset. As antibody titers rise, immune complex formation decreases, and soluble complexes are eventually cleared provided that antigen administration is not sustained. Treatment of underlying infectious substrates may hasten resolution of the glomerulonephritis.

CASE 110

A. This patient's suspicion that her arthralgias may be explained by lupus is supported by a high prevalence of SLE among African American women—approximately 1 in 250—as well as her family history of this disorder. In fact, if a mother has SLE, her daughters' risk of developing the disease is 1 in 40, considerably higher than the risk in the general population. However, to make the diagnosis with reasonable certainty, 4 of 11 diagnostic criteria should be met, supported by a strong clinical impression: (1) malar rash, (2) discoid rash, (3) photosensitivity, (4) oral ulcers, (5) arthritis, (6) serositis, (7) renal disease, (8) neurologic disease, (9) hematologic disorders (eg, hemolytic anemia, thrombocytopenia), (10) immunologic abnormalities (eg, antibodies to native DNA), and (11) positive anti-nuclear antibody (ANA).

B. A number of drugs (eg, procainamide, hydralazine, isoniazid) have been implicated in provoking a lupus-like syndrome. A helpful clue in distinguishing the drug-induced form from SLE is that withdrawal of the offending drug typically results in improved clinical features and resolution of abnormal laboratory values.

C. These mechanisms include (1) subendothelial deposition of immune complexes, in which antigens are derived from damaged or dying cells; (2) autoantibody binding to extracellular molecules in the target organs (eg, skin, joints, kidneys, blood elements), which activates inflammatory effector functions and induces damage at that site; and (3) induction of cell death by autoantibodies.

D. The natural history of SLE is characterized by a relapsing, remitting course. Flares reflect immunologic memory, sparked by rechallenge of a primed immune system with antigen. Numerous stimuli such as viral infections, ultraviolet light exposure, and endometrial and breast epithelial involution may induce apoptosis, which resupplies immune inciting antigens. Despite this course, 10-year survival rates commonly exceed 85%.

CASE 111

A. The pathophysiology of rheumatoid arthritis is centered around the synovial linings of joints. The normal synovium is one to three cell layers thick. In rheumatoid arthritis, the synovium is markedly thickened and contains inflammatory cells in the interstitium, including T cells, B cells, and macrophages. This inflammatory tissue can invade adjacent bone and cartilage, accounting for the bony erosions and joint destruction.

B. Rheumatoid arthritis is thought to arise when an environmental factor (such as an infection) triggers an autoimmune response to antigens present in the synovium and elsewhere in the body. However, the specifics have not been identified. No definite infectious agents have been identified as causal agents in rheumatoid arthritis. The autoimmune mechanisms involved in the triggering and maintenance of the rheumatoid inflammatory response have also not been definitively identified, although tumor necrosis factor (TNF) plays a central role. Genetic factors have been found, arising from the observation that twins have a 15–35% concordance rate of developing rheumatoid arthritis. A specific subset of MHC class II alleles have been found that determine disease severity.

C. For many years, the mainstay of treatment for rheumatoid arthritis involved nonspecific immunosuppressant agents. With the recognition of the central role of TNF in the autoimmune response in rheumatoid arthritis, TNF inhibitors have found widespread use in its treatment. These inhibitors sequester TNF so that it cannot maintain the inflammatory response. They either are soluble TNF receptors or monoclonal antibodies that bind the free TNF and clear it from the body.

Subject Index

Note: Page numbers in **boldface** indicate a major discussion. Page numbers followed by *f* indicate figures; those followed by *t* indicate tables.

XYY male syndrome, 638

Y

Y chromosome, microdeletions of, 638–639, 639*f*
Yersinia, infections caused by, 61

Z

ZAP-70. *See* Protein tyrosine kinase ZAP-70
Zollinger-Ellison syndrome, 337, 347–348
Zona fasciculata, 571
Zona glomerulosa, 571

Zona reticularis, 571
Zoonotic hosts or reservoirs in infectious diseases, 57
Zygote, 610
Zymogens, 414, 414*f*, 415

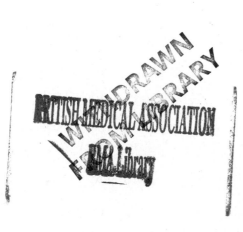